PRIMARY CARE OF THE

Child with a Chronic Condition

PRIMARY CARE OF THE

Child with a
Chronic Condition

Second Edition

PATRICIA LUDDER JACKSON, MS, RN, PNP

Clinical Professor, Associate Program Director,
Advanced Practice Pediatric Nursing Program,
Director, Primary Health Care
Department of Family Health Care Nursing,
School of Nursing, University of California, San Francisco,
San Francisco, California

JUDITH A. VESSEY, PhD, RN,C, DPNP

Professor, Program Director,
Advanced Practice Nursing Program,
Johns Hopkins University, School of nursing,
Baltimore, Maryland

with 72 illustrations

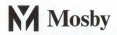 Mosby

St. Louis Baltimore Boston Carlsbad Chicago Naples New York Philadelphia Portland
London Madrid Mexico City Singapore Sydney Tokyo Toronto Wiesbaden

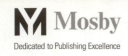
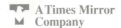

Mosby

Dedicated to Publishing Excellence

A Times Mirror
Company

Publisher: *Nancy L. Coon*
Senior Editor: *Sally Schrefer*
Associate Developmental Editor: *Michele D. Hayden*
Project Manager: *Linda McKinley*
Production Editor: *Rich Barber*
Designer: *Judi Lang*

A NOTE TO THE READER:

The author and publisher have made every attempt to check dosages and nursing content for accuracy. Because the science of pharmacology is continually advancing, our knowledge base continues to expand. Therefore we recommend that the reader always check product information for changes in dosage or administration before administering any medication. This is particularly important with new or rarely used drugs.

SECOND EDITION

Printed in the United States of America
Composition by Clarinda Company
Printing/binding by R.R. Donnelly & Sons Company

Mosby–Year Book, Inc.
11830 Westline Industrial Drive
St. Louis, Missouri 63146

Library of Congress Cataloging in Publication Data
Primary care of the child with a chronic condition / [edited by]
   Patricia Ludder Jackson, Judith A. Vessey. — 2nd ed.
          p.   cm.
      Includes bibliographical references and index.
      ISBN (invalid) 0-8151-4851-9 (hard cover)
      1. Chronic diseases in children—Treatment.   2. Chronic diseases in children—
   Nursing.   I. Jackson, Patricia Ludder.   II. Vessey, Judith A.
      [DNLM: 1. Chronic Disease—in infancy & childhood.   2. Primary Health
   Care.   WS 200 P952 1996]
   RJ380.P75   1996
   618.92—dc20
   DNLM/DLC
   for Library of Congress   95-50750
                                                                                   CIP

96 97 98 99 00 / 9 8 7 6 5 4 3 2 1

To Bruce whose memory lives on

To Heather, who has blossomed beautifully into womanhood

To Robert, whose struggles, challenges, and triumphs were the inspiration for this book

To Scott, whose devotion, hugs, and kisses have made motherhood so rewarding

And to Larry whose love, attention, and home cooking have helped keep us all together.

PLJ

To Kimberly and Matthew, who share with me the joys of childhood and

To Cheryl, who first taught me how special differently-abled children are.

JAV

Contributors

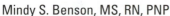

Mindy S. Benson, MS, RN, PNP
Coordinator, Pediatric Care
Bay Area Perinatal AIDS Center
San Francisco General Hospital
University of California-San Francisco
San Francisco, California

Elizabeth Ann Boland, MSN, RN, CS, PNP
Project Coordinator
Yale University, School of Nursing
New Haven, Connecticut

Barbara A. Carroll, MN, RN, CPNP
Clinical Nurse Specialist
Pediatric Hematology
Children's Center for Cancer and
Blood Disorders
Children's Hospital at Richland Memorial
Columbia, South Carolina

Elizabeth H. Cook, MS, RN,C, PNP
Pediatric Cardiology Clinical Nurse
Specialist
Children's Hospital-Oakland
Oakland, California

Beverly Corbo-Richert, PhD, RN
Lecturer
West Virginia University School of Nursing
Morgantown, West Virginia;
Adjunct Assistant Professor
University of Pittsburgh School of Nursing
Pittsburgh, Pennsylvania

Amy Cronister, MS, RN
Genetic Counselor
Dixon, New Mexico

Ginny Curtin, MS, RNC, PNP
Clinical Nurse Specialist
Craniofacial Center
Children's Hospital-Oakland
Oakland, California

Mary Alice Dragone, MS, RNC, PNP, CPON
Pediatric Nurse Practitioner
Pediatric Hematology/Oncology
Georgetown University
Washington, D.C.

Mary Jo Dunleavy, BSN, RN
Level III Staff Nurse;
Coordinator, Myelodysplasia Program
The Children's Hospital
Boston, Massachusetts

Rita Fahrner, MS, RN, PNP
Clinical Nurse Specialist
Occupational Infectious Disease Program
San Francisco General Hospital;
Assistant Clinical Professor
Department of Physiologic Nursing
University of California-San Francisco
San Francisco, California

Judith A. Farley, MSN, RN, CNRN
Director of Nursing and Patient Services and
Pediatric Neuroscience
The Children's Hospital
Boston, Massachusetts

Candace E. Gettys, BA, RN, CCTC
Senior Liver Transplant Coordinator
Stanford University Hospital
Palo Alto, California

Diane J. Goldman, MS, RN, PNP
Associate Clinical Professor
University of California-San Francisco
School of Nursing
San Francisco, California

Steven L. Goldman, MD
Direction, Neonatology Training Program
Department of Pediatrics
California Pacific Medical Center;
Associate Clinical Professor of Pediatrics
University of California-San Francisco
San Francisco, California

Margaret Grey, DrPH, FAAN, CPNP
Independence Foundation Professor of Nursing;
Associate Dean, Research & Doctoral Studies
Yale University, School of Nursing
New Haven, Connecticut

Randi J. Hagerman, MD
Professor of Pediatrics;
Section Head, Developmental & Behavioral
Pediatrics
University of Colorado Health Sciences Center;
Child Development Unit
The Children's Hospital
Denver, Colorado

Joyce Harvey, MS, RNC, PNP
Clinical Nurse Specialist
Pediatric Neurosurgery
University of California-San Francisco
San Francisco, California

Kayla Harvey, MS, RN, PNP
Pediatric Nurse Practitioner
Pediatric Pulmonary and Cystic
Fibrosis Center
California Pacific Medical Center
San Francisco, California

Sarah S. Higgins, PhD, RN, FAAN
Assistant Professor
School of Nursing
University of San Francisco
San Francisco, California;
Clinical Nurse Specialist
Adult Congenital Heart Disease Program
Children's Hospital-Oakland
Oakland, California

Toshiko Hirata, MD
Chief, Division of Neonatology
Department of Pediatrics
California Pacific Medical Center;
Clinical Professor of Pediatrics
University of California-San Francisco
San Francisco, California

Susan Karp, MS, RN
Nurse Coordinator
Hemophilia Program
University of California-San Francisco
San Francisco, California

Gail M. Kieckhefer, PhD, RN, CS, PNP
Associate Professor
Department of Family and Child Nursing
University of Washington
Seattle, Washington

Elizabeth A. Kuehne, MSN, RN, PNP
Instructor of Clinical Nursing
Columbia University School of Nursing
New York, New York

Carole A. Low, MS, RN, CCRN, CPNP
Child Neurology Clinical Nurse Specialist
University of California-Davis Medical Center
Sacramento, California

Margaret M. Mahon, PhD, RNC, PNP
Assistant Professor
University of Pennsylvania
School of Nursing
Philadelphia, Pennsylvania

Ellen A. McFadden, PhD, RN
Professor
California State University, Northridge
Northridge, California

Gail R. McIlvain-Simpson, MSN, RN, CS
Clinical Nurse Specialist
Pediatric Rheumatology
Alfred I. duPont Institute
Wilmington, Delaware

Ann Hix McMullen, MS, RN, CPNP
Senior Advanced Practice Nurse;
Pediatric Nurse Practitioner
Pediatric Pulmonary Center
University of Rochester Medical Center;
Assistant Professor of Clinical Nursing
University of Rochester School of Nursing
Rochester, New York

Eileen McNamara, BSN, RN
Assistant Director of Nursing
American Red Cross of Northern California
San Jose, California

Wendy M. Nehring, PhD, RN
Assistant Professor and Coordinator
Undergraduate Pediatric Nursing Program
University of Illinois at Chicago
College of Nursing
Chicago, Illinois

Roberta S. O'Grady, DrPH, RN
Lecturer and Field Program Supervisor
Program in Maternal and Child Health
School of Public Health
University of California-Berkeley;
Regional Nurse Consultant
Maternal and Child Health Branch
California Department of Health Services
Berkeley, California

Nancy A. Pike, MN, RN, CCRN
Clinical Nurse Specialist
Pediatric Cardiothoracic Surgery;
Pretransplant Coordinator
Lucile Salter Packard
Children's Hospital at Stanford
Stanford University Medical Center
Palo Alto, California

Veronica Perrone Pollack, MSN, RN
Assistant Professor
Yale University School of Nursing;
Clinical Nurse Specialist,
Pediatric Gastroenterology
Yale-New Haven Hospital
New Haven, Connecticut

Nancy B. Rabin, MN, RN, CRNP
Pediatric Clinical Instructor;
Pediatric Nurse Practitioner
University of Maryland School of Nursing
Baltimore, Maryland

Marijo Ratcliffe, MN, RN
Clinical Nurse Specialist
Children's Hospital and Medical Center;
Lecturer
Family and Child Nursing
University of Washington
Seattle, Washington

Marianne Warguska Reilly, MSN, RN, CPNP
Pediatric Nurse Practitioner
Newborn Nursery
Columbia Presbyterian Medical Center;
Adjunct Faculty
Columbia University
New York, New York

Judith A. Ruble, MS, RNC, PNP
Pediatric Nurse Practitioner
Children's Hospital-Oakland
Oakland, California

Cindy Hylton Rushton, DNSc, RN, FAAN
Clinical Nurse Specialist in Ethics
The Johns Hopkins Children's Center
Baltimore, Maryland;
Nurse Ethicist
Children's National Medical Center
Washington, D.C.

Janice Selekman, DNSc, RN
Professor and Chair
College of Nursing
Department of Nursing
University of Delaware
Newark, Delaware

Margaret Shepard, PhD, RN
Assistant Professor
University of Rochester
Rochester, New York

Marybeth M. Snyder, MS, RN
Instructor
College of Nursing
University of Delaware
Newark, Delaware

Jane Ryburn Starn, PhD, RN
Professor of Nursing
University of Hawaii;
Researcher, Center for Youth Research
Honolulu, Hawaii

Shirley Steele, PhD, RNC, PNP
Nursing Consultant
United Cerebral Palsy of Greater Birmingham
Birmingham, Alabama

Margo Swanson, MNSc, RNP, CSN
Practice Manager
Kids' Spot
Little Rock, Arkansas

Judy H. Taylor, MPH, RN, CNN
Pediatric Nephrology Nurse Coordinator
University of South Florida
Department of Pediatrics, Nephrology Section
Tampa, Florida

Kathleen Schmidt Yule, MS, RN
California Newborn Screening Program
Coordinator
Department of Pediatrics
Division of Medical Genetics
University of California-San Francisco
San Francisco, California

Reviewers

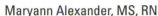

Maryann Alexander, MS, RN
Clinical Nurse Specialist
Rush-Presbyterian-St. Lukes Medical Center
Chicago, Illinois

Patricia Beierwaltes, MSN, RN, CS
Clinical Nurse Specialist, Pediatric
Neurology
Children's Hospital of Michigan
Detroit, Michigan

Julie Bushnell, MS, RN, PNP
Pediatric Nurse Practitioner
Pediatric Pulmonary and Cystic Fibrosis Center
California Pacific Medical Center
San Francisco, California

Arlene Butz, ScD, RN, CPNP
Associate Professor
Johns Hopkins University School of Nursing
Baltimore, Maryland

Karen L. Carlson, PhD, RN,C
Associate Professor
College of Nursing
University of Arkansas for Medical Science
Little Rock, Arkansas

Patricia D. Chibbaro, MS, RN, CPNP
Pediatric Nurse Practitioner;
Coordinator
Craniofacial, Cleft Lip/Palate, and
Microtia Teams
Institute of Reconstructive Plastic Surgery
New York University Medical Center
New York, New York

Lisa Anne Crupi, MS, RN, CNS
Clinical Nurse Specialist
Pediatric Immunology/Rheumatology
University of California-San Francisco
San Francisco, California

Angie S. Elser, MNSc, RN
Staff Nurse
Arkansas Children's Hospital
Little Rock, Arkansas

Michele M. Einloth, MS, RN, PNP
General Hematology Nurse Coordinator
Children's Hospital-Oakland
Pediatric Hematology Department
Oakland, California

Agatha M. Gallo, PhD, RN, CPNP
Associate Professor;
Coordinator
Pediatric Nurse Practitioner Speciality
University of Illinois at Chicago
Department of Maternal-Child Nursing
Chicago, Illinois

Theresa M. Giglia, MD
Cardiologist
Children's National Medical Center
Washington, D.C.

Rosemary Grant, BSN, RN
Nurse Coordinator, Division of Urology
The Children's Hospital
Boston, Massachusetts

Betsy Haas-Beckert, MS, RN, PNP
Clinical Nurse Specialist
Pediatric Gastroenterology/Nutrition
Pediatric Clinic
University of California-San Francisco
San Francisco, California

Carrie Goren Ingall, RN, MSN, PNP
Clinical Manager
Department of Cardiology
Children's National Medical Center
Washington, D.C.

Richard Koch, MD
Professor of Pediatrics
University of Southern California
School of Medicine;
Attending Physician
Division of Medical Genetics
Children's Hospital of Los Angeles
Los Angeles, California

Beverly Kosmach, MSN, CRNP
Adjunct Instructor
University of Pittsburgh School of Nursing;
Clinical Nurse Specialist
Transplant Services
Children's Hospital of Pittsburgh
Pittsburgh, Pennsylvania

Pam Laramie, MNSc, RN
Nurse Manager
Arkansas Children's Hospital
Neuroscience/Progressive Rehabilitation Units
Little Rock, Arkansas

Mira Lessick, PhD, RN
Associate Professor and
Practitioner-Teacher
Rush University College of Nursing
Chicago, Illinois

Jane E. Lowell, MS, RN, CPNP
Pediatric Nurse Practitioner
San Francisco General Hospital
San Francisco, California

Margaret M. Mahon, PhD, RNC, PNP
Assistant Professor
University of Pennsylvania
School of Nursing
Philadelphia, Pennsylvania

Maureen McGrath, MS, RN, PNP
Diabetes Nurse Educator
University of California-San Francisco
Diabetes Center;
Head Nurse/Educator
Bearskin Meadow Camp;
Education Director
Diabetic Youth Foundation
San Francisco, California

Sylvia Nagulko, MA, RN
Clinical Nurse Specialist
Division of Behavioral & Developmental
Pediatrics
University of California-San Francisco
San Francisco, California

Wendy M. Nehring, PhD, RN
Assistant Professor and Coordinator
Undergraduate Pediatric Nursing Program
University of Illinois at Chicago
College of Nursing
Chicago, Illinois

Cindy A. Nelson-Purdy, MPH, RN, CPNP
Pulmonary Nurse Specialist;
Pediatric Nurse Practitioner
Children's Hospital-Oakland
Pulmonary Medicine Department
Oakland, California

Kathy Perko, MS, RN, CPNP
Pediatric Hematology/Oncology
Clinical Nurse Specialist;
Nurse Practitioner
Sutter Memorial Hospital
Department of Pediatrics
Sacramento, California

Mary Smellie-Decker, MS, RN
Clinical Nurse Specialist, Neurosurgery
Myelomeningocele Care Center
Children's Hospital of Michigan
Detroit, Michigan

Foreword

Chronic conditions are here to stay. They will not vanish, despite the significant advances in medical knowledge and technology. The dramatic medical advances in the last few decades have resulted in an increased number of children with chronic conditions, who previously would have died much earlier from their disability. For example, there is evidence of a sevenfold increase in survival to age 21 among children with cystic fibrosis and of twofold or greater increases in survival for children with spina bifida, leukemia and congenital heart disease. Data from the National Health Interview Survey estimates that 31% of children under the age of 18 years have one or more chronic conditions. The task now is to enhance their lives and those of their families.

This book is important for many reasons. It comes at a time in our history in which major changes are taking place in the health care system. Increasingly nurses will play an important role in providing primary health care to children with chronic conditions and their families. Major changes have also taken place in educational settings. Legislation (PL 99-457/102-119) requires that educational systems provide comprehensive and individualized services to all preschool children with disabilities. As a result, the least restrictive environmental provisions of PL 94-142 (now known as IDEA) must be applied to young children as well as to those of school age. Health care providers must be able to address the needs of these children. This book does an important job by providing state-of-the-art knowledge for providers to enable them to make sensible decisions about care for children.

But most importantly, this book represents a recognition of the many factors that interact with one another when planning care for a child with a chronic condition. In fact, the authors have had the vision to structure the book around mutually interacting areas: specific condition, treatment, associated problems, developmental issues, and family concerns. In this way, the reader gains an understanding of the complexities involved, as well as how the various elements fit together.

The authors have presented clear and concise descriptions of selected chronic conditions and the assessment and management of those conditions for students and faculty who have accepted the challenge of caring for children with special needs and their families. This book should deepen the provider's understanding of the special challenges these children and their families face and of the opportunities the providers have to help them.

Bonnie Holaday, DNS, RN, FAAN
Professor and Chair
School of Nursing
Wichita State University

Preface

GROWING UP

I've got shoes with grown up laces,
I've got knickers and a pair of braces,
I'm all ready to run some races.
Who's coming out with me?

I've got a nice new pair of braces,
I've got shoes with new brown laces,
I know wonderful paddly places.
Who's coming out with me?

Every morning my new grace is,
"Thank you, God, for my nice braces:
I can tie my new brown laces."
Who's coming out with me?

A.A. Milne

"Growing up" is not easy. Seemingly limitless potential is juxtaposed with devastating possibilities. Medical advances over the past 50 years have dramatically decreased the mortality and morbidity rates in children, especially from infectious diseases that in previous decades killed thousands annually. With many devastating illnesses controlled, pediatric health care providers shifted their focus of care from illness management to prevention with the goal of maximizing each child's potential through health promotion, disease and injury prevention, and growth and development counseling.

During this same period, however, a new childhood morbidity profile has emerged. Children with chronic conditions who decades ago would have died as a result of their condition are now surviving. Their medical care is often complex, frequently requiring multiple treatment modalities. In addition, treatments that were previously only provided in acute care hospitals by professionals are now being provided in the home by family members, shifting medical responsibilities from hospital professionals to community providers.

In an attempt to keep pace with the rapid developments in medical and surgical treatment for children with chronic conditions, care has often become specialized, focusing on the disease process instead of holistic care for the child. In part, this has happened because primary care providers are hesitant to care for a child with a serious chronic condition for fear of not knowing how to manage the chronic condition well, and the specialist is reluctant to provide care above and beyond care needed for the chronic condition for fear of not knowing how to competently manage the child's primary health care needs. Consequently, children with chronic conditions often do not receive the primary health care provided their nonaffected peers.

"Growing up" with a chronic condition is inherently more difficult; a child's growth and development may be compromised by the stress of the illness and treatments and a child's susceptibility to common childhood illnesses, behavioral dysfunctions, and injuries may be increased as a result of the chronic condition. Many children with chronic conditions also come from improvised families with little or no access to preventive health care, further increasing the potential morbidity from the chronic condition, as well as general health risks. The purpose of this book is to provide pediatric health care professionals with the knowledge necessary to, in turn, provide comprehensive primary care to those children with special needs and their families.

Part I addresses the major issues common to care of all children with chronic conditions: the role of the primary care provider, the impact of a chronic condition on the child's development, on the family, school issues, ethical and cultural concerns, and the financial resources, or lack thereof, available and needed to support the care of a child with a chronic condition. This knowledge is generic in that it is not condition specific but forms the framework for delivery of care to all children with chronic conditions.

Part II identifies 26 chronic conditions found in children that necessitate alterations in standard primary care practices as a result of the chronic condition. Each condition-specific chapter was written and reviewed by health care professionals with extensive experience in caring for the complex needs of children with the identified chronic condition. The first part of each chapter reviews the etiology, incidence, clinical manifestations at the time of diagnosis, treatment, recent and anticipated advances in diagnosis and management, and associated problems of the condition and prognosis. The second part of each condition-specific chapter presents the primary care management for a child with the condition. This part is subdivided into two parts: health care maintenance and developmental issues. Under health care maintenance, growth and development, diet, safety, immunizations, health screening, common illness management, and drug interactions specific to the condition are presented along with the provider's role in promoting optimal health in these areas. Under developmental issues, the authors provide the reader with information on how this particular condition affects the child's sleep pattern, toileting, discipline, child care, schooling, sexuality, and transition into adulthood. The condition-specific chapters each end with a brief presentation on special family concerns and resources unique to this condition. Each chapter follows the same format for ease of reading with highlight boxes for key points of reference, and the primary care needs are summarized at the end of each chapter for quick reference.

Decisions as to which chronic conditions were to be included in this text were based on two criteria. First, the prevalence of the condition needed to be at least 1 in 10,000 or would likely reach this level if underreporting were not a problem. For conditions that are relatively new in children, such as organ transplantation or HIV infection, the decision to include them was based on how rapidly the incidence was increasing. The second criterion for inclusion was that the condition require significant adaptations in primary care.

Whenever possible, inclusive language regarding the primary care provider has been used throughout the text. We have extended this terminology to include nurse practitioners, physicians, and other health care providers, because individuals with a variety of professional preparations provide primary care to children with chronic conditions. The reader will also note that the terms patient and chronic illness are rarely used and whenever possible, the wording "the child with (condition name)" rather than the "(condition name) child" has been used. Although we recognize that this sometimes makes for awkward grammar, it reflects our philosophy that children be children first rather than be defined by their condition, and that wellness and illness are relative.

It would be presumptuous to edit such a text without acknowledging its scope and limitations. First, assumably the reader has a basic knowledge of growth and development and of common pediatric conditions and their management. Second, it is impossible to provide detailed information on treatment options for all secondary problems that may occur in conjunction with those highlighted. Wherever possible, the reader is referred to another chapter of this text. If this was not feasible, the reader should consult the general pediatric literature for management protocols. Third, a decision was also made to exclude pediatric psychiatric conditions. In part, this was due to the broad range of relatively uncommon conditions, the limited adaptations required in primary care, and the disparity in treatment regimens currently used.

The preparation of this text has been a professionally challenging and personally rewarding endeavor for us. As with any text, its successful completion depended on the help of numerous others. We wish to extend our gratitude to the contributors and reviewers for their excellent, careful and timely work. We would like to thank the clinical practitioners who used the first edition of this book and provided us with recommendations for additions and changes in the second edition. Our sincere thanks is also extended to our research assistants, Favrin M. Smith and Wanda Blevins Stephens, and our secretarial support staff, Peggy Absure, Kelly L. Wilson, and Danielle Rankin. Support for this project from the University of California, San Francisco Department of Family Health Care Nursing, the University of Arkansas for Medical Sciences, Johns Hopkins University School of Nursing, and grant support from the Bureau of Health Professions, Division of Nursing, Nurse Practitioner and Nurse Midwifery Program Grants number ID24 NU00394 and Bureau of Health Professions, Division of Nursing, Advanced Nurse Education Grant number ID23 NU01161, were all essential for its completion. The assistance and support of the Mosby–Year Book staff—editors, Sally Schrefer and Shelly Hayden, project manager Linda McKinley and production editor Rich Barber, are also greatly acknowledged and appreciated.

In summary, we hope the information provided in this book will help children with chronic conditions to receive more holistic primary care that will promote their growth and development and maximize their potential in all areas. This can only be done if health care professionals are willing to say "I will come out with you" and to assume the challenge of assisting these children in "growing up."

Patricia Ludder Jackson
Judith A. Vessey

Contents

CONCEPTS IN PRIMARY PEDIATRIC CARE

The Primary Care Provider and Children with Chronic Conditions

1

Patricia Ludder Jackson

A chronic health condition has been defined as one that is long term and is either not curable or has residual features that result in limitations in daily living requiring special assistance or adaptation in function (Jessop and Stein, 1988). Stein and colleagues (1992) have further defined chronic conditions as ongoing health conditions that at the time of diagnosis, or during the expected trajectory of the condition, will produce one or more of the following current or future long-term sequelae: limitation of functions appropriate for age and development; disfigurement; dependency on medication or special diet for normal function or control of condition; dependency on medical technology for functioning; current need for medical care or related services above the usual for the child's age, or special ongoing treatments at home or in school.

The exact number of children who have a chronic condition and the relative severity of their condition is unknown. The National Health Interview Survey on Child Health (NHIS-CH) conducted by the National Center for Health Statistics in 1988 estimated 31% of children under 18 years of age, or almost 20 million children nationwide had one or more chronic conditions, not including mental health conditions, based on parent report (Aday, 1992; Newacheck, McManus, and Fox, 1991; Newacheck and Taylor, 1992). See Table 1-1 for conditions and incidence. These statistics are based on parental report, not diagnostic criteria. Respondents are more likely to report conditions that have some impact on their child's activities but less

likely to report conditions that are associated with embarrassment or stigma (Newacheck and Taylor, 1992). Respondents with frequent contact with the health care system are more likely to have identified and labeled health conditions than those with limited health care.

The majority of the children (66%) in the NHIS-CH study were reported to have only mild conditions that resulted in little or no "bother" or activity limitation. The high incidence of reported respiratory, skin, and digestive allergies would probably account for this significant number of mild chronic conditions. Twenty-nine percent of the children experienced more than occasional "bother" or limitation of activity and 5% were reported to be bothered or limited by their condition often or all the time. Children in the severely affected group were reported to have an average 2.6 chronic conditions, to have spent 10 days in bed and missed 11 days of school annually. Sixteen percent of these children were hospitalized in the preceding year.

In this same NHIS-CH study, 17% of the children were identified as having a developmental disability with a prevalence rate range of 0.2% for cerebral palsy to 6.5% for learning disabilities (Boyle, Decouflé, and Yeargin-Allsopp, 1994). These children also were reported to have increased hospitalizations and to miss twice as many days of school than nonaffected children with 31% reporting the need to repeat a grade in school. Although the majority of children in this national study were

Table 1-1.   **PREVALENCE OF SPECIFIED CHRONIC CONDITIONS AMONG CHILDREN UNDER 18 YEARS OF AGE, 1988**

Condition	Cases per 1000	White	Black	Hispanic	Cases in 1000s
All children with chronic conditions	307.6				19,556
Impairments					
Musculoskeletal impairments	15.2	15.8	10.6	15.2	967
Deafness and hearing loss	15.3	18.0	6.0	15.2	975
Blindness and vision impairment	12.7	13.8	8.7	13.3	810
Speech defects	26.2	24.0	34.5	35.4	1666
Cerebral palsy	1.8	1.7	0.4	3.2	112
Diseases					
Diabetes	1.0	1.3	0.1	0.3	64
Sickle cell disease	1.2	0.1	7.1	0.3	74
Anemia	8.8	8.9	9.2	7.5	557
Asthma	42.5	42.0	51.3	35.1	2700
Respiratory allergies	96.8	114.7	53.6	47.4	6155
Eczema and skin allergies	32.9	36.7	21.7	19.2	2088
Epilepsy and seizures	2.4	1.9	2.4	6.2	151
Arthritis	4.6	4.8	5.4	2.0	290
Heart disease	15.2	18.3	7.7	10.0	965
Frequent or repeated ear infections	83.4	94.2	53.8	69.7	5304
Frequent diarrhea/bowel trouble	17.1	17.7	12.9	18.5	1085
Digestive allergies	22.3	27.0	9.9	8.4	1419
Frequent or severe headaches	25.3	28.4	21.1	14.7	1606
Other	19.8	23.6	10.2	9.2	1256

Adapted from Newacheck PW, Taylor WR: Childhood chronic illness: prevalence, severity and impact, *American Journal of Public Health 82*(3):364-371, 1992.

Newacheck PW, Stoddard JJ, and McManus M: Ethno cultural variations in the prevalence and impact of childhood chronic conditions, *Pediatrics 91*(5):1031-1038, 1993.

minimally affected by their reported chronic condition, the shear numbers of children affected by a chronic disorder is staggering. Expressed another way, 20% of U.S. children experienced mild chronic conditions, 9% experienced chronic conditions of moderate severity, and 2% of children experienced severe chronic conditions in 1988 (Newacheck and Taylor, 1992.)

The percentage of the pediatric population with a chronic condition is increasing as the patterns of childhood morbidity and mortality have changed with advanced technology, improved treatment of previously fatal infectious diseases, and implementation of public and preventive health measures that

have saved the lives of infants and children who previously would have died (Newacheck and Taylor, 1992). Mortality rates have fallen from 870 per 100,000 children aged 1 to 14 years in 1900 to 33 per 100,000 in 1987 (Newacheck and Taylor, 1992). This dramatic drop in mortality rates is not mirrored in the incidence of chronic conditions.

The overall incidence of most childhood chronic conditions has not changed significantly over the past 20 years. But in contrast to these relatively stable incidence rates, estimates of survival of children with a variety of chronic conditions have shown considerable change during the same time period. Dr. James Perrin (American Academy of Pediatrics Special Report, 1989) estimates that 20 years ago, 80% of children with chronic illness died. Today most of these children survive, requiring continued, often complex, care. For example, children with cystic fibrosis now frequently survive into adulthood (see Chapter 16). Improved surgical intervention and control of urinary tract infections have greatly prolonged the life expectancy of children with spina bifida (see Chapter 27). Newborn screening programs and early dietary intervention have dramatically improved the quality of life and reproductive capability of children with phenylketonuria (see Chapter 29).

New categories or groupings of childhood chronic conditions are also emerging. Infants surviving extreme prematurity or very low birth weight are posing new medical and management problems (see Chapter 30). A large population of infants and children with prenatal drug exposure present new challenges to the health care and educational systems (see Chapter 31). The number of children with acquired immune deficiency syndrome (AIDS) has increased dramatically during the past 10 years (see Chapter 22). The health care system, with its advanced technology, has created a spectrum of children with chronic iatrogenic conditions, such as infants with bronchopulmonary dysplasia (see Chapter 10), children with immune suppression as a result of drug therapy following organ transplantation (see Chapter 28), and survivors of childhood leukemia who later suffer the residual effects of treatment (see Chapter 11).

Not all children in the United States are equally affected by chronic conditions. Poverty and ethnicity play important roles in both the incidence and severity of chronic conditions. The Children's Defense Fund (Teitelbaum 1995) reports 16 million children in the United States live in poverty. This is the highest incidence since 1964 and means 1 in 5 children and 1 in 4 preschoolers live in impoverished families. Minority children are three times as likely to live in poverty than white children. Children living in poverty frequently have inadequate health care, housing, food, and education. Poverty is also associated with increased incidence and severity of many health problems (Crain et al, 1994; Gortmaker et al, 1990; Starfield, 1991). See Table 1-2.

Ethnicity and family culture play a significant role more in chronic condition management than

Table 1-2.
RELATIVE FREQUENCY AND SEVERITY OF HEALTH PROBLEMS IN LOW-INCOME CHILDREN COMPARED WITH OTHER CHILDREN

Frequency	
Low birth weight	Double
Delayed immunization	Double
Asthma	Double
Bacterial meningitis	Double
Rheumatic fever	Double-triple
Lead poisoning	Triple
Mild retardation	Double

Severity	
Neonatal mortality	1.5x
Post natal mortality	Double-triple
Child deaths due to:	
Accidents	Double-triple
Disease-related	Triple-quadruple
Diabetic ketoacidosis	Double
Complications of bacterial	
meningitis	Double-triple
% with conditions limiting	
school activity	Double-triple
Missed school days	Double
Severely impaired vision	Double-triple
Severe iron-deficiency anemia	Double

Adapted from Starfield B: Childhood morbidity: comparisons, clusters, and trends, *Pediatrics* 88(3):519-526, 1991.
Crain EF et al: An estimate of the prevalence of asthma and wheezing among inner-city children, *Pediatrics* 94(3):356-362, 1994.
Yeargin-Allsopp M et al: Mild mental retardation in black and white children in metropolitan Atlanta: a case-control study, *American Journal of Public Health* 85(3):324-328, 1995.

incidence (see Chapter 4). Newacheck, Stoddard, and McManus (1993) studied prevalency rates for chronic conditions in children from white, black, and Hispanic families. Overall, white children were identified as having considerably more chronic conditions than either black or Hispanic children, but their conditions were mild. The overall prevalence of chronic conditions among white children may be attributable to more frequent identification and reporting of common, but clinically minor conditions, such as hay fever or repeated ear infections. Reports of severe chronic conditions were not found to be statistically different across ethnic groups. The authors found the minority children experienced a disproportionate share of financial barriers to health care services even though their need for care was equal or greater than their white counterparts. Minorities experienced higher rates of being uninsured and a greater reliance on Medicaid versus private insurance (McManus and Newacheck, 1993). In addition, minority children with chronic conditions were found to use emergency rooms as their primary source of illness care 2 to 3 times as frequently as white children (Newacheck, Stoddard, and McManus, 1993).

Many children with chronic conditions receive the majority of their medical care in specialty clinics that do not provide routine health care management (Stein, 1992). Shuffled from specialist to specialist, the child often misses the screening, developmental assessment, anticipatory guidance, and even immunizations that healthy children of the same age receive. This lack of routine health care appears to cross disease categories. Jessop and Stein (1994) interviewed mothers of children with a variety of chronic conditions and found that although 56% could identify a usual source of care, few could identify a provider who would listen to their concerns (27%), provide them with general advice about the child's condition (24%), or facilitate case management services with other agencies (22%). (See Table 1-3.)

The development of medical specialization, which has improved the disease control and life expectancy of these children, has also resulted in fragmentation of health care delivery and increased medical costs (Liptak and Revell, 1989; Perrin, 1990). The families of these children, far more than other families, have to interact with multiple institutions providing some aspect of care for their child, such as early intervention programs, equipment vendors, social services, special education programs, and federal, state, or private financial providers of care. In addition, there are often multiple medical subspecialists whose expectations may or may not be realistic for the family or child and whose demands are sometimes conflicting, uncoordinated, and incomprehensible to the family (Jessop and Stein, 1988).

BARRIERS TO OPTIMAL HEALTH CARE

Children with chronic conditions have unique health and social needs. Chronic illness in children is often not stable but subject to acute exacerbations and remissions that occur superimposed on the child's changing growth and development. If the impact of the chronic illness is to be minimized and the child allowed to develop to his or her maximum potential, comprehensive family centered, community based and coordinated care must be provided (Committee on Children with Disabilities, 1993; Fox and Newacheck, 1990; Perrin, 1990).

Many barriers have to be overcome to provide comprehensive quality health care to children with chronic conditions. The American Academy of Pediatrics (AAP Special Report, 1989) identified three categories of barriers for families: financial barriers, system barriers, and knowledge barriers. Liptak and Revell (1989) surveyed community physicians and found they identified similar barriers to providing complete care to children with chronic conditions. The barriers identified were lack of payments, lack of time, lack of knowledge regarding resources, and unfamiliarity with new techniques.

Financial Barriers

In 1993, 13.6% of children (9,452,000) under the age of 18 were without insurance for the whole year with an additional 1% (806,000) without insurance for part of that year (Teitelbaum, 1994). Seventy-six percent of the children with chronic conditions in the NHIS-CH study discussed before had private insurance coverage, 11% had Medicaid coverage, and 12.8% had neither private insurance nor Medicaid coverage (Aday, 1992). Black and Hispanic children in this study were much more likely to be covered by Medicaid than their white counterparts. The Hispanic children (24%) were twice as likely as the non-Hispanic children (12%) to have no insurance coverage. Children with disabilities who were covered by health insurance were more likely to receive physician care than those children not covered by insurance (Butler, Rosenbaum & Palfrey, 1987). Though health status is an important predictor of children's use of services, for example, the sicker the child, the more frequent the use of health ser-

Table 1-3.   HEALTH SERVICES PROVIDED TO FAMILIES
WITH CHILDREN WITH CHRONIC CONDITIONS
AND THE QUESTIONS USED TO ELICIT THEM

Area	Question	% Indicating services currently provided
1. Usual source of care	Is there a place you usually go for care and a particular person you usually see there?	56%
2. Coordination with specialists	Does this provider make arrangements if the child needs to see a specialist?	50%
3. Coordination with other agencies	Does this provider talk to other agencies (e.g., school, day care center, Medicaid)?	22%
4. General advice	Does anyone give general advice about your child and such things as special schooling, handicaps, behavior problems, and things to expect later in childhood or adulthood?	24%
5. Family risk	Does anyone discuss with you whether the child's illness runs in the family or could occur in other family members?	38%
6. Listen to concerns	Does anyone listen to your concerns about your child and understand the problems of raising a child with an illness?	27%
7. Explanation of illness	Has the child's illness been explained to you?	62%
8. Intercurrent illness	Is there someone you go to when the child has a fever or an ear infection or something like that?	72%
9. Health care maintenance	Does anyone measure the child's height and weight, and talk about development, eating, etc.?	80%

Adapted from Jessop DJ, Stein REK: Providing comprehensive health care to children with chronic illness, *Pediatrics* 93(4):602-607, 1994.

vices, poor, minority, uninsured children, and children living only with their mother were most likely to experience barriers to access or were less apt to seek care than other children with comparable needs (Aday et al, 1993; Cunningham and Hahn, 1994; Wood, et al, 1990). The National Association of Children's Hospitals and Related Institutions found uninsured children received 40% less health care than their insured peers (Sealing, 1989). In children with chronic conditions, this lack of regular care fre-

quently results in aggravation of the chronic condition, although public programs such as Medicaid and Supplemental Security Insurance have improved access to health care for many poor families during the past 2 decades, Medicaid eligibility regulations and benefits remain restrictive and vary significantly from state to state (see Chapter 7). In addition, families receiving Medicaid have limited access to providers, having to depend on publicly financed clinics where continuity of care is almost nonexistent. This lack of continuity frequently results in poor identification of disabilities and subsequent lack of appropriate referrals (Butler, Rosenbaum, and Palfrey, 1987).

If the child is covered by private insurance, access to care is usually improved, but out-of-pocket medical expenses may still have a significant impact on family finances. A national survey of group health insurance policies (Fox and Newacheck, 1990) found widespread coverage for inpatient hospital care, outpatient physician services, medical supplies, prescription medications, and laboratory services but less frequent coverage for services such as physical therapy, speech therapy, occupational therapy, and mental health services. More than two thirds of the insurance policies offered limited comprehensive home health services in lieu of more expensive inpatient care. Long-term skilled nursing care was covered by only one third of the insurance policies. In addition, the proportion of insurance policies requiring copayments by families for nonhospital expenses and substantial individual or family deductible payments has increased dramatically in the past 5 years, resulting in greater medical costs for families (Fox and Newacheck, 1990).

The cost of caring for a child with a chronic condition is not limited to medical expenses (Hobbs, Perrin, and Ireys, 1985). Additional expenses may include transportation costs, special diets, clothing, day care or respite care, dental and visual services, or home remodeling. Frequently the care required by the child necessitates that one parent be at home with the child, reducing time at work with subsequent loss of income and possibly insurance coverage. The cost to the family in terms of medical expenses, time, and psychosocial stress is just beginning to be identified.

Because of limitations of insurance coverage, the increased needs and complexities of health care for these children can also financially affect the primary care provider (Liptak and Revell, 1989; Shoemaker, 1989; Wissow et al., 1988). Adequate reimbursement schedules that compensate the primary care provider for additional training and for the time they must spend to provide health care maintenance to children with complex needs does not currently exist. The advent of capitated managed care systems will further aggravate this problem (Altemeier, 1995; Newacheck, 1994). It is more cost effective for the practitioner to see two or three well children with minor acute illnesses than it is to see one child with a chronic condition. Subspecialists receive reimbursement at a much higher rate than primary providers, and this may be one reason care is often shifted to the tertiary care centers.

System Barriers

System barriers to optimal health care include the complex maze of federal, state, and private agencies designed to provide services, each with its own confusing bureaucracy and set of limitations and regulations (see Chapter 7) (Gale, 1989). Unfortunately, access to needed services is generally more dependent on geographic availability and the active involvement of medical personnel or disease-oriented voluntary organizations than it is on the needs of families (Blancquaert et al, 1992; Hobbs, Perrin, and Ireys, 1985). Living in a rural or inner-city community where few appropriate services are available requires the family to travel great distances for care and may result in a major barrier to obtaining adequate health care. This lack of available appropriate health care has resulted in a population of medically homeless children who are at greater risk for poor health outcomes (Sealing, 1989).

Health care providers also find the maze of bureaucratic regulations overwhelming. When a child in their practice develops special needs, it may take an inordinate amount of time to identify and refer that child to appropriate agencies in the community for needed services or the provider's request for referral may be denied by the health care organization (Cartland and Yudkowsky 1992; Sulkes 1995). Agencies and regulations keep changing, making it difficult to keep abreast of resources unless the provider has other clients with similar chronic conditions or access to a community social worker who can identify and make the appropriate referrals for the provider. In addition, many independent practices or managed care systems routinely schedule brief visits with inadequate time for the provider to assess a child with complex needs. If the practitioner has little control over the practice schedule or support from the agency for this type of complex care, seeing children with chronic conditions may be very frustrating.

Knowledge Barriers

Knowledge barriers to optimal health care can be present for both the family and the practitioner. Not knowing the need for or value of early intervention may delay initiation of care. Not knowing how to access services with proper referrals and eligibility identification may prevent the family from obtaining care they are entitled to receive. And not being sensitive to the families cultural heritage may inadvertently undermine the use of resources available to the family (Anderson and Fenichel, 1989) (see Chapter 4).

Because of the explosive growth of medical knowledge and technology, it is difficult for practitioners to keep abreast of the current management techniques for children with chronic conditions. The specific condition, condition severity, availability of specialists in the community, and parental request all affect the primary care providers perceived ability and role in caring for children with chronic conditions (Blancquaert, et al, 1992; Young, Shyr, and Schork, 1994). This recognition of knowledge limitations, possibly coupled with concern over potential legal consequences if subtle but important changes in a chronic condition are not recognized early, has been cited as the reason practitioners do not wish to assume medical or health care responsibilities for children with chronic conditions (Hobbs, Perrin, and Ireys, 1985; Liptak and Revell, 1989). Lack of specialist support for the role of the primary care provider was also identified as a barrier to care (Young, Shyr, and Schork, 1994).

ROLE OF THE PRIMARY CARE PROVIDER IN CARING FOR CHILDREN WITH CHRONIC CONDITIONS

Very few professionals would argue that the specialist, with advanced training and skills gained from caring for many children with similar conditions, is not the best professional to deal with the medical complexities of many chronic conditions. On the other hand, if the broader needs of the child and family are seen as the major focus of care—the common needs of education, support, advocacy, and health promotion, needs that families have regardless of the specific chronic condition—there is an obvious role for the primary care provider.

The primary care provider should be an integral part, if not the leading force, in the care of children with chronic conditions for multiple reasons. First, holistic health care of the child requires the child be viewed first, and primarily, as a child, with all the normal health care and developmental needs of any child. Second, the family must be seen as an integral part of the child's growth and development and recognized for its individual strengths and weaknesses (Briskin and Liptak, 1995; McDaniel, Campbell, and Seaburn, 1990). Third, health promotion, disease prevention, and anticipatory guidance have even greater significance when the child already has a condition that puts him or her at increased risk. Subspecialists are experts in their area of disease management but frequently have limited knowledge of normal growth and development and standard health care practices for health maintenance. Fourth, the primary provider most likely knows the family's community resources better than a subspecialist who may have a practice in a tertiary center many miles from the family's home. This knowledge of community resources is extremely important in helping families receive optimal care and support for their child.

In our rapidly changing health care system, financing of care, access to care, provision of care, and place of care are all in flux. Health care reform continues, if at a slower pace than originally anticipated. It is apparent more families will be insured under health maintenance organizations and capitated managed care systems than in previous years to control health care costs (see Chapter 7). The role of the identified primary care provider as the "gatekeeper" to specialist services will be expanded. Whether or not these changes in the health care system will alter our current disease-focused medical model is unknown. It is well recognized that less care will be provided in hospitals and much more care will be community and home based.

Caring for children with chronic conditions is a challenging, rewarding, and time-consuming proposition. It requires a commitment to service beyond that required for routine ambulatory pediatric care, increased knowledge about children with chronic conditions, and additional interpersonal communication and organizational skills necessary to provide optimal patient and family care.

Levels of intervention in the primary care of children and the knowledge base and skills needed by the primary care provider at each level of intervention are outlined in the box on pp. 11-12. These levels of intervention are cumulative; that is, level 3 intervention cannot be attained until the knowledge base and skills of levels 1 and 2 are mastered. As the levels increase, so do the commitment of the provider and the completeness of care for the child and family. This model of care was inspired by work done in the area of family-centered care by Doherty and Baird (1987).

Level 1 care is defined as the provision of routine health care maintenance and common illness management to healthy children and their families. Some health care providers may elect not to care for children with chronic conditions because of practice restrictions, a knowledge base limited to the care of normal children, or the lack of skills necessary to adequately manage more complex medical and psychosocial problems. Optimal care can be provided at level 1, but only to children and families without complex health care needs.

Level 2 care is task-oriented care requiring minimal interaction with the child or family and no commitment to continuity care. Level 2 care is not primary care but may be used to supplement primary care when a certain task needs to be accomplished. The knowledge base and skill level needed for this task-oriented care is limited to that which is necessary to complete the task efficiently, effectively, and safely. Examples of this level of care would include the primary care provider administering immunizations, ordering laboratory tests, or performing a prehospitalization physical examination, all at the request of the managing subspecialist.

Level 3 care is provided when the health care professional offers routine primary care to children with chronic conditions recognizing the unique health care needs of the child and family. The provider is able to assess the child's chronic condi-

tion but refers this care to other individuals or agencies. Because of the complexity of some conditions, personal interest or knowledge base of the provider, or practice restriction, the primary care provider may elect to manage some children with chronic conditions at this level while he or she manages children with other conditions at a higher level.

Level 4 care represents comprehensive primary health care incorporating the unique complexities of the chronic condition, the child, and the family. At this level the practitioner assumes the primary health care responsibilities of the child and family and uses consultation or referral for complex situations. He or she works collaboratively with the subspecialist to manage the chronic condition, common childhood illnesses, and routine health care maintenance. The practitioner does not abdicate care to the specialist but works with the specialist and the family to provide optimal care. As the health professional with the greatest knowledge of the family, the child, and the community, the primary care provider assumes a leadership role in providing comprehensive continuity care.

Level 5 care takes the role of the primary provider one step further, to that of case manager. A case manager is a person who assumes ongoing responsibility for service planning, assuring access to services, monitoring service delivery, advocating for child and family needs, and evaluating service outcomes, all while being concerned about cost effectiveness (Weil and Karls, 1985). The role of the case manager changes over time with levels of professional involvement increasing or diminishing based on the needs of the child and family (Jessop and Stein, 1991). It is the responsibility of the case manager to enhance the coordination, continuity, integration, and communication of services and to actively engage the family and child in this process (Harbin, 1989). The case manager must be able to perform a needs assessment of the child and family; plan, negotiate, and arrange for medical and nonmedical services; facilitate and coordinate services, including the education and training of community providers; assume responsibility for follow-up to monitor services and client progress; and facilitate empowerment of children and their families through counseling, education, training, and advocacy (Liptak, 1995; Kaufman, 1992; Liptak and Revell, 1989).

HIERARCHICAL INTERVENTION FRAMEWORK FOR PRACTITIONERS CARING FOR CHILDREN WITH CHRONIC CONDITIONS

Level 1

Ongoing health care and illness management for children without chronic conditions

Knowledge base needed

- Routine health care maintenance and common illness management for children without chronic conditions and their families

Skills needed

1. The ability to collect subjective and objective data related to child health maintenance and common pediatric illnesses
2. The ability to elicit relevant family data related to family structure, medical history, and current health problems and concerns
3. The ability to listen effectively
4. The ability to assess the information obtained
5. The ability to identify a treatment plan for an individual nondisabled child and family
6. The ability to effectively communicate the treatment plan to the child and family
7. The ability to identify those children with more complex needs requiring additional services

Level 2

Task-oriented care for children with chronic conditions; primary care needs and specialty care needs managed by other professionals

Additional knowledge base needed

- Task-related knowledge

Additional skills needed

1. Performance of task in efficient, correct manner

Level 3

Management of routine health care needs for children with chronic conditions; collaboration or referral for care related to the chronic condition

Additional knowledge base needed

- Basic pathophysiology of chronic conditions
- Child and family reactions to the stress of chronic conditions
- Collaborative role function
- Community agencies, tertiary care centers, and other professionals assuming responsibility for care of child's chronic condition

Additional skills needed

1. The ability to work with family members in their efforts to manage the child's normal growth and development
2. The ability to assess the child with a chronic condition identifying change requiring consultation or referral
3. The ability to identify family dysfunction requiring referral
4. The ability to communicate physical or psychosocial changes in the child or family to the appropriate professional

Level 4

Primary care of children with chronic conditions and their families

Additional knowledge base needed

- In-depth pathophysiology of chronic conditions
- Unique primary care needs of children with chronic conditions
- Common associated problems found in chronic conditions
- Differential diagnosis for common pediatric illnesses occurring in children with chronic conditions
- Community resources available to assist child and family
- Specific stressors for child and family of chronic condition

Additional skills needed

1. The ability to systematically assess the medical condition and health care needs of the child with a chronic condition

Continued.

HIERARCHICAL INTERVENTION FRAMEWORK FOR PRACTITIONERS CARING FOR CHILDREN WITH CHRONIC CONDITIONS—cont'd

2. The ability to plan and implement primary health care, including common illness management that is individualized for the child, the family, and the chronic condition
3. The ability to identify complications of the chronic condition requiring more complex care and to make appropriate referrals
4. The ability to educate the family on special complex needs of the child with a chronic condition
5. The ability to work with families to plan short- and long-term care consistent with medical needs and family function
6. The ability to assist parents and child in problem solving both medical and family concerns
7. The ability to help families recognize the needs of individual members and balance these needs during times of family stress and assist families in planning services and activities to reduce stress during these periods
8. The ability to make interdisciplinary referrals communicating child and family needs and expectations
9. The ability to provide consistent, available, long-term care

Level 5

Case management of families and children with chronic conditions

Additional knowledge base needed

- Service network available to child and family
- Cost-effective use of resources
- Service planning and systems coordination
- Eligibility requirements, referral process, and utilization measures for agencies or services that might benefit the family and child

Additional skills needed

1. The ability to develop an alliance with family and child to work together to provide optimum care
2. The ability to actively involve the family and child in the decision-making process for comprehensive care
3. The ability to make a comprehensive needs assessment for child and family
4. The ability to plan and initiate appropriate and successful referrals for services
5. The ability to coordinate services and personnel working with the family and child
6. The ability to monitor family and child progress
7. The ability to evaluate services used and make changes as necessary
8. The ability to communicate findings from multiple interdisciplinary sources to family, child, and other involved personnel or agencies
9. The willingness to function as child and family advocate

NEED FOR CASE MANAGEMENT

As the complexity of medical management increases with knowledge and technology and the health care financial system becomes overtaxed with health care costs, service efficiency and cost effectiveness will be central concerns. In the past, practitioners have been more likely to emphasize the quality of services and intensive care needs of clients, whereas administrators and funding sources often viewed service efficiency and cost effectiveness as more important (Weil and Karls, 1985). With the advent of new federal health care programs and managed care organizations based on a cost containment model, providers will have to be effective child and family advocates to obtain necessary services. Primary care providers, functioning as case managers, must learn to assess and document the effectiveness of treatment programs used by their clients to support the continuation of these programs in this era of shrinking health care dollars and rising incidence of chronic conditions in children.

The case manager role has been incorporated into Public Law 99-457, the Early Intervention Program for Infants and Toddlers with Handicaps. Reimbursement for these services will be provided, but the extent of reimbursement and the funding service source will vary from state to state. This formal federal recognition of the benefits and necessity of case management for children with chronic conditions and the need for reimbursement for those services hopefully portends more movement in this direction.

SUMMARY

Primary care providers working with children with complex needs must identify their role and the roles of other health care professionals working with the child and family and communicate this role to all concerned, including the family. If they plan to intervene only at levels 1 to 3, the family must be informed of this decision and an appropriate professional identified to provide level 4 and 5 care.

If the chronic condition is medically complicated, uses complex technology, or requires prolonged use of resources housed in a tertiary care center, the primary specialist (often more than one specialist is working with a child) may be the appropriate professional to assume the leadership role in total health care management for the child. In this situation the specialist would be required to consult with or refer to a primary practitioner for normal health care maintenance appropriate for the child. Many specialty clinics are now using advanced nurse practitioners knowledgeable in both the specialty area and primary care to help facilitate communication and care between the specialty clinic, primary provider, and family (Frauman and Morton, 1988; Davis and Steele, 1991; Jessop and Stein, 1991; Liptak and Revell, 1989; Martinez, Schreiber, and Hartman, 1991; Uzark et al, 1994; Wissow et al, 1988; Ziring et al, 1988).

But most chronic conditions of childhood are not so complex that the general practitioner, with additional knowledge about the chronic condition, its implications for primary care, and a commitment to effective communication, cannot assume a leadership role in health care management. Providers of pediatric health care have long embraced the philosophy that pediatric health care encompasses much more than disease management (Green, 1994). Regionalized systems of care that link high quality specialized health services with community-based primary care services are needed to coordinate the special needs of children with chronic conditions (Perrin et al, 1994). The primary care provider must play a key role in establishing, organizing, and participating in these systems if they are to exist and provide the holistic family-centered health care maintenance needed to ensure the maximum health and potential of each child (Committee on Children with Disabilities, 1993). Care rather than cure assumes greater meaning when one is working with children with chronic conditions, and there is much care to be provided that is common with the care needed by all children and their families.

The goal of health care maintenance for these children is to promote normal growth and development, to assist in maximizing the child's potential in all areas, to prevent or diminish the behavioral, social, and family dysfunction frequently accompanying a chronic condition, and to confine or minimize the biologic disorder and its sequelae (Stein 1992; Committee on Children with Disabilities, 1993). The primary care provider who knows the child and family well, knows the resources of the community, and is a specialist in health care maintenance is most often the appropriate health care professional to assume leadership in the often complex care and case management of these children.

REFERENCES

Aday LA: Health insurance and utilization of medical care for chronically ill children with special needs: health of our nation's children, United States, 1988, *Advanced Data from the Centers for Disease Control/National Center for Health Statistics* 215:1-8, August 18, 1992.

Aday LA et al: Health insurance and utilization of medical care for children with special health care needs, *Medical Care* 31(11):1013-1026, 1993.

Altemeier WA: Managed care for children with neuro developmental disabilities, *Pediatr Ann* 24(5):230-231, 1995.

American Academy of Pediatrics Special Report: *Barriers to care: why millions of children live in the shadows, unable to receive appropriate health care,* Elk Grove, Ill, 1989, The American Academy of Pediatrics.

Anderson PP, Fenichel ES: *Serving culturally diverse families of clinical infants and toddlers with disabilities,* Washington, DC, 1989. National Center for Infant Programs.

Blancquaert IR et al: Referral patterns for children with chronic diseases, *Pediatrics* 90(1):71-74, 1992.

Boyle, CA, Decouflé P, and Yeargin-Allsopp M: Prevalence and health impact of developmental disabilities in U.S. children, *Pediatrics* 93(2):399-403, 1994.

Briskin K, Liptak GS: Helping families with children with developmental disabilities, *Pediatr Ann* 24(5):262-266, 1995.

Butler JA, Rosenbaum S, and Palfrey JS: Ensuring access to health care for children with disabilities, *N Engl J Med* 317:162-165, 1987.

Butler JA, et al: Health insurance coverage and physician use among children with disabilities: findings from probability samples in fill metropolitan areas. *Pediatrics* 79:89-98, 1987.

Cartland JDC, Yudkowsky BK: Barriers to pediatric deferral in managed care symptoms, *Pediatrics* 89(2):183-192, 1992.

Committee on Children with Disabilities: Pediatric services for infants and children with special health care needs, *Pediatrics* 92(1):163-165, 1993.

Crain EF et al: An estimate of the prevalence of asthma and wheezing among inner-city children, *Pediatrics* 94(3):356-362, 1994.

Cunningham PJ, Hahn BA: The changing American family: Implications for children's health insurance coverage and use of ambulatory care services—in the future of children: Critical health issues for children and youth, *Center for the Future of Children, the David and Lucile Packard Foundation USA* 24-42, 1994.

Davis BD, Steele S: Case management for young children with special health care needs, *Ped Nurs* 17(1):15-19, 1991.

Doherty W, Baird MA: *Family centered medical care: a clinical casework,* New York, 1987, Guilford Press.

Fox HB, Newacheck PW: Private health insurance of chronically ill children, *Pediatrics* 85:50-57, 1990.

Gale CA: Inadequacy of health care for the nation's chronically ill children, *J Pediatr Health Care* 3:20-27, 1989.

Gortmaker SL et al: Chronic conditions, socioeconomic risks and behavioral problems in children and adolescents, *Pediatrics* 85(3):267-276, 1990.

Green, Morris (Ed.): *1994 Bright futures: National guidelines for health supervision of infants, children, and adolescent,* Arlington, Va, 1994, National Center for Education in Maternal and Child Health.

Harbin G: Issues in case management: a national perspective, *Early Childhood Update* 5(2):6, 1989.

Hobbs N, Perrin JM, and Ireys HT: *Chronically ill children and their families,* San Francisco, 1985, Jossey-Bass.

Jessop D, Stein R: Who benefits from a pediatric home care program? *Pediatrics* 88(3):497-505, 1991.

Jessop DJ, Stein, REK: Providing comprehensive health care to children with chronic illness, *Pediatrics* 93(4):602-607, 1994.

Jessop DJ, Stein RK: Essential concepts in the care of children with chronic illness, *Pediatrician* 15:5-12, 1988.

Kaufman J: Case management services for children with special health care needs: a family centered approach, *Journal of Case Management* 2:53-56, Summer 1992.

Liptak GS: The role of the pediatrician in caring for children with developmental disabilities: overview, *Pediatr Ann* 24(5):232-237, 1995.

Liptak GS, Revell GM: Community physician's role in case management of children with chronic illnesses, *Pediatrics* 84:465-471, 1989.

Martinez NH, Schreiber MC, and Hartman EW: Pediatric nurse practitioners: primary care providers and case managers for chronically ill children at home, *Journal of Pediatric Health Care* 5(6):291-298, 1991.

McDaniel SH, Campbell TL, and Seaburn DB: *Family-oriented primary care: a manual for medical providers,* New York, 1990, Springer-Verlag New York.

McManus MA, Newacheck P: Health insurance differentials among minority children with chronic conditions and the role of federal agencies and private foundations in improving financial access, *Pediatrics* 91(5):1040-1047, 1993.

National Center for Health Statistics: *Prevention profile. Health, United States, 1989,* Hyattsville, Md: Public Health Service, 1990.

Newacheck P et al: Children with chronic illness and medicaid managed care, *Pediatrics* 93(3):497-500, 1994.

Newacheck PW, McManus MA, and Fox HB: Prevalence and impact of chronic illness among adolescents, *Am J Dis Child* 145:1367-1373, 1991.

Newacheck PW, Stoddard JJ, and McManus M: Ethnocultural variations in the prevalence and impact of childhood chronic conditions, *Pediatrics* 91(5):1031-1039, 1993.

Newacheck PW, Taylor WR: Childhood chronic illness: Prevalence, severity, and impact, *Am Public Health* 82(3):364-371, 1992.

Perrin, JM: Children with special health needs: a United States perspective (Part II), *Pediatrics* 86(6):1120-1123, 1990.

Perrin JM et al: Health care reform and the special needs of children, *Pediatrics* 93(3):504-506, 1994.

Sealing PA: *Profile of child health in the United States,* Alexandria, Va, 1989, National Association of Children's Hospitals and Related Institutions.

Shoemaker FW: Are pediatricians intimidated by children with disabilities? *Calif Ped* 30:30, 1989.

Starfield B: Childhood morbidity: comparisons, clusters, and trends, *Pediatrics* 88(3):519-526, 1991.

Stein REK: Chronic physical disorders, *Pediatr Review* 13(6):224-229, 1992.

Sulkes SB: MD's DD basics: Identifying common problems and preventing secondary disabilities, *Pediatr Ann* 24(5):245-254, 1995.

Teitelbaum M: *Children's health insurance coverage update, Children's Defense Fund.* Draft Report, December, 1994.

Weil M, Karls J: *Case management in human service practice,* San Francisco, 1985, Jossey-Bass.

Wissow LS, et al: Case management and quality assurance to improve care of inner-city children with asthma, *Am J Dis Child* 142:748-752, 1988.

Wood DL et al: Access to medical care for children and adolescents in the United States, *Pediatrics* 86:666-673, 1990.

Uzark K et al: The pediatric nurse practitioner as case manager in the delivery of services to children with heart disease, *J Pediatr Health Care* 8(2):74-78, 1994.

Yeargin-Allsopp M, et al: Mild mental retardation in black and white children in metropolitan Atlanta: a case-control study, *American Journal of Public Health* 85(3):324-328, 1995.

Young PC, Shyr Y, and Schork MA: The role of the primary care physician in the care of children with serious heart disease, *Pediatrics* 94(3):284-290, 1994.

Ziring PR, et al: Provision of health care for persons with developmental disabilities living in the community: the Morristown model, *JAMA* 6:1439-1444, 1988.

Chronic Conditions and Child Development

2

Judith A. Vessey and Margo N. Swanson

Development does not exist in a vacuum; children's developmental domains are often significantly influenced by their physiologic state, psychological competence, and external environment. Children with chronic conditions may experience developmental lags in acquiring cognitive, communicative, motoric, adaptive, and social skills compared with their unaffected peers. These maturational alterations may range from minor to all encompassing, transient to permanent. The presence of a chronic condition does not necessarily connote the presence of developmental disturbances, however. The development of many children with chronic conditions progresses without interruption.

The maturational alterations that accompany chronic conditions may be characterized in several ways (Finn, 1982). Some alterations are manifested within a single area of development, such as motoric difficulty seen in a child with mild cerebral palsy. Other developmental alterations, such as those seen in a child with Down syndrome, are more global in nature. Alterations may also be classified as delayed or deviant. Children with delayed development will advance through the normal sequence of milestones but at a rate slower than that of their peers of the same chronologic age. Such is the case of a child with an uncorrected congenital heart defect. Deviant development, occurring from unevenly developed or damaged neurologic processes, involves a disruption in the normal developmental sequences. The child with poorly managed phenylketonuria is one such example.

The risks of children experiencing significant negative developmental sequelae increase exponentially for those with conditions of greater severity or multisystem involvement. Variables that contribute to the occurrence and severity of maturational alterations associated with chronic conditions include the natural history of the condition, personal characteristics of the child, and the larger social support networks.

CONDITION'S NATURAL HISTORY

The severity, pathophysiology, and prognosis of the condition, as well as any iatrogenic insults that may have occurred, all influence a child's developmental outcome.

Severity and Pathophysiology

Numerous specific pathophysiologic mechanisms, including chronic hypoxemia, swings in serum glucose levels, and malabsorption, are known to alter development, although the correlation between disease severity and developmental consequences is not very robust. Many pathophysiologic changes lack sufficient severity or are ameliorated by treatment so that the child readily adapts to them, and the potential for developmental insult is minimized. The existence of conditions marked only by occasional exacerbations or limited visibility or that appear to cause only marginal problems may be ignored or denied by children and their families.

This denial is often motivated by an effort to normalize the child's condition. Unfortunately, data suggest that these children may have poorer developmental outcomes if these behaviors interfere with symptom recognition or ongoing management regimens (Stein and Jessop, 1985).

Developmental sequelae secondary to prolonged disease states are also emerging. As research continues to advance health care technology, the mortality previously associated with many chronic conditions has been reduced. All too often, reductions in mortality initially result in escalating morbidity. For example, a decade ago infants diagnosed with HIV/AIDS survived only for months, dying before developmental lag could occur or was of significance. Today their life expectancy continues to increase dramatically with many children living into adolescence or beyond (Lewis, Haiken, and Hoyt, 1994). (See Chapter 22.)

Other developmental limitations are secondarily imposed by the condition's pathophysiology and management. Tremendous exertion may be needed to cope with intensive treatment protocols or time-consuming activities of daily living. Children with cystic fibrosis, for example, may spend more than 3 hours each day receiving pulmonary care. Additional energy is also required in adjusting to new or exacerbated symptoms. For children who are technologically dependent, their activities are often limited by the physical constraints and by the time needed to care for ventilators, infusion pumps, and the like. Such expenditures of time and energy may limit children's opportunities to engage in recreational activities or predispose them to significant fatigue because participation requires too much effort (Mearig, 1985).

Prognosis

Maturational progression is superimposed on the natural course of the condition. In conditions associated with increasing symptoms leading to a poor prognosis, children may initially achieve milestones but lose them as the condition worsens. It is always noted when there is progressive degeneration of the neurologic system, as with Tay-Sachs disease, but it is also a problem with any seriously compromised physiologic state. Even in nonprogressive conditions, developmental lags often become noticeable as children mature and

developmental expectations are higher. In part, the ability to sustain development is dependent on managing the disease's symptoms effectively and promoting the child's functional status and psychosocial adjustment when deterioration cannot be curtailed.

Another area of concern is for children who have a limited or uncertain future or whose significant others (family, teachers, etc.) consider the child's prognosis for reaching adulthood poor. These children may be deprived of a past-present-future perspective of learning about one's cultural heritage or forming goals and personal aspirations. This longitudinal perspective plays an integral role in shaping cognitive processes (Mearig, 1985). If individuals are misguided into thinking that such information is not worth transmitting or would be unduly upsetting, especially for the child who recognizes his or her potentially diminished longevity, this lack of information limits the child's ability to learn. Predicting prognoses is a risky business in light of rapid advances in medical science (Van Dyke and Lin-Dyken, 1993); the life expectancies for children with cystic fibrosis, organ transplantation, cancer, and many other conditions continue to increase at dramatic rates. If a poor prognosis is communicated to the family in the absence of a broader perspective for the child's future, it may become a self-fulfilling prophecy.

Iatrogenic Insults

Selected treatment protocols may cause temporary or permanent developmental changes. Developmental iatrogeny refers to those health care interventions that hinder children from progressing through their normal developmental milestones (Vessey, Farley, and Risom, 1991). Therapeutic interventions commonly associated with developmental iatrogeny are the associations between aminoglycosides and hearing loss (Kravitz and Selekman, 1992), cancer therapy and late effects, (Moore and Klopovich, 1989), and oxygen administration and retinopathy of prematurity (Weakley and Spencer, 1992). Numerous other interventions, however, directly or indirectly influence development. Many classes of drugs, such as anticonvulsants and asthma preparations, have been shown to alter cognitive performance and behavior (Bender et al, 1991; Bender, Lerner, and Poland, 1991).

CHARACTERISTICS OF THE CHILD

Age

The limitations imposed by chronic conditions have definite implications for each age group (Perrin, 1992). The age of onset of a condition will affect progression from one stage of development to the next. Achieving a developmental task that has never been acquired is very different from regaining a skill previously mastered and now lost. Overall, children with congenital conditions have greater developmental plasticity; they adjust more readily to condition-imposed limitations as greater adaptive mechanisms come into play (Pless, 1984).

The major developmental tasks of infancy include establishing trust and learning about the environment through sensorimotor exploration. For infants with congenital chronic conditions, these tasks may be difficult to accomplish. Parents who are mourning the loss of their perfect child may find that they have little energy. Yet these infants may be very wearisome to care for, and parents may find little gratification in trying to meet their basic needs despite their best efforts. Parents may begin to view their children as vulnerable because of the extensive care required; this attitude can affect future development (Goldberg, 1990). A poor prognosis may also lead some parents to emotionally divorce themselves from their infants in an effort to insulate themselves from further emotional hurt. Infants subjected to prolonged or frequent hospitalizations may encounter repeated separations, the unpredictability associated with numerous care givers, potentially unreliable or inadequate care, and painful experiences. All of these factors can inhibit attachment and subsequent development of a trusting relationship. For infants whose condition is physically limiting or painful, they are unable to explore and interact with their environment. This too can curtail development.

The major developmental tasks of toddlerhood include acquiring a sense of autonomy, developing self-control, and forming symbolic representation through the acquisition of language. If a child's chronic condition requires careful limit setting and control of activities of daily living, parents may not be able to encourage their children's independence in tasks such as toileting, feeding, or acquiring larger social networks. For example, toddlers who are immunosuppressed need to be restricted in their social contacts and play arenas. Mandatory prolonged dependency can create difficulty in separating and contribute to a tenuous self-image. Developmental tasks that have just been mastered are often easily lost in toddlers experiencing acute exacerbations of disease, with or without hospitalization. This behavioral regression is a means of social and emotional adaptation whereby children revert to earlier, previously abandoned stages when they do not have the necessary psychic energy to maintain functioning at already achieved developmental levels (Freud, 1966). Behavioral regression is exacerbated by stress, including stresses associated with separation and pain. Although regression can happen at any point along the developmental continuum, it is most commonly noted in this age group.

Acquiring a sense of initiative to successfully meet the challenges of their ever-expanding worlds is the primary developmental task for preschoolers. Preschoolers with chronic conditions may not have the physical energy or resources to design and perform such activities; opportunities for learning about the environment, developing social relationships, and cultivating self-confidence and a sense of purpose are diminished. They may have difficulty in forming a healthy body image and sexual identity, particularly if most of their body awareness is associated with disability and discomfort. Preschoolers are egocentric, engage in magical thinking, and use correlational rather than causal reasoning, all of which directly influence their interpretation of their condition. They are likely to think some unrelated behavior they engaged in has caused their condition, and often tell elaborate stories to explain what has happened to them. If such misconceptions are not corrected and children are permitted to assume responsibility for their condition, their developing self-esteem and motivation to undertake new tasks may be compromised.

For school-aged children, increasing independence and mastery over their environment are important developmental landmarks. A lack of physical stamina may prevent children with chronic conditions from participating in school and extracurricular activities. Such activities are known to contribute to gaining social skills, developing a sense of accomplishment, learning to effectively cope with stress, and acquiring those skills that result in self-sufficiency. Children with a condition that is not highly visible may try to hide its existence when they recognize that it makes them different from their peers until forced by circumstances to admit otherwise. If not provided with the skills needed to communicate information about their conditions to peers, these children may withdraw and their self-concept diminish. Moreover, enforced dependency, whether required by the treatment regimen or instituted by overprotective parents, creates additional social and emotional barriers between children with chronic conditions and their nonaffected peers.

Adolescents, in the transitional period from childhood to adulthood, should become increasingly independent of their parents. Those pursuing this developmental task may feel obligated to assume total responsibility for their care despite their relative inexperience. For other adolescents, their extensive care needs may preclude this from happening. Adolescents need to begin to make decisions about future career and personal goals. For an adolescent who requires complex care or who has a limited life expectancy, these developmental tasks may go unmet. Adolescents are prone to two dangers in planning for the future: (1) they may overemphasize the potential barriers that accompany their condition and succumb to a sense of futility or despair, or (2) they may deny realistic limitations and set themselves up for failure by holding forth unrealistic expectations. Puberty, always a time of rapid change and uncertainty for adolescents, further confounds this complex period for teens with chronic conditions. Integrating limitations into one's changing body image and self-concept is difficult. Delayed puberty accompanies many conditions, emphasizing the differences between affected and nonaffected adolescents. Adolescence is a particularly difficult time to be viewed as different by one's peers, and some adolescents may withdraw from those social activities and relationships with the opposite sex that promote healthy psychosexual development.

Individualism

Despite great odds, many children have been bestowed with intrapsychic and interpersonal resources that allow them to conquer virtually any disability and excel in life. A child's individualism, or the rubric of those relatively stable emotional attributes that underlie a child's behavior—temperament, motivation, hardiness, intellect, attitudinal qualities, and interpersonal skills—influence developmental attainment.

Children with chronic conditions display the same scope of individual differences as children without chronic conditions. Some behavioral traits, such as temperament, are present at birth, whereas others, such as self-concept, develop over time. A child's individualism is influenced by environmental factors, although there is no direct correlation between familial attitudes and practices and the child's psychologic development. A strong self-concept, or a positive interpretation of one's own individualism, is developed through successfully mastering a variety of physical, intellectual, social, and emotional tasks (Sinnema, 1991). At a somewhat higher risk for developing a vulnerable personality secondary to a poor self-concept in the presence of a chronic condition, many children develop an appropriately positive self-concept and approach life's challenges with aplomb. They learn to rapidly identify threats to their integrity, respond with justifiable anger to those who are prejudiced against them, and reject biased individuals as inferior to themselves. Simultaneously, these children will often work to educate those around them, dispelling myths and inaccuracies that might interfere with their own developmental competence. A vulnerable personality linked with critical developmental periods does not bode well for physical or socioemotional health.

Children at increased risk are those with multiple chronic conditions (Newacheck and Stoddard, 1994); although surprisingly, the severity of a single condition does not appear to affect a child's psychological outcome. Factors known to place children at greater risk for psychological co-morbidity are: (1) having a poor self-concept, (2) having a dysfunctional family, and (3) living in an isolated area and/or poverty (Hertzig, 1992). Moreover, selected therapeutic interventions, such as behavioral and cognitive effects of medications, can affect psychological well-being. Children at greatest risk are those with neurological conditions (Perrin, 1992). Psychological co-morbidity can be reduced when comprehensive preventive care is provided for the child and family (Stein and Jessop, 1991).

The interrelationships of a child's positive self-esteem, perceived autonomy, easy temperament, internal locus of control, at least normal intelligence, adequate perceptual and communication skills, and an accurate cognitive appraisal of the condition in conjunction with environmental and family support all increase the child's therapeutic adherence (Pidgeon, 1989; Luthar and Zigler 1991; Carey 1992). Therapeutic adherence is enhanced when the child actively participates in health care decisions. Practitioners who gradually involve children and adolescents in participating in decisions about their care improve therapeutic adherence and self-care abilities (Deatrick, Woodring, and Tollefson, 1990; Brady, 1994). For example, a child who has a low activity level, is given appropriate autonomy, and adapts easily to new situations is more likely to readily comply with a regimen of bedrest and nutritional restrictions than a very active child who has difficulty adapting to new situations.

ROLE OF FAMILY AND SOCIAL NETWORKS

Development depends on repeated and varied interactions between the growing child and the environment. Such reciprocity results in a spiral of mutually effective interactions. A child's parents are the most important influence on development during early childhood. Most parents are tremendously resilient despite the demands made by the child's condition and effectively assume their role in parenting the child, thus promoting his or her development. For a small minority of parents, the converse is also true. Parental guilt or despair, or unfinished grief work over the loss of the fantasied child may negatively affect the child's development. Other factors include maternal depression, "nerves", and/or poor self-esteem and a chronically stressful environment (Cadman et al, 1991). Well-functioning families enhance their child's development, whereas those with discordant functioning curtail it (see Chapter 3).

Differing cultural orientations and social class also influence development in children with chronic conditions. As these orientations vary, so

do the symbolic and semantic significance of the events, their perceived origins, and the potential consequences (Brookins, 1993; Geber and Latts, 1993; Groce and Zola, 1993). Although to date little research has been done in this area, practitioners working with children from varied circumstances need to recognize the variations in intrafamily communication patterns, temporal orientation, religiosity, and the value placed on childhood because these are known to influence development. (See Chapters 3 and 4).

As children mature, there is a natural expansion of their environment and social network, and extended family members, teachers, friends, and acquaintances influence their developmental attainment. Individuals who offer practical tangible support, provide intellectual stimulation, plan activities that help the child excel, and take pride in the child's accomplishments truly serve as the child's advocates. Unfortunately, some individuals have had few experiences with children with special needs, and they may overcompensate for or reject the child's limitations. For children whose conditions are associated with disfigurement, their development may be unwittingly at risk because of the reactions of others. Many uninformed individuals automatically assume that physical handicap is associated with cognitive impairment. Children may be spoken about as if they were not present, or questions may be addressed to nearby family members or peers. The damage that can be done to a child's sense of self-worth is inestimable. The family can be helped to educate significant others about the child's strengths and limitations, encouraged to mainstream their child into community activities, and offered suggestions about effective methods for working with insensitive individuals.

DEVELOPMENTAL PERSPECTIVES OF THE BODY, ILLNESS, MEDICAL PROCEDURES, AND DEATH

Children's perspectives about their bodies, illness, and death differ depending on their age. These perspectives need to be taken into account when children are taught about their condition and their help is enlisted in therapeutic adherence.

Understanding of the Body

By the preschool period children have well-defined concepts of their external body and the relationships between its parts. Their understanding of the internal body's structure and function, however, remains primitive and is in keeping with cognitive and perceptual abilities. Early school-aged children can name three to six body parts, with the heart, brain, bones, and blood the most common. Their descriptions of the parts and how they function tend to be global, undifferentiated, and laced with fantasy, although there is a great deal of variation among children about their specific ideas. Interrelationships among the parts and their functions are equally hazy. Physiologic processes are seen as a series of static states, with each organ having a singular, autonomous function. By middle to late school age, when children's causal reasoning and ability to differentiate matures, they begin to understand the complexities of anatomy and physiology. Levels of the body's organization are differentiated and hierarchically integrated with each other (Crider, 1981).

Children with chronic conditions hold a slightly different, though not more sophisticated, view of their internal bodies than that of their unaffected peers. They tend to focus on the affected part of the body but identify fewer other organ systems. Evidence also indicates that these children do not develop the increasing differentiation seen in children without chronic conditions but remain more fixated on their defective part (Offord and Aponte, 1967). Children's use of advanced terminology often confounds others into thinking that their comprehension far exceeds what normally would be expected. For example, one 4-year-old stated that he was receiving "methotrexate intravenously" yet thought his blood filled an empty body cavity because blood vessels remained an unknown entity.

Understanding of Illness

Children's self-concepts, interpersonal abilities, and therapeutic adherence to treatment regimens are related to the beliefs they hold about illness. For those who perceive their chronic condition as totally negative and restricting, functional status,

school performance, and psychosocial competence are more likely to be compromised. If children are considered to be sick by their parents, their developing views and personalization of illness will significantly influence how they interpret their condition. As children mature and their view of illness evolves, the primary care practitioner along with significant others are in the position to assist the child in developing a positive image of his or her condition.

Most research investigating how children conceptualize illness uses a developmental approach (Eiser, 1989; Gochman, 1988; Burbach and Peterson, 1986). Infants are concerned about illness only as it directly interferes with their comfort and attachment to their parents. By the toddler period, children begin to have an understanding of the concept of illness. For children with chronic conditions, this is usually interpreted by how the condition interferes with desired activities. Many condition-specific tasks such as injections of insulin or wearing a seizure helmet are particularly onerous for this group.

As children mature, they begin to form and articulate their feelings about illness. Preschoolers' cognitive processes remain dominated by prelogical thought, which is manifested in their views of illness. Phenomenism, the most simplistic form, occurs when illness is attributed to any external concrete phenomenon regardless of its relationship to illness. It is later replaced by contagion, or ascribing the causes of illness to other temporally occurring events. Recently diagnosed preschoolers, for example, will often view their condition as punishment for having misbehaved.

As children reach school age, their view of illness begins to reflect their evolving causal thought. Illness is initially perceived as occurring from contamination or physically coming in contact with the causal agent. Over time this view matures, and the cause of illness is believed to be external, such as germs that enter the body. With the development of formal operations in adolescents, illness causation is seen as a complex, multifaceted process. Physiologic explanations initially emerge as the basis for illness. These later evolve into psychophysiologic explanations, and the relationship of behavior and emotion to illness are acknowledged.

A second paradigm explaining how children learn about illness has recently been proposed. In this framework, learning about illness is not as dependent on a cognitive level as on previous experience (Yoos, 1994). Children with chronic conditions may develop expertise about selected illnesses within the range of their experiences and beyond that expected by their cognitive levels; yet, they may hold less sophisticated views about general concepts of illness (Perrin, Sayer, and Willett, 1991). New studies support this view (Rubovits and Siegel, 1994).

Understanding of Medical Procedures

Children's misconceptions of medical procedures closely parallel their thoughts about the body and illness. Initially infants and young children have no specific understanding of procedures; they are interpreted only in light of how they intrude on personal comfort. By preschool age, children's comprehension of medical procedures is marked by magical thinking, transductive reasoning, and overgeneralization. A procedure's purpose is independent of a child's health status, and little discrimination as to its diagnostic or therapeutic purpose is made except for those who have undergone repetitive procedures. All procedures are designed to make you "better" or "sicker." Because preschoolers' understanding of body boundaries are not well developed, virtually all invasive procedures are perceived as threats to their body integrity. Health care personnel are identified by their clothes, and curative powers are attributed to their actions (Steward and Steward, 1981).

As children mature, their view of medical procedures evolves from overgeneralization, through overdiscrimination, to correct identification of their functions. Multistep procedures and their purposes can be comprehended by school age; these children are able to classify and order variables. Information, however, is usually interpreted quite literally, and misunderstandings can occur if the content taught is not validated. Children of school age respect health care personnel and their hierarchical position, but expressions of affection are often ambivalent. School-aged children, often intrigued with understanding medical procedures, are usually pleased when asked to participate in their own care (Steward and Steward, 1981).

Adolescents are capable of understanding the efficacy of specific medical procedures and the relationships between procedures and their health status. Informed decisions about alternative treatments are possible. Adolescents view the health care provider's authority as extending only as far as their willingness to adhere to the therapeutic regimen. Although the need for therapeutic adherence is understood, treatments are not automatically affectively and behaviorally assimilated into an adolescent's daily activities (Steward and Steward, 1981).

Understanding of Death

Death is the ultimate experience in separation and loss for children and their families. Children's understandings of death are formed along a developmental progression and reflect their cognitive maturation (Mahon, 1993). Infants do not comprehend death itself but react to those phenomena, such as pain and separation, that are associated with death. By late toddlerhood and preschool age, children may talk freely about death but may describe its occurrence and attributes with magical thinking and from an egocentric viewpoint. They may perceive their impending death as punishment; yet, they do not view death as permanent but rather as "sleep" or a departure from the family. The permanence of death is not realized until the school-aged period, when the concepts of reversibility and irreversibility are learned. Children in this age group tend to personify death as the bogeyman or some kind of monster. For children who are dying, this newly found knowledge can enhance their fears of the unknown. Adolescents, with their new metacognitive abilities, conceptualize death as a process of the life cycle, readily comprehending the emotional, social, and financial implications of the loss that occurs from death for themselves and their families. Of all age groups, adolescents have the most difficulty in dealing with death.

Children with chronic conditions are often subjected to numerous intrusive and painful experiences and may have experienced the death of friends in the hospital. These experiences often exacerbate their anxieties about death. Depending on individual experience, a child's understanding of death may not follow the projected trajectory. Although information as to how affected children's views of death differ from their nonaffected peers is limited, it appears that the fears associated with death are remarkably similar to the fears of hospitalization and intrusive procedures. Even in preschool-aged children, fear of separating may be expressed despite the fact that death may not yet be conceptualized as irreversible.

For the dying child, how issues such as separation, mutilation, and loss of control are handled play an important role in their personal conceptualization of death. Care must be taken to help these children maintain their autonomy, sense of mastery, and other developmental skills whenever possible. (See Chapter 6 for additional information.)

PRIMARY CARE PROVIDER'S ROLE IN PROMOTING DEVELOPMENT

Because cure is not possible for many chronic conditions, the practitioner must focus on care. The goal of care is to minimize the manifestations of the disease and maximize the child's physical, cognitive, and psychosocial potential.

Realizing this goal will be facilitated if a family-centered approach to care is used. Family-centered care recognizes that the family is the constant in the child's life and as such, is vital to the child's success in meeting his or her potential. Practicing family-centered care requires professionals to: (1) recognize and respect a family's strengths and individuality, (2) promote a family's confidence and competence in caring for their child, and (3) empower the family to advocate for their child as they interface with the health care system.

In addition, adopting a noncategorical approach that focuses on those commonalities that children with chronic conditions share with each other rather than just on the disease process is useful (Perrin et al, 1993). This approach, incorporated with discrete dimensions of the disease, such as its onset, course, and manifestations, provide a nexus on which to develop a holistic management plan. A good maxim to follow is to generalize developmental information across diagnostic groups, then individualize it for each child and family (Stein and Jessop, 1989).

Assessment and Management

Maturational alterations are rarely immutable and should not be thought of as such. Children with chronic conditions require comprehensive habilitation if they are to achieve their optimal level of functioning (Curry and Duby, 1994). This requires a developmental surveillance program be established. Developmental surveillance is a broader approach than detection. It is comprehensive, continuous, and contains several components. These include: (1) general and condition-specific screening, (2) child and parental observation, (3) identification of concerns, and (4) general primary care guidance (Dworkin, 1989; Frankenburg, 1994). Although developmental surveillance falls under the primary care provider's purview, it can involve the input from an interdisciplinary group of professionals. The composition of the group is dynamic and will vary depending on the child's age, disability, level of impairment, familial involvement, and environmental resources. Coordination is critical if omissions and duplications of services are to be prevented (Smith, Layne, and Garell, 1994). Involvement of the primary care provider will help ensure consistency across the disciplines.

Ideally, children at risk for developmental lags should be identified as soon as possible and followed closely. The goal for the primary care provider is to anticipate and, whenever possible, vigorously intervene before significant aberrations occur. This is best accomplished by identifying and initiating treatment in the preclinical period, that time when slight indications of developmental impairment may be detected, but gross manifestations are not yet evident. A "wait and see" attitude is not warranted because these children are known to be at developmental risk. Early intervention may prevent or ameliorate many secondary problems or those that result from neglect or mistreatment of the original condition. Although a child may suffer hearing loss from aminoglycosides, for example, subsequent language and cognitive delays may be prevented with aggressive intervention. Because a chronic condition generally persists throughout a child's lifetime, ongoing surveillance of physical development and psychosocial adjustment is helpful.

Assessment of the child's physical development normally consists of evaluating basic indicators of health including growth measures and vital signs, performing a comprehensive physical examination, and noting any changes in the status of the chronic condition. An additional dimension, rating the child's functional status, should also be an integral part of the assessment. Functional status evaluation provides information about the child's ability to engage in activities of daily living known to heavily influence developmental outcomes.

Although the tendency may be to focus attention on the child's physical status, assessment of the child's psychosocial adjustment is of critical importance. Not all of the psychosocial stresses experienced by children with chronic conditions are caused by their condition, nor do only affected children experience stress. This population, however, has a higher percentage of psychologic difficulties, much of which can be attributed to the child's condition (Weiland, Pless, and Roghmann, 1992). It is estimated that 1½ to 3 times as many children with chronic conditions have behavioral problems as their nonaffected peers. Moreover, 30% to 40% of these children also have school-related problems, only one half of which are directly related to their condition (Andrews, 1991; Goldberg and Simmons, 1988).

Assessment has traditionally focused on identifying how the child with a chronic condition differs from nonaffected peers. This information is useful for developing an explanatory theory about the effects of chronic conditions but does little to help the child. Evaluating whether the child is effectively coping with the condition and successfully adjusting to school, peer groups, and the like provides guidelines on which interventions can be based.

Standardized assessment instruments are useful, necessary adjuncts to a complete history and physical examination for a comprehensive developmental evaluation. When used at regular intervals, they provide objective data so small developmental changes can be detected. Considering the ever-growing number of children with special needs being cared for in the community, the primary care practitioner needs to have a compendium of readily administered standardized instruments from which to draw (Table 2-1) and not rely only on first level or basic screening instruments like the DDST II. These first level instruments are designed to iden-

tify global delay rather than provide in-depth information about the type and severity of developmental problems (Bennett and Nickel, 1995). Second level or focused instruments provide more in-depth information about functional abilities and are a useful part of in-depth evaluation.

Care must be taken in choosing instruments and interpreting results because most of these did not include children with chronic conditions when the norms were determined. Others are invalid if they are measuring one developmental construct based on the performance in a different arena of development. For example, the cognitive development of a child with a tracheostomy should not be assessed by an instrument requiring verbal responses. Timed tests may also bias results, particularly if a child has a motor or learning deficit. If a child fatigues easily, it is best to perform developmental assessments in short intervals so as not to obscure the child's true capabilities.

In general, children with chronic conditions who are at risk for developmental deviations but where no indications of developmental deviations are apparent should participate in similar developmental surveillance programs as their nonaffected peers. For those who are exhibiting warning signs of developmental problems, more frequent assessments are appropriate. Too frequent assessments of at-risk but nonsymptomatic children, however, may alter parents' perceptions so that they believe their child is unduly vulnerable, creating a self-fulfilling prophecy (Chamberlin, 1987). The practitioner needs to walk the fine line between errors of commission and omission when deciding the frequency and intensity of assessment. The best defense is to place efforts on prevention rather than detection.

When untoward developmental manifestations are detected, the primary care provider can either provide treatment or, more likely, refer the child to specialists with expertise in the area of concern. Ideally referrals should be made to such individuals who are a part of the specialty team or within the child's school setting. However, additional local referrals may be necessary if the specialty team is geographically distant or school services are inadequate. Adding another layer of care providers requires exquisite coordination of services if the child is to receive appropriate care free of overlaps or gaps and avoid becoming fatigued by too many demands.

Obtaining services may require that the child's condition and associated problems be diagnostically labeled, although recent legislation has lessened the need. Providing a label may help validate the concerns of children and families and provide direction for future interventions and activities. However, it must be done judiciously. Labeling often sets the child apart from his or her peers and may result in different treatment by family members, teachers, and significant others. Diagnostic labels assigned in childhood follow children into adulthood, possibly preventing them from pursuing selected careers, joining the military, or being eligible for insurance. Although it is usually feasible to label specific disease entities, care should be taken in labeling associated with developmental manifestations.

The ultimate long-term goal of care is for the child to reach and sustain optimal levels of functioning. Developing precise, measurable, short-term goals will help ensure that optimal functioning is obtained.

Education

Two objectives of primary care, in addition to providing health maintenance, are to help prepare children in self-care behaviors and develop self-advocacy skills for dealing with the health care community. This is important for children and adolescents with chronic conditions because they will likely engage the health care system frequently throughout their lives. The transition between pediatric and adult care is never easy, especially for those who have conditions that used to be fatal in early childhood. Providers of adult care often have little experience with these conditions and their management. Educating children and adolescents will help empower them as they negotiate the health care system. Such education helps empower children and adolescents to do so effectively.

For children to accomplish these objectives, they must initially have a basic understanding of the workings of their body, characteristics of their condition, and the intricacies of the health care system. Unfortunately, it is often assumed that children are well versed about these topics because they know the jargon, often appear quite comfort-

able with the health care environment, and have been diagnosed "for years." As mentioned earlier, however, on closer examination much of this apparent sophistication is superficial (Carraccio, McCormick, and Weller, 1987); children may merely be mimicking vocabulary they have heard repeatedly. Children may also misinterpret or forget information, or advanced material may not be presented as they mature.

Developmentally appropriate teaching guides need to be incorporated into the primary care of all children with chronic conditions because learning is more likely to occur in a nonthreatening environment when the child is in a comparatively good state of health than when sick and hospitalized. A comprehensive plan, to be managed by the primary care provider in conjunction with parents and specialty providers, will help ensure that this learning occurs. Teaching methods need to be altered to fit the child's developmental age. Children will learn best when the material presented to them remains within one level above their current cognitive functioning.

A multisensory approach—one that brings all of the child's senses to bear on the learning task at hand—is more likely to be effective with preschool and school-aged children than more traditional methods. For example, using anatomic rag dolls to explain anatomy and physiology (Vessey, 1988) or doll hospitals for explaining various procedures has been shown to be highly effective with this population. A variety of options, including books, discussion, videos, and interactive computer programs, are appropriate for use with older children who are free of cognitive deficits.

Many commercially available materials are excellent and useful adjuncts to the individualized teaching plan. The practitioner is cautioned to examine all materials in advance to ascertain whether the information presented will correspond to the child's own experiences. The language of all materials needs to be carefully evaluated for age appropriateness and content validity. There is little sense of providing cute, albeit inaccurate, information to a child because these myths will only need to be dispelled as the child matures (Vessey, Braithwaite, and Wiedmann, 1990). For younger children who have not developed causal reasoning, who engage in fantasy, and who tend to interpret their

Text continued on p. 37

Table 2-1.   INSTRUMENTS USED IN DEVELOPMENTAL ASSESSMENT

Types of screening tools	Test/source	Age level	Method	Comments
General development	Battelle Developmental Inventory (BDI) (1984) Author: J Newborg, J Stock, L Wnek, J Guidubaldi, and J Svinicki Source: Riverside Publishing Co 8420 Bryn Mawr Ave Chicago, IL 60631	Birth-8 years	Structured test format Parent and teacher interview Observation	• Includes a screening test that can be used to identify areas of development in need of a complete comprehensive BDI • Full BDI consists of 341 test items in five domains: personal-social, adaptive, motor, communication, and cognitive 1-1½ hours to administer • Screening test consists of 96 items taking 20-35 minutes to administer *
	Bayley Scales of Infant Development-Second Edition (1993) Author: N Bayley Source: The Psychological Corp Harcourt, Brace, Jovanovich, Inc 6277 Sea Harbor Dr Orlando, FL 32887	1-42 months	Observation/demonstration	• Evaluates motor, mental, and behavior of the infant and toddler • Diagnoses normal *vs.* delayed development • New scoring procedures allow the examiner to determine a child's developmental age equivalent for each ability domain • Requires a qualified practitioner to examine and evaluate the infant
	Bender Visual Motor Gestalt Test Author: L Bender Source: American Orthopsychiatric Association, Inc Seventh Ave, 18th Floor New York, NY 10001	≥3 years	Demonstration	• Used as an evaluation tool for developmental problems in children, learning disabilities, retardation, psychosis, organic brain disorders • 10 minutes to administer
	Brigance Diagnostic Inventory of Early Development (Revised) (1991) Author: A Brigance	1 month-7 years	Performance task by child	• Assesses skills in all areas required for P.L.101-476 eligibility • Criterion and normative referenced, curriculum based

Instrument / Author / Source	Age range	Method	Features
Source: Curriculum Associates, Inc 5 Esquire Rd North Billerica, MA 01862-2589			• May be administered by paraprofessional with supervision • Does not require special equipment for testing
Developmental Profile II Author: G Alpern, T Boll, and M Shearer Source: Western Psychological Services 12031 Wilshire Blvd Los Angeles, CA 90025-1251	Birth-9½ years	Parent or teacher report	• Screens children for delays in 5 domains: physical (motor and muscle development), self-help, social, academic, communication • 186 items takes 20-30 minutes to administer • Can be computer scored
Hawaii Early Learning Profile (HELP) (1979) Author: SF Furuno, KA O'Reilly, CM Hosaka, TT Inatsuka, TL Allman, B Zeisloft, and S Parks Source: Vort Corporation PO Box 60880 Palo Alto, CA 94306	Birth to 36 months	Observation Parent interview	• 685 developmental tasks used to assess 6 domains: cognition, language, gross motor, fine motor, social-emotions and self-help • Criterion referenced, curriculum based • Each domain takes 15-30 minutes to administer. Domains may be selected for individual use *
Minnesota Infant Development Inventory (1988) Minnesota Early Child Development Inventory (1988) Minnesota Preschool Development Inventory (1984) Author: H Ireton and E Thwing Source: Behavior Science Systems PO Box 1108 Minneapolis, MN 55458	Birth-15 months 1-3 years 3-6 years	Observation/interview Parent report True/False	• A first level screening tool • Measures the infant's development in 5 domains: gross motor, fine motor, language, comprehension, and personal-social • Provides a profile of the child's strengths and weaknesses • 60-80 items on each inventory *
Rapid Developmental Screening Checklist Author: Committee on Children with Handicaps, American Academy of Pediatrics	1 month-5 years	Checklist	• Requires minimal time allotment *

Continued.

*Can be administered by professional or nonprofessional. Some special training required. Needs to understand testing procedures and be capable of developing rapport with children.

Table 2-1.   INSTRUMENTS USED IN DEVELOPMENTAL ASSESSMENT—cont'd

Types of screening tools	Test/source	Age level	Method	Comments
General development	Source: MJ Giannini, MD Director, Mental Retardation Institute New York Medical College Valhalla, NY 10595			
	Riley Motor Problems Inventory (RMPI) Author: GD Riley Source: Western Psychological 12031 Wilshire Blvd Los Angeles, CA 90025	≥ 4 years	Performance tasks by the child	• Provides a quantified system for observation and measurement of neurologic signs that lead to problems in speech, language, learning, and behavior • Needs to be administered by a qualified clinician
General	Wheel Guide to Normal Milestones of Development Author: U Hayes Source: A Developmental Approach to Case Findings, ed 2 US Dept of Health and Human Services Superintendent of Documents Washington, DC 20402	1-3 years	Observation	• Assesses basic reflexes and developmental milestones • Reinforces the normal growth and development patterns of children
Adaptive behavior	AAMR Adaptive Behavior Scale-School, ed 2 ABS-S:2 (1981-1993) Author: N Lambert, K Nihira, and H Leland Source: PRO-ED, Inc 8700 Shoal Creek Blvd Austin, TX 76758-6897	3-21 years	Performance tasks, observation, and parent report	• Used as a screening tool and for instructional planning • Can be an indicator in assessing children whose adaptive behavior indicates possible mental retardation, learning difficulties, or emotional disturbances. Provides 16 domain scores. • Previously called AAMD Adaptive Behavior Scale • Software for scoring available

	AAMR Adaptive Behavior Scale Residential and Community, ed 2 ABS-RC:2 (1969-1993) Author: K Nihira, H Leland, and N Lambert Source: PRO-ED, Inc 8700 Shoal Creek Blvd. Austin, TX 78758-6897	3-21 years	Performance task, observation, and parent report	• Similar to AAMR-School • Provides scores in 18 domains including: independent functioning, language development, social behavior, and physical development • Software for scoring available
	Vineland Adaptive Behavior Scales Author: SS Sparrow, DA Balla, and DV Cicchetti Source: American Guidance Services Inc 4201 Woodland Rd Circle Pines, MN 55014-1796	Birth-adult	Semi-structured interview with observation caregiver, observation	• Assesses adaptive behavior in four sectors: communication, daily living skills, socialization, and motor skills • Can be used with mentally retarded and disabled individuals • 20-40 minutes to administer • *
Temperament	Temperament Assessment Battery for Children (TABC) (1988) Author: RP Martin Source: Clinical Psychology Publishing Co, Inc #4 Conant Square Brandon, VT 05733	3-7 years	Structured test format	• Measures basic personality-behavioral dimensions in the areas of: activity, adaptability, approach/withdrawal, intensity, distractibility, persistence • 10-20 minutes to administer
	Carey and McDevitt Revised Temperament Questionnaire: Toddler Temperament Scale Author: W Fullard, SC McDevitt, and WB Carey Source: W Fullard, PhD Dept of Educational Psychology Temple University Philadelphia, PA 19122	1-3 years	Interview	• Provides an objective measure of the child's temperament profile • Fosters more effective interactions between parent and child • 95 items, 6-pt frequency scale • *

*Can be administered by professional or nonprofessional. Some special training required. Needs to understand testing procedures and be capable of developing rapport with children.

Continued.

Table 2-1.   INSTRUMENTS USED IN DEVELOPMENTAL ASSESSMENT—cont'd

Types of screening tools	Test/source	Age level	Method	Comments
Temperament	Carey and McDevitt Revised Temperament Questionnaire: Behavior Style Questionnaire Author: SC McDevitt and WB Carey Source: SC McDevitt, PhD Dev Profile II Devereaux Center 6436 E Sweetwater Scottsdale, AZ 85254	3-7 years	Interview	• Provides an objective measure of the child's temperament profile • Fosters more effective interactions between parent and child
	Infant Temperament Questionnaire (ITQ) Author: WB Carey and SC McDevitt Source: WB Carey, MD 319 West Front Street Media, PA 19063	4-8 months	Interview Parent Report	• Provides an objective measure of the infant's temperament profile • Fosters more effective interactions between parent and infant *
Vision	Allen Picture Card Test of Visual Acuity Author: HF Allen Source: LADOCA Project and Publishing Foundation E 51st Ave and Lincoln Street Denver, CO 80216	3-6 years	Observation	• Preschooler screening test for visual acuity • Trained volunteers/screeners can conduct the testing • Teach child names of pictures before testing
	Denver Eye Screening Test (DEST) (1973) Author: WK Frankenberg, AD Goldstein, and J Barker	3 years	Observation	• Identifies children with acuity problems • Good for preschool-age children unable to respond to the Snellen Illiterate E Test

	Source: LADOCA Project and Publishing Foundation E 51st Ave and Lincoln St Denver, CO 80216			

	HOTV (Matching symbol test)
	Author:
	O Lippmann
	Source:
	Wilson Ophthalmic Corp
	PO Box 496
	Mustang, OK 73064
		>3 years	Flashcards	• Good for young children or those who
				  don't like to verbalize
				• Children name the four letters H, O, T,
				  and V on a chart for testing at 10–20 feet
				  and match them to a demonstration
				  card
				• Avoids the problem with image reversal
				  and eye-hand coordination that can
				  occur with the letter E
				  *

	Picture Card Test
	(Adaptation of the Pre-school Vision
	   Test)
	Author:
	HF Allen
	Source:
	LADOCA Project and Publishing
	Foundation
	E 51st Ave and Lincoln St
	Denver, CO 80216
		≥ 2½
		years
			Interview/"name the
			picture"
				• Identifies children with acuity problems
				  *

	Snellen Illiterate E Test
	Author:
	H Snellen
	Source:
	National Society for Blindness
	79 Madison Ave
	American Association of
	   Ophthalmology
	1100 17th St NW
	Washington, DC 20036
		≥ 3 years	Observation using two
			persons as a team in
			screening
				• Intended as a screening measure for
				  central acuity of preschool-aged children
				  and of other children who have not
				  learned to read
				  *

Speech and
language
	The Bzoch-League Receptive
	Expressive Emergent
	Language Scale (REEL)
	Author:
	KR Bzoch and R League
		Birth–3
		years
			Paper-pencil inventory
			Parent interview
				• Identifies children needing further
				  follow-up in language
				• 15–20 minutes to administer
				  *

*Can be administered by professional or nonprofessional. Some special training required. Needs to understand testing procedures and be capable of developing rapport with children.

Continued.

Table 2-1.   INSTRUMENTS USED IN DEVELOPMENTAL ASSESSMENT—cont'd

Types of screening tools	Test/source	Age level	Method	Comments
Speech and language	Source: University Park Press 360 N Charles St Baltimore, MD 21201			
	Denver Articulation Screening Exam (DASE) (1971-1973) Author: AF Drumwright and WK Frankenburg Source: Denver Developmental Materials, Inc PO Box 6919 Denver, CO 80206-0919	2½-6 years	Observation	• Designed to identify significant developmental delay in the acquisition of speech sounds • Good for screening children who may be economically disadvantaged and have a potential speech problem with articulation—pronunciation • Administered by a qualified professional; special training required for the nonprofessional • 10-15 minutes to administer
	Emergent Language Milestone Scale (ELM) (1984) Source: Education Corporation PO Box 721 Tulsa, OK 74101	Birth-36 months	Interview/observation	• Screening instrument for auditory expressive, auditory receptive, and visual components of language *
	Peabody Picture Vocabulary Test, Revised (PPVT-R) (1981) Author: LM Dunn and LM Dunn Source: American Guidance Service 4201 Woodland Rd Circle Plains, MN 55014-1796	2½-40 years	Individual "Point to" response test	• IQ used to assess receptive vocabulary, not a measure of speech and language skills • Measures hearing vocabulary for standard American English • Used with non-English-speaking students to screen for mental retardation or giftedness • Requires a qualified practitioner to administer • 10-20 minutes to administer

Category	Test/Author/Source	Age	Method	Description
	Riley Articulation and Language Test, Revised (RALT-R) Author: GD Riley Source: Western Psychological 12031 Wilshire Blvd Los Angeles, CA 90025	≥ 4 years	Performance tasks by the child	• 2-3 minute screening test, identifies children in need of speech therapy • Provides a quantified system for observation and measurement of neurologic signs that lead to problems in speech, language, learning, and behavior • Needs to be administered by a qualified clinician
Hearing	Noise Stik Author: LH Eckstein Source: Eckstein Bros, Inc 4807 W 118th Place Hawthorne, CA 90250	Birth-3 years	Behavioral response to auditory stimulation	• Handheld free-field screener for use in the early detection of infant hearing loss *
Child behavior and cognition	Kaufman Brief Intelligence Test (K–BIT) (1990) Author: AS Kaufman and NL Kaufman Source: American Guidance Service 4201 Woodlawn Rd Circle Pines, MN 55014-1796	4-90 years	Structured test format	• Quick measure of intelligence, may not be substituted for comprehensive measure of intelligence • Assess expressive vocabulary, definitions, matrices • 15-30 minutes to administer *
	Brazelton Neonatal Behavioral Assessment Scale Author: TB Brazelton Source: JB Lippincott, Co 227 Washington Square Philadelphia, PA 19106-3780	3 days-4 weeks		• Used as a predictive tool in clinical practice and research for behavioral and neurologic assessment • Tests 27 behavioral items in the areas of habitation, orientation, motor maturity, variation, self-quieting, and social • Requires a trained examiner and 20-30 minutes to administer
	Child Behavior Checklist Author: TM Achenbach Source: Center for Children, Youth, and Families University of Vermont 1 S. Prospect St Burlington, VT 05401	4-18 years	Observation/interview	• Provides an overview of the child's behavior • Parent and teacher forms available

*Can be administered by professional or nonprofessional. Some special training required. Needs to understand testing procedures and be capable of developing rapport with children.

Continued.

Table 2-1.   INSTRUMENTS USED IN DEVELOPMENTAL ASSESSMENT—cont'd

Types of screening tools	Test/source	Age level	Method	Comments
Child behavior and cognition	Pediatric Symptom Checklist Author: M Murphy and M Jellinek Source: Dr. Mike Jellinek Child Psychology Service Mass General Hospital in Boston ACC725 Boston, MA 02114	6-18 years	Parent completed	• Used to screen for areas of weakness requiring more detailed diagnostic testing in scholastic achievement • Parent completed form • A child self-report version • Version for 2-5 years also available • 5 minutes to administer
	Peabody Individual Achievement Test: Revised (PIAT-R) (1970-1989) Author: LM Dunn and FC Markwardt, Jr Source: American Guidance Service 4201 Woodland Rd Circle Pines, MN 55014-1796	K-12 grade	Interview and written test	• Used to screen for areas of weakness requiring more detailed diagnostic testing in scholastic achievement • Must be administered by a psychologist • 50-70 minutes to administer • Assesses reading recognition such as reading comprehension, total reading, mathematics, spelling, written expression
	Riley Preschool Developmental Screening Inventory (RPDSI) Author: CMD Riley Source: Western Psychological 12031 Wilshire Blvd Los Angeles, CA 90025	3-5 years	Observation	• For children who have the tendency for academic problems • Requires a qualified clinician to administer • Used to screen for emotional, learning, and behavioral problems
	Wide Range Achievement Test (WRAT)3(1940-1993) Author: GS Wilkinson	5-75 years	Paper-pencil subtests	• Used for education placement, vocational assessment, and job placement training • Large print edition is available

Category	Test / Source / Author	Age range	Administration	Description
	Source: Jastak Associates, Wide Range Inc PO Box 3410 Wilmington, DE 19804-0250			• Measures the skills needed to learn reading, spelling, and arithmetic • 15-30 minutes to administer
Stress anxiety	State-Trait Anxiety Inventory for children (STAIC) (1970-1973) Author: CD Spielberg, CD Edwards, RE Lushene, J Montuori, and D Platzek Source: Consulting Psychologists Press, Inc 3803 E Bayshore Rd Palo Alto, CA 94303	4-6 grades	Group or individual Self-administered	• Measures anxiety in elementary school children • Title on test is "How I Feel Questionnaire" • 20 minutes to administer
	State—Trait Anxiety Inventory (STAI) (1968-1984) Author: CD Spielberger, RL Gorsuch, R Lushene, PR Vagg, and GA Jacobs Consulting Psychologists Press, Inc 3803 E Bayshore Road Palo Alto, CA 94303	9-16 years and adults	Group administration, test booklet Spanish and English available	• Designed to assess anxiety as an emotional state (S-Anxiety) and individual differences in anxiety proneness as a personality trait (T-Anxiety) • 10-20 minutes to administer
	Stress Response Scale (SRS) (1979-1993) Author: LA Chandler Source: Psychological Assessment Resources, Inc PO Box 998 Odessay, FL 33556	5-14 years	Group or individual structured test	• Designed to identify behavior or emotional problems: Impulsive (acting out), passive aggressive, impulsive (overactive), repressed, or dependent • Software available for scoring • 5 minutes to administer
Self-concept	Piers-Harris Children's Self-Concept Scale (The Way I Feel About Myself) (PHCSCS) (1969-1984) Author: EV Piers and DB Harris	8-18 years	Descriptive statements Used by group or individual	• 80 questions requiring yes-no response • Assesses a raw self-concept score plus cluster scores for behavior, intellectual and school status, physical appearance and attributes, anxiety, popularity, happiness, and satisfaction

*Can be administered by professional or nonprofessional. Some special training required. Needs to understand testing procedures and be capable of developing rapport with children.

Continued.

Table 2-1.   **INSTRUMENTS USED IN DEVELOPMENTAL ASSESSMENT—cont'd**

Types of screening tools	Test/source	Age level	Method	Comments
Self-concept	Source: Western Psychological Services 12031 Wilshire Blvd Los Angeles, CA 90025			• 15-20 minutes to administer *
Family function	Feetham Family Functioning Survey (FFFS) (1982) Author: Feetham and Humenick Source: Nursing Systems and Research Children's National Medical Center 111 Michigan Ave, NW Washington, DC 20010	Family	Self-reporting instrument	• 25 questions evaluating six areas of functioning: household tasks, child care, sexual and moral relations, interaction with family and friends, community involvement, and sources of support • 10 minutes to administer • Used for identifying specific areas of dysfunction in a stressed family *
	Home Observation for Measurement of the Environment (HOME) (1984) Author: R Bradley and B Caldwell Source: Center for Research on Teaching & Learning University of Arkansas at Little Rock 2801 S University Ave Little Rock, AR 72204-1099	Birth-3 years 3-6 years	Interview and direct observation of the interaction between the caretaker and the child	• Two separate instruments designed to assess the quantity and quality of social, the emotional, and cognitive support available to a child within his home • The inventory for children birth to 3 contains 45 items; the inventory for 3-6 year-old children contains 55 items • Each inventory takes about 1 hour *

environment from a singular perspective, this is of particular significance.

Advocacy

Numerous professions are called on to care for the complex needs of children with chronic conditions. Although all hold the same goal, to help the child reach maximum potential, conflicts may arise as to the best approach for realizing it. The primary care provider is in the unique position to advocate for the child, inform the child and family of available resources, and help coordinate these interdisciplinary services. (See Chapter 1.)

Hospitalization. Hospitalizations are not uncommon with this population of children, and during this time care is usually transferred to the specialty team. The primary care provider can be instrumental in assisting in a smooth transition. In addition to communicating information about the child's physical condition, parents need to be encouraged to provide information to the specialty team about developmental stimulation programs or schooling that the child is receiving. If the hospitalization is planned, every effort should be made for hospital-based educators or tutors to confer with school officials before the child's admission so that schooling is not interrupted. Properly preparing the child and family, especially for new situations, also helps in adjusting to hospitalization. Preparation needs to include procedural information about situations they will encounter, definitions of medical jargon specific to their condition, and opportunities to process (either through play, role playing, or discussion) new situations they may experience. For families who are nonassertive or overly aggressive, the primary care provider can assist in appropriately empowering the child and family members for self-advocacy by working through these tasks.

Monitoring the child's adjustment to hospitalization and future effects it may have on the child's development is also an important component of advocacy. Children's individualism and the severity of their condition are known to affect their adaptation to hospitalization. For many children with chronic conditions, hospitalization is an unwelcomed intrusion into their lives. Other children have positive memories of previous hospitalizations and may see the hospital as a safe environment. They may perceive the staff as friends and are frequently relieved

to have a temporary respite from school stresses, harassment of other children, or the demands of daily activities. Although uncommon, the primary care provider needs to recognize children will occasionally try to become hospitalized to remove themselves from home or school situations that have become particularly onerous.

In today's climate of cost constraint, children are being discharged earlier, and often sicker, than before. This places increased care demands on family members who may feel unprepared to handle these increased responsibilities. The primary care provider is in an ideal position to provide assistance during this transition.

Schooling. The role of the educational arena should not be undervalued. Participating in school provides a measure of independence and opportunities for self-mastery and self-esteem building that are not readily achieved at home (Sylva, 1994; Weitzman, 1984). The primary care provider can promote the benefits garnered from schooling in numerous ways. Suggestions for altering treatment protocols and medications that interfere with school activities may be offered. Attempts to schedule appointments around the school day should be made so that unnecessary absenteeism does not occur. A careful history of absenteeism needs to be collected. If it seems excessive for the child's condition, an interdisciplinary conference should be called.

After hospitalization, the primary care provider can facilitate the child's transition to school by helping parents provide information about the condition and its ramifications for school participation to school authorities (Andrews, 1991; Committee on Children with Disabilities and Committee on School Health, 1990). Although they may be reluctant to do so, parents should be encouraged to interface with their child's teacher and school nurse unless there is a good reason not to do so. Suggesting methods for preparing classmates for the return of the child is equally important, especially for the child with noticeable physical changes (Sexson and Madan-Swain, 1993). "Sanctioned staring," or encouraging classmates to preview the new appearance of the child without fear of recrimination or causing embarrassment, is conducive to a child's acceptance on returning to school. This can be facilitated by suggesting the child share hospital experiences with classmates by writing a letter and including his or her picture or making a video-tape to send to school. Because many teachers have little knowledge of chronic conditions, offer-ing the address and telephone number of specialty agencies such as the American Cancer Society initially provides an important source of useful information.

Counseling. Because children with chronic conditions have a higher percentage of psychoso-cial problems, careful attention must be paid to the child's mental and emotional health (Gizynski and Shapiro, 1990; Gortmaker et al, 1990). Growing up is difficult, and the incidence of alcoholism, drug abuse, suicide, and other self-destructive behaviors among all children continues to climb.

Children with chronic conditions, especially if they have problems with their self-esteem, may be particularly vulnerable. Having an ongoing rela-tionship with child and family members and taking careful histories is the best way of assessing psy-chosocial health; standardized assessment tools tend to perform poorly with populations of children with chronic conditions (Canning et al, 1992; Can-ning and Kelleher, 1994).

Proactive efforts to prevent psychosocial prob-lems from occurring include: (1) encouraging nor-mal life experiences, (2) improving coping abili-ties, (3) helping the child empower himself or her-self, (4) expanding social support networks, and (5) coordinating care (Committee on Children with Disabilities and Committee on Psychosocial As-pects of Child and Family Health, 1993; Patterson and Geber, 1991).

Some children will benefit from counseling. Referral may also be appropriate in helping a child adapt to a new diagnosis or deteriorating prognosis, to deal with school, family, and peer group issues, or to clarify interpersonal and career goals. These are usually very private concerns for older children and adolescents. Seeking such help while maintain-ing their privacy may be difficult if their ability to move about the community is limited. The primary care provider can be instrumental in facilitating such help.

Dying. Some children will die despite every-one's best efforts. The primary care provider can be of great assistance in planning for and providing psychologic care during this difficult and poignant

time. One of the key roles is to encourage and facili-tate the family's ability to provide this care (Koocher and Gudas, 1992). Children's emotional needs and fears need to be addressed from their perspective. The primary care provider can help family members with this by modeling ways to communicate these sensitive issues and offering insights as to how a child's developmental level affects his or her ability to conceptualize death. Many times children's ques-tions are upsetting to parents, such as when a 6-year-old requests detailed information about death rituals or a preschooler wants to know, "Who will read me stories after I die?" Helping family members and other significant individuals communicate effec-tively with the child and each other will make death easier to bear.

Many children want to die at home, where they are in familiar surroundings, where separation is minimized, and care is individualized, and where they are able to remain in great control of their sit-uations. Other children may feel insecure at home and prefer to be hospitalized, surrounded by profes-sionals they trust. Home care and hospitalization both have advantages and disadvantages, and the decision of which to pursue needs to be made in concert with the child's wishes and the family's ca-pabilities. The primary care provider can be instru-mental in facilitating either of these options in con-junction with local hospice services.

SUMMARY

Children with chronic conditions are at a higher risk for negative developmental sequelae than their nonaffected peers. The severity of the condition, in-dividualistic traits of the child, and the available network for social supports all influence the child's developmental outcomes. Comprehensive prospec-tive care, however, can eliminate or significantly ameliorate negative outcomes. Careful assessment using an interdisciplinary approach will help iden-tify potential or emerging problems associated with the child's disease progression, functional status, social interactions, or global development. Individ-ualized intervention strategies including therapeu-tic management, education, counseling, and advo-cacy can then be designed and implemented to as-sist children with chronic conditions in reaching their developmental potential.

REFERENCES

Andrews SG: Informing schools about children's chronic illness: parents' opinions. *Pediatrics* 88:306-311, 1991.

Bender BG et al: Psychologic change associated with theophylline treatment of asthmatic children: a 6-month study. *Pediatr Pulmonol* 11:233-242, 1991.

Bender BG, Lerner JA, and Poland JE: Association between corticosteroids and psychologic change in hospitalized asthmatic children, *Ann Allergy* 66:414-419, 1991.

Bennett FC, Nickel RE: Developmental screening surveillance, presented at *The Child with Special Needs,* San Francisco, April 1995.

Brady TJ: Patient control of treatment is essential. *Arthritis Care and Research* 38(Pt 2):195-202, 1994.

Brookins GK: Culture, ethnicity, and bicultural competence: implications for children with chronic illness and disability, *Pediatrics* 91:1056-1062, 1993.

Burbach D, Peterson L: Children's concepts of physical illness: a review and critique of the cognitive-developmental literature, *Health Psychol* 5:307-325, 1986.

Cadman D et al: Children with chronic illness: family and parent demographic characteristics and psychosocial adjustment, *Pediatrics* 87:884-889, 1991.

Canning EH, Kelleher K: Performance of screening tools for mental health problems in chronically ill children, *Arch Pediatr Adolescent Med* 148:272-278, 1994.

Canning EH et al: Mental disorders in chronically ill children: parent-child discrepancy and physician identification, *Pediatrics* 90:692-696, 1992.

Carey WB: Early health crises and vulnerable children. In MD Levine, WB Carey, and AC Crocker, editors: *Developmental-behavioral pediatrics,* ed 2, Philadelphia, 1992, WB Saunders.

Carraccio CL, McCormick MC, and Weller SC: Chronic disease: effect on health cognition and health locus of control, *J Pediatr* 110:982-987, 1987.

Chamberlin RW: Developmental assessment and early intervention programs for young children: lessons learned from longitudinal research, *Pediatr Rev* 8:237-247, 1987.

Committee on Children with Disabilities and Committee on Psychosocial Aspects of Child and Family Health. Psychosocial risks of chronic health conditions in childhood and adolescence, *Pediatrics* 92:876-877, 1993.

Committee on Children with Disabilities and Committee on School Health. Children with health impairments in schools, *Pediatrics* 86:636-638, 1990.

Crider C: Children's conceptions of the body interior. In R Bibace and M Walsh, editors: *New directions for child development: children's conceptions of health, illness, and bodily functions,* San Francisco, 1981, Jossey-Bass, No 14, pp 85-103.

Curry DM, Duby JC: Developmental surveillance by pediatric nurses, *Ped Nurs* 20:40-44, 1994.

Deatrick JA, Woodring BC, and Tollefson TL: Children should be seen and heard, *Health Progress* 71(3):76-79, 1990.

Dworkin PH: Developmental screening—expecting the impossible? *Pediatrics* 83:619-622, 1989.

Eiser C: Children's concepts of illness: towards an alternative to the "stage" approach, *Psychology and Health* 3:93-101, 1989.

Finn K: The hospitalization of children with developmental disorders, *Child Health Care* 10:131-134, 1982.

Frankenberg WK: Preventing developmental delays: is developmental screening sufficient? *Pediatrics* 93:586-593, 1994.

Freud A: *The ego mechanism of defense,* rev ed, New York, 1966, International Universities Press.

Geber G, Latts E: Race and ethnicity: issues for adolescents with chronic illness and disabilities. An annotated bibliography, *Pediatrics* 91:1071-1081, 1993.

Gizynski M, Shapiro VB: Depression and childhood illness, *Child and Adolescent Social Work* 7:179-197, 1990.

Gochman DC: Assessing children's health concepts. In P Karoly, editor: *Handbook of child health assessment: biosocial perspectives,* New York, 1988, John Wiley & Sons.

Goldberg S: Chronic illness and early development: parent-child relationships, *Pediatr Ann* 19:35, 39-41, 1990.

Goldberg S, Simmons RJ: Chronic illness and early development, *Pediatrician* 15:13-20, 1988.

Gortmaker SL et al: Chronic conditions, social-economic risks, and behavioral problems in children and adolescents, *Pediatrics* 85:267-276, 1990.

Groce NE, Zola IK: Multiculturalism, chronic illness and disability, *Pediatrics* 91:1048-1055, 1993.

Hertzig ME: Mental health and developmental problems of children in poverty, *Bull NY Acad Med* 68:25-31, 1992.

Jessop DJ, Stein R & K: Uncertainty and its relation to the psychological and social correlates of chronic illness in children. *Social Science Medicine* 20:993-999, 1985.

Koocher GP, Gudas LJ: Terminal illness in childhood. In MD Levine, WB Carey, AC Crocker, editors: *Developmental-behavioral pediatrics,* ed 2, Philadelphia, 1992, WB Saunders, pp 327-336.

Kravitz L, Selekman J: Understanding hearing loss in children, *Ped Nurs* 18:591-594, 1992.

Lewis SY, Haiken HJ, and Hoyt LG: Living beyond the odds: a psychosocial perspective on long-term survivors of pediatric human immunodeficiency virus infection, *Dev Behav Pediatr* 15:512-517, 1994.

Luthar SS, Zigler E: Vulnerability and competence: a review of research on resilience in childhood, *Am J Orthopsychiatry* 61:6-22, 1991.

Mahon MM: Children's concept of death and sibling death from trauma, *J Pediatr Nurs* 8:335-344, 1993.

Mearig JS: Cognitive development of chronically ill children. In N Hobbs and JM Perrin, editors: *Issues in the care of children with chronic illness,* San Francisco, 1985, Jossey-Bass, pp 672-697.

Moore IM, Klopovich PM: Late effects of cancer treatment in children and adults, *Semin Oncol Nurs* 5:1-3, 1989.

Newacheck PW, Stoddard JJ: Prevalence and impact of multiple childhood chronic illnesses, *J Pediatr* 124:40-48, 1994.

Offord DR, Aponte JF: A comparison of drawings and sentence completion responses of congenital heart children with normal children, *J Project Techniques Personality Assess* 31:57-62, 1967.

Patterson JM, Geber G: Preventing mental health problems in children with chronic illness or disability, *Children's Health Care* 20:150-161, 1991.

Perrin EC et al: Issues involved in the definition and classification of chronic health conditions, *Pediatrics* 91:787-793, 1993.

Perrin EC, Sayer AG and Willett JB: Sticks and stones may break my bones...reasoning about illness causality and body functioning in children who have a chronic illness. *Pediatrics*, 88:608-619, 1991.

Perrin JM: Chronic illness. In Levine MD, Carey WB, and Crocker AC (editors): *Developmental-behavioral pediatrics,* ed 2, Philadelphia, 1992, WB Saunders.

Pidgeon V: Compliance with chronic illness regimens: school-aged children and adolescents, *J Pediatr Nurs* 4:36-47, 1989.

Pless IB: Clinical assessment: physical and psychological functioning. *Pediatric Clinics of North America* 31:189-209, 1984.

Sexson SB, Madan-Swain A: School re-entry for the child with chronic illness, *Journal of Learning Disabilities* 26:115-125, 1993.

Sinnema G: Resilience among children with special health care needs among their families, *Pediatr Ann* 20:483-485, 1991.

Smith K, Layne M, and Garell D: The impact of care coordination on children with special health care needs, *Children's Health Care* 23:251-266, 1994.

Stein REK, Jessop DJ: Long-term effects of a pediatric home care program, *Pediatrics* 88:490-496, 1991.

Stein REK, Jessop DJ: What diagnosis does not tell: the case for a noncategorical approach to chronic illness in children, *Social Science Medicine* 29:769-778, 1989.

Steward MS, Steward DS: Children's conceptions of medical procedures. In R Bibace and M Walsh, editors: *New directions for child development: children's conceptions of health, illness, and bodily functions,* San Francisco, 1981, Jossey-Bass, No 14, pp 67-83.

Sylva K: School influences on children's development, *J Child Psychol Psychiatry* 35:135-170, 1994.

Van Dyke DC, Lin-Dyken DC: The new genetics, developmental disabilities, and early intervention, *Infants and Young Children* 5:8-19, 1993.

Vessey JA: Comparison of two teaching methods on children's knowledge of their internal bodies, *Nurs Res* 37:262-267, 1988.

Vessey JA, Braithwaite KB, and Wiedmann M: Teaching children about their internal bodies, *Pediatr Nurs* 16:29-35, 1990.

Vessey JA, Farley JA, and Risom LP: Iatrogenic developmental effects and pediatric intensive care, *Pediatr Nurs* 17:229-232, 1991.

Weakley DR, Spencer R: Current concepts in retinopathy of prematurity, *Early Human Development* 30:121-130, 1992.

Weiland SK, Pless IB, and Roghmann KJ: Chronic illness and mental health problems in pediatric practice: results from a survey of primary care providers, *Pediatrics* 89:445-449, 1992.

Weitzman M: School and peer relations, *Pediatr Clin North Am* 31:59-70, 1984.

Yoos HL: Children's illness concepts: old and new paradigms, *Pediatr Nurs* 20:134-140, 145, 1994.

Chronic Conditions and the Family

3

Margaret P. Shepard and Margaret M. Mahon

THE FAMILY

Caring for a child with a chronic condition also involves caring for the child's family. Sometimes the family is identified as the context of care and other times it is identified as the unit of care. Defining the family is not as easy as it once seemed because a majority no longer exists that can define a "traditional family." The family is a unique human group that can be represented by many different configurations of its members. Although there are still nuclear families, a variety of family structures are now common. These include single-parent families by choice or as a result of death or divorce, blended families, multigenerational families, children raised by gay or lesbian parents, children living in foster or adoptive homes, and children living with grandparents, aunts or uncles, older siblings, or nonrelatives.

When working with a child and family, the practitioner must ascertain who they define as the family and work within those parameters. This information must be updated over time, recognizing the high rate of flux within families today.

The definition of family and the expectations of family members vary from culture to culture. Any definition of the family should include the following concepts: generational and permanent relationships, a nurturing and caregiving orientation, emotional intensity, a mixture of qualitative and quantitative purposes, altruistic values, and a nurturing form of governance (Burr, Bahr, and Herrin, 1989).

"The family generally creates an environment in which the basic needs necessary to sustain life and growth are met. When a family functions in a manner supportive of, or enabling the growth of its members, it is said to be functioning well" (Thomas, 1987). Moreover, the family influences individual members' expressions of illness and health through the processes of socialization and the transmission of basic values, beliefs, attitudes, hopes, and aspirations.

These unique aspects of family might be considered ideal. They may not always be apparent at the same time in all families. The bonds that tie can be those of obligation or ambivalence rather than affection (Yost, Hochstadt, and Charles, 1988). For example, the ever-increasing numbers of infants abandoned in newborn nurseries by substance-abusing mothers represent parents who do not feel this bond or who are drawn more strongly by other forces.

Stability of family life is not ensured. Families of children with chronic conditions have needs and concerns that extend far beyond the health care system. The needs of families are diverse and change over time (Hostler, 1991). Death, divorce, and separation of legally or nonlegally sanctioned relationships all lead to the stress of family members (Johnson, 1986; McCubbin, 1993). Children may also experience instability if their parent or parents are substance abusers, are emotionally or physically abusive, or suffer from other chronic conditions (Blackford, 1988; Dura and Beck, 1988;

Meyers and Weitzman, 1991). Some children who have been removed from their biologic families and adopted or placed in foster care experience a lack of cultural continuity associated with family life.

Changes in family structure do not necessarily mean weaker families, but these changes do require the practitioner to have a greater awareness and sensitivity to differences within individual families and within society. Relationships within the family, rather than structure or type of family, are much greater predictors of outcomes for children (Visher and Visher, 1995). Each family is defined by individual differences, and has ethnic and cultural influences. The role of each family member should be identified, as well as the family's perceived strengths and weaknesses.

FAMILY CRISIS AND THE CHILD WITH A CHRONIC CONDITION

All families experience crises. Generally crises can be categorized into two types—developmental and situational. Developmental crises are experienced as an expected part of the developmental process of individuals and families, for example, marriage, birth of a child, toilet training, starting school, or leaving home. Situational crises are not universal in that even though all families experience situational crises, they do not necessarily experience the same crises. Having a child with a chronic condition is an example of a situational crisis. In all crises family coping is challenged and the family must learn to adapt. The way the family perceives the situation, problem-solving strategies, coping repertoire, and usual patterns of functioning will moderate the family's ability to adapt to the new situation (McCubbin, 1993). Any crisis, whether developmental or situational, changes the family. The attempt to adapt leaves the family stronger, weaker, or dissolved.

In assessing the impact of a chronic condition on a family, the practitioner must consider the situational crisis in the context of any concomitant or proximal developmental crisis. For example, the family whose newborn has a condition necessitating surgery or other treatment is dealing with the birth of a newborn *and* the newborn's chronic condition.

It is also essential that a practitioner not assume the family's functional level will be static; rather, the functional level may fluctuate over time. Highs and lows relate presumably to those stresses that impinge on the system and to crisis resolution (Kazak, 1989; McCubbin, 1993). These stresses are not solely the result of a chronic condition. Families in which a child has a chronic condition are subject to the same stresses as other families. "The additions of other children to the family, divorces, deaths of grandparents, financial problems, relocation, and inclusion of nonblood kin in the family system are all 'normal' events families experience that will affect the way in which the child's illness is perceived and handled over time" (Kazak, 1989). Periodic evaluation of both the family's level of functioning and of the accumulation of stresses the family is experiencing will ultimately contribute to better adaptation for the child and the family as a whole.

Much of what is known about chronic conditions of childhood is from disease-specific studies (Feetham, 1984; Pless and Nolan, 1991). This complicates the task of drawing broad conclusions about the effects of chronic childhood illness on family functioning. Some generalizations are possible, which, together with the disease-specific information, can help to explain the range of responses to chronic conditions.

Any family member's situation has an effect on all other family members. A chronic condition in a child not only affects that child but has ramifications for all members of the family system (Kazak, 1989). Having a child with a chronic condition is stressful (Hobbs, Perrin, and Ireys, 1985; Jessop, Reissman, and Stein, 1988; Kazak, 1989; Thomas, 1987). Despite family experiences causing greater stress, however recent studies suggest that families who have a child with a chronic condition do not suffer a noticeable excess of dysfunction relative to control group families (Cadman et al, 1991; Hostler, 1991). Families are not only managing the specific event that brings them to the attention of the health care system, but they are also managing other stresses from all areas of work and family life. Preliminary investigations suggest the accumulation of family demands will adversely affect family adaptation (McCubbin, 1993; Patterson and McCubbin, 1983). These generalizations underscore the importance of working with families to identify the stress they are experiencing regarding both the care burden of the child with the chronic condition and other stresses the family may be experiencing. Until recently relatively little research has been done regarding the stress experienced by a child with a chronic condition relative to other stresses.

The term *chronic condition* is appropriate because it recognizes that children with a variety of deviations from the norm are not always "ill children." Families often define their children as "normal" even though to observers this is not the case (Anderson, 1981; Deatrick, Knafl, and Walsh, 1988). Despite a history of morbidity, parents consider most of their children to be in good to excellent health (McCormick et al, 1988). Moreover, ratings by the health care provider regarding the burden of care of the child has no relationship to the mother's psychologic status (Jessop, Reissman, and Stein, 1988). It is essential, as with the definition of family, to work within the framework given by the family.

The definition of chronic illness, as developed by the 1949 National Commission on Chronic Illness (and as used in Chapter 1), reveals that a wide range of conditions qualify as chronic. The condition need not be permanent, serious, or obvious. On the other hand, some chronic conditions are irreversible, serious, and require comprehensive care.

The reality is that a child may be seriously impaired from birth, may have a transitory condition from which recovery is complete, or may have any degree of severity in between. Furthermore, a diagnosis is not always indicative of the severity of a child's condition. For example, asthma, the most common chronic condition of childhood, may severely affect a child's ability to function on a daily basis or may cause only occasional short-term disability.

FAMILY RESPONSES TO THE DIAGNOSIS OF A CHRONIC CONDITION

The diagnosis of a chronic condition is a time of extreme distress (Goldberg and Simmons, 1988) and disequilibrium (Thomas, 1987) for a family. Many factors affect the family's responses. The identification of a diagnosis might cause a response that is not necessarily congruent with presenting symptoms, health of the child, or interventions required as a result of the diagnosis (Goldberg and Simmons, 1988). This suggests that family response, especially parental response, is based more on preconceived ideas about a chronic condition. A child previously thought of as healthy may now be thought of as ill.

Chronic conditions in newborns are either congenital (e.g., cleft lip or palate), genetic (e.g., trisomy 21), vertically transmitted from the mother (e.g., pediatric HIV infection), or a function of prematurity. In each of these situations the parents are likely to grieve the healthy newborn they envisioned (Solnit and Stark, 1962; Meyers and Weitzman, 1991). Initial reactions may include shock, disbelief, and denial (Holaday, 1984), which may translate to thoughts that the newborn is not their newborn but that there has been some kind of mix-up or mistake. If the condition is genetic, some parents will feel guilty that they caused this condition in their newborn (Goldberg and Simmons, 1988). For some parents this grieving might mean that they are not immediately able to respond to their newborn or that they respond by distancing themselves. This temporary distancing is not necessarily inappropriate and should not be treated as maladaptive.

Pediatric HIV has been identified as the "newest chronic illness of childhood" (Meyers and Weitzman, 1991; Sherwen and Boland, 1994). Often the diagnosis of HIV in a newborn is associated with the new diagnosis of other family members. Parental concerns for the child may include the knowledge of a parent's diminished health and impending death. Care concerns may be further complicated by parental guilt and continued addiction or other compromised lifestyle behaviors. Care for the child with HIV infection is certainly complex, but it is essential for the primary care provider to maintain a child-centered, family-focused, and community-based framework for treatment (Meyers and Weitzman, 1991).

As with newborns, the diagnosis of a chronic condition in a child requires the family to adapt to the situation. Initial efforts at family adjustment may result in disequilibrium for the family system (McCubbin, 1993; Thomas, 1987). The family response may include shock, disbelief, denial (Holaday, 1984), disgust, relief, guilt, despair, hate, rage, or confusion (Hobbs, Perrin, and Ireys, 1985).

"Disruption of the family depends on the nature, severity, length, prognosis of illness and parental coping: support systems, fiscal resources, educational background, previous experience with illness and a variety of individual definitions" (Andrews and Nielson, 1988). One major difference that occasionally occurs with the diagnosis of a chronic condition in older children is a sense of relief at finally having a diagnosis. The suspicions of the parents are confirmed, the uncertainty is over, and interventions may now begin. The child and family may also become eligible for a range of services for which they previously were not eligible (Goldberg and Simmons, 1988).

The diagnosis sets some parents on a search for causes of the condition, whether physiologic or environmental (Lipman, 1988). This quest for information is usually very appropriate and should be supported as part of the family's efforts to cope. The parent or parents are obtaining knowledge about the condition, which is the first step in having some control over the situation (Hobbs, Perrin, and Ireys, 1985). In some parents, however, the search for information is a denial of the reality of their child's situation. For example, some parents will read medical books and talk with a variety of specialists and subspecialists. This self-education can allow them to make informed choices or can be the beginning of a search exclusively for a cure, resulting in the child not receiving the immediate medical care needed.

Besides looking for facts about the condition, some parents search for religious or philosophic reasons for what has happened (Holaday, 1984). Family functioning is enhanced when parents are able to give a more positive than negative interpretation and are able to define the chronic condition and resultant situations within a previously existing personal, medical-scientific and/or religious philosophy of life (Venters, 1981). This sometimes takes the form of "why me" questions. Parents also worry about the health of their other children and begin to search for means to prevent the condition from occuring in these other children (Lipman, 1988).

The prognosis of the condition may affect the response of the parents, especially if the condition is potentially life threatening (Goldberg and Simmons, 1988). Similarly, the family's subjective perception of the impact of the illness on the family system may affect the level of family functioning (Shepard, 1992).

Other factors that affect the responses of parents and others are the visibility of the condition, the presence or absence of mental retardation, the expectation of pain for the child, the uncertainty about changes in the condition, the parents' experience with others who have chronic conditions, and the preconceptions about the condition, whether correct or incorrect (Burr, 1985; Jessop and Stein, 1985).

RESPONSES TO TREATMENT AND CHRONICITY

Role of the Primary Care Provider

When a chronic condition is diagnosed, the focus of the family often becomes narrow and very disease oriented. Whether caring for a newborn or an older child, the primary care provider should consider several important guidelines. *First,* be concrete. Provide as much information as is immediately needed but not much more. Parents should participate fully in the decision-making process and should receive information in sufficient time to make informed decisions. Answer specific questions asked by the family. Provide information in writing or tape record discussions about the condition so the parents and child can read or hear the explanations repeatedly. Children should be given developmentally appropriate information. Periodically assess how the parents and child are responding to and utilizing the information provided.

Second, provide resources, such as the primary care provider, or a subspecialist, a clinical nurse specialist, and/or a resource group. The family should be supplied information about "what comes next." Again, if possible, do this in writing. *Third,* help the family put the diagnosis in perspective. This may be hard to do but can be very helpful for families. The first step is to ascertain what expectations the parent or parents already have. If there are misconceptions, clarify them. In addition, find something normal and positive about this child. For example, comment on the alertness of an infant born with myelomeningocele or on the infant's strong grasp. This is not an attempt to minimize the seriousness of the situation but to focus on the child as an individual with many of the same needs as other children. In fact, the process of parent-infant attachment may be enhanced when parents are able to identify aspects of normality and strengths in their infant (Drotar et al, 1975).

There are no right or wrong responses for family members at the time of diagnosis. The coping strategies of families are rich and diverse. They may reflect ethnic or other cultural values unfamiliar to the primary care provider. Different cultural and religious belief systems need to be understood and accepted by the primary care provider (Hostler, 1991). The primary care provider should look for cues from the family concerning their readiness to learn, their difficulty accepting the diagnosis, or their unique fears or stressors. The primary care provider should respond to these cues in a supportive manner. Supportive efforts may also include referral of the family for mental health counseling to prevent some of the emotional sequelae that can occur for both the child and the family (Pless and Nolan, 1991). Any family system evaluation should help the family identify strengths, coping styles, and patterns of behavior that might facilitate or impede adjustment to the chronic condition (Sholevar and Perkel, 1990). Every interaction at this critical juncture should end with a statement concerning what to expect next and when the family will be seen again.

When the diagnosis of a chronic condition is made by someone other than the primary care provider, the family will often turn to the primary care provider for information, help, or advice. In some cases the practitioner is available but inaccurate (Hobbs, Perrin, and Ireys, 1985) concerning the details or treatment of the condition. It is important for the practitioner to consult with the specialist to facilitate the family's understanding of the diagnosis and treatment. The practitioner needs to help establish a team approach to care that *includes* the family because the ultimate responsibility for care of the child lies with the family (Horner, Rawlins, and Giles, 1987; Hostler, 1991). This requires knowing and building on family strengths and considering potential stressors in planning for care. Most important, it means using and respecting the knowledge the family has acquired, not only about the condition, but also about the child and his or her individual responses.

The relationship of the family with the primary care provider often, and appropriately, changes over time as the locus of expertise shifts to the family. It is essential that the primary care provider recognize the acquisition of increasing knowledge by the family and the management behaviors and styles of the family (Deatrick, Knafl, and Guyer, 1993).

Family Roles and Responsibilities

The management of a chronic condition rarely falls equally on family caregivers. It is now well-documented that the mother is usually identified as the one primarily responsible for the day-to-day care and management of the child (Breslau, 1983; Glazer 1990; Howlin, 1988; Jessop, Reissman, and Stein, 1988; Kazak, 1989; Moyer, 1989). Some mothers give up their jobs to care for their child perhaps because of the demands of medical treatment (Stein et al, 1989). Because of limited day care for children with chronic conditions, some mothers who might otherwise be employed outside the home are forced to stay at home (Hobbs, Perrin, and Ireys, 1985; Stein et al, 1989). The chronic condition or resultant treatments may bring about behavioral changes that affect the parental relationship with the child. Such changes have been observed in response to the blood testing and insulin injections required for a child with diabetes (Goldberg and Simmons, 1988). The gender of the child may also affect how mothers perceive the burden of caring for the child. Compared with mothers of daughters, mothers of sons with sickle cell disease were usually more involved in caregiving, more likely to intervene to protect their child's health, and expressed more anxiety over their child's health. Mothers of sons were also more likely to describe their child's health as fragile, and they were more likely to supervise closely and restrict their son's activities (Hill and Zimmerman, 1995). Although there can be numerous stressors, many women evaluate their caregiving experience as very positive.

Parents also may be negatively affected by these care demands. Some parents of children with chronic conditions are depressed and have decreased self-esteem, psychologic pain (Schlomann, 1988), and somatic conditions (Sabbeth and Leventhal, 1984). Some mothers experience depression, fatigue, headaches, insomnia, and loss of appetite, whereas fathers experience depression, fatigue, ulcers, headaches, and obesity (Hobbs, Perrin, and Ireys, 1985). The rate for seeking treatment for "nerves" is two to three times higher for both mothers and fathers of children with chronic conditions in comparison to parents of well children (Cadman et al, 1991). Mothers may have more symptoms than fathers (Jessop, Reissman, and Stein, 1988), possibly because mothers are more frequently the subject of research. Although it has been suggested that the functional status of the child is correlated with the mother's symptoms, maternal symptoms may have a stronger relationship to the stresses experienced than to the child's actual functional level (Jessop, Reissman, and Stein, 1988).

Many mothers say it is very helpful to have someone with whom they can talk (Jessop, Reissman, and Stein, 1988). Because this person may not necessarily be a family member (Kazak, Reber, and Carter, 1988), support groups may help meet this need (Horner, Rawlins, and Giles, 1987; Hostler, 1991). These groups are often most helpful to families near the time of diagnosis, probably because of the need for concrete information that is shared among the relatively small number of people who are in a similar situation. After the initial crisis period and during periods of acute hospitalizations, parents may find they are without support from friends and family. This can result in social isolation (Andrews and Nielson, 1988). In one study, 49% of the respondents said they needed help in finding community resources, and 34% asked for help in finding recreational activities for their children with chronic conditions (Horner, Rawlins, and Giles, 1987; Williams, 1993).

Families perceive the chronic condition, its effects, and its implications in a variety of ways. Some families are able to integrate the condition as just another part of the daily routine, whereas others perceive it as a feared and loathsome intrusion into their lives. Knafl and others (1993) categorized families' views of chronic illness as a "manageable condition," an "ominous situation," a "hateful restriction," or that the family had a "limited understanding of the condition." Interestingly, these authors explored parents' views of their children and parenting philosophies, since these views interact with each other. There is also an interactive effect between the views of those involved in parenting and caregiving.

Normalization. Normalization is a management process used by some families of children with a chronic condition. Normalization involves acknowledging the chronic condition, defining the life of the family as normal, defining the social effects of having a child with a chronic condition as minimal, and engaging in behaviors that demonstrate to others that this is a normal family (Knafl and Deatrick, 1986). Normalization is an ongoing process of actively accommodating the child's evolving physical, emotional, and social needs (Deatrick, Knafl, and Walsh, 1988). The child is integrated into the mainstream to the greatest extent possible (Holaday, 1984).

Acknowledging the condition is essential as the foundation of normalization. There is no denial involved, rather the family is making a statement that "this child is a part of our family, and our family is just like every other family." The child's age and the condition's severity affect the ability of the family to use the process of normalization (Knafl and Deatrick, 1986).

Krulik (1980) described several antecedent principles necessary for the normalization process: (1) those involved in the care of the child, including the child, are prepared for the effects of the condition and treatment; (2) the child is involved in self-care and the decisions made about that care; (3) the child with a chronic condition is treated as a part of the family, not differently; (4) the child's condition is not treated as something to be kept secret, rather information is shared; and (5) recognition of the parents' preexisting role in managing care decreases feelings of passivity and uncertainty.

Normalization is important because it focuses on the child, not on the condition. Most parents who have used normalization techniques have discovered these techniques on their own. The process, however, involves some concrete steps that can be taught. The primary care provider can demonstrate some of these steps by recognizing the normalcy, the strengths, and the weaknesses of the family system, by being open and supportive concerning the child's condition and treatment, and by actively involving the family in all aspects of care. Reinforcing the family's successful use of these tactics can improve self-esteem and motivate further development.

Siblings. The impact of the chronic condition on siblings can be analyzed in much the same way as other childhood stressors. Having a sibling with a chronic condition may engender feelings of isolation, rejection, anxiety, helplessness, resentment, guilt, or depression. These feelings frequently stem from emotional realignment within the family, where there are periods of physical and emotional separation, a lack of information, and disrupted communication (Kramer, 1981; Krener and Adelman, 1988). A lack of balance between the needs of the affected child and of siblings is also disrupting (Krener and Adelman, 1988). Some researchers have found no significant difference in social and behavior problems between siblings of children with chronic conditions and a normative sample (Gallo et al, 1993).

Parents may have difficulty accurately perceiving how their children are coping with the additional family stress. Furthermore, if problems do exist, it may be difficult to distinguish if these problems *are* related to the sibling's chronic condition (Gallo et al, 1993). It is often helpful for the primary care provider to ask how the sibling or siblings are doing and what they understand about the recent changes in the family. Siblings may be uninformed about the nature of the condition for several weeks or much longer (Kramer, 1981). Parents may not have been able to take the time to explain the recent changes to the sibling.

Siblings are directly and immediately affected by the diagnosis of a chronic condition but often lack the power to have any impact on the many and perhaps serious changes within the family. What makes this more difficult is that siblings often guess about the chronic condition and the resulting health status, in part because of the absence of the affected sibling or the parents and the influx of visitors or increased number of telephone calls. What they overhear or piece together is often much worse than the reality. If the parents are unable to talk to the siblings, it is important to find someone else, such as the primary care provider, who can speak with the siblings in a developmentally appropriate way.

Worries or fears of the siblings can, to a certain extent, be predicted based on their developmental level. Children in the operational stage of development are likely to have fears based on egocentrism. They must be told specifically that they were not responsible for the condition. Siblings whose conceptual ability is at the level of concrete operations are likely to be afraid of catching the condition. For example, a sibling of a child who was being treated for cancer began to scrub the toilets in the house thoroughly. When asked about this by his mother, he explained that because the cancer cells were coming out in the urine, he did not want to catch it when he went to the bathroom. In this case the sibling received some appropriate teaching, but took the information and integrated his fears at his current level of understanding.

Siblings also often imagine gruesome things about the experiences associated with illness, hospitalization, and treatment. If possible, siblings should be allowed to see the hospital, treatment rooms, and perhaps treatments if it is acceptable to the sibling with the chronic condition.

The effects of a condition or treatment, such as hair loss, flatulence, or copious secretions, may be embarrassing for siblings of school age and older. At the same time, children also want to protect their affected sibling from the derisive statements or stares of others (Trahd, 1986). These feelings of shame and embarrassment are usually not severe (Howlin, 1988), though they can engender simultaneous or subsequent feelings of guilt.

Siblings often feel that the discipline for the child with a chronic condition is not as strict as it is for them (Howlin, 1988); in fact, this is often the case. Some parents are not aware that they are treating their children with different standards. Quittner and Opipari (1994) concluded that there were both qualitative and quantitative differences in parenting when a child with cystic fibrosis (CF) was in the family, despite the parents' lack of awareness. It is appropriate for the primary care provider to question families about methods and consistency of discipline.

Siblings are usually very aware of their negative feelings, which may include anger, feelings of being neglected, fears of causality, contagion, or responsibility, and other founded and unfounded feelings (Howlin, 1988; Kramer, 1981). As a result of their negative feelings, they may experience guilt. Children need to be told that their emotions are acceptable, but at the same time misconceptions need to be clarified. This may be a time-consuming process calling for self-realization—a difficult task for some families. For example, a sibling's perception that he or she has been receiving less attention can be confirmed. The child should also be told that it is okay to feel angry about receiving less attention. This can be very difficult if sharing emotions is not usually done by a particular family.

The developmental level of siblings, both physical and psychosocial, must be considered in the plan for care of the affected child at home. If a child is to be cared for at home and needs the use of equipment and medications, recognizing and planning for sibling safety are required. Andrews and Nielson (1988) reported several cases of children injuring or potentially injuring themselves or their siblings by changing intravenous flow rates or by not understanding the danger of electrical equipment.

Siblings have also described many positive effects from having a sibling with a chronic condition, including being well adjusted, having a positive self-concept, being more mature, being more tolerant, and being capable of handling greater responsibility than their peers (Howlin, 1988; Kramer, 1981; Lynn, 1989). Siblings of children with chronic conditions have been reported to be cooperative and cognitively able to master situations earlier than their peers (Lynn, 1989).

Several factors predict adjustment. The most important factor is parental attitude about the child (Howlin, 1988). Siblings in a two-child family may be at greater risk because the bond with the affected child forms the sole sibling relationship (Trahd, 1986).

Relative birth order and gender are also significant. In one study among siblings younger than their affected brother or sister, boys were more impaired than girls; among siblings older than their affected brother or sister, girls were psychologically more distressed (Breslau, Weitzman, and Messenger, 1981). These authors believed this was most likely to be the case if the condition were congenital. The possibility of more difficult adaptation by older sisters is congruent with the finding of Howlin (1988) because girls were more likely to have care-giving demands placed on them. Older sisters might be called on more often than younger sisters to perform care-giving tasks. Williams, Lorenzo, and Borja (1993) found that siblings of children with chronic conditions had significantly more responsibilities at home, involving both housework and child care. Siblings' perceptions of the home environment are likely to differ from the impressions of their parents (Feeman and Hagen, 1990).

There is some disagreement about the degree to which siblings should be involved in the care of a child with a chronic condition. One consideration is "what would be expected of siblings if a chronic condition were not involved." Two areas should be considered—the developmental abilities of the siblings and their desire to be involved. Gender-biased expectation of siblings does occur but should be avoided if possible. The most important consideration is consistency, for example, are demands being made regardless of whether a chronic condition is present or absent in any particular child? For those siblings who want to be involved in the care of the child with the chronic condition, this altruism should not be discouraged (Howlin, 1988).

Throughout the course of the chronic condition, information for the siblings needs to be updated for two primary reasons. First, what is known about the condition changes, both as the affected child and parents learn more about the condition and because the manifestations of the condition in this particular child might change. Second, the developmental level of the siblings change, thereby changing their ability to integrate information. Primary care providers are often in an ideal position to provide the impetus for further teaching, both as more is known about the condition and as the siblings progress developmentally.

Finances. Some chronic conditions place large financial demands on the family (Jacobs and McDermott, 1989), though costs vary a great deal depending on the condition and even among individuals with the same condition (Hobbs, Perrin, and Ireys, 1985). There are many additional expenses beyond those directly involved in the care of the child with the chronic condition.

Additional costs for families include food required by special diets, transportation, baby-sitters for siblings while a child receives treatment or other care, time lost from work or school, cosmetics, wigs or clothing to hide the effects of the disease or treatment; and incidentals such as bandages, test kits, diapers, and bed pads—the costs of which accumulates quickly (Hobbs, Perrin, and Ireys, 1985). Other financial requirements arise because of structural modifications to the home, counseling and mental health services, and respite homemaker services (Gale, 1989). Not all of these are covered by most third-party payers. If these costs are covered, there is likely to be a limitation placed on the amount of reimbursement (see Chapter 7).

Differences in the type of insurance or health care coverage can result in differences in access to care, continuity, comprehensiveness, and coordination of care. Common types of insurance include health maintenance organizations (HMOs), independent practice associations (IPAs), and fee-for-service coverage (Safron, Tarlov, and Rogers, 1994). Furthermore, in some of these agencies the people responsible for or involved in teaching may have little or no pediatric expertise or experience with this child's condition.

Of children with chronic conditions, 2% to 5% are candidates for home health services, which might include monitoring equipment, phototherapy, oxygen and tracheostomy care, enteral and parenteral therapy, artificial ventilation, and dialysis (Andrews and Nielson, 1988). Primary care providers are likely to be caring for a child and family who are the recipients of such services. Home care teaching is usually done by nurses or a representative from a home care agency while a child is hospitalized. Many families have found that the teaching they received does not meet their needs once the child comes home. This may not be a reflection of inadequate teaching, rather a reflection on the lack of a frame of reference for the parent or parents learning the care or of the person doing the teaching. Also, the anxiety associated with providing care at home might interfere with parents' ability to learn. The first two weeks at home are often the hardest (Andrews and Nielson, 1988).

Though parents usually deliver much of the care of children with chronic conditions who are at home, the trend towards shorter hospital stays has resulted in children being at home sometimes sicker and with more complex care demands. Sometimes children return home with nurses or other caregivers. Having "outsiders" in the home on a regular basis can be very stressful for families. Also, the increase in acuity and the number of care providers requires more vigilant efforts in communication between care providers.

Because of some families' inability to provide care, some children with chronic conditions are in need of medical foster care. The need for families capable of providing this service has dramatically increased in recent years. When foster care is not available, these children sometimes become boarder infants in hospitals at great financial cost to the hospital and the public and at significant personal risk to the children. These children do not need the level of care a hospital provides; instead, they require a family environment for nurturance (Yost, Hochstadt, and Charles, 1988). Placing children in medical foster care results in a 40% to 98% savings in monetary terms and provides a home environment for the children (Yost, Hochstadt, and Charles, 1988).

Social Support

A primary need of most families is emotional support and practical help (Holaday, 1984). At the time of diagnosis there is often an influx of concerned people, possibly too many. The family may have difficulty using these resources. Types of support that families have found helpful include transportation for siblings, having siblings stay with friends during hospitalizations, providing meals, doing the laundry, running errands, or baby-sitting in the home so that the parents can have some time for themselves. This latter form of assistance may entail learning care such as cardiopulmonary resuscitation (CPR), use of monitors, or emergency care. It is extremely important that someone in addition to the mother be able and willing to do this. Improved social supports benefit the entire family (Hamlett, Pelligrini, and Katz, 1992; Wallander and Varni, 1989).

Mothers may perceive and use social supports differently from fathers (Kazak, Reber, and Carter, 1988). In one study, fathers and older parents were less likely to want to join support groups than mothers and younger parents (Winkel, 1988). Race and ethnicity may also influence the ways families perceive and utilize social supports. In a comparison study of black families and white families, white families were more likely to identify affective support (e.g., support conveying empathy and understanding) as their primary type of support, whereas black families identified instrumental assistance (e.g., help with other children or transportation) as the primary means of support from friends and families (Williams, 1993). Primary care providers can facilitate family support by identifying the types of support that may be most helpful for the family and by being knowledgeable about community resources and parents' groups.

If the condition the child has is relatively common or well understood, that child is less likely to face societal prejudice (Garrison and McQuiston, 1989). This issue of familiarity with the condition is one reason some parents turn to support groups; parents do not have to explain and reexplain the condition because the support group members experience similar situations themselves.

School

The transition to school can be a difficult time for families. Although attendance at school is an indication that the child is "like other children" and well enough to attend school, many obstacles may need to be overcome in starting and maintaining school participation. Families often think teachers and others in the school system are not ready for the challenge of school attendance (Johnson, Lubker, and Fowler, 1988). Teachers support this by reporting they feel inadequately prepared to care for children with chronic conditions.

The implications for teachers of having a child with a chronic condition in their class range from minimal to overwhelming. For example, the teacher of a child with diabetes should know what to do for a child who is having a hypoglycemic reaction. The teacher of a child with heart disease should know CPR. The teacher of a child with epilepsy should know what to do if the child has a seizure. It is unrealistic to expect that care of children with chronic conditions can be handled by a school nurse; often a school nurse divides time between several schools and would be unable to respond to an emergency in a timely manner.

Therefore, families in which a child has a chronic condition are left in a very difficult position. Optimally their child should be in school, but often the school, and specifically the teacher, is inadequately prepared to properly care for the student. From the teacher's point of view, caring for the student would, at the least, take time away from other students and, at worst, could result in a dangerous situation for those students left unattended while the teacher is caring for the affected student. Because there is no ideal solution at this time, each situation should be planned for in advance, before the child begins in the classroom. This planning stage offers an ideal opportunity for the school nurse and primary care provider to cooperate with the family and teacher so that all concerned feel comfortable having the child in the classroom.

LONG-TERM ADAPTATION

Initial responses of the family system to a chronic condition are often similar to an acute illness. After living with the condition and learning its nuances and management, the family has a more thorough understanding of chronicity. The depth and breadth of understanding usually do not extend beyond the immediate family. Relatively simple things such as going out for a meal become difficult, require a great deal of planning, and may be time limited if a child cannot be away from suctioning and oxygen for an extended period.

The amount of time that has elapsed since diagnosis is directly related to the family's involvement in all aspects of care. The longer the child has had the condition, the greater the duration of the chronicity, the more likely the family is to be involved in all aspects of the care. Over time family members gain greater understanding of the interplay of the condition with the individuality of the child. The expectations of the family become more realistic as experience with the condition is acquired (Goldberg and Simmons, 1988).

Selected aspects of some chronic conditions are frequently viewed by the parents as disruptive to their relationship with their child (Goldberg and Simmons, 1988). Examples include parents of children with CF who must perform postural drainage, the decreased physical contact that might be required if the child has osteogenesis imperfecta, or the blood testing and insulin injections required by children with diabetes who are too young for self-care. Parenting a child with a chronic condition "involve[s] qualitatively different work than parenting a child" without a chronic condition (Deatrick, Knafl, and Walsh, 1988). There is often the assumption that "different" has negative connotations. It is essential to differentiate between assuming that having a child with a chronic condition is inherently negative and specifying which aspects of the situation are problematic (Knafl and Deatrick, 1987).

Parental concerns are often the same as those of parents whose child does not have a chronic condition. In a study about the concerns of parents who have children with diabetes, the parents wanted information about diet, the child with diabetes marrying and having children, diabetes itself, care of minor illnesses, normal growth and development, and management of child behavior (Moyer, 1989). All of these concerns were readily addressed by the primary care provider. All parents worry; the extent to which the parent of a child with a chronic condition worries cannot be predicted from the severity of symptoms (Stein et al, 1989).

Many parents are concerned not only about the effect of a chronic condition on the family as it exists at the time of diagnosis but also about the implications for future children. A major factor is whether or not the chronic condition has a genetic component. If, for example, a family has a child with Tay-Sachs disease, the parents might choose not to have more children or might choose to use prenatal screening to assess if the fetus is affected. If the condition is genetic but not a mendelian inheritance, such as trisomy 21 with a translocation defect that might have a 3% to 15% recurrence rate, the family might be more willing to risk having another child. In this case as well the family can avail themselves of prenatal diagnosis. Parents who felt guilty about having a child with a genetically transmitted chronic condition will need to deal with this again if they consider having another child (Goldberg and Simmons, 1988) and later in life when their children reach child-bearing age.

Another common concern for parents is that of parental (usually maternal) workload; can they physically and fiscally care for another child? Again, these concerns are often the same as those families in which there is no child with a chronic condition. Moreover, anecdotal evidence suggests that many families rise to the challenge of providing for a child with a chronic condition (Cadman et al, 1991).

As the ill child with a chronic condition gets older, the concerns about the ability to have children become his or her own. For example, with the increased survival time of people with CF, more women are surviving to childbearing age. Fertility for some of these women is unaffected by CF (MacMullen and Brucker, 1989), which has implications not only for these women but also for the

family and for primary care providers. Education and contraceptive counseling are specific areas of intervention.

Marital Relations

Some people have assumed that because the presence of a chronic condition increases the stress in a family, the rate of family dissolution is greater. On the contrary, carefully controlled studies have indicated neither differences in marital functioning nor differences in the rates of divorced or single-parent families among families of children with chronic conditions (Cadman, et al 1991; Kazak, 1989; Spaulding and Morgan, 1985). In fact, several studies indicated that in families of children with spina bifida, increased severity of the illness was related to higher levels of marital satisfaction for both mothers and fathers (Kazak and Clark, 1986; Martin, 1975). Although divorce is not more prevalent, tension and stress are more common than in families without a child who has a chronic condition (Hobbs, Perrin, and Ireys, 1985). All families have issues and stressors, and when families have a child with a chronic condition, it is easier to overemphasize the causal role of the child's condition in any problems that do exist (Howlin, 1988).

Chronic sorrow. Olshansky (1962) first described the phenomenon of "chronic sorrow" as an ongoing process differing from grief. Olshansky's description came as a result of working with children with mental retardation. Chronic sorrow refers to *the recurrence of parents' feelings engendered by the recognition that their child is "different."* These feelings include sadness, anger, guilt, and failure. Chronic sorrow persists throughout the child's life. This does not mean parents are always sad or that the family does not feel happiness or satisfaction and pride from the child with the chronic condition. Those positive feelings are present, sometimes with great intensity, just as they are for parents whose child does not have a chronic condition.

Parents are likely to experience the surges of emotion associated with chronic sorrow at times of expected developmental milestones such as when the child would have started walking or started school, when younger siblings surpass their sibling, and when the child turns 21 years of age. Chronic sorrow also resurges at unpredictable times, times that likely would have been shared with significant ceremony or otherwise marked had the child not had a chronic condition (Wikler, Wascow, and Hatfield, 1981).

Other researchers have generalized the use of the term "chronic sorrow" to apply to children with chronic physical alterations (Jackson, 1985; Lawson, 1977; Neill, 1979; Tenbrink and Brewer, 1976; Young, 1977). Much of the work that has been done is not research based, but has been adopted because clinicians sensed an intuitive fit with the responses of families in which a child has a chronic condition.

Chronic sorrow does not necessarily occur uniformly within families. Damrosch and Perry (1989) found "clearcut differences in maternal and paternal patterns of overall adjustment. Although 83% of the fathers depicted their adjustment as steady, gradual, and timebound, 68% of the mothers perceived their own adjustment as chronic, periodic crises." The authors stressed the need not to assess family functioning and adaptation as a unit, but also to recognize the responses of individuals within that unit.

THE DYING CHILD AND FAMILY

Most pediatric primary care providers do not frequently deal with the death of a child. Because trauma is the leading cause of death in children, pediatric primary care providers are likely to have more experience with survivors (e.g., parents and siblings) than with a terminally ill child. At the same time, the return of much chronic care to the community is increasing the exposure of primary care providers to many facets of dying and death. Primary care providers might be called on to provide care for a child with a terminal condition who has been treated at a tertiary care facility but is returning home to die. For the primary care provider the death of a child can be a painful and awkward situation.

Parents often turn to the practitioner for advice on communicating with the ill child or the siblings concerning death. A good guideline to use in working with families is to answer the question the child asks, though it also is important to understand why the child is asking the question. Often the subtext is "who will take care of me?" or "does it hurt to die?" The inclination of parents and primary care providers may be either to avoid answering the questions altogether or to inundate children with information. If the primary care provider is open to questions, that is, takes the time to listen and is clearly willing to respond, the child will most often ask what he or she is ready to hear.

One exception is in the area of blame. Children of all ages often inappropriately assume some responsibility for the death or feel guilty about their responses to the death (Mahon and Page, 1995). The child should be told that he or she had no responsibility for the death. As is true with all crucial issues of development, information will probably have to be repeated several times.

Parents

Once a child's condition has reached the terminal phase, the focus of care should switch from cure to amelioration of symptoms and provision of comfort (Edwardson, 1983). Often by this time, the parents have become experts in providing complete care for their child. With time, the focus switches from cure to facilitating a good death, though this is often a difficult and painful transition. The actual care given is likely to be based on several areas of input, including objective information, the wishes of the child, options the parents are given about the child's death, and personal and professional support the parents receive (Edwardson, 1983). When the decision as to whether the child should die at home or in the hospital is being made, it is essential to get the input of the child who is dying (Martinson, 1983).

Children who have been sick for a long time often have an understanding of sickness and death well beyond their chronologic age. These children are also able to judge who is comfortable dealing with their impending death and who is not. Dying children may use the way caregivers have handled other deaths as a test. For example, if a child and family are seen regularly in a clinic, they get to know other children and families. This bond increases if simultaneous hospitalizations occur. If a friend dies, the child is likely to use the response of staff and other families to gauge how his or her own death will be handled and to measure how helpful others are likely to be in the process of preparing for death. The dying child, then, individualizes interactions based on an assessment of those with whom he or she is interacting. Children "maintain an open awareness with those who can handle it, and at the same time maintain mutual pretense with those who want to practice it" (Bluebond-Langner, 1978).

To be honest with the child and family does not mean to take away hope; hope should be interwoven throughout the course of the illness. The focus of hope, however, changes in the same way that increased knowledge and varying patient responses result in modification of plans of care (Gyulay, 1989). As the inevitability of death becomes clearer, the focus of the hope changes, perhaps from cure to minimal pain and control in the process of dying.

Pain control is an extremely important issue as a child is dying. Pain control in children is not as well understood as in adults largely because of underestimation of and misconceptions about the child's ability to feel pain. The guideline should be to treat the symptoms (Meehan, 1989). It is important to realize that symptoms and coping are likely to be different in children than in adults. Assessment of pain also must be different from techniques used with adults. Because a child is able to play with a video game for 30 minutes without complaining does not mean the child is not in pain. It is more likely that the child has excellent self-distraction abilities.

It is important to maintain the usual activities of childhood, such as playing and reading. Play is important because it enhances the child's feelings of control (Gray, 1989; Vessey and Mahon, 1990). Though the dying child may be less able to participate in familiar and favorite activities, usually modifications can be made if this is something the child really wants to do. For example, someone else can roll dice and move a game piece. If the child is no longer able to read his or her own books, many children love to have books read to them. These are both ideal ways to involve siblings. Music is also a favorite distraction for children. Even very young children of 1 or 2 years of age have favorite tapes.

Older children may want to be involved in planning their own funeral. This is often very difficult for the family, but it is the last act of control for some children. In the past, children have chosen particular readings or music for their funerals. One child asked that balloons be released in the church "to go up in the same way his spirit would go."

Dying children often seem ambivalent about the role of those around them. They may be adamant about not being left alone, but they are also likely to be selective about who they want with them. It may seem that their world is becoming progressively smaller. The child is likely to become less verbal because of decreased energy and perhaps because of a physical inability to talk. The child might also be in a coma, depending on the condition. If the latter is the case, parents can be encouraged to continue physical and verbal contact with the child. The presence of a few people and physical contact when possible are very important to the child. Some parents or families are never able to acknowledge the reality of a child's impending death. This can be very hard for the dying child and can be draining for the rest of the family.

The death of a child is the most painful loss an individual can experience. It is likely to take 3 years before parents regain the energy level they had before the child's death (Arnold and Gemma, 1983), although a person never "gets over" the death of a child. Parents are likely to be preoccupied. There is not one specific right thing to say to support parents, but there are wrong responses. Parents should never be told "at least you have other children," "at least he was young enough so you didn't have time to know him well," "You're young. You can have more children," or worst, "I know how you feel." Even those who have experienced the death of a child will not experience the same responses.

Within families there will also be variation in response to the death of a child. Mothers are more likely to receive social support and recognition of the depth of their loss. Fathers are expected to support the mothers. This may help to explain why fathers grief is different from that of mothers (Hogan, 1988).

Many families have found it helpful to have contact with the primary care provider about 1 month or more after the death. By this time, friends and relatives may be expecting the family members to manage their grief, but family members' pain is still fresh. Not uncommonly, many parents want to learn more about their child's death. The primary care provider may be the person best able to answer any questions the parents have about the death, especially any last words, or whether or not the child was in pain, particularly if it was a sudden death or the parents were not present at the time of death.

Meeting with parents serves another purpose. It shows the family that someone does remember how recent the death was and how acute the pain is. Even with the death of a newborn, it is increasingly common for a parent to have found a pediatric care provider before their child's birth. With the death of an infant, the mother is likely to feel guilt or even rejection (Novak, 1988). These feelings must be acknowledged and realistic explanations given for the death. They might not immediately ameliorate negative feelings the mother has, but the information can serve as an accurate standard against which incorrect or irrational beliefs can be checked and can ultimately facilitate the grieving process.

Siblings

Siblings are likely to feel extremely isolated while the child is dying, especially if that child is hospitalized. If the child is hospitalized, it is very important that the sibling be kept informed about the child's condition. Again, hospital visits are ideal but should not be forced.

If the child is dying at home, it is possible for the siblings to have a more active role in the dying process. This does not necessarily mean a task orientation, though doing tasks can help siblings feel less isolated. Siblings should be prepared for what is likely to happen at the time of death. Home hospices or visiting nurse agencies can be very helpful in this concrete preparation.

After the child dies, the siblings' reactions are based not just on their own feelings but also on the grief reactions of their parents. Children are used to depending on their parents, and to see them in such pain exposes a vulnerability not previously evident. This is painful for the child and can even evoke fear. As a result, siblings might act cheerful in an effort to spare the parents pain. Parents may misinterpret this response and believe the sibling is not grieving. This can increase tension at an already difficult time (Hogan, 1988).

A child's concept of death moderates the response to death. A child's concept of death is comprised of an understanding of finality, universality, and inevitability. This means the child recognizes death as permanent, the end of bodily functioning,

something that happens to everyone, and something that will eventually happen to the child. A child's concept of death is acquired gradually. In one study, 46% of 5-year-olds and ≥60% of 6- to 8-year-olds had an accurate concept of death (Mahon, 1993). This is younger than predicted in earlier studies. In the same study, children who had experienced the death of a sibling from trauma did *not* have a more accurate concept of death than children who had not experienced sibling death.

The primary care provider may be helpful during this time of crisis. Parents are often so overwhelmed with grief it is difficult for them to support and understand the grief work of their surviving children. Children are often reluctant to talk to their parents about their deceased sibling or matters related to the death for fear of causing their parents more pain. The practitioner can offer support and guidance for parents and concrete information and reassurance for the surviving children. Counseling services should be offered to all family members and are often available through the local hospice agency.

SUMMARY

The family unit, varied in structure and composition, is the primary unit of care and support for the child. A chronic condition in a child alters the roles and expectations of all family members by creating stressors to which the family must learn to adapt. The primary care provider can be instrumental in assisting the child and family to cope with a chronic condition by supporting individual coping strategies, by providing accurate, understandable information on the condition and on all aspects of the child's care, by implementing preventive health measures to minimize complications of the condition and promote optimal well-being, by accessing needed services for the family, and by offering support for the long-term emotional needs of each family member.

REFERENCES

Anderson JM: The social construction of illness experiences: families with a chronically ill child, *J Adv Nurs* 6:427-434, 1981.

Andrews MM, Nielson DW: Technology dependent children in the home, *Pediatr Nurs* 14:111-114, 1988.

Arnold JH, Gemma PB, editors: *A child dies: a portrait of family grief,* Rockville, MD, 1983, Aspen.

Blackford KA: The children of chronically ill parents, *J Psychosoc Nurs Ment Health Serv* 26:33-36, 1988.

Bluebond-Langner M: *The private worlds of dying children,* Princeton, NJ, 1978, Princeton University Press.

Breslau N: Care of disabled children and women's time use. *Med Care* 21:620-629, 1983.

Breslau N, Weitzman M, and Messenger K: Psychologic functioning of siblings of disabled children, *Pediatrics* 67:344-353, 1981.

Burr CK: Impact on the family of a chronically ill child. In N Hobbs and JM Perrin, editors: *Issues in the care of children with chronic illness,* San Francisco, 1985, Jossey-Bass.

Cadman D et al: Children with chronic illness: family and parent demographic characteristics and psychological adjustment, *Pediatrics* 87:884-889, 1991.

Damrosch SP, Perry LA: Self-reported adjustment, chronic sorrow, and coping of parents of children with Down syndrome, *Nurs Res* 38:25-30, 1989.

Deatrick JA, Knafl KA, and Guyer K: The meaning of caregiver behaviors: inductive approaches to family theory development, 1993.

Deatrick JA, Knafl KA, and Walsh M: The process of parenting a child with a disability: normalization through accommodations, *J Adv Nurs* 13:15-21, 1988.

Drotar D et al: The adaptation of parents to the birth of an infant with a congenital malformation: a hypothetical model, *Pediatrics* 56:710-717, 1975.

Dura JR, Beck SJ: A comparison of family function when mothers have chronic pain, *Pain* 35:79-89, 1988.

Edwardson SR: The choice between hospital and home care for terminally ill children, *Nurs Res* 32:29-34, 1983.

Feeman DJ, Hagen JW: Effects of childhood chronic illness in families, *Soc Work Health Care* 14(3):37-53, 1990.

Feetham SL: Family research: issues and directions for nursing, *Annu Rev Nurs Res* 2:3-25, 1984.

Gale CA: Inadequacy of health care for the nation's chronically ill children, *J Pediatr Health Care* 3:20-27, 1989.

Gallo AM et al: Well siblings of children with chronic illness: parents' reports of their psychological adjustment, *Pediatric Nursing* 18:23-27, 1992.

Gallo AM et al: Mothers' perceptions of sibling adjustment and family life in childhood chronic illness, *J Pediatr Nurs* 8:318-324, 1993.

Garrison WT, McQuiston S: *Chronic illness during childhood and adolescence,* Newbury Park, CA, 1989, Sage Publications.

Glazer NY: The home as workshop: women as amateur nurses and medical care providers, *Gender & Soc* 4:479-499, 1990.

Goldberg S, Simmons RJ: Chronic illness and early development, *Pediatrician* 15:13-20, 1988.

Gray E: Emotional and play needs of the dying child, *Issues Compr Pediatr Nurs* 12:207-224, 1989.

Gyulay J: Home care for the dying child, *Issues Compr Pediatr Nurs* 12:33-69, 1989.

Hamlett KW, Pelligrini DS, and Katz KS: Childhood chronic illness as a family stressor, *J Pediatr Psychol* 17:33-47, 1992.

Hill SA, Zimmerman MK: Valient girls and vulnerable boys: the impact of gender and race on mothers' caregiving for chronically ill children, *J Marriage and Fam* 57:43-53, 1995.

Hobbs N, Perrin JM, and Ireys HT: *Chronically ill children and their families,* San Francisco, 1985, Jossey-Bass.

Hogan NS: The effects of time on the adolescent sibling bereavement process, *Pediatr Nurs* 14:333-335, 1988.

Holaday B: Challenges of rearing a chronically ill child, *Nurs Clin North Am* 19:361-368, 1984.

Horner MM, Rawlins P, and Giles K: How parents of children with chronic conditions perceive their own needs, *MCN* 12:40-43, 1987.

Hostler SL: Family-centered care, *Pediatr Clin North Am* 38:1545-1560, 1991.

Howlin P: Living with impairment: the effects on children of having an autistic sibling, *Child Care Health Dev* 14:395-408, 1988.

Jackson PL: When the baby isn't perfect, *Am J Nurs* 85:396-399, 1985.

Jessop DJ, Reissman CK, and Stein REK: Chronic childhood illness and maternal mental health, *J Dev Behav Pediatr* 9:147-156, 1988.

Jessop DJ, Stein REK: Uncertainty and its relation to the psychological correlates of chronic illness in children, *Soc Science and Med* 20:993-999, 1985.

Johnson JH: *Life events as stressors in childhood and adolescence,* Newbury Park, CA, 1986, Sage Publications.

Johnson MP, Lubker BB, and Fowler MG: Teacher needs assessment for the educational management of children with chronic illnesses, *J Sch Health* 58:232-235, 1988.

Kazak AE: Families of chronically ill children: a systems and social-ecological model of adaptation and challenge, *J Consult Clin Psychol* 57:25-30, 1989.

Kazak AE, Clark MW: Stresses in families of children with myelomeningocele, *Dev Med Child Neurol* 17:757-764, 1986.

Kazak AE, Reber M, and Carter A: Structural and qualitative aspects of social networks in families with young chronically ill children, *J Pediatr Psychol* 13:171-182, 1988.

Knafl KA, Deatrick JA: How families manage chronic conditions: an analysis of the concept of normalization, *Res Nurs Health* 9:215-222, 1986.

Knafl KA, Deatrick JA: Conceptualizing family response to a child's chronic illness or disability, *Fam Relat* 36:300-304, 1987.

Knafl KA et al: Family response to a child's chronic illness: a description of major defining themes. In S Funk and E Tornquist, editors: *Key aspects of caring for the chronically ill: home and hospital,* New York, 1993, Springer.

Kramer RF: Living with childhood cancer: healthy siblings' perspective, *Issues Compr Pediatr Nurs* 5:155-165, 1981.

Krener P, Adelman R: Parent salvage and parent sabotage in the care of chronically ill children, *Am J Dis Child* 142:945-951, 1988.

Krulik T: Successful "normalization" tactics of parents of chronically ill children, *J Adv Nurs* 5:573-578, 1980.

Lawson BA: Chronic illness in the school-aged child, *MCN* 2:49-55, 1977.

Lipman TH: What causes diabetes? *MCN* 13:40-43, 1988.

Lynn MR: Siblings' response in illness situations, *J Pediatr Nurs* 4:127-129, 1989.

MacMullen NJ, Brucker MC: Pregnancy made possible for women with cystic fibrosis, *MCN* 14:196-198, 1989.

Mahon MM (1993). Children's concept of death and sibling death from trauma. *Journal of Pediatric Nursing 8*, 335-344.

Mahon MM, Page ML, (1995). Childhood bereavement after the death of a sibling. *Holistic Nursing Practice, 9*[(3)] 15-26.

Martin P: Marital breakdown in families of patients with spina bifida cystica, *Dev Med Child Neurol* 17:757-764, 1975.

Martinson I: Home care for the child with cancer. In JE Schoewalter et al, editors: *The child and death,* New York, 1983, Columbus University Press.

McCormick MC et al: Preliminary observations on maternal rating of health of children: data from three subspecialty clinic, *J Clin Epidemiol* 41:323-329, 1988.

McCubbin MA: Family stress theory and the development of nursing knowledge about family adaptation. In SL Feetham et al, editors: *The nursing of families: theory/research/education/practice,* Newbury Park, CA, 1993, Sage Publications.

Meehan J: Pain control in the terminally ill child at home, *Issues Compr Pediatr Nurs* 12:187-197, 1989.

Meyers A, Weitzman M: Pediatric HIV disease: the newest chronic illness of childhood, *Pediatr Clin North Am* 38:169-191, 1991.

Moyer A: Caring for a child with diabetes: the effect of specialist nurse care on parents' needs and concerns, *J Adv Nurs* 14:536-545, 1989.

Neill K: Behavioral aspects of chronic physical disease, *Nurs Clin North Am* 14:443-456, 1979.

Novak S: In moments of crisis, *MCN* 13:349-351, 1988.

Olshansky S: Chronic sorrow: a response to having a mentally defective child, *Soc Casework* 43:190-193, 1962.

Patterson J, McCubbin H: The impact of family life events on the health of chronically ill children, *Family Relations* 32:255-264, 1983.

Pless B, Nolan T: Revision, replication and neglect-research on maladjustment in chronic illness, *J Child Psychol Psychiatry* 32:347-365, 1991.

Quittner AL, Opipari LC: Differential treatment of siblings: interview and diary analysis comparing two family contexts, *Child Dev* 65:800-814, 1994.

Sabbeth BF, Leventhal JM: Marital adjustment to chronic childhood illness: a critique of the literature, *Pediatrics* 73:762-768, 1984.

Safron DG, Tarlov AR, and Rogers WH: Primary care performance in fee-for-service *AMA* 271:1579-1586, 1994.

Schlomann P: Developmental gaps of children with a chronic condition and their impact on the family, *J Pediatr Nurs* 3:180-187, 1988.

Shepard MP: *The identification of the family system responses to the perceived impact of chronic illness which promote adaptation in a child with a chronic illness.* (Doctoral Dissertation, University of Pennsylvania, 1992). Dissertation Abstracts International.

Sherwen LN, Boland M: Overview of psychosocial research concerning pediatric human immunodeficiency virus infection, *J Dev Behav Pediatr* 15:s5-11, 1994.

Sholevar GP, Perkel R: Family system intervention and physical illness, *Gen Hosp Psychiatry* 12:363-372, 1990.

Solnit A, Stark M: Mourning the birth of a defective child, *Psychoanal Study Child* 16:523-536, 1962.

Spaulding BR, Morgan SB, (1986). Spina bifida children and their parents: A population prone to family dysfunction? *Journal of Pediatric Psychology 11*, 359-374.

Stein A et al: Life threatening illness and hospice care, *Arch Dis Child* 64:697-702, 1989.

Tenbrinck M, Brewer P: The stages of grief experienced by parents of handicapped children, *Ariz Med* 33:712-714, 1976.

Thomas RB: Family adaptation to a child with a chronic condition. In MH Rose, RB Thomas, editors: *Children with chronic conditions: nursing in a family and community context,* Orlando, FL, 1987, Grune & Stratton.

Trahd GE: Siblings of chronically ill children: helping them cope, *Pediatr Nurs* 12:191-193, 244, 1986.

Venters M: Family coping with chronic and severe childhood illness: the case of cystic fibrosis, *Soc Science and Med* 15a:289-297, 1981.

Vessey JA, Mahon NM: Therapeutic play and the hospitalized child, *J Pediatr Nurs* 5:328-333, 1990.

Visher JS, Visher EB: Beyond the nuclear family: resources and implications for pediatricians, *Pediatr Clin North Am* 42:31-46, 1995.

Wallander JA, Varni JW: Social support and adjustment in chronically ill and handicapped children, *Am J Community Psychol* 17:185-201, 1989.

Wikler L, Wascow M, and Hatfield E: Chronic sorrow revisited: parent vs. professional depiction of the adjustment of parents of mentally retarded children, *Am J Orthopsychiatry* 51:63-67, 1981.

Williams HA: A comparison of social support and social networks of black parents and white parents with chronically ill children, *Soc Science and Med* 37:1509-1520, 1993.

Williams PD, Lorenzo FD, and Borja M: Pediatric chronic illness: effects on siblings and mothers, *Matern Child Nurs J* 21:111-121, 1993.

Winkel MF: Juvenile rheumatoid arthritis—parent support groups: do parents perceive a need? *Pediatr Nurs* 14:131-132, 1988.

Yost DM, Hochstadt NJ, and Charles P: Medical foster care: achieving permanency for seriously ill children, *Child Today* 17(5):22-26, 1988.

Young RK: Chronic sorrow: parents' response to the birth of a child with a defect, *MCN* 2:38-42, 1977.

Family Culture and Chronic Conditions

4

Jane Ryburn Starn

THE CHANGING FACE OF AMERICA

America is a pluralistic country with rapidly increasing numbers of ethnic minorities and recent immigrants. Since 1975 more than one million legal refugees have immigrated from Southeast Asia, Mexico, Central America, and Eastern Europe (Frye, 1991). Countless others have entered the country without legal authority. Unofficial estimates from the U.S. Census Bureau put the total number of immigrants in the United States who do not have legal authority at approximately four million in 1993 (Mendoza, 1994). Racial and ethnic minorities are becoming a greater portion of the population. By the year 2000 nearly one third of all the school-age children will be from minority populations (The Center for the Study of Social Policy, 1991). In some states, especially states in the Southwest, white children are expected to be in the minority by the year 2000. This is partially because of the increased fertility rates of nonwhite women between the ages of 15 and 44 years old in the United States (Mendoza, 1994). "As the population of culturally diverse groups increase, health care providers must strive to understand the interface of culture, ethnicity, child development, chronic disability, and family systems" (McPherson, 1993) (see box definition of terms). This chapter will outline dominant vs. minority values and the cultural implications for the care of children with chronic conditions.

DEFINITION OF TERMS

Culture: Shared beliefs, which are learned through socialization during childhood, that form a group identity. culture is dynamic and ever-changing.
Ethnicity: Shared linguistic, social, and/or cultural customs or backgrounds.
Race: Shared geographic and genetically transmitted physical characteristics.

DOMINANT VS. MINORITY VALUES

The definitions of chronic conditions and disability have often been grounded in the dominant Euro-American values of socially and psychologically defined uniformity, normative behaviors, and responses to stress and illness. The Euro-American philosophy of predestination/social Darwinism evolved into the belief that being different from the majority of the population was harmful to the community. This view led to a social intolerance or stigmatization of children with chronic conditions, especially those who have visible differences or whose condition is known to the community (Gallo et al, 1991). Since the latter part of the nineteenth century the dominant culture's view has assumed that phenomena must be observable or measurable to be real, that health is the absence of disease, and that mind, body, and spirit are separate entities. The dominant culture in the United States values physical attractiveness and health (Gallo et al, 1991).

Minority views of nontechnologic societies and Eastern cultures are more likely to be intuitively based on experiences, feelings, sentiments, and the belief that mind, body, and spirit are inseparable (Larson-Presswalla, 1994; Leininger, 1991; Wuest, 1991). Ethnocentrism, a belief that one's own values are superior, and the continuing prevalence of racism in America leave the impression that deviation from dominant, white middle-class values is abnormal (Patterson and Blum, 1993). Yet there are noticeable perceptual differences between the dominant white culture and the multiple ethnic groups regarding chronic conditions and health care. Ethnic differences are found in beliefs concerning kinds and causes of diseases, behaviors to practice and avoid when ill, appropriate kinds of treatment, patterns of accessing care, types of primary care providers preferred, and patterns of decision making within the family (Frye, 1991).

These variations are further complicated by grouping people into broad subgroups, such as Asian, African-American, or Hispanic. Grouping people into these subgroups assumes a similarity or homogeneity in each subgroup that does not exist. There are a wide variety of Hispanic cultures with differing points and times of entry into the United States. Among Native American groups, tribal differences continue. There are broad differences among Japanese-, Korean-, and Chinese-Americans, as well as differences based on the length of time or the number of generations since original immigration. Within these subgroups, much variation exists across educational and socioeconomic status. More similarity exists by class and education than by specific culture, especially if the family has lived in the United States for a long time (McCubbin et al, 1993; Patterson and Blum, 1993; Starn, 1991). For example, more highly educated and acculturated minorities may be unaware of or discount folk belief systems that are prominent with new immigrants or less-educated citizens of the same ethnic group (Groce and Zola, 1993).

Primary care providers caring for families who have children with special needs must constantly strive for cultural competence (see box accompanying). Cultural competence and sensitivity is essential in multiethnic populations so primary care providers do not unintentionally alienate the parents or families by inappropriate or unacceptable suggestions or behavior (McCubbin et al, 1993). According to Friedman (1990), the failure to understand culture is the root of poor communication, tension, inaccurate assessments, and inappropriate intervention. The misunderstanding of language may lead to problems at all stages of health care; for example, "independent living" may signify living alone, which may be a culturally unacceptable goal, rather than signify an ability to achieve a level of self-care. Misunderstandings may occur unless terms are carefully defined when working cross-culturally (Patterson and Blum, 1993; Ahmann, 1994).

THEORETICAL CONCEPTS OF CULTURE AS RELATED TO PEDIATRIC CHRONIC CONDITIONS

Culture is learned through socialization during childhood. It is based on shared beliefs and patterns that form a group identity that adapts to the environment and is dynamic and ever-changing (Boyle and Andrews, 1989). Ethnicity is a group's shared linguistic, racial, and cultural customs and

COMPONENTS OF CULTURAL COMPETENCE

Cultural Competence Requires:
1. Awareness and acceptance of cultural differences
2. Self-awareness
3. Understanding the dynamics of cultural differences
4. Knowledge of the client's family culture
5. Adaptation of services to support the client's culture

background (Ramer, 1992). On the other hand, race is the local or global geographic population distinguished as a group by genetically transmitted physical characteristics. Linguistic and cultural backgrounds are not necessarily similar among all members of a race. In the multicultural United States there are fundamental differences among ethnic groups based on roles, communication, and cognitive styles. Thus primary care providers must learn cultural relativity or have an understanding of child and parental values, behavior, and beliefs based on the context. Primary care providers should avoid becoming ethnocentric, believing that their own culture and practices are superior to others.

Conversely, the primary care provider must not assume that by studying a particular culture or ethnicity each family automatically fits into the common patterns of that culture. Each family develops a paradigm which describes its ". . . fundamental beliefs, convictions, or core assumptions shared by family members about the nature of the social environment and the family's place within it" (Campbell, 1991). Understanding family celebrations, traditions, and patterns such as daily routines and the division of labor helps determine how the family functions. The family's stage of development, socioeconomic and educational status, and degree of acculturation account for vast differences within ethnic groups (Friedman, 1990; Phillips and Crowell, 1994). Proficiency in the English language and a higher level of education is often associated with greater acculturation than that shared by newly immigrated families with minimal competence in the English language.

A first step for those persons acquiring transcultural understanding is to become aware of their own cultural beliefs, values, and practices. This self-assessment includes determining their citizenship, ancestral roots, and family-identified geographic region of origin (e.g., German-American Midwesterner, Columbian-American Californian). The box found on p. 61 is an assessment guide designed to assist the primary care provider in identifying cultural characteristics as determined by family of origin or as practiced in the present family. Table 4-1 identifies some common conditions that are currently found more frequently in minority or immigrant populations in acquiring transcultural understanding.

A second step in acquiring transcultural understanding is to recognize ways culture can influence families. Groce and Zola (1993) have identified three concepts essential to understanding a family's approach to a child with a chronic condition.

1. The culturally perceived cause of a chronic illness or disability plays a significant role in the attitudes of the family and community. Some families view chronic disease or disability as a curse by a "supreme being" for violation of a taboo. Southeast Asians who believe in reincarnation may view the disability as the result of a transgression committed in a past life. Irish-Americans who live in the Southern or Eastern parts of the United States may believe that merely thinking about a disability occurring in their child may "mark" or cause the disability to occur. Samoans may believe that licking icing or coconut dessert off of a knife may cause a cleft lip. Native Americans, Cambodians, and Mayans are more likely to believe that a chronic condition results from disharmony with nature (Frye, 1991; Phillips and Hoban, 1990). Fetal alcohol syndrome among Native Americans who drink excessively during pregnancy illustrates a disharmony with nature and has very serious consequences for the unborn child. Immigrants from the Caribbean, Pacific Basin, and Mediterranean countries may believe that a disability is caused by witchcraft or the "evil eye." As a result, pregnant women are protected from exposure to anger or harm and not allowed to attend funerals or other rituals where perceived harm may come to their babies. A pregnant woman could attend a funeral only by attaching a mirror to her enlarged abdomen to reflect and ward off evil spirits. In contrast, Mexican-Americans believe that, to a certain extent, disabilities just happen. They also believe that families who have a disabled child are given that role because of their past kindnesses to others (Groce and Zola, 1993). Thus chronic conditions do not carry as much of a stigma for these families as in other cultures in which people deem the condition a failure or punishment.

2. When a family or community views a chronic condition as a punishment rather than in biomedical terms, there is likely to be much less support available to that family because the family is thought to be responsible for the chronic condition. Parents who hold themselves or their be-

CULTURAL ASSESSMENT

Rate yourself or a client family on each of the following cultural categories. Indicate the frequency of the practice in your family of origin or the client's family. A low score (i.e., less than 30 out of a possible 80 points) indicates affiliation with Western norms, whereas a high score (i.e., over 50) indicates affiliation with non-Western norms. The more discrepant the rating between yourself (the primary care provider) and the client family, the higher the potential for cultural misunderstanding and conflict.

Range of occurrence

5	4	3	2	1
very often	often	sometimes	infrequent	rarely

Cultural category	Score
Affection: Demonstrative vs. reserved	_____
Emotions: Demonstrative regarding physical and emotional pain vs. stoic	_____
Self-Care: Use of home remedies, preventive care, native healers, acupuncturists vs. going to the physician	_____
Values Regarding Children:	
Children are equals vs. children are to be seen and not heard	_____
Children are gifts from God vs. children are secondary to adult needs and activities	_____
Children need to be nurtured at home vs. children need to be sent to schools and institutions for training	_____

	Score
A child with a congenital condition is punishment for parental misdeeds or a gift from God vs. the result of a genetic deviation	_____
Values Regarding Time:	
Time is taken within the context of other activities such as family needs vs. time is relative	_____
Directness vs. Vagueness:	
Vague answers are seen as a way to avoid confrontation and embarrassment vs. vague answers are dishonest	_____
Direct questions are intrusive and rude vs. direct questions are the best way to gain information	_____
Eye contact is disrespectful or intrusive vs. eye contact demonstrates interest and attention	_____
Calling an adult, not well known by first name is friendly vs. disrespectful	
Direct or Indirect Locus of Control:	
One does not control one's own destiny vs. one does control one's own destiny	_____
Decisions are influenced by God or other deities vs. decisions result from group/family process	_____
Independence vs. Familial Supremacy:	
One must act in a way to support the needs of the family vs. the individual's needs come first	_____
Total Score	_____

Modified from Ramer L: *Culturally sensitive caregiving and childbearing families,* White Plains, NY, 1992, March of Dimes Birth Defects Foundation.

havior responsible for the disability of their child may not seek services designed to help them. The family sincerely may not understand that early stimulation or therapy can enhance the development of a child with a disability. They may keep the child hidden at home because the family is embarrassed by the child, or they may try to protect the child from being teased by others (Serpell, Mariga, and Harvey, 1993). Child neglect may occur in the form of failing to nurture, provide education, care, or emotional support. Immigrants from Eastern European countries may hide their child to prevent the child from being removed from the family's care and institutionalized without their

Table 4-1.   **CONDITIONS FOUND MORE FREQUENTLY IN MINORITY OR IMMIGRANT POPULATIONS**

Ethnic groups	Condition	Screening tests	Age of child
All immigrants	Tuberculosis	PPD	Newborn to adult
All immigrants	PKU	Guthrie	Newborn to adult
All immigrants	Iron deficiency anemia	Hgb/Hct	>6 months
All immigrants and high-risk teens	STDs	Examination/laboratory serology	High-risk newborn/teenager
All immigrants	Vitamin A deficiency	Serum test for vitamin A deficiency	All children
Asian	Anencephaly	Imaging studies,	Newborn
	VSD, PDA	examination, ECG, echo-	Newborn, child
	Down syndrome	cardiogram, amniocentesis, MSAFP, chromosome analysis	Fetus, newborn
	Cleft lip	examination	Newborn
	Congenital hip	examination, x-ray	Newborn
African-Americans	Sickle Cell disease	Hgb electrophoresis	All ages
African-American, Mediterranean, Jewish, Thai Filipino/Chinese	G6PD	Assay for enzyme	Newborn
African-American	Prematurity	Early prenatal care	Fetus, newborn
	perinatal drugs	toxicology screen	Newborn
	alcohol/drugs	toxicology screen	Teenager
	microcephaly	examination, imaging	Newborn
	PDA and pulmonary artery stenosis	examination, x-ray, ECG	Child
French Canadian	Tyrosinemia (1)	Serum tyrosine	High-risk newborn
Filipino	Gout	Serum uric acid	Symptomatic infant/child
Hispanic/ Puerto Rican	Low birth weight prematurity	Prenatal care	Newborn
	obesity, low SES	Growth chart	Preschoolers/teens
Jewish	Tay-Sachs disease	Amniocentesis chromosome analysis	Fetus, newborn/child
Mediterranean	Thalassemia	Hemoglobin electrophoresis	All children
Native American (including Eskimos)	Low birth weight	Prenatal care	Fetus Neonate
	SIDS	Apnea monitor	Infant
	Persistent otitis	Otoscopy, tympanometry	Infant/school age
	Juvenile diabetes	Blood glucose	School age/teenager
	Fetal alcohol syndrome	Toxicology, examination	All ages
	Alcohol/inhalants	Drug screens,	Teenager
	PDA, valve stenosis /atresia	Examination, x-ray, ECG	Neonate/child
	Cleft lip	Examination, amniocentesis	Newborn
	Hydrocephalus	Amniocentesis, examination	Newborn
	Congenital hip	Examination	Infant

Continued.

Table 4-1.   CONDITIONS FOUND MORE FREQUENTLY IN MINORITY OR IMMIGRANT POPULATIONS—cont'd

Ethnic groups	Condition	Screening tests	Age of child
Southeast Asian Pacific Islander and Haitian	Parasites/ diarrhea	Corneal scars, stool for O & P, peripheral eosinophilia	All children
	Malaria	Blood smear/parasitemia	All ages
	Hepatitis	Hepatitis surface antigen	All ages
	Hemoglobinopathy	CBC with RBC indices	Any child
Caucasian	Cystic fibrosis	Sweat test	School age
	Club foot	Examination	Newborn
	Congenital hip	Examination, x-ray	Newborn
	Hypospadias	Examination	Newborn
	Allergic rhinitis	Esophilia, examination	Preschoolers, school age
	Asthma	Examination, x-ray	Postnewborn
British	Neural tube defect	MSAFP amniocentesis	Fetus, newborn

Alexander MA, Sherman JB, and Clark L, 1991; Groce NE and Zola IK, 1993; Hewvada A and Newman D, 1992; Hoekelman RA et al, 1992; Nelson, 1987, Niederhouser L, 1989; Palafox N and Warren A, 1980; Ramer L, 1992; Wuest J, 1991.

consent, since this frequently occurred in their home countries.

3. Expectations for survival critically affect care and the amount of effort expended on a child. If it is thought that the child with a severe disability will not live, then services are more likely to go to the child who is healthy and to the child who is less in need. This pattern may manifest itself in different ways. Euro-Americans are more likely to believe in technology and want "everything possible" to be done (Finn, 1994). Families with strong religious beliefs may keep waiting for a miracle cure to happen that can thwart long-term planning for the care of their disabled children. Families from countries where there are few services for children with special needs may genuinely think that nothing more can be done to help them.

Families with a strong gender bias favoring male children may want extensive services, schooling, and training for their sons but not for their daughters (Frye, 1991; Kendall, 1990). In such families, daughters may be seen as contributing to the family by doing housework, cooking, and taking care of children, all of which do not require outside educa-

tion (Groce and Zola, 1993). In families for whom family loyalty is a central value, such as Arabian or Italian families, outside training or schooling may be refused, especially if a residential program is involved (Meleis and LaFever, 1984). Also, families with a more deferential rather than assertive or independent value, may not be upset with children whose development is delayed; indeed, they may not view their children's development as abnormal. Native Americans may hold this belief, viewing the child as perhaps a little different, but acceptable, therefore not needing additional services.

CULTURAL VARIATIONS IN DECISION MAKING

Varying cultural values affect decision making regarding the care of children with special health care needs. Primary care providers often believe critical pediatric decisions must be made by the parents, despite the fact that only 6% of the world's families exist in the isolated nuclear mode (Groce and Zola, 1993). As discussed earlier, it is important to determine who the family considers to be members, and who among these members makes the decisions. African-Americans are more likely to consult family and friends about care for their children; these extended family members share the responsibility for decision making (Russell and Jewell, 1992; Serpell, Mariga, and Harvey, 1993). Do not assume that typical patterns of decision making for well children will be followed for a child with a chronic condition. For example, although Cambodian fathers rarely intervene in the care of well children, they are the central decision makers when long-term, chronic problems occur in their children (Frye, 1991). Thus failure to consult the father in these instances may result in the family's alienation from the health care team.

Family members from a nondominant culture who view primary care providers as authority figures may not understand their own role in the decision-making process because these family members expect the "authority" to tell them what to do for their child. Out of respect these family members may also nod "yes" to all instructions, but have no intention of following through. This happens because the suggestions make no sense in their belief or value systems. For example, Native Americans value harmony with nature, accept life stoically, and may not be upset with a child who is "different" from others. They may act as if they intend to enroll their child in an infant stimulation program but do not follow through because it does not make sense to send the child for remedial stimulation when the child is acceptable as is (Jacobson, 1994). In contrast, some privileged immigrant families, such as wealthy Middle Easterners, may see primary care providers as inferior and may expect preferential treatment. This viewpoint can lead to conflict if the nurse gives instructions rather than the physician. Wealthy Europeans who pay extra for private health care in their countries may also be offended by having to wait for services or by not being treated deferentially as they are in their home countries (Ryburn, 1995).

CULTURAL COMPETENCE

Cultural competence entails five components—awareness and acceptance of cultural differences, self-awareness, understanding the dynamics of cultural differences, basic knowledge about a family's culture, and adaptation of services to respond to

that family's culture (Davis and Voegtle, 1994). Culturally competent primary care providers are those who understand and embrace their own personal and professional cultures while acknowledging the cultures of their clients by learning and accepting the others' beliefs as necessary for functioning effectively (Brookins, 1993). Primary care providers are more effective when they respect individuals from other cultures, make continued attempts to understand the others' views, are open to learning, are flexible, have a sense of humor, and tolerate ambiguity (Lynch and Hanson, 1992). Table 4-2 is a cross-cultural assessment tool to guide primary care providers in collecting cultural information in order to develop the child's management plan.

The primary care provider must assess the level of initial crisis as the child is diagnosed with a chronic condition, as well as assess the subsequent day-to-day coping as the family adjusts to the ongoing care of their child with special needs. The primary care provider needs to determine the modalities the family uses for care and healing. See Table 4-3 for a list of common folk-healing practices the family may use instead of or in conjunction with Western medical practices. Insensitivity to the family's belief in folk practices may drive the family away from Western medical care. If the family believes that a combination of traditional and technologic medicine is the most therapeutic, then the child suffers unnecessarily if cultural bias or ethnocentrism is shown by the primary care provider.

Cultural competence is essential to prevent mistakes such as inadvertently teaching interventions that lead children to develop behaviors inconsistent with their family's culture. Teaching children to express their feelings openly, to ask questions of adults, or even to speak English may result in cultural conflict within the family (Chang and Pulido, 1994; Phillips and Crowell, 1994).

It is important to understand the emotional meaning of language in addition to the nonverbal body language, gestures, personal space, and use of touch within the culture (Almonte, 1994). Cultural competence in care is also necessary to prevent legal suits caused by neglect or insensitivity toward cultural needs (Leininger, 1990).

The characteristics of culturally sensitive caregiving systems are based on an asset model vs

Table 4-2.   CROSS-CULTURAL ASSESSMENT OF A FAMILY WITH A CHILD WITH A CHRONIC CONDITION

Family Demographics	Who lives in your family (i.e., members, ages, sexes)?
	What kind of work do members of the household do?
	What is your family's socioeconomic status?
	What kind of health insurance coverage do you have?
	Which family members are covered?
	Which child are you seeking care for today?
	What chronic conditions or symptoms does the child have?
	How would you describe the problems that have brought you here today?
	Who is the primary care taker in your family?
Orientation	Where were the members of the family born?
	What is the ethnic background of the family members?
	How many years have family members lived in the United States? (NOTE: Only ask if appropriate.)
	In your family is it important to be on time for an appointment or to get to an appointment when possible based on everyone's schedule for that day?
	Why do you think your child has (the above-named) chronic condition (e.g., punishment for a parent's past behavior such as conceiving a child out of wedlock, the result of a genetic problem, or a gift given because of the family's patience and love)?
Communication	What language(s) and dialect(s) are spoken at home?
	Who reads English in the family? If no one reads English, in what language would you prefer printed materials?
	Do parents and children look when spoken to or do they look down? To whom should questions be addressed?
	What can be asked of the child directly? (NOTE: Avoid using the child as a translator, if at all possible, because of the strain this task imposes.)
Family Relationships	Besides the immediate household, who else makes up the members of this family?
	Who makes the decisions in this family (e.g., mother-in-law, father, both partners, other family or friends, group decision)?
	Who cares for the child and the child's medical needs?
	What are the housing arrangements (e.g., space, number of rooms, members living in the home)?
	What is the child's or family's usual daily routine like?
	To whom do you turn when you need help with or have questions about your child?
Beliefs about Health	What is the present health status of family members?
	What illnesses or conditions are present in the current family members?
	What illnesses or conditions were present in deceased family members?
	How often and for what reasons have family members used western medicine in the past?
	What complimentary therapies are used by your family routinely and specifically for the child (e.g., acupuncture, healers, prayer, massage)?
	What do you do when your child is in pain?
	Who takes care of the child if the child is hospitalized?
	Is it important to keep the child at home or to use institutional placement?
	What do you think will help clear up the problem?
	Are there things that help your child get better that the doctors should know?
	What problems has your child's illness caused your family?

Continued.

Table 4-2.　　**CROSS-CULTURAL ASSESSMENT OF A FAMILY WITH A CHILD WITH A CHRONIC CONDITION—cont'd**

Education	How much schooling have members of the family completed?
	What ways are the best for you to learn about your child's condition (e.g., pamphlets, videos, direct patient teaching, home visits, return demonstrations)?
	From whom are you most comfortable learning about your child's condition (e.g., doctor, nurse, social worker, home health aide, other family members)?
Religion	What religion(s) are practiced in your family?
	What religious things do you do to help your child (e.g., pray, meditate, attend a support group, practice the laying on of hands)?
	What things does your religion say you should *not* do for this child (e.g., have blood transfusions, allow strangers or dangerous circumstances to affect child)?
Nutrition	When are usual mealtimes for your family?
	With whom does the child eat?
	What foods does the child usually eat?
	What special foods does the child eat when the child is sick?
	What foods do you *not* give the child and when?

Davis B and Voegtle K, 1994; Fong CM, 1985; Jacobson SF, 1994; Lynch FW and Hanson MJ, 1992; Ramer L, 1992; Zagorsky E, 1993

Table 4-3.　　**FOLK HEALING PRACTICES**

Practice name	Ethnicity	Practice procedure	Purpose
Acupuncture	Asian (Chinese)	Needles in meridians (energy lines), herbs	Pain, sinus problems, injuries, stress, stroke, deafness, epilepsy, and so on
Cao Gio	Vietnamese, Cambodian	Coining produces ecchymosis, petechiae	Coughing, congestion, fever
Curanderismo	Hispanic	Bleeding, herbs, emetics, diuretics, prayers, penance, miracles	Physiologic or psychologic problems, social maladjustment
Folk practitioners	Haitian	Poltices, voodoo	Evil eye lifted
Hilot	Filipino	Faith healing through prayer, herbal medicine, massage, manipulation of bones and tissues	Most illness
Medicine men	Native American	Meditation, sweat lodges, herbal medicine, ritual	Any disease caused by an imbalance with nature
Moxa	Chinese	Burning of a plant on the skin	Mumps, convulsions, epistaxis
Root doctor	African-American	Herbs, laying on of hands	Any illness
Spiritual healer	White	Laying on of hands	Physiologic, psychologic, or social problems

Brennan BA, 1987; Capers CF, 1985; DeSantis L and Thomas JT, 1990; Harpur T, 1994; Kirkpatrick SM and Cobb AK, 1990; Lenart JC, St. Clair PA, and Bell MA, 1991; Orque MS, Bloch G, and Murray LS, 1983; Spector RE, 1991.

a deficit model of family assessment. Community and ethnic involvement should be incorporated into planning and implementing health care services targeted to communities with diverse populations. When possible the primary care providers and staff should mirror the cultural and ethnic diversity of the families they serve. If necessary, translaters must be made available and trained in medical translations and in the importance of confidentiality. Information necessary for cultural assessment must be obtained from the family and used when developing family care plans. See the box below for hallmarks of a culturally sensitive caregiving system.

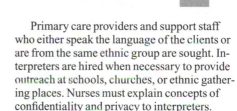

HALLMARKS OF CULTURALLY SENSITIVE CAREGIVING SYSTEMS

1. An asset model based on recognizing cultural differences in child rearing, family strengths, and culturally based coping methods should be used.

   The primary care provider gathers data based on reviewing previous health care records, reading about the specific culture to learn about basic beliefs and values, and asking family members questions (see Table 4-3). This model asks what the family's strengths are (e.g., family members present, ways the family cares for their child, types of complementary therapies the family has used, ways family members find support or coping techniques, shared caregiving by all family members). These strengths are then built on by the primary care provider to foster care for the child with a chronic condition.

2. Primary care providers seek community participation in all stages of program design, development, implementation, outreach, policy making, problem solving, and evaluation.

   Informal and formal community leaders need to be involved in and approve of assessment and intervention approaches. This means talking to church leaders, various traditional healers, and elders who are respected in each ethnic community to learn what they think is culturally appropriate and sensitive care. Primary care providers may also seek out leaders of support groups for children with special needs.

3. Community outreach to families is ongoing and culturally appropriate.

   Primary care providers and support staff who either speak the language of the clients or are from the same ethnic group are sought. Interpreters are hired when necessary to provide outreach at schools, churches, or ethnic gathering places. Nurses must explain concepts of confidentiality and privacy to interpreters. Nurses should also look at the client/parent when the interpreter is translating, unless direct eye contact is contraindicated in the culture (e.g., Native American or Filipino cultures).

4. Intake systems are sensitive to family and cultural values.

   Primary care providers should ask the family appropriate questions about the family's culture (see Table 4-3). However, intake may take several visits if privacy and mistrust of outsiders are issues that must be resolved before effective service can begin. Limit the number of professional care providers present. Encourage the family to have those family members who are important to them and the interpreter present. Conduct the meeting in either an informal or a formal manner based on the family's values.

5. Families are involved directly in the family treatment and service plan.

   Families help prioritize the goals. The family decision makers are consulted in determining the plan. The family's orientation to primary care providers as authority figures or joint decision makers is determined before attempting to develop the service plan. Family caregivers and decision makers are involved in the ways that the family deem acceptable when developing the individualized service plan.

Continued.

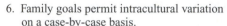

HALLMARKS OF CULTURALLY SENSITIVE CAREGIVING SYSTEMS—cont'd

6. Family goals permit intracultural variation on a case-by-case basis.

   Standard care plans are altered based on family needs to include alternative modes of therapy such as healers, acupuncture, or other practices of importance to the family.

7. Emphasis is placed on maintaining and improving the self-esteem, cultural identification, and goal-setting ability of each family to foster self-sufficiency.

   Family decision makers and the caregivers are acknowledged. Family strengths are praised.

8. The teaching of parent-child interaction patterns must fit ideal family cultural values.

   For example, a Filipino or Native American child is not pushed to look at authority figures or to speak up in a disagreement; deference and avoidance of eye contact are culturally appropriate.

9. Team members have ongoing, culturally appropriate training.

   Team members are either of the same cultural background and speak the same language as the family or they have taken workshops given by ethnic leaders or others with expertise in the cultural group receiving care.

10. Educational materials, media, evaluation, and monitoring instruments are field-tested for cultural appropriateness and congruency in language content and emotional meaning.

11. Typical cultural and familial celebrations and symbolism are incorporated within services. Special holidays may be acknowledged by families sharing native foods and holiday traditions with care providers and other families.

12. Continuous evaluation is mandated to ensure cultural appropriateness and program effectiveness. The child's progress is monitored internally and by external evaluators. Assess the family's perceptions of the intervention. Determine whether the family is meeting goals and prioritizing these goals.

Adams EV, 1990; Bernstein HK and Stettner-Eaton B, 1994; Leininger M, 1991b; Lowenthal B, 1994; Lynch EW and Hanson MJ, 1992; Russell K and Jewell N, 1992; Slaughter-Defoe DT, 1993.

IMPLICATIONS FOR RESEARCH

The United States is in the middle of a paradigm shift from the "melting pot" theory that all people should adopt dominant cultural values, beliefs, language, and practices to recognition of the richness of cultural diversity. This new paradigm has been called "chunky stew" by Ahmann (1994) because a stew is savored for all of its individual parts (ethnocultural differences) and the blending of flavors (social integration). Culturally competent and multicultural researchers need to be involved in designing and evaluating programs and innovative models for primary care providers in minority communities. There continues to be limited research "linking cultural and ethnic factors to the ways in which families respond and cope with childhood illnesses and disabilities" (McCubbin et al, 1993).

Cross-cultural research challenges the validity of assumptions made by the dominant culture, such as concepts of normality and risk. For example, teen childbearing in Puerto Rico and childbearing out of wedlock in Ireland are not associated with negative outcomes when extended family support, which is common to these cultures, is present (Greene et al, 1989; Nugent, 1994). Developmental practices such as the Native American cradleboarding of infants may be thought to confine and limit development. Research that used the Brazelton Neonatal Assessment Scale, however, found that Native American newborns have well-modulated infant states, cry little, and have low activity—all traits that encourage cradleboarding. The cradleboard is hung near the mother while she works. This increases stimulation in the upright position and facilitates development (Chisholm, 1989). Dreher, Nugent, and Hudgins (1994) studied

Jamaican infants whose mothers were heavy marijuana users, a condition usually associated with poor infant development. They found the infants were more alert, were less irritable, and had better self-regulation than a control sample. The more nurturing home environment and better educated mothers from higher socioeconomic classes among the marijuana users appeared to override the drugs effects when compared to the nondrug using, but poor control group.

Researchers must adopt a multicultural model rather than a deficit model that shows differences from dominant culture as inferior (Friedman, 1990). The effects of chronic conditions by disease categories across multiethnic groups have not been adequately studied; the interventions and environmental characteristics most likely to foster optimal development have also not been adequately studied. The Caldwell Home Observation for the Measurement of Environments (HOME) has a long history of use to determine the environmental effects of families with children who have special needs (Bradley et al, 1992); however, not many other assessment instruments are specifically available for this special population and few have been cross-culturally tested.

A body of current research focuses on resiliency or the ability of the child to attain optimal development despite biopsychosocial stressors (Garmezy, 1991; Werner, 1988). Maternal depression, a greater sense of caregiver burden, perception of the child's temperament or condition as difficult, increased family stress, lack of adequate child care, and lack of one stable, caring adult are all associated with less optimal outcomes for at-risk children (Bradley et al, 1992; Goldberg, 1990; Gross, 1989; Klein, 1989; Werner, 1988). The specific meaning of these concepts, however, may vary among ethnic groups and families based on their view of the world and family patterns of functioning (McCubbin et al, 1993). Research into what fosters resiliency in different cultures needs to be done.

SUMMARY

Public policy has mandated culturally competent care for families who have a child with a chronic condition. Caregivers can no longer provide care based on their own values and schemas if they are to be effective in the multicultural United States.

Primary care providers must first understand their own cultural beliefs, values, and biases and then learn the cultural beliefs and values of the multicultural families for whom they are caring. Genuine interest in and skilled assessments of these families are important to learning how to better understand their beliefs and values. Intervention must integrate professional knowledge and values with the values of each community and family if effective and sensitive care is to be offered.

REFERENCES

Adams EV: *Policy-planning for culturally comprehensive special services: bureau of maternal and child health,* Washington, DC, 1990, US Department of Health and Human Services.

Ahmann EL: "Chunky stew": appreciating cultural diversity while providing health care for children, *Pediatr Nurs* 20(3):320-322, 1994.

Alexander MA, Sherman JB, and Clark L: Obesity in Mexican-American preschool children—a population group at risk, *Pediatr Health Nurs* 8(1):53-58, 1991.

Almonte DE, Professionalization as culture change: Issues for infant/family community workers and their supervisors. *Zero to Three*: National center for Clinical Infant Programs. Oct/Nov 1994 15(2):18-23.

Bernstein HK, Stettner-Eaton B: Cultural inclusion in part H: systems development, *Infant-Toddler Intervention* 4(1):43-50, 1994.

Boyle J, Andrews M: *Transcultural Concepts in Nursing Care,* Glenview, IL, 1989, Scott, Foresman/Little, Brown College Division.

Bradley RH et al: The HOME inventory: a new scale for families of pre- and early-adolescent children with disabilities, *Res Dev Disabil* 13:313-333, 1992.

Brennan BA: *Hands of Light,* Toronto, 1987, Bantam Books.

Brookins G: Culture, ethnicity, and bicultural competence: implications for children with chronic illness and disability, *Pediatrics* 91(5):1056-1062, 1993.

Campbell DW: Family paradigm theory and family rituals: implications for child and family health, *Nurse Pract* 16(2):22-31, 1991.

Capers CF: Nursing and the African-American client, *Topics in Nursing* 7(3):11-17, 1985.

Champion VI, Austin JK, and Tzing OCS: Relationship between cross-cultural health attitudes and community health indicators, *Public Health Nurs* 7(4):243-250, 1990.

Chang HN, Pulido D: The critical importance of cultural and linguistic continuity for infants and toddlers, *Zero to Three* (Oct/Nov):13-17, 15(2):1994.

Chisholm J: Biology, culture, and the development of temperament. In JK Nugent, BM Lester, TB Brazelton, editors: *The cultural context of infancy,* vol 1, Norwood, NJ, 1989, Ablex.

Davis B, Voegtle K: *Culturally competent health care for adolescents,* Chicago, 1994, American Medical Association.

DeSantis L, Thomas JT: The immigrant Haitian mother: trancultural nursing perspective on preventive health care for children, *Journal of Transcultural Nurs* 2(1):2-15, 1990.

Dreher M, Nugent JK, and Hudgins R: Prenatal marijuana exposure and neonatal outcomes in Jamaica: an ethnographic study, *Pediatrics* 93(2):254-260, 1994.

Finn JM: Culture care of Euro-American women during childbirth: using Leininger's theory, *J Transcultural Nurs* 5(2):25-37, 1994.

Fong CM: Ethnicity and nursing practices, *Top Clin Nurs* 7(3):4, 1985.

Friedman M: Transcultural family nursing: application to Latino and Black families, *J Pediatr Nurs* 5(3):214-222, 1990.

Frye BA: Cultural themes in health-care decision making among Cambodian refugee women, *J Community Health Nurs* 8(1):33-44, 1991.

Gallo AM et al: Stigma in childhood chronic illness: a well-sibling perspective, *Pediatr Nurs* 7(1):21-25, 1991.

Garmezy N: Resilience in children's adaptation to negative life events and stressed environments, *Pediatr Ann* 20(9):459-466, 1991.

Goldbergh S: Chronic illness and early development: parent-child relationships, *Pediatr Ann* 19(1):35-41, 1990.

Greene S et al: Contraceptive practices of married and single first-time mothers, *J Biosoc Sci* 21:379-385, 1989.

Groce NE, Zola IK: Multiculturalism, chronic illness, and disability, *Pediatrics* Vol.1 #5, May (suppl 5):1048-1055, 1993.

Gross D: Implications of maternal depression for the development of young children, *Image J Nurs Sch* 21(2):103-107, 1989.

Harpur T: *The uncommon touch: an investigation of spiritual healing,* Toronto, 1994, McClelland & Stewart, Inc.

Hervada A, Newman D: Weaning: historical perspectives, practical recommendations, and current controversies, *Curr Probl Pediatr*(May/June) 22(5):223-240, 1992.

Hoekelman RA et al: *Primary pediatric care,* ed 2, St Louis, 1992, Mosby.

Jacobson SF: Native American Health, *Annu Rev Nurs Res* 12:193-213, 1994.

Kendall K: Maternal and child care in an Iranian village, *J Transcultural Nurs* 4(1):29-36, 1990.

Kirkpatrick SM, Cobb AK: Health reliefs related to diarrhea in Haitian children: building transcultural nursing knowledge, *J Transcultural Nurs* 1(2):2-12, 1990.

Klein SRS: Caregiver burden and moral development, *Image J Nurs Sch* 21(2):94-97, 1989.

Larson-Presswalla: Insights into Eastern health care: some transcultural nursing perspectives, *J Transcultural Nurs* 5(1):21-24, 1994.

Leininger M: Biases, questions, and concerns related to the nursing diagnosis cultural movement from a transcultural nursing perspective, *J Transcultural Nurs* 2(1):23-31, 1990.

Leininger M: Becoming aware of types of health care practitioners and cultural imposition. *Journal of Transcultural Nursing* 1991, 2(2):32-39.

Leininger M: *Culture care diversity and universality: a theory of nursing,* New York, 1991b, National League for Nursing.

Leininger M: Culturally competent care: visible and invisible, *J Transcultural Nurs* 6(1):23-25, 1994.

Lenart JC, St. Clair PA, and Bell MA: Childrearing knowledge, beliefs, and practices of Cambodian refugees, *J Pediatr Health Care* 5:299-305, 1991.

Lowenthal B: The service coordinator and the home visitor: competencies for the dual role, *Infant-Toddler Intervention* 4(1):43-58, 1994.

Lynch EW, Hanson MJ: *Developing cross-cultural competence: a guide for working with young children and their families,* Baltimore, 1992, Paul H. Brookes Publishing Co.

McCubbin HI et al: Culture, ethnicity, and the family: critical factors in childhood chronic illnesses and disabilities, *Pediatrics* Vol. 1 #5 May (suppl 5):1063-1070, 1993.

McPherson M: General comments, *Pediatrics* 91(5):1023-1024, 1993.

Meleis AI, LaFever CW: The Arab-American and psychiatric care, *Perspect Psychiatr Care* 22(2):72-86, 1984.

Mendoza FS: The health of Latino children in the United States, *The Future of Children* 4(3):43-72, 1994.

Nelson: *Textbook of pediatrics,* Philadelphia, 1987, WB Saunders Co.

Niederhouser V: Health care of immigrant children: incorporating culture into practice, *Pediatr Nurs* 15(6):569-574, 1989.

Nugent JK: Cross-cultural studies of child development: implications for clinicians, *Zero to Three* 15(2):1-8, 1994.

Orque MS, Bloch G, and Murray LS: *Ethnic nursing care: a multicultural approach,* St Louis, 1983, Mosby.

Palafox N, Warren A: *Cross-Cultural caring: a handbook for health care professionals in Hawaii,* Honolulu, 1980, Transcultural Health Care Forum, John A. Burns School of Medicine, University of Hawaii.

Patterson JM, Blum RS: A conference on culture and chronic illness in childhood: conference summary, *Pediatrics* 91(suppl 5):1025-1030, 1993.

Phillips D, Crowell N, editors: *Cultural diversity and early education,* Washington, DC, 1994, National Academy Press.

Phillips S, Hoban SL: Literature summary of some Navajo child health beliefs and rearing practices within a transcultural nursing framework, *J Transcultural Nurs* 1(2):13-20, 1990.

Ramer L: *Culturally sensitive caregiving and childbearing families,* White Plains, NY, 1992, March of Dimes Birth Defects Foundation.

Russell K, Jewell H: Cultural impact of health care access: challenges for improving the health of African-Americans, *J Comm Health Nurs* 9(3):161-169, 1992.

Russell K, Jewell K: Cultural impact of health-care access: Challenges for improving the health of African Americans. *Journal of Community Health Nursing* 9(3):161-169, 1992.

Ryburn J: Personal communication, 1995, Salzburg, Austria.

Serpell R, Mariga L, and Harvey K: Mental retardation in African countries: conceptualization, services, and research, *Int Rev Res Mental Retardation* 19:1-35, 1993.

Slaughter-Defoe DT: Home visiting with families in poverty: introducing the concept of culture. In RE Behrman, editor: *The future of children: home visiting,* 1993, David and Lucille Packard Foundation.

Spector RE: Culture, health, and illness. *In Cultural Diversity of health and illness,* Norwalle, CT, Appleton Century Crofts:1-154.

Starn J: Culture childbearing, *Int J Childbirth Ed,* 1991 6(3):38-39.

Werner EE: Individual differences, universal needs: a three-year study of resilient high-risk infants, *Zero to Three* 8(4):1-5, 1988.

Wuest J: Harmonizing: a North American Indian approach to management of middle ear disease with transcultural nursing implications, *J Transcultural Nurs* 3(1):5-14, 1991.

Zagorsky E: Caring for families who follow alternative health care practices, *Pediatr Nurs* 19(1)71-75, 1993.

School and the Child with a Chronic Condition

5

Judith A. Vessey, Patricia Ludder Jackson,
Nancy Rabin, and Ellen McFadden

The role of school should not be underestimated in a child's life. School provides opportunities for social, emotional, and cognitive development. In addition to the family, school is the major context in which children develop their sense of self and understanding of their place in relation to peers. More importantly, most children genuinely enjoy school, despite their protestations. This may be particularly true for children with chronic conditions, because they may have fewer opportunities to socialize outside of the school setting. Another positive benefit of including children with chronic conditions in school activities is that nondisabled children have the chance to develop attitudes of acceptance and respect for their peers with special needs.

Integration of children with chronic needs into the school setting, however, is not without problems. These children and their families may experience community resistance and resentment. Moreover, many schools have inadequate resources to educate the child, despite the fact that educational services are mandated by law. Parents' fears, guilt, and values need to be carefully assessed because these play critical roles in their children's school success. This chapter will initially examine the legislative underpinnings of special education and then explore ways the primary care provider can facilitate the child's school experience.

LAWS REGARDING THE EDUCATION OF CHILDREN WITH CHRONIC CONDITIONS

Legislative and judicial rulings over the past 25 years have dramatically changed the role of public educational institutions in providing services to children with chronic conditions (see box on legislative ruling p. 73). The change in public policy actually started with the civil rights movement when the landmark decision in *Brown v. Board of Education* (1954) banned segregated schools and affirmed education as a right of all Americans. The principle of "separate-is-not-equal" was used almost 20 years later in the *Pennsylvania Association for Retarded Citizens v. Pennsylvania* (1972) to challenge the state's right to exclude children with mental retardation from public education (Burns and Thornan, 1993). The Supreme Court that same year ruled that a free, public education must be provided regardless of disability or degree of impairment to all school-age children (Mills v. Board of Education of the District of Columbia, 1972). This landmark Supreme Court decision paved the way for the federal government to enact legislation supporting public education for all children regardless of their health or ability.

MAJOR LEGISLATIVE
RULINGS REGARDING
EDUCATION FOR
CHILDREN WITH
DISABILITIES OR CHRONIC
CONDITIONS

- Brown v. Board of Education, 1954.
- Public Law 93-112, 1973, The Civil Rights Act, Rehabilitation Act, Section 504.
- Public Law 94-142, 1975, The Education for All Handicapped Children Act.
  Amended by Public Law 99-457, 1986, The Education of Handicapped Amendments.
  Became Public Law 102-119.
- Public Law 100-407, 1988, The Technology Related Assistance for Individuals With Disabilities Act.
- Public Law 101-476, 1990, Individuals With Disabilities Education Act (IDEA).
  Amended by Public Law 102-119, 1991, The Individuals With Disabilities Education Act Revisions of 1991.
- Public Law 101-336, 1992, Americans With Disabilities Act.

GOALS OF PUBLIC LAW
94-142

Goals of Public Law 94-142, The Education of All Handicapped Children Act of 1975 are to provide:
1. A free and appropriate education for all children.
2. An education in the least restrictive environment based on individual needs.
3. An assessment of needs that is racially and culturally unbiased and is given in the individuals native language or mode of communication.
4. An individualized education program (IEP) prepared by a team of professionals that includes parents.
5. Due process and a procedure for complaints to ensure the rights of the individual.

cludes school health services, social work services in schools, and parent counseling and training" (PL 94-142, 1975b).

Public Law 94-142 was amended in 1986 by Public Law 99-457, which extended services to children from birth to 21 years of age and required interagency and interdisciplinary collaboration, development of a child identification system, a family designated care manager, the development of an individualized family service plan (IFSP) for children birth through 2 years, analogous to the IEP for the child, and a broader definition of developmental delay including children "at risk" (PL 99-457, 1986). This amendment dramatically increased the school systems' role in providing services to young children. In 1990 and 1991, these laws were amended further under the Individuals With Disabilities Education Act (IDEA), Public Law 101-476 (PL 101-476, 1990) and Public Law 102-119, The Individuals With Disabilities Education Act Revisions (PL 102-119, 1991).

The intent of these legislative acts is honorable and certainly an improvement over previous inequities and lack of services for children with

In 1975 Congress passed Public Law 94-142, the Education for All Handicapped Children Act as an educational bill of rights for children 5 to 18 years of age (see box on the goals of public law). Public Law 94-142 entitles children to a "free and appropriate public education" including "special education and related services provided at public expense, under public supervision and direction, without charge, which meet the standards of the state educational agency, and are provided in uniformity with the Individualized Educational Program (IEP)" (PL 94-142, 1975a).

The term "related services" includes "transportation and other developmental, corrective, and supportive services, including speech pathology and audiology, psychological devices, physical and occupational therapy, recreation, early identification and assessment of disabilities in children, counseling services, and medical services for diagnostic or evaluative purposes. The term also in-

disabilities. Problems exist with interpretation, funding, responsibility for services, and the actual provision of services to the targeted child. Public Law 94-142 and 99-457 identified only certain chronic health conditions as handicapping and as being eligible for special education and related services (see box on disabling conditions). To be eligible for special education, the child must test at or below a designated level of performance, often 1.5 to 2.0 standard deviations below the norm in specific or multiple areas of function. Children with milder handicaps or chronic conditions that do not

---

CONDITIONS IDENTIFIED AS DISABILITIES IN CHILDREN UNDER THE INDIVIDUALS WITH DISABILITIES EDUCATION ACT, 1990

A. *Disabilities as defined for children 5 to 21 years of age:*

1. *Autism:* A developmental disability significantly affecting verbal and nonverbal communication and social interaction.
2. *Deaf-blindness:* Children with both deafness and blindness; communication with others is severely impaired.
3. *Deafness:* Children with hearing deficiency that impairs process of linguistic information through hearing with or without amplification.
4. *Hearing Impairment:* Permanent or fluctuating hearing loss that adversely affects the child's educational process.
5. *Mental Retardation:* Significant subaverage general intelligence existing with deficits in adaptive behavior.
6. *Multiple Disabilities:* Concomitant impairments other than deaf-blindness resulting in severe educational problems that cannot be addressed in a special education program solely for one impairment.
7. *Orthopedic Impairments:* Severe orthopedic impairments that adversely affect the child's educational performance.
8. *Other Health Impairments:* Limited strength, vitality, or alertness due to chronic or acute health problems that affect the child's educational performance.
9. *Serious Emotional Disturbance:* A child who exhibits over a prolonged period of time one or more of the following characteristics: an inability to learn that cannot be explained by intellectual, sensory, or health factors; an inability to build or maintain satisfactory interpersonal relationships; inappropriate behavior or feelings; depression or unhappiness; and a tendency to develop physical symptoms or fears associated with personal or school problems.
10. *Specific Learning Disability:* A disorder in one or more of the psychological processes involved in understanding or using spoken or written language. This term does not apply to children who have learning problems primarily due to other disabilities listed previously or environmental, cultural, or economic disadvantages.
11. *Speech or Language Impairment:* A communication disorder due to impaired articulation, problems with language development, or voice impairment that adversely affects a child's educational performance.
12. *Traumatic Brain Injury:* Acquired injury to the brain resulting in total or partial functional and/or psychosocial impairment.
13. *Visual Impairments (including blindness):* Visual impairments, including correctable ones that can be corrected, that adversely affect a child's educational performance.

B. *Disabilities as defined for children 3 to 5 years of age:*

Children experiencing developmental delays, as defined by the state, in one or more of the following developmental areas: physical, cognitive, communication, social, emotional, or adaptive.

Adapted from Publication 99-457, Individuals With Disabilities Education Act (IDEA), Part B.

result in significant disability in a given functional area, such as speech, learning, motor function, or cognition are not eligible for special education. The 1990 Individuals With Disabilities Education Act, Part B, limited "related services" to only children eligible for special education, thereby limiting services to many children with milder disabilities who would also benefit from services to support their learning (Committee on Children With Disabilities, 1993). Section 504 of the Rehabilitation Act of 1973 (PL 93-112) protects individuals with physical or mental impairment from discrimination in education or employment. This federal law has been used in the courts to extend "related services" to children with milder disabilities not eligible for special education designation (Ballard, 1977). Children protected under Section 504 of the Rehabilitation Act must receive services required for them to participate in the educational system, but these services must be paid for with general education funds and not special education funds.

Lack of adequate funding to support public education and services for children with special needs is the basis for most controversies. Federal programs mandate services but do not adequately provide the financial resources to supply the services to all children who would benefit from them. States are mandated to provide the services to "eligible" children, not to all children who would benefit, setting up a complex mechanism for establishing eligibility. This often results in an adversarial relationship between parents seeking services for their children and the educational departments of school systems functioning under severe budgetary constraints. Those states that actively embrace the call for early case finding and intervention may indeed increase their financial obligations without receiving additional money from the federal government. School districts that identify therapeutic interventions for children with special needs in the IEP process are generally required to pay for the services, although Medicaid or other public funding frequently can be billed (Committee on Children With Disabilities, 1993). Private insurance will usually not cover services provided in the school setting. School systems' inability to collect revenue for services provided often results in minimal services. As a result, parents feel they have to fight for each service provided.

Because educational systems are responsible for the "related services" or therapies provided children in the school setting, they have become overseers of medical care, often quite independent of the child's primary or specialty care providers. The medical role, as determined under Public Law 94-142, is to determine a child's medically related handicapping condition, that results in the need for special education and related services (PL 94-142, 1975c). This limited role may further fragment health care delivery, resulting in duplicated or omitted services and puts the responsibility of health care on an institution designed to provide education not health care (Committee on Children With Disabilities, 1993; Palfrey, et al, 1990).

As children with chronic conditions live longer and medical technology enables them to participate in school, concern has surfaced about the qualifications of school personnel to provide services to children with special needs (Krier, 1993). Public Law 94-142 identified "a qualified school nurse or other qualified person" as the appropriate person for the provider of school health services (PL 94-142, 1975d). As the complexity of health conditions increase, the number of school nurses has decreased. Over 90,000 public schools currently exist, but the number of school nurses has dropped to 26,000 (Igoe, 1993). The number of school-based clinics operating in elementary, middle, and high schools is approximately 300 with an additional 20 school-linked clinics (Passarelli, 1994). Obviously, professionally educated primary care providers are not adequately represented in the school setting to directly provide services to all children with special health care needs. Procedures such as tracheotomy care, ileostomy care, gavage feedings, and intermittent clean catheterization are all procedures done routinely in school settings now, often by unlicensed health care personnel (Harrison, Faircloth, and Yaryan, 1995; Krier, 1993). Krier found that educators were performing medical procedures such as medication administration (35%), tube feeding (12%), ostomy care (5%), catheter care (2%), and tracheostomy care (1%). Of the educational staff, 68% felt unprepared to care for medically fragile children, and only 30% had any training in health care procedures including first aid or CPR (Krier, 1993).

Public Law 100-407, the Technology-Related Assistance for Individuals With Disabilities Act, defines technology assistance as any item or equipment that is used to increase, maintain, or improve a disabled person's functional capabilities (PL 100-407, 1988). Under the Individuals With Disabilities Education Act, Public Law 101-476, schools must provide "assistive technology services" to eligible students if these services are identified as necessary to assist a child to benefit from the special education program (Parette and Parette, 1992). Assistive technology may be as simple as an adapted spoon designed to support independent feeding or as complex as a laser-operated computer to establish communication with a severely disabled but cognitively intact child. School systems are financially responsible for providing the necessary equipment to support the child's educational program but can attempt to obtain reimbursement or funding from other resources such as Crippled Children Services, Medicaid, or other private health insurance plans. Cooperative funding arrangements may be negotiated to pay for equipment used across environments (Parette and Parette, 1992). The high cost of many modern technological assistive devices has put a major financial strain on the already underfunded special education programs.

SPECIAL EDUCATION SERVICES

Special education services can be provided in a regular classroom, special classroom or facility, home, private nonprofit preschool, college, hospital, and even state prison. Children eligible for services attending private school are still eligible through the public school system, but the parents will need to bring the child to the public school for services.

"Mainstreaming" is the term used when a child receiving special education services is in a regular day care, preschool, or school program (Sarzynski, 1994). This environment is seen as the least restrictive, providing the child the fullest educational potential (see Fig. 5-1). Most children in special education are in regular classes, either receiving their special services directly in the classroom or in another location for periods of time to receive speech, or other occupational, physical therapy services.

Children with severe disabilities or who are medically fragile will require services in special classrooms, often found within regular school set-

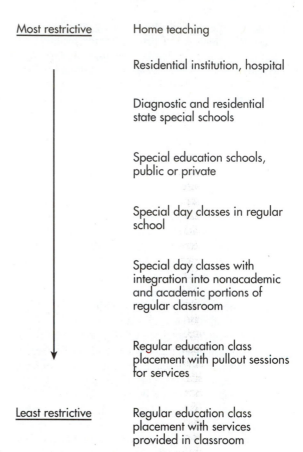

Fig. 5-1. Most to least restrictive environment for educational services.

tings or in special schools, institutions, hospitals, or at home if the individual is unable to attend other facilities. Special day classes usually fall into four categories and serve children with various severe disabilities (see Table 5-1, p. 77). Even the profoundly handicapped are required by law to receive educational services for a designated period of time each week. Depending on the size of the school district and the population served, these special classes may be available in the child's actual school district or in adjoining school districts that contract out services. In some situations, school districts will contract services for special education to private institutions or programs.

Although the momentum has been toward full inclusion or mainstreaming of children with special

Table 5-1.
CATEGORIES OF SPECIAL DAY
CLASSES

Special day classes	Diagnostic category
Learning Handicapped (LH)	Severely learning disabled Educably mentally handicapped Mildly mentally handicapped
Communicatively Handicapped (CH)	Severe disorder of language Hearing handicapped Language delayed Severely learning disabled
Physically Handicapped (PH)	Orthopedically handicapped Physically handicapped/disabled Multihandicapped Visually impaired/handicapped or disabled
Severely Handicapped (SH)	Severely/profoundly or mentally handicapped Severely mentally handicapped Moderately mentally handicapped Severely emotionally disturbed Autistic Multihandicapped Orthopedically handicapped

needs, additional research is needed to determine its degree of benefit or detriment to the child with special needs and the other children in the classroom. Hopefully, including children with special needs will increase the public's awareness and acceptance of individuals with chronic conditions. Although this has been found to occur (York, et al, 1992), discrimination continues (Turner-Henson, et al, 1994). Children with mild to moderate disabilities have been found to gain more from integrated classes, or mainstreaming, than severely disabled children (Cole, et al, 1990; Jenkins, Odom, and Speltz, 1989). Each child must be assessed carefully during the IEP process, and the classroom assignment best suited for them should be identified and evaluated over time. (See box on assessment questions, p. 79.)

THE ROLE OF THE HEALTH PROFESSIONAL IN THE INDIVIDUALIZED EDUCATION PROGRAM (IEP)

The Individualized Education Program (IEP) is the cornerstone of the Education for All Handicapped Children Act. The legislation requires that each child referred to special education follow a predetermined process to ensure compliance with the law in a timely manner (see Fig. 5-2). Each child must be evaluated by a multidisciplinary team comprised of appropriately chosen professionals. This team is responsible for writing the IEP that contains specific educational goals and therapeutic strategies. It is therefore imperative that its membership include the professionals needed to determine the best possible plan for the child. This team will propose the teaching environment for the child under the principle of "the least restrictive environment" with the knowledge of programs available in the school system. Their plan will also identify the related services including the technological assistive devices required to support the child's educational goals. Specific measurable goals and a time line for attaining those goals is built into the plan. There should be a yearly evaluation of the plan that may be initiated earlier if indicated. The IEP is a contract for services that must be provided and paid for by the school system (Decker, 1992).

The primary care provider's role starts with early identification and assessment of "children at risk" for disability. If the primary care provider identifies a child at risk, the family should be referred to the school district's special education office to determine the appropriate public agency for evaluation of the child. Children in the birth to 2 year age range may be evaluated through the local regional center, whereas most older children will be evaluated through the school district.

In order to initiate the IEP process, the parents or caretaker must request a special education assessment in writing. A written letter by the primary care provider is critical because it provides medical documentation to evaluate and support that request. The IEP assessment plan is determined by this initial request, so it is important to identify all areas of delay or potential risk.

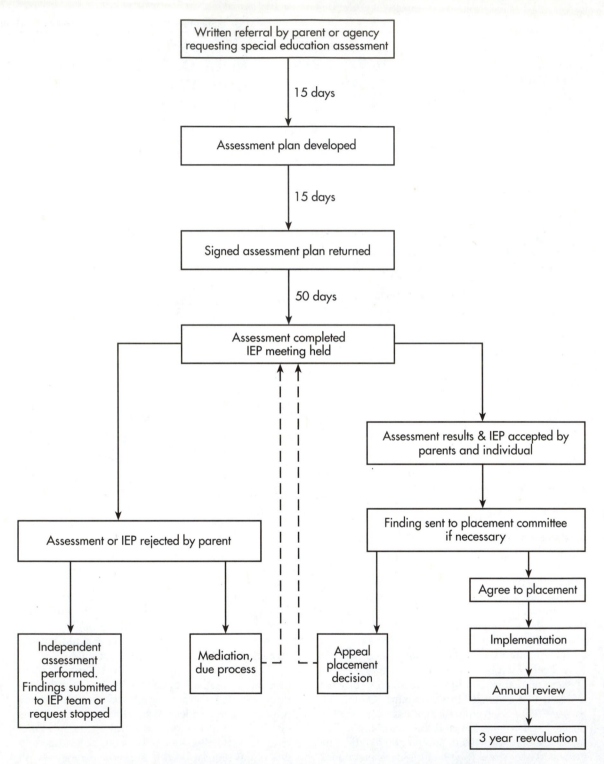

Fig. 5-2. Identification and assessment procedure for Individualized Educational Program (IEP).

QUESTIONS TO ASK WHEN PERFORMING A SCHOOL ASSESSMENT

1. What does the child know about the condition? How much of the care is the child responsible for?
2. Is the child's general health stable, improving, or worsening? Is the child terminally ill?
3. Are any classes or school activities contraindicated by the child's condition?
4. Is preferential seating in the classroom recommended?
5. What modifications in diet exist? Will the child be bringing his or her own lunch or will he or she be participating in the school meals program?
6. What physical restrictions and exercise limitations exist? How are they best managed at home? Are assistive devices required?
7. What medications and/or treatments does the child receive during the school day? Can dosage times be modified around school hours?
8. Does the child require counseling, special therapies (e.g., occupational, physical, or speech), adaptive equipment, or protective devices?
9. Does the child need assistance with any activities of daily living?
10. What precautions and first aid interventions should school personnel be familiar with? Does the child wear a medic-alert bracelet?

The primary care provider is part of the comprehensive multidisciplinary assessment process by providing health records and physical findings with parental consent to the IEP team. The primary care provider may participate in additional assessments or in referrals to other specialists. Although the IEP team is responsible for explaining the assessment findings to the parents and child, the primary care provider may be able to offer additional insight or interpretation.

The school district has 50 days to complete the assessment process and establish the educational plan. The primary care provider can be very helpful in reviewing the plan with the family to determine its appropriateness for the child. If the provider and family feel the plan is not sufficient to meet the child's developmental and cognitive needs, then the plan can be rejected and additional recommendations made to the IEP team. Recommendations supported by assessment findings or relevant literature are more likely to be accepted and incorporated into the plan. The primary care provider should act as an advocate for the parents and child when there is evidence of inappropriate or incomplete planning by the IEP team (Committee on Children with Disabilities, 1992).

FACILITATING THE SCHOOL EXPERIENCE

Many chronic conditions affect children's development, either directly in some conditions or indirectly by diminishing the child's opportunity to participate in developmentally appropriate activities (see Chapter 2). An important developmental task of children 5 years and older is to move beyond the family sphere into the school community where academic achievement, social competence, and regular attendance are major goals (Fowler, Johnson, and Atkinson, 1985).

The primary care provider can facilitate a child's adjustment to school. Although the school district is the lead agency for services provided in the school setting, school personnel often welcome coordination of medical services by the child's primary care provider. If the school district has a nurse assigned to oversee the health care services for children with chronic conditions, it is advisable for the primary care provider to establish a link with that individual so that changes in the child's condition or medical management can be easily communicated. The clinician can be very helpful in serving as a resource to the school by offering in-service education sessions on the child's health care needs, teaching specific therapy techniques, or demonstrating the appropriate use of assisted technology.

To best assist the child, it is important to obtain a detailed history regarding the student's capabilities in performing daily living skills and assessing the student's stamina. This information is invaluable in helping the child cope with limitations that may be encountered in school while simultaneously assisting the child to maintain independence (Page-Goertz, 1989).

Before initiating discussion with the school, it is important for the primary care provider to seek the permission of the child and the family before medical information is released to the school district or before any dialogue occurs with school personnel. Although this will not be a problem for most families, the need to establish open communication with the school district may be a need to be explored. If a condition is mild and not visible, families may not want information about the condition conveyed to school personnel because they do not want their child labeled as "different." In other cases, families genuinely fear ostracism or reprisal from the school community, as has been documented with many children infected with HIV. The family's wishes should be respected if at all possible. However, when withholding information about a child places that child at risk, the family must be counseled about the risks and benefits of disclosure and appropriate legal action must be taken. For example, withholding information about an adolescent with epilepsy who is enrolling in driver's education is both dangerous and illegal.

PROMOTING THE CHILD'S SELF-CONCEPT

Developing a healthy self-concept is of paramount importance for children with chronic conditions if they are to succeed in school and later activities. Many normative school activities, such as instruction in nutrition or sex education, teach children health-promoting behaviors that can help build healthy self-concepts. Helping these children to develop wholesome relationships and to share their talents with other children is also beneficial; children who excel in a specific academic area or participate in sports and other extracurricular activities are more likely to be successful. Participating in these activities not only helps build self-esteem but also enhances other spheres of development (Walsh and Ryan-Wenger, 1992).

Unfortunately, developing self-esteem of children with chronic conditions in the school setting is not without difficulty. These children are likely to be teased; some may experience bullying or even ostracism (Vessey, Swanson, and Hagedorn, 1995). Children with chronic conditions will benefit from interventions to strengthen their coping abilities that help them deal constructively with peer rejection, loneliness, or isolation that results from such discriminatory practices (Turner-Henson, et al, 1994). Incorporating social skills training into the IEP is one way to assist the child and family in becoming more confident in their interactions with others and in their use of appropriate behaviors when dealing with discrimination. School personnel can assist by dealing with inappropriate behavior of other students and developing an awareness of what it is like to have a chronic condition.

Parents, teachers, and school professionals need to acknowledge that children with chronic conditions experience the same developmental stressors as their peers and therefore need to be treated similarly and taught the same coping skills. Using a variety of techniques to assist these children in normalizing their school experience will be beneficial to developing their self-concept (Walsh and Ryan-Wenger, 1992).

Administering Medications and Treatments

If medications are required during the school day, the general guidelines and criteria of each state and school district must be followed: (1) a legal prescriber must authorize the medication, (2) parents must give written permission for medication to be given, (3) the mediation should be properly labeled, (4) the medication must be stored in a locked area, and (5) the school needs to document that the medication was administered. If it is likely that a child will need to take medications ordered on a prn basis, arrangements for their administration should be made.

Whenever possible, the clinician should alter treatment protocols to occur around school schedules. There are several pragmatic reasons for this. The child with a chronic condition wants to be considered normal. Requiring the child to go to the nurse for medications may be met with resistance, particularly in this era of "Just say NO to drugs." Moreover, even in the best of circumstances, there may not be adequate time or qualified personnel within the school to administer or oversee treatments. As children enter adolescence, it is often appropriate to explore ways to help children develop self-care behaviors, such as self-medication, intermittent clean catheterizations, or testing blood glucose levels. Such activities will help children become more autonomous, an important developmental goal.

Promoting Mobility

Limited mobility is an issue for many children with chronic conditions. Mobility is affected by physical impairments, diminished strength, and fatigue. Regardless of the cause, limited mobility can affect students' ability to achieve and compete. Physical changes can limit some children from participating fully in gym, recess, sports, and afternoon activities (Chekryn, Deegan, and Reid, 1986; Ahmann and Rollins, 1995). In the worst case scenario, limited mobility will hinder children from participating in critical learning activities.

If mobility is a problem, this needs to be discussed and appropriate adaptations planned for need to be addressed in the child's IEP meetings. Two major approaches are used to facilitate a child's mobility—structuring the environment and improving mobility. When choosing a school is an option, consideration of the physical layout (e.g., one floor, width of hallways, presence of elevators, location of bathrooms) needs to be considered. Providing the child with two sets of books, one for the classroom and one for home, eliminates the problem of transporting them. Scheduling a study hall or lunch after physical education class will give the student more time to change and to avoid tardiness for the next class.

The child's mobility will be improved and normalization promoted if appropriate assistive devices are used. For example, an adolescent in a large high school may prefer to use a wheelchair when traveling long distances between classes rather than limiting the class schedule to those that are near each other. Adaptive aids can help children write, reach books on library shelves, or respond to questions in the classroom. For children who need a raised toilet seat or handrails, efforts should be made to locate a toilet where these adaptations can be installed.

Managing Fatigue

It is important to set reasonable expectations for children. Fatigue is an integral part of many chronic conditions. Sometimes this is a symptom of the disease, such as in heart disease; other times it is associated with time-consuming therapies, such as with cystic fibrosis; or it is a side effect of medications such as those given for epilepsy (Walker and Jacobs, 1984). Fatigue also may occur as a result of induced physiologic changes, such as in children undergoing chemotherapy.

There are several strategies for reducing fatigue; most focus on structuring the child's educational experience in a way that is not physically taxing. For example, the child could be encouraged to use a tape recorder for note taking, serve as score keeper rather than participating in vigorous activity during physical education, or be assigned easy classroom chores such as sharpening pencils with an electric sharpener. Classes that are located close together require less travel and reduce fatigue. This is particularly important in very large schools or those with several buildings. Scheduling a study hall period immediately after lunch provides an opportunity for the child to nap (ideally in a different setting!) without missing class time. Another strategy is arranging the child's schedule so that the most important classes are either in the morning or in the afternoon. That way, if the child can only attend for half-day sessions, he or she still learns the most important content. Homework demands of various courses should be taken into account when planning a child's schedule. It is better to defer one class rather than have the child embark on a rigorous schedule that sets him or her up for failure. Extra courses can be taken during summer school to help lighten a child's academic load. Ideally, this will be planned as part of the IEP, because many schools have limited offerings in the summer.

Ensuring Safety

There are numerous safety issues to consider. Environmental safety is paramount. Ramps need to be installed where necessary. Electrified adaptive equipment must be periodically inspected. For children using life-sustaining equipment such as ventilators; a reserve generator needs to be available. Provisions for transporting a student with a physical disability during emergencies, such as fires and earthquakes, need to be determined and disseminated to all school personnel. School buses may need to be retrofitted with appropriate safety devices such as seat belts or wheelchair locks (Committee on Injury and Poison Prevention, 1993).

Many chronic conditions place children at greater risk for infection and illness. Clarify the school's policy on notifying parents about possible exposure to contagious diseases. Depending on the child's chronic condition, specific areas of concern may include strep throats, measles, mumps, meningitis, hepatitis A and B, salmonella, or shigella infections (McMillan, 1995). Other chronic conditions such as asthma can be aggravated by chemicals used in chemistry class, cleaning fluids, chalk dust, and many other substances (Swanson and Thompson, 1994).

Physical and mental disabilities may hinder participation in sports and place the child at higher risk for injury (Ahmann and Rollins, 1995). Care must be taken to use appropriate safety equipment and have good supervision. Strengthening exercises will also help prevent injury.

School Absenteeism and Reentry

Parents need to clearly communicate their expectations about school to their child and whenever possible, facilitate their child's attendance. The more school absences a child experiences, the greater the risk of poor academic achievement (Walker and Jacobs, 1984). Studies indicate that school absences are significantly higher among children with chronic conditions. Although all absences place a child at risk, frequent short-term interruptions are more disruptive than a single, longer absence (Perrin, 1992). Exacerbations in the child's condition, side effects from various interventions, fatigue, and health care appointments are the primary reasons for absenteeism (Passarelli, 1992); however, if psychosocial problems co-exist, such as behavior or family difficulties the child is at greater risk for high absenteeism (Fowler, Johnson, and Atkinson, 1985). For example, parental guilt and anxiety can foster school phobia and subsequent absenteeism. Repeated absenteeism not only affects academic performance but may create a downward spiral in the child's self-concept, peer relations, and family functioning.

Illness alone is rarely a suitable excuse for school failure. Families and professionals need to work together to reduce absenteeism. Whenever possible, health care visits should be scheduled around school hours. If this is not possible, it is better to schedule several appointments on one day rather than miss several half days of class.

If a prolonged absence is anticipated, parents need to arrange for home instruction. School policies vary widely and delays as a result of child ineligibility, poor coordination of services, or unavailable teachers may be encountered before homebound education is initiated (Passarelli, 1992). If schools are not approached before the requisite length of absenteeism (usually 2 to 4 weeks) is met, additional delays are likely to be encountered before services are arranged (Walter and Jacobs, 1984). Many schools, however, are willing to proactively work with families in maintaining their child's education by providing the child with homework assignments, communicating with hospital-based teachers, helping parents become informal tutors, and arranging for tutorial services to begin as soon as the child is eligible. If frequent hospitalizations or prolonged, lengthy absences are anticipated, a specific objective should be included in the child's IEP that anticipates and plans for uninterrupted schooling.

The decision to repeat a grade needs to be made with great care. This setback can cause feelings of shame, inadequacy, and inferiority; however, the decision to remain in the same grade can also enhance feelings of success because the work requirements may be easier. New classmates provide a second chance for forming friendships (Wong, 1995).

Successful school reentry for children who have had prolonged absences or disfigurement must occur to avoid impeding the child's development. A positive reentry experience can provide the child with a sense of accomplishment and social acceptance, strengthen faltering self-esteem, and lessen maladaptive emotional responses to his or her condition (Chekryn, Deegan, and Reid, 1986). The primary care provider can help promote a smooth transition for such children by helping the family proactively determine strategies that facilitate school reentry (Rabin, 1994). The two primary goals are to help the child and family anticipate situations they may encounter; and the second is to prepare the teachers and classmates for the child's return.

One helpful approach for preparing the child for reentry is role playing, where the primary care provider plays the role of the classmate while the child plays himself or herself (Rabin, 1994). The purpose is to act out a variety of scenarios that may occur during the first day back at school. This activity enables the child to develop answers to potentially embarrassing questions or situations he or she may encounter. Another useful strategy is to ask close friends to accompany the child and serve as a buffer on returning to school. Parents may also bring the child for several "drop in visits" or sponsor a "welcome back" class party designed to promote peer acceptance.

A variety of approaches can be used to help teachers and classmates adjust. The child may be encouraged to write a letter or record a videotape about his or her experiences. This is then shared with teachers or classmates several days before the child's return. Providing visual images of a child, either on videotape or in a snapshot, allows time for "sanctioned staring," or time for classmates to ask questions or express their concerns without fear of recrimination. This is particularly important if the child has undergone major physical changes, such as alopecia secondary to chemotherapy or scarring from burns. Roleplaying is another helpful strategy. Two classmates can act out the scenario, with the teacher or the primary care provider guiding the experience. Science projects, literature assignments, and video presentations also can be used by the teacher to promote understanding and acceptance within the child's peer group. Careful advance planning will improve the likelihood of success for the student returning to school.

EDUCATING THE TERMINALLY ILL STUDENT

School remains an appropriate activity for many children who are terminally ill because it provides opportunities for socialization and personal achievement (Davis, 1989). Depriving the child of these opportunities may cause increased stress. For children to have a successful school experience, several issues must be considered. First, the devel-

opmental level of the child and peer group must be considered in deciding on the "who, what, where, and how" information about the child's condition is shared with the child, peers, school personnel, and other parents. Second, flexibility in planning the child's educational program will be needed if his or her condition deteriorates. Third, efforts to help the child maintain a positive self-concept and body image are important. This may be very difficult when a child begins to lose weight, cough productively, or have skin changes. Fourth, academic programming needs to be tailored for the child. For example, an adolescent enrolled in a college preparatory curriculum needs to be helped in developing achievable objectives rather than giving up all hope for the future (Davis, 1989). Lastly, children who are dying often need to exhibit more control over their lives and their environments. Whenever possible, efforts need to be made to assist children in reaching the goals that they have set for themselves.

It is not enough to focus attention only on the dying child and his or her family. Many students have not had to confront death and dying and feel that they do not know how to act or know the appropriate thing to say. Strategies that were suggested in the school reentry section of this chapter are equally appropriate for helping students deal with the death of a peer.

The effect that a dying child has on school personnel also needs to be considered. The attitudes of school personnel toward illness and death, as well as their ability to individualize instruction, their concern or need to protect the dying child, and their fear of an emergency arising in the classroom are all areas that can influence their effectiveness (Davis, 1989). Flexibility and realistic expectations are needed if the school experience is to be a successful one for the child who is terminally ill.

Do Not Resuscitate Orders

Comprehensive planning for end-of-life care for a child with a terminal condition may include promulgating the family's wishes that the child not be resuscitated should a cardiac arrest occur. A comprehensive approach to responding to do not resuscitate (DNR) orders in the school requires school personnel to develop a protocol or set of guidelines, to follow when a child attends school with a "do not resuscitate" DNR order.

The National Education Association (NEA) (1994) has developed guidelines for DNR orders in the schools (in the event a school district decides to honor a DNR) emphasizing that it was *not* establishing a policy. The NEA has suggested the following minimum conditions if a school board is to honor DNR: that the request should be submitted in writing and be accompanied by a written order signed by the student's physician; that the school establish a team to consider the request and all available alternatives, and if no other alternative exists, to develop a medical emergency plan; and that staff receive training, and staff and students receive counseling. In its statement, the NEA delineated the following elements of the medical emergency plan: (1) the student's teacher specifies actions that he or she should take if the student suffers a cardiac arrest or other life-threatening emergency, (2) other school employees who supervise the student receive briefing sessions, (3) the student wears an ID bracelet indicating he/she is subject to a DNR order, (4) the parents execute a contract with the local emergency medical service and send a copy to the superintendent, and (5) the team reviews the plan annually.

Minimally, schools should develop a protocol for responding to DNR orders. Guidelines such as those suggested by the NEA must be implemented in a spirit of collaboration, respect, and sensitivity. Parents, educators, support personnel, and members of the health care team must be committed to a process that is flexible and responsive to the changing needs of the child. Essential to the process are ongoing forums where parents and educators can discuss their concerns, share their values and preferences about how certain situations should be handled, and define or revise plans. Within these discussions, it is crucial to define the range of possible scenarios that are likely to occur for the child and to build contingency plans for how they are to be handled (Rushton, Will, and Murray, 1995).

SUMMARY

Primary care providers must not lose sight of the fact that school provides opportunities for social, emotional, and cognitive development (Rabin, 1994). The primary care provider may assume the role of coordinator, bringing together the child, parents, peers, and school personnel, and fostering open communication. A team approach is the only way to guarantee that educational and health care needs are met (Davis, 1989). Innovative school health programs based on delivering primary care in the school and linking it to the school program need to be encouraged.

REFERENCES

Ahmann E, Rollins J: Family-centered care of the child with special needs. In D Wong, editor: *Nursing care of infants and children,* ed 5, St Louis, 1995 Mosby.

Baker C: School health: policy issues, *Nurs Healthcare* 15(4):179-184, 1994.

Ballard J: *Public law 94-142 and section 504—understanding what they are and are not,* Reston, VA, 1977, Governmental Relations Unit, The Council for Exceptional Children.

Brown v Board of Education. US Supreme Court 347 US 483, Washington, DC, 1954, US Supreme Court.

Burns M, Thornan CB: Broadening the scope of nursing practice: federal programs for children, *Pediatr Nurs* 19(6):546-552, 1993.

Chekryn J, Deegan M, and Reid J: Normalizing the return to school of the child with cancer, *Ped Oncol Nurses* 3:20-24, 34, 1986.

Cole KN et al: Effects of preschool integration for children with disabilities, *Exceptional Child* 58:36-45, 1991.

Committee on Children with Disabilities. Pediatrician's role in the development and implementation of an individual evaluation plan (IEP) and/or individual family service plan (IFSP), *Pediatrics* 89:340-342, 1992.

Committee on Children with Disabilities. Provision of related services for children with chronic disabilities, *Pediatrics* 92(6):879-881, 1993.

Committee on Injury and Poison Prevention. School bus transportation of children with special needs, *AAP News* 9(11), 1993.

Davis K: Educational needs of the terminally ill student, *Issues in Compr Pediatr Nurs* 12:235-245, 1989.

Decker B: A comparison of the Individualized Education Plan and the Individualized Family Service Plan, *Am J Occupational Therapy* 46:242-252, 1992.

Fowler M, Johnson M, and Atkinson S: School achievement and absence in children with chronic health conditions, *J Pediatr* 106(4):683-687, 1985.

Harrison BS, Faircloth JW, and Yaryan L: The impact of legislation and litigation on the role of the school nurse, *Nurs Outlook* 43:57-61, 1995.

Igoe JB: School-linked family health centers in health care reform, *Pediatr Nurs* 19:67-68, 1993.

Jenkins JR, Odom SL, and Speltz ML: Effects of social integration on preschool children with handicaps, *Exceptional Child* 55:311-320, 1989.

Krier JJ: Involvement of educational staff in the healthcare of medically fragile children, *Pediatr Nurs* 19(3):251-254, 1993.

McMillan JA: Control of infections in schools, *Pediatr in Rev* 16:283-88, 1995.

Mills v Board of Education of the District of Columbia. US Court of Appeals 348F, Supp. 866, Washington, DC, 1972, US Court of Appeals.

National Education Association: Executive committee, *Policy on do not resuscitate orders,* June, 1994.

Page-Goertz S: Even children have arthritis, *Pediatr Nurs* 15(1):15-16, 30, 1989.

Palfrey JS et al: Providing therapeutic services to children in special educational placements: an analysis of the related services provisions of Public Law 94-142 in five urban school districts. *Pediatrics* 85(4):518-525, 1990.

Parette HP, Parette PC: Young children with disabilities and assistive technology: the nurse's role on multidisciplinary technology teams, *J Pediatr Nurs* 7:237-245, 1992.

Passarelli C: Case management of chronic health conditions of school-age youth. In HM Wallace, K Patrick, GS Parcel, and JB Igoe, editors: *Principles and practices of student health: school health,* vol 2, Oakland, CA, 1992, Third Party Publishing Co, pp 350-389.

Passarelli C: School nursing trends for the future, *J Sch Health* 64(4):141-148, 1994.

Pennsylvania Association for Retarded Citizens v Pennsylvania. US Court of Appeals 343 F, Supp. Philadelphia, PA, 1972, US Court of Appeals.

Perrin J: *Developmental-behavioral pediatrics,* ed 2, Philadelphia, 1992, WB Saunders.

Public Law 93-112 The Vocational Rehabilitation Act, Section 504, 29 USC, 45CFR, Washington, DC, 1973. US Government Printing Office.

Public Law 94-142. The Education for All Handicapped Children Act 20 USC Sec 11 404 [18], Washington, DC, 1975a, US Government Printing Office.

Public Law 94-142. The Education of the Handicapped Act 20 USC Sec 121a, 13[4], Washington, DC, 1975b, US Government Printing Office.

Public Law 94-142. The Education of the Handicapped Act 20 USC Sec 121a, 13[4], Washington, DC, 1975c, US Government Printing Office.

Public Law 94-142. The Education of the Handicapped Children Act 20 USC Sec 121a, 13[10], Washington, DC, 1975d, US Government Printing Office.

Public Law 99-457. The Education of the Handicapped Act Children Amendments of 1986, Washington, DC, 1986, US Government Printing Office.

Public Law 100-407. Technology-Related Assistance for Individuals with Disabilities Act of 1988, Washington, DC, 1988, US Government Printing Office.

Public Law 101-476. The Individuals with Disabilities Education Act of 1990, Washington, DC, 1990, US Government Printing Office.

Public Law 102-119. The Individuals with Disabilities Education Act Revisions of 1991, Washington, DC, 1991 US Government Printing Office.

Rabin N: School reentry and the child with a chronic illness: the role of the pediatric nurse practitioner, *J Pediatr Health Care* 8:227-232, 1994.

Rushton CH, Will J, and Murray M: To honor and obey: DNR orders in the schools, *Pediatr Nurs* 20(6):581-585, 1995.

Sarzynski A: Pediatric nurse practitioners and educational mainstreaming. *J Pediatr Health* 8:27-32, 1994.

Swanson MN, Thompson PE: Managing Asthma Triggers in School, *Pediatr Nurs* 20(2):181-184, 1994.

Turner-Henson A et al: The experiences of discrimination: challenges for chronically ill children. *Pediatr Nurs* 20(6):571-577, 1994.

Vessey JA, Swanson MN, and Hagedorn M: Teasing Who says names can never hurt you, *Pediatric Nursing,* 21:297-299, 342, 1995.

Walker D, Jacobs F: Chronically ill children in school, *Peabody J Educ* 61:28-74, 1984.

Walsh M, Ryan-Wenger N: Sources of stress in children with asthma, *J of School Health* 62(10):459-463, 1992.

Wong O: *Nursing care of infants and children,* St Louis, 1995.

York J et al: Feedback about integrating middle-school students with severe disabilities in general education classes, *Exceptional Child* 58:244-258, 1992.

Ethics and the Child with a Chronic Condition

6

Cindy Hylton Rushton*

DECISION MAKING ALONG THE TRAJECTORY OF CHRONIC CONDITIONS

The trajectory of a chronic condition is likely to include diagnosis and treatment, periods of recovery, exacerbations, stability, or instability, and in some cases, deterioration and death. These phases are often punctuated by recurring ethical questions. These include: (1) defining what constitutes a life worth living, (2) recognizing the threshold for certainty in diagnosis and treatment, (3) choosing a decision maker who decides about treatment or nontreatment, (4) determining the role of minors in making treatment decisions, (5) deciding whether to pursue experimental or innovative therapies, and (6) knowing how to resolve conflicts. The range of chronic conditions in childhood and adolescence is paralleled by the range of values held by people with, or caregivers of, those with chronic conditions. Competing ethical obligations can create a set of problematic situations for children, families, and health care providers.

*Portions of this chapter are excerpted from the following publications with the permission of the publishers: Rushton CH, Glover J: Involving parents in decisions to forgo life-sustaining treatment for critically ill infants and children, *AACN Clinical Issues in Critical Care Nursing* 1(1):206-214, 1990; Rushton CH, Lynch MA: Dealing with advance directives for critically ill adolescents, *Critical Care Nurse* 12(5):31-37, 1992; and Rushton CH: Ethical decision making: the role of parents, *Capsules and Comments in Pediatric Nursing* 1(2):1-10, 1994.

The Ethical Domain

Ethics is concerned with what "ought to be" and the ways individuals think about and discuss "what ought to be." Ethics is concerned with the behavior, choices, and character of individuals and groups. Ethical questions arise alongside, but differ from, fundamental social, legal, political, professional, and scientific questions. For example, public policies and laws such as the death penalty set boundaries for human behavior but do not necessarily correspond to an individual's sense of "what ought to be." It is within this context that ethical discourse occurs.

There are many ways of discerning the ethical dimensions of an issue or quandary. The process of discernment is complex and is influenced by emotions, scientific facts, values, interpersonal relationships, culture, religion, the essence of who we are, and a myriad of situational factors. All of these elements converge to shape the way ethical questions are framed. Ethical questions arise because an individual is unsure about what is the right thing to do or what is the proper outcome to pursue. Primary care providers, for instance, may be concerned about whether to offer an experimental treatment protocol to a family when the likelihood of altering the natural course of the child's condition is remote and pursuing the therapy will require that the family pay out of pocket for the treatment. Ethical questions may also arise because there are genuine value conflicts about what is the right thing to do or what are the proper outcomes to pursue. For instance, primary care providers and families may disagree about whether it is justified to continue aggressive treatment for a child with end-stage cystic fibrosis. The providers may reason, for example, that continued treatment is burdensome and will prolong death. In contrast, parents may believe extending life despite the burden endured by the child is the appropriate goal to be pursued. In both instances, careful consideration of the judgments that are made and the justifications that are used to defend one's position and behavior is warranted.

Ethical deliberation involves a process of discernment, analysis, and articulating ethically defensible positions, and then acting upon them. Ethical thinking helps give a reasoned account of an ethical position and move beyond intuitions or emotions. The goal of ethical deliberations is not to achieve absolute certainty about what is right, but rather to achieve *reliability* and *coherence* in behavior, choices, character, process, and outcomes.

Ethical theories and principles provide a foundation for ethical analysis and deliberation (see box on normative ethical theories). They offer a guide for organizing and understanding ethically relevant information in a dilemma or conflict situation. They also suggest direction and avenues for resolving competing claims, and supply reasons for justifying moral action. Ethical principles are universal in nature but they are *not* absolute. Each case involves particular principles and values integral to the decision-making process. A person must balance the claims generated from competing principles relevant to a particular case. Moreover, factors such as family dynamics, the nature of relationships, contextual features, integrity, and faithfulness to commitments are also morally relevant to the decision-making process. Even when a person chooses a morally justifiable course of action, there will always be unmet obligations; hence, there will always be a "moral remainder" when resolving ethical dilemmas.

Ethical theories and principles must be applied systematically within the decision-making process. Ethical analysis is enhanced by using a framework that provides a systematic process of decision making and avoids making mistakes by using only logic and reason (see box on examining ethical conflicts, p. 88). In addition, because some decisions such as those to withhold or withdraw certain therapies help to determine the timing and consequences of

---

NORMATIVE ETHICAL THEORIES AND PRINCIPLES

Teleological theories—determine an action to be right or wrong based on the consequences the action produces. For example, in utilitarianism, the principle of utility or maximizing the good or minimizing harm is the central criterion for action.

Deontological theories—focus on doing one's duty. The intrinsic quality of the act itself or it's conformity to a rule determines whether an act is right or wrong, not its consequences.

Selected ethical principles

Beneficence—the duty to do good; to promote the welfare of the individual
Nonmaleficence—the duty not to harm or burden
Respect for persons—recognizing another person as sharing a common human destiny

Derivative principles

Autonomy—self determination
Veracity—the duty to tell the truth
Fidelity—the duty to keep one's promise or word
Justice—fairness; giving every person what they are entitled. Distributive justice refers to the equitable distribution of benefits and burdens under conditions of scarcity and competition.

Adapted from Beauchamp and Childress, 1989

---

death, there are also other important social, ethical, and religious values that come into play.

A MORAL FRAMEWORK FOR DECISION MAKING WHEN CARING FOR CHILDREN

A specific framework provides a mechanism for individuals, families, and providers dealing with the ethical dimensions of difficult situations. For adults, a morally defensible framework for decision making is relatively straightforward and widely accepted (President's Commission for the Study of

FRAMEWORK FOR EXAMINING ETHICAL CONFLICTS

Questions to consider

1. What are the significant medical factors in the case?
2. What are the significant human factors in the case? This may include relationships, contextual features, culture, religion, etc.
3. What values/duties/rights are at stake for the individual? Are those values/duties/rights in conflict with others?
4. What is the ethical problem in this case? Which moral principles are in conflict?
5. What are the possible courses of action that could be pursued in this case and potential consequences of each?
6. How do you weigh conflicts among the stakeholders' values, duties, rights, principles? Is it more important to preserve or protect some values, duties, rights, or principles over others? State justification for your position.
7. Considering all of the above, what ought to be done in this case?
8. Prioritize various courses of action.
9. What competing values might affect your willingness to take moral action?
10. What kinds of objections might be raised about your decision? How can you explain your decision in a way that addresses those objections?
11. Identify possible strategies for resolving the issue.

Adapted from Duckett et al, 1986.

A MORAL FRAMEWORK FOR DECISION MAKING

Beneficence
  Balancing benefit and burden
Respect for persons
  Informed consent
Justice
  Macro- and microallocation of resources
  Individual vs society needs
An ethic of care

Ethical Problems in Medicine and Biomedical and Behavioral Research, 1983) (see box on moral framework for decision making). Consistent with a western view of autonomy, treatment options should promote the well-being of the individual according to that individual's own understanding of well-being. When individuals lack the capacity to make choices for themselves, someone else must represent that individual's particular values and preferences. Ethical decision making is a process with multiple contributors; it is a combination of expertise of the health provider concerning available choices and expertise of the individual or surrogate concerning what choices best promote the individual's life goals and values. This decision-making process is also influenced by the family system, culture, religious and spiritual affiliations, and personal values and preferences (Grodin and Burton, 1988).

Ethical decision making for children is more complex because most children lack the capacity to make informed, independent decisions. Children have not formulated life goals and values upon which such decisions would be based. Although the capacity to be involved in decision making varies according to the child's level of maturity, it is generally assumed that children need surrogate decision makers (American Academy of Pediatrics Committee on Bioethics, 1994). Decisions made on behalf of children lack a key feature of the moral framework for adults—the individual's unique assessment of his own well-being. Despite this, minors can be involved in meaningful ways in decisions about their own health care (see section on respect for persons, p. 90). The moral principles involved in adult decision making do, however, provide a valuable framework when making decisions on behalf of children (American Academy of Pediatrics, 1994).

Beneficence

The primary principle involved in decision making is beneficence (doing good) and it's corollary nonmaleficence (avoiding or minimizing harm). Treatment options should include those that benefit the infant or child and clearly outweigh the associated burdens and harms. This "best-interest" standard is often used as a hallmark when making decisions for children. This standard establishes a presumption in favor of life, since existence is usually required for other interests to be advanced. Generally, life should be saved when possible. When life cannot be saved or the chance of survival is minimal, treatment regarded as burdensome should not be provided (Macklin, 1982). Burdens for children with chronic conditions might include, for example, repeated pain and suffering associated with invasive procedures, symptoms, or disability; or emotional distress caused by fear, immobilization, prolonged hospitalization, or isolation from family and friends. Decisions concerning a child whose chances of dying are great might reasonably focus on the comfort associated with dying, rather than on therapies to prolong life.

An additional standard, the "relational potential" standard, has also been suggested as an adjunct to the best interest standard when balancing the benefit and burden of various courses of action (McCormick, 1974). This standard focuses on the child's cognitive and intellectual capacities, the degree of neurologic impairment, prognosis regarding reversibility of the neurologic condition, and whether the outcome of the condition can be altered through treatment or therapy. Infants or children who are permanently unconscious, for example, have no capacity to feel either pleasure or pain. Their "interests" are limited to prolongation of biologic life. Because such children cannot be burdened in the usual sense, and most of the reasons for treatment are gone—better function, fewer symptoms, the opportunity for human relationships or greater opportunity to achieve life's goals— many would argue that treatment may be futile (Paris and Fletcher, 1987). The Baby Doe regulations (Child Abuse Amendments, PL 98-457, 1984), for example, regard permanent unconsciousness as a condition that does not require life-sustaining treatment. Yet, there are a wide range of views regarding the degree of neurologic impairment that justifies limiting or foregoing treatment.

The challenge for children, parents, and health care providers is to understand the unique meaning of the concepts of health, sickness, disability, suffering, care, and death for the child in a particular situation. The meaning that these concepts give to an individual's life is influenced by their values, interests, aims, rights, and duties. A holistic understanding of a child's life, a recognition of important values that give direction to treatment decisions, and the tenor of the professional-client relationship evolve and change over time; hence, discovering the threshold for balancing benefits and burdens in a particular case may change as the child's condition changes. For example, the initial goals for a newborn with multiple congenital anomalies resulting in neurologic impairment and severe physical disability may be to understand the extent of the child's condition and to preserve life. In this instance, parents and professionals may agree to tolerate a high degree of burden to the child in order to diminish the uncertainty surrounding diagnosis and prognosis. Two years later, after the diagnosis and prognosis have been clarified, parents and professionals may have a different view of how much burden the child must tolerate to sustain life, particularly when continued treatment will not alter the prognosis and may impose significant burdens.

Beneficence is promoted by assisting the child and family to construct a meaningful life by balancing the burdens of the condition with the positive dimensions of living. Beneficence is expressed by identifying individualized care outcomes that enhance the child's well-being. These objectives include adequately managing symptoms, accommodating to limitations imposed by the chronic condition, and maximizing functional capacities. Treatment interventions must therefore be designed to contribute to individualized goals that enhance quality of life and promote the child's sense of integrity despite the limitations related to her condition.

Parents and professionals must openly discuss uncertainty in diagnosis and prognosis and explore the extent of certainty needed for both parental and professional decision making. At times, the need for greater certainty by either parents or professionals may result in burdensome diagnostic evaluations that do not contribute to the child's well-being or outcome. Alternatively, parents may accept uncertainty when professionals are compelled to seek further evidence to support their recommendations. The dynamic nature of the condition's trajectory may create special challenges for caregivers and parents. Ideally a shared vision and a common understanding of the balance of benefit and burden that is acceptable for a particular child is created.

The introduction of experimental or innovative therapies for children with chronic conditions often raises ethical concerns. Primary care providers, children, and families must consider the balance of benefit and burden of experimental therapies. To address these challenging situations, parents and caregivers should engage in ongoing, open discussions regarding poorly tested therapies or experimental treatments. For example, when an innovative surgical procedure is considered for a young child with an orthopedic deformity, the health care provider must disclose the uncertainty surrounding its effectiveness.

Respect for Persons

A second principle involved in decision making is respect for persons. Respect for persons means respecting another person as sharing a common human destiny (Curtin, 1986). Adult decisions focus on the unique life goals and values of the individual out of respect for that individual and for the integrity of his or her life. The uniquely human freedom of each person to create a meaningful life is highly valued. Even though children are neither autonomous nor self-determining, respect is still required because children's lives also have unique meanings. To treat individuals with respect is to acknowledge and value who they are outside of a medical context, rather than to only treat them in accordance to how professional goals and values are advanced. Most children live in families that provide nurturance and care. The relationships that arise within families are inherently valuable to the well-being of children. To respect a child is to acknowledge the importance of the child's world and the relationships that are central to it. Unilateral decision making by health care professionals based solely on "medical indications" would deny the fullness of a child's life, and the value of the relationships that also benefit and sustain the child.

A central problem associated with parental or other surrogate decisions is the inherent difficulty of judging the quality of a child's life and the bene-

fits and burdens that he or she experiences. The child, the family members, and health care providers all may attach unique, but different, meanings to the child's life. Although life itself is regarded as valuable, professionals and surrogate decision makers cannot consider the prolongation of life exclusively. Decisions need to benefit and respect the child as an individual but recognize the child's unique position of reliance on the family for nurturance and physial care. The values that parents place on their parenting role may make it difficult for them to separate the benefits and burdens of parenting a child with special needs from the benefits and burdens experienced by the child. For primary care providers, these decisions are even more complex as they attempt to discern what is best for the child in the context of the family. The choice of interventions can positively or negatively affect the comfort or ease with which a child lives life.

Respect for others is enhanced and evidenced by nonjudgmental attitudes and behaviors. It is important to stress that being nonjudgmental does not mean relinquishing values or being blind or indifferent to personal principles. Rather, the goal is openness to different ways of viewing and acting upon personal commitments and life circumstances. An essential dimension of nonjudgmental behavior is resisting imposing personal judgments on others.

The standard of informed consent is derived from the principle of respect for persons. Autonomy, or self-determination, is the central moral value expressed through the process of informed consent. Legally, informed consent requires disclosure, comprehension, and voluntary agreement or consent by the competent individual or the surrogate. Relevant information about diagnosis and treatment including a description of the nature and purpose of treatment or procedure, the benefits and risks, the problems related to recovery, the likelihood of success, and the alternative treatments must be discussed with the surrogate and the child to every extent possible. The person giving consent, usually the parent, must have the ability to understand relevant information, to reason and deliberate according with his or her values and preferences and the perceived values and preferences of the child, and the ability to communicate the choices to others. Finally, consent must be given voluntarily without coercion. The informed consent process must be evaluated as the child matures and altered as necessary to include the child's expressed decisions or concerns.

Justice

Justice pertains to fairness and equity in the treatment of others. Justice refers to an individual's access to an adequate level of health care and to the distribution of available health care resources. Caregivers promote the principle of justice by being fair in the provision of care and attention to children and their families. The Code for Nurses, for example, focuses on the delivery of care with respect for human dignity, which is not to be defined in terms of personal attributes, socioeconomic status, or the nature of an illness (American Nurses Association, 1985). This provision requires that a criterion such as age, gender, wealth, religious beliefs, or social unacceptability of a condition should not be a factor in deciding between or among individuals competing for the same treatment. This provision strives for a genuine impartiality, equal respect for all persons, and a refusal to create a hierarchy of worth of individuals. Prejudicial treatment on the basis of personal or other attributes constitutes a violation of a moral norm and ideal that has been precious to the nursing profession for generations.

Consistent with the ethical obligations of justice, children with chronic conditions are legally protected from discriminatory treatment through the enactment of state and federal laws. Section 504 of the Rehabilitation Act of 1973 (PL 93-112) grants protection from discrimination based on disability, whereas the Education for All Handicapped Children Act (EHA) of 1975 (PL 94-142), now known as the Individuals with Disabilities Education Act (IDEA), creates access for children with disabilities to education by establishing a federal grant program to assist states to provide a free and appropriate public education to all students in need of special education. The Americans with Disabilities Act (ADA) (1990) gives civil rights protection to individuals with disabilities by guaranteeing equal opportunity to public accommodations, employment, transportation, state and local government services, and telecommunications. Such laws create important obligations for both parents and health care providers and must be considered within the ethical analysis of troubling cases.

Health policies for children with chronic conditions address some of the same concerns encompassed in the principle of justice. These policies include strategies to avoid discrimination, stigmatization, and the exploitation of dependence. Additionally, strategies to support family-centered service delivery, health insurance reform, access to employment and educational opportunities, and the community's role in offering support to children and their families are consistent with a justice perspective.

Issues involving the just distribution of health care resources arise at two levels. The *macroallocation level* refers to the share of societal resources allocated to specific societal goods such as health. Resources allocated to support the health, development, and education of children with chronic conditions are a reflection of society's values and willingness to recognize and address the unique circumstances and needs of these children. For example, proposed national health care reform legislation rarely includes habilitation-rehabilitation services for children. Furthermore, access to long-term care and other services (such as home nursing, some durable and nondurable equipment, and habilitation services) are usually highly limited. Eligibility is often restricted and is based on income or physical, mental, or emotional disabilities. Additionally, by not establishing uniform eligibility requirements for Medicaid from state to state, a child who depends on Medicaid for support services and care in one state may not be able to obtain those same services if he moves to another state. These issues reflect some of the challenges of devising national health policy that supports the interests of children with chronic conditions.

Within health care, macroallocation refers to the division of a resource, such as money, among various services, such as transplantation programs, critical care, or outpatient services (Beauchamp and Childress, 1989; Reigle, 1989). This issue becomes particularly relevant at the institutional level where costs and priorities for allocation of scarce resources are determined. In an era of cost containment and downsizing, institutions and programs providing specialized services to children with chronic conditions may be particularly vulnerable.

Providers may reason, for example, that the expenditures for specialized services for children with cystic fibrosis consume a disproportionate share of the overall budget for pediatric care. They may conclude that greater numbers of children can be helped if money is spent on preventive services. Such reasoning focuses on the consequences of actions by evaluating their utility based on their ability to maximize the benefits and outcomes for the greatest number of children. Focusing on a single criterion such as utility may not account for other important moral values such as the protection of vulnerable populations or existing obligations toward those in the greatest need of services.

The term *microallocation* is applied at the individual level; these decisions involve determining the distribution of a specific resource. In general, the professional's main concern is for the individual; however, especially during periods of shortages of human and material resources, the needs of others may impinge on an individual's care. Health care providers participate in microallocation decisions when determining which child needs the greatest amount of care, thereby limiting care to others who are perceived as less needy. Microallocation issues arise when resources are limited and there is insufficient quantity of the resource to provide for all who need it.

The ethical principles of beneficence and justice are central to issues of resource allocation and rationing. The principle of beneficence requires the health care provider to help others and to promote good. This principle is evident on two levels—the individual level and the societal level (Beauchamp and Childress, 1989). Each level includes different considerations regarding the allocation of limited resources. On the individual level, the health care provider fulfills the duty of beneficence by allocating resources based on individual needs. Scarce resources are distributed to those with immediate needs without regard to the needs of other potential clients or the community at large. For example, when an infant is born with spina bifida, currently a cadre of medical, developmental, educational, and social resources are mobilized regardless of socioeconomic status, cultural, or religious heritage, or ability to pay. This initial commitment to provide equitable and fair services for all families may not be sustained. Cost constraints, lack of available resources, and accessibility to resources may limit services for some children and their families as they mature.

Realizing beneficence at the societal level involves allocating resources based on the needs of society and considering the greatest good for the entire community, a utilitarian perspective. The focus shifts from crisis care and doing good for the individual to preventive care and actions that benefit society. This is particularly important for children with chronic conditions because greater emphasis on prevention may result in diminished specialized services designed to meet their needs. As resources become more scarce, difficult decisions will need to be made to balance the needs of individuals, particularly those with chronic conditions, with the needs of society.

An Ethic of Care

Traditional ethical reasoning requires providers to ascertain the rights of the individual and to weigh the ethical principles in order to resolve conflicting obligations. Applying ethical principles alone cannot resolve the clinical quandaries that arise in the care of a child with a chronic condition. The language and method used to analyze a particular case can either clarify or confound the situation. When the rights of children are held in opposition to the rights of their parents, for example, an adversarial tension can be established that may polarize discussion. In contrast, if it is recognized that most parents are motivated to promote their child's interests, such polarity may be avoided. Considering other aspects of the moral life, such as virtue and individual experience, may reduce adversarial tensions between the rights of children and their parents and allow for a more comprehensive appreciation of the attitudes, values, and moral commitments of decision makers within the context of family relationships. This perspective is often referred to as an "ethic of care."

From the care perspective, the resolution of ethical quandaries is focused on the child's needs in the context of the family, and the provider's corresponding responsibilities within the context of the provider-client relationship. The primary care provider can focus on the special circumstances and context of the specific situation where moral action occurs instead of merely considering the individual's interests and preferences in isolation. In other words, the uniqueness of individuals and particular dynamics of their relationships are endorsed as essential components of moral decision making (Carse, 1991). Such a model supports efforts to assist children and their families in finding unique meaning or purpose in their living or their dying and in assisting them to realize goals that promote a meaningful life or death.

The values and expectations involved in certain roles and relationships are seen as primary from this vantage point. Therefore, being an advocate for a child with a chronic condition involves appreciating the relationships significant to the child and understanding how those relationships affect care. Children with chronic conditions develop an intricate web of relationships that support and sustain them throughout their lives. In keeping with a family-centered philosophy of care, families are viewed as essential partners in children's treatment and care. Professionals must recognize and respect these interconnections as central to the well-being of the child. A care perspective also emphasizes the interrelationships of the members of the health care team. It recognizes that nurses, physicians, and other caregivers work collaboratively to advance the interests and goals of children with chronic conditions.

Ethical principles (beneficence, nonmaleficence, respect for persons, and justice) and an ethic of care provide a framework for approaching ethical questions occurring in clinical practice. It must also be acknowledged that these are not the only principles that may have relevance to a particular case. The challenge for primary care providers is to discern how these and other principles can assist to illuminate the ethical issues and provide guidance in resolving competing obligations.

THE PROCESS OF DECISION MAKING

Shared Decision Making

Traditionally, a model of shared decision making is based on the assumption that decisions are shared between children if capable, parents, and professionals. Treatment decisions must represent a combination of the individuals' expertise in order to se-

lect choices that best promote the life goals and values for the child. Parents do not have the expertise to act as surrogate health care professionals nor can health care professionals replace the expertise of parents. Shared decision making means that parents and professionals should agree about general treatment goals, but professionals should make decisions about which treatment modalities are necessary to advance the mutually agreed upon goals.

Endorsement of a model of shared decision making in an ideal sense means that parents, or if able, children, engage fully in the process by understanding the range of possibilities for treatments and their consequences, and by sharing in a meaningful way in the dialogue about their goals, values, and aspirations. Such a model goes beyond the legal requirements for disclosure, comprehension, and voluntary consent (King, 1992). Although in theory professionals embrace the ideal of shared decision making as the desired model of parent-professional decision making, it is rarely accomplished in reality (King, 1992).

The Role of Parents in Treatment Decision Making

Based on the moral framework of shared decision making described above, it is necessary for someone to represent the interests of the child. There is a strong presumption that parents should make judgments about what is in the best interest of the child (King, 1987). Parents are identified as appropriate surrogates because strong bonds of affection and commitment are likely to yield the greatest concern for the well-being of their children. Parents are obligated to protect their children from harm and to do as much good for them as possible (Fletcher, 1983).

There is a direct connection between the well-being of parents and their children; the identity of each is inextricably linked. A woman who defines herself as a mother, for example, regards her own welfare partly in terms of the welfare of her child. Harm to the child constitutes personal harm to the mother. Such relationships are valuable to both parents and children, and society needs to limit its interference into this private realm (Caplan and Cohen, 1987). Furthermore, parents are identified as primary decision makers because of the importance of the family institution. Families play an essential role in maintaining the integrity of society. Children learn values of cooperation and commitment within the family context that then can be generalized to other members of society.

Parents must be involved in treatment decisions for their infants and children because there are lifelong consequences of these decisions. Parents will be responsible for the ongoing physical, emotional, medical, and financial care of the infant or child who survives with serious disabilities (Reiser, 1986). They also will live with the consequences of decisions to forego treatment. Long after health care professionals are likely to have forgotten a case, the family will be remembering and incorporating these momentous decisions into the fabric of their lives.

Limits to Parental Authority

Children are not only members of their immediate families, but of the broader community as well. A moral community shares an interest in the life and well-being of each member. There are certain community standards of best interest, like the preservation of life, that may override a family's interpretation of a child's best interest. Although there are compelling reasons to support parents' decision-making authority, such authority is not absolute. The interests of the parents and the family must take a high priority but do not override the fundamental respect for the best interest of the infant or child (Hastings Center Research Project on the Care of Imperiled Newborns, 1987).

Even when there is a presumption of shared responsibility on the part of both parents and professionals to promote the well-being of a child, there will be times when parents should be disqualified as primary decision makers. This parental disqualification may be the result of incapacity or choice of a course of action clearly against the child's best interest (President's Commission, 1983). If a parent has a known psychiatric condition and is behaving irrationally or there has been a documented history of child abuse or neglect, the primary care provider may question parental capacity to advocate on behalf of the child. If there is a dispute about the parents' intentions or capacity to function as decision makers, it is incumbent upon those who would substitute another decision maker to show convincing evidence why the parents should be disqualified.

For example, even though respect for religious beliefs is an important community value, so is the value of life. Although adults who are Jehovah's Witnesses can choose to forgo a life-saving blood transfusion for themselves, they are often not permitted to make a similar decision on behalf of their children. Moreover, children are entitled to grow up and make independent assessments of their own religious beliefs.

In such circumstances health care providers must be advocates for children and uphold the community standard of best interest. Clearly, there will always be cases where such assumptions are challenged; however, these will likely be few in number. It is incumbent upon those who would challenge parents' motives and commitments to prove that parents should be disqualified as decision makers instead of parents having to prove their motives and commitments are authentic. Safeguards to protect the interests of children, families, and professionals will continue to be necessary and prudent (Rushton, 1994). The process of assessing when community standards should outweigh a family determination is extremely difficult.

Whether the disqualification of parents always requires court intervention is the source of much current debate (Hastings Center, 1987; President's Commission, 1983). When parents are disqualified, a surrogate decision maker should have knowledge of all relevant facts and the ability to perceive and represent the feelings and interests of those involved. They should also be free of serious conflicts of interest that may bias a decision. Often a court appointed guardian *ad litem* serves as a surrogate decision maker.

The Role of Minors in Treatment Decision Making

Professionals who care for children and adolescents with chronic conditions are increasingly concerned about the role minors play in making decisions about their health care. Many adolescents experience catastrophic physical and mental problems associated with severe disabilities, malignancies, or cardiac, pulmonary, and hepatic organ disease without having the legal right to decide about their treatments.

As client advocates, primary care providers must be concerned with how to promote the interests of adolescents in decisions about their health care. The concerns of adolescents escalate when parents and primary care providers appear to disregard the adolescent's previously expressed preferences or they embark on a course of treatment that is inconsistent with the adolescent's life goals and values. Many health professionals are questioning the adequacy of current decision-making models and are searching for creative solutions, perhaps through the advent of advance directives for minors.

From a moral viewpoint, minors with decision-making capacity have a legitimate claim to be involved in decisions about their health care. Their claim is based on a respect for persons that recognizes that adolescents and young adults can be self-determining and therefore, should have a voice in their care and the extent of medical interventions to be provided. Such respect for them as individuals and as members of families and society compels primary care providers to take seriously their preferences when treatment decisions are made. Moreover, adolescents' particular interpretations of the benefits and burdens of treatment should be considered.

The standards for determining decision-making capacity for minors are the same as those for adults: (1) the ability to comprehend essential information about their diagnosis and prognosis, (2) the ability to reason about their choices in accordance with their values and life goals, and (3) the ability to make a voluntary informed decision which includes being able to recognize the consequences of various courses of action (President's Commission, 1983). Based on our knowledge of conceptual development, most children do not reach this level of maturity until they are 11 or 12 years of age (Piaget, 1969), although there is wide variation. These standards are straightforward, but their application in clinical practice will require clinicians to become more skilled in systematically assessing and documenting the decision-making capacity of minors.

Despite the importance of self-determination and well-being in justifying the participation of minors in treatment decisions, there is another competing value at stake—the interests of parents in making decisions for their minor children. Traditionally, it has been assumed that minors require surrogates to make decisions on their behalf. Parents are generally identified as the appropriate surrogate for their children and have been afforded considerable discretion in making treatment decisions. Currently, treatment decisions for adolescents are made through a joint determination by the physician-health care team and the parent or guardian for the child. Joint decisions to withhold or withdraw therapeutic interventions are difficult to formulate for parents as well as for health care providers. Parents may seek any possible intervention that will prolong their child's life regardless of the burdens to be endured. Alternatively, they may wish to relieve their child's suffering by forgoing certain life-sustaining treatments. The physician-health care team and the parent or guardian may have a different agenda for either continuing or initiating certain therapeutic interventions or instead, forgoing certain interventions. Yet both groups may interpret their decisions as being in the best interest of the child. Despite their assessments, neither group may truly understand the adolescent's perspective. In many cases, the adolescent may already understand the pain and consequences of treatment options, including the finality of death. Unfortunately, parents and health care providers may be hesitant to consider the adolescent as a legitimate decision maker regarding medical treatment.

As the model of decision making enlarges to include a definitive role for minors with decision-making capacity, health care providers must recognize that such a departure will also challenge the traditional process of decision making and may create conflicts between minors and their parents. The potential for such moral and legal conflicts will require the development of a mechanism for resolving disputes.

Legal Viewpoint Regarding the Role of Minors in Decision Making

The legal system has determined that adolescents in certain circumstances have specific rights and responsibilities associated with their decision-making capabilities for health care (Cohn, 1991). Emancipated minors are children less than 18 years of age who are totally self-supporting financially and who have renounced their parents' rights and responsibilities for caretaking (Blacks Law

Dictionary, 1988). The majority of states have formulated legislation recognizing the rights and responsibilities of an emancipated minor. Emancipation is rarely determined by the courts, and is generally implied through factors such as marital status, pregnancy or parenthood, and financial self-sufficiency. Emancipated minors do not need parental consent for medical treatment and have a similar right as adults to refuse medical treatment (Cohn, 1991).

The courts have also classified some adolescents as mature minors in relation to their decision-making capacity for seeking and accepting health care interventions. These mature minors are at least 15 years of age and are believed to have the capacity to understand the nature and risk of the medical interventions. Adolescents classified as mature minors may consent to treatment that is of benefit to them and does not involve any substantial risk (Cohn, 1991).

State statutes generally support a minor's (14 to 17 years old) rights to consent to ordinary medical care. For example, some state statutes support the right of minors to consent to specific medical treatment, such as contraceptive therapies, without parental notification and consent; however, the rights to consent to abortions are complex and varied. The Omnibus Reconciliation Act of 1990, also called the Patient Self-Determination Act (PSDA) of 1990, supports the right of adults (≥ 18 years old) who are admitted to health care facilities to accept or refuse medical treatment. This age limit is based on the belief that only adults have the capacity and the right to determine what should be done to their bodies, even if executing that right means implementing their right to die. It is crucial, however, that health care providers not ignore the plight of thousands of adolescents (ages 12 to 17 years old) who face similar catastrophic and terminal conditions but who are not given this legal right.

Although the PSDA was created only for adults, the spirit of the PSDA creates an opportunity to examine the potential role for minors in their treatment decisions and ultimately their right to determine the circumstances of their death. It is likely that many young children and adolescents do have the capacity to assist in making their own treatment decisions and determining what is in their best interest. There has been minimal guidance by the courts or through legislation regarding a minor's rights to refuse life-saving medical care. In the few decisions that have been rendered, the application of the mature minor status was used in supporting the minor's decision-making capacity to refuse treatment and understand the consequences of this decision. Unfortunately, since there are minimal and vague legal guidelines available to support a minor's rights to refuse treatment, health care providers are reluctant to intervene and support the minor's decision to withhold treatment particularly if it is in opposition to the parents' wishes.

Involving minors in treatment decision making will require families and professionals to join together to create a system that supports their participation. Such a system must include comprehensive guidelines aimed at assessment, intervention, and ongoing revision (McCabe, Rushton, and Glover, 1994).

Making Shared Decision a Reality

Regardless of the age of the child, family composition, or professional involvement, resolution of ethical concerns is supported by an authentic model of shared decision making that accommodates the diverse ways children and families choose to participate. To accomplish this, it is necessary to move beyond a procedural model of informed consent to an authentic partnership with parents where parents, the child, and professionals create an alliance that promotes the child's interests. The foundation for this alliance is a mutual understanding of each other's aspirations and goals, their perspectives on what makes life meaningful for the child, and their concepts of benefit and burden. In addition, parents need to share their goals, their values, and their definition of being good parents, and professionals must share their uncertainties and identify boundaries of their professional responsibility.

Shared decision making requires a vision that results from collaboration and open, effective communication using language free from technical terminology and jargon. One reason success in achieving shared decision making fails is that professionals may focus primarily on the decision itself, rather than on the process. Parents also may have difficulty separating emotions from facts. A revised model of shared decision making would focus more on the context of the situation—especially the relational dimensions, the parents' unique concept of good parenting, and the factors that mediate decision making—rather than on the decision itself.

Professionals must begin to appreciate the parents' perspective in decision making and not attempt to force them into a traditional, rational, step-wise model that is incongruent with their perspective. This means the goals of the parent-professional relationship, the outcomes of the process, and the process itself must be closely scrutinized. If, for example, the goal of the relationship with families is to get them to see the world in the same way as the professional, then dissenting views cannot be articulated or respected. Parents should be engaged early in a variety of choices about their child's care, rather than reserving their involvement for required consents for treatment or decisions about life-sustaining treatment. Parents need and want professionals to be partners in the care of their child regardless of the outcome and they want the professionals to assist them to be good parents in the process. Sharing in decision making must, therefore, begin early in the condition's management.

Authentic shared decision making does not mean differences will not exist or that everyone will come to the same conclusion about when and how to advance the child's interests. Nor does it mean that all participants will have the same skills, abilities, or preferences. Shared decision making is a process whereby differences are discussed, where differing opinions can be valued, and where ultimately the quality of care provided to the child and family will be enhanced.

STRATEGIES FOR ETHICAL DECISION MAKING

Increase Knowledge of Ethics, Law, and Policies

Professionals can enhance their effectiveness in resolving ethical conflicts by seeking opportunities to enhance knowledge and skills in ethical analysis and identifying resources to assist them in resolving dilemmas. Furthermore, knowledge of legal, public, and professional policies is advantageous. In particular, primary care providers who care for children with chronic conditions should be aware of pertinent state statutes and case laws that may affect their health care. Primary care providers must be particularly aware of institutional policies regarding the relinquishment of life-sustaining treatment if policies exist, and participate in policy development if they do not. Institutional policies that permit withholding information from parents or that effectively deny parental access to divergent medical opinions should also be examined and challenged.

Proactive Dialogue, Assessment, and Planning

Children with chronic conditions and their families often have a high level of personal interaction with primary care providers. Because many chronic conditions persist over a lifetime, there are many natural opportunities to examine, revise, or abandon various goals or dimensions of the treatment plan. With proactive planning, it is also possible and desirable to anticipate the ethical conflicts that accompany the treatment plan. Wharton and colleagues (1994) have developed a Child Health Advisory Plan, a clinical tool used to assist parents and providers in engaging in a process to generate and support decisions that are in the child's best interest (Wharton et al, 1994). Ongoing dialogue about these issues is essential for optimal planning and must not be reserved for crisis situations associated with acute episodes or illness, deteriorating conditions, or death.

Many children with chronic conditions and their families and providers will confront difficult decisions regarding treatment that will create significant moral tensions for each of them. For example, questions such as using psychoactive medications to treat children with learning disabilities, or deciding to try an experimental protocol for treating cancer may arise in primary care of children with chronic conditions. Morally difficult decisions such as these are best made when there is adequate time for education, discussion, and reflection. Hence ethical issues should be anticipated and discussions begun early.

Strategies for Dealing with Conflict

Even when communication among children, parents, and professionals is optimal, conflicts arise. In fact, good communication may illuminate points of real ethical dispute. Frequently, participants prioritize values differently and employ different processes to reach morally defensible conclusions. Therefore activities that promote multidisciplinary sharing, analysis, and decision making in an atmosphere of openness, objectivity, and diversity can lead to a greater tolerance of the views of others.

When moral disagreements occur, strategies for resolution include: (1) obtaining the most current, factual information regarding points of controversy, (2) reaching consensus about the language used for concepts or definitions, (3) agreeing on a common framework of moral principles to guide discussions, and (4) engaging in a balanced discussion of the positive and negative aspects of a viewpoint.

Mechanisms for institutional review of difficult or disputed cases include institutional ethics committees and other means to efficiently access legal, governmental, and consultative services. An internal review process can serve several purposes. These include: (1) verifying the facts of the case, (2) confirming the propriety of decisions, (3) resolving disputes, or (4) making referrals to public agencies when appropriate. Frequently, institutional ethics committees function as a consultant to staff and families experiencing ethical conflict. Multidisciplinary membership including a parent provides a broad representation of different viewpoints. In general, the actions of these committees are primarily consultative without any binding authority; however, the opportunity for uninvolved parties to assist in the review of difficult cases can provide constructive recommendations for resolution.

Mechanisms to resolve conflicts between minors and their parents must be developed as the process of involving minors in treatment decisions unfolds. Based on a model of family-centered care, mechanisms supporting individual self-determination within the context of the family system will be necessary. Strategies also will be needed to support families as they allow more involvement of their minor children in decision making. Mechanisms for examining family decision-making patterns and the role of children and parents in other types of decisions within the family also will be necessary. Finally, strategies to prepare minors to participate in decisions about

health care through community-school educational programs and as part of routine health care encounters are important prerequisites (Rushton and Lynch, 1992).

SUMMARY

The resolution of ethical conflicts requires that health care professionals recognize there is a moral problem, use a systematic process of moral reasoning, and take action. As a prerequisite to such analysis, primary care providers who care for children with chronic conditions and their families must examine their own values regarding the content and structure of treatment decisions. Such clarification will be necessary to ensure that the ideal of authentic shared decision making becomes a reality.

REFERENCES

American Academy of Pediatrics Committee on Bioethics: Guidelines for forgoing life-sustaining medical treatment, *Pediatrics* 93(3):532-536, 1994.

American Nurses Association: *Code for nurses with interpretive statements,* Kansas City, 1985, The Association.

Americans with Disabilities Act of 1990, 42 USC 12101 et seq, 1990.

Beauchamp TL, Childress JF: *Principles of biomedical ethics,* ed 3, New York, 1989, Oxford University Press.

Blacks law dictionary, St Paul, 1988, West Publishing Co.

Caplan A, Cohen C: *Ethics and the care of imperiled newborns: a report by the Hastings Center's research project on ethics and the care of imperiled newborns,* Briarcliff Manor, NY, 1987, The Hastings Center.

Carse A: The voice of care: implications for bioethical education, *J Med Philos* 16:5-28, 1991.

Cohn SD: The evolving law of adolescent health care, *NAACOG's clinical issues* 2:201-207, 1991.

Curtin L: The nurse as advocate: a philosophical foundation for nursing. In PI Chinn, editor: *Ethical issues in nursing,* Rockville, MD, 1986, Aspen Systems.

Duckett et al: Ethics education project, University of Minnesota School of Nursing, Minneapolis, MN, 1986.

Fletcher JC: Ethics and trends in applied human genetics, *Birth Defects* 19(5):143-158, 1983.

Grodin M, Burton LA: Context and process in medical ethics: the contribution of family-systems theory, *Family Systems Medicine* 6:435-445, 1988.

Hastings Center Research Project on the Care of Imperiled Newborns: Imperiled newborns: a report, *Hastings Cent Rep* 17(6):5-32, 1987.

King N: Federal and state regulation of neonatal decision making. In R McMillian, H Englehardt, and H Specker, editors: *Euthanasia and the newborn: conflicts regarding saving lives,* Dordrecht, 1987, Reidel Publishing.

King N: Transparency in neonatal intensive care, *Hastings Cent Rep* 18-25, 1992.

Macklin R: Return to the best interests of the child. In W Gaylin and R Macklin, editors: *Who speaks for the child: the problems of proxy consent,* New York, 1982, Plenum Press.

McCabe MA, Rushton CH, and Glover JJ: *Operational guidelines for involving adolescents in health care decisions,* Washington, DC, 1994, Children's National Medical Center.

McCormick R: To save or let die: the dilemma of modern medicine, *JAMA* 229(2):172-176, 1974.

Omnibus Reconciliation Act [Patient Self-Determination Act (PSDA)], Title IV, Section 4206, h12456-h12457, *Congressional Record,* October 26, 1990.

Paris J, Fletcher J: Withholding of nutrition and fluids in the hopelessly ill patient, *Clin Perinatol* 14:367-377, 1987.

Piaget J: The intellectual development of adolescents. In G Caplan and S Levovici, editors: *Adolescence: psychological perspective,* New York, 1969, Basic Books, Inc.

President's Commission for the Study of Ethical Problems in Medicine and Biomedical and Behavioral Research: *Deciding to forgo life-sustaining treatment,* Washington, DC, 1983, US Government Printing Office.

Public Law 93-112. Section 504 of the Rehabilitation Act of 1973,Washington, DC, 1973, US Government Printing Office.

Public Law 94-142. Education for All Handicapped Children Act 29 USC 1400 et seq,Washington, DC, 1975, US Government Printing Office.

Public Law 98-457. The Child Abuse Amendments 42 US Code, 101, Interpretative guidelines (45 CFR Part 1 1340.15 et eq.), Washington, DC, 1984, US Government Printing Office.

Public Law 101-476. Individuals with Disabilities Education Act (IDEA), Washington, DC, 1990, US Government Printing Office.

Reigle J: Resource allocation issues in critical care nursing, *Nurs Clin North Am* 24:1009-1015, 1989.

Reiser S: Survival at what costs? origins and effects of the modern controversy on treating severely handicapped newborns, *Journal of Health Policy* 11(2):199-213, 1986.

Rushton CH: Ethical decision making: the role of parents, *Capsules and Comments in Pediatric Nursing* 1(2):1-10, 1994.

Rushton CH, Glover J: Involving parents in decisions to forgo life-sustaining treatment for critically ill infants and children, *AACN Clinical Issues in Critical Care Nursing* 1(1):206-214, 1990.

Rushton CH, Lynch MA: Dealing with advance directives for critically ill adolescents, *Crit Care Nurse* 12(5):31-37, 1992.

Wharton RH et al: Parental wishes regarding participation in critical health care planning for children with disabilities (abstract) *Pediatr Res* 35:47A, 1994.

Financing Health Care for Children with Chronic Conditions

7

Roberta S. O'Grady

Care for children with chronic conditions in the United States is financed by complex methods that are generally categorized as follows: (1) private health insurance, including prepayment arrangements; (2) public programs, such as Medicaid, the Title V Program for Children with Special Health Care Needs, and other federal and state categorical programs; (3) private, philanthropic sources; and (4) the family's own funds (Perrin, Shayne, and Bloom, 1993). A child's health care may be supported by one or a combination of these methods. The source of financial coverage depends on a number of factors, including type of health condition, family income, parents' employment, state and county of residence, availability of a voluntary organization for the specific condition, and the availability to the family of persons in the health care system and the legal system who have the knowledge to advocate for the child's rights to specific sources of financial assistance.

Both private and public sources of funding for the general population are undergoing reform to control costs of care while providing universal access to care. These reforms are of particular interest to the families of children with chronic conditions and their primary care providers because there is evidence that the reforms may be insensitive to the interests of children (Jameson and Wehr, 1993).

PRIVATE HEALTH INSURANCE

The role of private health insurance in paying the costs of care for children with chronic conditions is substantial but difficult to comprehend because of great variation in patterns of coverage and scope of benefits (Rowland, 1989). Private health insurance is generally categorized by the method of reimbursement. The fee-for-service plans are those that pay after the service is provided (see the box on private health insurance). That is, the payers, either patients or insurers, agree to pay the fee set by the provider. The fee is determined by a variety of market forces, including custom, altruism, profit, and administrative costs. Prepayment plans, which are also called managed care plans, offer services in exchange for an all-inclusive payment to a provider or group of providers. This payment is set in advance of need or request for services.

Fee-for-Service Plans

Blue Cross/Blue Shield arose from nonprofit, voluntary prepayment programs to cover unexpected hospital expenses and physician fees for treatment of conditions in the office or hospital, laboratory tests, and other services. Commercial health insurance is provided by profit-making organizations that sell all types of insurance.

Benefits that are likely to be covered by Blue Cross/Blue Shield and commercial insurance are hospital room and board, miscellaneous hospital expenses, surgery, physicians' nonsurgical services rendered in a hospital, and outpatient diagnostic x-ray examination and laboratory expenses. Room and board in an extended care facility may be included when there is proof that continued medical

PRIVATE HEALTH INSURANCE

Fee-for-service plans

Nonprofit prepayment programs (Blue Cross/Blue Shield)

Coverage for hospital care and physician services
Deductible
Coinsurance costs

Major medical policies

Coverage for catastrophic medical expenses
Large deductible

Limitations of policies

Preexisting conditions may not be covered
Preventive health care may not be covered
Limited home services available

care is required, as opposed to custodial care (Health Insurance Association of America [HIAA], 1994).

The insured person may pay a fee, or deductible, before insurance benefits are realized. The insured individual may also pay another portion of the cost of care, called *coinsurance,* of approximately 20% of physician, hospital and other related fees. In addition, there may be a stop-loss provision, which is the amount that a family must pay out of pocket in a calendar year before the plan pays 100% of further covered charges. There may also be a maximum lifetime benefit. Two million dollars is a typical lifetime benefit for a commercial insurance company.

Separate from general health insurance policies, major medical expense policies are available which cover a broad range of catastrophic medical expenses. The cost of major medical insurance is controlled by a deductible fee that ranges from $2000 to $15,000 or more and a coinsurance fee of 20% of those medical expenses that exceed the deductible. Maximum benefits are usually limited to $250,000 per person within a benefit period of 1 to 3 years, but there may be no limit to coverage

within the benefit period (HIAA, 1994). Major medical plans do not necessarily have advantages for children with chronic conditions. The health care needs of these children are likely to be long term and repetitive and therefore do not fit into a benefit structure of 1 to 3 years (Jameson and Wehr, 1993).

The problems faced by families who depend on fee-for-service health insurance to finance care for a child with a chronic condition are evident by looking at the exclusions and limitations of these health care policies. The insurer usually does not pay for preexisting conditions. Thus if a family was not adequately covered before their child acquired the chronic condition, a fee-for-service plan often will not cover the medical expenses related to the chronic condition. Other common exclusions are payments for preventive health care, such as routine physical examinations, rehabilitation services, hearing aids, glasses, and expenses associated with the birth of an infant up to the first 30 days of life.

Health insurance was designed to cover medical expenses; consequently, coverage for health needs defined as nonmedical, such as special education, mental health services, transportation to health care facilities, and home renovations to care for a child with a chronic condition, may not be included in fee-for-service plans offered by Blue Cross/Blue Shield or commercial health insurance. A survey of 259 members of The American Spinal Injury Association demonstrated that requests for durable medical equipment deemed medically necessary for mobility and transfer, adaptations to bathrooms for toileting and bathing, functional equipment to enable persons to feed themselves or turn the pages of a book, and special seating for functional posture are routinely denied by most types of fee-for-service plans (Donovan, Carter, and Wilkerson, 1987).

Fox and Newacheck (1990) studied the adequacy of fee-for-service health insurance coverage for children with chronic illnesses. These findings are based on a telephone survey, conducted in 1987, of 150 randomly selected employers representing small, medium, and large firms. Information was requested only for traditional insurance plans and preferred provider organizations. Prepaid plans were excluded from the survey. The response rate was 99%. All medium and large firms offered health insurance, but only 80% of small firms provided this coverage. Approximately one fourth of these firms did not offer either Blue Cross/Blue Shield or commercial insurance, but chose instead to offer self-insured plans. This is an important fact to note for those persons caring for children with chronic conditions. The self-insured plans are not governed by the same laws as other private health insurance plans. They may offer even fewer benefits to children than other fee-for-service plans, which are subject to the statutory and common law doctrines regulating insurance. Self-insured plans are governed by the Employee Retirement Income Security Act of 1974, called *ERISA,* which makes the plans exempt from state and federal insurance regulations and allows employers to establish, modify, and cancel employee medical benefits without state or federal interference (Jameson and Wehr, 1993). The children of employees on self-insured plans can be left without coverage for costly conditions, and the families have no legal recourse for protection against denial of claims or cancellation of policies.

Typical coverage provided in the insurance plans surveyed by Fox and Newacheck (1990) included hospital care and physician services for diagnosis and treatment of illness or injury. Approximately 60% of plans covered some preventive services. Care coordination, or case management, which is highly beneficial for children with a chronic condition who must frequently use more than one provider, was covered in about 20% of plans. Coverage was good for medical supplies and equipment, but other therapies, such as physical therapy, speech, and hearing, were less likely to be covered. Less than 10% covered nutrition services. Long-term care was often covered with limitations placed on the number of in-home services or days of service. Home care was only approved if the care was tied to an immediate prior hospitalization. Of the firms surveyed, 69% had plans that included a comprehensive home-care benefit, including skilled nursing, home health aids, physical therapy, respiratory therapy, and medical social work. The current trend in employer-based insurance is to authorize a wide range of community-based and home-based services when it can be shown that the total cost of these services is less than hospitaliza-

tion. Mental health services may also be covered with limitations on the number of visits and the type of provider. In summary, employer-based plans typically provide good coverage for hospital care and physician services. Coverage for special therapies and mental health is less comprehensive. Employees of small firms have more limited coverage than those of large firms. To control costs, private insurance companies and employers expect their employees to share more of the cost of using health care services.

Managed Care Plans

The nonprofit voluntary associations, Blue Cross/ Blue Shield, and commercial insurance companies offer both fee-for-service and managed care plans (see the box on managed care plans). In a managed care arrangement, the insured individual or family has access to selected providers who have agreed to furnish a defined set of health care services at a lower than usual fee, called the *capitation rate,* which is paid by the insurance company. There are two basic types of these managed care plans— preferred provider organizations and point-of-service plans. The forms, financial incentives, and utilization management of the plans are described by Freund and Lewitt (1993). Both types of managed care plans provide the insured with a list of primary care providers. The insured chooses a provider and goes to this provider for all routine care, paying little or nothing out of pocket. When the insured wishes to go outside the plan for care,

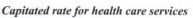

MANAGED CARE PLANS

Capitated rate for health care services
Preferred provider organizations
Point-of-service plans

Health maintenance organizations

Limitations of policies
Limited specialist services
Limited ancillary health care services

he or she has to pay a significantly higher share of the cost. The provider may also suffer financially by referring the insured to more costly specialty services. This is because the insurance company may allow providers to keep the difference between the capitated rate and actual patient costs or otherwise share in any profit made by restricting the use of more costly health services.

Other managed care plans are health maintenance organizations (HMOs). There are four models of HMOs: (1) the staff model, which provides services directly through primary care providers who are salaried employees of the plan; (2) the group model, in which the HMO contracts with an independent group of primary care providers; (3) the network model in which the HMO contracts with two or more provider group practices; and (4) the Independent Practice Association (IPA), in which the HMO contracts with individual providers in private practice (Freund and Lewitt, 1993). These plans have the potential of providing more comprehensive services to children with chronic conditions because they may include, on staff or by contract, pediatric specialty physicians, pediatric nurse practitioners and clinicians, and nutrition and social service workers with expertise in various problems of living with a chronic condition. Other advantages are that the monthly premiums are generally paid by the employer, preexisting conditions are not excluded, and there may be no deductible or coinsurance provision. Services that are provided are similar to those offered in fee-for-service plans, including limited skilled nursing facility and home health service. In contrast to most private insurance companies, HMOs provide preventive health services as a covered benefit. HMOs have a strong incentive to keep their enrollees healthy, because the agency is at financial risk if more costly health services are required. There is little evidence, however, that it is less expensive to provide care to children or that care is of higher quality in HMOs, a fact that has been measured by use of hospitals, emergency services and primary care, and by adherence to preventive care protocols (Freund and Lewit, 1993).

The HMOs may restrict access to specialty health care in the interest of controlling overall health plan costs, in the same way as the preferred provider organizations and point-of-service plans. Access to pediatric specialty care is restricted either by requiring the family to bear a higher share of the total cost of out-of-plan services or by penalizing the primary care provider for referral to specialists. The primary care provider is penalized by deducting the cost of specialty care from the overall profit of the plan or the fees paid to the provider; either way of imposing restrictions may not be in the best interests of a child with a chronic condition. The primary care provider may not be as knowledgeable regarding either the diagnosis or the treatment of rare conditions as would a pediatrician or pediatric specialist. The child may be at further risk by not having easy access to ancillary health care services, such as physical therapy or in-home care, which may greatly enhance the quality of life for the child and family.

Parents of children with chronic conditions must consider their options for health insurance carefully to get the best coverage for their particular needs. A publication for parents that may facilitate an understanding of these options is available through the Association for the Care of Children's Health (McManus, 1988). Once the policy is purchased or obtained through employment, careful attention must be given to accuracy in filling out claims and filing them promptly, working with the claims agent who understands the family's problems, and following up rejected claims with convincing evidence of the importance of the treatment or piece of equipment to the well-being of the child (Jones, 1985). The primary care provider can be of great help to the parents by supporting their legitimate insurance claims and completing insurance forms accurately and in a timely manner.

GOVERNMENT HEALTH CARE PROGRAMS

There are public health care financing programs for individuals and families who do not have access to employer-based health insurance or who cannot afford to purchase private insurance (see the box on government health care programs). These programs may be entirely supported by federal money, such as health care for Native Americans, military personnel and federal civilian employees and their dependents, or may be jointly administered and funded by the federal government and the states. States may also have revenue sharing agreements with counties or other local health jurisdictions to

GOVERNMENT HEALTH CARE PROGRAMS

Eligibility for government health care programs
Medicaid

Designated health services for eligible persons
    Aid to Families with Dependent Children
    Supplemental Security Income
    Case Management Services (PL 101-329)
    Early Periodic Screening, Diagnostic, and
      Treatment Program

Medicaid managed care

Selected provider care
Coordinated continuity care possible

Medicaid waiver programs

Case management
Homemaking services
Home modifications
Therapy

Supplemental security income

Change in condition eligibility definition
Financial eligibility complex

Medicare end-Stage renal disease program

Civilian Health Medical Program of the Uniformed Services

Fee-for-Service Care
Managed Care Service—TRICARE

Indian Health Service

Maternal Child Health Block Grant—Title V

Federal-state program for children with special
  needs

Linkage to other children's health services

MCH block grants (SPRANS)

Generic disease testing and counseling services

Hemophilia treatment centers

Pediatric AIDS

provide financial coverage for health care through public revenues.

Persons who do not have health insurance are not necessarily unemployed or living at or below the national poverty level.[1] Over 60% of persons without access to private health insurance are steadily employed or members of a family with a steadily employed adult. Of this group, 39% have incomes that are greater than twice the federal poverty level (Health Insurance Association of America [HIAA], 1994). Uninsured workers are usually employed in small businesses or are self-employed. An employed person may lose health insurance if he or she or a family member acquires a chronic condition with high medical costs, and the employer cancels the worker's coverage. Other ways that employers avoid the high cost of insuring their employees is to rely on part-time workers or contract work out to small firms, neither of which require employers to offer insurance benefits. Of all uninsured persons, 20.3% are unemployed, and 26.3% are children (HIAA, 1994). Undocumented residents are another group who are at risk for being uninsured. They may not wish to be identified as working in the United States and therefore may accept positions without health insurance coverage or other work-related benefits. The number of uninsured individuals in the United States is estimated to be over 38 million, and these individuals are potential users of public health care programs (HIAA, 1994).

Medicaid

Medicaid (Title XIX of the Social Security Act) is the largest public medical program in the United States. It is administered by the Health Care Financing Administration (HCFA) in the U.S. Department of Health and Human Services (USDHHS). Medicaid is a program that gives federal grants to states to pay for designated health services for eligible persons. In this group are children with chronic conditions in eligible families. Medicaid was established in 1965 and soon surpassed any other federally funded public health care program serving children.

---

[1]The poverty index is based on a determination by the U.S. Department of Agriculture that families spend approximately one third of their incomes on food. The poverty level is therefore set at three times the cost of the economy food plan, which includes specific amounts of meat, vegetable, and other commodities. As of February, 1995, a family of four meets the federal poverty guideline (stated as 100% of poverty) if their annual income is $15,149.

In 1993, Medicaid served approximately 16.3 million children, which was 49% of all persons eligible for Medicaid (U.S. Department of Health and Human Services, Health Care Financing Administration, 1994). However, children's share of total Medicaid expenditures is only 16.5 billion dollars; for example 16% of total expenditures.

Eligibility and available services vary from state to state because states are permitted to add services and enhance eligibility over and above the requirements of the federal law. The primary criterion for eligibility is that the individual must receive welfare, such as Aid to Families with Dependent Children (AFDC), or Supplemental Security Income (SSI) for old age, blindness, or other disability. In 1992, income eligibility for AFDC, expressed as a percentage of the federal poverty level, ranged from 44.3% in Mississippi, to 99.3% in Hawaii, with a national (state) average of 68.1% (Center for the Study of Social Policy, 1993). That is, a family of four could earn no more than $6711 per year in Mississippi or $15,043 in Hawaii, with a national (state) average of $10,317, to be eligible for AFDC and Medicaid (Federal Register, February 9, 1995).

It is important to look at state requirements for AFDC because of the wide disparity in defining eligibility, which disqualifies approximately one third of children defined as poor by the federal government from receiving Medicaid coverage for health care through AFDC. Other eligible groups are infants born to mothers eligible for Medicaid; children under 6 years of age; pregnant women who are financially up to or at 133% of the federal poverty level; recipients of adoption assistance and foster care under Title IV-E of the Social Security Act; and groups defined by the state as "medically needy," which may include two-parent families with a disabled or unemployed head of the household, infants up to 1 year of age, and pregnant women who are financially up to or at 185% of the federal poverty level.

It is very important for families of children with chronic conditions and their primary care providers to be informed about Medicaid service rights and entitlement programs that pertain to the state in which the child resides. All states that receive funds from the Developmentally Disabled Assistance and Bill of Rights Act of 1978, the Protection and Advocacy for Mentally Ill Individuals Act of 1986, the Protection and Advocacy of Individual Rights Act of 1992, and the Technology-Related Assistance for Individuals with Disabilities Act of 1988 are required to have a protection and advocacy organization to inform persons with disabilities of their rights to payment for health care through Medicaid.

A full range of preventive-related and illness-related services are covered by Medicaid. These are inpatient hospital care, physician and other out patient services, and laboratory and skilled nursing services. States may choose to cover the costs of dental care, eye glasses, drugs, inpatient psychiatric care, and home health care. Of importance to children is the Early Periodic Screening Diagnosis and Treatment Program (EPSDT), which is a preventive health program that was added to Medicaid in 1972. This program enables children who are eligible for Medicaid to receive health screening. If health problems are identified in an EPSDT screen, the law requires referral for diagnosis and treatment (PL 101-329, 1989).

Federal law (PL 101-329, 1989) further stipulates that children enrolled in Medicaid are entitled to case management, rehabilitative services, psychologic counseling, and recuperative and long-term residential care as deemed necessary by a primary care provider. States must now include in their Medicaid benefit package all ambulatory health care services offered to Medicaid beneficiaries receiving care in community and migrant health centers that are funded by the federal Public Health Services Act. The law also encourages the use of pediatric and family nurse practitioner services in rural health clinics by mandating states to cover their services as long as they are practicing within the scope of state law, regardless of whether they are under the supervision of or associated with a physician. Obstetricians and pediatricians may be reimbursed at rates that are higher than prevailing Medicaid rates to enlist enough providers to serve eligible families. Otherwise, physicians may choose not to accept these families if reimbursement is not as high as that of private insurance for a given geographic area. When a family cannot find a provider who will accept them, they are forced to go to emergency rooms and hospital outpatient departments for needed health care services. This is costly to Medicaid, but more importantly, the family may not be able to establish a relationship with a single provider who understands their family members' particular needs.

Other provisions of Public Law 101-329 (1989) encourage referral of mothers eligible for Medicaid and infants at nutritional risk to the Special Supplemental Food Program for Women, Infants, and Children (WIC), which is funded by the Department of Agriculture. Some long-standing deficiencies in the EPSDT have also been corrected. Although many states have periodicity standards for all types of health screening, the law now requires that states establish these standards for medical, vision, hearing, and dental screenings, and further requires that services must be furnished at other than scheduled intervals when medically necessary to treat a suspected illness or condition. In addition, states must offer necessary health services to correct or ameliorate a condition found in the EPSDT screen, whether or not such services are covered by the state plan.

In most states, eligibility for Medicaid for individuals and families is determined by the Department of Social Services in the counties. Social workers in hospitals, public health, child welfare, and other human services agencies can assist families with children with chronic conditions to determine if they are eligible for Medicaid coverage. Social workers can also help primary care providers to remain informed of health services that are covered by Medicaid. Receiving Medicaid coverage for health care does not preclude receiving assistance from other federal programs for services and equipment not covered by Medicaid.

The provider who is familiar with Medicaid law can serve as an advocate for the family who may be denied services to which they are entitled. The provider should also know the local protection and advocacy staff and parent advocacy groups who stay abreast of issues regarding the various laws affecting both private and public health insurance plans, and who are able to protect the civil, legal, and service rights of children with chronic conditions.

Medicaid managed care As the costs of Medicaid rise, states are adopting certain strategies to conserve funds (USDHHS, HCFA, 1993). These strategies deny eligibility to the medically needy groups whose eligibility is not mandated by federal law, or require eligible families to join Medicaid managed care plans. These managed care plans are like those plans described earlier for private insurance. The individual or family receiving Medicaid has access to selected providers who have agreed to furnish a defined set of health care services at a set fee, called the capitation rate, which is paid by the state Medicaid agency. Managed care should reduce the overall cost of health care to Medicaid by providing access to a health care provider who will offer less expensive medical services, such as preventive health care, early treatment for acute conditions, and control referral to the more expensive specialty services. When families can depend on seeing a primary care provider, it is more likely that they will reduce their use of costly emergency services for routine health care.

Joining a managed care plan could be of benefit to children with chronic conditions because a wider range of preventive health services and other therapies may be available and better coordinated than under the traditional Medicaid fee-for-service plan. It is not yet known, however, if Medicaid managed care will provide access to necessary specialty providers and services. The capitation rate may be too low to refer a child to pediatric specialty providers outside the plan or to have pediatric specialty providers and services available within the plan. Newacheck and others (1994) reviewed the research on the effects of Medicaid-managed care for children. They urged that the reimbursement rate for children with chronic conditions be carefully considered and that norms for appropriate treatment be defined to monitor quality of care.

Medicaid waiver programs. Children who are dependent on ventilators, parenteral nutrition, or other technologies and cannot be discharged from the hospital without skilled nursing and other health services may be eligible for coverage of home care under the Medicaid Model Home and Community-Based Waiver. These services were initially authorized in 1981 in the Omnibus Budget Reconciliation Act, Section 2176 (PL 97-35). The current purposes of the program are to reduce the cost of care to Medicaid resulting from lengthy hospitalizations and to avoid unnecessary institutionalization of children. The program provides case management, homemaker services, home modifications, and other therapies. In a recent study of home-care costs and cost-effectiveness of home care as an alternative to institutionalization (Fields et al, 1991), the investigators found that for six children on mechanical ventilation, the annual savings to the state Medicaid program was 79,000, and for four with tracheostomies, the annual savings was $83,000. Qualification for coverage and services for home care varies among states. States may remove parental income and assets as an eligibility consideration, or may raise the Medicaid income standard. Conditions that are designated as eligible may differ, and some states require that the child be discharged from an institution immediately before applying for the waiver (Leonard, Brust, and Choi, 1989). Primary care providers who wish to determine if this program is appropriate for a Medicaid-eligible or medically needy client, and available in their state, should request information from the state agency responsible for implementation of the Medicaid program, which is usually the Department of Social Services in the clients county of residence. The local protection and advocacy office (Protection and Advocacy, Inc, 1995) will also explain a family's rights to have a child cared for under home care Medicaid waiver programs and will help the family plead their case when a waiver is denied by the local Medicaid agency.

Supplemental Security Income

The Supplemental Security Income program (SSI), Title XVI of the Social Security Act, was established by Congress in 1972 for aged, blind, and disabled adults; and in 1976 for children under 16 years of age with disabilities. This is an income support program to help recipients become as self-sufficient as possible within the limits of their disability. This program does not pay directly for costs of health care of a child with a chronic condition. However, SSI recipients are eligible to receive health care services through Medicaid, regardless of other state Medicaid eligibility requirements. It can be of great financial help to a family with a child with a chronic condition to have that child become eligible for SSI and thus receive Medicaid coverage for costly health care.

Eligible adults and children are those with specific disabilities who live in low-income households. Adults must show that they have an impairment that is on the federal list of impairments. If the adult's impairment does not meet or equal those on the list, the claimant's functional limitations may be assessed.

Before 1990, children with disabilities were less likely than adults with disabilities to be eligible for SSI, because children's impairments had to meet or equal those on the list. No other assessment of residual functional capacity was allowed (Jameson and King, 1989). This definition of disability for children seeking SSI was contested in the courts. On February 20, 1990, the Supreme Court upheld a lower court ruling that the policy for determining SSI eligibility for children was unfair and inconsistent with the statutory standards of comparable severity. At that time, approximately 50,000 children with disabilities had been denied SSI. This ruling has enabled lower courts to reopen cases where a child had earlier been denied benefits.

The financial requirements for eligibility for SSI are complex. The first requirement is that the applicant must be beneath the maximum income level. In 1994, eligibility for federal SSI was set at 74% of the poverty level (Social Security Administration, 1994). The amount of SSI paid to an individual and the administration of the program varies by state, because states have the option of supplementing the payments. About half the states administer their own supplementary payments, and the recipients receive this payment separately from that of the federal program. Other states elect to have the federal Social Security Administration issue the federal payment and the state supplement in one check. Applications for SSI payments are made at district offices of the Social Security Administration where supporting documentation on age, income, and assets is examined (Social Security Administration, 1994).

The second step in determining financial eligibility is to know the cash value of the applicant's resources. For children, this involves determining portions of the parents' income that is available to the child. The regulations must be studied carefully to understand how the amount of available income is calculated (Association of Maternal and Child Health Programs, 1991; Protection and Advocacy Inc, 1994). In 1994, the monthly federal SSI payment made to an individual in his or her own household with no other countable income was $446 (Social Security Administration, 1994). Countable income, which is the amount of parental income determined to be available to the child or any income earned by the child, would reduce this amount and state supplements would increase it.

Medicare's End-Stage Renal Disease Program

Medicare is authorized under Title XVIII of the Social Security Act. Children are generally not entitled to any health care benefits under Medicare because it provides health insurance protection for persons over 65 years of age and persons under age 65 who are collecting Social Security or Railroad Retirement Benefits. Children with end-stage renal disease, however, may be eligible to receive health care benefits to cover costs of peritoneal dialysis or hemodialysis and related services in the hospital or home.

Civilian Health and Medical Program of the Uniformed Services

Medical treatment at any Department of Defense installation is available to all active military personnel and their dependents. The Civilian Health and Medical Program of the Uniformed Services (CHAMPUS) is a program of medical benefits provided by civilian primary care providers for military families who are unable to use government medical facilities because of distance, overcrowding, or unavailability of appropriate medical treatment (HIAA, 1994). CHAMPUS resembles a traditional health insurance plan in that beneficiaries must pay a deductible, may have out-of-pocket costs, and may also be limited to a preferred provider panel of physicians (Hosek et al, 1987). Military organizations provide families of children with chronic conditions with information, financial assistance, and health care within the military community or through local community, state, and federal agencies. Health benefits advisors located on military bases facilitate access to both military and public programs in coordination with the multidisciplinary medical and social service support from the Army's Exceptional Family Member Program, the Air Force's Children Have Potential Program, and the Navy's Family Support Program. Of importance to eligible families with children with chronic conditions are the extensive benefits for home care, including physician visits, skilled nursing care and visiting nurse services, provision of durable medical equipment, drugs and supplies, and physical and occupational therapy (Helton, 1988).

The Civilian Health and Medical Program of the Uniformed Services is also being reformed to decrease the cost to the federal government. The Pentagon calls this health care reform plan *Tricare,* because it offers three managed care plans. The first plan is similar to an HMO, in which the client pays an annual enrollment fee and uses the plan exclusively. Another option provides a discounted share of costs if the client uses a provider who is part of a network of providers who agree to accept a fee set by CHAMPUS. The third option is the same as the present CHAMPUS, allowing unrestricted choice but requiring copayments and deductibles. The effect of these plans on access to care for military dependents with chronic conditions is not yet known.

Indian Health Service

The Indian Health Service (IHS) is an organization within the Public Health Service, U.S. Department of Health and Human Services. Its purpose is to ensure the availability of a comprehensive health care delivery system to American Indians and Alaskan Natives, including hospital and ambulatory medical care, preventive and rehabilitation services, and community and environmental health programs. The IHS integrates health services delivered directly through IHS facilities, with those services purchased by the IHS through contractual arrangements with other providers. The extent to which children with chronic conditions are well served in this system depends on the skill of the staff at the local IHS unit in determining the family's eligibility for third-party payment for health services, in making appropriate referrals, and in providing culturally sensitive counseling and education. The IHS interacts with other federal and state agencies and public and private institutions in developing ways to deliver health services, stimulate consumer participation, and apply resources. These include IHS, tribal-operated hospitals and health centers, and rural and urban health programs that receive both state and federal funding and are subject to regulations of Medicaid and private health care insurance (USD-HHS, IHS, 1993). Information on eligibility and the location and health care programs of the local IHS unit may be obtained from Indian Health Services Headquarters in Washington, DC, Headquarters West in Albuquerque, New Mexico, or through one of eleven service area offices (see appendix for IHS area offices).

The Maternal and Child Health Block Grant—Title V

The federal-state program for children with special health care needs was established by Title V of the Social Security Act of 1935. Title V provided three grants-in-aid programs to states—maternal and child health, children with special health care needs, and child welfare. The program for children with special health care needs was called Services for Crippled Children until approximately 1987.

Title V legislation grew out of increased recognition that the federal government should bear some responsibility for the well-being of mothers and children, and that federal assistance to state health departments would enable the states to provide needed services on the local level. Data demonstrating poor maternal care, an infant mortality rate that exceeded other industrialized countries, and lack of access to health care for children with disabilities, (particularly those in rural areas), gave further impetus to Congress to pass the Act. This data was gathered by the U.S. Children's Bureau, established in 1912, under the direction of the Maternity and Infancy Act (Sheppard-Towner) of 1920 to 1929. The Sheppard-Towner Act set a precedent for federal assistance to states for services for pregnant women and for infants and children with disabilities or conditions that might lead to a disability. Although the Sheppard-Towner Act only survived 8 years, states had the opportunity to establish a public health unit for mothers and children, improve birth registration, and increase public health nursing services. These positive experiences with federal support of state public health programs helped to lessen resistance to federal intervention in health care on the part of private practitioners of medicine, and enabled passage of Title V (Lesser, 1985).

In 1981, with passage of the Omnibus Reconciliation Act (PL 97-35), Title V programs were continued in the Maternal and Child Health (MCH) Block Grant. The MCH Block Grant is administered by the Bureau of Maternal and Child Health, Health Resources, and Services Administration of the Public Health Service in the Department of Health and Human Services. The MCH Block Grant, as amended in 1989 (PL 101-329), continues the original purpose of the 1981 Act, but with provisions that strengthen connections between health services for mothers and children on Medicaid and the Medicaid children's prevention program, EPSDT. As previously noted, these programs are supported by the Health Care Financing Administration. The 1989 MCH Block Grant legislation also specified connections between the infants' and children's immunization programs of the U.S. Public Health Service, Centers for Disease Control; and the supplemental feeding program for low-income women, infants, and children (WIC) in the Department of Agriculture (US Code, 1989).

The purpose of the block grant is to improve the health of all mothers and children, to be consistent with the applicable health status goals and national health objectives for the year 2000.[2] For the fiscal year 1994, $687 million was authorized to be appropriated to the states (Maternal and Child Health Bureau, 1994). Each state's share of the total allocation is based in part on the number of births and the percentage of the nation's low-income children residing in each state. A rural birth counts twice that of an urban birth, which is a concept that goes back to 1935 when children who were born in rural areas were more likely to be isolated from health services. Other determinants of a state's allocation are the amounts spent on Title V and other maternal and child health programs before 1981. The states are required to match each $4 of federal funds with $3 in cash or kind. The goals of the program are to:

1. Reduce infant mortality and the incidence of handicapping conditions among children;
2. Increase the number of children appropriately immunized against disease;
3. Increase the number of low-income children receiving health assessments and follow-up diagnostic and treatment services;
4. Provide and ensure access to comprehensive perinatal care for women;
5. Provide and ensure access to preventive and primary child care services;
6. Provide and ensure access to comprehensive care, including long-term care services, for children with special health care needs;

---

[2]*Healthy people 2000: national health promotion and disease prevention objectives,* Washington, D.C., 1990, Public Health Service, U.S. Department of Health and Human Services.

7. Provide and ensure access to rehabilitation services for blind and disabled children under 16 years of age who are eligible for Supplemental Security Income (SSI);
8. Facilitate the development of comprehensive, family-centered, community-based, culturally competent and coordinated care systems of services for children with special health care needs and their families.

The MCH Block Grant also includes a program of discretionary grants, financed by 15% of block grant funds for special projects of regional and national significance (SPRANS). These discretionary programs are as follows:

• Maternal and Child Health (MCH) research
• Training of health professionals for public health practice in MCH
• Genetic disease testing, counseling, and information dissemination
• Hemophilia diagnostic and treatment centers
• Maternal and child health improvement projects

States have certain authority to prioritize how they will meet the goals of the program, but are required to allocate 30% of Title V funds for children with special health care needs. No more than 10% of the state allocation may be spent on administrative costs.

The Maternal and Child Health Block Grant—programs for children with special health care needs. The program for children with special health care needs mandated by the Omnibus Reconciliation Act, Title V legislation, requires that federal funds in combination with state matching funds be used to provide services for locating these children and for providing medical, surgical, corrective and other services, and facilities for diagnosis and treatment for chronic conditions or for conditions that may become chronic. States have different service delivery systems that are funded by this program. The delivery systems may provide services directly through program-funded clinics that are staffed by program providers, or they may be a source of reimbursement for services rendered in the private sector by medical specialists, selected by the state program as qualified to offer services on a fee-for-service basis. Many states have elements of both systems (Ireys and Eichler, 1989).

In general, children who are likely to be eligible for care under this program have chronic conditions that are correctable, such as a broad range of orthopedic conditions, conditions requiring plastic or orthodontic reconstruction, eye and ear conditions that if untreated would lead to loss of vision or deafness, and other congenital anomalies that can be corrected or ameliorated with medical and surgical intervention. In addition to the eligible condition, most states require that the family income not exceed a specified amount. This amount varies according to family size and tends to be set at 100% to 200% of poverty. Another criterion for eligibility may be that the child's parents be legal residents of the county or state in which they apply for assistance. This makes some children of undocumented persons ineligible.

The covered benefits are (1) diagnostic services; (2) comprehensive treatment by the appropriate pediatric medical and surgical specialties, including nursing, social work, physical and other therapies; and (3) case management, to enable the child and family to benefit from the multidisciplinary services. Case management includes the skilled services of a professional who is able to evaluate the psychosocial needs of the family and approve authorized services and interpret these to the family. As states have received less money for this program, some case management has been taken over by persons trained on the job and supervised by the program administrator, nurse, or social work consultant. These persons are paid less than the health professionals but are able to approve authorized services and give advice on the location of such services. In general, they do not provide other counseling.

Children with mental retardation, mental illness, and those with illness for which there is little curative or corrective intervention available are generally not eligible for this program. In recent years, with the development of new therapies, some state programs have broadened the definition of a child with a chronic condition to include those children with neoplasms, with conditions of the nervous system, and with endocrine and metabolic disorders. Primary care providers must continually update themselves on the types of conditions covered by the states in which they practice through consultation with the state office responsible for Title V programs. In most states, this office is located in the state health department; however, the agency may be found in a university medical center, the state welfare department, or the state education department.

Other Programs for Children with Chronic Conditions Funded by the Maternal and Child Health Services Block Grant

Genetic disease testing and counseling service. The Maternal and Child Health Block Grant includes the funding for screening, education, and counseling for persons at risk for or afflicted with sickle cell disease under Public Law 92-294, The National Sickle Cell Control Act of 1972, and education, counseling, and medical referral for all genetic disorders mandated by Public Law 95-626, Title XI of the Public Health Services Act, 1978. This program supports genetic service grants and sickle cell clinic grants in some states. The program also supports (1) the National Clearinghouse for Human Genetic Diseases for the collection and dissemination of informational materials (2) a laboratory support program in hematology, cytogenetics, and biochemistry to develop laboratory standards, provide training, and conduct proficiency testing (3) and a system to collect and analyze epidemiologic data on genetic disease. Regional genetic networks are also supported to promote coordination and communication among genetic services providers and to demonstrate ways to address emerging issues in genetic testing and service delivery.

There are no direct payments to families for genetic counseling, fetal diagnosis, and other services under this program. Clinics serving pregnant women and families of children with genetic diseases must seek third-party payment for their clients to be financially self-supporting (Bernhardt et al, 1987).

Screening programs for newborns exist in all states, but states differ in disorders screened. All states screen for hyperphenylalaninemia (phenylketonuria) and hypothyroidism. Many states also screen for galactosemia and hemoglobinopathies. Other screening tests that may be offered are for maple syrup urine disease, homocystinuria, and biotinadase (Council of Regional Networks for Genetic Services [CORN], 1994).

Hemophilia treatment centers. The purposes of this program are to establish comprehensive hemophilia diagnostic and treatment centers, including clinical services; to provide training of professional and paraprofessional personnel in research, diagnosis, social, and vocational counseling; and to provide comprehensive individual care plans for those affected with hemophilia. Once the center is established, third-party payment for services to individuals must be sought to enable the center to be financially solvent. Persons with hemophilia are represented by the National Hemophilia Foundation, which is a nationally coordinated health agency with local chapters to promote education and to change the restrictive policies of third-party payment programs to better cover treatment (Hilgartner, Aledort, and Giardina, 1985).

Pediatric AIDS The Maternal and Child Health Bureau administers Title IV of the Ryan White Comprehensive AIDS Resources Emergency (CARE) Act, which is called the Pediatric/Family HIV Health Care Demonstration Program. Through this program, funds are provided to communities for information and training, and to organize and improve patient access to care. Funds are also used to pay for the care of children participating in clinical trials of the new treatments.

Federal Programs for Individuals with Mental Retardation and Developmental Disabilities

Mental retardation is defined as significantly subaverage intellectual functioning with an IQ of 75 or below, existing concurrently with deficits in at least two areas of adaptive behavior, and manifested during the developmental period from birth to 18 years of age (Luckasson, 1992). The term "developmental disabilities" was introduced in the 1970s to enable children with cerebral palsy, epilepsy, autism, and learning disabilities to benefit from federal programs directed at children with mental retardation and other functional problems that inhibited their entry into school, employment, and mobility in the community. By the 1980s, the definition of developmental disabilities changed from the above categories to a functional description. The new definition required a limitation in at least three of seven areas of major life activities; self-care, receptive and expressive language, learning, mobility, self-direction, capacity for independent living, and economic self-sufficiency (Braddock, 1987).

Third-party payment for preventive and illness care of children with mental retardation and developmental disabilities does not differ from that of other children with chronic conditions. Eligibility for private health insurance will depend on the parents' access to comprehensive health insurance through employment. Medicaid eligibility is determined on a state-by-state basis by household income in relation to the federal poverty guidelines and the Medicaid regulations. Eligibility for financial support of medical and surgical treatment through the MCH Block Grant, Title V, and Program for Children with Special Health Care Needs, will depend on the state definition of an eligible condition, family income, and access to other third-party payments of medical expenses.

The history of federal programs for individuals with mental retardation and developmental disabilities is reviewed by Braddock (1987) (see box on federal programs for individuals with disabilities). Care of children with these diagnoses was traditionally the responsibility of states and counties and voluntary associations. The programs for mothers and infants in Title V of the Social Security Act of 1935 were intended to prevent mental retardation. However, the care and reha-bilitation of these children was considered to be beyond the scope of Title V. Children with mental retardation have been excluded from these state programs to the present time, unless they have an eligible condition in addition to mental retardation.

FEDERAL PROGRAMS FOR INDIVIDUALS WITH MENTAL RETARDATION AND DEVELOPMENTAL DISABILITIES

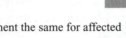

Third-party payment the same for affected children
PL 88-164 Mental Retardation Facilities and Community Mental Health Centers Construction Act, 1963.
PL 91-517 Developmental Disabilities Services and Facilities Construction Act, 1970
PL 94-142 Education for All Handicapped Children Act, 1975
Americans with Disabilities Act, 1990

Funds for research in mental retardation and demonstration of services and personnel training were provided by several congressional bills throughout the 1950s. In the early 1960s, President John F. Kennedy's panel on mental retardation contributed to the passage of Public Law 88-164, the Mental Retardation Facilities and Community Mental Health Centers Construction Act of 1963, thus beginning the modern era of the federal government's mental retardation and financial assistance programs. This law enabled the establishment of research centers, a mental retardation branch at the National Institute of Child Health and Human Development, and 18 university-affiliated facilities for the provision of clinical services and training of personnel in the care of children with mental retardation.

Public Law 91-517, the Developmental Disabilities Services and Facilities Construction Act of 1970, extended services to individuals with cerebral palsy and epilepsy in addition to those with mental retardation. To receive federal funds under this Act, states were required to establish developmental disabilities councils to promote coordinated planning and service delivery. Other significant legislation during this decade included Public Law 92-603, the Social Security Amendments of 1972, which added Title XVI, Supplemental Security Income; Public Law 92-223, the Social Security Amendments of 1971, which permitted the reimbursement for active treatment of those with developmental disabilities in intermediate care facilities (ICF); Section 504 of the Rehabilitation Act of 1973, which prohibited discrimination against individuals with developmental disabilities in any activity or place of employment receiving federal assistance; Public Law 93-647, the Social Security Amendments of 1974, which consolidated social services grants to states under a new Title XX of the Social Security Act to provide states with funds to develop alternatives to institutional care; and Public Law 94-142, Education for All Handicapped Children Act of 1975, which ensures that children with developmental disabilities or any chronic illness would have access to public education in the least restrictive environment.

By the 1980s the definition of developmental disabilities required a limitation in at least three of seven areas, as previously described. The Omnibus

Reconciliation Act of 1981 reduced federal funding of all social programs, and for several years there was no growth in developmental disabilities services. However, the Medicaid waiver program for home-based and community-based care was included in the Omnibus Reconciliation Act to discourage the use of the more expensive intermediate care facilities.

In the area of civil rights legislation for all persons with disabilities, including those with mental retardation, the Americans with Disabilities Act, passed in 1990, extended federal protection in the private and public sectors in employment, transportation, public accommodations, and communication. This law required changes in physical plants to accommodate employees with disabilities; for example, buses, trains and subway cars, hotels, and retail stores and restaurants should be accessible; and telecommunications devices on ordinary telephones should enable hearing-impaired and voice-impaired persons to place and receive calls (United Cerebral Palsy Associations, 1990).

Given the complexity of both federal and state laws that govern the availability and accessibility of services for individuals with developmental disabilities, it is often difficult for families to know their rights in regard to treatment, education, and employment of a child with a developmental disability. Protection and Advocacy, Inc. provides advocacy and education for parents and primary providers who are determining the legal entitlements and service benefits for children with developmental and mental disabilities. *Rights Under the Lanterman Act* (Protection and Advocacy, 1994) is an example of a manual written for parents that explains in simple and concise language the service rights and entitlement programs for these children and adults in California. Social workers in agencies serving those with developmental disabilities, public health nurses in programs for children with special health care needs, teachers in special education programs in public schools, voluntary organizations for individuals with mental retardation and other diagnoses leading to developmental disabilities, and members of local developmental disabilities councils are all sources of information.

Individuals with Disabilities Education Act

For providers who care for children with chronic conditions, programs of interest that link health and educational benefits are the 1990 Education of the Handicapped Amendments, Public Law 101-476. This law amended both Public Law 94-142, Education for All Handicapped Children Act of 1975, with amendments to expand early intervention services for preschool-age children, 3 to 5 years of age; and Public Law 99-457, the 1986 amendments to provide early intervention services to infants and toddlers with disabilities or at risk for disability. The new law is the Individuals with Disabilities Education Act (IDEA).

The Education for All Handicapped Children Act resulted from legal decisions establishing that children with disabilities had a constitutional right to a publicly funded education in the least restrictive environment. The Education for the Handicapped Amendments of 1986, Public Law 99-457, Part H, extended the benefits of Public Law 94-142 to handicapped children, birth through 2 years of age. This Act designated funds for the development of a statewide comprehensive, coordinated, multidisciplinary interagency system to provide early intervention services.

The Individuals with Disabilities Education Act defines handicapped children as those who require special education and related services because they have a learning disability, mental retardation, emotional disturbance, or specified physical handicaps. Other services that must be provided if determined necessary to the educational program are transportation and developmental, corrective or other support services required for the child to benefit from education. These services

---

INDIVIDUALS WITH DISABILITIES EDUCATION LAWS

PL 94-142 Education for All Handicapped Children Act, 1975

PL 99-457 Early Intervention Services for Infants and Children, 1986

PL 101-476 Education of the Handicapped Amendments, 1990

may include therapy for problems with speech and hearing, psychologic services, physical and occupational therapy, recreation, counseling, and social work and medical services. A parent has the right to participate in planning her child's educational program and the right to appeal a school system's decision about his or her child's education. State education agencies are responsible for implementing the law.

Children served in this program must have an Individualized Education Plan (IEP), which is reviewed annually. The IEP includes a statement of the child's current educational performance, short-term objectives and long-term goals, and a description of services to be provided (Federal Register, October 27, 1992). Primary care providers are encouraged to participate in the development of the IEP, although the law does not specify the extent of their involvement.

Eligible infants are those who are experiencing developmental delays in cognitive, physical, language and speech, psychosocial and self-help skills, or who have a diagnosed physical or mental condition that has a high probability of resulting in developmental delay. States may also include in their definition children they determine to be at risk for developmental delay if early intervention services are not provided.

Services to eligible infants and toddlers may include family training (counseling and home visits) special instruction, speech and hearing therapy, occupational and physical therapy, psychosocial services, case management services, medical services restricted to diagnosis or evaluation, early identification (screening and assessment) and health services necessary to enable the recipient to benefit from the other early intervention services. The services must be provided by qualified personnel in conformity with an individualized family service plan (Center for Policy Research, 1987).

The main purpose of this program is not to fund direct services but to support interagency service coordination. States designate a lead agency to receive the funds, and have in place a policy to provide appropriate early intervention services to all infants and toddlers who have or who are at risk for handicapping conditions in the state. Typical lead agencies are human services agencies, departments of education, or health departments.

One of the barriers to service coordination is that payment of direct services, regardless of the extent to which they are coordinated and comprehensive, are generally under the control of public or private third-party payers. The method of payment for services ultimately determines what services are received. Bringing an interagency collaboration initiative to fruition under the present fragmented system of paying for health services is a complex and labor-intensive process. Typical state programs publish directories of early intervention resources by health jurisdiction and fund local interagency coordination efforts and family resource centers or networks.

FUTURE TRENDS IN FINANCING HEALTH CARE FOR CHILDREN WITH CHRONIC CONDITIONS

Following the failure in the 103rd Congress in 1994 to pass a national health care reform act, a reform of the way health care is organized, administered, and financed in the United States for the population at large and for persons with chronic conditions has now been taken up by employers, insurance companies, managed care networks, and the states. These health care reform initiatives will affect both private and public financing of health care. It is evident from the review of the benefits of private health insurance and public programs for children with chronic conditions that there are gaps in funding for both primary and specialty care. Quality, comprehensive coverage by private health insurance companies has been a long-standing problem. In today's climate of rapidly accelerating health care costs and emphasis on cost-containment, private insurance is turning to managed care. The dilemma faced by health care providers and children's advocates is how to support the highest quality of pediatric care in a managed care environment. The issues of quality of care for children in managed care are just being defined. Research will be a priority of agencies implementing private and public managed care plans and the Title V program for children with special health care needs to determine the effect on access to specialty care and the outcomes of care.

In the absence of national health care reform, there are few solutions to providing either primary or specialty care for uninsured children with chronic conditions. They will depend on incremental reform in Medicaid (Oberg and Polich, 1990). For example, states are permitted to separate eligibility for Aid to Families with Dependent Children from Medicaid eligibility. This enables children up to age 6 in families with incomes up to 133% of poverty to be eligible for Medicaid. Medicaid coverage may also be extended for families ineligible for Aid to Families with Dependent Children as a result of beginning employment.

SUMMARY

Private and public programs and agencies for financing care for children with chronic conditions are examining ways to provide adequate health care and at the same time reduce the costs of care. The major approach is to implement various managed care features, such as capitation, in which the insured has access to a primary provider who acts as a gatekeeper to specialty services and financial penalties born by the primary provider or by the family for referral to providers outside the health plan. The immediate future of health care for children with chronic conditions is marked by limitations in choice of specialty providers and services. Primary providers, both physicians and nurse practitioners, will find that they are increasingly limited in their abilities to advocate for quality care for those children in their case loads who have chronic conditions. Families will be advocating for their children by joining together, becoming informed of their rights under the law, and using the legal system for access to care. To add to the complexity of seeking health care for children with chronic conditions are the inequalities in implementing private and public health care programs among counties both within a state and among states. Federal programs are implemented by states; the states may choose to follow the law by providing just the required state match of federal funds or may choose to overmatch to enrich the program by adding services or broadening coverage to include more diagnoses. Access to private insurance is favorable for those who are steadily employed in large businesses or who are members of strong labor unions that can negotiate comprehensive benefit packages.

Primary care providers must be informed regarding the means that families of children with chronic conditions in their case loads are paying for care, and regarding access to specialty services under the various payment plans, for families to realize the benefits for which they are eligible. Referral for help in purchasing appropriate insurance or in gaining access to a federal-state public benefit requires dedication and persistence on the part of the family and primary care provider and is crucial to implementing the plan of care.

APPENDIX OF USEFUL REFERENCES ON FINANCIAL COVERAGE FOR CHILDREN WITH CHRONIC CONDITIONS

1. National Center for Clinical Infant Programs (NCCIP): *Meeting the medical bills,* (25-minute videotape), Washington, DC, 1988, NCCIP. Available from the National Information Center for Handicapped Children and Youth (NICHCY), P.O. Box 1492, Washington, DC 20013.

   This 25-minute videotape discusses Medicaid waivers that finance home care for children with special health needs, Supplemental Security Income (SSI), and how parents can work with private insurance companies to obtain the best possible coverage for children.

2. McManus MA: *Understanding your health insurance options: a guide for families who have children with special health care needs,* Washington, DC, 1988, Bureau of Maternal and Child Health and Resources Development. Available from the Association for the Care of Children's Health, 3615 Wisconsin Ave NW, Washington, DC 20013.

   This guide is designed to help families who have children with special health care needs understand their health insurance options and select plans that are most suited to their needs. Important concerns in private and public insurance plans are also addressed.

3. Griffiths B, Peterson RA: *Families forward: health care resource guide for children with*

special health care needs, Madison, WI, 1993, Center for Public Representation. For reprint permissions or ordering contact Publications Department, Center for Public Representation, 121 Pinckney St. Madison, WI 53703, or call 1-800-369-0388.

This book is for parents and others who are responsible for the health care of a child with a chronic illness or disability. Information is provided on private and public health care coverage to enable parents to make decisions on financing treatment and obtaining services. This guide is specific to health insurance and services in Wisconsin, but any interested reader would benefit from the discussions on legal rights, resolving disputes, accessing public programs, and many other financial issues.

4. Protection and Advocacy, Inc: *Medi-Cal: service rights 2 and entitlement programs affecting Californians with disabilities,* Sacramento, CA, 1995, Protection and Advocacy, Inc, Available from Protection and Advocacy, Inc., 100 Howe Ave, Suite 185-N, Sacramento, CA 95825; or call (916) 488-9950.

This manual provides general information for persons with disabilities in California seeking information regarding their specific legal entitlements and service benefits under Medicaid, Medicaid and managed care, Medicaid and private health benefit plans, and Medicaid waivers. The manual is of interest to persons in other states because of its focus on advocacy skills for the consumer and basic definitions of federal Medicaid laws.

5. *Indian Health Service Administrative Offices:* Headquarters:
Indian Health Service
Office of Health Programs
Parklawn Building, Rm 6A-55
5600 Fishers Lane
Rockville, MD 20857
(301) 443-3024
Headquarters West-Albuquerque
Indian Health Service
5300 Homestead Road, NE
Albuquerque, NM 87110
(505) 837-4101

REFERENCES

Association of Maternal and Child Health Programs: *Supplemental Security Income (SSI) for Disabled Children.* In *MCH related federal programs: legal handbooks for program planners.* Washington, DC, August, 1991, The National Maternal and Child Health Clearinghouse.

Bernhardt BA et al: The economics of clinical genetics services: a time analysis of a medical genetics clinic, *Am J Hum Genet* 41(4-6):559-565, 1987.

Braddock D: *Federal policy toward mental retardation and developmental disabilities,* Baltimore, 1987, Paul H. Brookes.

Center for Policy Research: Getting it together for handicapped and at-risk infants and toddlers, *Capital Ideas* June 1, 1987.

Center for the Study of Social Policy: *Kids count data book: state profiles of child well-being,* Washington, DC, 1993, Center for the Study of Social Policy, Annie E. Casey Foundation.

Council of Regional Networks for Genetic Services (CORN): *National newborn screening report—1991,* New York, July, 1994, The Council of Regional Networks for Genetic Services.

Department of Education: Assistance to states for the education of children with disabilities program and preschool grants for children with disabilities; correction, final rule, *Federal Register* 57(208):48694, October 27, 1992.

Donovan WH, Carter RE, and Wilkerson MA: Profiles of denials of durable medical equipment for SCI patients by third-party payers, *Am J Phys Med* 66:238-243, 1987.

Fields AI et al: Home care cost-effectiveness for respiratory technology-dependent children, *Am J Dis Chil* 145:729-733, July, 1991.

Fox HB, Newacheck PW: Private health insurance of chronically ill children, *Pediatrics* 85:50-57, January, 1990.

Freund DA, Lewitt EM: Managed care for children and pregnant women: promises and pitfalls. In *The future of children: health care reform* 3(2) Summer/Fall, 1993.

Health Insurance Association of America: *Source book of health insurance data,* ed 33, Washington, DC, 1994, Health Insurance Association of America.

Helton, JD: Comments before the task force of technology dependent-children. In *Fostering home and community-based care for technology-dependent children: report of the task force on technology-dependent children,* vol 1, Health Care Financing Administration Pub No 88-02171, Washington, DC, 1988, US Government Printing Office.

Hilgartner MW, Aledort L, and Giardina PJV: Thalassemia and hemophilia. In Hobbs and Perrin, editors: *Issues in the care of children with chronic illness,* San Francisco, 1985, Jossey-Bass.

Hosek SD et al: *Plan for the evaluation of the CHAMPUS reform initiative,* Santa Monica, 1987, The RAND Corporation.

Ireys HT, Eichler RJ: Program priorities of crippled children's agencies: a survey, *Public Health Rep* 103:77-83, 1989.

Jameson E, King SC: The failure of the federal government to care for disabled children: a critical analysis of the supplemental security program, *Columbia Human Rights Law Review* 20(2):309-342, Spring, 1989.

Jameson E, Wehr E: Drafting national health care reform legislation to protect the health interests of children, *Stanford Law and Policy Review* 5(1):152-176, Fall, 1993.

Jones ML: *Home care of the chronically ill or disabled child,* New York, 1985, Harper & Row.

Leonard BJ, Brust JD, and Choi T: Providing access to home care for disabled children: Minnesota Medicaid Model Waiver Program, *Public Health Rep* 104:465-472, 1989.

Lesser AJ: The origin and development of maternal and child health programs in the United States, *Am J Public Health,* 75:590-598, 1985.

Luckasson R, editor: *Mental retardation: definition, classification and systems of support,* ed 9, Washington, DC, 1992, American Association on Mental Retardation.

Maternal and Child Health Bureau: *Fact pack,* Rockville, MD, January, 1994, Health Resources and Services Administration, Department of Health and Human Services.

McManus MA: *Understanding your health insurance options: a guide for families who have children with special health care needs,* Washington, DC, 1988, Bureau of Maternal and Child Health and Resource Development.

Newacheck PW et al: Children with Chronic Illness and Medicaid Managed Care, *Pediatrics* 93(3):497-500, 1994.

Oberg CN, Polich CY: Medicaid: entering the third decade, *Health Aff* 7:83-96, 1990.

Perrin JM, Shayne MW, and Bloom SR: *Home and community care for chronically ill children,* New York, 1993, Oxford University Press.

Protection and Advocacy, Inc: *Memorandum: how to determine how much income is attributed or deemed from the parents to the disabled child and how to determine whether the disabled child qualifies for any SSI,* Sacramento, January 10, 1994, Protection and Advocacy, Inc.

Protection and Advocacy, Inc: *Rights under the Lanterman Act:*

service rights and entitlement programs affecting Californians with disabilities, revised ed, Sacramento, 1994, Protection and Advocacy, Inc.

Protection and Advocacy, Inc: *Medi-Cal: service rights and entitlement programs affecting Californians with disabilities,* Sacramento, January, 1995, Protection and Advocacy, Inc.

Public Law 97-35: Omnibus Budget Reconciliation Act of 1981, Section 2176.

Public Law 101-329: Omnibus Budget Reconciliation Act of 1989, Section 6403.

Rowland D: *Financing of care: a critical component.* In Stein REK, editor: *Caring for children with chronic illness: issues and strategies,* New York, 1989, Springer.

Social Security Administration: *Annual statistical supplement to the social security bulletin,* Washington, DC, August, 1994, Social Security Administration.

United Cerebral Palsy Associations: *Word from Washington,* New York, April/May, 1990, United Cerebral Palsy Associations.

US Annual update of the US poverty guidelines, US Department of Health and Human Services, Office of the Secretary of Health and Human Services: *Federal Register* 60:7772, Feb. 9, 1995.

US Code: *Congressional and administrative news, 1st Session, Public Laws,* St. Paul, MN, 1989, West Publishing.

US Department of Health and Human Services, Indian Health Services: *Regional differences in Indian health,* Washington, DC, 1993, US Government Printing Office.

US Department of Health and Human Services, Health Care Financing Administration: *National summary of state medicaid managed care programs,* Baltimore, June 20, 1993, Medicaid Bureau, USDHHS.

US Department of Health and Human Services, Health Care Financing Administration: *Medicaid statistics, FY 1993,* Pub No 10129, Baltimore, October, 1994, Medicaid Bureau, USDHHS.

CHRONIC CONDITIONS

PART

II

Asthma

8

Gail Kieckhefer and Marijo Ratcliffe*

ETIOLOGY

The exact etiology of asthma remains equivocal. Although a familial tendency has long been recognized, environmental factors are now thought to contribute to the presence of clinically recognized asthma (Morgan and Martinez, 1992). In the past, asthma has been characterized as obstructive airway disease caused primarily by bronchoconstriction (smooth muscle contraction); however, over the last decade the roles of inflammation and mucous secretion have become increasingly recognized.

The current definition of asthma includes three components:
1. Airway obstruction that can be reversed
2. Airway inflammation
3. Increased (hyperreactivity) airway responsiveness to stimuli (Hilman, 1993)

Asthma episodes have at least two response phases to an affending trigger. Cockroft (1990) describes the two different responses that can occur in a child's airway, based on the two types of triggers: (1) inflammatory triggers such as allergens, chemical sensitizers, viral infections; and (2) noninflammatory triggers such as dust, cold air, and other irritants. Inflammatory triggers are considered asthmogenic insofar as they actually cause asthma by increasing the frequency and severity of airway smooth muscle contraction and enhance airway responsiveness through inflammatory mechanisms. Noninflammatory triggers cause a bronchospastic response which may become more severe depending upon the existing level of responsiveness in the airway.

Within the first 10 to 20 minutes of the early response phase when an inflammatory trigger is encountered, an acute reaction will occur when an antigen binds to the specific immunoglobulin-E surface on the mast cell and a cell mediator, such as histamine, is released. This early response causes bronchospasm even though inflammatory mediators are involved and can spontaneously remit within 60 to 90 minutes. When treatment is required, however, a bronchodilator such as a β_2-adrenergic agonist is effective as a result of the underlying pathophysiology of bronchospasm.

During the late phase response which occurs 3 to 4 hours later, the initial bronchospastic reaction has subsided and the cellular phase of inflammation will peak around 4 to 8 hours, even up to 12 hours later. This is most likely due to the early phase release of chemotactic factors that recruit inflammatory cells, such as eosinophils and neutrophils, to the submucosa of the large and small airways. Subsequently, histamine and other mediator levels increase again, causing a bronchospastic component in addition to the inflammatory reaction. This response can cause a continuing cycle with both inflammatory and bronchospastic components requiring treatment with antiinflammatory and β_2-adrenergic medications.

*The editors and authors would like to acknowledge the work done by Nanci L. Larter on this chapter in the first edition of the book.

Airway hyperreactivity to stimuli is noted in all children with asthma, but is particularly correlated with the individuals experiencing the late phase response. "The degree of hyperresponsiveness also correlates with the severity of asthma, as measured by reduced airway caliber and the amount of medication required to control symptoms" (Cockroft, 1990). Therefore, the child with asthma may have heightened sensitivity to nonallergic stimuli which will more readily exacerbate the airway obstruction. This airway responsiveness may persist for weeks to months (Boulet et al, 1983).

The nature of the child's response—early, late, or dual (early and late)—and the severity of the long-term hyperresponsive phase, will direct therapeutic modalities.

INCIDENCE

Respiratory disease remains the major cause of hospitalization in young children. Cumulative prevalence rates of wheezing in young children range from 30% to 60%, with the recent U.S. report of 4.3% of children under 17 years having diagnosed asthma (Halfron and Newacheck, 1993). When the presence of recurrent wheezing is considered in addition to formal diagnosis, prevalence increases to over 6% (Bloomburg and Strunk, 1992). With even more liberal criteria, others quote up to 15% prevalence rates in school-age children (Cypcar, Stark, and Lemanske, 1992).

Reports on the incidence of asthma indicate an increase in the diagnosis over the past decade, with an even greater increase in reported morbidity and mortality (Rachelefsky, 1995). Whether the increase in asthma is the result of a rise in the disease or in improved diagnostic screening is unknown. Asthma is more common in boys than girls, with a ratio of 2:1.5 until puberty.

CLINICAL MANIFESTATIONS AT TIME OF DIAGNOSIS

Many children with asthma initially have wheezing associated with or following an upper respiratory infection (URI). Other conditions that may lead to the diagnosis of asthma include recurrent pneumonia, sinusitis or otitis media, or chronic cough in the absence of wheezing, and nocturnal cough or

CLINICAL MANIFESTATIONS

I. Symptoms
   - Wheezing
   - Nocturnal cough and wheeze
   - Recurrent pneumonia, sinusitis, otitis
   - Shortness of breath on exercise (EIB)
II. Family history
III. Pattern recognition
   - Follow URI or exercise
   - Seasonal presentation
IV. Response to therapy

wheeze. In children and teenagers, decreased ability to exercise with complaint of shortness of breath, chest pain or pressure, and a history of cough or wheeze after exercise are indicative of exercise-induced bronchospasm, or EIB (see box for clinical manifestations).

Because children have a variety of symptoms, with asthma, other diseases must be ruled out. Children who have recurrent pneumonia or sinusitis, even with no evidence of malabsorption, should have a quantitative pilocarpine iontophoresis (sweat chloride test) for cystic fibrosis (see Chapter 16). In young children monophonic expiratory wheezing or expiratory stridor (sometimes difficult to distinguish from one another) may indicate foreign body aspiration, tracheal compression, stenosis, or tracheomalacia. Referral to a pulmonologist or otolaryngologist for bronchoscopy may be necessary for diagnosis.

Usually the diagnosis of asthma is made when the child has been seen repeatedly for wheezing or coughing episodes, especially when there is a positive family history of asthma or the episodes are responsive to bronchodilator therapy. Many children seen during acute exacerbations of asthma have a history of URI. Symptoms typically include a 2- to 3-day history of rhinitis and slight fever. As these common URI symptoms persist, a cough, wheeze, or both begin. Some children respond more quickly to asthma triggers, and thus exacerbations occur within a short period after exposure. These children may have tachypnea, increased use of accessory muscles (nasal flaring, retractions), and prolonged expiratory phase or wheeze (or both). Children with sternocleidomastoid contraction and supraclavicular indrawing most often have severe airway obstruction and need rapid assessment of their cardiorespiratory status, including pulse oximetry if available in the office setting, and interventions immediately initiated. Observations regarding degree of dyspnea, retractions, body position, use of abdominal muscles to expel air, and mental status should also be noted. Auscultation for adventitious sounds will elicit the following and represent increasing airway obstruction: prolongation of the expiratory phase, expiratory wheeze, inspiratory and expiratory wheeze, and absence or distancing of breath sounds, an ominous sign indicative of little air exchange and possible impending respiratory arrest (American Academy of Pediatrics Provisional Committee on Quality Improvement, 1994).

TREATMENT

The current approach to asthma treatment is changing to reflect the understanding that airway inflammation appears to be evident in most phases of the illness. Although therapy must be individualized to the particular child, it is now recognized that prevention of symptoms due to underlying inflammation must be treated in addition to treatment of the acute symptoms due to bronchoconstriction (Stempel and Szefler, 1992) (see box on treatment).

In the treatment of the child with asthma, the primary goal is to allow the child to live as normal a life as possible. The child should be able to participate in normal childhood activities, experience exercise tolerance similar to peers, and attend school to grow intellectually and develop socially. Treatments to obtain these goals should be blended into family schedules, and if possible, side effects should minimally interfere with achievement of goals.

Shared Management

Educating the family and maturing child to become effective partners with the primary care provider in the day-to-day management of asthma is a primary treatment goal (Rachelefsky, 1995; Wigal et al, 1990). Instruction in shared management is a necessary cornerstone in regular health care and requires

TREATMENT

Shared management programs

I. NHLBI Asthma Education Program
II. Components (see box on p. 124):
III. Lifelong learning
IV. Treatment plans
   A. Recognition of early warning signs
      Treatment appropriate to level of severity
      Mild asthma
      Moderate asthma
      Severe asthma
   B. Management of chronic condition
V. Medications
   A. Bronchodilators
      β_2-andrenergic agonist
      Methylxanthines
   B. Antiinflammatory agents
      Short acting—steroid burst
      Long acting—cromolyn, nedocromil
   C. Anticholinergic agents
   D. Methotrexate

age-appropriate sharing of responsibilities among family members and the primary care provider. The purposes of shared management education are to help prevent episodes of asthma exacerbation, minimize the severity of episodes that cannot be prevented, enhance the family's ability to understand and implement treatment strategies, and respond to life changes that may be necessitated by asthma.

Family education in shared management should promote a sense of teamwork. The foundations should be laid early, with the primary care provider drawing the family into treatment decisions as their basic knowledge and skills increase.

Individual providers or community organizations recruiting families from a variety of providers have offered formal education programs and developed and extensively tested curricular guides for several programs, which are useful, relatively inexpensive, and easy to implement (Howell, Flaim, and Lung, 1992; Wigal et al, 1990). Other approaches have successfully used games and camp experiences, most commonly coupled with one of the formal education programs listed at the end of this chapter.

Most asthma education programs contain information on the basic physiology of asthma exacerbation and information on controlling triggers, knowing early warning signs that signal the onset of a problem, managing an exacerbation (including when to contact the primary care provider), knowing strategies for relaxation and controlled breathing, altering medications according to set guidelines, and solving problems. Programs have demonstrated effectiveness in reducing child and family anxiety, increasing asthma management behavior, improving school attendance, and reducing costly emergency room and hospital use. Before a program is implemented or a child is referred to a program, it is imperative that the primary care provider review the program to ensure it is consistent with the provider's treatment philosophy, know whether it is an individualized or group approach, and identify the age, child, or type of family for whom the program has previously worked best. When the provider is knowledgeable about the shared management program and can reinforce learning during routine health care visits with the family, a true child-parent-provider partnership is enhanced to ultimately improve the child's overall health status.

Education must be viewed in the context of lifelong learning. Changes in the child's and family's capabilities and in treatment modalities will necessitate ongoing evaluation and provision of further education. This ongoing education will help ensure that as the family gains experience in managing the child's asthma, the depth of their knowledge and skills is enhanced and keeps pace with treatment guidelines.

When the asthma diagnosis is made during an acute exacerbation, the family will first need education regarding immediate care, signs of improvement or deterioration which require immediate contact with the provider, immediate environmental changes that could be implemented, and action and side effects of medications. Subsequent return to a comprehensive education program can follow. Families have noted it takes them up to a year to gain any sense of ease with the full perspective of asthma management. The components of an asthma education program suggested by the National Heart, Lung, and Blood Institute (NHLBI) (1991) are listed in the following box.

NHLBI ASTHMA EDUCATION PROGRAM

Components

- Definition of asthma
- Signs and symptoms of asthma
- Characteristic changes in the airways of children with asthma and the role of medications
- Asthma triggers and how to avoid, eliminate, and control them
- Treatment
- Parent/child fears concerning medication
- Use of written guidelines
- Correct use of inhalers
- Criteria for premedicating to prevent onset of symptoms
- Criteria for detecting the onset of symptoms and initiating treatment
- Indications for emergency care
- Optimal use of home peak expiratory flow rate (PEFR) monitoring
- Fears and misconceptions
- Family understanding and support
- Communication with the child's school or child care center
- Feelings about asthma

Specific treatment modalities will depend on the age of the child, severity of disease, medication tolerance, and ability of the child or family to implement the treatment regimen. A detailed history is necessary when various medications and schedules are considered. The frequency and severity of the episodes will direct intermittent vs. continuous treatment. Children who quickly develop severe airway obstruction when exposed to a trigger must initiate a plan of treatment immediately. Identification of triggers assists in development of a plan for avoidance, pretreatment with medications before exposure (e.g., exercise-induced asthma), or initiation of treatment with early symptomatology (e.g., begin bronchodilators with signs of respiratory tract infection). Clearly documenting presenting or persistent symptoms over time helps to identify specific components of asthma. Some children have primarily a bronchospastic component, whereas others have more of an inflammatory response similar to the early or late phase responses.

Treatment of a Child with Asthma

Because asthma is a chronic disease with episodic symptoms, asthma management entails treatment based on the needs or severity of the child's underlying airway pathology. A child with "mild" asthma may have symptoms with exercise or cough and wheezing 1 to 2 times per week at night that respond to bronchodilators. The child with mild asthma does not need corticosteroids and has normal pulmonary function values with good exercise tolerance. Moderate asthma is described as presence of cough and/or wheeze more than 2 times a week and 2 to 3 times per week at night, symptoms between exacerbations, spirometric evidence of airflow obstruction with limitations in exercise and activity, daily medication requirement and periodic systemic corticosteroid use. Children with severe asthma have daily symptoms of wheeze and cough, frequent nighttime sleep disruptions, significant spirometric airflow obstruction and variability with poor exercise tolerance, frequent need for emergent medical care with exacerbations, and multiple daily medications including systemic corticosteroids (National Asthma Education Program, National Heart, Lung, and Blood Institute [NHLBI], 1991).

Timely treatment of an asthma exacerbation requires recognition of early warning signs of an acute exacerbation in a child and treatment appropriate to the level of severity. These early warning signs may be unique to a particular child (e.g., tickle in the throat, frequent yawning or sighing) or may be fairly common symptoms, such as a cough, especially at night, tightness in the throat with URI symptoms of a runny nose and congestion, and a decreased peak expiratory flow rate (PEFR) if the child can perform this maneuver. Later symptoms will usually include wheezing, shortness of breath, and chest pain or tightness.

After reviewing their child's usual early warning signs with their primary care provider, parents can be instructed to evaluate their child's respiratory rate, breathlessness, use of accessory muscles, alertness and color, and have a mutually agreed upon individualized plan of action to initiate treatment of the exacerbation (NHLBI, 1991). For example, a treatment plan might be: (1) begin or increase Albuterol medication up to every four hours at home, (2) start oral steroid "burst" at prescribed dose, and (3) notify primary care provider of progress. This type of action plan is meant to reduce the severity, and hopefully the length of the exacerbation, so that emergent medical care is not needed (Stemple and Redding, 1992). Just as one would not watch a small fire that began in their home to see if it was going to get worse, the same holds true for an asthma exacerbation. Immediate treatment of the "fire" will impact its damage and severity.

If a child's symptoms do not respond to home management, the child will need further evaluation and treatment in a primary care provider's office if appropriate monitoring and treatment equipment is available, or in an emergency room or hospital setting. These settings offer the added ability to monitor the child's air movement, oxygenation and/or blood gases, administer O_2 as needed, perform spirometry, monitor cardiac and respiratory status continually, and give medications intravenously in a controlled environment. Delineated treatment modalities for management of mild, moderate, and severe asthma are available to facilitate decision making in any setting (NHLBI, 1991; Rachelefsky, 1995) as well as management of acute exacerbations in the office setting (American Academy of Pediatrics, 1994).

Medications

With regard to the current understanding of the pathogenesis of airway obstruction caused by inflammation and the subsequent hyperresponsiveness, asthma therapy has changed to reflect the need to combine bronchodilatory medications with antiinflammatory medications. The three types of medications used are: (1) bronchodilators, which include β_2-adrenergic agonist agents, long- and short-acting preparations and methylxanthines (theophylline preparations); (2) antiinflammatory agents such as cromolyn sodium, nedocromil sodium, and inhaled or systemic corticosteroids; and (3) anticholinergic agents such as ipratropium bromide. The accompanying box lists commonly used medications grouped by primary action.

For most children the first medication chosen for symptomatic treatment of cough or wheeze is a

MEDICATIONS

I. Antiinflammatory agents
  A. *Corticosteroids*
     Prednisone
     Prednisolone (Prelone and Pediapred)
     Methylprednisolone
     Triamcinolone acetonide (Azmacort)
     Beclomethasone dipropionate (Vanceril)
  B. Cromolyn sodium inhalation aerosol
     (Intal)
     Nedocromil sodium (Tilade)
II. Bronchodilators
   β-adrenergic agents
   Metaproterenol (Alupent and Metaprel)
   Albuterol (Proventil and Ventrolin)
   Terbutaline (Brethaire, Bricanyl, and
      Brethine)
   Salmeterol (Seravent)
   Methylxanthines
   Quick release: (Elixophyllin, Slo-Phyllin)
   Sustained release: (Slo-Bid, Slo-Phyllin,
      Theo-Dur Sprinkles)
   Ultra-sustained release: (Uniphyl)
III. Anticholinergics
    Ipratropium bromide (Atrovent)
    Atropine
IV. Methotrexate

β-adrenergic agent such as albuterol, which inhibits the early phase asthmatic response. All β-adrenergics can cause increased heart rate and may cause tremor of the fingers or hands. Hyperactivity, irritability, and sleeplessness are also noted by some parents of young children. Using an air compressor with an updraft nebulizer to deliver a β-adrenergic medication is common; however, children as young as 4 years of age may be able to use a metered dose inhaler (MDI, or puffer) if a spacer is used with the MDI. A spacer is a chamber that attaches to the MDI, allowing the medicine to be puffed into the chamber. The child can then inhale from the spacer to receive the medication, which avoids having to coordinate compressing the MDI while slowly inhaling. A new delivery device, the rotocap, is now being used for delivery of β-adrenergics. It involves inhaling a powdered form of the medication but does not require a coordinated effort like the MDI.

Nebulized treatments offer several advantages, including (1) direct deposition of aerosolized medication in the respiratory tract, (2) decreased side effects, (3) better delivery than MDI when the tidal volume is reduced during an acute episode, and (4) the ability to mix β-adrenergic medications with other medications such as cromolyn sodium or atropine. Oral syrups containing β-adrenergic agents are also available, but they cause hyperactivity in many children. For convenience, some older children prefer to take a pill rather than use an MDI and compliance may be improved if adolescents are given this choice.

When a child experiences exercise-induced bronchospasm (EIB), either a $β_2$-agonist or an antiinflammatory agent such as cromolyn can be used to block the symptoms that inhibit the child's continued exercise (Hilman, 1993). These agents should be taken approximately 15 minutes before participation in scheduled exercise.

Antiinflammatory agents are used as the first choice preventive medication for asthma because they inhibit both the early and the late phase response (Goldenhersh and Rachelefsky, 1989). These agents are best known as mast cell stabilizers, but there may be other inhibitory effects on inflammatory cells. Cromolyn delivered by nebulizer or MDI is given 2 to 4 times per day. One treatment per day is not sufficient for maintenance therapy. Cromolyn is compatible when mixed with β-adrenergics or anticholinergics for delivery by a hand-held nebulizer (Drug Evaluations, 1993).

Corticosteroids inhibit the late phase asthmatic response and are used to treat inflammation and edema associated with asthma. Those children not responding adequately to β-adrenergics and cromolyn will require long-term corticosteroid therapy. Children on maintenance asthma therapy will probably require corticosteroid treatment when asthma is exacerbated by exposure to triggers such as a URI, irritants, or allergens (e.g., smoke, air pollution, pollen). Those children who need corticosteroid therapy more than once every 6 weeks to manage symptoms may require a continuous, every other day treatment program with corticosteroids (Ellis, 1988; NHLBI, 1991). Reevaluation is needed every 3 to 4 months. Children by 4 to 6 years of age may be able to use aerosolized corticosteroids via MDI with a spacer and reduce their need for systemic treatment.

When a child is receiving continuous corticosteroid therapy, complications may occur. These include the development of a cushinoid appearance, growth suppression, eye abnormalities (e.g., glaucoma or cataracts), osteoporosis with development of pathologic vertebral fractures, hypertension, glycosuria, menstrual disturbances, and peptic ulceration. A thorough history is necessary to determine any adverse effects from corticosteroid therapy. In addition, growth and blood pressure should be monitored at each well-child visit. Other tests such as urinalysis or ophthalmic examination are indicated when a child is on long-term corticosteroid therapy. Referral to the pulmonary-allergy specialist is warranted when adverse side effects of corticosteroid therapy are detected.

Anticholinergic agents, such as ipratropium bromide and atropine, block cholinergic reflex bronchoconstriction and may be most useful in children with bronchitic symptoms of increased mucous secretion. They are not particularly helpful against allergic challenges, do not block late phase response, and do not inhibit mediators from mast cells. Ipratropium bromide is the only anticholinergic drug currently approved for treatment of airway disease. Delivery of ipratropium is by MDI and has fewer side effects than atropine. Atropine sulfate is absorbed rapidly when given via aerosol and can be mixed with albuterol and cromolyn sodium for the convenience of providing three medications with one aerosol treatment. Side effects include dry mucous membranes, cutaneous flush, and fever. Behavioral and neurologic symptoms can occur with central nervous system toxicity (Gross, Boushey, and Gold, 1988).

Although not commonly used by primary care providers, methotrexate is utilized as a steroid sparing therapy for children with steroid dependent refractory asthma. This complex treatment modality requires comanagement with a pulmonary specialist and a primary care provider.

Some children will require the addition of theophylline if asthma is not controlled by antiinflammatory and β-adrenergic agents. Methylxanthines in combination with β-adrenergics work synergistically to produce bronchodilation and may improve control of asthma symptoms. Metabolism of theophylline varies greatly among individuals and age groups, as does serious toxicity with possible permanent central nervous system side effects; therefore, the dose must be individually adjusted by monitoring theophylline blood levels. Usual therapeutic levels are 10 to 20 μ/ml (Hilman, 1993). For children in the ambulatory setting, a level of 15 μ/ml should be the upper limit because theophylline metabolism is affected by many factors and this level provides a safe buffer should the theophylline level rise. Some children have a therapeutic response with a level lower than 10 μ/ml and will not need an increase in their maintenance dose.

Theophylline levels should be obtained every 6 to 12 months (Redding, Larter, and Brown, 1989). The theophylline dose is significantly adjusted when there are signs of toxicity or when the child experiences persistent or recurring asthma episodes on maintenance medications. Side effects of theophylline include nausea, hyperactivity and restlessness. Signs of toxicity that indicate an immediate need to determine the theophylline level include severe headaches, abdominal pain, vomiting, or any combination of these. Seizures are a sign of severe toxicity and require immediate intervention and hospital admission.

RECENT AND ANTICIPATED ADVANCES IN DIAGNOSIS AND MANAGEMENT

The greatest number of advances in children's asthma care are in the area of pharmacology. A new β₂-adrenergic medication has been recently approved for children over 12 years of age. Serevent (Salmeterol xinafoate) is administered via an MDI twice daily, approximately 12 hours apart, for individuals experiencing daily asthma symptoms, especially nocturnal symptoms, and individuals who need long-lasting protection against exercise-induced symptoms. It is *only for routine use* and not for treatment of exacerbations. The addition of short-acting β₂ medications such as albuterol is still required for intervening symptoms. (Mirgalia de Guidudici, et al, 1995).

Nedocromil sodium is a nonsteroidal, antiinflammatory medication unique in its chemical structure and appears to have a synergistic effect with inhaled steroids (Rebuck et al, 1990). Nedocromil inhibits the release of inflammatory chemotactic and smooth muscle contracting mediators from eosinophils, neutrophils, and mast cells. In some individuals it has been more effective than cromolyn sodium with regard to antigen and exercise-induced symptoms and should be considered as part of a preventive therapeutic plan. Although usually well tolerated, the most significant disadvantage to nedocromil has been its undesirable taste and is best administered with a spacer to minimize this effect. Recommended dosage is 2 puffs qid or tid initially, then based on the response, may be reduced to bid (Rebuck et al, 1990).

Budesonide (under investigation for approval) and Fluticasone are two new inhaled corticosteroids that appear to reduce airway obstruction, reduce the number of inflammatory cells in the airways, and reduce the number of asthma exacerbations (Dahl et al, 1993; Varsano et al, 1990). Both are highly potent corticosteroids that have lower systemic bioavailability as measured by plasma cortisol levels, compared to the current inhaled medications prescribed (Fabbri et al, 1993). Budesonide is currently under investigation in clinical trials in a 5-year multicenter controlled study comparing it to nedocromil and placebo. One advantage of budesonide is that it can be nebulized for children under 4 or 5 years of age who are unable to reliably use an MDI with a spacer and must currently take oral steroids for antiinflammatory effects.

ASSOCIATED PROBLEMS

Allergies

All children who have allergies do not have asthma, but approximately 50% to 75% of children with asthma have allergies (Smith, 1988). These can be in the form of atopic dermatitis or allergic rhinitis. Allergic triggers may include foods like peanuts or less frequently, cow's milk, soy, egg, wheat, or fish (Mahan and Arlin, 1992). Animal dander, pollens from trees, grasses, or weeds, or a variety of other substances (e.g., feathers, lamb's wool, and house dust mites) are also common allergens. If there is a strong history of allergic reactions associated with

---

ASSOCIATED PROBLEMS

Additional allergies
Aspirin sensitivity
Gastrointestinal reflux

---

respiratory symptoms, testing to determine specific problematic allergens may be beneficial. Avoidance techniques and allergy immunotherapy may then be helpful. Antihistamines for treatment of allergic rhinitis also may help relieve postnasal drip or sinusitis symptoms, which can trigger an asthma episode.

Medications

Aspirin and nonsteroidal antiinflammatory agents may precipitate an asthma episode in some children (NHLBI, 1991). These substances should be avoided and parents taught about reading over-the-counter drug labels because aspirin can be combined with other substances in certain drugs, particularly cold remedies.

Gastroesophageal Reflux

Gastroesophageal reflux (GER) can be found in many children with chronic lung disease. Reflux of gastric secretions into the esophagus can initiate a vagal response with an increased production of airway secretions. Theophylline is known to increase gastric secretion and decrease esophageal pressure and thus may aggravate GER in some children (Johannesson et al, 1985). Management of GER includes upright positioning following thickened feedings for infants and use of medications that reduce acidity or increase gastric motility.

PROGNOSIS

Many children with mild to moderate asthma can be well controlled. Some will have refractory asthma, which may be caused by poor implementation of the treatment plan, extremely severe asthma, or corticosteroid resistance. Psychosocial difficulties in families also can complicate asthma and its management. Chronic uncontrolled asthma may lead to persistent airway inflammation and fibrosis. Although some children seemingly outgrow their asthma, some who experience a disappearance of symptoms during the teen years or early adulthood will have symptoms return and increase in severity with increasing age (Weiss, 1995).

Mortality from asthma is increasing again after a slight fall between 1989 and 1990. Death rates have increased in all age groups with the highest mortality occurring in blacks and the greatest proportional increase in the 10- to 14-year age group (Sly, 1994). Many factors may contribute to the increased rate of reported mortality, including increased severity of the disease, under treatment or misuse of pharmacologic treatment, failure to recognize severity of asthma symptoms, delay in initiating treatment, and psychosocial factors.

Primary Care Management
HEALTH CARE MAINTENANCE
Growth and Development

There is evidence that asthma is not outgrown; persistent changes remain in the pulmonary tract of adults with asthma who have been free of symptoms for many years. Therefore asthma must be considered a chronic condition that may affect growth and development throughout the life span. As always, it is essential that the practitioner consistently measure height and weight and record these measurements on the child's National Center for Health Statistics growth grid. Any major deviation from the population norms (less than the 10th percentile) or departure (two or more zones) from the child's individualized curve should be noted and assessed in further detail. Smaller alterations may need to be monitored. During a series of acute exacerbations of asthma, the primary care provider may note a plateau or small drop in weight; however, with improvement in health status, catch-up growth should occur. If it does not occur, the cause of the weight loss should be further explored. Genetic, social, and nutritional factors potentially unassociated with asthma must be considered.

Asthma should have no direct influence on growth, although it has been associated with delay in the onset of puberty (Reid, 1992). There remains some controversy on whether or not medications used in the treatment of asthma may also diminish growth velocity (Crowley et al, 1995; Furukawa, 1993). Of asthma medications, corticosteroids are most frequently thought to be associated with delayed growth. Further research is needed in this area, but multicenter studies have shown significant dose-related suppression of unstimulated diurnal glucocorticosteroids even with inhaled corticosteroids (Zora, 1989). Primary care providers should be concerned if a child in prepuberty uses inhaled steroids in greater than 12 puffs per day (Stemple and Szefler, 1992).

Although the adolescent growth spurt may be slightly delayed, maximal height attainment is thought to be possible in children with asthma, given optimal management of the disease. The better the daily management and control of acute exacerbations, the more likely full height will be obtained at the age-appropriate time.

Standard infant, child, and adolescent assessment tools are appropriate for use in assessing development (see Chapter 2). Research has documented both normal and delayed development, with delayed development related not necessarily to the physiologic severity of the asthma, but to the imposed limitations placed on the child's experiences (Newacheck and Taylor, 1992). Limitations typically involve reductions in physical activity and social experiences, including day care and school attendance. Therefore the practitioner should encourage normalization of experiences whenever possible to reduce the unnecessary negative impact on development (Perrin et al, 1992).

If there are instances where normal experiences must be discouraged to avoid specific asthma triggers, the primary care provider should assist the parent and child to identify alternative experiences that could provide developmental stimulation. For example, if the child cannot play competitive soccer because of grass allergy, the child and family should be assisted in identifying an alternate sport, such as basketball or swimming; either allows the child to exercise and participate in a competitive team sport, and the opportunity to engage in an age-appropriate social and skill-building activity.

Without normalized experiences the child's self-image, self-esteem, perception of bodily control, and overall level of health are likely to be reduced and anxiety, fear, and dependency behavior increased (Creer et al, 1992).

Parents and children may limit strenuous activity because of repeated exacerbations, or fear of exacerbations. If this is done frequently, the primary care provider should assist family members in building an exercise habit into their daily routine. This will help avoid a sedentary life pattern, which may lower the child's sense of physical accomplishment and result in unwanted weight gain.

Unnecessary limitation of the child's activity may be particularly harmful because children connect activity with health (Kieckhefer, 1988) and may limit activity even further, possibly producing a downward spiral in self-perception. Integration of children into sports programs has been associated with positive clinical outcomes even up to 12 months following the program (Huang et al, 1989). Helping the child find an enjoyable sport should be a significant goal for the primary care provider.

There are reports of impaired cognitive development in children with repeated brief school absences. Similar impairment has been linked to some medications used to manage asthma. However, the demonstrated negative effect of medications on cognitive capabilities is not universal and is still being investigated (Weldon and McGeady, 1995). Clearly, prevention and swift, adequate management of exacerbations will reduce the number and length of school absences and thus limit what is thought to contribute most to the impairment of cognitive development.

Diet

Today's children and families eat many meals away from home, so dietary restrictions could effect family habits. Sulfites, previously used to enhance the appearance of many fresh foods, have been implicated in severe asthma exacerbations in some children. Though now banned by the FDA for fresh fruits and vegetables, sulfites may still be found in processed potatoes, shrimp, dried fruits, molasses, nonfrozen lemon and lime juices, and in labeled bulk preparations of fruits and vegetables (Rachelefsky, 1995; Mahan and Arlin, 1992). There are no other special dietary requirements for the

child with asthma unless the child has concurrent food allergies. When food allergies are present, the primary care provider needs to be familiar with alternative sources of the nutrients in the eliminated foods. If local grocery stores do not carry the alternative food sources, health food stores, dairy councils, or American Lung Association affiliates may be of assistance in locating the necessary items. Alternatively, the primary health care provider may refer the family to a local nutritionist for consultation. When the child has multiple food allergies, this referral is critical.

Safety

All age-appropriate family safety precautions must be similarly considered for the child with asthma. The primary care provider furnishes anticipatory guidance in this area and should be familiar with age-typical risks. Equipment and medications that are used to prevent or treat asthma exacerbations in the home may present additional concerns for safety.

Electrical burns are possible when equipment such as nebulizers are run in the child's presence. Infants and young children should never be left alone where they can reach the equipment, cord, or open socket. School-age children and adolescents should be properly instructed in the safe use of electrical equipment and should demonstrate their use to parents or the primary care provider before being encouraged to use the equipment independently.

Medications kept in the home must be safely stored in their original containers, in a locked location, inaccessible to the infant and young child. Since the child will ultimately need to become responsible for self-medication, the family should be assisted in making an age-appropriate plan to help the child with the medication regimen.

Practitioners can help parents identify their child's developmental capabilities and limits for safely assisting in the medication regimen by providing age-normative suggestions. For example, when the child is an infant or toddler, the parents need to speak about the medications as such, not as candy. With maturation, the toddler can be taught how to help take medicine from a spoon or hold the nebulizer mask to assist in therapy. The preschool-age child typically has the manual dexterity to take part in the medicinal therapy by helping the parent pour the medication or, in the parent's presence, take the capsule from the container. The young school-age child may be asked to get the medication and take it in the presence of the parent. When older school-age children can tell time, they can assume greater responsibility to prompt the parent when the medication is needed, get the medication, take the medication in the parent's presence, and return it to its proper storage place. The school-age child should also become increasingly responsible for taking needed medication while at school. Parents can monitor and encourage safe and knowledgeable use by discussing or having the child count and record on a calendar the number of times medication was taken as required. As the child grows to adolescence, more autonomy should be given for independently purchasing, taking, and replenishing both routine and prn medication. However, parents need to be reminded that one consistent finding in successful adolescent compliance with prescribed regimens is the continued support and age-appropriate assistance of their parents (Gaut and Kieckhefer, 1988). This support is not shown by "doing for" or "nagging" the adolescents, but by demonstrating faith in their capabilities and offering assistance with any problems that arise. Thus parents can maintain an interested, interdependent attitude to best assist the adolescent in growing in self-management of asthma.

Over the past 10 years there has been concern about the safe use of MDIs by persons of all ages. This concern is greatest for children too young to fully appreciate temporal relationships. Although MDIs are considered safe and uniquely effective in delivering a therapeutic dose of medication directly to the target organ, their use by children must be monitored by the family and the primary care provider. The child's skill in using the inhaler should be observed at each visit with the practitioner. Even many adults have difficulty in this maneuver. Up to 50% of children who do not receive such monitoring and corrective prompting for proper technique do not use the inhaler effectively (Baciewicz and Kyllonen, 1989). Use of spacers with MDIs for all age groups lessens these problems and enhances proper medication deposition (NHLBI, 1991).

With age and increasing time spent away from parents, children need to independently recognize when their treatment is not as effective as expected

and to seek the assistance of their parent or another adult. An episode that does not respond to treatment in the manner expected may herald a particularly severe exacerbation requiring medical assistance. Simple mnemonic devices have been found helpful in this regard. A rhyme of "twice is nice but three needs more than me" could be a mnemonic device used to teach children their individual asthma plan. Perhaps they can try the inhaler twice, but if symptoms persist and they feel the need to use it a third time, they should discuss it with a parent or the health care provider.

Immunizations

Although it has been suggested by some that vaccination with live virus vaccines may lead to airway inflammation and therefore increased hyperresponsivity in the child with asthma (Vermere, Demedts, and Yernault, 1988), the standard schedule of immunizations is recommended. If the child has egg sensitivity, vaccines using alternative media must be considered, even though some vaccines grown in chick embryo have been found devoid of allergenic components. Skin testing may be warranted. Treatment equipment for anaphylactic reactions should be readily available in the office.

Although infants and children with asthma may have signs of respiratory infection more frequently, these signs should not alone, in the absence of specific contraindication, be the basis for deferring immunizations (Committee on Infectious Diseases, 1994). Inadequate immunization with subsequent risk of infection is of great concern. Individualized assessment of the child with respiratory symptoms, including progressive signs of pulmonary dysfunction, should guide decisions regarding immunization. Delayed immunizations should be rescheduled as soon as possible. Special brief appointments, when the child is afebrile, may be needed to ensure adequate immunization during early childhood.

Children with asthma may experience complications with influenza, such as increased wheezing, fluctuating theophylline levels, bronchitis, pneumonia, increased school absences, and increased medical care visits. Therefore it is recommended that children with moderate to severe asthma annually receive an influenza vaccine after the age of 6 months (Committee on Infectious Diseases, 1994). The subviron (split) vaccine is given to children less than 13 years of age in the fall before the influenza season. Children without prior vaccination may require two doses to develop a satisfactory antibody response. If the child has had a related strain vaccine previously, one dose is thought adequate to confer protection.

Children with severe, anaphylactic reaction to chicken or eggs should not generally receive the immunization given the risk, need for yearly vaccination, and availability of chemoprophylaxis (Committee on Infectious Diseases, 1994). Before 6 months of age and in the presence of contraindications to influenza vaccination, alternative treatment methods should be considered. These include immunization of contacts or treatment of influenza with amantadine or rimantadine if the child is more than 1 year of age (Committee on Infectious Diseases, 1994).

Influenza vaccine may be given at the same time as measles-mumps-rubella (MMR), DTP or DTaP, varivax Hepatitis A and B, and oral polio vaccine. A different site and separate syringe are needed if two vaccines are given parenterally.

There is no research on the efficacy of giving children with asthma pneumococcal vaccine; thus pneumococcal immunization is not currently recommended. The primary care provider will need to keep informed of new research in this area as it becomes available.

Screening

Vision. Routine screening is recommended unless the child is taking daily high-dose corticosteroids because these drugs are known to cause inflammatory changes, cataracts, and glaucoma. If abnormal findings are identified during an eye examination the child should be referred to an ophthalmologist.

Hearing. Routine screening is recommended.

Dental. Routine screening is recommended.

Blood pressure. Blood pressure should be evaluated at each visit because sympathetic stimulation secondary to medications may occur, especially with β-adrenergic agents.

Hematocrit. Routine screening is recommended.

Urinalysis. Routine screening is recommended unless the child is taking high-dose corticosteroids daily, which may cause glycosuria. If glycosuria is

SCREENING
Routine childhood screening
Vision—see text
Hearing—routine
Dental—routine
Blood pressure—see text
Urinalysis—see text
Tuberculosis—routine
Condition-specific screening
Lung function
Theophylline levels
Allergic triggers

present the child should be referred to a pulmonary allergy specialist for evaluation.

Tuberculosis. Routine screening is recommended.

Condition-specific screening

LUNG FUNCTION. Monitoring lung function is essential to assess immediate function as well as to identify long-term trends. Pulmonary function testing should be done to establish lung function baseline levels when the child is well. Referral to a specialist for spirometry in children with moderate or severe disease may be warranted to monitor lung function and thus direct appropriate treatment. Spirometry, recording the forced expiratory flow in 25 to 75 seconds (FEF 25-75) and the forced expiratory flow in 1 second (FEV) assess severity of airway obstruction. Table 8-1 lists pulmonary function norms. Peak flow meters are more commonly used in the primary care office to measure the greatest rate of air flow during a forced exhalation. This measurement is labeled the peak expiratory flow rate (PEFR). PEFR, however, is effort dependent. Thus, if the child is obviously in respiratory distress or unwilling to cooperate, a PEFR may not be obtainable. Measurements of PEFR over time will establish an individual's baseline best effort for continuous assessment and may or

Table 8-1.   **PULMONARY FUNCTION NORMS**

Height		FVC (L)		FEV$_1$(L)	PEFR (L/mn)	FEF 25-75 (L/sec)
cm	in	Boys	Girls			
100	39.4	1.00	1.00	0.70	100	0.90
102	40.2	1.03	1.00	0.75	110	0.99
104	40.9	1.08	1.07	0.82	120	1.08
106	41.7	1.14	1.10	0.89	130	1.16
108	42.5	1.19	1.19	0.97	140	1.25
110	43.3	1.27	1.24	1.01	150	1.34
112	44.1	1.32	1.30	1.10	160	1.43
114	44.9	1.40	1.36	1.17	174	1.51
116	45.7	1.47	1.41	1.23	185	1.60
118	46.5	1.52	1.49	1.30	195	1.69
120	47.2	1.60	1.55	1.39	204	1.78
122	48.0	1.69	1.62	1.45	215	1.86
124	48.8	1.75	1.70	1.53	226	1.95
126	49.6	1.82	1.77	1.59	236	2.04
128	50.4	1.90	1.84	1.67	247	2.12
130	51.2	1.99	1.90	1.72	256	2.21
132	52.0	2.07	2.00	1.80	267	2.30
134	52.8	2.15	2.06	1.89	278	2.39
136	53.5	2.24	2.15	1.98	289	2.47
138	54.3	2.35	2.24	2.06	299	2.56
140	55.1	2.40	2.32	2.11	310	2.65
142	55.9	2.50	2.40	2.20	320	2.74
144	56.7	2.60	2.50	2.30	330	2.82
146	57.5	2.70	2.59	2.39	340	2.91
148	58.3	2.79	2.68	2.48	351	3.00
150	59.1	2.88	2.78	2.57	362	3.09
152	59.8	2.97	2.88	2.66	373	3.17
154	60.6	3.09	2.98	2.75	384	3.26
156	61.4	3.20	3.09	2.88	394	3.35
158	62.2	3.30	3.18	2.98	404	3.44
160	63.0	3.40	3.27	3.06	415	3.52
162	63.8	3.52	3.40	3.18	425	3.61
164	64.6	3.64	3.50	3.29	436	3.70
166	65.4	3.78	3.60	3.40	446	3.78
168	66.1	3.90	3.72	3.50	457	3.87
170	66.9	4.00	3.83	3.65	467	3.96
172	67.7	4.20	3.83	3.80	477	4.05
174	68.5	4.20	3.83	3.80	488	4.13
176	69.3	4.20	3.83	3.80	498	4.22

Adapted from Polgar G and Promadhar V: *Pulmonary function testing in children: techniques and standards,* Philadelphia, 1971, WB Saunders.

may not reflect average PEFR values as listed in Table 8-1.

Children who cannot or will not recognize airway obstruction or those with very labile asthma can use a home peak flow meter to monitor their asthma. Indeed, most primary care providers now advocate the systematic use of peak flow meters for all children with moderate to severe asthma (NHLBI, 1991). These meters are inexpensive, are fairly easy to use, and provide a detailed record of airway reactivity in the morning and evening. These objective data are used to individualize the child's treatment plan, often in the form of a three-zone action plan as recommended in the NHLBI, Asthma Management Kit for Clinicians (1992). See Table 8-2 for a graphic depiction.

THEOPHYLLINE LEVELS. Since theophylline preparations come in quick-release (every 6 to 8 hours), sustained-release (every 8 to 12 hours), or ultra–sustained-release (every 24 hours) forms, monitoring theophylline levels will be determined by the preparation or reason for the level. In general, it is best to follow the manufacturer's guidelines for measuring theophylline levels. The level should be drawn at the same time (e.g., al-ways 4 hours after the dose of a sustained-release preparation) to ensure continuity in level monitoring. In the case of suspected theophylline toxicity, levels should be ordered immediately. See Table 8-3.

ALLERGIC HISTORY. A biannual review of possible allergens and irritants in the home is helpful. In addition to identification of asthma triggers, it provides a time to discuss other health issues such as parent or adolescent smoking, avoidance of triggers, dust control, or desirability of allergy skin testing. Asthma shared-management education can be updated at this time to ensure increasingly mature understanding of the condition and its management.

COMMON ILLNESS MANAGEMENT

Differential Diagnosis

Wheezing. It is well known that all wheezing is not asthma, so when a child presents with recurrent or persistent cough or wheeze, other diagnoses should be considered. These include foreign body aspiration (particularly in the infant or toddler), vocal cord dysfunction, infections such as bronchitis, bronchiolitis, or pneumonia, other underlying airway diseases such as cystic fibrosis or bronchiectasis, structural abnormalities such as a vascular ring, or aspiration as a result of a primary swallowing disorder or secondary to underlying neuromuscular disease.

Table 8-2.
ZONE ACTION PLAN

Zone	PEFR (Best or predicted for age)	Action
Green	80%-100%	All clear, continue regular management plan.
Yellow	50%-80%	Caution, implement action plan predetermined with primary care provider.
Red	<50%	Medical alert, implement action plan predetermined with primary care provider and call provider if PEFR does not return to yellow or green zone.

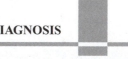

DIFFERENTIAL DIAGNOSIS

Wheezing—may not be asthma only
Respiratory infections—trigger asthma exacerbation
Vomiting and diarrhea—may indicate theophylline toxicity
Headache—may indicate sinusitis or theophylline toxicity
Fever—not associated with asthma unless underlying infection present

Respiratory infections. Viral respiratory infections are the most common cause of asthma exacerbations in children. Treatment is usually supportive and parents will need to know to give antipyretics for fever, provide extra fluids, and that a change in asthma therapy medications may be necessary. For example, the child who only receives cromolyn sodium via nebulizer for asthma control may need to temporarily add albuterol to the nebulized treatments for control of cough or wheeze during an exacerbation.

Vomiting and diarrhea. Children with asthma who present with vomiting should be evaluated for theophylline toxicity if they are on theophylline preparations, especially if the vomiting is associated with headache or stomachache. When gastroenteritis occurs in the child with asthma, the usual supportive care is required. The child should remain on the usual asthma therapy but may have difficulty with oral medications because of vomiting and may be at increased risk for mucus plugging if dehydration occurs. Controlling the respiratory symptoms with nebulized medications and providing extra fluids should be considered. Hospitalization may be necessary if the child's asthma worsens, medications cannot be tolerated orally or by nebulizer, or fluid intake is extremely reduced.

Headache. Sinusitis can present as a headache especially if associated with complaints of purulent nasal drainage, fetid breath odor, or nighttime cough. Since sinusitis can trigger an asthma episode, there may also be increased wheezing. When diagnosed, sinusitis must be treated aggressively and early to minimize the occurrence of asthma exacerbations. The common cold and symptoms of allergic rhinitis do not, however, require antibiotic treatment.

If the child with asthma (on a theophylline preparation) presents with complaint of headache, theophylline toxicity should be ruled out especially if gastrointestinal upset, stomachache, and vomiting are also occurring.

Fever. Asthma exacerbations are not associated with fever unless there is an underlying infection such as sinusitis, pneumonia, or otitis media. The cause of the fever needs to be evaluated by the usual methods. Increased fluids should be given to keep the child well hydrated to avoid mucus plugging which can occur with asthma.

Drug Interactions

Several factors cause theophylline levels to rise or fall and should be considered when the child's overall health care plan is assessed (see Table 8-3).

Table 8-3.   FACTORS AFFECTING SERUM OF THEOPHYLLINE LEVELS

	Factors increasing serum levels due to decreased clearance	Factors decreasing serum levels due to increased clearance
Age	Infants	12 mo-12 yr
Medications	Erythromycin—alone or in combination	Phenobarbital
	Azithromycin (Zithromax)	Phenytoin (Dilantin)
	Clarithromycin (Biaxin)	Rifampin (Rifadin)
	Cimetidine (Tagamet)	
	Oral contraceptives	
	Propanolol (Inderal)	
	Carbamazepine (Tegretol)	
Illnesses	Liver or heart dysfunction	
	Acute viral illnesses	
	Fever for over 24 hours	
Other	Obesity	Cigarette or marijuana smoking

Medications that affect theophylline clearance should be avoided or the theophylline dose appropriately adjusted and levels monitored.

Cough suppressants should generally be avoided because they may mask asthma signs or symptoms and delay diagnosis and appropriate treatment. Occasionally cough suppressants are helpful to control nighttime or continuous postviral cough where coughing itself is a trigger for increased cough because of irritation of the trachea and bronchi. In these cases over-the-counter cough medicines will probably be inadequate for cough control.

Antihistamines are now available without medical prescription and may be helpful in relieving allergic rhinitis. Antihistamines are thought not to contribute to drying or inspissation of secretions in the well-hydrated child. A history of use by the child is important in planning a treatment regimen. More recently developed antihistamines such as Seldane, Hismanal, and Claritin bring the advantage of little or no sedation (American Medical Association Division on Drugs and Toxicology, 1992). Although children with asthma are frequently atopic and receiving topical steroids in addition to inhaled steroids, no special concerns have yet been documented with this combined steroid regimen.

DEVELOPMENTAL ISSUES

Sleep Patterns

The sleep of young children is often disrupted during asthma exacerbations. Even when an exacerbation is not evident, the child may routinely awaken with wheezing and coughing during the night or early morning hours. This tendency for early morning problems probably represents the normal circadian rhythm in airway caliber and steroid production (DuBuske, 1994). Because the symptom pattern represents an exaggeration of existing bronchial hyperresponsivity, optimizing daytime control and reducing environmental irritants in the sleeping room minimizes the symptoms. Persistent difficulty may necessitate an evening dosage of a short-acting theophylline preparation (DuBuske, 1994) or use of a long-acting time-release preparation in school-age children, or adolescents.

Parents have reported that some medications disrupt their children's sleep, but systematic documentation is scarce. Most providers attempt an alternative medication regimen if the sleep disturbance does not resolve within 1 or 2 weeks of beginning a medication. Young children find a nighttime ritual soothing. This is accentuated in the child with asthma. Thus the primary care provider should help parents establish a bedtime ritual that is relaxing and can be easily implemented by their family. A consistent bedtime is also helpful because frequent deviation of more than 30 minutes may cause difficulty in both settling the child and bringing on sleep.

Toileting

Toileting needs typically are not altered by the child's asthma. Bowel and bladder training is achieved at the expected ages. Clinicians have noted that a small proportion of children experience problems with enuresis when taking theophylline preparations, possibly because of its diuretic action. The exact incidence, however, remains undocumented. If standard behavioral interventions are not effective in eliminating enuresis, most primary care providers seek an alternative medication regimen to manage the asthma.

Discipline

Parents frequently report they find it difficult to deal with discipline for fear of upsetting the child and initiating an asthma exacerbation. Given current estimates that up to 40% of the children with asthma will experience some degree of bronchospasm with intense crying (Schwam, 1987), parental concern is realistic and understandable. Crying probably cannot be entirely avoided, but the parent should be reassured that most discipline can be implemented by rewarding desirable behaviors if this is done routinely and begun early in the child's life. Inconsistent limit setting for undesirable behavior only confuses the child and makes it more difficult to learn and internalize the limits chosen by the parents.

Another parental concern is that the child's irritability, refusals, or acting-out behavior is caused by illness or medications. Medications and illness may influence the child's behavior, but consistency of expectations is of greater importance. Blaming the illness on medication does not remove the necessity to assist the child to develop behaviors desired by the family and social networks.

Ultimately the child will need to develop a strong sense of internal control to participate effectively in self-management. Early consistent positive expectations set by the parents will form the foundation for the child's later self-discipline and sense of mastery and control. Avoiding discipline early in the child's life will not make the ensuing years more pleasant for the parent or aid the child in learning socially expected behaviors. Thus primary care providers should initiate discussion regarding positive discipline early during an infant's first year of life, assuring parents that with time this issue should become less burdensome as the child is able to verbally express emotion without excessive crying leading to bronchospasm.

Child Care

Most families will find it necessary to use child care services on either a regular or sporadic basis. Having a child with asthma should not prohibit use of child care. Because URIs trigger exacerbations of asthma in many children under 5 years of age, a smaller day care with less chance of exposure to these infections may reduce the number of illnesses. With proper communication and explanation, child care can be safely used with a responsible, interested caretaker. Whether child care is at a center or is home based, provided by a relative, neighbor, or professional, information must be shared by the parent to ensure success.

Parents must be responsible for providing all relevant information to the caretaker—what triggers the child's asthma, early warning signs of an impending asthma episode, what the caretaker should do first and what should be done next if the last action is not effective, how the parent and other responsible party (including health care provider) can be reached, and what information must be passed on to emergency personnel should they need to be called. The best way to provide this information is in a written format. A laminated card with detailed instructions on one side and the primary care provider's name and telephone number on the reverse side has proved helpful for many families.

If the child care provider is to give any treatments, the parent must demonstrate the procedures and observe the provider's repeat performance. In addition, center-based programs may require written prescriptions from the primary health care provider and written permission of the parent for the child care provider to perform the treatment. Parents must maintain close contact with the child care provider to learn about changing triggers, medications, or early warning signs. Anyone in repeated contact with the child who observes responses to treatments should also relay that information to the parent. The information can then be integrated into the overall routine reevaluation of the treatment plan. Any treatment changes should be related immediately to the child care provider so that a consistent approach is provided to the child regardless of setting. Frequent and open communication is the key to successful child care arrangements.

Schooling

Surveys of children with asthma report an average of 18 days lost from a typical 180-day school year (Redding et al, 1994). Often these days are scattered throughout the year. This pattern of frequent, brief absences historically has been felt to be more harmful to academic progress than infrequent long absences, and efforts should be made to avoid this tendency.

Parents report that communicating with school personnel is essential but often difficult. Many fears and misconceptions regarding children with asthma still exist in the general public. Many teachers do not recognize cough as a symptom of asthma. They may believe the child has an infectious disease restricting school attendance. Teachers and administrators may attempt to limit the child more than the parent or primary care provider believes necessary, especially in regard to sports participation. With proper therapy and education, only those with severe asthma should need to consider limitations (American Academy of Pediatrics Committee on Sports Medicine and Fitness, 1994). With proper warmup, pacing, and preventive pharmacologic therapy, almost all will be able to participate in sports activities.

Scheduling an annual parent-teacher conference to discuss the child's current treatment regimen is essential. Teachers should have the same written information suggested for child care providers. In addition, the teacher should be informed of the skills the child has for shared management. The school nurse may provide support to the parent during annual conferences and should be informed of all emergency treatment requirements that might be needed. Provider-prescribed emergency medications that may be needed should be given to the nurse or designate. If the school personnel hesitate to assume this responsibility, the parents or primary care provider should discuss with them their legal responsibility to allow all children access to medications they need to enable school attendance. Mutual problem solving is essential to finding a workable solution.

Fitting in with school peers and maintaining positive peer relationships are essential to the child's full development. The parent can actively arrange peer gatherings, encourage the child to join clubs or organizations, and allow the child age-appropriate independence in visiting friends to ensure social experiences. Friends may question why the child is taking medications or has special equipment in the home. Simple explanations about the child's asthma should be given with the assurance that asthma is not contagious. This might also be done in school as a class presentation with the teacher's assistance. Parents are encouraged to discuss their child's asthma with parents of their child's peers so that all may have an honest understanding of the child's condition and abilities as well as any limitations.

Sexuality

As noted earlier, sexual development may be delayed if the asthma has not been adequately controlled to allow regular growth. Systemic corticosteroids historically have been associated with delay in sexual development because of their effect on the adrenal glands and corticosteroid production. Current treatment regimens that rely on inhaled corticosteroids or every other day, morning dosage schedules appear to have reduced the adverse effect on general and sexual growth patterns.

If the adolescent becomes sexually active and wishes to use contraceptives, drug interactions must be considered. It is known that oral contraceptives may interfere with the breakdown of theophylline, thus increasing the likelihood of toxicity. As new asthma management drugs continue to be developed, their impact on the efficacy of any pharmacologic means of birth control must be explored. If there is a strong family pattern of asthma, pregnancy counseling would include promoting subsequent breast feeding to potentially decrease or delay allergy in the newborn (Morgan and Martinez, 1992).

Transition into Adulthood

As youth with asthma enter adulthood it is important that they continue to increase and periodically update their understanding of asthma and its management. Reviewing and updating the education might take place before a move to college or a switch in primary care provider. If persons with a history of moderate to severe asthma is currently without symptoms, they should be reminded to inform their new provider of this history because symptoms may return in later life. Maintaining a smoke-free work environment is essential. Some vocations that involve inhaled irritants or allergens, overexposure to known triggers such as work with laboratory animals, cleaning fluids, bakery or painting products, may be best avoided (NHLBI, 1991).

SPECIAL FAMILY CONCERNS AND RESOURCES

Because of the familial nature of asthma, some family members express guilt during the child's flare-ups. Parents should be reminded that there is nothing they could have done to prevent asthma and that in regard to acute exacerbations, hindsight is always better than foresight. Eliminating all exacerbations may be an ideal but impossible goal to achieve. A more realistic goal is to limit the number and extent of flare-ups and to learn something about prevention or management from each episode.

If many family members have a history of asthma, the family may retain outdated beliefs and habits regarding the treatment of asthma. The primary care provider needs to respect the family history but also stress new knowledge and discuss the development of new therapies. This should encourage the family to take advantage of current information.

Given the familial nature of asthma, cultural and ethnic considerations are important. Minority ethnicity and poverty have been linked to increased prevalence, reduced access to care, lower quality of care provided, and reduced implementation of recommended care with subsequent higher risks of morbidity and mortality (Finkelstein et al, 1995; Halfon and Newacheck, 1993). Primary care providers need to consider their role in changing this reality. Providers must be child advocates to reduce environmental exposures of children to causes of asthma and its exacerbation (e.g., smoke, preterm birth, housing projects with poor ventilation, mold and mildew, early URI). Providers can continue to support policy and legislation that ensures access to health care by all. Exploring values, beliefs, and health practices of the families should enable the creative primary care provider to individualize critical elements of practice guidelines to the individual family. This individualization may help to ensure the greatest acceptance and implementation of the recommended care by tailoring the management program to the cultural realities of the child and family. It is within the ongoing trusting relationship of the family and caregiver that further information regarding cultural beliefs and practices can be discussed.

Most parents express ambivalence regarding long-term medication regimens. Although most parents acknowledge the effectiveness of these regimens, the majority also hold the belief that long-term medication can be harmful to their child (Donnelly, Donnelly, and Thong, 1987). Helpful approaches for supporting parents include acknowledging and discussing these common feelings while presenting the fact that the most detrimental effects of asthma seem to come from poor management. It is also useful to reinforce that the program will continue to be tailored to their child, trying to decrease medication to the minimum amount needed for control.

Asthma does cause disruption in the life of the child's primary caretaker, most often the mother. This disruption is most marked when the child is young but can be minimized by actively involving the other parent or another family member in concrete, daily management tasks (Wasilewski et al, 1988).

Smoking by a family member continues to be associated with increased asthma flare-ups (Evans et al, 1987; Murray and Morrison, 1993; Sander and Boyer, 1992), but changing smoking habits of family members is difficult. When advising families to eliminate smoke from their child's environment, the practitioner should convey resources for smoking cessation. In severe cases, in-home smoking can be viewed as child endangerment. Parents must be reminded to only smoke outside (not in another room or near an open window) and wear a "smoking jacket," an outer layer to prevent smoke retention on clothes.

Resources

Primary care providers should become familiar with the local offices of national organizations (see the list that follows) to identify community-based services in their clients' local areas that can complement their health care services. Many of these community-based services have programs that are useful to children and parents in managing day-to-day effects of asthma. These programs typically offer education about asthma and training in shared management skills for the child and parents.

If the primary care provider's practice is large enough, educational programs for age-similar children with asthma have been effectively implemented in private practices (Alexander et al, 1988). Having a well-stocked lending library of reading materials on asthma assists parents and children in learning how to manage asthma. It is imperative that the practitioner provide families with information on how they may obtain these materials for their own use.

Information materials
Self-management curricular guides
Available from National Heart, Lung, and Blood Institute: *AIR WISE, AIR POWER, Open Airways, and Living with Asthma.*
Available from Asthma and Allergy Foundation of America: *Asthma Care Training for Kids (ACT).*
Available from the American Lung Association: *Super Stuff. Open Airways for Schools.*
Newsletters
Allen and Hanburys Respiratory Institute: *Air Currents,* PO Box 1409, West Caldwell, NJ 07007-1409.
Sander N, (editor): *Mothers of Asthmatics Newsletter,* 5316 Summit Dr, Fairfax, VA 22030.
Media
A Kids Guide to Asthma: Making Compliance Fun (VHS), 1994. Available from Devilbiss Health Care Inc, PO Box 635, Sommerset, PA 15501-9986.

Books

American Lung Association: *Let's talk about asthma: a guide for teens,* 1990. Available from your local ALA.

Mendoza, A: *Peak performance: a strategy for asthma self-assessment.* Hawthorne Community Medical Group, Los Angeles, 1987.

Mendoza G, Sander N, and Scherrer D: *A user's guide to peak-flow monitoring,* Fairfax, VA, 1988, Mothers of Asthmatics.

Plaut T: *Children with asthma: a manual for parents,* ed 2, Amherst, MA, 1988, Pedipress.

Sander N: *So you have asthma and I'm a meter reader,* Fairfax, VA, 1988, Glaxo. Provided as a public service by Glaxo Inc. Available from Allergy and Asthma Network and Mothers of Asthmatics, 3554 Chain Bridge Rd, Suite 200, Fairfax, VA 22030-2709. Phone: 1-800-878-4403

Sander N: *A parent's guide to asthma,* ed 2, New York, 1994, Doubleday.

Organizations

American Lung Association and local or state affiliates. (Check your telephone book for the chapter nearest you.)

Asthma and Allergy Foundation of America, 1125-15th St NW, Suite 502, Washington, DC 20005. Phone: 202-466-7643

National Heart, Lung, and Blood Institute Information Center, PO Box 30105, Bethesda, MD 20824-0105. Phone: 301-251-1222.

National Jewish Center, 1400 Jackson St, Denver, CO 80206.

A variety of hospitals and clinics in your area may have ongoing support groups. Telephone their public relations department for information.

Telephone lines

Allergy Information Line, 1-800-822-ASMA.

Asthma and Allergy Foundation of America, 1-800-7-ASTHMA.

National Jewish Center Lung Line, 1-800-222-LUNG.

SUMMARY OF PRIMARY CARE NEEDS FOR THE CHILD WITH ASTHMA

Health care maintenance

Growth and development

Delayed adolescent growth is associated with poor control with exacerbations or oral corticosteroids.

Delayed development is noted only when unnecessary limitations are imposed on child.

Impaired cognitive development is most clearly linked to repeated school absences.

Diet

Children may have allergies to sulfites or foods.

Safety

Electrical burns are possible from nebulizers or steamers.

Medication safety varies with developmental age. Caution is needed on repeated use of MDIs.

Immunizations

Routine immunizations are recommended.

If child has documented egg sensitivity, vaccines using other media must be considered.

Influenza vaccine is recommended for children with moderate to severe asthma who are more than 6 months of age. Pneumococcal immunization is not currently recommended.

Screening

Vision

Routine screening is recommended unless daily highdose corticosteroids are taken which may result in cataracts or glaucoma, then referral to opthalmologist is required for any eye changes.

Hearing

Routine screening is recommended.

Dental

Routine screening is recommended.

Blood pressure

Should be evaluated at each visit due to possible sympathetic stimulation from medications.

Hematocrit

Routine screening is recommended.

Urinalysis

Routine screening is recommended unless daily doses of corticosteroids are taken which may result in glycosuria. If glycosuria present refer for reevaluation of asthma management.

Tuberculosis

Routine screening is recommended.

Condition-specific screening

Corticosteroid Therapy: Additional assessments are necessary to monitor glycosuria, osteoporosis, blood pressure, cataracts, glaucoma, and growth delay.

Lung Function Tests: Testing of PEFR should be done at each primary care office visit and on a routine schedule in the home based on individualized management plan.

Theophylline Levels: Should be monitored with change in therapy, growth, and illness.

Allergy Testing: Skin testing may be indicated depending on history and therapy response.

Common illness management

Differential diagnosis

Recurrent or persistent cough or wheeze: Rule out infection, aspiration, structural anomalies, and cystic fibrosis.

Viral respiratory infections: URI may require change in asthma therapy to prevent or modify exacerbation of asthma.

Gastrointestinal symptoms: Rule out theophylline toxicity.

Headache: Rule out theophylline toxicity and sinusitis.

Fever: Not associated with asthma alone. When fever present, prevention of dehydration is important to prevent mucus plugs.

Drug interactions

Antihistamines are not contraindicated.

Medications such as erythromycin, cimetidine or oral contraceptives will raise theophylline levels.

Continued.

SUMMARY OF PRIMARY CARE NEEDS FOR THE CHILD WITH ASTHMA—cont'd

Phenobarbital will decrease theophylline levels.
Cough suppressants may mask symptoms of asthma.

Developmental issues

Sleep patterns

Exacerbation may interfere with sleep.
It is important to reduce environmental allergens in sleep area.
If medications disturb sleep, an alternative regimen should be tried.

Toileting

Toileting is routine.
Few children experience enuresis while on theophylline.

Discipline

Concern over discipline initiating asthma attack.
Rewarding desirable behavior should be encouraged.
The influence of medication and illness on behavior is a concern.
Consistency of expectation is important.

Child care

Child care workers need to be provided with information on asthma triggers, early warning signs of asthma, treatment, emergency contacts, and medications used in day care.

Schooling

Repeated school absences may interfere with academic performance.
School personnel must be educated to evaluate child's symptoms and use of medications.
There is concern over peer acceptance of child with chronic condition.
Maintain sports participation.

Sexuality

Sexual development may be delayed in severe cases or with prolonged corticosteroid use.
Oral contraceptives may interfere with breakdown of theophylline.

Transition into adulthood

Update knowledge.
Inform new primary care provider.
Vocational issues

Special family concerns

Familial nature of asthma may lead to outdated beliefs of treatment.
Parents may be ambivalent regarding long-term medication regimens.
Smoking in home is detrimental to children with asthma. Parents who smoke need support and assistance in quitting.
Ethnic minority and poverty have been linked with increased prevalence, morbidity and mortality.

REFERENCES

Alexander SJ et al: Effectiveness of a nurse-managed program for children with chronic asthma, *J Pediatr Nurs* 3:312-317, 1988.

American Academy of Pediatrics Committee on Sports Medicine and Fitness. Medical conditions affecting sports participation, *Pediatrics* 94(5):757-760, 1994.

American Academy of Pediatrics Provisional Committee on Quality Improvement. Practice parameter: the office management of acute exacerbations of asthma in children, *Pediatrics* 93:119-126, 1994.

American Medical Association. Department of Drugs. *AMA*

Drug Evaluations, Littleton, MA, 1993, Pub Sciences Group.

American Medical Association Division on Drugs and Toxicology. *Drug Evaluations,* 1992.

Baciewicz A, Kyllonen K: Aerosol inhaler technique in children with asthma, *Am J Hosp Pharm* 46:2510-2511, 1989.

Bloomburg G, Strunk R: Crisis in asthma care, *Pediatr Clin North Am* 39(6):1225-1241, 1992.

Boulet LP et al: Asthma and increases in nonallergic bronchial responsiveness from seasonal pollen exposure, *J Allergy Clin Immunol* 71:170-177, 1983.

Cockroft DW: Airway hyperresponsiveness in asthma, *Hosp Pract* 1:111-129, 1990.

Committee on Infectious Diseases. *Report of the committee on infectious diseases,* ed 23, Elk Grove Village, IL, 1994, American Academy of Pediatrics.

Creer TL et al: Behavioral consequences of illness: childhood asthma as a model, *Pediatrics* 90(5), (suppl) 808-815, 1992.

Crowley S et al: Growth and the growth hormone axis in children in prepuberty with asthma, *J Pediatr* 126(2):297-303, 1995.

Cypcar N, Stark J, and Lemanske R: The impact of respiratory infections on asthma, *Pediatr Clin North Am* 31(6):1259-1276, 1992.

Dahl R et al: A dose-ranging study of fluticasone propionate in adult patients with moderate asthma. International study group, *Chest* 104(5):1352-1358, 1993.

Donnelly JE, Donnelly WJ, and Thong YH: Parental perceptions and attitudes toward asthma and its treatment: a controlled study, *Soc Sci Med* 24:431-437, 1987.

DuBuske LM: Asthma: diagnosis and management of nocturnal symptoms, *Compr Ther* 20(11):628-639, 1994.

Ellis E: Asthma: current therapeutic approach, *Pediatr Clin North Am* 35:1041-1052, 1988.

Evans D et al: The impact of passive smoking on emergency room visits of urban children with asthma, *Am Rev Respir Dis* 135:567-572, 1987.

Fabbri L et al: Comparison of fluticasone propionate with beclomethasone dipropionate in moderate to severe asthma treated for 1 year. International Study Group [see comments], *Thorax* 48(8):817-823, 1993. Comment in *Thorax* 49(4):385, 1994.

Finkelstein JA et al: Quality of care for preschool children with asthma: the role of social factors and practice setting, *Pediatrics* 95(3):389-394, 1995.

Furukawa CT: Stepping up the treatment of children with asthma, *Pediatrics* 92:144-145, 1993.

Gaut D, Kieckhefer G: Assessment of self-care agency in chronically ill adolescents, *J Adolesc Health Care* 9:55-60, 1988.

Goldenhersh M, Rachelefsky G: Childhood asthma: management, *Pediatr in Review* 10:259-267, 1989.

Gross N, Boushey H, Gold W: Anticholinergic drugs. In Middleton E Jr, Reed CE, Ellis EF et al: *Allergy: principles and practice,* ed 3, St Louis, 1988, Mosby.

Halfon N, Newacheck PW: Childhood asthma and poverty: differential impacts and utilization of health services, *Pediatrics* 91(1):56-61, 1993.

Hilman B (editor): *Pediatric respiratory disease: diagnosis and treatment,* Philadelphia, 1993, WB Saunders.

Howell H, Flaim T, Lung C: Patient education, *Pediatr Clin North Am* 39(6):1333-1361, 1992.

Huang S et al: The effects of swimming in asthmatic children—participants in a swimming program in the city of Baltimore, *J Asthma* 26:117-121, 1989.

Johannesson N et al: Relaxation of lower esophageal sphincter and stimulation of gastric secretion and diuresis by antiasthmatic xanthines, *Am Rev Respir Dis* 131:26-31, 1985.

Kieckhefer G: The meaning of health to children with asthma, *J Asthma* 25:325-333, 1988.

Mahan KL, Arlin M: *Food, nutrition and diet therapy,* ed 8, Philadelphia, 1992, WB Saunders, pp 653-669.

Middleton Jr E et al: (editors:) *Allergy: principles and practice,* St Louis, 1993, Mosby.

Mirgalia de Guidudici M et al: Salmeterol vs. theophylline in asthmatic children, *Respir Crit Care Med* 151(4):A270, 1995.

Morgan W, Martinez F: Risk factors for developing wheezing and asthma in childhood, *Pediatr Clin North Am* 39(6):1185-1203, 1992.

Murray AB, Morrison BJ: The decrease in severity of asthma in children of parents who smoke since the parents have been exposing them to less cigarette smoke, *J Allergy Clin Immunol* 91 (1 Pt. 1):102-110, 1993.

National Asthma Education Expert Panel Guidelines for the Diagnosis and Management of Asthma. *National asthma education program expert panel report,* Anonymous, US Department of Health and Human Services, Publication No 91-3042, 1991.

National Asthma Education Program, National Heart, Lung, and Blood Institute. *Teach your patients about asthma: a clinician's guide,* US Department of Health and Human Services, Publication No 92-2737, October 1992.

Newacheck PW, Taylor WR: Childhood chronic illness: prevalence, severity, and impact, *Am J Public Health* 82(3):364-371, 1992.

Perrin JM et al: Improving the psychological status of children with asthma: a randomized controlled trial, *J Dev Behav Pediatr* 13(4):241-247, 1992.

Rachelefsky GS: Asthma update: new approaches and partnerships, *J Pediatr Health Care* 9(1):12-21, 1995.

Rebuck AS et al: A 3-month evaluation of nedocromil sodium in asthma: a randomized, double blind, placebo controlled trial of nedocromil sodium conducted by a Canadian multicenter study group, *J Allergy Clin Immunol* 85:612-617, 1990.

Redding GJ, Larter N, and Brown G: Guidelines for care of children with chronic lung disease, *Pediatr Pulmonol* 19 (suppl 3), 19, 1989.

Redding GJ et al: Prevalence and impact of diagnosed asthma among primary-school children, *Am Rev Respir Dis* (Abstract), 1994.

Reid M: Complicating features of asthma, *Pediatr Clin North Am* 39(6):1327-1341, 1992.

Sander N: *A parent's guide to asthma,* New York, 1989, Doubleday.

Sander N, Boyer JG: The National Allergy and Asthma Network Report. Interesting observations from households with and households without smokers and pets, *Am J Asthma Allergy Pediatricians* 5(2):110-113, 1992.

Schwam JS: Assisting the parent of a child with asthma, *J Asthma* 24:45-54, 1987.

Sly RM: Changing asthma mortality, *Ann Allergy* 73(3):259-268, 1994.

Smith L: Etiology and pathogenic factors in allergic diseases, In *Allergic disease from infancy to adulthood,* ed 2, Philadelphia, 1988, WB Saunders.

Stempel DA, Redding GJ: Management of acute asthma, *Pediatr Clin North Am* 39:1311-1325, 1992.

Stempel DA, Szefler SJ: Management of chronic asthma, *Pediatr Clin North Am* 39:1293-1310, 1992.

Taylor WR, Newacheck PW: Impact of childhood asthma on health, *Pediatrics* 90(5):657-662, 1992.

Varsano I et al: Safety of 1 year of treatment with budesonide in young children with asthma, *J Allergy Clin Immunol* 85:914-920, 1990.

Vermere P, Demedts M, and Yernault J, (editors): *Progress in asthma and COPD,* New York, 1988, Elsevier North Holland.

Wasilewski Y et al: The effect of paternal social support on maternal disruption caused by childhood asthma, *J Community Health* 13:33-42, 1988.

Weiss S: Early childhood asthma: what are the questions: long-term outcome, *Am J Respir Crit Care Med* 151:suppl 6, 1995.

Weldon DP, McGeady SJ: Theophylline effects on cognition, behavior, and learning, *Arch Pediatr Adolescent Med* 149(1):90-93, 1995.

Wigal JK et al: A critique of 19 self-management programs for childhood asthma, Part I: development and evaluation of programs, *Pediatr Asthma Allergy Immunol* 4:17-39, 1990.

Zora J: The use of corticosteroids in childhood asthma, *J Asthma* 26:159-165, 1989.

Bleeding Disorders

9

Mary Alice Dragone and Susan Karp

ETIOLOGY

Hemophilia and von Willebrand's disease are the most common inherited bleeding disorders resulting from deficiencies or abnormalities of specific coagulation proteins. The von Willebrand protein is activated when the endothelium is damaged. It promotes formation of an initial platelet plug by enabling platelet adhesion. Multiple coagulation proteins, including those that are deficient in hemophilia, are critical components of the secondary or intrinsic hemostatic mechanism that is activated when collagen fibers are exposed in a damaged blood vessel. These proteins are required for the formation of the final fibrin clot (Hilgartner Corrigan, 1995; Montgomery and Scott, 1993).

Hemophilia

Hemophilia involves a defect in the intrinsic hemostatic mechanism (Fig. 9-1). Factor VIII deficiency (classic hemophilia, hemophilia A) accounts for approximately 80% of hemophilia cases, whereas factor IX deficiency (Christmas disease, hemophilia B) accounts for 20% (Lanzkowsky, 1995; Hilgartner and Corrigan, 1995). Less common factor deficiencies exist, although they are not specifically discussed in this chapter. Severity of hemophilia is defined by the percentage of activity of the deficient coagulation protein as presented in Table 9-1.

Hemophilia is inherited in an X-linked pattern. Most frequently, female carriers pass the disorder to their sons. The severity of hemophilia remains constant within families, although clinical symptoms may vary based on lifestyle and treatment regimens. Although at least 30% of all hemophilia cases are sporadic (e.g., negative prior family history), recently available genetic testing shows that many of the mothers of these isolated cases of hemophilia are carriers (Peake et al, 1993). A woman is considered to be an obligate carrier if hemophilia has been diagnosed in either her father, two of her sons, or in one son and one other relative. Carriers of hemophilia A or B would be expected to have, on average, factor VIII or IX levels that are approximately 50% of normal. However, because of lyonization, some carriers have very low factor levels, with resultant symptoms of excessive or unusual bleeding (Greer et al, 1991; Peake et al, 1993). This validates the need for determination of factor VIII/IX coagulant levels even in obligate carriers.

von Willebrand's Disease

Generally a mild bleeding disorder, von Willebrand's disease is closely related to hemophilia. The von Willebrand protein's primary action is to facilitate platelet adhesion (Fig. 9-1). This protein also helps to stabilize factor VIII, and when it is deficient, the amount of circulating active factor VIII may also be reduced. Most children with von Willebrand's disease have prolonged bleeding times when they injure cutaneous tissue.

Three main variants of the disorder exist (Triplett, 1991; Hilgartner and Corrigan, 1995). In the most common variant, type I, the total amount

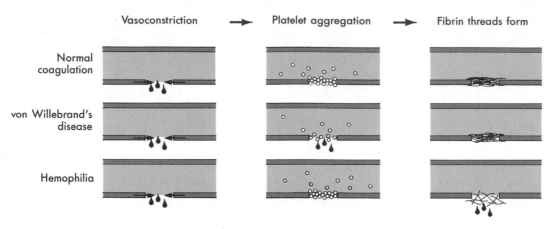

Fig. 9-1. Comparison of the defect in hemophilia and von Willebrand's disease with normal coagulation after a break occurs in a vessel wall. Defect in von Willebrand's disease is in platelet aggregation. Defect in hemophilia is in fibrin thread formation.

Table 9-1. **SEVERITY OF HEMOPHILIA**

Severity	Factor VIII and IX coagulant activity (%)	Frequency and type of bleeding
Severe	<1	By school age, often several bleeding episodes that require treatment occur each month.
		Bleeding may be spontaneous or the result of injury.
Moderate	1-5	Frequency of bleeding is variable.
		Spontaneous bleeding is less common.
Mild	>5	Generally bleeding is excessive only as a result of trauma or surgery.

Note: normal factor VIII and IX coagulant levels are generally >50% (>50 U/dl) but vary slightly between laboratories.

of the protein is decreased and both large and small forms (multimers) of the von Willebrand protein are present. Its inheritance is autosomal dominant. In type II the large and intermediate multimers are absent in the plasma and platelets. Of note are the potential for thrombocytopenia with desmopressin use in type IIB, in which the large multimers are absent in the plasma, and the autosomal recessive inheritance of the more rare type IIC, in which the large multimers are absent in the plasma and platelets. Type III is a severe autosomal recessive form of the disorder and is marked by the absence of detectable von Willebrand protein.

INCIDENCE

Hemophilia occurs in all ethnic groups, with an incidence of 1 in 7500 males (Goldsmith, 1994). Although the true incidence of von Willebrand's disease is not known, it is believed to be the most common inherited bleeding disorder. Many scientists estimate that von Willebrand's disease is present in over 1% of the general population (Montgomery and Scott, 1993; Mannucci, 1992; Miller, Lenzi, and Breen, 1989). Many cases are not diagnosed because of the mild nature of many of the symptoms.

CLINICAL MANIFESTATIONS AT TIME OF DIAGNOSIS

By 18 months of age, most children with severe hemophilia are diagnosed because of positive family history or unusual bleeding (see box on clinical manifestations). Before diagnosis, parents often are questioned regarding child abuse because of excessive bruising. Diagnosis in infancy most commonly occurs because of a positive family history confirmed by cord blood coagulation assays, intracranial hemorrhage, excessive bruising with hematomas, cephalohematoma, or bleeding following circumcision and venipuncture. Bleeding from the umbilical cord stump is indicative of factor XIII deficiency. Intracranial hemorrhage is life threatening and occurs in 1% to 5% of newborns with moderate to severe hemophilia (Michaud, Rivard and Chessex, 1991; Yoffe and Buchanan, 1988). Michaud and colleagues (1991) recommend that male newborns of known carriers be tested for hemophilia by cord blood sampling if not diagnosed prenatally. If a child has a positive prenatal diagnosis of hemophilia by cord blood analysis, they also recommend follow-up with Computerized tomography (CT) or ultrasonography in the first 24 hours of life, even after cesarean section. Cesarean section is not routinely recommended in nontraumatic deliveries. Although factor VIII levels generally rise to greater than 50% during pregnancy, carriers whose baseline levels are less than 50% are at particular risk for postpartum hemorrhage (Greer et al, 1991). The inheritance pattern for hemophilia is shown in Fig. 9-2.

When a newborn has a family history of hemophilia, circumcision, heel sticks, and immunizations should ideally be delayed until a definitive diagnosis is made. Vitamin K may be given subcutaneously. Diagnosis is performed prenatally or by using cord blood to test factor levels.

Children who first show signs later in childhood or in adolescence more frequently have mild to moderate hemophilia. A frequent misconception is that children with hemophilia can bleed to death from a typical childhood cut or scratch. They may, however, demonstrate joint bleeding (hemarthrosis), muscle hematomas, excessive postoperative bleeding, or excessive or prolonged oral bleeding following frenulum tears, lost deciduous teeth, tooth eruption, and dental extractions.

CLINICAL MANIFESTATIONS AT THE TIME OF DIAGNOSIS

Hemophilia

- Bleeding following circumcision
- Excessive bruising
- Hematomas after venipuncture or minimal injury
- Bleeding from the umbilical cord stump
- Intracranial bleeding
- Cephalohematoma
- Prolonged oral bleeding (after frenulum tear, dental extraction, tooth loss)
- Hemarthrosis (generally not the first symptom)

Von Willebrand's disease

- Prolonged oral bleeding
- Prolonged or repeated epistaxis
- Prolonged or excessive menstrual bleeding
- Gastrointestinal bleeding

Von Willebrand's disease is commonly manifested by bleeding from the mucous membranes. Although epistaxis is most frequently noted, excessive oral, gastrointestinal (GI), and menstrual bleeding also occur. Additional findings may include excessive bruising with hematomas, oozing following circumcision, or excessive postoperative bleeding (Aledort, 1994). Diagnostic testing is often requested in the presence of a positive family history of the disorder or when an increased partial thromboplastin time is obtained during routine preoperative screening. Because the level of the von Willebrand protein and factor VIII vary over time, coagulation testing may need to be repeated to establish a diagnosis (Triplett, 1991). Despite the relatively high incidence of this disorder, persons are frequently not diagnosed because the common symptoms of epistaxis and heavy menstrual bleeding are often not brought to medical attention.

Hemophilia Carrier Testing

A single performance of carrier testing for hemophilia using a factor VIII coagulant-antigen ratio

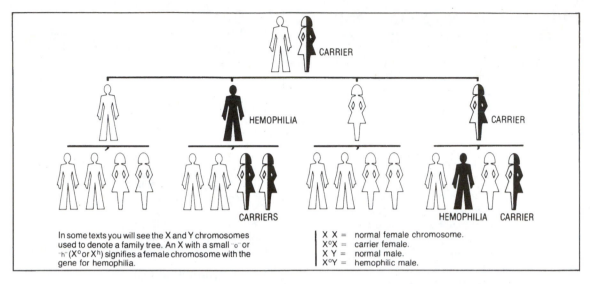

CARRIER

HEMOPHILIA

CARRIER

CARRIERS

HEMOPHILIA   CARRIER

In some texts you will see the X and Y chromosomes used to denote a family tree. An X with a small "o" or "h" (X°or Xʰ) signifies a female chromosome with the gene for hemophilia.

X X = normal female chromosome.
X°X = carrier female.
X Y = normal male.
X°Y = hemophilic male.

Fig. 9-2.   Inheritance pattern for hemophilia. *(From Eckert EF:* Your child and hemophilia, *New York, 1990, © The National Hemophilia Foundation.)*

has an accuracy rate of 80% to 90%, which increases when the test is repeated (White and Shoemaker, 1989). The use of DNA testing to detect carriers has an estimated accuracy of 95% to 99%, depending on the number of probes used; however, it is expensive and requires blood samples from multiple family members including an affected male (Kemahli et al, 1994). A newly discovered genetic defect found in approximately 50% of persons with severe hemophilia A is called an *inversion* and occurs when the distal end of the X chromosome containing part of the factor VIII gene flips over so that the factor VIII message is interrupted by irrelevant genetic material. If the affected male has this inversion, all female relatives who are carriers will also have it. This inversion test has 100% accuracy (Lakich et al, 1993). Carrier testing for factor IX hemophilia using DNA probes is also now available (Ketterling et al, 1991).

Prenatal diagnosis may be performed by amniocentesis as early as 13 to 16 weeks' gestation, by chorionic villus sampling at 8 to 12 weeks' gestation, or by fetal blood sampling at 18 to 20 weeks' gestation using percutaneous umbilical blood sampling. Male fetuses can be diagnosed as having hemophilia in utero by using DNA probes or by the

inversion test. In the event that percutaneous umbilical blood sampling is performed, the hemophilia diagnosis is made by means of a specialized test called factor VIII or factor IX clotting antigen (Koerper, 1990).

TREATMENT

Comprehensive Care

The standard of care in hemophilia is a collaborative interdisciplinary approach facilitated by local hemophilia treatment centers (HTCs). These centers, funded in part by the federal government, provide comprehensive management of inherited coagulation disorders, namely hemophilia and von Willebrand's disease. The core team consists of a pediatric hematologist, nurse coordinator, and social worker. Other integral team members are the genetic counselor and physical therapist. Consultative services are provided by a pediatric dentist and orthopedic surgeon. With the advent of human immunodeficiency virus (HIV), HTCs have also been mandated by the government to either provide or procure comprehensive management for their clients exposed to HIV. Services of the HTC include interdisciplinary comprehensive evaluations,

---

TREATMENT

- Factor replacement products (see Table 9-2)
- Desmopressin acetate (vWd and mild hemophilia)
- Prophylactic factor treatment (hemophilia)
- Estrogen therapy (vWd)
- Oral antifibrinolytic agents
- Topical hemostatic agents
- Physical therapy
- Surgery: synovectomy, joint replacement

---

counseling and support services, carrier detection, access to new technology treatment products through clinical trials, and home infusion instruction for those with severe hemophilia.

All children and adolescents with hemophilia and von Willebrand's disease should receive regular comprehensive evaluations at the nearest HTC. The frequency of evaluations is every 6 months to 1½ years, depending on the severity of the child's bleeding disorder, use of prophylaxis, and immune status. At these visits, children and their families are routinely seen by the members of the interdisciplinary team. Families and the primary care provider receive updated information on the status of the child's health and development, treatment options, and readiness for home therapy. The centers work closely with primary care providers to give care that is comprehensive, coordinated, and accessible, and rely on them to provide day-to-day management of pediatric health care.

General Guidelines

The goals of treatment are to rapidly initiate clotting when bleeding occurs, prevent bleeding during high-risk procedures, and in many persons with severe hemophilia, to prevent joint bleeding through prophylactic infusions of factor concentrate (see box on treatment).

The treatment product of choice should be decided in consultation with the child's hematologist (Table 9-2). This information should be updated yearly, incorporating rapid changes in available technology. It recently has been shown that CD4 counts may be more stable in persons with HIV infection who use ultrapure factor concentrates when compared with those using intermediate purity concentrates (Hilgartner et al, 1993; Hoots, 1994; Serementis et al, 1993). This information should be considered when recommending factor concentrates for child use (Medical and Scientific Advisory Committee, 1992).

Some families who are not on home therapy keep a supply of the preferred concentrate in their home refrigerators to expedite treatment of their child in local emergency rooms. Factor concentrate need not be kept at school unless infusions are performed there.

Bleeding episodes frequently requiring hospital admission and hematologic consultation are significant head trauma or bleeding into the iliopsoas muscle (retroperitoneal), hip, GI tract, neck, or posterior pharynx. Consultation is also recommended for bleeding that requires more than two treatments, (i.e., concern that an inhibitor may be developing), and when there is any doubt as to the need to treat an injury or bleeding episode. However, when in doubt, it is safest to treat a suspected bleeding episode.

Providers are frequently asked by school personnel and families to recommend first-aid measures that can be instituted while the child is waiting for evaluation and possible infusion. For soft tissue, joint, and muscle bleeding, elevation of the affected area and the application of an elastic bandage and ice may help to reduce swelling. The child should be allowed to fully rest the affected joint. Firm pressure applied over a clean dressing is often sufficient to stop bleeding from surface lacerations in children with both hemophilia and von Willebrand's disease. Firm pressure applied to the nares is recommended for nose bleeding. Universal precautions must be used whenever blood or body secretions are encountered. Although ice may help to reduce the superficial swelling from a head hematoma, it should never replace a medical evaluation, because intracranial bleeding is unaffected by its application.

Hemophilia

In the early 1970s clotting factor concentrates revolutionized the treatment of hemophilia because of

Table 9-2. **TREATMENT PRODUCTS AND GENERAL GUIDELINES FOR USE**

Protein purification process and viral inactivation methods	Manufacturer or distributor	Product
Factor VIII concentrates		
Recombinant DNA	Miles	Kogenate
	Baxter Hyland	Recombinate
	Armour	Bioclate, Helixate
Immunoaffinity Purified (Ultrapure Products)		
Pasteurized	Armour	Monoclate P
Solvent-detergent	Baxter Hyland	Hemofil M
	American Red Cross	Coagulation FVIII, Method M
Intermediate and High Purity Products		
Solvent Detergent and Affinity Chromatography	Alpha	Alphanate
Solvent-detergent	Alpha	Profilate OSD
	Miles	Koate HP
Pasteurized	Armour	Humate P

Dosage: To increase factor VIII activity 2% (2 percentage points, or 2 U/dl), give 1 U/kg. Example: To treat an intracranial hemorrhage, 100% factor VIII activity is desired (dose = 50 U/kg for a child with a baseline level of <1% factor VIII).

Factor IX concentrates		
Coagulation Factor IX (purest)		
Solvent detergent	Alpha	Alphanine SD
Ultrafiltration Sodium Thiocyanate	Armour	Mononine
Factor IX Complex Concentrates		
Wet heat	Alpha	Profilnine HT
Dry heat	Miles	Konyne 80
	Baxter Hyland	Proplex T
Vapor heated	Immuno	Bebulin

Dosage: To increase factor IX activity 1% (1 percentage point, or 1 U/dl), give 1 U/kg. Example: To treat an intracranial hemorrhage, 100% factor IX activity is desired (dose = 100 U/kg for a child with a baseline level of <1% factor IX).

Inhibitor treatment products		
Factor VIII Products	As above	
Factor IX Complex Concentrates	As above	
Activated Factor IX Complex Concentrates		
Vapor treated	Immuno	FEIBA
Dry heat	Baxter Hyland	Autoplex
Porcine Factor VIII	Porton Products	Hyate C
Recombinant FVIIa (in clinical trials)	Novo Nordisk	NovoSeven

Adapted from Goldsmith J: *Hemophilia: current medical management,* New York, 1994; National Hemophilia Foundation, Medical and Scientific Advisory Committee of the National Hemophilia Foundation: *Recommendations concerning HIV infection, hepatitis, and other transmissible agents in the treatment of hemophilia (Medical Bulletin #226)* New York, 1995, National Hemophilia Foundation.

Continued.

Table 9-2.   **TREATMENT PRODUCTS AND GENERAL**
                    GUIDELINES FOR USE—cont'd

Desmopressin Acetate (DDAVP)
    Dosage: 0.3 micrograms/kg IV in 30-50 ml of normal saline.
    Administration: give over 15-30 minutes. Take blood pressure and pulse every 10 minutes during infusion.
        Decreased response if given more frequently than every 48 hours.
Stimate (desmopressin acetate) nasal spray (1.5 mg/ml) (150 μg/0.1 ml spray).
    Dosage: if patient weighs <50 kg, give 1 spray into one nostril only (total dose 150 μg).
        If patient weighs >50 kg, give 1 spray into each nostril (total dose 300 μg).
    Administration: intranasal. Decreased response if given more frequently than every 48 hours.
    Side effects (Applies to both IV and intranasal forms):
        Common: flushing, headache; enhancement of clot lysis (give with an antifibrinolytic agent when mouth or
           nose bleeding is being treated) (Bowie, 1984; Poole, 1987).
        Less common: tachycardia, hypertension, hyponatremia.
        Uncommon: seizures secondary to hyponatremia (more common if <2 yr of age)(Smith et al, 1989).

Oral antifibrinolytic agents
    ε-Aminocaproic acid (Amicar)
      Dosage: approximately 50-100 mg/kg/dose by mouth every 6 hours until site of bleeding is healed (dose
        guidelines vary greatly; consult child's hematologist).
      Supplied as 500-mg tablet and 250 mg/1 ml elixir.
    Tranexamic acid (Cyklokapron)
      Dosage: approximately 25 mg/kg/dose by mouth or 10 mg/kg IV every 8 hours.
      Supplied as 500-mg tablet, IV solution (100 mg/cc).
    Interactions: do not give in the presence of hematuria (enhances renal clot formation). Give at least 12 hours after
      or 6 hours before an activated PCC dose (otherwise may induce hypercoagulation).

their ease of administration, fewer allergic side effects, and ease of home storage compared with fresh frozen plasma and cryoprecipitate. Each vial of these same factor concentrates, contains the plasma of thousands of donors. Initial production methods did not inactivate HIV. Although there have been isolated cases of HIV seroconversion with the use of some unscreened or dry heat-treated products after 1987, there have been no seroconversions in viral safety studies of the concentrates that are currently available (Fricke et al, 1992). Although there have been no seroconversion to hepatitis B or C using products that are currently available, one cannot assume that the risk of hepatitis transmission has been completely eliminated (Kasper et al, 1993).

Large amounts of extraneous proteins in earlier products first led to the development of higher purity products using affinity purification techniques. The newest technologic advance in factor replacement is the use of recombinant DNA techniques to clone the human factor VIII gene (Kasper et al, 1993); this synthetic factor VIII is theoretically free of all human viruses.

Advanced technologic products for factor IX generally become available a few years after introduction of similar factor VIII concentrates (see Table 9-2). There are presently two types of factor IX products available for use: prothrombin complex concentrates, also known as factor IX complex concentrates, and the newer coagulation factor IX products. The prothrombin complex concentrates contain clotting factors II, VII, IX, and X and are known to be thrombogenic when given frequently and in large doses. The coagulation factor IX products contain only factor IX and do not induce thrombosis. Therefore those children who are having surgery, have experienced trauma, or are having a severe bleeding episode and require factor IX therapy more than once a day for several days in a row should be treated with one of the coagulation factor IX products. There have been no reported cases of thrombosis with these products (Goldsmith et al, 1992; Kim et al, 1992; Thompson, 1993).

Desmopressin acetate (DDAVP) is also effective in raising the levels of factor VIII in many children with mild factor VIII deficiency (Furie, Limentani, Rosenfield, 1994; Goldsmith, 1994). Its benefits include relatively few major side effects and the lack of viral contaminants, because it is not derived from human blood. DDAVP is discussed in greater detail in reference to von Willebrand treatment options.

Studies in the United States (Aledort et al, 1994), Sweden (Petrini et al, 1991; Nilsson et al, 1992), and Germany (Schramm, 1993) have documented that prophylactic factor treatment can maintain normal joint function when begun early and may prevent further deterioration even when arthropathy is present. Some dosing schedules are 20 to 40 units/kg/dose administered 3 times each week for children with hemophilia A, and 25 to 40 units/kg/dose administered 2 times each week for children with hemophilia B. A large prospective randomized study is planned to more accurately define the costs and benefits of prophylactic treatment when compared with traditional on-demand therapy (Bohn and Avorn, 1993).

Use of implanted venous access devices (IVAD) has been helpful when prophylactic or frequent treatment is needed in children with poor venous access. IVADs have been used successfully in many children with hemophilia with a relatively low incidence of sepsis and catheter occlusion (Zappa et al, 1994; Ljung et al, 1992).

Recent studies have shown that as many as 20% to 30% of persons with factor VIII deficiency will develop an inhibitor, or antibody, to infused factor VIII (Addiego et al, 1993; Ehrenforth et al, 1992). Most persons who will develop an inhibitor do so at an early age, after an average of 9 treatment days. A much smaller percentage, less than 5%, of persons

with factor IX deficiency will develop an inhibitor (Brettler, 1995). Many inhibitors are transient, or levels may be so low as to be clinically insignificant. However, half of these persons with inhibitors do develop significant inhibitors and cannot be treated with conventional factor VIII or IX therapy (Bray et al, 1994; Lusher, 1994; Lusher et al, 1993; Scharrer and Neutzling, 1993; White, 1994). Treatment options include immune tolerance regimens, high doses of certain factor concentrates that can bypass part of the standard clotting cascade (Kasper, 1989; Lusher, 1994), porcine factor VIII (Brettler et al, 1989; Hay et al, 1994), and a recombinant factor VIIa product which is still in clinical trials (Hedner, 1990; Serementis, 1994). The use of immune tolerance regimens, however, is becoming a more commonly accepted and desirable option (Kruetz et al, 1993; Mariani et al, 1994; Nilsson, 1994; Scheibel et al, 1987). These treatment regimens call for large doses of factor VIII or IX to be given daily in an effort to suppress or eradicate the inhibitor. When laboratory measurements indicate that suppression has been achieved, the frequency of administration and dosage of factor concentrate can be tapered. Success rates have been reported at 60% to 90% (Mariani, Ghirardini, and Bellocco, 1994). Some children, particularly those with high titer inhibitors, may also be given cyclophosphamide and intravenous gamma globulin to hasten the suppression of the inhibitor (Nilsson, Berntorp, and Zettervall, 1988).

The unit of measurement for products that replace the deficient factor protein is calculated in international units of factor VIII or IX activity. Choice of a particular dose is based on the type of hemophilia, severity of the bleeding episode, half life of the chosen product, the child's weight, occurrence in a chronically affected joint, and the likelihood of follow-up by the child and family within 24 hours (Table 9-3). Repeat doses may be given if significant improvement has not occurred.

Treatment is initiated as soon as a bleeding episode is identified. For bleeding of a joint, treatment may begin as early as the point at which a child notices the onset of tingling in the joint. Many have come to know this as the first indicator of oozing blood in that area. For another child, loss of range of motion of a joint, mild swelling, or mild pain may be the first recognizable indicators. In still

Table 9-3.   **ASSESSMENT AND TREATMENT OF COMMON
BLEEDING EPISODES***

Site of bleeding	Signs and symptoms	Treatment
Subcutaneous/soft tissue	Mild: not interfering with ROM, not enlarging	Ice, Ace wrap
	Moderate: occurring in wrist, volar surface or forearm, plantar surface of foot; interferes with ROM or is enlarging	Ice, splint/Ace wrap FVIII 20-30 U/kg or desmopressin† FIX 30-40 U/kg
	Severe: pharyngeal; areas listed in "moderate" category accompanied by change in neurologic signs	Admit to hospital FVIII 50 U/kg and follow-up doses FIX 80-100 U/kg and follow-up doses
Joint	Earlier: moderate swelling, mild to moderate pain, warmth, stiffness, limited motion	Rest, splint/crutches FVIII 20-25 U/kg or desmopressin† FIX 30 U/kg
	Later: tense swelling, moderate to severe pain, marked decrease in ROM; hip bleeding: limited abduction or adduction	Rest, splint/crutches PT plan May need repeat doses FVIII 30-40 U/kg FIX 40-50 U/kg Ultrasound follow-up for hip bleed
Muscle	Mild: swelling does not greatly affect ROM, mild discomfort	Rest, ±crutches, PT plan Ice, splint/Ace wrap FVIII 20-30 U/kg or desmopressin† FIX 20-40 U/kg
	Severe: swelling with neurologic changes, decreased ROM	Rest, splint/Ace wrap PT plan FVIII 50 U/kg and follow-up doses FIX 80-100 U/kg and follow-up doses
	Iliopsoas: abdominal, inguinal, or hip area pain, limited hip extension, numbness from nerve compression	Strict bed rest/hospitalization May need repeat doses FVIII 50 U/kg FIX 80-100 U/kg
Nose	Mild: <10 min	Pressure to nares
	Severe: prolonged or recurrent	Collagen hemostat fibers and nasal pack vWd desmopressin, EACA/TXA FVIII 20 U/kg or desmopressin† FIX 20 U/kg

Modified from: Hilgartner M, Corrigan J: Coagulation disorders. In Miller D, Baehner R, editors: *Blood diseases of infancy and childhood,* St. Louis, 1995, Mosby.
Note: Specific dosages may vary for individual patients; consult with child's hematologist.
*ROM, range of motion; FVIII, factor VIII hemophilia; FIX, factor IX hemophilia; U/kg, units of factor VIII or IX per kilogram (factor concentrate vials contain a given number of FVIII or FIX activity units); PT, physical therapy; vWd, von Willebrand's disease; EACA/TXA, antifibrinolytics: ε-aminocaproic acid and tranexamic acid; cryo, cryoprecipitate.
†Desmopressin may be used if, after a test dose, the child with mild hemophilia has achieved a factor VIII coagulant level equal to the level that would be achieved after the recommended dose of factor VIII concentrate. Example: For a moderate soft tissue bleed in the calf, a dose of 20-30 U/kg should raise a child's factor VIII level to 40% to 60%. If after desmopressin the child reached a peak of only 25%, it is likely desmopressin would not be beneficial.

Continued.

**Table 9-3.   ASSESSMENT AND TREATMENT OF COMMON
                    BLEEDING EPISODES*—cont'd**

Site of bleeding	Signs and symptoms	Treatment
Oral areas	Dental extractions; regional blocks; frenulum, tongue, or lip bleeding	Topical hemostatic agents EACA/TXA (caution with PCCs) May need follow-up doses May need hospitalization if hard to control or severe anemia vWd desmopressin FVIII 30-40 U/kg or desmopressin FIX 30-40 U/kg
Gastrointestinal system	Abdominal pain, hypotension, blood in emesis, tarry or red stools, weakness	Hospitalization likely vWd desmopressin/FVIII product with high level vWd FVIII 50 U/kg and follow-up doses FIX 100 U/kg and follow-up doses
Central nervous system	Head, neck, or spinal injury; presence of blurred vision, headaches, vomiting, unequal pupils, change in speech or behavior, drowsiness; if no symptoms yet significant injury, treat and observe	Hospitalization and/or rapid consult with hematologist depending on injury CT scan vWd desmopressin/FVIII product with high level vWd factor FVIII 50 U/kg for at least 1 wk FIX 80-100 U/kg for at least 1 wk
Urinary tract	Gross hematuria (bright red to brown); if clots present, more likely to infuse with factor concentrate	Push oral fluids, rest ±prednisone (2 mg/kg/day, maximum 60 mg/day) ±factor concentrate EACA/TXA *contraindicated*

FOLLOW-UP: By daily telephone contact or office visits through resolution of bleeding episode. If family is on home therapy, they should have telephone or office consultation if head, neck, or throat injury occurs, if >2 treatments are needed, or if bleeding occurs in hip, iliopsoas muscle, or urinary tract.

other children with high pain tolerances or little self-awareness of bodily changes, the bleeding episode may not be recognized until there is severe swelling, major limitation of joint motion, and severe pain. Joint and bone x-ray examinations are generally not needed unless the child has a history of trauma. Treatment is usually given on demand as soon as bleeding is identified but may be given prophylactically to facilitate healing when bleeding is recurrent or severe or before high-risk procedures such as surgery, dental extractions, and physical therapy of a chronically affected joint.

Vials of factor concentrate come in various concentrations. The number of *whole* vials that, at

a minimum, provide the desired dose is always given because of the cost of wasted medication and the lack of adverse sequelae from a dose slightly higher than that originally prescribed. Most concentrates may be given by slow intravenous (IV) push over 5 to 10 minutes. Because these concentrates are blood products, those who reconstitute the lyophylized factor should always wear gloves and dispose of supplies that contact the factor in approved infectious waste containers.

High-purity products, such as the recombinant and affinity purified factor VIII and IX concentrates, cost 3 to 4 times as much as the intermediate-purity products (Abramowicz, 1993).

For persons with severe hemophilia using at least 40,000 U/year, a 1-year supply of recombinant or ultrapure product would cost more than $40,000.

von Willebrand's Disease

The standard treatment for this disorder encompasses both synthetic and plasma-derived products. The primary care provider is urged to consult with the child's hematologist and the National Hemophilia Foundation for the most current recommendations.

Desmopressin acetate (see Table 9-2), a synthetic analog of vasopressin, is the treatment of choice for persons with von Willebrand's disease, excluding subtype IIB (Hilgartner and Corrigan, 1995). Although the mechanism of action is not completely understood, it is postulated that desmopressin releases stores of factor VIII and the von Willebrand protein from the endothelial lining of the blood vessels (Mannucci, 1992). Stores, however, may be depleted (see Table 9-2) if treatment is repeated more frequently than every 24 hours (Mannucci, Bettega, and Cattaneo, 1992).

Use of this medication for various bleeding episodes depends on the rise in coagulation protein activity or decrease in bleeding time after a test dose. Peak response is generally obtained 30 minutes after IV infusion is complete. Individuals tend to show consistency in the degree of response over time (Rodeghiero et al, 1989). Desmopressin has also been given subcutaneously with good results in some children (Köhler et al, 1989).

A concentrated intranasal form of desmopressin is now available as Stimate Nasal Spray (1.5 mg/ml). Its peak effect is obtained 1 hour after administration. A 300 µg dose given intranasally raises the factor VIII and ristocetin cofactor two- to threefold, an increase equivalent to a 0.2 µg/kg intravenous dose (Rose and Aledort, 1991). Studies have shown significant clinical response with the use of this intranasal form in children with mild hemophilia A and von Willebrand's disease who responded well to the intravenous form (Rose and Aledort, 1991; Lethagen and Tennvall, 1993). If a child has had prior desmopressin testing with the intravenous form, repeat laboratory testing with the intranasal form is still indicated before its clinical use.

If a blood product is needed to control bleeding in children with von Willebrand's disease, virally inactivated high-purity or intermediate-purity factor VIII concentrates containing von Willebrand factor are preferable to cryoprecipitate, which cannot be virally inactivated (Mannucci, 1992). Humate-P in particular has been clinically effective in controlling bleeding (Czapek et al, 1988).

Estrogens may be useful in the management of excessive menstrual and other types of bleeding because of their ability to increase levels of factor VIII and the von Willebrand protein (Aledort, 1991).

Oral Antifibrinolytic Agents

Children with hemophilia and von Willebrand's disease often have oral bleeding that requires additional medication to keep the clot stable once it has formed. Because of the presence of digestive enzymes in the saliva that lyse fibrin clots, antifibrinolytic agents should be given orally for 7 to 10 days or until the site of oral bleeding has completely healed (Hilgartner and Corrigan, 1995). Two such medications are ε-aminocaproic acid (Amicar) and tranexamic acid (Cyklokapron) (see Table 9-2).

Topical Hemostatic Agents

Collagen hemostat (Avitene) fibers can be applied to nasal packing or salt pork pledgets to control epitaxis or at the site of frenulum tears or tooth extraction. When nasal packing is used, it is generally left in place for 24 to 36 hours to promote stable clot formation. Nose bleeds frequently can be diminished by using petroleum jelly or antibiotic ointment in the nares or by humidification of room air.

Less conventional topical agents have been used successfully in the treatment of oral bleeding. Moistened tea bags containing tannic acid provide local hemostasis, and commercially available superbonding glue has also been effective in sealing tongue lacerations without concurrent bonding between mucous membrane surfaces (Rothman, 1990).

Fibrin glue has been used to promote local hemostasis in some circumcisions (Martinowitz et al, 1992). Cryoprecipitate is the source of fibrinogen in this treatment.

Pain Management

Uncontrolled bleeding into a joint or muscle can produce significant pain. Prompt replacement of the deficient coagulation protein is the most effective way to prevent significant pain and to relieve current pain. Mild pain may be treated with acetaminophen (not aspirin), ice, and elevation of the affected extremity. If pain is moderate or severe, acetaminophen with codeine every 4 to 6 hours is recommended. Pain medication is generally not necessary after the first day of factor replacement. Continued pain may suggest ineffective control of bleeding because of inadequate dosing of the factor concentrate, development of an inhibitor, or synovitis. Pain caused by irritation of the synovial lining may be more effectively treated with a nonsteroidal antiinflammatory agent. These agents should be used with caution, however, because they can cause GI bleeding secondary to interference with platelet aggregation.

Physical Therapy

Splinting and immobilization for 1 to 2 days after acute bleeding often aid resolution of the episode (Koch, 1985). A resting splint that extends the extremity in a comfortable position is recommended for night use for up to several days following a significant hemarthrosis to prevent further bleeding during sleep (Koch, 1985). Following severe bleeding or prolonged immobilization, a physical therapy program should be prescribed, thus enabling the child to achieve his or her baseline range of motion and to regain muscle mass. Factor replacement is often needed with vigorous physical therapy.

Surgical Intervention

Destruction of a joint secondary to repeated bleeding episodes can result in significant pain, decreased strength and range of motion, and an impaired ability to use the affected extremity. Several orthopedic procedures have been successful in individuals with hemophilia and can provide the individual with significantly reduced joint pain and greater range of motion and endurance (Luck and Kasper, 1989). Open synovectomy is successful in reducing pain and bleeding episodes; however, mobility is often lost and progression of the arthropathy continues (Greene, 1994; Teigland et al, 1994). Arthroscopic synovectomy reduces the pain and frequency of bleeding episodes without loss of mobility. A newer procedure, injection of a radioactive isotope into the affected joint to eradicate abnormal

synovium, has been quite successful in improving range of motion and decreasing bleeding episodes in those individuals who are not surgical candidates (Siegel et al, 1994). Once the child is fully grown and the epiphyseal plates are closed, total joint replacements, particularly of the knee, have been quite successful in individuals with hemophilia as measured by increased function and decreased pain and frequency of bleeding episodes (Teigland et al, 1993).

RECENT AND ANTICIPATED ADVANCES IN DIAGNOSIS AND MANAGEMENT

As previously discussed in greater detail, more accurate diagnosis of factor VIII hemophilia carrier status has been advanced by the discovery of a genetic defect found in approximately 50% of persons with severe hemophilia A. This genetic inversion has led to the development of a carrier detection test that is 100% accurate for families in whom the person with hemophilia carries this gene (Lakich et al, 1993). Factor IX hemophilia carrier testing has also become more accurate through the use of DNA probes (Ketterling et al, 1991).

Recent treatment advances include the availability of recombinant factor VIII concentrates that have a theoretical absence of the viral contamination risks of plasma-derived products, coagulation factor IX products that do not induce thrombosis when used frequently, and a concentrated intranasal form of DDAVP for the treatment of some children with mild hemophilia A and von Willebrand's disease.

In 1994, the Medical and Scientific Advisory Council of the National Hemophilia Foundation recommended that prophylactic factor treatment be considered "optimal therapy" for children with severe hemophilia. Routine preventive treatment, given 2 to 3 times per week, has demonstrated a significant reduction in the incidence and degree of joint deterioration. In addition, individuals on prophylaxis lose far fewer days from work or school and spend fewer days in the hospital (Aledort et al, 1994; Manco-Johnson et al, 1994).

Immune tolerance regimens have become the standard of treatment for the development of inhibitors. In addition, newer products, such as re-combinant Factor VIIa, are being developed to help bypass the inhibition of coagulation.

Attainment of a cure for hemophilia has been explored through liver transplantation and gene insertion therapy. Liver transplantation has been found to cure both hemophilia A and B because both factor VIII and factor IX are synthesized in the liver. However, liver transplantation is both an extremely costly and high-risk procedure and requires immunosuppressive therapy for life (Bontempo et al, 1987). Successful gene insertion therapy in the future may well provide a cure for hemophilia or, at the very least, convert persons with severe hemophilia to a milder form of the disorder. Research is currently underway in an attempt to find the best vector for gene expression and to define the best animal model for research (Hoeben et al, 1993; Lozier and Brinkhous, 1994).

ASSOCIATED PROBLEMS

Hematologic Problems

Anemia is found in some children with hemophilia in part because of sequestration of blood in joints and muscles during bleeding episodes. Significant anemia can also occur as a result of slow persistent oozing from oral bleeding or pooling of blood in muscle hemorrhages. In persons with von Willebrand's disease, excessive or prolonged menstrual bleeding or persistent or recurrent epistaxis can be problematic.

Neurologic Problems

Intracranial hemorrhage is the most frequent cause of death in children with hemophilia (Dietrich et al, 1994). If left untreated, it can result in spastic quadriplegia, developmental delay, or death. In some cases of intracranial bleeding, no known prior injury is identified. For this reason, any injury or neurologically related symptom should be treated aggressively. There may be significant intracranial bleeding without the presence of a "goose egg" because the most significant bleeding occurs from internal shearing of the brain and cranium. However, the presence of a hematoma indicates that the cranium may have met with significant force. Because of the high risk of rebleeding after intracranial bleeding, prophylactic factor treatment is contin-

ASSOCIATED PROBLEMS

- Anemia
- Neurologic deficits from intracranial hemorrhage
- Airway obstruction as a result of bleeding
- Hepatitis
- Gastrointestinal bleeding
- Inhibitor development
- HIV
- Arthropathy/arthritis
- Genital urinary bleeding
- Pain

ued for an extended period of time. Those with von Willebrand's disease also are at increased risk for this type of bleeding. Bleeding within or around the spinal column can also produce enough pressure to produce neurologic damage. Compartment syndrome resulting from nerve compression may occur following untreated bleeding into the forearm or calf.

Respiratory Problems

Posterior pharyngeal bleeding, increasing the potential for asphyxia, can result from a traumatic throat culture, bronchoscopy, or from dental extractions or deep injection of anesthetic without pretreatment with factor concentrates or desmopressin. Arterial blood gases should only be drawn after pretreatment with factor concentrate.

Hepatitis/Gastrointestinal Problems

In the past, exposure to blood products resulted in a high incidence of infection with hepatitis B and C in the hemophilia population. Approximately 75% of persons with hemophilia have been exposed to hepatitis B; approximately 8% are chronic carriers. Of the individuals with hemophilia, 80% to 90% have been exposed to hepatitis C (Blanchette et al, 1994; Kumar et al, 1993; Troisi et al, 1993). With the use of the hepatitis B vaccine series, the incidence of hepatitis B has been greatly reduced. In addition, the factor products currently on the market are considered to have a negligible risk of hepatitis transmission as a result of current screening and processing methods (Medical and Scientific Advisory Council of the National Hemophilia Foundation, 1994).

There are limited treatment options for both hepatitis B and C. Interferon Alfa-2b has approximately a 50% success rate in returning ALT values to normal and improving liver histology, but unfortunately, relapse is common after treatment (Davis et al, 1989; Korenman et al, 1991; Telfer et al, 1995). In persons who are coinfected with HIV and hepatitis C, it has been found that the HIV-induced immune dysfunction may increase hepatitis C replication and promote an increased incidence of liver disease and liver failure (Eyster et al, 1994).

Bleeding into the GI tract may occur in children with von Willebrand's disease and in those with hemophilia. The fragile mucous membrane-lined digestive system is prone to bleeding that can result from ulcers, gastritis, hemorrhoids, rectal fissures, and endoscopic procedures. This type of bleeding should be considered when there is either an unexplained drop in hemoglobin levels or abdominal pain.

Immunologic Problems

As many as 20% to 30% of persons with factor VIII deficiency will develop an inhibitor, or alloantibody, to infused factor VIII at an early age, after an average of 9 treatment days. Less than 5% of persons with factor IX deficiency will develop an inhibitor. Approximately half of inhibitors are transient, or levels are so low as to be clinically insignificant (Addiego et al, 1993; Brettler, 1995; Ehrenforth et al, 1992; Lusher, 1994; Scharrer and Neutzling, 1993; White, 1994). Level of inhibitor severity is measured in Bethesda units. Bleeding episodes are much more difficult to control and treatment options more limited when alloantibody formation occurs. There appears to be a genetic predisposition to the development of inhibitors.

Although the incidence varies greatly from center to center, approximately 70% of those exposed to untreated factor concentrates between 1978 and 1985 have developed HIV infection (Brettler and Levine, 1989). The incidence of HIV infection in persons with von Willebrand's disease who were exposed to cryoprecipitate is much lower, however, because of the smaller size of the donor pool.

Musculoskeletal Problems

The normally smooth synovial lining of a joint produces synovial fluid that with the cartilage serves as a shock absorber for the joint (Fig. 9-3). The synovium is also supplied with many blood vessels. When bleeding into a joint ceases with the administration of the deficient coagulation protein, enzymes clear away the blood from the synovial fluid. These enzymes, however, do not seem to focus their destruction solely on the unwanted blood cells; they begin to eat away at the smooth synovial lining, producing breaks in the surface that can make it easier for bleeding to recur in that joint. Eventually the cartilaginous surface of the bones may undergo destruction by these enzymes (Arnold and Hilgartner, 1977; Pettersson, 1993). The more blood that accumulates in the joint capsule, the more enzymes that are released. This destructive process can ultimately lead to fusion of the joint. A single hip hemarthrosis can produce aseptic necrosis of the femoral head if bleeding is not fully resolved. When bleeding recurs in a specific joint, it may be referred to as a "target joint." Thus a strong case is made, minimally, for early detection and treatment of bleeding episodes, and ultimately, for the use of prophylactic treatment for children with severe hemophilia (Aledort et al, 1994; Gilbert, 1993).

The nonintact synovial lining can cause the synovium to produce abnormal amounts of fluid in an inflammatory response, which is known as *synovitis*. Even when actual bleeding into the joint does not occur, the joint may become swollen and stiff. Synovitis is differentiated from a hemarthrosis by its gradual onset, mild or absent pain, and fuller range of motion.

Genitourinary Problems

If a boy has bleeding into the testicle that is not treated promptly, future fertility and maintenance of a patent urinary tract may be compromised. This type of bleeding can result from riding on an adult's shoulders, performing bicycle stunts, or taking part in vigorous play on a rocking horse or playground toy.

Hematuria occurs most commonly in adolescents with hemophilia, is usually not a result of trauma, is of short duration, and often stops spontaneously (Lusher and Warrier, 1991). Clots can

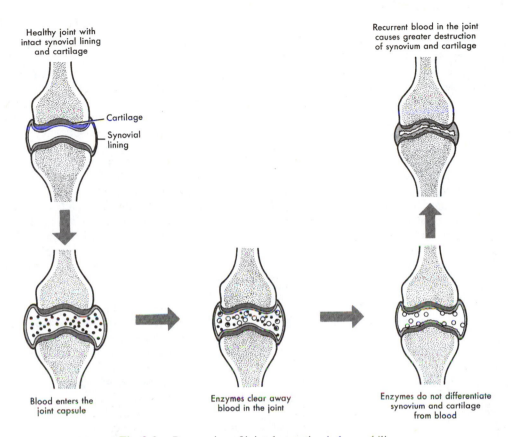

Fig. 9-3.   Progression of joint destruction in hemophilia.

sometimes cause renal or ureteral obstruction with temporary renal colic and, at times, hydronephrosis.

PROGNOSIS

The major factors contributing to morbidity in hemophilia are neurologic sequelae of intracranial bleeding, disability from chronic joint disease (arthropathy), liver disease secondary to hepatitis, and HIV infection. Intracranial bleeding that occurs at or soon after birth may result in spastic quadriplegia and brain damage, whereas bleeding that occurs later in life may affect the achievement of developmental milestones. Because of the availability of clotting factor concentrates, disabling arthropathy in childhood is now much less common. However, those who are affected by it often have visible deformities, increased school absen-

teeism, and more difficulty finding suitable employment. Before the use of heat-treated concentrates, approximately 75% to 90% of those treated were exposed to hepatitis B, with 5% to 10% becoming chronic carriers (Brettler and Levine, 1989; Troisi et al, 1993. It is also believed that 90% to 100% of those who received untreated products have been exposed to hepatitis C (Brettler and Levine, 1989; Troisi et al, 1993). The incidence of hepatitis should decrease with the use of more highly purified products and use of the hepatitis B vaccine. The rate of HIV infection among adolescents with hemophilia in the United States ranges between 22% and 75% depending on the type of clotting factor received and the treatment center surveyed (Brady and Humphries, 1990).

By the mid- to late 1970s, life expectancy of persons with hemophilia approached that of the general population (Hilgartner, Aledort, and

Giardina, 1985). HIV-related disease is now the leading cause of death in persons with hemophilia, accounting for 55% of deaths from 1987 to 1989. However, in those not affected with HIV, the leading causes of death are circulatory disease and bleeding, especially from intracranial hemorrhage (Chorba et al, 1994). These were the leading causes of death for all persons with hemophilia between 1979 and 1985.

Data regarding morbidity and mortality of persons with von Willebrand's disease are not readily available; however, because of the generally mild nature of the disorder, life expectancy is postulated to be normal. The relatively small number who have been infected with HIV or hepatitis through infusions of cryoprecipitate have a decreased life expectancy.

Primary Care Management
HEALTH CARE MAINTENANCE
Growth and Development

Monitoring a child's weight is particularly important because obesity places added stress on joints and muscles. Limb length may be increased by bony overgrowth of the epiphysis from chronic arthropathy. Gait disturbances caused by scoliosis may predispose an individual with hemophilia to joint or muscle bleeding.

A thorough baseline and ongoing assessment of developmental parameters and neurologic status is useful in follow-up for head trauma and for screening of potentially undiagnosed or unreported intracranial bleeding. Normal development is anticipated unless there has been a history of intracranial bleeding.

Diet

It is especially important for children with bleeding disorders to meet the recommended requirements for protein and calcium intake because of their role in bone and muscle formation. A nonconstipating diet may prevent rectal bleeding that can occur when hard stools are passed. When a child has mouth bleeding, a soft diet and avoidance of hot foods, those with sharp edges (chips), and straws (because the sucking action can disturb the clot), are recommended.

Safety

Protection against head injury is of primary importance. A protective helmet for children with hemophilia who are learning to walk may reduce the risk of head injury. However, use of a helmet is controversial because helmets also restrict peripheral vision and can provide the child and parent with a false sense of security. Knee pads may be used in the pants of toddlers prone to knee hematomas. High-top leather sneakers and shoes are suggested for children at risk for hemarthroses from the time they start to walk.

Contact sports such as football, soccer, hockey, wrestling, boxing, and vigorous competitive basketball are strongly discouraged because of the increased chance of head trauma. However, appropriate physical activity is encouraged to maintain strong muscles that promote joint stability and to promote normal social adjustment. Swimming is an ideal aerobic activity. Although recommended for all children, helmets are of particular importance for those with bleeding disorders when they are riding bikes or scooters or using rollerskates/blades. In addition, knee and elbow pads are recommended for roller skating/blading. Skateboarding is not recommended even with the use of a helmet.

Use of a medical identification emblem that includes diagnosis, treatment product, and blood type is required for safety. Infants can have the emblem pinned to their car seats or jackets when traveling. Older children who grow up wearing an emblem become accustomed to it. A wallet identification card may be used if the child or adolescent refuses to wear the emblem. Medical information should be checked yearly and updated as necessary.

Families participating in a home infusion program should follow accepted guidelines for infection control, including both use of gloves to mix and administer factor concentrates, and the disposal of infectious wastes in approved containers that are then disposed of at the hospital or picked up by a home care company.

Immunizations

Routine injectable vaccines should be given subcutaneously, when possible, because intramuscular injections may cause muscle bleeding. Several sources state that some vaccines should be given intramuscularly because subcutaneous injection can cause severe local skin reactions with tissue damage. These vaccines are the hepatitis B, DPT, and Pedvax HIB [PRP-OMP] vaccines (Eckert, 1990; Committee on Infectious Diseases, 1994). While Evans and Shaw (1990) could show no adverse sequelae from giving the hepatitis B vaccine intramuscularly to persons with hemophilia, Santagostino and colleagues (1993) continue to recommend that it be given subcutaneously. When any injectable vaccine is given, the following interventions can help to prevent hematoma development: applying firm pressure to the site for 5 minutes, use of a 25-gauge needle, and use of factor concentrate before intramuscular injection.

Before the oral polio vaccine is given, it is important to obtain a history of exposure to HIV and determine potential contact with others who are infected with HIV. Even if the child is not at risk for HIV infection, those with hemophilia are likely to have close family contacts who also have hemophilia and who may be infected with HIV. If children or adolescents were exposed to blood products before 1985 and test positive for the HIV antibody, have not yet been tested, or have close household contact with a person with HIV infection, they should receive the inactivated polio vaccine.

The hepatitis B vaccine series is recommended for all children likely to be exposed to blood products. If the at-risk child did not receive the vaccine as an infant, the vaccine may be administered immediately and again at 1 month and 6 months after the first dose. Santagostino and colleagues (1993) studied the effects of an accelerated vaccine series, given subcutaneously, for persons with hemophilia in which the vaccine was given immediately and again at 2 weeks, 6 weeks, and 24 weeks after the first dose. Protective titers were produced in 80% of participants by week 8 and in 93% by week 24. The investigators felt that the fourth (booster) dose was needed because titers were lower than those achieved when giving the vaccine intramuscularly. Although there are currently no recommendations for routine booster doses (Committee on Infectious Diseases, 1994; Greenberg, 1993), many providers feel that persons at high risk for blood product exposure should have antibody titers checked and booster doses given if titers are low (Tedder, Zuckerman, and Brink, 1993; Lunn, 1993).

The newly available hepatitis A vaccine has been recommended for use in persons with bleeding disorders who are at least 2 years of age and who are seronegative for the hepatitis A virus (Medical and Scientific Advisory Committee, 1995). Recommendations for those children under 2 years of age is still pending FDA approval. Currently, a two-dose series is recommended for adults (at 0 and 6 to 12 months) and a three-dose series for children 2 years of age and older (at 0, 1, and 6 months). Revaccination may be needed in those persons who have lost immunity to the hepatitis A antigen.

Screening

Vision. Following an eye injury, referral to an ophthalmologist is recommended, with follow-up until resolution is obtained. Otherwise, routine office screening and attention to the fundal examination are sufficient.

Hearing. Routine screening is recommended.

Dental. Invasive dental procedures can often be prevented through careful oral hygiene (including flossing under parental supervision) and regular dental evaluations. An initial dental evaluation is recommended by 2 to 3 years of age (Eckert, 1990), in part to help the child establish a positive relationship with the dentist, and to impress upon parents the importance of preventive care. Pediatric dentists with expertise in the management of persons with bleeding disorders are often associated with the local hemophilia treatment center. If needed, local dentists can manage most procedures with consultation. Prophylactic treatment with desmopressin or factor concentrate may not be necessary for routine dental cleaning or anesthetic infiltrates close to the gum line. For dental extractions and regional blocks, desmopressin, factor concentrate, an antifibrinolytic, or a combination of these is recommended (Hilgartner and Corrigan, 1995). If the child has an implantable port, external venous catheter, or joint replacement, some treatment centers advocate the use of subacute bacterial endocarditis (SBE) antibiotic prophylaxis, although these indications are not specifically noted in the American Academy of Pediatrics' 1994 edition of *The Red Book: Report of the Committee on Infectious Diseases.*

Blood pressure. Routine screening is recommended.

Hematocrit. Annual screening for anemia is recommended. Nosebleeds that are short in duration but occur frequently may not be regularly reported by families and may lead to significant anemia. If venipuncture is required, a 23-gauge butterfly needle should be used and firm pressure should be applied to the site for at least 5 minutes to prevent hematoma formation. Trauma may be reduced if a skilled pediatric phlebotomist performs venipuncture.

Urinalysis. An annual urinalysis is recommended to screen for microscopic hematuria.

Tuberculosis. Routine screening is recommended. No factor pretreatment is needed for tine or PPD skin testing.

Condition-specific screening. Children who have received any blood products in the past year should have liver function studies performed. For those with hemophilia, a factor VIII or IX inhibitor screen should also be administered, but these tests are usually performed during comprehensive evaluations at the hemophilia treatment center. HIV antibody testing with pretest and posttest counseling are recommended for children and adolescents exposed to blood products before 1986.

COMMON ILLNESS MANAGEMENT

Differential Diagnosis

Headaches and head injury. Intracranial bleeding must be ruled out whenever there is a history of injury within the past several days, focal headaches, or vomiting without GI distress. A CT scan is often helpful in ruling out intracranial bleeding. However, providers in consultation with the hemophilia team will often treat the child with factor concentrate or desmopressin prophylactically to achieve a factor VIII or IX level of 100% if either significant history or physical symptoms are present. This conservative approach is often adopted because of the serious implications of a delay in diagnosis. Therapy may cease after the resolution of symptoms if scans remain normal. If bleeding is documented, the child would need hospitalization and factor replacement regularly for several weeks or longer.

Visual disturbance. In the presence of acute changes in visual acuity, it is necessary to rule out intraocular bleeding by performance of a thorough funduscopic examination. In the presence of documented bleeding, ocular injury, or persistent visual changes, referral to an ophthalmologist is warranted.

Fever. When children with indwelling venous access devices develop a fever, blood cultures should be drawn and intravenous antibiotics begun until the cultures are shown to be negative. These indwelling devices present a significant risk for infection even in children whose immune systems are not suppressed.

If pretreated with factor concentrates, children with hemophilia may have lumbar punctures performed safely (Silverman et al, 1993), should they be required for a sepsis work-up.

Sore throat. If a throat culture is indicated, extreme caution must be exercised because of the potential for posterior pharyngeal bleeding. A throat culture should not be attempted in an uncooperative child. If streptococcal pharyngitis is suspected, a course of penicillin should be initiated based on history and physical findings.

Mouth bleeding. Although oral bleeding may not appear profuse in children with hemophilia, persistent slow oozing can cause a significant drop in hemoglobin levels. Bleeding is often not well controlled with the use of topical measures and antifibrinolytics alone. In most cases, factor replacement or the use of desmopressin is also required. Rebleeding in the first week can be prevented by use of a soft diet and avoidance of straws, hot foods, chips, and toys placed in the mouth.

Abdominal pain. In children with hemophilia or von Willebrand's disease, the primary care practitioner should have a high index of suspicion for GI bleeding in the presence of acute abdominal pain or significant drop in hemoglobin levels in the absence of other bleeding. Testing stool or emesis for blood can easily be done in the office as a screening tool. In hemophilia, iliopsoas bleeding (i.e., combination of the iliacus muscle [origin, iliac fossa; insertion, greater trochanter] and psoas muscle [origin, thoracic and lumbar vertebrae; insertion, lesser trochanter]) can cause pain in the abdomen or in the inguinal area. Psoas bleeding can result in a large amount of blood loss and in nerve damage necessitating hip joint replacement in some men. Hospital admission is often required for iliopsoas and GI bleeding.

Gait disturbance. Gait disturbance may be the result of scoliosis or bleeding in or around the ankle, knee, hip, or iliopsoas muscle. Inability to fully extend the hip, and later, leg paresthesias are characteristics of iliopsoas bleeding. Ultrasonography is useful for confirmation. Bleeding into the hip socket, which is rare in children, is characterized by limitation of hip abduction and adduction. Hospital admission is often required for severe hip or iliopsoas bleeding.

Dysuria and hematuria. Pressure within the urinary tract can cause dysuria. It is necessary to rule out testicular bleeding. Frequently, bleeding into the testicular area is quite pronounced, with obvious bruising and swelling. Hospitalization may be required for aggressive therapy and bed rest. Hematuria may be spontaneous and related directly to the bleeding disorder. However, whenever it occurs, the origin of bleeding within the urinary tract and potential infection should be considered. Increased fluid intake, bed rest, and avoidance of antifibrinolytic agents, as these may cause obstructive clots, are routinely recommended as part of a treatment plan. The benefits of treating with factor concentrate or corticosteroids, however, are debated among clinicians.

Heavy menstrual bleeding. Women who are hemophilia carriers or who have von Willebrand's disease may have heavy menstrual flow resulting in anemia. Once other causes have been ruled out, these women may benefit from treatment with estrogen therapy in the form of oral contraceptives or the use of intranasal DDAVP.

Numbness, tingling, and pain. Compression of nerves caused by deep or superficial hematomas should be suspected in individuals with changes in sensation or focal pain. Bleeding in or near the calf, volar surface of the forearm, spine, buttock, and iliopsoas muscle can lead to neurologic changes.

Drug Interactions

All products that contain aspirin are contraindicated. Caution should also be exercised with prolonged use of other medications that can affect platelet aggregation, such as antihistamines, guaifenesin (cough medications), dextromethorphan (cough medications), and nonsteroidal antiinflammatory agents. Because of the proliferation of over-the-counter medications, a list of those that can affect bleeding may be obsolete soon after compilation. It is more helpful to educate parents about how to read medication labels, for example, choosing those with acetaminophen rather than those with acetylsalicylic acid, and how to enlist the help of the pharmacist when they are in doubt about the use of a particular product.

Oral antifibrinolytic agents (e.g., Amicar and Cyklokapron) and prothrombin complex concentrates ideally should not be given within the same 24 hours because of an increased risk of hypercoagulation.

DEVELOPMENTAL ISSUES

Sleep Patterns

Standard developmental counseling is advised.

Toileting

Standard developmental counseling is advised.

Discipline

Some families tend to overprotect the child with a bleeding disorder and may be more strict with unaffected siblings. Age and developmentally appropriate, positive disciplinary techniques that do not include physical punishment should be recommended for all children. Pulling a child with a bleeding disorder by the arm is a specific action that may result in serious shoulder bleeding and radial head subluxation. The primary care provider should evaluate the disciplinary style of the parents and offer counseling on alternative discipline measures if potentially injurious methods are used.

Child Care

Contact with the proposed source of child care can help allay fears and clarify the caretaker's responsibilities with regard to the prevention and management of bleeding episodes. Hemophilia treatment center personnel or the primary care provider may provide this service. For children with hemophilia, it is helpful to emphasize that early recognition of bleeding (mild swelling or slight change in range of motion) and rapid access to medical evaluation and treatment are of primary importance. Spontaneous bleeding may occur, however, despite diligent safety efforts. Child care providers should be discouraged from trying to make treatment decisions without the input of the parents. This is especially applicable when seemingly mild head "bumps" occur. To find the safest environment possible, parents may be encouraged to seek out sources of child care that have smaller numbers of children per provider, those with protective ground cover under outside activity spaces, and a staff that is willing to learn about the special needs and activity requirements of a child with a bleeding disorder. Some facilities may be fearful of admitting children with bleeding disorders because of their fear of liability or potential HIV infection.

Schooling

The teacher, school nurse, and athletic coaches should be informed of the child's bleeding disorder. Families and children may be reticent to disclose the diagnosis to others, fearing discrimination because of the connection between hemophilia and HIV. The most frequent concerns of school personnel are prevention of bleeding (which may not be possible), emergency management, and fear of HIV infection. Many HTCs offer school visits by the program's nurse coordinator and social worker. These educational visits are most helpful on entrance to a new school and should be done with the permission and, most ideally, the participation of the child and parent or parents. It is not uncommon for children and adolescents with hemophilia to encounter peer disbelief that the disability and the need for crutches or a sling created by an acute bleeding episode can resolve in 1 to 2 days.

Alterations in body image and self-esteem may be precipitated by chronic joint arthropathy or limitations on physical activity caused by the bleeding disorder. From the time of diagnosis, parents may be assisted in guiding their child toward skills, careers, and sports that place lower stress on joints and are not associated with high rates of injury. It is critical that the child have activities and skills at which he/she can excel. The advent of prophylaxis has enabled more "normal" active play without the fear of increased injury and bleeding.

Children with learning problems resulting from intracranial bleeding must be fully evaluated and provided with appropriate support.

Sexuality

Safe-sex counseling, including decision-making skills, values clarification, and instruction in the use of condoms to prevent transmission of HIV, hepatitis B, and other sexually transmitted diseases, should be offered to all adolescents. Some adolescents who test HIV-antibody positive may avoid sexual relationships because of fear of rejection once their status is known to a potential partner.

The genetic counselor at the HTC interacts with children beginning with basic education regarding the inheritance of the bleeding disorder and eventually including a discussion of reproductive options.

Transition into Adulthood

The transition from adolescence to adulthood can be particularly stressful for some individuals with bleeding disorders. When they approach adulthood, many individuals with bleeding disorders have their comprehensive Hemophilia Treatment Center medical care transferred from the pediatric hematology service to the adult hematology service. Some young men experience feelings of anger and rejection because of the need to develop relationships with new providers, while severing the nurturing relationships they have had since infancy with the pediatric team. This is usually the time when the responsibility for medical care is transferred from parents to the young adult. In addition, choice of college may be influenced by availability of specialized medical care in the area, and career choice may be influenced by physical limitations.

As adolescents make the transition into adulthood, they may no longer be eligible for medical coverage under their parent's policy and may have difficulty finding coverage that will accommodate their disorder. In many states, there are special programs that cover individuals with hemophilia, or the individual may be eligible for a federal government program such as Medicare, Medicaid, or Supplemental Security Income (SSI) as a result of disability.

SPECIAL FAMILY CONCERNS AND RESOURCES

If the child with a bleeding disorder has excessive bruising before and after diagnosis, parents will frequently encounter questions regarding suspected child abuse from health care providers, or stares from friends, relatives, teachers, and strangers. Compounding the distress of the parents may be guilt regarding the inheritance of the bleeding disorder.

It is difficult for parents to cope with their inability to prevent bleeding episodes despite diligent efforts to prevent injury. Fear of injury to the infant may even interfere with parent-infant bonding. When the child does require an infusion of blood products to stop bleeding, parents often continue to question the viral safety of the product despite current data on product safety. Although most children and adolescents exposed to HIV have been tested for the antibody, families may continue to fear future positive test results.

Reimbursement for factor replacement has reached crisis proportions as adults and in some cases children reach maximum lifetime amount of insurance reimbursement and medical providers debate the cost-effectiveness of ultrapure products.

The societal myth that bleeding disorders constitute a "white man's disease" has led to feelings of isolation among many minority groups. Persons with hemophilia may receive little understanding from their own ethnic community and may even encounter racial bias in the delayed diagnosis of a hemarthrosis. Imagine this true incident in which an African-American man is assumed to be having a sickle cell episode when he presents with a swollen joint rather than being treated with a prompt infusion of factor concentrate. In many Asian cultures, it is a sign of weakness to tell others about an illness or disease. A Latino outreach worker has commented that many Latinos are hesitant to join organized support networks for their disorder because they fear stigmatization. Women are another minority group that has been overlooked regarding the impact of bleeding disorders or carrier status (National Hemophilia Foundation, 1994; Odubiyi, 1994).

The National Hemophilia Foundation (NHF) has made an effort to reach out to minority groups through CODP (Chapter Outreach Demonstration Projects) grants to local chapters. These grants are funded in part by the Maternal Child Health Bureau and the Centers for Disease Control. The NHF has a listing of chapters and organizations who have active CODP programs. There is also a specific support network for men (MANN: Men's Advocacy Network of NHF), and one for women (WONN: Women's Outreach Network of NHF).

Organizations

The National Hemophilia Foundation* and its local chapters disseminate information regarding recent advances in therapy not only for hemophilia and von Willebrand's disease but also for HIV infection. Its active membership includes consumers, their families, and health care providers at hemophilia treatment centers. The local chapters provide educational programs and support services to meet the members' needs.

HTCs also provide educational programs and support groups for children and adolescents with bleeding disorders and their families. A list of HTCs is available from the National Hemophilia Foundation.

---

*National Hemophilia Foundation, Soho Bldg, 110 Greene St, Suite 303, New York, NY, 10012 (212) 219-8180.

SUMMARY OF PRIMARY CARE NEEDS FOR THE CHILD WITH BLEEDING DISORDERS: HEMOPHILIA AND VON WILLEBRAND'S DISEASE

If the child or adolescent with a bleeding disorder also has HIV infection, please see additional guidelines given in Chapter 22.

Health care maintenance

Growth and development

Developmental screening should be done as a follow-up for head trauma or to screen for undiagnosed or unreported intracranial bleeding.

Diet

Adequate protein and calcium intake is of particular importance because of the role of both in bone and muscle formation.
Obesity should be avoided because it places extra stress on joints.

Safety

May recommend a protective helmet for children who are learning to walk to reduce the risk of head injury. Use of a helmet is controversial because it restricts peripheral vision.
Knee pads in the pants of toddlers may decrease knee hematomas.
Recommend high-top sneakers and shoes (not canvas type) for children at risk for hemarthroses from the time they start to walk.
Encourage participation in noncontact sports.
Recommend wearing a medical identification emblem that includes information regarding diagnosis, treatment product, and blood type. The information should be updated annually. .
Discourage activities that increase the chance of testicular bleeding, particularly in boys with moderate or severe hemophilia.
Families participating in a home infusion program should follow accepted guidelines for universal precaution and disposal of infectious wastes.

Immunizations

Some sources recommend that the hepatitis B, DPT, and PedVax HIB vaccines be given intramuscularly, despite risk of bleeding, whereas other sources recommend giving all immunizations subcutaneously.

Hepatitis A vaccine is recommended for persons 2 years of age or older.
Some children may require factor replacements before immunization injections.
Injectable vaccines should be given with a 25-gauge needle.
Firm pressure should be applied over the immunization site for 5 minutes.
Because of potential contact with family members who may have hemophilia and HIV infection, inactivated polio vaccine may be needed. Inactivated vaccine is also indicated when the child is untested for HIV but has been exposed during risk years.
The hepatitis B vaccine series is recommended for all children likely to be exposed to blood products.

Screening

Vision
Examination for eye injury should be done by an ophthalmologist. Routine office screening with attention to funduscopic examination is recommended.
Hearing
Routine screening is recommended.
Do not curette wax aggressively.
Dental
Initially, teeth should be evaluated at 2-3 years of age, followed by regular routine examinations. Hygiene should include flossing under supervision. Factor replacement or desmopressin is recommended for regional blocks; an antifibrinolytic should be added for dental extractions.
Blood pressure
Annual screening is recommended.
Hematocrit
Annual screening is recommended.
Use a 23-gauge butterfly needle for venipuncture in persons of any age.
Urinalysis
Annual screening for microscopic hematuria is recommended.

Continued.

SUMMARY OF PRIMARY CARE NEEDS FOR THE CHILD WITH BLEEDING DISORDERS: HEMOPHILIA AND VON WILLEBRAND'S DISEASE—cont'd

Tuberculosis
Routine screening is recommended.
Condition-specific screening
If blood product has been received in the past year, a factor VII or IX inhibitor screen (specifically for persons with hemophilia) and liver function studies are indicated. HIV antibody testing with precounseling and postcounseling are recommended for those exposed to blood products before 1986.

Common illness management

Differential diagnosis

Headaches and head injury
Rule out intracranial bleeding, especially with concurrent vomiting and absence of GI symptoms.
Visual disturbance
Rule out intraocular bleeding.
Fever
If indwelling venous access device is present, blood cultures must be drawn and intravenous antibiotics started.
Sore throat
Throat cultures present a risk for posterior pharyngeal bleeding. Cultures should not be taken from an uncooperative child.
Mouth bleeding
Mouth bleeding often requires factor replacement in addition to topical measures and antifibrinolytic agents.
Abdominal pain
Rule out GI bleeding. Rule out iliopsoas muscle bleeding with groin pain and decreased hip extension.
Gait disturbance
Rule out scoliosis and bleeding in and around the ankle, knee, hip, and iliopsoas muscle.
Dysuria and hematuria
Rule out testicular bleeding, renal or ureteral bleeding, and infection.
Heavy menstrual bleeding
May occur in hemophilia carriers or women with von Willebrand's disease. DDAVP or estrogen therapy may be helpful.

Numbness, tingling, and pain
Rule out nerve compression caused by bleeding.

Drug interactions

Products that contain aspirin are contraindicated.
Prolonged use of other substances that can affect platelet aggregation such as antihistamines, guaifenesin, dextromethorphan, and nonsteroidal antiinflammatory agents should be avoided.

Developmental issues

Sleep patterns

Standard developmental counseling is advised.

Toileting

Standard developmental counseling is advised.

Discipline

Recognize the potential for overprotection of the affected child and the use of deferential disciplinary methods when compared with unaffected siblings.
Pulling a child by the arm may result in shoulder joint bleeding.
Physical punishment may result in internal bleeding.

Child care

Contact with the proposed source of care by the primary health care provider or hemophilia treatment center staff is often useful to allay fears and clarify responsibilities with regard to prevention and management of bleeding episodes and trauma. The importance of early recognition and treatment of bleeding should be stressed.
Recognize that the child care provider may have fears regarding potential HIV infection.

Schooling

School visits are most helpful on enrollment in a new school and ideally include the child and parent or parents.
Because of the difficulty in understanding acute onset and resolution of bleeding episodes, peer acceptance may initially be poor.

Continued.

SUMMARY OF PRIMARY CARE NEEDS FOR THE CHILD WITH BLEEDING DISORDERS: HEMOPHILIA AND VON WILLEBRAND'S DISEASE—cont'd

Acknowledge potential fear of HIV infection among school personnel, and educate regarding transmission.

Recognize potential alterations in body image and self-esteem because of chronic joint arthropathy or limitations on physical activity.

Intracranial bleeding may result in learning problems.

Sexuality

Delay circumcision until the child with a positive family history is screened for bleeding disorders.

Safe-sex counseling is recommended to prevent sexually transmitted diseases.

Transition into adulthood

The transfer of medical care from a pediatric center to an adult hemophilia center may be difficult.

Educational and career opportunities may be restricted because of physical limitations and the need to be near a treatment center.

Obtaining health care coverage for a bleeding disorder may be difficult and may limit employment opportunities. The individual may be eligible for SSI if disabilities are significant.

Special family concerns

Child abuse may be suspected.

Parents may experience guilt regarding hereditary nature of a bleeding disorder.

The fear of injury to an infant may decrease parent-infant bonding.

Parents may fear the inability to prevent bleeding episodes despite attempts to prevent injury.

The potential for undiscovered HIV infection may be a concern.

The family may experience uncertainty regarding the viral safety of blood products.

Insurance crises may occur as children and adults reach lifetime maximum amounts of reimbursement.

REFERENCES

Abramowicz M, (editor): Recombinant antihemophilic factor, *The Med Letter Drug Therapeut* 35:51-52, 1993.

Addiego J et al: Frequency of inhibitor development in haemophiliacs treated with low-purity factor VIII, *Lancet* 342:464-464, 1993.

Aledort L: Treatment of von Willebrand's disease, *Mayo Clin Proc* 66:841-846, 1991.

Aledort L et al: A longitudinal study of orthopaedic outcomes for severe factor-VIII-deficient haemophiliacs, *J Intern Med* 236:391-399, 1994.

Arnold W, Hilgartner M: Hemophilic arthropathy, *J Bone Joint Surg* 59A:287-305, 1977.

Blanchette V et al: Hepatitis C infection in patients with hemophilia: results of a national survey, *Transf Med Rev* 8:210-217, 1994.

Bohn R, Avorn J: Cost-effectiveness—can it be measured? *Semin Hematol* 30:20-23, 1993.

Bontempo F et al: Liver transplantation in hemophilia A, *Blood* 69:1721-1724, 1987.

Bowie E: von Willebrand's disease, Clin Lab Med 4:303-317, 1984.

Brady R, Humphries R: Pediatric HIV infection and AIDS: AIDS and adolescents, *Semin Pediatr Infect Dis* 1:156-162, 1990.

Bray G et al: A multicenter study of recombinant factor VIII (Recombinate): safety, efficacy, and inhibitor risk in previously untreated patients with hemophilia A, *Blood* 83:2428-2435, 1994.

Brettler D: Inhibitors of factor VII and IX, *Hemophilia* 1:35-39, 1995.

Brettler D et al: The use of porcine factor VIII concentrate (Hyate:C) in the treatment of patients with inhibitor antibodies to factor VIII, *Arch Intern Med* 149:1381-1385, 1989.

Brettler D, Levine P: Factor concentrates for the treatment of hemophilia: which one to choose? *Blood* 73:2067-2073, 1989.

Chorba T et al: Changes in longevity and causes of death among persons with hemophilia A, *Am J Hematol* 45:112-121, 1994.

Committee on Infectious Diseases: *1994 red book: report of the committee on infectious diseases,* Elk Grove, IL, 1994, American Academy of Pediatrics.

Czapek E et al: Humate-P for treatment of von Willebrand disease, *Blood* 72:1100, 1988.

Davis G et al: Treatment of chronic hepatitis C with recombinant interferon alfa, *N Engl J Med* 321:1501-1506, 1989.

Dietrich A et al: Head trauma in children with congenital coagulation disorders, *J Pediatr Surg* 29:28-32, 1994.

Eckert E: *Your child and hemophilia,* New York, 1990, National Hemophilia Foundation.

Ehrenforth S et al: Incidence of development of factor VIII and factor IX inhibitors in haemophiliacs, *Lancet* 339:594-598, 1992.

Evans D, Shaw A: Safety of intramuscular injection of hepatitis B vaccine in haemophiliacs, *Br Med J* 300:1694-1695, 1990.

Eyster E et al: Increasing hepatitis C virus RNA levels in hemophiliacs: relationship to human immunodeficiency virus infection and liver disease, *Blood* 84:1020-1023, 1994.

Fricke W et al: Human immunodeficiency virus infection as a result of clotting factor concentrates: results of the Seroconversion Surveillance Project, *Transfusion* 32:707-709, 1992.

Furie B, Limentani S, and Rosenfield C: A practical guide to the evaluation and treatment of hemophilia, *Blood* 84:3-9, 1994.

Gilbert M: Prophylaxis: musculoskeletal evaluation, *Semin Hematol* 30:3-6, 1993.

Goldsmith J: *Hemophilia: current medical management,* New York, 1994, National Hemophilia Foundation.

Goldsmith J et al: Coagulation factor IX: successful surgical experience with a purified factor IX concentrate, *Am J Hematol* 40:210-215, 1992.

Greenberg D: Pediatric experience with recombinant hepatitis B vaccines and relevant safety and immunogenicity studies, *Pediatr Infect Dis J* 12:438-445, 1993.

Greene W: Synovectomy of the ankle for hemophilic arthropathy, *J Bone Joint Surg* 76A:812-819, 1994.

Greer I et al: Haemorrhagic problems in obstetrics and gynaecology in patients with congenital coagulopathies, *Br J Obstet Gynaecol* 98:909-918, 1991.

Hay CR et al: Porcine factor VIII therapy in patients with congenital hemophilia and inhibitors: efficacy, patient selection, and side effects, *Semin Hematol* 31:20-25, 1994.

Hedner U: Factor VIIa in the treatment of hemophilia, *Blood Coagul Fibrinolysis* 1:307-317, 1990.

Hilgartner M, Aledort L, and Giardina P: *Thalassemia and hemophilia.* In Hobbs N, and Perrin JM, (editors): *Issues in the care of children with chronic illness,* San Francisco, 1985, Jossey-Bass, pp 299-323.

Hilgartner M et al: Purity of factor VIII concentrates and serial CD4 counts, *Lancet* 341:1373-1374, 1993.

Hilgartner M, Corrigan J: *Coagulation disorders.* In Miller D, and Baehner R (editors): *Blood diseases of infancy and childhood,* St Louis, 1995, Mosby, pp 924-986.

Hoeben R et al: Toward gene therapy for hemophilia A: long-term persistence of factor VIII-screening fibroblasts after transplantation into immunodeficient mice, *Human Gene Ther* 4:179-186, 1993.

Hoots K: Who should use recombinant factor VII? *Ann Hematol* 68:S65-S68, 1994.

Kasper C: *Treatment of factor VIII inhibitors.* In Coller BS, (editor): Progress in hemostasis and thrombosis, vol 9, Philadelphia, 1989, WB Saunders, pp 57-86.

Kasper C, Lusher J, and The Transfusion Practices Committee: Recent evolution of clotting factor concentrates for hemophilia A and B, *Transfusion* 33:422-434, 1993.

Kemahli S et al: Value of DNA analysis with multiple DNA probes for the detection of hemophilia A carriers, *Pediatr Hematol Oncol* 11:52-62, 1994.

Ketterling R et al: Direct carrier detection for hemophilia B: experience with 140 families. Abstract presented at the meeting of the National Hemophilia Foundation, Tampa, FL, October 1991.

Kim H et al: Purified factor IX using monoclonal immunoaffinity technique: clinical trials in hemophilia B and comparison to prothrombin complex concentrates, *Blood* 79:568-576, 1992.

Koch B: Rehabilitation of the child with joint disease. In G Molnar, (editor): *Pediatr Rehab,* Baltimore, 1985, Williams & Wilkins, pp 263-271.

Koerper M: Prenatal diagnosis of hemophilia in the United States. In Kasper C, (editor): Recent advances in hemophilia care, New York, 1990, Alan R Liss Inc, pp 13-17.

Köhler M et al: Subcutaneous injection of desmopressin (DDAVP): evaluation of a new, more concentrated preparation, *Haemostasis* 1:38-44, 1989.

Korenman J et al: Long-term remission of chronic hepatitis B after alpha-interferon therapy, *Ann Intern Med* 114:629-634, 1991.

Kruetz W et al: Factor VIII inhibitors in hemophilia-rapid and successful induction of immune tolerance after early and continuous high-dose factor VIII, *Thromb Haemost* 69:1101A, 1993.

Kumar A et al: Serologic markers of viral hepatitis A, B, C, and D in patients with hemophilia, *J Med Virol* 41:205-209, 1993.

Lakich D et al: Inversions disruption the factor VII gene area a common cause of severe haemophilia A, *Nature Genet* 5:236-241, 1993.

Lanzkowsky P: *Manual of pediatric hematology and oncology,* New York, 1995, Churchill Livingstone.

Lethagen S, Tennvall GR: Self-treatment with desmopressin intranasal spray in patients with bleeding disorders: effect on bleeding symptoms and socioeconomic factors, *Ann Hematol* 66:257-260, 1993.

Ljung R et al: Implantable central venous catheter facilitates prophylactic treatment in children with haemophilia, *Acta Pediatr* 81:918-920, 1992.

Lozier J, Brinkhous K: Gene therapy and the hemophilias, *JAMA* 271:47-51, 1994.

Luck J, Kasper C: Surgical management of advanced hemophilic arthropathy: an overview of 20 years' experience, *Clin Orthopaedics Related Res* 242:60-82, 1989.

Lunn JA: Hepatitis B vaccination, *BMJ* 307:732, 1993.

Lusher J: Summary of clinical experience with recombinant factor VIII products—Kogenate, *Ann Hematol* 68:S3-S6, 1994.

Lusher J: Use of prothrombin complex concentrates in management of bleeding in hemophiliacs with inhibitors—benefits and limitations, *Semin Hematol* 31:49-52, 1994.

Lusher J et al: Recombinant factor VIII for the treatment of previously untreated patients with hemophilia A, *New Engl J Med* 328:453-459, 1993.

Lusher J, Warrier I: Hemophilia, *Pediatr Rev* 12:275-281, 1991.

Manco-Johnson M et al: Results of secondary prophylaxis in children with severe hemophilia, *Am J Hematology* 47:113-117, 1994.

Mannucci PM: von Willebrand's disease and its management, *Br J Haematol* 82:210-212, 1992.

Mannucci PM, Bettega D, and Cattaneo M: Patterns of developmental of tachyphylaxis in patients with haemophilia and von Willebrand disease after repeated doses of desmopressin (DDAVP), *Br J Haemotol* 82:887-893, 1992.

Mariani G, Ghirardini A, and Bellocco R: Immune tolerance in hemophilia-principal results from the international registry, *Thromb Haemost* 72:155-158, 1994.

Mariani G et al: Immunetolerance as treatment of alloantibodies to factor VIII in hemophilia, *Semin Hematol* 31:62-64, 1994.

Martinowitz U et al: Circumcision in hemophilia: the use of fibrin glue for local hemostasis, *J Urol* 148:855-857, 1992.

Medical and Scientific Advisory Committee of the National Hemophilia Foundation: MASAC resolution concerning product selection for persons who are HIV positive (Medical Bulletin #188), New York, 1992, National Hemophilia Foundation.

Medical and Scientific Advisory Committee of the National Hemophilia Foundation: MASAC recommendations concerning prophylaxis (Medical Bulletin #193), New York, 1994, National Hemophilia Foundation.

Medical and Scientific Advisory Committee of the National Hemophilia Foundation: Recommendations concerning HIV infection, hepatitis, and other transmissible agents in the treatment of hemophilia (Medical Bulletin #226) New York, 1995, National Hemophilia Foundation.

Michaud JI, Rivard G, and Chessex P: Intracranial hemorrhage in a newborn with hemophilia following cesaerean section, *Am J Pediatr Hematol Oncol* 13:473-475, 1991.

Miller C, Lenzi R, and Breen C: Gene frequency in von Willebrand disease. Abstract presented at the meeting of the American Society of Human Genetics, Baltimore, MD, November 1989.

Montgomery R, Scott JP: *Hemostasis: diseases of the fluid phase.* In Nathan D and Oski F (editors): *Hematology of infancy and childhood,* Philadelphia, 1993, WB Saunders, pp 1605-1637.

National Hemophilia Foundation. Perspectives, *HANDI Quarterly* 2-3, 6-7, 1994.

Nilsson I: Immune tolerance, *Semin Hematol* 31:44-48, 1994.

Nilsson I et al: Twenty-five years' experience of prophylactic treatment in severe hemophilia A and B, *J Intern Med* 232:255-32, 1992.

Nilsson I, Berntorp E, and Zettervall O: Induction of immune tolerance in patients with hemophilia and antibodies to factor VIII by combined treatment with intravenous IgG, cyclophosphamide, and factor VII, *N Engl J Med* 318:947-950, 1988.

Odubiyi M: Cultural awareness in the world of hemophilia, *HANDI Quarterly* 5:1, 7, 1994.

Peake I et al: Haemophilia: strategies for carrier detection and prenatal diagnosis, *Bull World H Org* 71:429-458, 1993.

Petrini P et al: Prophylaxis with factor concentrates in preventing hemophilic arthropathy, *Am J Pediatr Hematol Oncol* 13:280-287, 1991.

Pettersson, H: Radiographic scores and implications, *Semin Hematol* 30:7-9, 1993.

Rodeghiero F et al: Consistency of responses to repeated DDAVP infusion in patients with von Willebrand's disease and hemophilia A, *Blood* 74:1997-2000, 1989.

Rose E, Aledort L: Nasal spray desmopressin (DDAVP) for mild hemophilia A and von Willebrand disease, *Ann Intern Med* 114:563-568, 1991.

Rothman D: Personal communication, April 23, 1990.

Santagostino E et al: Accelerated schedule of hepatitis B vaccination in patients with hemophilia, *J Med Virol* 41:95-98, 1993.

Scharrer J, Neutzling O: Incidence of inhibitors in haemophiliacs: a review of the literature, *Blood Coagul Fibrinolysis* 4:753-758, 1993.

Scheibel E et al: Continuous high-dose factor VIII for the induction of immune tolerance in haemophilia A patients with high responder state: a description of 11 patients, *Thromb Haemost* 58:1049-1052, 1987.

Schramm W: Experience with prophylaxis in Germany, *Semin Hematol* 30:12-15, 1993.

Serementis S: The clinical use of factor VIIa in the treatment of factor VIII inhibitor patients, *Semin Hematol* 31:53-55, 1994.

Serementis S et al: Three-year randomised study of high-purity or intermediate-purity factor VIII concentrates in symptom-free HIV seropositive haemophiliacs: effects on immune status, *Lancet* 342:700-703, 1993.

Siegel J et al: Hemarthrosis and synovitis associated with hemophilia: clinical use of P-32 chromic phosphate synoviorthesis for treatment, *Radiology* 190:257-261, 1994.

Silverman R et al: Safety of lumbar puncture in patients with hemophilia, *Ann Emerg Med* 22:1739-1742, 1993.

Smith T et al: Hyponatremia and seizures in young children given DDAVP, *Am J Hematol* 31:199-202, 1989.

Tedder RS, Zuckerman M, and Brink N: Hepatitis B vaccination, *BMJ* 307:732, 1993.

Teigland J et al: Synovectomy for haemophilic arthropathy: 6 to 21 years of follow-up in 16 patients, *J Intern Med* 235:239-243, 1994.

Teigland J et al: Knee arthroplasty in hemophilia, *Acta Orthop Scand* 64:153-156, 1993.

Telfer P et al: Alpha interferon for hepatitis C virus infection in haemophilic patients, *Haemophilia* 1:54-58, 1995.

Thompson A: Factor IX concentrates for clinical use, *Semin Thromb Hemost* 19:25-34, 1993.

Triplett K: Laboratory diagnosis of von Willebrand's disease, *Mayo Clin Proc* 66:832-840, 1991.

Troisi C et al: A multicenter study of viral hepatitis in a U.S. hemophilic population, *Blood* 81:412-418, 1993.

White G: Summary of clinical experience with recombinant factor VIII products—Recombinate, *Ann Hematol* 68:S7-S8, 1994.

White G, Shoemaker C: Factor VIII gene and hemophilia A, *Blood* 73:1-12, 1989.

Yoffe G, Buchanan G: Intracranial hemorrhage in newborn and young infants with hemophilia, *J Pediatr* 113:333-336, 1988.

Zappa S et al: Implantable intravenous access devices in children with hemophilia, *Arch Pediatr Adolesc Med* 148:327-330, 1994.

Bronchopulmonary Dysplasia

10

Kayla Harvey*

ETIOLOGY

Bronchopulmonary dysplasia (BPD) was first described by Northway, Rosan, and Porter (1967) in a review of chest radiographs of premature infants who were treated with positive pressure ventilation and oxygen for respiratory distress syndrome (RDS). When they first described the disease, they used a four-stage classification. Stage 1 described the first 2 to 3 days, with a radiograph similar to that showing RDS. Stage 2 evolved over the next 4 to 10 days, with a chest radiograph revealing complete opacification of lung fields. Stage 3, from 10 to 20 days, was marked by small round cystic lesions on x-ray film. Stage 4, the final and most severe stage, showed small bubbles of radiolucency on x-ray film, enlarging to form a hyperaerated cyst. Infants in this group had mechanical ventilatory support for greater than 1 month.

Philip (1975) broadened the definition to include nonradiographic findings and management. They included: (1) institution of positive pressure ventilation within the first week of life for a minimum of 3 days, (2) clinical findings of tachypnea, rales and retractions persisting beyond 28 days of life, (3) an oxygen requirement to maintain arterial oxygen pressure (PaO_2) greater than 55 mm Hg for more than 28 days, and (4) chest radiographs showing persistent strands of densities with areas of normal and hyperlucency in bilateral lung fields.

As advances in the study, diagnosis, and treatment of BPD progress, these early classification systems are used less frequently. Today BPD is often classified as mild, moderate, or severe.

Respiratory failure at birth is critical to the etiology of BPD because it requires treatment with supplemental oxygen and mechanical ventilation (Northway, 1990). Respiratory failure may be a result of several different causes, but most often from respiratory distress syndrome (Northway, 1990). Other contributing conditions to the development of BPD include hyaline membrane disease, meconium aspiration, congenital heart disease, patent ductus arteriosus, fluid overload, pulmonary air leak, and edema in the newborn period (Bancalari and Sosenko, 1990).

The BPD process is initiated through cellular injury to the immature lung. Infants born before 28 to 32 weeks' gestation have an insufficient amount of pulmonary surfactant. *Surfactant* is a lipoprotein that lowers the surface tension of the air-alveolar surface and allows lung expansion, thus maintaining the patency of alveoli and preventing atelectasis. Synthetic surfactant given in the first 24 hours of life has been shown to decrease neonatal mortality but not significantly reduce the incidence of BPD (Long et al, 1991).

Rozycki and Kirkpatrick (1993) describe BPD pathogenesis in the following sequence: (1) expo-

---

*The editors and authors would like to acknowledge the work done by Virginia H. Conte on this chapter in the first edition of the book.

172

sure to damaging stimuli, such as barotrauma and oxygen, (2) local cellular damage and death from oxygen radicals and lung stretch, (3) mediators initiate the inflammatory process, (4) persistent alveolitis, (5) proliferation of fibroblasts with subsequent fibrosis, and (6) epithelial metaplasia and inflammation followed by smooth-muscle hypertrophy. Figure 10-1 outlines the pathogenesis of BPD.

Risk factors that are key indicators for infants prone to develop BPD include lung immaturity, oxygen toxicity, positive pressure ventilation with lung stretch, inflammation (from neonatal pneumonia), and family history of asthma (Hazinski, 1990).

INCIDENCE

There are an estimated 7000 to 10,000 new cases of BPD diagnosed each year (Farrell and Palta, 1986; Hoekstra et al, 1991). Bronchopulmonary dysplasia is the leading cause of chronic lung disease in infants in the United States (Farrell and Palta,

1986). Parker, Lindstrom, and Cotton (1992) reported a 22% rise in the incidence of BPD in the past decade.

The reported incidence of BPD varies because of the lack of a consistent definition of the disease. As medical technology progresses, some suggest the increase in BPD is a result of an increase in the survival of premature and very-low-birth-weight newborns (e.g., less than 1500 g) (Parker, Lindstrom, and Cotton, 1992).

CLINICAL MANIFESTATIONS AT TIME OF DIAGNOSIS

Clinical manifestation of BPD varies depending on the age of the child at onset and the severity of the disease. The severity can range from a child having some pulmonary symptoms that require bronchodilator treatment and diuretics to a child requiring a tracheostomy and mechanical ventilatory support for prolonged periods of time, both in the hospital and at home.

The infant with BPD displays significant alteration in lung mechanics. Compliance is diminished by a combination of: (1) fibrosis secondary to alveolar injury, (2) increased lung fluid as a result of damage at the alveolar-capillary membrane, and (3) overdistention because of injury to alveolar-supporting structures, which causes airway collapse and subsequent air-trapping (Ackerman,

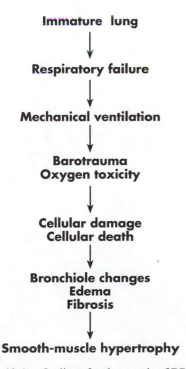

Immature lung

↓

Respiratory failure

↓

Mechanical ventilation

↓

Barotrauma
Oxygen toxicity

↓

Cellular damage
Cellular death

↓

Bronchiole changes
Edema
Fibrosis

↓

Smooth-muscle hypertrophy

Fig. 10-1.   Outline of pathogenesis of BPD.

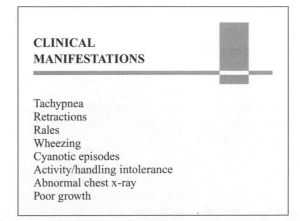

CLINICAL MANIFESTATIONS

Tachypnea
Retractions
Rales
Wheezing
Cyanotic episodes
Activity/handling intolerance
Abnormal chest x-ray
Poor growth

1994). An increase in airway resistance is found secondary to fibrosis, airway edema, and bronchoconstriction (Ackerman, 1994). The combination of decreased lung compliance and increased airway resistance produces clinical findings such as tachypnea, wheezing, and increased work of breathing. Fluid leak from cellular damage manifests as inspiratory and expiratory rales.

Chest x-rays of infants with BPD reveal increased interstitial markings, including cystic changes or fine, lacy densities with or without hyperinflation (Alpert, Allen, and Schidlow, 1993). The degree of abnormality in x-rays of children at 1 month of age can provide some insight to prognosis (Greenough, 1990).

An abnormal respiratory examination is the key finding in the diagnosis of BPD (see Fig. 10-2). On visual examination, the respiratory rate may be elevated by as much as 20 to 30 breaths/minute above the baseline for the child's age. With respiratory distress, the primary care provider will observe a prolonged exhalation with increased use of abdominal and accessory muscles. Umbilical or inguinal hernias may occur as a result of increased abdominal pressure from high airway resistance and use of accessory muscles (Hazinski, 1990).

Other clinical manifestations of the preterm infant with BPD include poor gas exchange, bronchospasms, mucus plugging, and poor physical growth. Cyanosis and activity intolerance with feeding and handling are common findings (Hagedorn and Gardner, 1989). Ultimately the task of breathing robs these infants of precious calories needed for physical growth and development.

TREATMENT

Treatment for BPD primarily focuses on accelerating lung maturation. Treatment also focuses on enhancing the infant's natural healing process, thereby avoiding further complications often associated with BPD. A "tincture of time" is the primary force that leads to stabilization of BPD. In the interim, support is employed until physiologic maturation of lung tissue can support oxygen needs. Such treatment modalities include oxygen therapy, diuretics, bronchodilators, and corticosteroids.

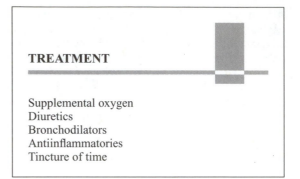

TREATMENT

Supplemental oxygen
Diuretics
Bronchodilators
Antiinflammatories
Tincture of time

Oxygen

The need for supplemental oxygen varies with the severity of lung dysfunction. Infants who require oxygen after hospital discharge rarely require more than 1 to 2 L/min delivered by nasal cannula. These children who are on oxygen must be followed at frequent intervals to assess for hypoxia by physical examination and by oxygen and carbon dioxide readings. Ideally, these readings can be obtained via pulse oximeter or transcutaneous oxygen monitoring instead of arterial blood samples. Oxygen and carbon dioxide measurements must be done during periods of rest and activity to accurately determine the child's continuing supplemental oxygen needs (Singer et al, 1992). When the child appears clinically stable, is gaining weight, and is not anemic, gradual weaning from oxygen is initiated by the neonatal pulmonary team. A typical weaning schedule is presented in Table 10-1. To avoid significant oxygen desaturation during sleep, the child with BPD, continue nighttime supplemental oxygen until daytime oxygen saturations equal or exceed 92% in room air (Zinman, Blanchard, and Vachon, 1992).

Diuretics

Diuretics are frequently used in the care of infants with BPD. These medications correct fluid retention, prevent fluid overload, decrease pulmonary resistance, and increase pulmonary compliance (Brem, 1992) (see box on diuretics, p. 176). Furosemide (Lasix) is a commonly used diuretic effective in eliminating excess fluid in the lungs that accumulates as a result of a disruption in lymph

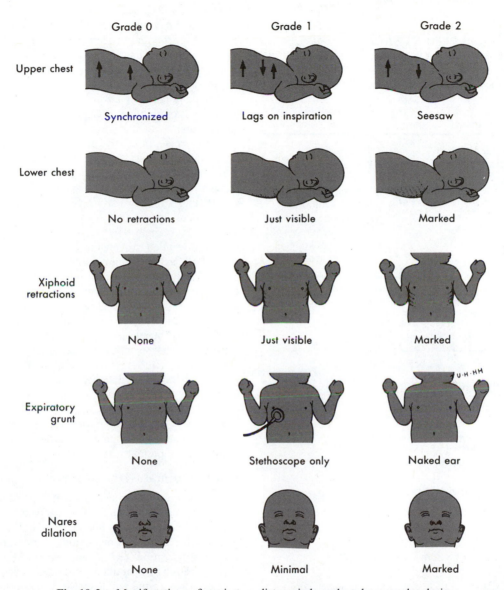

	Grade 0	Grade 1	Grade 2
Upper chest	Synchronized	Lags on inspiration	Seesaw
Lower chest	No retractions	Just visible	Marked
Xiphoid retractions	None	Just visible	Marked
Expiratory grunt	None	Stethoscope only	Naked ear
Nares dilation	None	Minimal	Marked

Fig. 10-2. Manifestations of respiratory distress in bronchopulmonary dysplasia.

drainage and increased capillary permeability (Brem, 1992). In moderate to severe BPD, potassium sparing spironolactone (Aldactone) and chlorothiazide (Diuril) is often needed for additional diuresis. Because of the potential electrolyte imbalance associated with diuretic therapy, children with BPD must have serum electrolyte values monitored and are frequently given potassium chloride supplements (Brem, 1992). Serum electrolytes should be monitored monthly with supplements adjusted to maintain chloride greater than 92 mEq/L and potassium greater than 3.5 mEq/L (Ackerman, 1994). Nutritional requirements must be balanced with fluid restriction to avoid overloading the already stressed cardiopulmonary system.

Table 10-1.
WEANING A PATIENT FROM
SUPPLEMENTAL OXYGEN:
SAMPLE SCHEDULE

Time	Amount of oxygen (per min)
At hospital discharge	0.5 L at all times
1 month after discharge*	0.5 L during feedings and sleep; 0.25 L when awake
2 months*	0.25 L at all times
3 months*	0.25 L during feedings and sleep; room air when awake
4 months*	Room air at all times

From Bernbaum JE, Friedman S, Hoffman-Williamson M, et al: Preterm infant care after hospital discharge, *Pediatr Rev* 10:195-208, 1989.
*Assumes clinical stability, adequate weight gain, and proof of adequate oxygen saturation (intervals may vary).

DIURETICS USED
TO TREAT BPD

Furosemide (Lasix)

1-4 mg/kg/dy   in 1-2 divided doses

Chlorothiazide (Diuril)

30-40 mg/kg/dy   in 2 divided doses

Spironolactone (Aldactone)

2-4 mg/kg/dy   in 1-2 divided doses

Data from Ackerman VL: Bronchopulmonary dysplasia. In GM Loughlin, H Eigen, (editors): Respiratory disease in children: diagnosis and management, Baltimore, MD, 1994, Williams & Wilkins; Truog WE: Bronchopulmonary dysplasia: issues in long-term management, *J Resp Diseases* 14:130-145, 1993.

Bronchodilators

Infants with BPD may be predisposed to bronchial hyperreactivity and bronchospasm from neonatal lung injury and hyperplasia of smooth muscle (Rush and Hazinski, 1992). Bronchodilator therapy is used to reduce the effects of bronchoconstriction by relaxing smooth muscle in the airways. The outcome is improved gas exchange through a decrease in air-flow resistance and gas-trapping (Wilkie and Bryan, 1987). A positive response from this therapy is demonstrated clinically by a decrease in wheezing, coughing, or in supplemental oxygen requirements.

Three categories of bronchodilators are β-adrenergic agonists (albuterol), anticholinergics (atrovent), and methylxanthines (theophylline). Albuterol is commonly used via inhalation at a dose of 0.02 to 0.1 ml/kg/dose (maximum 0.5 ml) every 4 to 6 hours depending on response and disease severity (Ackerman, 1994). Use of nebulized ipratropium bromide (atrovent) in combination with albuterol can enhance pulmonary function in infants with BPD. Ipratropium bromide antagonizes muscarinic receptors in the airways resulting in bronchodilation (Brundage et al, 1990; Greenough, 1990). Theophylline is an oral bronchodilator that has the added benefit of providing respiratory drive stimulation; however, theophylline has numerous side effects including feeding intolerance, tachycardia, irritability, diarrhea, increased gastroesophageal reflux (GER), and lowered seizure threshold (Rossing, 1989). As a result, the role of theophylline in bronchodilator therapy is diminished but may be indicated in infants with BPD with apnea of prematurity.

Antiinflammatories

Corticosteroids have been used in the acute and chronic phases of BPD disease. Steroid treatment with dexamethasone has been effective in weaning infants with BPD from mechanical ventilation during hospitalization (Rush and Hazinski, 1992). Corticosteroids can reduce pulmonary edema and inflammation in the small airways, and potentiate the effects of bronchodilators (Truog, 1993). Prednisone (1 to 2 mg/kg) given for 3 to 5 days can be effective for acute exacerbations. Watterberg and Scott (1995) speculate that infants with BPD have a decreased ability to secrete cortisol in response to stress, leaving them more vulnerable to inflammatory lung injury. Infants with severe BPD may require a prolonged course of corticosteroids with a slow taper of the drug treatment over weeks. A gradual decrease in dosage every 3 to 7 days followed by a change in frequency to every other day at twice the daily dose is a common weaning schedule (Truog, 1993; Kountz, 1989). Infants using this type of therapy are at risk for adrenal suppression. They should receive an increase in their usual steroid dose during significant biophysical stressors such as moderate-severe infection or surgical procedures (Kountz, 1989). The primary care provider should consult with a pulmonologist when caring for an infant of such high risk.

Cromolyn sodium (Intal) is an inhaled nonsteroidal antiinflammatory that can be beneficial to infants and children with BPD (Ackerman, 1994; Truog, 1993). Cromolyn sodium reduces airway hyperreactivity by preventing release of inflammatory mediators into the airways. Cromolyn sodium (20 mg) given via inhalation 2 to 4 times a day may be indicated for empirical trial in those infants with a significant reactive airway disease component (Rush and Hazinski, 1992).

RECENT AND ANTICIPATED ADVANCES IN DIAGNOSIS AND MANAGEMENT

Bronchopulmonary disease is often associated with asthma. Control of airway inflammation has been limited to oral steroids or nebulized cromolyn sodium. The use of inhaled corticosteroids and their effectiveness on controlling inflammation has been documented in children with asthma (Konig, 1988). Recent studies reviewed the efficacy and safety of nebulized steroids in infants and children with BPD. Preliminary results indicated a decrease in number of days of hospitalization and ability to decrease oral corticosteroid therapy (Cloutier, 1993; Konig et al, 1992).

Respiratory syncitial virus (RSV) infection causes significant mortality and morbidity in infants with BPD. Researchers are investigating the efficacy of administering immunoglobulins specific for RSV to decrease the incidence and severity of RSV infection in children with BPD (Groothuis et al, 1993).

Machines used to administer aerosolized medications can be cumbersome and inconvenient. Spacer devices have become a portable alternative for older children and adults with airway obstruc-

tion. Studies on infants indicate a spacer with a mask is an effective means of administering aerosolized bronchodilators (Conner et al, 1989).

Some clinicians speculate that BPD can be prevented by supplementing nutrients that are deficient in premature neonates. Vitamin E (for reduction of oxygen-free radicals) and vitamin A (to promote healing) have been given to infants considered to be at high risk for BPD without uniform success (Rozycki and Kirkpatrick, 1993). Further research is needed to investigate treatment modalities that will reduce BPD severity.

Medical and technologic advances in neonatology have resulted in an increase in the survival rates of very-low-birth-weight infants (less than 750 g) contributing to the increased incidence of BPD (Parker, Lindstrom, and Cotton, 1992). Prevention of premature births through improved prenatal care is the key to decreasing the incidence of BPD.

ASSOCIATED PROBLEMS

Airway Complications

Structural damage to the infant's premature respiratory tree frequently occurs as a result of endotracheal intubation and positive pressure ventilation (Alpert, Allen, and Schidlow, 1993). Upper airway anomalies including subglottic stenosis, granuloma, tracheal scarring, and polyp formation can occur immediately after extubation or as a late

ASSOCIATED PROBLEMS

Airway complications
Infection
Poor growth and nutrition
Gastroesophageal reflux
Cardiac conditions
Neurodevelopmental complications
Ophthalmologic sequelae
Renal conditions
Rickets
Stoma care
Otitis media/sinusitis

presentation (Hazinski, 1990). Infants presenting with homophonous wheezing, hypoxia, and brady-cardia (cyanotic "BPD spells") should be evaluated for lower airway anomalies such as tracheomalacia and bronchomalacia (Alpert, Allen, and Schidlow, 1993); Duncan, 1991.

Infants who require prolonged ventilatory support and infants who develop respiratory failure from an upper airway obstruction will need a tracheostomy. Children with a tracheostomy are now quite commonly cared for at home. The most frequent complications are infection of the tracheostomy, obstruction by secretions, or accidental decannulation (Bernbaum et al, 1989). Parents and primary care providers must be competent in tracheostomy care. This includes the knowledge and skills necessary for maintenance of tracheostomy patency, stoma care, and performance of tracheostomy tube changes.

Airways of infants with BPD exhibit significant loss of cilia and denudation of airway lining resulting in the absence of the normal cleansing abilities of the lung (Hazinski, 1990). Daily chest physiotherapy (CPT) and postural drainage facilitate the mobilization of secretions to allow for removal from the airway by coughing or suctioning if an artificial airway is present. During a viral or bacterial illness, secretion production increases and more frequent CPT and drainage may be necessary.

Infection

Infants with BPD are at increased risk of lower respiratory tract infections in the first year of life (Tammela, 1992). Infection is the major cause of rehospitalization, late morbidity, and mortality in children with BPD (Cunningham, McMilan, and Gross, 1991). Therefore early evaluation and close follow-up are recommended for children with BPD with *any* upper respiratory illness or cold. Community-acquired viruses can exacerbate BPD with worsening hypoxia, edema, bronchoconstriction, and secondary bacterial infection (Hazinski, 1990). Treatment for stabilization of such episodes includes an increase in supplemental oxygen, extra doses of diuretics (Lasix), and administration of aerosolized bronchodilators (Hazinski, 1990). Broad-spectrum antibiotic treatment and a septic work-up are indicated for the febrile infant with BPD. Nasopharyngeal aspirate for immunofluores-

cence may be helpful in identifying particularly harmful viruses such as RSV, adenovirus, and influenza (Southhall, 1990).

Poor Growth and Nutrition

Growth patterns overall in children with BPD depend on the severity of the lung disease and nutritional status. Growth retardation in infants with BPD occurs most commonly as a result of an inability to match caloric intake with energy expenditure (Rozycki and Kirkpatrick, 1993). The combination of fluid restrictions, frequent respiratory infections, and an elevated metabolic rate often result in poor weight gain (Hazinski, 1990). Feeding disorders such as oral aversion can occur in infants with BPD as a result of exposure to negative oral stimuli (endotracheal tubes and suctioning), and as a result of deprivation of positive oral feeding-sucking experiences (Alpert, Allen, and Schidlow, 1993). Furthermore, infants with BPD who have labored breathing at rest often have difficulty coordinating their rapid respirations, suck, and swallow (Truog, 1993). Other potential causes of growth failure in infants with BPD include hypoxemia, heart failure, gastroesophageal reflux, and rickets of prematurity (Alpert, Allen, and Schidlow, 1993).

Total parenteral nutrition early in treatment is often necessary, followed by supplementation of breast or bottle feedings with gavage feedings. In infants with severe BPD and feeding problems, a gastrostomy tube may be necessary. Caloric requirements are high, up to 150 to 200 kcal/kg per day. Most infants require formula with a caloric concentration of 24 to 30 kcal/30 m/s (1 oz) or greater to achieve optimal catch-up growth (Ackerman, 1994; Hazinski, 1990). Formula may be fortified with vegetable oil, tryglycerides, or glucose polymers to increase the calories per ounce (Hazinski, 1990).

Gastroesophageal Reflux

Gastroesophageal reflux (GER) is a common gastrointestinal dysfunction seen in children with BPD, which is caused by an incompetent lower esophageal sphincter that allows acidic gastric contents to pass back up into the esophagus. Symptoms of GER include emesis, apnea, bradycardia, recurrent pneumonia, delayed growth, and esophagitis (Armentrout, 1995).

Abnormal lung mechanics leading to abnormal pressure gradients between the chest and abdomen may contribute to the occurrence of GER in infants with BPD (Hazinski, 1990). Esophageal pH probe monitoring over an 18 to 24 hour period is used to confirm the diagnosis of GER (Armentrout, 1995; Alpert, Allen, and Schidlow, 1993). Theophylline decreases lower esophageal sphincter tone and should therefore be avoided in infants with both BPD and GER. Ranitidine (Zantac) and cimetidine (Tagamet) help to buffer the acidity of the stomach after meals and decrease the episodes of bronchospasm caused by gastric content irritation. If these medications are not effective in controlling symptoms, metoclopramide (Reglan) and cisapride (Prepulsid) should be considered to promote gastric emptying and prevent residuals from refluxing.

Thickening food with rice cereal and using reflux precautions (keeping head of bed elevated 30 degrees with infant in prone position) are effective adjunct therapies (Goldson, 1990; Armentrout, 1995). The last option considered if symptoms and the clinical picture do not demonstrate any improvement is Nissan fundoplication surgery (Armentrout, 1995).

Cardiac Conditions

Chronic cardiac changes persist in children with BPD who have suffered numerous hypoxic insults or who have been maintained at a low PaO_2. Pulmonary vasoconstriction occurs in response to alveolar hypoxia resulting in pulmonary hypertension (Rush and Hazinski, 1992). The mainstay treatment of pulmonary hypertension is supplemental oxygen (Ackerman, 1994). Maximum pulmonary vasodilation occurs when oxygen saturations are maintained between 92% and 95% (Goodman et al, 1988).

Progression of pulmonary hypertension can lead to right ventricular hypertrophy, cor pulmonale, and congestive heart failure (Alpert, Allen, and Schidlow, 1993). Congestive heart failure can present as unexplained weight gain and significant liver enlargement (>7 cm span) (Alpert, Allen, and Schidlow, 1993).

Refractory hypoxemia or sudden fluctuations in PaO_2 may represent the presence of a cardiac defect (Alpert, Allen, and Schidlow, 1993). Patent ductus arteriosis, incompetent foramen ovale, or septal defect can cause congestive heart failure or pulmonary hypertension (Alpert, Allen, and Schidlow, 1993; Hazinski, 1990).

Diagnostic tests including echocardiogram and cardiac catheterization are utilized to confirm cardiac complications.

Neurodevelopmental Complications

Children with BPD are at high risk for developmental delays. All aspects of development can be affected: physical, cognitive, language, and sensorimotor skills. Mild gross motor sequelae including hypotonia, hypertonia, and delayed motor development are frequently seen in the first year of life (Tammela and Koivisto, 1992). The presence of an intraventricular hemorrhage, periventricular leukomalacia, or echodensity in the newborn period are all predictors for poor developmental outcome (Luchi, Bennett, and Jackson, 1991; Ackerman, 1994). Regular assessment with early intervention involving a physical therapist, an occupational therapist, and a developmental specialist (or neurologist) is necessary for optimal development (Ackerman, 1994). Regular screening exams for vision and hearing are important in a population prone to retinopathy of prematurity and recurrent ear infections (Goldson, 1990).

Seizures

Hypoxic insults and intraventricular hemorrhages occurring in the newborn period predispose the infant to seizures. Even with anticonvulsant therapy the onset of new seizures can be triggered at any time by an infection with a high fever or a hypoxic insult. Children with BPD who have been free of seizures for a minimum of 1 year with electroencephalograms free of epileptiform activity can be considered for weaning of anticonvulsants (see Chapter 19).

Ophthalmologic Sequelae

The incidence of retinopathy of prematurity (ROP) has decreased as the toxic effects of oxygen have become known. Central blindness can occur with repeated incidence of severe hypoxia and severe intraventricular hemorrhage.

All infants weighing less than 1500 g should be screened for ROP (Moore, 1990). Infants with BPD that are diagnosed with ROP should be followed closely by an ophthalmologist because of a risk of strabismus and amblyopia (Moore, 1990).

Renal Conditions

One half of infants with BPD who receive chronic furosemide (Lasix) therapy will develop renal calcification (Greenough, 1990). Infants on IV furosemide for longer than 2 weeks should have a renal ultrasound (Greenough, 1990). Thiazides (Diuril) decrease calcium excretion and may help prevent nephrocalcinosis (Alpert, Allen, and Schidlow, 1993). If renal stones are identified, furosemide should be discontinued as soon as possible to allow the calcium to reabsorb.

Rickets

Infants with BPD often develop rickets secondary to prolonged parenteral nutrition and difficulty absorbing calcium and phosphorus. The population most at risk are those infants with a birth weight less than 1000 g. Long-term furosemide administration can also contribute to a negative calcium balance, inhibiting normal bone formation. This condition is reversible with dietary management and use of alternate diuretics such as spironolactone and hydrochlorothiazide (Alpert, Allen, and Schidlow, 1993).

Stoma Problems

Children with tracheostomy tubes are at risk for irritation around the tracheostomy stoma. Secretions that ooze from tracheostomy stomas may irritate the skin. Meticulous regular care to the tracheostomy stoma will generally maintain skin integrity.

Skin lacerations on the neck can be caused by fastening tracheostomy ties too tightly. A small premeasured protective patch of skin barrier may be placed over the laceration to allow it to heal without continued direct contact with tracheostomy ties or the flange of the tracheostomy tube.

Some children may develop areas of granulation tissue on and around the tracheostomy stoma. If left unattended, the tissue will continue to grow and can impede or block insertion of the tracheostomy tube into the stoma. Occasionally the tissue forms a tight band around the tracheostomy stoma. Application of silver nitrate to the site will promote shrinkage and eliminate tissue. In extreme cases the child will

need to be referred to an otorhinolaryngologist for possible surgical excision under anesthesia.

Similar difficulties with granulation tissue occur with gastrostomy stomas and the same treatment applies. Leakage of feeding around the gastrostomy tube causes irritation of the skin on the abdomen. Usually the cause is mechanical. Some families are instructed to change gastrostomy tubes on a regular basis because over time the stomach acid alters the integrity of the tube within the stomach.

The primary care provider should examine the tube to determine its type and how it is inserted. Foley catheters, Malecot tubes, and gastrostomy button devices may be used as gastrostomy tubes. Some tubes may be placed securely with a fluid-inflated balloon. The amount of fluid in the balloon should be documented in the discharge plan. If the amount contained within the balloon is less than the prescribed amount, it can contribute to leakage. It is important to ensure that the internal balloon is pulled up close to the internal abdominal wall to prevent leakage.

When leakage is persistent, some practitioners insert a larger tube into the stoma. This technique is controversial because over time the stoma will only expand and the problem will recur. The less the tube is manipulated, the longer the stoma will remain intact. Secure fastening procedures can help minimize movement of the gastrostomy tube.

Otitis Media/Sinusitis

Often the same bacteria that colonize the lower airways also colonize the upper airways and precipitate upper respiratory infections. Recurrent otitis media is frequently seen in this population, resulting in the need for antibiotic prophylaxis, placement of bilateral myringotomy tubes, or both. Hearing loss can occur as a result of chronic infection and chronic intravenous use of furosemide and aminoglycosides.

Sinusitis is prevalent in children with chronic lung disease and children who have required or continue to require nasogastric tube feedings. There is a persistent unilateral or bilateral off-colored drainage from the nares. Postnasal drainage results in coughing and throat clearing, especially after waking from sleep. Severe sinusitis causes coughing throughout the day and is unrelieved by bronchodilator therapy or frequent suctioning of an artificial airway. Radiographs of the sinuses confirm the presence of infection and degree of involvement. Oral antibiotics taken for a minimum of 3 weeks clear most infections, but prolonged therapy may be needed to treat severe cases.

PROGNOSIS

Survival rates and outcomes are steadily improving for infants with BPD. Expert medical care is now available for these infants through easier access to tertiary care personnel. Improvements in prenatal care and technologic advances in diagnostic and treatment techniques have greatly improved the outcome for infants with BPD.

Even with these new advances, mortality is approximately 25% for infants with BPD (Ackerman, 1994). Ventilator parameters (peak inspiratory pressure and ventilator rate) on day 28 may be predictive of survival outcomes in infants with severe BPD (Gray et al, 1993). Higher peak inspiratory pressure (720) and ventilator rate (740) were associated with nonsurvival of infants requiring prolonged ventilation (Gray et al, 1993).

For infants with BPD who survive, growth and developmental delay improve over time. However, when compared to their peers as young children, adolescents, and young adults, the effects of BPD appear to linger. Infants and children with BPD are found to have a lower mean weight and less subcutaneous tissue than their peers (Robertson et al, 1992). Reduced height and weight (25% to 35% are below the 10th percentile) can persist into middle childhood and adolescence (Robertson et al, 1992; Northway et al, 1990; Vrlenich et al, 1995). Catch-up growth of a child's head circumference in the first year of life may be a predictor of neurodevelopmental outcome. Hack et al (1991) found that infants with subnormal head growth persisting at 8 months of age had poor academic performance, lower IQ, and less speech-language skills at 8 to 9 years of age. However, for children without perinatal central nervous system insult, the neurodevelopmental outcome was good. By age 10 to 12 years, more than 60% of children with BPD were developmentally normal (Vohr et al, 1991).

Overall, school age children with a history of BPD when compared to their peers demonstrated academic delays (Robertson et al, 1992). Assessments often reveal attention deficit disorders, perceptual-motor integration problems, and language delays (Bernbaum et al, 1989; Hack et al, 1991).

Although the effects of BPD on the respiratory system diminish in time, 70% of adolescents with BPD demonstrate continued airway obstruction and 52% have persistent airway hyperreactivity (Ackerman, 1994).

Primary Care Management
HEALTH CARE MAINTENANCE

Growth and Development

Height and weight measurements, corrected for gestational age, should be obtained and plotted monthly while the child is hospitalized and with each subsequent ambulatory care visit. Growth measurements taken before the child is discharged from the hospital will help establish growth trends in the newly discharged infant. Even minor illness in children with BPD may result in weight loss because of their high caloric needs.

The head shape of the premature infant often appears boxy, and the head circumference must be measured and recorded carefully on standardized growth curves for premature infants or corrected for gestational age and plotted on National Center for Health Statistics graphs. The corrected age should be used for 2½ years, or until the sutures are normally fused. A head circumference percentile that is significantly higher than weight or height percentile suggests the possibility of intraventricular hemorrhage or poor nutritional status with head sparing (Gardner and Hagedorn, 1992). Careful physical examination and documentation of caloric intake should indicate if a cranial ultrasound is needed.

Developmental screening by the primary care provider can be accomplished using the child's corrected age and standard screening tools. Even with correction for prematurity, these infants often exhibit developmental lag during the first year of life. Most infants with transient developmental delays will test normal after they are 1 year of age. If developmental delays are significant or persist after the first year of life, referral for further assessment and therapeutic intervention is recommended. Early intervention for children who are high risk and control of secondary pulmonary problems offer the best prospect for optimal long-term prognosis.

Diet

The high caloric requirements caused by prematurity and the increased work of breathing with BPD require creative ways of providing adequate nutrition in an appealing, tasteful manner that does not require high expenditure of energy to consume or create fluid overload in the infant who is compromised. It is important for the primary care provider to assess weight gain on a regular basis and evaluate nutritional needs. It is beneficial to maintain contact with the nutritionist from the discharging hospital and ask for assistance in maintaining adequate caloric intake. As mentioned before, children with severe BPD or feeding problems may require supplemental feedings via gavage or gastrostomy tube.

The introduction of solid foods is generally initiated between 4 and 6 months of corrected age or when the infant weighs 6 to 7 kg (Bernbaum et al, 1989). Oral tactile hypersensitivity as a result of oral trauma from passage of nasogastric or orogastric tubes, endotracheal tubes, or repeated suctioning may make it difficult for the child to feed adequately. Early recognition of the problem and intervention by trained health care providers such as nurses, the speech pathologist, or the occupational therapist can facilitate feeding and decrease parental frustration and feelings of failure.

Safety

Children with BPD who are tethered by oxygen or ventilator tubing require close supervision. Respiratory equipment should have alarm systems because free-spirited toddlers will wander beyond the length of the tubing. Restricted and supervised areas of play need to be set up to create a safe environment for recreation. Children should be supervised at all times to prevent them from manipulating dials on their support equipment. Some devices have safety Plexiglass that cover control dials.

Children with tracheostomy tubes need virtually continuous observation. If they are not directly attended by caregivers, a noninvasive monitoring system with an oxygen saturation or apnea monitor should be in place. An accidental decannulation can cause death or serious physical and developmental sequelae. Security of the tracheostomy tube ties should be assessed every 4 to 8 hours and readjusted if greater than one finger-breadth insertion is found between the tracheostomy ties and the child's

neck. Family members should be taught CPR before the child is discharged from the hos-pital.

Families with toddlers must be warned against the insertion of small toys into ventilator tubing and artificial airways. Playful siblings can contribute to accidental airway decannulations and equipment disconnections when they are insufficiently supervised or educated. Older school-aged and adolescent children can be instructed to observe and intervene with specified responsibilities in emergency or routine situations.

Oxygen is a highly flammable gas and must be used with caution in the home. Parents and caretakers must be taught the necessary safety precautions, and the implementation of these safety measures should be evaluated whenever a home visit is made (see Table 10-2).

The primary care provider should review the use of aerosol cans and open flames in the home with the family. Fumes and smoke cause increased irritation to already sensitive airways and a fire hazard is present if oxygen is in use. Caregivers and visitors should be warned against smoking in the home and around the child.

Consideration for safety with the use of electrical equipment should be part of the discharge preparation from the hospital. Reinforcement from the primary care provider will help ensure safety. All medical equipment should be electrically grounded. Extension cords should not be used unless approved by the home care equipment vendor.

Before the child is discharged, contact with emergency services should be established. Contacts include fire, ambulance, police, electric, and telephone services. A review of this with families helps reinforce required actions. Inadvertent omission of an essential contact may be identified, thus avoiding needless anxiety or lack of attention in a true emergency (Southall and Samuels, 1990).

Immunizations

Infants with BPD should receive all standard immunizations at the appropriate chronologic age. This includes hepatitis B, hemophilus influenza (Truog, 1993), and varicella vaccine (Committee on Infectious Disease, 1994). Hepatitis B immunization is usually given to preterm infants at discharge if weight is 2 kg or more, or at 2 months of chronologic age (Red Book, 1994). Because of prolonged hospi-

Table 10-2.   SAFE USE OF OXYGEN AT HOME

Safety guidelines	Rationale
Secure oxygen tank in upright position.	Oxygen tanks are highly explosive; if a horizontally positioned tank explodes, the rapid release of oxygen can catapult it through animate (human bodies) and inanimate (walls) objects.
Keep oxygen tanks at least 5 ft from heat source and electrical devices (e.g., space heaters, heating vents, fireplaces, radios, vaporizers, and humidifiers).	
Ensure that no one smokes in the room or in the area of the oxygen tank.	Smoking increases the risk of fire, which could cause the tank to explode; escaped oxygen would feed the fire.
Use lemon-glycerin swabs to relieve dryness around the child's mouth; avoid oil or alcohol-based substances (e.g., petroleum jelly, vitamin A and D ointment, baby oil).	Both alcohol and oil are flammable and increase the risk of fire.
Have the child wear cotton garments.	Silk, wool, and synthetics can generate static electricity and cause fire.
Keep a fire extinguisher readily available.	It is necessary to put out fire immediately.
Turn off both volume regulator and flow regulator whenever oxygen is not in use.	If the volume regulator is on when oxygen is turned on, the child might receive a rapid, forceful flow of oxygen in the face that could be frightening and uncomfortable. Oxygen leakage, which might not be detected because oxygen is odorless, can cause fire.

From Hagedorn MI and Gardner SL: Physiologic sequelae of prematurity: the nurse practitioner's role. part 1. Respiratory issues, *J Pediatr Health Care* 3:288-297, 1989.

talizations and recurrent illnesses, however, infants with BPD are often delayed in their immunization schedule. Before immunizations are initiated in the primary care office, hospital records should be reviewed to determine if any immunizations were administered during hospitalization. If inactivated polio vaccine was given in the hospital, the practitioner may continue with this series or switch to trivalent oral polio vaccine. If the infant has a history of uncontrolled seizures, pertussis may be withheld until the seizures are controlled or diphtheria and tetanus vaccines may be given without pertussis (see Chapter 19). Infants and children with chronic BPD are at highest risk for serious morbidity with pertussis infection, so pertussis vaccination should not be withheld without cause. A cellular pertussis vaccine should be used when the child reaches the approved chronologic age for administration.

Administration of subvirion influenza vaccine during the fall or early winter months is recommended for children more than 6 months of age with BPD and their caretakers (Truog, 1993). Pneumococcal vaccine is recommended at 24 months of age (Truog, 1993; Red Book, 1994).

Screening

Vision. Evaluations for retinopathy of prematurity (ROP) should be done every 2 or 3 months by a pediatric ophthalmologist during the child's first year of life. If there is a question of blindness, a visual evoked response test can be requested. Routine eye examinations with Hirschberg, cover test, tracking, and fundoscopic examinations should be done at each primary care visit to follow the common problems of myopia and strabismus. Surgical correction for strabismus is often required.

Hearing. Infants with BPD are at risk for hearing loss as a result of prematurity and the IV administration of furosemide, corticosteroids, and aminoglycosides. A basal auditory evoked response

(BAER) test should be completed before discharge from the hospital, and routine screening for hearing should be conducted with each primary care visit. If recurrent otitis media is a problem, regular audiometry examinations should be conducted to identify hearing impairment and speech delays. Speech delays can be anticipated in children with long-term tracheostomies.

Dental. Routine dental care is recommended. Hypoplastic and discolored maxillary central and lateral incisors were found in more than 25% of infants with BPD in one study (Sauve and Singhal, 1985). Orally ingested ferrous sulfate may cause tooth staining, which can be remedied with good dental hygiene. Daily tooth brushing may be a challenge for parents because of the child's oral defensiveness. Primary care providers can recommend using toothettes or foam-tipped brushes, which are softer, and baking soda instead of toothpaste because of its milder taste.

Blood pressure. Measurements of blood pressure should be taken with every visit and routinely followed to detect early signs of progressive cardiac disease, pulmonary hypertension, or renal dysfunction.

Hematocrit. Premature infants are more susceptible to iron deficiency anemia than full-term infants and must be followed closely during their first year of life. Hematocrit values should be checked monthly for the first 6 months of life and bimonthly for the following 6 months (see Chapter 30). Anemia of prematurity may be further aggravated by erosive gastroesophageal reflux and frequent blood tests. Children with chronic hypoxia may have elevated hemoglobin and hematocrit values.

Urinalysis. Routine screening is recommended.

Tuberculosis. Routine screening is recommended.

Condition-specific screening

CHEST X-RAY FILMS. Chest x-ray studies should be ordered upon discharge from the hospital to establish lung disease severity, and then annually for evaluation and with acute illness as clinically indicated.

PULMONARY FUNCTION TESTS. Pulmonary function tests should be done upon discharge from the hospital to establish lung disease severity, and then annually for evaluation and with acute illness as clinically indicated.

COMMON ILLNESS MANAGEMENT

Differential Diagnosis

Respiratory distress. Respiratory distress is a common cause of urgent visits to the primary care practitioner. The child should be assessed for an elevated respiratory rate, increased work of breathing with substernal and intercostal retractions, nasal flaring, and a change in baseline breath sounds. Activity level and appetite may decrease. The child also should be assessed for sources of infection, such as a viral illness. Children dependent on respiratory support, either oxygen, aerosolized bronchodilators, or mechanical ventilation, may require an increased level of support to reverse hypoxia and hypercarbia during this period of respiratory workload.

A chest x-ray will determine if the child has atelectasis, aspiration pneumonia, an infectious pulmonary process such as viral-bacterial pneumonia, or increased pulmonary fluid. Respiratory distress with wheezing or prolonged expiratory phase which resolves after bronchodilator treatment indicates bronchospasm.

Significant respiratory distress in the infant with severe BPD may be cardiac in origin. Pallor, diaphoresis, and tachypnea may indicate congestive heart failure. Evaluation through an ECG will reveal right and left ventricular hypertrophy. The presence of a heart murmur in the infant with severe BPD necessitates an immediate cardiology consult to rule out patent ductus, foramen ovale, or septal defect.

Cough. Cough in the infant with BPD can indicate several possible processes. A productive, persistent, or moist cough without changes in lung sounds or chest x-ray may indicate sinusitis. Intermittent dry cough that is more pronounced after feedings and when the infant is in a supine position may result from undiagnosed or poorly controlled reflux. Cough associated with increased activity may indicate undertreated reactive airway disease. A new cough in combination with tachypnea and crackles without evidence of infection often indicates pulmonary edema. Sudden onset of a staccato cough (with or without apnea) that interferes with feedings may indicate pertussis. If this is accompanied by copious, clear rhinorrhea, RSV should be considered.

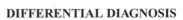

DIFFERENTIAL DIAGNOSIS

Respiratory distress

Pneumonia (viral-bacterial)
Pulmonary edema
Congestive heart failure
Cardiac defect
Bronchospasm

Cough

Sinusitis
Gastroesophageal reflux (GER)
Reactive airways
Pulmonary edema
Pertussis
Respiratory syncitial virus (RSV)

Gastrointestinal disturbances
(emesis, feeding intolerance, diarrhea)

Antibiotic therapy
Theophylline toxicity
Gastroesophageal reflux (GER)
Formula density intolerance
Gastroenteritis

Fever

Otitis media
Sinusitis
Respiratory tract infection
Urinary tract infection
Septicemia

Skin-mucosa changes

Candida dermatitis
Oral thrush

BPD unresponsive to therapy

Wilson-Mikity
Pulmonary interstitial emphysema
Congenital heart disease
Pulmonary hemorrhage
Viral pneumonia
Cystic fibrosis
Pulmonary lymphangiectasia

Fever. Otitis media and sinusitis are often causes of fever in infants with BPD, and their upper respiratory tract processes can lead to lower respiratory tract infection. Fever without respiratory tract symptoms may indicate urinary tract infection.

If an infant's body temperature persists above 101°F for more than 24 hours despite antipyretic administration, the primary care provider should consider further work-up with a complete blood cell count, secretion culture, and possible chest x-ray. The outcome of the culture and sensitivity test will determine the antibiotic of choice and the route of administration, either enteral or intravenous. An infant with BPD who exhibits a toxic or septic appearance should also have a blood culture drawn to rule out septicemia.

Gastrointestinal disturbances. Disturbances such as diarrhea, nausea, emesis, and feeding intolerances are common in this population. Gastrointestinal disturbances may be associated with a respiratory infection, antibiotic therapy, theophylline toxicity, feeding intolerance to formulas, or a change in osmotic load as a result of changes in caloric density of the formula. If these reasons have been reviewed and diarrhea persists, a stool specimen should be obtained to rule out bacterial or viral etiology. Frequent emesis may indicate the presence of gastroesophageal reflux. Hydration status must be monitored to avoid dehydration. The child may need to be hospitalized for fluid management.

Skin-mucosa changes. Candida infections are often contracted after a course of antibiotic treatment or prolonged systemic steroid treatment. Most sensitive are the warm, moist surfaces of the body, including diaper areas, oral mucosa, tracheostomy and gastrostomy stomas. Practicing good skin hygiene and keeping the skin dry prevent the spread of the rash. Topical treatment with antifungal creams such as Nystatin also is indicated. Nystatin suspension is the treatment for oral thrush.

BPD unresponsive to therapy. Occasionally an infant with diagnosed BPD will not respond to treatment as expected. If unresponsiveness occurs, consider other respiratory disorders related to the neonatal period. Conditions that may mimic BPD in infants include: (1) Wilson-Mikity syndrome, which presents as increasing respiratory distress in the premature infant at 2 to 6 weeks of life. Cystic changes make it pathologically different from BPD; (2) pulmonary interstitial emphysema, which appears similar to stage III BPD on radiograph; (3) congenital heart disease with left-to-right shunting, which can result in respiratory failure secondary to pulmonary edema. Congenital heart disease is easily differentiated from lung disease with an echocardiogram and cardiac catheterization; (4) pulmonary hemorrhage, which can cause complete opacification on chest x-ray, mimicking stage II BPD; (5) viral pneumonia, which is differentiated from BPD with titers and bronchial wash cultures; (6) cystic fibrosis (CF) in the neonatal period, which can present with respiratory distress and abnormal x-rays similar to BPD. A sweat chloride test will rule out CF; and (7) congenital pulmonary lymphangiectasia, which is an overgrowth of the lung lymphatic vessels. Unlike BPD, a chest x-ray of this condition shows mottling and hyperinflation at birth.

Drug Interactions

Cough suppressants are not recommended for the child with BPD; the cause of the cough should be evaluated and treated. Likewise, antihistamines are not recommended for the child with an artificial airway. The drying effect can cause thickening of airway secretions, presenting the potential for plugging of the smaller peripheral airways and the tracheostomy tube.

Theophylline is a commonly used bronchodilator. If doses are missed, the blood level and resulting effectiveness of the medication may be significantly altered. Theophylline may cause a number of adverse GI side effects, including gastric irritability, nausea, and vomiting. These can be prevented by administering certain preparations with food. If the child is already difficult to feed, this adds an additional challenge. Theophylline levels are altered by some commonly used medications (see Table on p. 185), and serum levels must be checked often when these medications are prescribed. (See Chapter 8 for additional asthma drug interactions.)

DEVELOPMENTAL ISSUES

Sleep Patterns

Most hospitals preparing to discharge a child with BPD attempt to arrange the child's care to provide for several hours of undisturbed sleep at night. The primary care provider should determine if there has been any change in the child's status as a result of the schedule adjustment. For example, bronchodilator treatments and CPT may be extended from 6 to 8 hours to promote the child's and parents' sleep. If schedules for home life have not been restructured, this is an appropriate time to discuss the schedule with the family and gradually implement changes.

The infant's and parents' sleep patterns may be altered because of the monitors placed in the home for children who require mechanical ventilation, receive oxygen therapy, or have a history of apnea. The primary care provider should inquire about the frequency of alarms and determine what type of alarm is appropriate for the child's condition. Readjustment of alarm limits may be warranted if there is a frequent number of false alarms; the limits are set within the physiologic range of the child's heart and respiratory rate. With increasing frequency, the pulse oximeter is the preferred monitor because of the simplicity of use and accuracy of measurement.

It is important to determine how audible the monitor alarm is to the family. If the alarm is so loud that it is very disturbing, the monitor can be placed on a cloth to absorb sound. If the sound is not sufficiently audible, the primary care provider can recommend a commercially available intercom system.

Toileting

Delayed bowel and bladder training may occur as a result of prolonged hospitalization, prematurity, or neurodevelopmental delay. The use of diuretics or theophylline may make bladder training more difficult because of increased frequency of urination. Parents must be assisted in identifying cues indicating the child's neurologic readiness for toilet training.

Discipline

Children with technologic support learn quickly that the sounding of alarms and monitors immediately summons a caregiver. Purposeful disconnections can easily become an attention maneuver. The child and family should be educated with regard to potential risks.

Parents need support and guidance from the primary care provider in recognizing that their children need reasonable, consistent discipline. The primary care provider can assist the family in developing consistent responses and discipline approaches that can be used by numerous caregivers, including parents, siblings, therapists, and nurses. Approaches should be based on the child's cognitive and developmental age, not chronologic age.

Child Care

Children requiring mechanical ventilation often have the support of nursing care during the night that is reimbursed by third-party payers. Children who have an artificial airway may or may not have this coverage; this will depend on third-party payer guidelines.

Children who do not require technologic support may not qualify for supportive care through insurance. This can present a problem for families who have limited budgets and cannot afford private in-home baby-sitters. Regular day care services are not recommended because of the increased exposure to infections (Thacker et al, 1992; Takala et al, 1995).

Traditional well-child day care centers are not equipped or trained to care for a child who is medically fragile (Fewell, 1993). There have been a few medical day care centers created by individuals or agencies that employ skilled nurses to provide high-quality child care (Porter, 1992).

The primary care provider can assist families in exploring child care options. Hospital discharge programs will often incorporate additional family members or neighbors into the teaching plans if requested.

The primary care provider should review the family support systems to determine if the systems are satisfactory to the well-being of the child and the family. Nursing care should be used to provide support for families during activity-intensive periods of the day (Folden and Coffman, 1993). Time without nursing support can be scheduled to incorporate activities and responsibilities within the context of the family structure and routine (Folden and Coffman, 1993).

Increasingly there is an awareness of the need for medical day care facilities that provide services for children requiring supportive treatments. Funding may be supported by insurance. The number of operating facilities is small, but the availability should increase as the need intensifies.

Schooling

All children with BPD should have a thorough developmental evaluation. Plans should be established for outpatient follow-up either at a community-based education center or within the home. This is in accordance with Public Laws 99-457 and 101-476. Parents will need ongoing support as the child grows and develops.

When the child is 3 years old, an individualized education plan (IEP) should be initiated by the parent with the help of the public school system. On entering the school system, the child may notice differences in physical build and exercise endurance. Body image and peer acceptance may become an issue. Children with attention deficit disorder or those that are put in special classes for the learning disabled may have difficulty developing social skills. Increased absences during the winter season from respiratory tract infections may further disrupt the school routine. Separation anxiety from the parents' perspective may develop from concern for the loss of control over their "fragile" child.

The primary care provider can assist in the transition from home to school by providing specific instructions to school personnel regarding the child's medical conditions and medications. Each school has a policy regarding medication administration during school hours. The ultimate goal is to encourage these children with special needs to take responsibility for self-care.

Sexuality

There are no specific sexuality problems related to BPD. The children with physical and developmental delays and handicaps will need referrals and follow-up appropriate to their needs. The earliest survivors of BPD are now approximately 30 years old, and to date there has been no documentation on any difficulties in the area of sexuality.

Children with BPD generally become adults with asthma. Pregnancy for women with BPD would bring a certain degree of stress on the respiratory system. Airway inflammation and bronchoconstriction should be controlled so both mother and baby receive an adequate oxygen supply (National Institute of Health [NIH] Executive Summary, 1993). Inhaled bronchodilators and antiinflammatories are considered safe for pregnant women (NIH, 1993).

Transition into Adulthood

Pulmonary dysfunction in adolescents and adults with a history of BPD is commonly seen. Airway obstruction, airway hyperreactivity, and hyperinflation persist in a significant percentage of persons with BPD (Ackerman, 1994). Anticipatory guidance including environmental control and possible future needs for asthma therapy is suggested. Vocational counseling should be provided regarding environmental irritants in the workplace (i.e., secondhand cigarette smoke, construction dust or particles, pollens, and factory smoke) and their relationship to asthma. Yearly influenza vaccine is recommended for individuals with BPD. An educational review during adolescence and again in young adulthood of the pathophysiology of airway disease, medication action and indication, use of a peak flow meter, use of a metered dose inhaler (MDI) or aerochamber, and signs and symptoms of distress that warrant immediate medical attention is essential for the older individual to assume self-care.

SPECIAL FAMILY CONCERNS

Education and Discharge Planning

Discharge planning ideally starts several weeks before the anticipated discharge date. Family members who will be caregivers must attend informal teaching sessions and hands-on practice sessions with the hospital nurses in order to safely care for the infant when at home.

Basic respiratory assessment skills, which include counting a sleeping breathing rate, and recognizing fluid overload (puffiness), retractions, flaring, and color changes, are essential for families to monitor their infants at home. The family members should have a basic understanding of the pathophysiology of BPD, its chronic nature, and the need for close follow-up. Caregivers at home should have an understanding of the infant's high nutritional needs balanced with an appreciation of the infant's low respiratory reserve. CPR instruction should be provided before the child is discharged from the hospi-

tal. The family must be able to demonstrate use of any medical equipment that will be in the home (i.e., oxygen, apnea monitor, pulmonaide).

Family members and friends should practice good hand washing and, when ill, avoid contact with the infant. Environmental control of airway irritants can be maximized in the home. A smoke-free, pet-free home without mold or mildew and with minimal dust is ideal.

Financial Responsibilities

Most third-party payers fund the cost of equipment and rehabilitative and nursing needs. Variations exist from state to state for children supported by Medicaid (see Chapter 7). Financial strains created by numerous visits from medical and rehabilitative care practitioners (McAleese, Knopp, and Rhodes, 1993) can stress family budgets. Equipment such as mechanical ventilators, compressors, and monitors increase the use of electricity. Calls to physicians, therapists, vendors, and nursing services increase telephone bills. Some utility companies have programs for families with special needs. Other hidden costs such as medications, special formulas, corrective glasses, rehabilitative equipment, and higher electricity and heat bills can create further financial burden. Loss of parental wages because of a leave of absence from work in order to care for a fragile infant causes families further financial burden.

Privacy

The increased amount of people in the home environment, including nurses, vendors, respiratory therapists, and rehabilitative therapists, can seriously limit family privacy. When the family appears capable of assuming care safely and voices concerns about the lack of privacy, and if the needs of the child are stabilized, the primary care provider in conjunction with the pediatric respiratory team can suggest decreasing some of this support (Folden and Coffman, 1993).

Once a child has been discharged from the hospital, the reality of the developmental delay may become apparent. Families will need ongoing emotional support to face and adjust to this problem. The primary care provider can assist with investigation of appropriate educational and rehabilitative programs (Folden and Coffman, 1993).

SUMMARY OF PRIMARY CARE NEEDS FOR THE CHILD WITH BRONCHOPULMONARY DYSPLASIA

Health care maintenance

Growth and development

Height and weight are less than average in the majority of children even at 2 years of age.

Plot head circumference, height, and length corrected for gestational age with each visit.

Review caloric intake for adequacy.

Developmental delay is often seen during the first year of life. Continued delay may be seen in children of very low birth weight or with a history of severe BPD. Learning disabilities are often evident during school years.

Diet

Adequate caloric intake is important for optimal lung repair and growth and development.

Difficulties may arise with oral motor function. Oral feedings may need to be supplemented with enteral feedings.

Early referral to a pediatric nutritionist can prevent long-term problems.

Safety

Beware of accidental disconnections from respiratory support and accidental decannulations.

Use caution with oxygen use in home.

Electrical safety requires grounded equipment.

Establish emergency service contact before the child is discharged home.

Immunization

Many children are delayed in receiving immunizations because of prolonged hospitalization.

Children should be immunized according to routine schedule based on the chronologic age, not gestational age.

Hospital records must be reviewed.

Pertussis vaccine should be withheld only with just cause because of the high risk of significant morbidity with active disease in children with BPD. Use Acellular pertussis if age appropriate.

Inactivated polio vaccine may be administered in the hospital before discharge.

Influenza vaccine is recommended yearly for children with chronic lung disease.

Pneumococcal vaccine and varicella vaccine are recommended.

Screening

Vision

Evaluation by a pediatric ophthalmologist should be done every 2 to 3 months during the first year of life to rule out ROP. Cover test and tracking ability should be screened at each visit.

Myopia and strabismus are common and must be followed in the primary care office and by a pediatric ophthalmologist.

Hearing

A BAER test should be done before discharge from the hospital.

There is a risk of hearing loss because of prematurity and medications.

Age appropriate screening should be done at each office visit.

Audiometry screening should be done with recurrent serous otitis media.

Speech delays are anticipated in children with tracheostomies.

Dental

Routine screening is recommended.

Hypoplastic and discolored teeth are common.

Oral defensiveness may make dental hygiene difficult.

Blood pressure

Blood pressure should be taken at each visit. Children with abnormal BP findings should be referred to a pulmonologist.

Hematocrit

Because of prematurity, iron deficiency anemia is common.

Hematocrit screening must be done frequently during the first year of life.

Chronic hypoxia may cause elevated hemoglobin levels.

Urinalysis

Routine screening is recommended.

Tuberculosis

Routine screening is recommended.

Continued.

SUMMARY OF PRIMARY CARE NEEDS FOR THE CHILD WITH BRONCHOPULMONARY DYSPLASIA—cont'd

Condition-specific screening

CHEST X-RAY

Radiographic examinations of the lung should be done at discharge then annually and prn clinical indication.

PULMONARY FUNCTION TESTS

Pulmonary function tests should be done at discharge, annually and prn clinical indication.

Common illness management

Differential diagnosis

Respiratory distress

Rule out bacterial or viral infection, atelectasis, pneumonia, bronchospasm, pulmonary edema, heart failure, and sinusitis. During November to March, consider RSV infections.

Cough

Rule out sinusitis, GER, reactive airway disease, pulmonary edema, pertussis and RSV.

Fever

Rule out otitis media, sinusitis, upper or lower respiratory tract infection, UTI and septicemia.

Rule out respiratory tract infection, otitis media, and viral infection.

Gastrointestinal disturbances

Consider feeding intolerances, bacterial and viral infections, GER, or theophylline toxicity.

Skin

For skin problems around tracheostomy and gastrostomy stomas, and diaper areas, consider candida infection and cellulitis.

Drug interactions

Theophylline interacts with other medications (see Table on p. 135).

Cough suppressants may mask an underlying condition. They are not recommended.

Do not use antihistamines with children with tracheostomy tubes because of the thickening of airway secretions.

Developmental issues

Sleep patterns

Attempt to evaluate the child's schedule of care to decrease disturbances and provide for the whole family.

Evaluate functioning of monitors.

Toileting

Delayed bowel and bladder training may occur as a result of prolonged hospitalization and the use of diuretics and theophylline.

Discipline

Children should receive discipline appropriate to their developmental level of understanding.

A consistent plan should be followed.

Child care

Recommend that children not supported by oxygen and mechanical ventilation attend home or small day care centers to reduce exposure to infection.

Children with mechanical support may be eligible for nursing support from third-party payers.

Schooling

Assist family with developmental evaluations and planning early intervention programs.

Assist families with adjustment to developmental delays.

Sexuality

Care is routine unless associated problems warrant additional care.

Transition into adulthood

Abnormal pulmonary function frequently persists into adulthood. Counsel regarding possible environmental irritants in workplace or school. Review and educate concerning disease process and management.

Special family concerns

Financial responsibilities are great even with insurance coverage.

There may be a lack of privacy in the home because of the need for medical caregivers.

Developmental outcome is uncertain. The potential for developmental delay and persistent medical problems result in great emotional strain on parents.

REFERENCES

Ackerman VL: Bronchopulmonary dysplasia. In Loughlin GM and Eigen H, (editors): *Respiratory disease in children: diagnosis and management,* Baltimore, MD, 1994, Williams & Wilkins.

Alpert BE, Allen JL, and Schidlow, DV: Bronchopulmonary dysplasia. In Hilman B, (editor): *Pediatric respiratory disease: diagnosis and treatment,* Philadelphia, 1993, WB Saunders.

Anderson AH et al: Systemic hypertension in infants with severe bronchopulmonary dysplasia: associated clinical factors, *Am J Perinatol* 10:190-193, 1993.

Armentrout D: Gastroesophageal reflux in infants, *The Nurse Practitioner* 20:54-63, 1995.

Bancalari E, Sosenko I: Pathogenesis and prevention of neonatal chronic lung disease: recent developments. *Pediatric Pulmonol* 8:109-116, 1990.

Bernbaum JE et al: Preterm infant care after hospital discharge, *Pediatr Rev* 10:195-208, 1989.

Brem AS: Electrolyte disorders associated with respiratory distress syndrome and bronchopulmonary dysplasia, *Clin Perinatol* 19:223-232, 1992.

Brundage KL et al: Bronchodilator response to ipratropium bromide in infants with bronchopulmonary dysplasia, *Am Rev Dis* 142:1137-1142, 1990.

Cloutier MM: Nebulized steroid therapy in bronchopulmonary dysplasia, *Pediatr Pulmonol* 15:111-116, 1993.

Committee on Infectious Disease. Report of the committee on infectious disease, ed 23, Elk Grove Village, IL, 1994, American Academy of Pediatrics.

Conner WT et al: Reliable salbutamol administration in 6- to 36-month-old children by means of a metered dose inhaler and aerochamber with mask, *Pediatr Pulmonol* 6:263-267, 1989.

Cunningham CK, McMilan JA, and Gross SJ: Rehospitalization for respiratory illness in infants of less than 32 weeks' gestation, *Pediatrics* 88:527-532, 1991.

Duncan S, Eid N: Tracheomalacia and bronchopulmonary dysplasia, *Ann Otol Rhinol Laryngol* 100:856-858, 1991.

Farrell PM, Palta M: Bronchopulmonary dysplasia. In PM Farrell and LM Taussing (editors): Bronchopulmonary dysplasia and isolated chronic respiratory disorders, Columbus, OH, 1986, Ross Laboratories.

Fewell RR: Child care for children with special needs, *Pediatrics* 91:193-198, 1993.

Folden SL, Coffman S: Respite care of families of children with disabilities. *J Pediatr Health Care* 7:103-110, 1993.

Gardner SL, Hagedorn MI: Physiologic sequelae of prematurity: the nurse practitioner's role, *J Pediatr Health Care* 6:263-270, 1992.

Goldson E: Bronchopulmonary dysplasia, *Pediatric Annals* 19:13-18, 1990.

Goodman G et al: Pulmonary hypertension in infants with bronchopulmonary dysplasia, *J Pediatr* 112:67-72, 1988.

Gray PH et al: Prediction of outcome of preterm infants with severe bronchopulmonary dysplasia, *J Paediatr Child Health* 29:107-112, 1993.

Greenough A: Bronchopulmonary dysplasia: early diagnosis, prophylaxis, and treatment, *Arch Dis Child* 65:1082-1088, 1990.

Groothuis JR et al: Prophylactic administration of respiratory syncitial virus immune globulin to high-risk infants and young children, *N Engl J Med* 329:1524-1530, 1993.

Hack M et al: Effect of very low birth weight and subnormal head size on cognitive abilities at school age, *N Engl J Med* 325:231-237, 1991.

Hagedorn MI, Gardner SL: Physiologic sequelae of prematurity: the nurse practitioner's role, part I, Respiratory issues, *J Pediatr Health Care* 3:288-297, 1989.

Hazinski TA: Bronchopulmonary dysplasia. In Chernick V and Kendig E, (editors): *Disorders of the respiratory tract in children,* ed 5, Philadelphia, 1990, WB Saunders.

Hoekstra RE et al: Improved neonatal survival following multiple doses of bovine surfactant in very premature neonates at risk for respiratory distress syndrome, *Pediatrics* 88:10-18, 1991.

Konig PK et al: Clinical observations of nebulized flunisolide in infants and young children with asthma and bronchopulmonary dysplasia, *Pediatr Pulmonol* 13:209-214, 1992.

Konig P: Inhaled corticosteroids—their present and future role in the management of asthma, *J Allergy Clin Immunol* ••:297-306, 1988.

Kountz DS: An algorithm for corticosteroid withdrawal, *Clinical Pharmacology* 39:250-254, 1989.

Long W et al: Effects of two rescue doses of a synthetic surfactant on mortality rate and survival without bronchopulmonary dysplasia in 700- to 1350-gram infants with respiratory distress syndrome, *J Pediatr* 118:595-605, 1991.

Luchi JM, Bennett FC, and Jackson JC: Predictors of neurodevelopmental outcome following bronchopulmonary dysplasia, *AJDC* 145:813-817, 1991.

McAleese KA, Knapp MA, and Rhodes TT: Financial and emotional cost of bronchopulmonary dysplasia, *Clin Pediatr* ••:393-400, 1993.

Moore A: Retinopathy of prematurity. In Taylor D, (editor): *Pediatric ophthalmology,* Boston, MA, 1990, Blackwell Scientific Publications.

National Institutes of Health Executive Summary: Management of asthma during pregnancy, National Asthma Education Program, National Heart, Lung and Blood Institute, National Institutes of Health, NIH publication no 93-3279A, March 1993.

1994 Red Book: Report of the committee on infectious diseases, ed 23.

Northway WH: Bronchopulmonary dysplasia: then and now, *Arch Dis Child* 65:1076-1081, 1990.

Northway WH et al: Late pulmonary sequelae of bronchopulmonary dysplasia, *N Eng J Med* 323:1793-1799, 1990.

Northway WH, Rosen RC, and Porter DV: Pulmonary disease

following respiratory therapy of hylane membrane disease., *N Eng J Med* 267:357-368, 1967.

Parker RA, Lindstrom DP, and Cotton RB: Improved survival accounts for most, but not all, of the increase in bronchopulmonary dysplasia, *Pediatrics* 90:663-668, 1992.

Philip AG: Oxygen plus pressure plus time: the etiology of bronchopulmonary dysplasia, *Pediatrics* 55:44-50, 1975.

Porter SA: Infant medical day care: a natural extension of home, *Caring Magazine* ••:90-94, 1992.

Robertson CMT et al: 8-year school performance, neurodevelopmental and growth outcome of neonates with bronchopulmonary dysplasia: a comparative study, *Pediatrics* 89:365-372, 1992.

Rossing TH: Methylxanthines in 1989, 110:502-504.

Rozycki HJ, Kirkpatrick BV: New developments in bronchopulmonary dysplasia, *Pediatr Ann* 22:532-538, 1993.

Rush MG, Hazinski TA: Current therapy of bronchopulmonary dysplasia, *Clin Perinatol* 19:563-590, 1992.

Sauve RS, Singhal N: Long-term morbidity of infants with bronchopulmonary dysplasia, *Pediatrics* 76:725-733, 1985.

Singer L et al: Oxygen desaturation complicates feeding in infants with bronchopulmonary dysplasia after discharge, *Pediatrics* 90:380-384, 1992.

Southall DP, Samuals MP: Bronchopulmonary dysplasia: a new look at management, *Arch Dis Child* 65:1089-1095, 1990.

Takala AK et al: Risk factors for primary invasive pneumococcal disease among children in Finland *JAMA* 273:859-864, 1995.

Tammela OKT: First-year infections after initial hospitalization in low-birth-weight infants with and without bronchopulmonary dysplasia, *Scand J Infect Dis* 24:515-524, 1992.

Tammela OKT, Koivisto ME: A 1-year follow-up of low-birth-weight infants with and without bronchopulmonary dysplasia: health, growth, clinical lung disease, cardiovascular and neurological sequelae, *Early Human Development* 30:109-120, 1992.

Thacker SB et al: Infectious diseases and injuries in child day care, *JAMA* 268:1720-1726, 1992.

Truog WE: Bronchopulmonary dysplasia: issues in long-term management, *J Resp Diseases* 14:130-145, 1993.

Vohr BR et al: Neurodevelopmental and medical status of low-birth-weight survivors of bronchopulmonary dysplasia at 10 to 12 years of age, *Develop Med Child Neurol* 33:690-697, 1991.

Vrlenich LA et al: The effect of bronchopulmonary dysplasia on growth at school age, *Pediatrics* 95:855-859, 1995.

Watterberg KL, Scott SM: Evidence of early adrenal insufficiency in babies who develop bronchopulmonary dysplasia, *Pediatrics* 95:120-125, 1995.

Wilkie RA, Bryan MH: Effect of bronchodilators on airway resistance in ventilator-dependent neonates with chronic lung disease, *J Pediatr* 111:278-282, 1987.

Zinman R, Blanchard, PW, and Vachon F: Oxygen saturation during sleep in patients with bronchopulmonary dysplasia, *Biol Neonate* 61:69-75, 1992.

Cancer

Mary Alice Dragone*

11

ETIOLOGY

An estimated 8200 children are diagnosed with cancer annually in the United States (American Cancer Society, 1994). Cancer results when there is a failure of the body to regulate cell production. A proliferation and spread of abnormal cells then occurs, which, if left unchecked, may lead to death of the host. Common sites of malignancy in children include the blood and bone marrow, bone, lymph nodes, brain, central nervous system (CNS), kidneys, and soft tissues (Table 11-1).

The causes of childhood cancers are poorly identified. It is frequently hypothesized that genetic and environmental influences play a role in the expression of malignancies.

INCIDENCE

The overall incidence of malignancy in children less than 15 years of age is approximately 14:100,000 per year (Bleyer, 1990). The incidence of malignancy among children worldwide varies with the exception of Wilms' tumor, which is remarkably uniform. A comparison of the incidence rates of the various childhood malignancies in the United States (see Table 11-1) illustrates a wide variation depending on site.

CLINICAL MANIFESTATIONS AT TIME OF DIAGNOSIS

The signs and symptoms of a malignant disease will depend on the interval between time of origin and diagnosis, as well as the type and location of the tumor. In general, cancer may manifest in one of three ways: (1) as a mass lesion, (2) with symptoms directly related to the tumor, or (3) with nonspecific symptoms. The presence of a mass lesion should alert the primary care provider to the possibility of a malignancy. The few mass lesions considered to be benign on the basis of location or physical appearance alone would include an inflamed lymph node, hemangiomas, thyroglossal duct cyst, fat necrosis, dermoid cysts of the eyebrow, prepubertal breast hyperplasia, lymphangiomas, and torticollis tumors (Altman and Schwartz, 1983). A biopsy of other lesions should be taken in a timely manner to rule out malignancy. Symptoms related directly to the tumor may include bony pain, limping (Sherry, 1990), unexplained bleeding, bruising or petechiae, morning headache and vomiting, hematuria, paleness, swelling in face or neck, white spot in pupil, airway or urinary tract obstruction, or endocrinologic symptoms from hormone production by the tumor. Nonspecific symptoms would include weight loss, diarrhea, low-grade fevers, malaise, or failure to thrive.

Text continued on p. 199.

*Previous author Elizabeth Dawes.

Table 11-1.   COMMON PEDIATRIC CANCERS

Type	Site	Incidence (<15 yr)	Etiology	Signs/symptoms	Treatment
Leukemia					
	Bone marrow	43.7 per 1 million white children per year 25.2 per 1 million black children per year	Genetic factors Constitutional chromosomal abnormalities Familial predisposition (ALL-infant identical twins)	Pallor Fatigue, headache Fever, infection Purpura, bruising Organomegaly Bone pain	
Acute lymphoblastic leukemia (ALL)		32.9 per 1 million white children per year 14.8 per 1 million black children per year	Environmental factors Ionizing radiation Chronic chemical exposure Use of alkylating agents for treatment of malignant disease (AML) Possible viral infection		Combination chemotherapy CNS prophylaxis Radiation therapy (for high risk patients) and intrathecal chemotherapy Combined intrathecal chemotherapy
Acute myelogenous leukemia (AML)		6.1 per 1 million white children per year 5.2 per 1 million black children per year			Combination chemotherapy CNS prophylaxis Single-agent intrathecal chemotherapy Bone marrow transplant in first remission
Central nervous system					
Infratentorial Medulloblastoma	Cerebellum/brainstem Midline cerebellar	24.9 per 1 million white children per year	Genetic factors Heritable disease (NF*) Familial	Early Decreased academic performance Fatigue Personality changes Intermittent headache	Anticonvulsants, if symptoms present Treatment of hydrocephalus Corticosteroids Shunting Surgical resection (if operable)
Ependymoma	Ependymal lining of ventricular system or/central cord of spinal cord	22 per 1 million black children per year	Environmental factors Chronic chemical exposure		

Type	Common Sites	Incidence	Etiology	Clinical Manifestations	Treatment
Brainstem glioma	Brainstem		Ionizing radiation Other primary malignancies Exogenous immunosuppression	Late Morning headache Vomiting Diplopia/visual changes Brainstem/cerebellar Deficits of balance/positioning	Radiation therapy Chemotherapy for some tumors Bone marrow transplant in rare cases
Supratentorial Astrocytomas	Ventricles, midline diencephalous, cerebrum			Supratentorial Nonspecific headache Seizures Hemiparesis	
Craniopharyngioma Gliomas Primitive neuroectodermal tumor or germ cell	Sella turcica Visual pathway Pineal region				
Non-Hodgkin's lymphoma Lymphoblastic lymphoma	Usually generalized Anterior mediastinum Lymph nodes Bone marrow	6.9 per 1 million white children per year 3 per 1 million black children per year	Multifactorial Immunodeficiency Exogenous immunosuppression Viral-associated with Ebstein-Barr virus	Generally rapid progression Lymphoblastic lymphoma Dysphagia, dyspnea Swelling of neck, face, upper extremities	Treatment of emergent symptoms Multiagent chemotherapy CNS prophylaxis
Small noncleaved lymphoma Burkitt's lymphoma Non-Burkitt's lymphoma	Abdomen Bone marrow Mediastinium (rare)			Supradiaphragmatic lymphadenopathy Respiratory distress Small noncleaved lymphoma Abdominal pain or swelling Change in bowel habits	Multiagent chemotherapy CNS prophylaxis

Continued.

Table 11-1.   COMMON PEDIATRIC CANCERS—cont'd

Type	Site	Incidence (<15 yr)	Etiology	Signs/symptoms	Treatment
Large cell lymphoma	Lymph nodes Cutaneous lesions Mediastinum Abdomen Head, neck			Nausea/vomiting GI* bleeding Rarely, intestinal perforation Inguinal/iliac adenopathy Intussuception Large cell lymphoma As cited earlier, depending on site	Multiagent chemotherapy
Hodgkin's lymphoma	Single lymph node or lymphatic chains Mediastinal mass Spleen	6.2 per 1 million white children per year 4.7 per 1 million black children per year	Genetic factors Familial predisposition Environmental influence Iatrogenic or acquired immunodeficiency Infectious etiology	Lymphadenopathy Organomegaly Fatigue Anorexia/weight loss/fever	Splenectomy, if surgical staging Multiagent chemotherapy Radiation therapy

Neuroblastoma	Anywhere along the sympathetic nervous system chain
	Most commonly
	  Adrenal gland
	  Paraspinal ganglion
	  Thorax
	  Neck
		12.5 per 1 million white children per year
		10.2 per 1 million black children per year
			Possible genetic factors
			Familial predisposition
			Associated with fetal alcohol syndrome and fetal hydantoin syndrome
				Dependent on primary site, site of metastases
				Metastases present in 70% of cases at diagnosis (especially in bone marrow)
				Presence of a mass (abdomen, thoracic, cervical, pelvic, liver)
				Symptoms from compression of mass (Horner's syndrome, edema of upper and
					Treatment of emergent symptoms
					Surgery (staging excision of tumor, evaluation of treatment)
					Radiation therapy
					Combination chemotherapy
					Bone marrow transplant, in some cases

	Location	Incidence	Etiology	Clinical manifestations	Treatment
				lower extremities secondary to vascular compression, hypertension caused by compression of renal vasculature, cord compression symptoms [paresis, paralysis, bowel/bladder dysfunction] Diarrhea from vasoactive intestinal peptides produced by tumor cells Skin or subcutaneous nodules (infants only) Nonspecific symptoms (fever, weight loss, failure to thrive, generalized pain) Rarely syndrome of opsoclonus-myoclonus	Surgical removal (if feasible) Radiation therapy for residual tumor Multiagent systemic chemotherapy
Soft tissue sarcomas Rhabdomyosarcoma Undifferentiated sarcoma	Head and neck (most common) Abdomen Anywhere in body	8.6 per 1 million white children per year 8.3 per 1 million black children per year	Genetic factors Associated with NF and maternal history of breast cancer Environmental factors Parental smoking, ingestion of animal organs Possible viral etiology	Dependent on location and size of tumor	
Kidney Wilms' tumor (nephroblastoma, renal embryoma)	Unilateral, bilateral	9.0 per 1 million white children per year 12.4 per 1 million black children per year	Genetic factors Associated with aniridia, NF, Beckwith-Wiedemann	Asymptomatic mass Malaise, pain Microscopic or gross hematuria Hypertension	Complete surgical excision (if bilateral, nephrectomy of more involved site, excisional biopsy/ partial nephrectomy)

Continued.

Table 11-1. COMMON PEDIATRIC CANCERS—cont'd

Type	Site	Incidence (<15 yr)	Etiology	Signs/symptoms	Treatment
			Familial predisposition Environmental factors Chronic chemical exposure (hydrocarbons/lead)		of smaller lesion in remaining kidney) Multiagent chemotherapy Radiation therapy
Bone tumors Osteosarcoma	Long bones of extremities	2.5 per 1 million white children per year 3.4 per 1 million black children per year	Genetic factors Familial predisposition (hereditary retinoblastoma)	Pain over involved area with or without swelling (often 3-6 mo. or longer)	Multiagent chemotherapy Surgical excision of tumor preserving as much function of primary site as possible
Ewing's sarcoma	Bones of pelvis, humerus, femur, generally axial skeleton	2.4 per 1 million white children per year 0.4 per 1 million black children per year	Genetic factors Associated with hereditary retinoblastoma Association with skeletal and genitourinary abnormalities	In presence of metastatic disease nonspecific symptoms (fatigue, anorexia, weight loss, intermittent fever, malaise)	Amputation may be necessary, if extent of disease or location does not allow complete excision Localized radiation therapy (Ewing's sarcoma)
Retinoblastoma	Eye	4.0 per 1 million white children per year 5.1 per 1 million black children per year	Genetic factors Gene mutation (nonhereditary) Autosomal dominant (all bilateral retinoblastoma and 15% of unilateral)	Leukocoria (cat's eye reflex) Squint Strabismus Orbital inflammation	Surgery (resection, enucleation with extensive disease; salvage of one eye attempted in bilateral disease) Radiation therapy Chemotherapy (usually palliative)

Incidence data modified from National Cancer Institute. Rie LA, Hankey BF, Miller BA, et al (eds): *Cancer Statistics Review 1973-1988*, Bethesda, NIH Publication No. 91-2789, 1991.
*GI, gastrointestinal
NF, neurofibromatosis

**CLINICAL MANIFESTATION
AT TIME OF DIAGNOSIS**

- Mass lesion
- Lymph node enlargement that is unresponsive to antibiotic therapy or is accompanied by nonspecific symptoms
- Unexplained bruising, bleeding, or petechiae
- Pallor
- Unexplained or persistent fevers
- Recurrent infection
- Bone pain or limping
- Morning headache or vomiting
- Swelling in face or neck
- White spot in pupil (leukocoria)
- Hematuria
- Airway or urinary tract obstruction
- Nonspecific symptoms: weight loss, diarrhea, failure to thrive, malaise, low-grade fevers

TREATMENT

- Surgery
  Biopsy
  Resection
  Palliation
- Chemotherapy
- Radiation
- Biologic response modifiers
- Bone marrow transplantation

Prompt referral to a pediatric cancer treatment center ensures specimens for staging are properly obtained and the child is enrolled in multiinstitutional treatment studies. The initial work-up is crucial to the accurate and timely establishment of a diagnosis. One large study of the "lag times" to diagnosis Krischner of pediatric solid tumors found that older children, and those with Ewing's sarcoma and osteosarcoma, had much longer "lag times" than young children and those with other tumors (Pollock, Krischner, and Vietti, 1991). Children with neuroblastoma had the shortest "lag time". After a thorough history and physical examination and laboratory tests, the work-up may include nuclear-radiological examinations, ultrasound, bone marrow aspirate-biopsy or lumbar puncture, depending on the type of tumor suspected and the most frequent sites for metastases.

Whenever a biopsy is being considered, the primary care provider should consult with an oncology treatment center before proceeding. Accurate staging is increasingly dependent on the molecular genetics and immunocytochemistry of initial diagnostic materials processed in specialty laboratories (Pizzo, 1990). Prompt referral to a pediatric cancer

treatment center will allow the child to be enrolled in multiinstitutional treatment studies.

TREATMENT

Cancer treatment involves the concurrent or sequential use of surgery, chemotherapy, radiation therapy, biologic response modifiers, and less frequently, bone marrow transplantation. Bone marrow transplantation is used both as an initial therapy of choice and as a salvage therapy when other therapies have failed.

State-of-the-art treatment is provided by multi-institutional cooperative study groups and by some specialty cancer treatment centers. These centers generally employ a multidisciplinary approach combining the expertise of physicians, nurses in advanced practice, social workers, art and child life therapists, and other specialists. The National Cancer Institute sponsors two groups that register over 60% of children with cancer in the United States for treatment: the Children's Cancer Group (CCG) and the Pediatric Oncology Group (POG) (Pizzo, 1990).

A child's treatment protocol, determined by the type of cancer and the extent of disease, consists of a schedule and combination of therapies shown to be effective in treating the condition. A particular disease protocol may have several treatment regimens ("arms") which are based on an accepted standard treatment with slight variations. Because no protocol regimen is known to be more effective than another, ongoing research investigates various therapies that maximize treatment efficacy while minimizing toxicity. Before a child is assigned to a particular protocol, informed consent is obtained from the parents and, if appropriate, the child. If a child is treated on a research protocol, the family may elect to withdraw the child from the study at any time and have the child treated according to standard therapy.

Surgical intervention is used to (1) obtain a biopsy specimen, (2) determine the extent of disease, (3) remove primary or metastatic lesions, (4) evaluate previously unresectable tumors, (5) provide a "second look" to evaluate the effect of chemotherapy and radiation on partially or nonresected tumors, and (6) relieve symptoms. Surgical procedures are also used in placing indwelling venous access devices and for displacing organs outside of the radiation field (e.g., ovaries during pelvic irradiation).

The goal of chemotherapy is to interrupt the cell cycle of proliferating malignant cells while minimizing the damage to normal cells. In combination chemotherapy, different drugs are used to disrupt the cell cycle at different phases. This increases the exposure of the malignant cells to cytotoxic agents.

Chemotherapeutic agents may be either cell-cycle phase specific or nonspecific. Cell-cycle specific drugs kill cells only in a certain stage of the cell's development and are most effective on rapidly growing cells. Along with malignant cells, the cells of the bone marrow, hair follicles, and intestinal epithelium are susceptible to damage from these drugs. Cell-cycle nonspecific drugs kill cells regardless of their stage of development. They act on dormant as well as dividing cells. Chemotherapeutic agents are further classified by their mechanism of action. The major classifications include alkylating agents, antimetabolites, vinca alkaloids, antibiotics, and corticosteroids. Side effects and toxicities vary depending on the specific agent (see Table 11-2).

Radiation therapy is often used in conjunction with surgery and chemotherapy. Radiation causes breakage of DNA strands, thus inhibiting cell division. The goal of radiation therapy is to destroy the cancer cells while minimizing complications and long-term sequelae. The role of radiation therapy may be definitive, adjunctive, or palliative. Defini-

tive treatment is given with curative intent to a tumor on which a biopsy has been performed or that has been partially resected. In adjunctive radiotherapy, a primary tumor, although totally resected, is at risk for a local recurrence. This area is then treated with a lower dose of radiation than what would be given to control the tumor without surgery. Palliative radiotherapy is used to relieve symptoms of incurable disease after more conservative methods have proved ineffective. Some children benefit from hyperfractionated radiation delivery. This method uses smaller individual doses of radiation twice daily, instead of the usual daily dose, to affect more of the rapidly dividing tumor cells. Overall, the total dosage of radiation used is higher. Early studies of its use in individuals with brain tumors have not shown greater toxicity (Freeman et al, 1988); however, long-term studies are needed to detect late effects.

The tumor's response to radiation is dependent on the type of tumor, type and dose of radiation delivered, and size of the area irradiated. These factors also influence the type and severity of side effects and long-term sequelae. Many side effects are similar to those of chemotherapy. However, rather than a systemic response, the side effects are generally related to the irradiated area. They include nausea and vomiting, diarrhea, mucositis, cataracts, skin changes, and growth and endocrine abnormalities.

The use of biologic response modifiers (BRMs) in the treatment of cancer is one of the newest available treatments and was previously described as immunotherapy. The goal of this therapy is to stimulate the body's natural immune system to selectively target and destroy malignant cells. BRMs encompass colony stimulating factors (CSFs), interleukins, interferons, tumor necrosis factor (TNF), and monoclonal antibodies. Their use has been more completely studied in adults and is currently being applied to children with cancer.

Bone marrow transplantation is used in treating relapsed acute lymphoblastic leukemia (ALL), acute nonlymphocytic leukemia (ANLL), neuroblastoma (Pinkel, 1993), Hodgkin's and non-Hodgkin's lymphoma, and is being investigated for use in recurrent Ewing's sarcoma and brain tumors (Ramsay, 1993). In some institutions, bone marrow transplantation is the initial therapy of choice for

Text continued on p. 208.

Table 11-2.   **SUMMARY OF CHEMOTHERAPEUTIC AGENTS USED IN THE TREATMENT OF CHILDHOOD CANCERS***

Agent/administration	Side effects and toxicity	Comments and specific nursing considerations
Alkylating agents		
	All alkylating agents: Azospermia, ovarian failure Secondary malignancy (AML)	Sperm banking, egg donation, if feasible
Mechlorethamine (nitrogen mustard, Mustargen) IV, Intracavitary	N/V§ (0-2 hrs later) (severe) BMD‖ (2-3 wks later) Alopecia Local phlebitis Anaphylaxis (rare)	Vesicant†
Cyclophosphamide (Cytoxan, CTX,¶ Endoxan) PO, IV, IM‡	N/V (4-12 hrs later) (severe at high doses) BMD (7-10 days later) Alopecia Hemorrhagic cystitis Severe immunosuppression Stomatitis (rare) Hyperpigmentation Transverse ridging of nails Cardiac toxicity (high dose) Pulmonary fibrosis (high dose) Syndrome of inappropriate secretion of antidiuretic hormone (SIADH)	BMD has platelet-sparing effect Give dose early in day to allow adequate fluids afterward Force fluids before administering drug and for 2 days after to prevent chemical cystitis; encourage frequent voiding even during night Warn parents to report signs of burning on urination or hematuria to practitioner MESNA given with high doses to protect bladder MESNA causes false ketonuria
Ifosfamide (IFEX, isophosphamide) IV	N/V (moderate) BMD (7-10 days later) Alopecia Renal tubular damage (Fanconi-like syndrome) Hemorrhagic cystitis Peripheral neuropathy Encephalopathy	See cyclophosphamide above MESNA is given with all doses to protect the bladder
Busulfan (Myleran) PO	N/V (mild) BMD (11-30 days later) Excessive dryness of skin and mucous membranes Gynecomastia (rare) Pulmonary fibrosis (long-term therapy)	Pulmonary function tests

Continued.

Table 11-2.   **SUMMARY OF CHEMOTHERAPEUTIC AGENTS
USED IN THE TREATMENT OF CHILDHOOD
CANCERS*—cont'd**

Agent/administration	Side effects and toxicity	Comments and specific nursing considerations
Procarbazine (Matulane) PO, IV (investigational)	N/V (moderate) BMD (3-4 weeks later) Lethargy Dermatitis Myalgia Arthralgia Diplopia Stomatitis Neuropathy Alopecia Diarrhea Amenorrhea	Central nervous system depressants (phenothiazines, barbiturates) enhance central nervous system symptoms Monoamine oxidase (MAO) inhibition sometimes occurs; therefore all other drugs are avoided unless medically approved; red wine, fava beans, broad bean pods, tea, coffee, cola, cheese, banana are to be avoided Give medication in evening to reduce nausea
Dacarbazine (DTIC-Dome) IV	N/V (especially after first dose) - (severe) BMD (3 weeks later) Alopecia Flulike syndrome Burning sensation in vein during infusion (not extravasation)	Vesicant (less sclerosive) Must be given cautiously in patients with renal dysfunction Decrease IV rate or use cold pack on IV site to decrease burning
Antimetabolites		
Cytosine arabinoside (Ara-C, CytosarU, Cytarabine) IV, IM, SC,‡ IT	N/V (within 2 hours of IT dose) (mild-severe dose dependent) BMD (7-14 days later) Mucosal ulceration Hepatitis (usually subclinical) Conjunctivitis (high dose) ARA-C syndrome: fever, myalgia, malaise, rash 6-12 hr after administration	Crosses blood-brain barrier Use with caution in individuals with hepatic dysfunction Corticosteroid ophthalmic drops to prevent conjunctivitis
5-Azacytidine (5-AZA) IV	N/V (moderate) BMD (7-14 days later) Diarrhea	Infuse slowly via IV drip to decrease severity of N/V Administer cautiously with liver disease or albumin <3.8 g/dl
Mercaptopurine (6-MP, Purinethol) PO (IV, IT-investigational	N/V (mild) Stomatitis BMD Dermatitis Elevated liver enzymes	6-MP is an analog of xanthine; therefore allopurinol (Zyloprim) delays its metabolism and increases its potency, necessitating a lower dose (⅓ to ¼) of 6-MP Take daily dose at bedtime, 2 hours after food/milk

Continued.

Table 11-2.   SUMMARY OF CHEMOTHERAPEUTIC AGENTS USED IN THE TREATMENT OF CHILDHOOD CANCERS*—cont'd

Agent/administration	Side effects and toxicity	Comments and specific nursing considerations
Methotrexate (MTX, Amethopterin) PO, IV, IM, IT. May be given in conventional doses (mg/m²) or high doses (g/m²)	N/V (moderate-severe at high doses) Diarrhea Mucosal ulceration (2-5 days later) BMD (10 days later) Dermatitis Photosensitivity Alopecia Hepatitis (fibrosis) Elevated liver enzymes Nephropathy Pneumonitis (fibrosis) Neurologic toxicity with IT use—arachnoiditis, leukoencephalopathy, seizures	Side effects and toxicity are dose related. Potency and toxicity increased by reduced renal function, salicylates, sulfonamides, and aminobenzoic acid; avoid use of these substances, such as aspirin and ibuprofen High dose therapy: Citrovorum factor (folinic acid or leucovorin) decreases cytotoxic action of MTX; used as an antidote for overdose and to enhance normal cell recovery following high-dose therapy; avoid use of vitamins containing folic acid during MTX therapy unless prescribed by physician IT therapy: Drug *must* be mixed with preservative free diluent Report signs of neurotoxicity immediately
6-Thioguanine (6-TG) PO, IV (investigational)	N/V (mild) BMD (7-14 days later) Stomatitis Dermatitis Liver dysfunction	Side effects are unusual
5-Fluorouracil (5-FU, Fluorouracil, Adrucil) IV, PO, intrahepatic artery	N/V (moderate) BMD (9-14 days later) Dermatitis Stomatitis Alopecia Hyperpigmentation of nail beds	For PO use, mix IV form with flavored water or soda; do not mix with acidic fruit juice Take at least 2 hours before or after food
Plant alkaloids Vincristine (Oncovin) IV	Neurotoxicity—paresthesia (numbness), ataxia, weakness, foot drop, hyporeflexia, constipation (adynamic ileus), hoarseness (vocal cord paralysis); abdominal, chest, and jaw pain Fever N/V (mild) BMD (minimal; 7-14 days later) Alopecia SIADH	Vesicant Report signs of neurotoxicity as this may necessitate cessation of drug Individuals with underlying neurologic problems may be more prone to neurotoxicity Monitor stool patterns closely; administer stool softener Excreted primarily by liver into biliary system; check bilirubin before administration

Continued.

Table 11-2.   **SUMMARY OF CHEMOTHERAPEUTIC AGENTS USED IN THE TREATMENT OF CHILDHOOD CANCERS*—cont'd**

Agent/administration	Side effects and toxicity	Comments and specific nursing considerations
Vinblastine (Velban) IV	Neurotoxicity (same as for vincristine but less severe) N/V (mild 4-12 hours later) BMD (especially neutropenia; 7-14 days later) Alopecia	Same as for vincristine
VP-16-213 (Etoposide, Ve-Pesid) PO, IV	N/V (mild) BMD (7-14 days later) Alopecia Hypotension with rapid infusion Diarrhea May reactivate erythema of irradiated skin (rare) Allergic reaction with anaphylaxis possible Secondary malignancy (AML)	Give slowly via IV drip over at least 1 hr with child recumbent Have emergency drugs available at bedside* Vital signs with blood pressure every 15 minutes during infusion
Antibiotics		
Dactinomycin (Antin-omycin D Cosmegen, ACT-D) IV	N/V (0-6 hours later) (moderate-severe) BMD (especially platelets; 2-3 weeks later) Mucosal ulceration Abdominal cramps Diarrhea Anorexia (may last few weeks) Alopecia Acne Erythema or hyperpigmentation of previously irradiated skin Fever Malaise	Vesicant Enhances cytotoxic effects of radiation therapy but increases toxic effects May cause serious desquamation of irradiated tissue

Doxorubicin (Adriamycin) IV	N/V (moderate)
	Stomatitis
	BMD (7-14 days later)
	Local phlebitis
	Alopecia
	Cumulative-dose toxicity includes
	  Cardiac abnormalities
	  ECG changes
	  Heart failure
	Hyperpigmentation of nailbeds
	Secondary malignancy (AML) when used in high doses with cyclophosphamide
		Vesicant (extravasation may *not* cause pain)
		Use only sterile distilled water as a diluent
		Observe for any changes in heart rate or rhythm and signs of failure; follow echocardiogram or MUGA (multiple gated arteriography) scan
		Cumulative lifetime dose must not exceed 450 mg/m^2
		Warn parents that drug causes urine to turn red (for up to 12 days after administration); this is normal, not hematuria

Continued.

Table 11-2.   **SUMMARY OF CHEMOTHERAPEUTIC AGENTS USED IN THE TREATMENT OF CHILDHOOD CANCERS*—cont'd**

Agent/administration	Side effects and toxicity	Comments and specific nursing considerations
Daunorubicin (Cerubidine, Daunomycin, Rubido mycin) IV	Similar to doxorubicin	Similar to doxorubicin
Bleomycin (Blenoxane) IV, IM, SC, Intracavitary	Allergic reaction—fever, chills, hypotension, anaphylaxis Fever (nonallergic) N/V (mild) Stomatitis Cumulative dose effects include Skin—rash, hyperpigmentation, thickening, ulceration, peeling, nail changes, alopecia Lungs—pneumonitis with infiltrate that can progress to fatal fibrosis	Should give test dose (IM) before therapeutic dose administered Have emergency drugs* at bedside Hypersensitivity occurs with first one to two doses May give acetaminophen before drug to reduce likelihood of fever Concentration of drug in skin and lungs accounts for toxic effects Cumulative lifetime dose no >400 units Pulmonary function test as baseline and in follow-up
Hormones		
Corticosteroids (prednisone most frequently used; many proprietary names such as Meticorten, Deltasone, Paracort, Dexamethasone also used) PO, IV	For short-term use, no acute toxicity Usual side effects: moon face, fluid retention, weight gain, mood changes, increased appetite, gastric irritation, insomnia, susceptibility to infection	Explain expected effects, especially in terms of body image, increased appetite, and personality changes Monitor weight gain Recommend moderate salt restriction Administer with antacid and early in morning (sometimes given every other day to minimize side effects) May need to disguise bitter taste (crush tablet and mix with syrup, jam, ice cream or other highly-flavored substance; use ice to numb tongue before administration; place tablet in gelatin capsule if child can swallow it) Observe for potential infection sites; usual inflammatory response and fever are absent
	Long-term effects of chronic steroid administration are mood changes, hirsutism, trunk obesity (buffalo hump), thin extremities, muscle wasting and weakness, osteoporosis, poor wound healing, bruising, potassium loss, gastric bleeding, hypertension, diabetes mellitus, growth retardation, acne	All of above; in addition, encourage foods high in potassium (bananas, raisins, prunes, coffee, chocolate) Test stools for occult blood Monitor blood pressure Test blood for sugar and urine for acetone Observe for signs of abrupt steroid withdrawal: flulike symptoms, hypotension, hypoglycemia, shock

Continued.

Table 11-2.   SUMMARY OF CHEMOTHERAPEUTIC AGENTS
USED IN THE TREATMENT OF CHILDHOOD
CANCERS*—cont'd

Agent/administration	Side effects and toxicity	Comments and specific nursing considerations
Enzymes		
Asparaginase (L-asparaginase, Elspar) IM, IV	Allergic reactions (including anaphylactic shock) Fever N/V (mild) Anorexia Weight loss Fibrinogenemia Liver dysfunction Hyperglycemia (transient) Renal failure Pancreatitis Somnolence, lethargy	Have emergency drugs at bedside* Record signs of allergic reaction, such as urticaria, facial edema, hypotension, or abdominal cramps Normally, BUN and ammonia levels rise as a result of drug—not evidence of liver damage Check urine for sugar and ketones. Treat with insulin as needed Check PT, PTT, Fibrinogen—may need fresh frozen plasma Check amylase levels
Nitrosoureas		
Carmustine (BCNU) IV Lomustine (CCNU) PO	N/V (2-6 hours later) (severe) BMD (3-4 weeks later) Burning pain along IV infusion (usually due to alcohol diluent) BCNU—flushing and facial burning on infusion —pulmonary infiltrates and/or fibrosis	Prevent extravasation; contact with skin causes brown spots Oral form—give on empty stomach Reduce IV burning by diluting drug and infusing slowly via IV drip Crosses blood-brain barrier Check pulmonary function tests
Other agents		
Hydroxyurea (Hydrea) PO	N/V (mild) Anorexia Rash, facial erythema BMD Mucosal ulceration	Must be given cautiously in children with renal dysfunction
Cisplatin (Platinol) IV	Renal toxicity (severe) N/V (1-6 hours later) (severe) BMD (2-3 weeks later) Ototoxicity Neurotoxicity (similar to that for vincristine) Nephrotoxicity-induced electrolyte disturbances, especially hypomagnesemia, hypocalcemia, hypokalemia, and hypophosphatemia	Renal function (creatinine clearance) must be assessed before giving drug Must maintain hydration before and during therapy (specific gravity of urine is used to assess hydration) Mannitol may be given IV to promote osmotic diuresis and drug clearance Mannitol will artificially increase specific gravity Monitor intake and output

Continued.

**Table 11-2.   SUMMARY OF CHEMOTHERAPEUTIC AGENTS
USED IN THE TREATMENT OF CHILDHOOD
CANCERS*—cont'd**

Agent/administration	Side effects and toxicity	Comments and specific nursing considerations
	Anaphylactic reactions may occur	Monitor for signs of ototoxicity (e.g., ringing in ears) and neurotoxicity; report signs immediately; ensure that routine audiogram is done before treatment for baseline and routinely during treatment
		Do not use aluminum needle; reaction with aluminum decreases potency of drug
		Monitor for signs of electrolyte loss; i.e. hypomagnesium—tremors, spasm, muscle weakness, lower extremity cramps, irregular heartbeat, convulsions, delirium
		Have emergency drugs at bedside*
Carboplatin (Paraplatin) IV	N/V BMD Ototoxicity (rare) Neurotoxicity Electrolyte disturbance: decreased sodium, potassium, calcium, magnesium Renal toxicity Anaphylaxis	As for Cisplatin

Sources:

Renick-Ettinger A: Chemotherapy. In G Foley, D Fochtman, and K Mooney, editors: *Nursing care of the child with cancer,* Philadelphia, 1993, WB Saunders, pp 81-116.

Balis F, Holcenberg J, and Poplack D: General principles of chemotherapy. In P Pizzo and D Poplack, editors: *Principles and practice of pediatric oncology,* Philadelphia, 1993, JB Lippincott, pp 197-245.

Perry M: Toxicity: 10 years later, *Semin Oncol* 19:453-457, 1992.

*Table includes principal drugs used in the treatment of childhood cancers. Several other conventional and investigational chemotherapeutic agents may be employed in the treatment regimen.

†Vesicants (sclerosing agents) can cause severe cellular damage if even minute amounts of the drug infiltrate surrounding tissue. Only nurses experienced with chemotherapeutic agents should administer vesicants. These drugs must be given through a free-flowing intravenous line. The infusion is stopped *immediately* if any sign of infiltration (pain, stinging, swelling, or redness at needle site) occurs. Interventions for extravasation vary, but each nurse should be aware of the institution's policies and implement them at once.

‡IV, intravenous; IT, intrathecal; PO, by mouth; IM, intramuscular; SC, subcutaneous.

§N/V, nausea and vomiting. Mild = <20% incidence; moderate = 20% to 70% incidence; severe = >75% incidence.

‖BMD, bone marrow depression.

¶Abbreviations stand for chemical compound.

*Emergency drugs include oxygen and parenteral preparations of epinephrine 1:1000, diphenhydramine or similar antihistamine, aminophylline, corticosteroids, and vasopressors.

children with high-risk (having clinical and laboratory features at diagnosis that are known to have a poor prognosis) ALL and acute myelogenous leukemia (AML). Bone marrow transplantation allows for potentially lethal doses of chemotherapy and radiation to be given to rid the body of all malignant cells. The donor marrow replaces the child's destroyed marrow and after engraftment should produce the donor's nonmalignant functioning cells.

There are four forms of bone marrow transplantation. Syngeneic transplantation uses genetically identical bone marrow from a twin. Allogeneic transplantation uses marrow from a tissue-identical donor who is preferably related to the recipient. Tissue-identical unrelated transplantation uses a donor from outside the immediate family who meets very specific tissue typing criteria. An autologus transplant is one in which the marrow is collected from the affected child. An autologus transplantation may be used when the tumor is not in the marrow or the marrow can be purged of all tumor cells.

Bone marrow transplantation is a promising treatment modality for certain malignancies in children. However, it must be realistically viewed in terms of the potentially fatal toxicities, developmental sequelae, and psychosocial and financial impact on the child and family. A second concern for the family is using an otherwise healthy sibling as the marrow donor. Although the marrow harvest itself entails little risk (Ramsay, 1993), the use of anesthesia has a small but increasing risk with decreasing age (Wiley and House, 1988).

RECENT AND ANTICIPATED ADVANCES IN DIAGNOSIS AND MANAGEMENT

Increasingly, cytogenetic studies have linked specific chromosomal changes with specific tumors or have identified inherited genetic abnormalities that place persons at risk for developing cancer. One example is the identified loss of the p53 or tumor suppressor gene that places an individual at risk for the development of specific types of cancer. Additionally, more biologic tumor markers (substances on the surfaces of tumor cells that identify them as

malignant) have been identified to assist in the diagnosis and staging of tumors as well as determining a response to therapy. Polymerized chain reaction (PCR) is increasingly used to detect minimal residual cancer cells with greater sensitivity. Advances in molecular genetics will help to refine prognostic groupings by identifying specific cell types in tumors that are associated with higher or lower rates of cure.

Treatment with chemotherapy is continuously being refined through the efforts of multiinstitutional and cooperative studies. Choice of agents, dosage, timing, and route of administration are more selective to increase effectiveness and decrease late effects of therapy. Future advances in chemotherapy will address the potential reversal of multidrug resistance in tumor cells. Advances in radiation include hyperfractionated radiation dosing (discussed earlier) and stereotactic radiation or radiosurgery. The latter uses CAT scans to focus radiation in a three-dimensional space to more specifically target the tumor. One method has been referred to as the "Gamma Knife" (Lunsford et al, 1989). Bone marrow transplant is being applied to more types of tumors and is being used as "rescue" therapy when very high doses of chemotherapy are needed to treat recurrent tumors.

As previously mentioned, biologic response modifiers (BRMs) are an exciting new addition to the multimodal treatment approach to curing childhood cancer and modifying treatment toxicities. Colony stimulating factors (CSF's) are cytokines that stimulate the body's production of different types of hematopoietic cells. For example, G-CSF stimulates the production of granulocytes (G); GM-CSF stimulates the production of both granulocytes (G) and macrophages (M); and erythropoietin stimulates the production of red blood cells. These substances have helped to reduce the bone marrow suppressive toxicities of chemotherapy. The use of interleukins, it is hoped, will augment the body's natural immune system response. Interleukin-2 shows the potential for destroying tumor cells while leaving nonmalignant cells intact. Tumor necrosis factor (TNF) disrupts the vascular supply to tumor cells resulting in hemorrhagic necrosis. Its use is being studied as a part of multimodal treatment for cancer. Monoclonal antibodies have the potential of working with chemotherapy agents to more specifically target tumor cells. The ability of interferon to prolong the cell cycle would allow other agents to destroy a greater number of cells. The side effect common to most BRMs is a flulike syndrome consisting of fever, chills, headache, fatigue, and muscle aches (McGuire and Moore, 1990; Woolery-Antil and Colter, 1993).

ASSOCIATED PROBLEMS

Vascular Access

Children receiving prolonged, intensive treatment are required to endure frequent venipunctures for laboratory tests, chemotherapy, administration of blood products, antibiotic therapy, and nutritional support. These children are often aided by the placement of a long-term indwelling central venous access device (VAD), which helps minimize the trauma of frequent needle sticks and vein irritation from the chemotherapy. Access devices include right atrial catheters (Broviac, Hickman) and a subcutaneous (SC) port or reservoir (Port-a-cath, Infus-A-Port, MediPort) (Marcoux, Fisher, and Wong, 1990).

The right atrial catheters are single or double lumen silicone catheters with a Dacron felt cuff that anchors the catheter under the skin and provides a barrier to infection (Hartman and Shochat, 1987). The right atrial catheter has an internal and external portion, whereas the SC port or reservoir is totally implanted below the skin. The catheter tip lies at the junction of the superior vena cava and the right atrium. The catheter is tunneled under the skin and attached to a port that lies in an SC pocket on the chest (Marcoux, Fisher, and Wong, 1990). Venous access is achieved by puncturing the skin above the reservoir and passing a specially designed needle through the silicone membrane into the port receptacle. Eutectic mixture of lidocaine and prilocaine, Astra (EMLA) cream may be applied to port sites for 1 to 2 hours before accessing is required to reduce discomfort and fear. (Goede and Betcher, 1994)

The patency of all long-term VADs is maintained through periodic flushing with heparinized saline. Care of these lines is taught to the child (when appropriate) and parents. Complications of the indwelling VADs include infection, occlusion of the catheter because of thrombus and fibrin formation, damage to the external portion of the catheter, and rarely, cardiac tamponade (Harms et al, 1992; Wickham, Purl, and Welker, 1992; Keegan-Wells and Stewart, 1992).

Because the child with cancer is at risk for profound neutropenia as a result of therapy, prompt and aggressive treatment of infection at the catheter site is necessary. Most external infections can be cleared with oral antibiotics; however, tunnel infections and septicemia require IV antibiotics and possible catheter removal.

Therapy-Related Complications

Nausea and vomiting. Nausea and vomiting are common side effects of chemotherapy and radiation. Nausea and vomiting can have a profound physiologic and psychologic impact on the child

---

ASSOCIATED PROBLEMS

- **Vascular access:** most children require the use of indwelling central VADs
  All lumens must be cultured if any fever
  SBE prophylaxis for dental procedures
- **Nausea and vomiting:** use antiemetics before and after chemotherapeutic administration, NOT on an "as needed" (PRN) basis
- **Anorexia and weight loss:** monitor weight regularly, early intervention
- **Bone marrow suppression:**
  Hemoglobin <7 to 8 g/dl, consider transfusion
  Platelets <10,000 to 20,000, consider transfusion
  ANC <500, high risk for infection
  Possible use of BRMs for treatment of anemia and neutropenia
- **Infection:** blood cultures for all fevers
  IV antibiotics for fever and neutropenia or for any child with an implanted central venous access device
- **Alopecia**
- **Late effects:** See Table 11-3

receiving therapy (Fricke et al., 1988). Problems including dehydration, chemical and electrolyte imbalances, and decreased nutritional intake can lead to decreased compliance or termination of treatment.

The mechanisms involved in nausea and vomiting are complex, and no single drug will consistently control these side effects. The situation is further complicated by the wide variation in response by the individual child to both the chemotherapeutic agent and the antiemetic. The antiemetic should be given before nausea and vomiting occur and should be continued until the symptoms have resolved. Generally nausea and vomiting related to the chemotherapy will not last longer than 48 hours after chemotherapy administration.

A new class of antiemetics exert their action by acting as serotonin antagonists. Ondansetron (Zofran) and Granisetron (Kytril) inhibit the binding of serotonin to receptors in both the central nervous system and the gastrointestinal system. These medications do not have the side effects associated with antiemetics that inhibit dopamine (drowsiness, extrapyramidal side effects) (Betcher and Burnham, 1991). Adjunctive methods such as hypnosis (Zeltzer et al, 1991) have had some positive effects when combined with antiemetic medications.

Anorexia and weight loss. During therapy, anorexia and weight loss are common and can be attributed to both the disease and its treatment. The psychologic impact of cancer and the tumor's metabolic influence can contribute to weight loss. Treatment-induced nausea and vomiting, and changes in taste acuity may lead to food aversion. Therefore it is imperative to closely monitor the child's weight throughout treatment. Oral supplements and, in some cases, nasogastric feedings or hyperalimentation may be necessary.

Bone marrow suppression. Bone marrow suppression is another side effect of chemotherapy and radiation. With chemotherapy, leukopenia, thrombocytopenia, and anemia begin within 7 to 10 days after drug administration, and the nadir (the point at which the blood cell counts are the lowest) occurs at approximately 14 days. The marrow then recovers by 21 to 28 days. The exact time of the nadir will vary depending on the specific chemotherapeutic agent. Close monitoring is necessary to determine the extent of marrow suppression.

Leukopenia refers to the presence of a low number of all white blood cells (WBCs), whereas neutropenia refers specifically to a low neutrophil cell count. Neutrophils are the body's main defense against bacterial infection. It is necessary to determine the absolute neutrophil count (ANC) (see box on calculating neutrophil count) because the incidence and severity of infection are inversely related to an ANC <500 (Katz and Mustafa, 1993).

Infections represent the major cause of morbidity and death in children with cancer (Gootenberg and Pizzo, 1991). The use of good handwashing techniques by the child, the parents, and the caregivers is paramount to reducing the spread of pathogens. Good personal hygiene by the child, including thorough dental care, is also important. The child with neutropenia should avoid individuals who are ill, crowded situations, and anyone with a communicable disease, especially chickenpox. Rectal temperatures and suppositories should also be avoided because abrading the rectal mucosa increases the risk of introducing bacteria into the bloodstream.

CALCULATION OF ABSOLUTE NEUTROPHIL COUNT (ANC)

White blood count (WBC) = 7400 (also expressed as 7.4 k/UL; $7.4 \times 10^3/mm^3$)
Neutrophils (poly. segs) = 40%
Nonsegmented neutrophils (bands) = 12%

Step 1: Determine total percent neutrophils (poly. segs + bands)
    40% + 12% = 52% (0.52)
Step 2: Multiply WBC by % neutrophils
    ANC = 7400 × 0.52
    ANC = 3848 (normal)

WBC = 900 (0.9 k/UL; $0.9 \times 10^3/mm^3$)
Neutrophils (poly. segs) = 7%
Nonsegmented neutrophils (bands) = 7%
Step 1: 7% + 7% = 14% (0.14)
Step 2: ANC = 900 × 0.14
    ANC = 126 (severely neutropenic)

The child who is thrombocytopenic may require transfusions of platelets because of the risk of serious hemorrhage. If the platelet count is less than 10,000 to 20,000 and/or in the presence of bleeding, cytomegalovirus (CMV)-negative, irradiated platelets should be administered.

A child whose hemoglobin level is less than 7 to 8 g and/or who is symptomatic (i.e., shortness of breath, headache, or dizziness) may require a transfusion of CMV-negative, irradiated packed red blood cells (RBCs). Any child who is a potential bone marrow transplant candidate and is CMV-negative should receive CMV-negative blood products.

Hair loss. A distinguishing therapy-related complication that is bothersome to children is alopecia. A temporary condition, it results from damage of the hair follicles by chemotherapy and radiation. The child can be reassured that the hair will grow back after therapy; however, initially the texture and color may be slightly different. Cutting the child's hair into a shorter style may help to reduce some distress when the hair begins to fall out. Younger children and some adolescents prefer to cover their heads with colorful hats, baseball caps, and scarves. Adolescent girls are more likely to consider the use of wigs.

Late Effects

As the survival rates continually improve, the long-term effects of therapy are becoming evident. The goal of current therapy is not merely improving survival but also reducing physiologic and developmental morbidity. A growing body of knowledge indicates that both chemotherapy and radiation have adverse effects on normal tissues that may not be manifested for months or years after therapy. The development of second malignancies, impaired growth, diminished cognitive functioning, and organ damage are the areas of greatest concern. Factors that appear to influence the development of late effects include the child's age and stage of development at the time of diagnosis, the primary tumor and extent of involvement, and the therapy used.

Secondary malignant neoplasms (SMN) are found with greater frequency in children with a genetic predisposition based on the primary tumor or as a result of chemotherapy and radiation therapy. The highest rate of SMN occurs in children with hereditary retinoblastoma. These children are at risk for the development of osteosarcoma. There may also be an increased risk of SMN in persons with the genetic forms of Wilm's tumor (bilateral), neuroblastoma, and other embryonal tumors. In children with Hodgkin's disease treated with radiation and chemotherapy, there is an increased incidence of SMN, especially AML (Meadows and Fenton, 1994). Treatment with alkylating agents and etoposide increases the risk of AML. Concurrent use of dose intensive anthracyclines with cyclophosphamide has been associated with an increased risk of SMN (Smith, Rubinstein, and Ungerleider, 1994; Pedersen-Bjergaard et al, 1992; Heyn et al, 1994).

Children receiving treatment directly to the CNS are at risk for negative neurologic and intellectual sequelae (Brown et al, 1992; Moore, Glasser, and Albin, 1988). Neurotoxicity is related to the number and sequence of treatment modalities used. Although the use of radiation and intrathecal chemotherapy for CNS prophylaxis in the child with ALL has greatly increased survival, neurotoxicity and learning disabilities have been reported (Ochs and Mulhern, 1988; Moore et al, 1991). The impact of late effects on the various organ systems is described in Table 11-3.

Relapse

Despite the advances in treatment of childhood cancer, some children will experience a relapse of their disease. Relapse, like diagnosis, is a crisis period for the family. It poses a challenge for the oncology team because the best methods of treatment were used at diagnosis. Relapse often requires more experimental modes of treatment. The primary care provider in cooperation with the oncology team can support the family and especially the child through this difficult time.

Death

There may come a time when all possible viable treatment options have been exhausted. The care of the child moves from focusing on a cure to providing comfort and providing as much quality time as possible. The collaboration between the primary care provider and the oncology team can be invaluable during this time. Families frequently seek guidance and support in making decisions that they

Text continues on p. 218.

Table 11-3. **ADVERSE EFFECTS OF ANTINEOPLASTIC THERAPY UPON BODY SYSTEM**

Body system	Adverse effects	Causative agent	Time interval	Signs and symptoms	Predisposing factors	Preventive therapeutic measures
Cardiovascular system	Cardiomyopathy	Anthracycline chemotherapy Cyclophosphamide (high dose) Radiation to mediastinum	Weeks to months	Abrupt onset of congestive heart failure; tachycardia; tachypnea; edema; hepatomegaly; cardiomegaly; gallop rhythms; pleural effusions; dyspnea	Anthracycline therapy; especially lifetime cumulative dose of >300 mg/m²	Careful monitoring with chest x-ray film ECG, Echocardiogram, MUGA scan Observation for shortness of breath, weight gain, edema Partial shielding of mediastinum
	Chronic constrictive pericarditis	Radiation to mediastinum	Few months to years	Chest pain; dyspnea; fever; paradoxic pulse; venous distention; friction rub; Kussmaul's sign	Radiation to heart Most common with doses of 4000-6000 cGy	Treatment with antiinflammatory agents Pericardial stripping
Pulmonary system	Pneumonitis followed by pulmonary fibrosis	Pulmonary radiation; Bleomycin, BCUU, high dose cytoxan	2-12 months following radiation	Increased dyspnea; decreased exercise tolerance; pulmonary insufficiency	Increased risk with Large lung volume in radiation field Therapy during period of pulmonary infection Concomitant mediastinal radiation Chemotherapeutic agents that act as radiation sensitizers Doses >4000 cGy	Careful monitoring of status with physical examination, chest x-ray film, and pulmonary function tests High-dose corticosteroids for severe cases Yearly influenza vaccine Pneumovax Avoid smoking Encourage frequent rest periods

System	Late Effect	Cause	Onset	Signs and Symptoms	Predisposing Factors/Doses	Management
Hematopoietic system	Long-term suppression of bone marrow function	Extensive radiotherapy to marrow-containing bones; Chemotherapy	Months to years following therapy	Fall in WBC and platelet counts; hypoplastic/aplastic bone marrow aspirates; diminished uptake of radioisotopes	Radiation doses: 3000-5000 cGy in older individuals; Concomitant use of chemotherapy	Limitation of areas of marrow irradiated; Monitoring of child's status with periodic bone marrow aspirates and peripheral blood cell counts
	Alterations in immune system	Radiotherapy to marrow-containing bones; Chemotherapy; Bone marrow transplant; Splenectomy	Months to years following therapy	Fall in WBC and platelet counts; hypoplastic/aplastic bone; marrow aspirates; predisposition to infection	Radiation doses: 3000-5000 cGy; Chemotherapy: high dose/extended periods	Pneumococcal vaccine and penicillin if splenectomized; Monitoring of child's status with periodic blood counts and tests of immune response
Gastrointestinal system	Hepatic fibrosis-cirrhosis	Chemotherapy	Months to years following therapy	Persistent elevation of liver function tests after cessation of therapy; hepatomegaly; cirrhosis; jaundice; spider nevi	Daily low doses of methotrexate by mouth for long periods; Long-term use of 6-mercaptopurine	Monitor child's status with liver function tests; Perform liver biopsy if liver function test results remain persistently abnormal
	Chronic enteritis	Radiation therapy	Months to years following therapy	Pain, recurrent vomiting; diarrhea; malabsorption syndrome; weight loss	Radiation doses >5000 cGy; Children with previous abdominal surgery; Chemotherapy with radiation sensitizers (actinomycin and adriamycin)	Avoid concomitant use of radiation sensitizers; Careful monitoring of height and weight; Supportive therapy when symptoms develop, including low residue, low-fat, gluten and milk-free diet
Kidney and urinary tract	Nephritis; Acute and chronic	Radiation to renal structures	Acute: 6-12 months following therapy; Chronic: months to years following therapy	May appear as benign or malignant hypertension. Acute: rapid decrease in renal function with BUN, proteinuria, anemia, hypertension, signs of congestive heart failure	Renal radiation of 2000-3000 cGy; Combined use of radiation and chemotherapy	Periodically monitor renal status during and after therapy, with blood pressure readings, urinalysis, and CBC, BUN, and creatinine; Radiation-induced hypertension spontaneously

Continued.

Table 11-3.   ADVERSE EFFECTS OF ANTINEOPLASTIC THERAPY UPON BODY SYSTEM—cont'd

Body system	Adverse effects	Causative agent	Time interval	Signs and symptoms	Predisposing factors	Preventive therapeutic measures
				Chronic: persistence of above or insidious development of anemia, azotemia, proteinuria, hypertension; may lead to chronic renal failure or cardiovascular damage		resolves when damage is unilateral Once progressive renal failure develops, treatment is supportive
	Chronic hemorrhagic cystitis	Chemotherapy: Cytoxan and Ifosfamide	Months to years	Sterile, painful hematuria; urinary frequency	Pelvic radiation >4000 cGy Inadequate hydration of chemotherapy patients	Sound radiotherapy techniques to reduce bladder exposure to radiation Frequent emptying of bladder during and 24 hrs after therapy Adequate hydration before, during, and after chemotherapy Concomitant use of MESNA with chemotherapy Treatment of bladder hemorrhage with formalin instillation and/or fulguration of bleeding sites
	Tubular dysfunction	Cytoxan and Ifosfamide		Low magnesium; Low phosphorus; glycosuria	None	Magnesium and phosphorus supplements

System	Late Effect	Causative Treatment	Time of Onset	Clinical Manifestations	Comments	Management
Musculo-skeletal system	Impaired skeletal growth	Radiation to skeletal structures and abdomen	Months to years following treatment	Growth retardation; reduction in sitting height; scoliosis; altered growth of facial skeleton	Effect of spinal irradiation to vertebral bodies in doses 1000-2000 cGy dependent on age of child; known damage >2000 cGy; Unilateral radiation results in asymmetric deformities; Symmetric growth delay during periods of chemotherapy	Careful monitoring of child's status with growth charts, x-ray studies, sitting and standing height; Dose radiation reduction during periods of rapid growth
	Delayed or arrested tooth development	Radiation to maxilla or mandible; Chemotherapy	Months to years	Teeth are small with pale enamel; malocclusion	Radiation during period of dental growth and development	Dental examinations every 6 months; Good oral hygiene including flossing; Flouride prophylaxis
Endocrine system	Thyroid gland dysfunction	Radiotherapy to thyroid gland, brain, and total body irradiation	Months to years	Hypothyroidism; may be asymptomatic and have abnormal thyroid function; nodular abnormalities	Reported with varying radiation doses: 2500-7000 cGy	Monitor thyroid function with T3, Free T4, and TSH; Hormonal replacement therapy for all patients with abnormal thyroid tests
	Injuries to gonads	Radiation field, including gonads; Chemotherapy (alkylating agents)	Months to years	Infertility; sterility, hormonal dysfunction, azoospermia; teratogenic during first trimester of pregnancy	Testicular radiation; ovarian radiation; Chemotherapy damage dependent on drug used, dose, duration of therapy, child's sex, and age	Tanner staging yearly; Protection of testes/ovaries from radiation field; Gonadal dysfunction from chemotherapy may be reversible; Males (14 y.o.) check LH, FSH, testosterone levels; Females (12 y.o.) check LH, FSH, estradiol levels

Continued.

Table 11-3.   ADVERSE EFFECTS OF ANTINEOPLASTIC THERAPY UPON BODY SYSTEM—cont'd

Body system	Adverse effects	Causative agent	Time interval	Signs and symptoms	Predisposing factors	Preventive therapeutic measures
Nervous system	Peripheral sensory or motor neuropathies	Radiotherapy to peripheral nerves; chemotherapy (Vincristine, VP-16, cisplatin)	Months to years	Deficit in function Pain Decreased tendon reflexes	Radiation doses: 5500-12,000 cGy Chemotherapy with vinca-alkaloids	Careful monitoring of patient status during and after therapy Vinca-alkaloid damage may be diminished or reversed by reducing or withholding therapy
	Central neuroendocrine dysfunction of hypothalamic pituitary axis	Cranial radiation; chemotherapy	Months to years	Growth hormone deficiency Panhypopituitarism with short stature; hypothyroidism; Addison's disease	Dependent on dose of radiation, age of child, and concomitant use of chemotherapy Younger children who receive >2400 cGy at greatest risk	Careful monitoring of patient status with growth charts, Tanner staging, Bone age at 9 yr then yearly to puberty Thyroid, hormone, insulin, and cortisol measurement may be necessary Treatment with replacement of deficient hormones
	Encephalopathy	Cranial radiation; chemotherapy	Months to years	May be asymptomatic but demonstrate abnormalities on head CAT scans May have overt symp-	Cranial radiation alone or with concomitant chemotherapy Frequency in-	Monitor patient status with careful physical examination, head MRI/ CAT* scans, psychometric testing

Intelligence deficits and/or neuropsychologic dysfunctions	Radiation; chemotherapy	Months to years	toms ranging from lethargy, somnolence, dementia, seizures, paralysis, and coma Abnormal psychologic tests with deficits in perceptual behavior, language development, and learning abilities Personality changes	creased with chemotherapy Less damage with cranial radiation <1800 cGy Younger children more vulnerable More common in younger children, those who received cranial irradiation >1800 cGy and concomitant chemotherapy Damage may occur in all individuals who receive CNS prophylactic or therapeutic cranial radiation and/or chemotherapy	Reduce chemotherapy dose when preclinical x-ray findings appear Careful monitoring with periodic neurocognitive/ psychological evaluations Early intervention with multidisciplinary approach and specialized education programs

Schwartz C et al: *Survivors of childhood cancer: assessment and management,* St Louis, 1994, Mosby.

Blatt J, Copeland D, and Bleyer A: Late effects of childhood cancer and its treatment. In Pizzo P and Poplack D, editors: *Principles and practice of pediatric oncology,* Philadelphia, 1993, JB Lippincott, pp 1091-1114.

*CAT, Computerized Axial Tomography/MRI, Magnetic Resonance Imaging

can live with long after the child's death. Knowledge of the community- and hospital-based hospice programs in their area can be beneficial in meeting many of the home care and support needs of families. All families need reassurance that they will not be abandoned at this time and that multidisciplinary resources will be made available to them as required.

PROGNOSIS

The prognosis of a malignancy is dependent on the age of the child, primary site, extent of the disease, and cell type. Over the past 20 years dramatic advances have been made in the treatment and potential cure of children with cancer (see Table 11-4). The current figures on ALL estimate a durable (defined as 5 years or greater) event-free survival to be 70% (Pui and Crist, 1994). The outcomes for ANLL

are estimated to be 35% to 40%. The prognosis for brain tumors is also steadily improving, with the 5-year survival rate approximating 59%. This is attributed to the combined therapy of surgical resection, radiation therapy, and multiagent chemotherapy.

Non-Hodgkin's lymphoma constitutes a wide variation in tumors. The estimated overall survival rate for this group is approximately 68%. Hodgkin's disease boasts approximately an 85% to 90% cure rate, but there is controversy over what constitutes the optimal therapy. The issues center around striking a balance between aggressive treatment with lower relapse rates, higher potential for second malignancies, and long-term sequelae as opposed to less aggressive therapy, with potentially higher relapse rates but fewer late effects.

An overall survival rate for those who have neuroblastoma is approximately 56%. When the survival rates are viewed by age group, there is a

Table 11-4.   TRENDS IN SURVIVAL OF CHILDREN WITH MALIGNANT DISEASE

Site	Relative 5-yr survival rates (%)				
			Yr of diagnosis		
	1960-1963*	1970-1973*	1974-1976†	1977-1980†	1981-1986†
All sites	28	45	55.1	61.6	66.8‡
Acute lymphocytic leukemia	4	34	53.4	67.9	72.8‡
Acute myeloid leukemia	3	5	16.1	25.4§	24.3§
Wilms' tumor	33	70	74.1	79.6	83.3
Brain and nervous system	35	45	54.5	55.9	59.0
Neuroblastoma	25	40	48.6	52.3	56.4
Bone	20	30	51.9§	47.1	53.8§
Hodgkin's disease	52	90	80.4	87.5	85.0
Non-Hodgkin's lymphomas	18	26	42.3	50.1	68.3‡

From American Cancer Society: Cancer statistics. *CA,* Statistics Branch, National Cancer Institute.*Rates are based on End Results Group data from a series of hospital registries and one population-based registry.

†Rates are from the SEER program. They are based on data from population-based registries in Connecticut, New Mexico, Utah, Iowa, Hawaii, Atlanta, Detroit, Seattle, Puget Sound, and San Francisco-Oakland. Rates are based on follow-up of patients through 1986.

‡The difference in rates between 1974-1976 and 1980-1986 is statistically significant ($p < 0.05$).

§The standard error of the survival rate is between 5 and 10 percentage points.

significantly higher survival rate for children less than 1 year of age. For children with stage I, II, and IVS disease, there is a 75% to 90% chance of survival. Those with stage III and IV disease have 2-year disease-free survival rates of 10% to 30% (Brodeur and Castleberry, 1993).

Children with Wilms' tumor have an estimated survival rate of more than 85% (Brodeur and Brodeur, 1991); the majority of these children have less advanced forms of the disease with a favorable histology. With rhabdomyosarcoma, children's overall survival rate is 65%, with 44% to 73% survival for children with less advanced disease compared with 25% for those with distant metastatic disease (Raney et al, 1993).

Children with bone cancers, including osteosarcoma and Ewing's sarcoma, have an approximately 60% survival rate for the former (Jaffe, 1991) and a 74% survival rate for the latter. Long-term disease-free survival is a reality for the majority of children with a malignant disease, but research needs to continue to focus on therapy for those children with more advanced disease.

Primary Care Management
HEALTH CARE MAINTENANCE
Growth and Development

Growth retardation secondary to chemotherapy appears to be temporary (Marcus et al, 1994). The effect of radiation, however, can be permanent. Radiation affects growth by damaging the epiphyseal plates of the long bones and by damaging the glands that are responsible for growth-related hormone production. The child's growth should be followed on a standardized growth curve, with growth patterns examined over time rather than as isolated measurements. Preferably both sitting and standing heights should be obtained. Growth rates should be followed every 1 to 3 months during therapy and for the first year after therapy; then measurements should be taken every 6 months until linear growth is completed. Because of the risk of significant weight loss, weight should also be monitored at each visit.

The primary care provider can play an invaluable role in providing anticipatory guidance for parents regarding the developmental changes the child with cancer will experience. Children with cancer are often limited in their opportunities for developing independence and autonomy. The limitations come from restrictions placed by treatment regimens, therapy-related complications, and protective parents.

Ongoing developmental assessment should be performed during and after therapy. Early identification and intervention is important in assisting the child in maintaining age-appropriate development. Neuropsychologic testing is recommended within the first 2 years after completion of therapy for children receiving cranial radiation or who were younger than 8 years at the time of diagnosis. Age-standardized tests should be used to measure intellectual ability, visual perception, visual-motor and motor skills, language, memory and learning, academic achievement, and behavior and social functioning (see Chapter 2). Neuropsychologic testing may need to be repeated to diagnose long-term effects.

Diet

Maintaining adequate nutrition while a child is receiving treatment is challenging because of the child's anorexia. Well-balanced, nutritious meals should be offered. Often small, frequent meals may be more appealing than the standard three meals each day. High-calorie, high-protein snacks may also be helpful.

Children receiving corticosteroids will often experience an increased appetite and weight gain, but because corticosteroids usually are administered for limited amounts of time, such symptoms generally are of short duration. Nutritious foods low in sodium should be encouraged.

Constipation and diarrhea are frequent side effects of chemotherapy. Constipation may be relieved by increasing the child's fluid intake and encouraging high-fiber foods and fruits. A stool softener or laxative may be necessary, especially with vincristine therapy. Enemas and suppositories should be avoided, especially if the child is neutropenic. Diarrhea should be monitored closely and the child evaluated for signs and symptoms of dehydration.

Often parents will inquire about the use of herbs, special diets, or other dietary interventions to speed the recovery of the blood cell counts or to combat the tumor. It is important to examine with the parents the intervention they desire to use. Herbs and vitamins must be viewed in terms of their potential for interacting with chemotherapeutic agents. The primary care provider can acknowledge and support the parents' desire to help their child while also acting in the best interest of the child.

Safety

Safety issues for the child with a malignant disease involves balancing normal participation in daily activities with taking appropriate precautions imposed by the treatment of a malignant disease. For the safety of all children, chemotherapeutic agents must be stored securely out of reach. Thorough handwashing should follow the handling of any chemotherapeutic agent. Pregnant women should avoid contact with the chemotherapeutic agents and the urine of children on chemotherapy. If circumstances make this impossible, gloves should be worn to avoid direct contact with the medication. Unused portions of chemotherapeutic drugs should be returned to the dispensing pharmacy for disposal with other potent chemicals.

Central VADs must have a clean dressing applied to the exit site and the line secured to the chest to minimize any excessive tension of the catheter. Needles, syringes, and other supplies used in the maintenance of the line should be stored properly out of reach of children. Needles should be disposed of carefully, without recapping, in a sharps container.

Children with these devices should also avoid lake or ocean swimming and hot tubs, because of potential infection, and should have an extra padded clamp available in case of damage to the catheter lumen.

If the child should have a fall or head injury, blood cell counts should be checked to determine the platelet count. Platelets should be given prophylactically if the level is less than 50,000. The child should be instructed not to roughhouse or play contact sports if the platelet count is less than 100,000.

Many of the chemotherapeutic agents will alter the skin's tolerance for sun exposure. It is important that children on chemotherapy take extra caution in using a p-aminobenzoic acid (PABA)-free sun-

block whenever prolonged sun exposure is anticipated. It is best to avoid sun exposure during the time of day when the child's shadow is shorter than the child's height. If the child has alopecia, a hat and sunblock should be worn to protect the scalp.

The primary care provider can play a key role in helping the child and family set realistic expectations and limitations on activities. Limitations are influenced by immunosuppression, hematologic compromise, or extremity dysfunction because of peripheral neuropathy induced by chemotherapy or as a result of amputation or limb salvage procedures.

Immunizations

Because of the immunosuppressive nature of treatment, the child's immune system may not be able to mount a response to vaccinations. Normal immunologic response usually returns between 3 months and 1 year after discontinuing immunosuppressive therapy (Committee on Infectious Diseases, 1994). There is great variation in immunization recommendations; therefore, it is best to consult with the child's oncology team for specific recommendations. The child recovering from a bone marrow transplant presents a special situation. Immunizations should be given according to the schedules and protocols established by the transplant center.

Diphtheria, tetanus, and pertussis. The schedule for diphtheria, tetanus, and pertussis (DTP) vaccines should be resumed after treatment, generally at 6 months off therapy (Bennetts, 1993).

Poliovirus. Children should not receive the Sabin (live) oral polio vaccine once therapy has been initiated and also for the first year off therapy. Siblings of the child should receive the Salk (inactivated) polio vaccine until the child has been off therapy for 1 year because the polioviruses are transmissible to the child who is immunocompromised (Committee on Infectious Diseases, 1994; Bennetts, 1993).

Measles, mumps, and rubella. The child's protection against these diseases must rely on herd immunity until 12 months after cessation of treatment, when the measles, mumps, and rubella (MMR) vaccine may be given. Children who have been previously immunized should have antibody titers done after therapy because many children lose protective titers with chemotherapy (Feldman et al, 1988). If the child is directly exposed to someone with a documented case of measles and the child is seronegative for the rubeola antibody, the child should receive prophylactic γ-globulin at a dose of 0.5 ml/kg, with a maximum dosage of 15 ml (Committee on Infectious Diseases, 1994). Siblings may receive the MMR vaccine without any special precautions.

Haemophilus influenzae type B. The *Haemophilus influenzae* type B vaccine may be given after therapy at the discretion of the child's pediatric oncology team. Children diagnosed with Hodgkin's disease should be immunized 2 weeks before starting chemotherapy or undergoing a splenectomy (Committee on Infectious Diseases, 1994).

Hepatitis B. Children who are at high risk to receive blood transfusions may be immunized with the hepatitis B vaccine. It has been suggested that children receive twice the usual recommended dose as a three-shot series in order to establish an adequate antibody response (Bennetts, 1993).

Varicella exposure prophylaxis and vaccination. If a child who is seronegative for antibody to the varicella virus has a direct exposure to a person with active chickenpox or to a person who develops lesions within 48 hours of the contact, the child must receive varicella-zoster immune globulin (VZIG). It is available with a physician's order through the regional distribution centers of the American Red Cross Blood Services. It should be administered within 72 to 96 hours of exposure. The dose of VZIG is 125 units/10 kg, with a maximum dosage of 625 units. Once a child is exposed to chickenpox, the child must be isolated from other children who are immunocompromised from day 7 to day 28 following the exposure.

According to the Committee on Infectious Diseases (1995), children with malignancies should not routinely receive the live attenuated varicella vaccine. However, use of the vaccine may be considered for children with ALL who have been in remission for at least 1 year and who have an absolute lymphocyte count over 700 and platelets over 100,000. In addition, the vaccine should not be administered within 5 months of the administration of blood products or any form of immune globulin. Vaccination of these children is being coordinated under research protocols and specific recommenda-

tions may vary between treatment centers. (Arbeter et al, 1990; Lawrence et al, 1990). No special precautions are required if healthy siblings who receive the vaccine do not develop a rash. If siblings develop a rash after vaccination, they should avoid contact with the child who is immunocompromised until the rash resolves.

Other immunizations. Children over 2 years of age with Hodgkin's disease should routinely receive the pneumococcal vaccine before a splenectomy is performed. Additionally, children 5 years of age and older should be maintained on twice daily penicillin therapy (250 mg twice daily) while those under 5 may receive penicillin (125 mg twice daily) or, as has been recommended, amoxicillin or trimethoprim/sulfamethoxazole (Committee on Infectious Diseases, 1994). Pneumococcal vaccine has also been recommended for persons who are at high risk for pulmonary fibrosis (e.g., received Bleomycin, BCNU).

Although there is limited research to validate the efficacy of giving routine influenza vaccines to either the child with a malignant disease or to their families, many centers do recommend vaccine use for children and their families for up to 1 year off therapy. Persons at risk for pulmonary fibrosis may benefit from use of the vaccine.

Screening

Vision. Routine vision screening is advised. A recurring brain tumor may manifest as impaired visual acuity caused by ocular nerve compression or increased intracranial pressure or as blurred vision caused by papilledema. There may be ptosis, visual disturbances, and sixth cranial nerve dysfunction with recurrent orbital rhabdomyosarcoma. Two classic signs of recurrent retinoblastoma are the white eye reflex in place of the normal red reflex and strabismus. Cataracts are also a late effect of radiation therapy. In addition, Vincristine and vinblastine may cause ptosis that can interfere with vision.

Hearing. Routine screening of hearing is advised. Unilateral hearing loss may be indicative of the presence of a mass. Children receiving radiation, cisplatin, or both are at increased risk for hearing loss; evaluation by an audiologist every 6 to 12 months is recommended.

Dental. Routine dental care is advised during treatment and after therapy. Both radiation therapy and chemotherapy place a child at risk for stomatitis, dental caries, and periodontal disease. Dental work requiring manipulation of the oral tissues should be avoided if the ANC is less than 1000 or the platelet count is less than 50,000. Prophylactic amoxicillin to prevent subacute bacterial endocarditis must be used for all children with central venous access devices (Altman et al, 1993) (see Chapter 15 for SBE guidelines). Daily brushing with a soft-bristled brush and flossing are recommended when counts are not compromised and stomatitis is not present. Daily fluoride rinses may be indicated in children with a high potential for caries. Good oral hygiene is important in preventing stomatitis and infection. In the presence of low blood cell counts or stomatitis, cleansing with a mild mouthwash (salt and bicarbonate of soda, half-strength hydrogen peroxide) and a gauze pad or sponge is recommended.

Blood pressure. Blood pressure should be measured at every visit because of possible hypertension from corticosteroids, potential renal toxicity of many chemotherapeutic agents, and cardiac toxicities from anthracyclines.

Hematocrit. Because of frequent hematologic analyses, routine hematocrit screening is not necessary while a child is on therapy. After therapy, routine screening is recommended.

Urinalysis. Routine urinalysis is advised because it may reveal RBCs in children with bladder or kidney tumors. Late effects of radiation therapy may include proteinuria. Children receiving cyclophosphamide (Cytoxan) may experience hemorrhagic cystitis, although symptoms may occur months to years after the drug has been discontinued. Particular care is required to screen for and treat urinary tract infections in children who have undergone a nephrectomy.

Tuberculosis. Routine screening for tuberculosis of children off therapy is advised. Children receiving therapy may be anergic to skin testing. The placement of controls (e.g., *Candida* and diphtheria-tetanus [dT]) will help assess the individual's responsiveness. A chest x-ray may be necessary if skin testing is unsuccessful.

Children receiving immunosuppressive therapy are at risk for tuberculosis. Children with documented tuberculosis should receive 9 to 12 months of therapy with at least two effective antituberculous agents (e.g., isoniazid [INH, Isoniazid] and rifampin [Rifadin]) (Freifield, Hathorn, and Pizzo, 1993).

Condition-specific screening. The primary care provider must keep in mind the possibility of abnormalities because of disease recurrence or the long-term effects of treatment (see Table 11-3). Screening for these complications should be done in consultation with either the pediatric oncology team or other subspecialty.

COMMON ILLNESS MANAGEMENT

Differential Diagnosis

Fever. Children receiving therapy will experience the same illnesses as their peers. The presence of an infection, however, adds a critical dimension in the face of neutropenia. If adequate therapy is not initiated immediately, septic shock may occur and quickly progress to death (Gootenberg and Pizzo, 1991). The first step in evaluating a fever is obtaining a complete blood cell count (CBC) with differential to determine if the child is neutropenic and blood cultures from all central venous access device (VAD) lumens.

Evaluation of the child who is febrile and nonneutropenic involves a thorough history and physical examination. Blood and urine cultures and a diagnostic work-up for any localized symptoms should be obtained. Antibiotic treatment is begun if the child has a central VAD.

The febrile child with a central VAD should have aerobic and anaerobic blood cultures obtained peripherally and from each lumen of the catheter or port (Gorelick et al, 1991). A broad-spectrum antibiotic should be started and continued until the culture results are final. If after 48 to 72 hours, the ANC is over 500 and the cultures are negative, the antibiotics may be stopped (Jones et al, 1994). If the cultures are positive, a full 10- to 14-day course should be administered.

If the ANC is less than 500 and a temperature is greater or equal to 38.5°C, the child must be admitted to the hospital. After cultures of the blood, urine, throat, sputum (with cough, tachypnea, or dyspnea), stool (in the presence of diarrhea), and any skin lesion and chest x-ray are obtained, an IV form of broad-spectrum antibiotics should be started immediately. Antibiotic choice is based on suspected organism and institutional-regional patterns of antibiotic resistance.

Viral infections. The human viruses affecting the child with a malignant disease are herpes simplex virus (HSV), varicella-zoster virus (VZV), and cytomegalovirus (CMV). Treatment of HSV infections in children with cancer is dependent on the site and severity of the infection. Mild lesions on the mucosal surface may resolve without intervention. Acyclovir (Zovirax) may be applied topically to speed the healing process of mild to moderate skin lesions (Committee on Infectious Diseases, 1994) or may be used orally in more severe or persistent lesions.

In the event that the child contracts a primary (chickenpox) or secondary (shingles) VZV infection, acyclovir (500 mg/m^2 every 8 hours) should be administered intravenously immediately and continued for at least 7 days or until all lesions have crusted. The child is closely monitored for evidence of systemic involvement. A chest x-ray is obtained to rule out pulmonary involvement. Aspartate aminotransferase (AST [SGOT]), alanine aminotransferase (ALT [SGPT]), and total bilirubin levels should be monitored for signs of liver involvement. Vigorous hydration and monitoring of BUN and creatinine during Acyclovir treatment is needed to prevent renal toxicity of the drug.

Cytomegalovirus infection may occur as reactivation of a child's own latent infection or from transmission of the virus through blood products. Signs and symptoms of an acute CMV infection include fever, hepatosplenomegaly, retinitis, pneumonia, colitis, CNS manifestations, and a rash. Antiviral therapy for CMV includes the use of gancyclovir and immune globulin intravenously.

Other infections. Candidiasis and aspergillosis are the two most common fungal infections in the child with a malignant disease. Candidiasis is more common and can involve the oral mucosa, GI tract, urinary tract, bone, lungs, and, less frequently, the blood. Meticulous oral care and prompt identification of lesions help to reduce morbidity from oral candidiasis. Prophylactic oral care regimens may include baking soda or normal saline mouth rinses, 0.1% chlorhexidine gluconate (Peridex), or antifungal suspensions or troches. Once an oral infec-

tion is documented, systemic oral antifungal agents may be used. Aspergillosis is seen most frequently in the respiratory tract, GI tract, and brain. Amphotericin B (Fungizone) is the most effective drug for systemic fungal infection; however, it has potent side effects.

The child who is immunocompromised and at risk for *Pneumocystis carinii* may take trimethoprim/sulfamethoxazole (Septra, Bactrim) prophylactically. The usual dose is 150 mg/m^2 divided and given twice daily for 3 consecutive days. The prophylaxis is continued for approximately 6 months after the completion of therapy. Parenteral or aerosolized Pentamidine given on a monthly or biweekly basis has been shown to be effective prophylaxis for the child with human immunodeficiency virus (HIV). Research is being conducted to evaluate its use in the child with cancer. Oral dapsone, given daily, may also be beneficial in young children who cannot tolerate Septra or Bactrim (Committee on Infectious Diseases, 1994). Pneumonitis is the most common clinical manifestation of *Pneumocystis carinii*. Symptoms include a dry cough, fever, tachypnea, cyanosis, and respiratory distress. Onset may be acute (few days) or insidious (months). All significant infections in children who are immunocompromised should be managed by the oncologist specialist.

Gastrointestinal symptoms. Nausea, vomiting, and diarrhea, common side effects of cancer treatment, may be difficult to distinguish from viral or bacterial illness. The primary care provider must establish the relationship of the symptoms to the administration of chemotherapy or radiation. During these periods, it is important to monitor fluid intake and avoid dehydration, especially in children who are currently receiving chemotherapy. In some cases IV fluid replacement and antiemetics may be necessary. Blood chemistry values, especially BUN, creatinine, AST, and ALT, must be monitored closely to avoid damaging vital organs from concentrated levels of the chemotherapeutics and from delayed excretion as a result of dehydration. Many families are taught how to administer antiemetics and IV hydration at home.

Vinca alkaloids predispose children to the development of constipation. If dietary intervention is not successful, supplementation with a stool softener or laxative will be needed to prevent paralytic ileus. This is most often needed when frequent repeated doses of vincristine are used. Suppositories and enemas should not be used without consultation with the oncology team because of the potential risk of infection related to reduced WBC counts.

Headaches. Headache pain, usually benign late in childhood and adolescence, is indicative of serious underlying difficulties in the young child. Morning headaches associated with vomiting and minimal nausea should always arouse suspicion of a brain tumor or CNS involvement. Headaches following a lumbar puncture, which resolve with lying down, may be caused by a slow cerebrospinal fluid leak. This type of headache is best treated by bed rest and adequate hydration. While taking a thorough history, the primary care provider should note onset, any precipitating factors or symptoms, location, severity, and what, if any, medication gives relief. A thorough neurologic examination is imperative. Many headaches may be treated at home with acetaminophen and rest; however, if the headache symptoms are unrelieved by medication, or there is any change in vision or neurologic function, immediate evaluation is necessary.

Pain. Pain in children is often difficult to assess and requires understanding of normal child development and age-appropriate verbal and behavioral cues. Most importantly, keep in mind that children rarely fabricate the presence of pain (Miser and Miser, 1989). The child with cancer poses additional challenges because of the multiple etiologies of pain, which may result from the malignancy, treatments, or procedures (e.g., bone marrow and spinal tap).

Tumor-related pain occurs with direct tumor invasion of the bone, with impingement of the tumor on nervous tissue, or by metastatic lesions. Compression of the spinal cord by a tumor may result in back pain and is accentuated by maneuvers such as coughing, sneezing, and flexion of the spine (Pack and Maria, 1987). Immediate evaluation is imperative, because an untreated cord compression can rapidly progress to irreversible neurologic damage. Treatment-related pain can occur from mucositis, infection, radiation-induced dermatitis, neurotoxicity from chemotherapy (vincristine), abdominal pain, or phantom limb pain following the amputation of a limb.

Pain resulting from procedures is greatly reduced with the use of conscious sedation (e.g., using one or more of the following agents: demerol, phenergan, thorazine, fentanyl, morphine, or versed) and topical anesthetics. Some children who experience great psychologic or physical pain during procedures may benefit from the use of short-acting general anesthetics such as propofol. EMLA cream, applied 2 to 3 hours before a procedure, can also significantly reduce the pain from lumbar punctures and bone marrow aspirates or biopsies. Although there is greater preparation time involved, the benefits to the child and family are significant. Art and play therapy can also assist children and adolescents in coping with the loss of control, pain, and uncertainty of a cancer diagnosis (Council, 1993; Walker, 1989).

Drug Interactions

Children receiving therapy need to avoid aspirin-containing products because they impair platelet function. Acetaminophen is generally recommended; however, its use during periods of neutropenia is discouraged because it may mask a fever. Multivitamins high in folic acid should be avoided because of the interference of folate with methotrexate. Vitamins low in folic acid are acceptable. Because of the number of drugs a child may be taking for therapy and the possibility of interaction, it is advisable that the primary care provider contact the pediatric oncology team before prescribing additional medications.

DEVELOPMENTAL ISSUES

Sleep Patterns

Disturbances in sleep patterns are common. The extent to which the child is affected will depend on the age at diagnosis, medication schedules, the frequency of hospitalizations, and the general coping patterns of the child. Maintaining a consistent bedtime ritual whenever possible provides security during a time when many things are disrupted. Parents should also be encouraged to accept transitional objects, such as a teddy bear or favorite blanket, because these may help the child with sleep during periods of hospitalization.

Toileting

Diarrhea and constipation may occur with certain chemotherapy agents. Toilet training may be delayed or regression may occur if treatment occurs during the toddler or preschool period.

Discipline

Discipline for the child with a cancer should be the same as for all children. A consistent approach in establishing expectations and setting limits is important to the child's sense of security. The parents should be supported in maintaining normal patterns of discipline, although they may initially be ambivalent about disciplining their child who is ill. Consistency in discipline among siblings is also important (Walker et al, 1993).

Child Care

The intensity of certain phases of therapy may make regular day care both impractical and potentially harmful to the child with cancer because of the increased risk of acquiring some infectious diseases in these settings (Thacker et al, 1992). When a child has begun less intensive therapy, a home or small group situation is recommended because it minimizes exposure to the various common pediatric illnesses. The caretaker must be educated about (1) the child's disease and instructed to notify the family immediately of any fever, signs and symptoms of infection, or increased bruising or bleeding; (2) reporting any communicable illness in the other children, especially chickenpox; and (3) any medication or oral chemotherapeutic agent that must be administered during child care hours. In addition, the importance of good handwashing should be emphasized, especially before and after toileting, food preparation, and meals.

Schooling

With advances in the treatment of children with cancer, more children are surviving into adulthood. The child who is too ill to participate in the regular classroom should be enrolled in a home study program. The role of health care providers, parents, and educators is to work as a team to assist the child in returning to school as soon after diagnosis as is medically possible. The return to school provides a sense of normalcy and contributes to the child's sense of hopefulness (Baysinger et al, 1993).

The child's school reentry must be carefully planned. To enhance the child's participation in school activities and prevent discrimination, anticipatory guidance should include attention to the balance between special precautions that need to be taken for the child's safety, learning needs, and avoidance of overprotectiveness (Turner-Henson et al, 1994). This can be achieved by mutual respect between parents and school personnel, a willingness to provide needed resources such as homebound education, and advocacy on the part of parents and the oncology team to educate school personnel as to the special needs created by hospitalizations, chemotherapy-induced side effects, and long-term sequelae of surgery, radiation, and chemotherapy on learning abilities.

Establishing an individualized educational plan (IEP) can help define and anticipate the special needs of the child. The teachers and the school staff must be informed of the child's illness and implications that will influence attendance, social interaction, educational capacity, and the restrictions or special needs dictated by medical care (Riley-Lawless, 1988). Early recognition of learning disabilities will enhance prompt assessment and intervention.

It is recommended that, with the family's and child's permission, the child's classmates be taught about the child's illness at an appropriate developmental level. The child will also need to be prepared to answer classmates' questions. The primary care provider can provide the family with support and resources to help ease the transition into school. See chapter 5.

Sexuality

The child with cancer often struggles with an alteration in body image because of hair loss, weight loss or gain, or disfiguring surgery. A major task of these children is learning to deal with this change, be it temporary or permanent. This is especially true in the adolescent who, in addition to treatment, may or may not be experiencing the normal pubertal changes. Ongoing monitoring of the child's development through the use of Tanner staging is important. Failure to progress through the stages warrants referral to a pediatric endocrinologist.

A young woman on chemotherapy may experience delayed development of secondary sexual characteristics and amenorrhea. Often after the cessation of therapy, development will occur and the menses will begin. Fertility status of children surviving childhood malignancies is variable depending on the type and extent of treatment. Transposition of ovaries from the radiation field has been shown to help preserve ovarian function (Thibaud et al, 1992; Leventhal and Kato, 1990). In 1991, Strong evaluated 2000 childhood cancer survivors and found that for those who were fertile, the chance of a normal pregnancy outcome was no different from that of their unaffected siblings. Ongoing long-term follow-up is required.

Sperm banking should be offered to pubescent males, if feasible, before therapy because sterility and mutagenicity can occur from cancer treatment (Voûte and deKraker, 1992). Ongoing assessment of appropriate sexual development and functioning (e.g., libido, impotence) is important. Peer support groups are often helpful in assisting the adolescent to deal with issues of sexuality and body image.

Transition into Adulthood

Because most children diagnosed with cancer are surviving into adulthood, pediatric cancer centers are attempting to create follow-up or "late effects" clinics that meet the needs of young adults or are referring them to adult oncologists who have remained current on issues specific to childhood cancer survivors. Follow-up including the same multidisciplinary approach used during treatment would benefit the young adult.

A recent survey indicated that job rejection rates were similar for childhood cancer survivors and their siblings except for application for military service (Hays et al, 1992). The Department of Defense generally does not allow cancer survivors to enlist but has provided waivers on a case-by-case basis when the individual has been off therapy with no recurrence for 5 years. To avoid job discrimination, it is advisable for young adults to apply for jobs for which they are clearly qualified, be honest with employers' questions but not volunteer a prior cancer history, and supply a letter from their primary care provider regarding prognosis and life expectancy should a question arise (Hoffman, 1994). Health insurance through large employers is much less likely to create a barrier to coverage than individual or small business policies.

SPECIAL FAMILY CONCERNS AND RESOURCES

Advances in medicine that have led to improved survival rates of children with cancer have also brought problems of chronic uncertainty. Chronic uncertainty "is experienced as an exquisitely heightened sense of vulnerability, accompanied by a compelling need to know the unknowable future" (Cohen and Martinson, 1988). The uncertainty faced by families centers around the basic issue of the child's survival. Family concerns will often reflect the phase of treatment they are experiencing. In the beginning, uncertainty is focused on whether or not remission will be obtained. If remission is achieved, will it be long term or will relapse occur? If relapse occurs, will the child enter remission again or die?

The goal of members of the health care team must be to help the families cope with uncertainty, not to focus on the unlikely goal of removing that uncertainty (Cohen and Martinson, 1988). Learning to cope with uncertainty is important to the health and well-being of all family members. Support for the child and family must be ongoing, not only at diagnosis but long after completion of therapy or death of the child.

The "intensity and agony" experienced by families while waiting for a definitive diagnosis should not be underestimated (Clarke-Steffen, 1993). At diagnosis, parents feel incredible guilt for not having brought the child to medical care sooner or for not being a more vocal advocate if providers did not realize the significance of the symptoms. The pediatric oncology team tries to support families through this difficult time by allowing opportunities for individual and family counseling. Siblings of the child with cancer benefit from an understanding of what happens during clinic and hospital visits and hopefully have opportunities to participate in art and play therapy activities.

Compliance becomes an issue when the child or adolescent's chemotherapy consists primarily of oral medications taken at home. A study of adolescents found, by laboratory testing, that approximately 50% were nonadherent to treatment with their oral medications. The factors correlated with poor compliance were poorer understanding of their illness and its prognosis without treatment, less perceived vulnerability, increased use of denial as a psychologic defense mechanism, and less future orientation (Festa et al, 1992; Tamaroff et al, 1992). Although adolescents should be specifically assessed regarding these issues, compliance in younger children usually encompasses a parent's inability to get the child to take the medication because of its taste or form. There are many innovative methods that can be shared with parents if they are given acceptance to express their difficulties in administering the chemotherapy.

Cultural issues related to how individuals regard and prepare for death are of particular interest in the care of children with cancer. In Korea, for example, dying outside of the home is considered very undesirable. This value has implications for the importance of home care for these children who are terminally ill. With regard to caretaking of children who are ill, most commonly mothers take on this responsibility in Korea, Japan, and in many Hispanic families, whereas in China, fathers often assume this role when the child is ill (Martinson et al, 1995). At an appropriate time, assessing such issues as the family's feelings about disclosure of information to the child, caretaking responsibilities, death rituals, and comfort with asking questions and voicing concerns and disagreement with health care providers is important.

The financial burden of a catastrophic illness is of monumental concern to the family. It not only affects the current financial status of the family but also has far-reaching implications for the child's future insurability. Insurance companies and health maintenance organizations vary in their reimbursement of medications and procedures they deem to be experimental. All of these factors place a tremendous amount of stress on an already taxed family unit.

Numerous local, regional, and national organizations provide information and educational resources about childhood malignant diseases. Local hospitals and cancer centers will often provide support groups for family members. Informal parent-to-parent interactions based on the sense of having a common understanding of parenting a child with cancer can be a powerful source of support. Identifying local resources will provide a much-welcomed service to these families.

Organizations

American Cancer Society, 1599 Clifton Rd, NE, Atlanta, GA 30329. Phone: 1-800-ACS-2345; in GA 404-320-3333. This is a volunteer organization offering educational programs, family services, rehabilitation support, and referral to local and regional resources.

Cancer Information Service, NCI, Blair Bldg, Rm 414, National Institute of Health, 9000 Rockville Pike, Bethesda, MD 20892. Phone: 1-800-4CANCER. This is a network of regional information centers that provides personalized answers to cancer-related questions from patients, families, the general public, and health care professionals. This organization also provides referral to local and regional resources.

Candlelighters Childhood Cancer Foundation, Inc, 7910 Woodmont Ave, Suite 460, Bethesda, MD 20814. Phone: 1-800-266-2223. This is an international organization of parents whose children have had cancer. This organization provides guidance and emotional support through local chapters, information, and referral to local and regional resources.

Leukemia Society of America, 600 Third Ave, New York, NY 10017. Phone: 1-212-573-8484. This is a volunteer organization offering educational programs, information, financial assistance, and referral to local and regional resources.

SUMMARY OF PRIMARY CARE NEEDS FOR THE CHILD WITH CANCER

Health care maintenance

Growth and development

Slowing of growth because of chemotherapy and radiation.

Closely monitored weight; child is at risk for significant weight loss because of disease and treatment.

Periodic developmental screening to assess for age-appropriate behaviors.

Neuropsychologic testing for children who received cranial radiation or who were less than 8 years old at the time of diagnosis.

Diet

Maintain an adequate diet. Offer small frequent meals if the child is experiencing anorexia. Low-sodium foods should be given to children on corticosteroid therapy. Increase fluid intake and high-fiber foods for constipation. Monitor diarrhea closely.

Safety

Ensure proper handling of chemotherapeutic agents at home and proper maintenance and protection of indwelling venous access devices. Use platelet prophylaxis for head injury or fall if counts are low. Minimize roughhousing and contact sports if the platelet count is less than 100,000. Because of photosensitivity, protect the child from sun. Use PABA-free sunblock.

Immunizations

No immunizations are recommended while the child is receiving therapy. Killed vaccines may be restarted after 6 months off therapy; live vaccines after 1 year off therapy.

Siblings and household contacts should not receive live polio vaccine because of transmissibility to child who is immunocompromised. Siblings and household contacts may receive MMR vaccine.

The varicella vaccine, although not routinely recommended for children with malignancies, is available for use in some children with ALL. Recommendations vary between cancer treatment centers.

Children recovering from bone marrow transplantation require special consideration in determining immunization schedule and protocol.

Children with Hodgkin's disease should be vaccinated with the pneumococcal and H. influenzae type B conjugate vaccines before splenectomy is performed.

Screening

Vision

Routine screening is recommended. Thorough assessment is warranted if visual abnormalities are detected.

Hearing

Routine screening is recommended. Children receiving ototoxic drugs should have regular evaluations by an audiologist.

Dental

Routine screening is recommended. A CBC should be done before an appointment to verify adequate ANC, platelet count. Meticulous oral hygiene is necessary to prevent infections. Oral SBE prophylaxis is needed for children with central VADs.

Blood pressure

Blood pressures should be taken at each visit to evaluate for hypertension as a result of drug toxicity.

Hematocrit

Hematocrit testing is routine and is done off therapy. It is done as needed while the child is on therapy. Critical levels are ANC less than 500, platelets less than 20,000, and hemoglobin less than 7 to 8 g/dl.

Urinalysis

Urinalysis is routine. Protein may be observed after radiation therapy, or hematuria may be seen after cyclophosphamide/ifosfamide therapy. Special caution when only one kidney is present.

Tuberculosis

Tuberculosis screening is routine and is done off therapy. Possible anergic status would require use of a control if tested on therapy.

Condition-specific screening

Close assessment is required for signs and symptoms of late effects of therapy or recurrence of malignancy (see Table 11-3).

Continued.

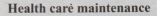

Health care maintenance

Common illness management

Differential diagnosis

Fever

Rule out neutropenia and infection. Do septic work-up as warranted. Prompt intervention is required with neutropenia or with presence of central VAD.

Viral and other infections

Treat mucosal lesions topically. Children without prior immunity should avoid exposure to chickenpox. Acyclovir is given intravenously for chickenpox in the immunosuppressed individual. Rule out dissemination of disease.

Give Pneumocystis carinii prophylaxis.

Gastrointestinal symptoms

For chemotherapy-induced constipation, ensure adequate hydration and begin stool softeners or laxatives as needed. Avoid suppositories and enemas.

For nausea and vomiting, determine the relationship to chemotherapy and radiation; rule out viral and bacterial infection. Give hydration fluid and antiemetics as needed.

Headaches

Perform a thorough neurologic examination. Consider possibility of a brain tumor, CNS involvement, sinusitis, and lumbar puncture cerebrospinal fluid leak.

Pain

Determine the source of pain; rule out cord compression.

Premedicate for procedures.

Drug interaction

No aspirin-containing products should be given. Acetaminophen is recommended except in times of neutropenia to avoid masking a fever.

Low folic acid multivitamins may be taken. Consult with the oncology team before prescribing additional medication because of the risk of drug interaction.

Developmental issues

Sleep patterns

Disturbances are common. Maintain consistent bedtime schedule and routine whenever possible. A transitional object may increase security during hospitalization.

Toileting

Standard developmental counseling is advised. Regression may occur.

Discipline

Use normal patterns of discipline; it is important to maintain consistency for all siblings.

Child care

Generally a small group setting is better than a large group to minimize exposure. The caretaker should know the signs and symptoms that pose a concern.

Schooling

The child should return to school as soon as possible. Ongoing communication between primary care providers and teachers is necessary. Education of school staff and classmates is crucial. Assist the family in the development of an IEP. Periodically assess for school problems and learning disabilities. If the child is unable to participate in a regular school program, arrange for home tutoring.

Sexuality

Give support for altered body image. Assess for appropriate Tanner staging. Sperm banking may be an option before the adolescent male begins chemotherapy or radiation.

Transition into adulthood

Need to transition care from pediatric oncology center to adult oncology center knowledgable on long-term survival of children with cancer.

Obtaining individual health care insurance coverage may be difficult and costly even after long-term survival.

Primary care providers may be of assistance in employment situations, if requested by client, by providing factual information concerning prognosis.

Special family concerns

Dealing with chronic uncertainty.

Insurance and catastrophic financial impact.

REFERENCES

Altman A et al: The prevention of infection. In Ablin A, (editor): *Supportive care of children with cancer,* Baltimore, 1993, Johns Hopkins University Press, pp 1-12.

Altman AJ, Schwartz AD: *Malignant diseases of infancy, childhood, and adolescence,* Philadelphia, 1983, WB Saunders.

American Cancer Society: Cancer facts and figures—1994, The American Cancer Society, pp 13-14.

Arbeter A et al: Immunization of children with acute lymphoblastic leukemia with live attenuated varicella vaccine without complete suspension of chemotherapy, *Pediatrics* 85:338-344, 1990.

Balis F, Holcenberg J, and Poplack D: General principles of chemotherapy. In Pizzo P and Poplack D, (editors): *Principles and practice of pediatric oncology,* Philadelphia, 1993, JB Lippincott, pp 197-245.

Baysinger M et al: A trajectory approach for education of the child/adolescent with cancer, *J Pediatr Oncol Nurs* 10:133-138, 1993.

Bennetts G: Immunization of patients with malignant disease. In Ablin A, (editor): *Supportive care of children with cancer,* Baltimore, 1993, Johns Hopkins University Press, pp 131-136.

Betcher D, Burnham N: Ondansetron, *J Pediatr Oncol Nurs* 8:183-185, 1991.

Blatt J, Copeland D, and Bleyer A: Late effects of childhood cancer and its treatment. In Pizzo P and Poplack D, (editors): *Principles and practice of pediatric oncology,* Philadelphia, 1993, JB Lippincott, pp 1091-1114.

Bleyer WA: The impact of childhood cancer on the United States and the world, *CA* 40:355-367, 1990.

Brodeur A, Brodeur G: Abdominal masses in children: neuroblastoma, Wilms' tumor, and other considerations, *Pediatr Rev* 12:196-206, 1991.

Brodeur G, Castleberry R: Neuroblastoma. In Pizzo P and Poplack D, (editors): *Principles and practice of pediatric oncology,* Philadelphia, 1993, JB Lippincott, pp 739-768.

Brown R et al: Chemotherapy for acute lymphocytic leukemia: cognitive and academic sequelae, *J Pediatr* 121:885-889, 1992.

Clarke-Steffen L: Waiting and not knowing: the diagnosis of cancer in a child, *J Pediatr Oncol Nurs* 10:146-153, 1993.

Cohen MH, Martinson IM: Chronic uncertainty: its effect on parental appraisal of a child's health, *J Pediatr Nurs* 3:89-96, 1988.

Committee on Infectious Diseases. Recommendations for using the live attenuated varicella vaccine, *Pediatrics* 95:791-796, 1995.

Committee on Infectious Diseases. Report of the committee on infectious diseases, ed 23, Elk Grove Village, IL, 1994, American Academy of Pediatrics.

Council T: Art therapy with pediatric cancer patients: helping normal children cope with abnormal circumstances, *Art Therapy* 10:78-87, 1993.

Feldman S et al: Measles and rubella antibody status in previously vaccinated children with cancer, *Med Pediatr Oncol* 16:308-311, 1988.

Festa R et al: Therapeutic adherence to oral medication regimens by adolescents with cancer. I. Laboratory assessment, *J Pediatr* 120:807-811, 1992.

Freeman CR et al: Hyperfractioned radiation therapy in brain stem tumors: results of Pediatric Oncology Group study, *Int J Radiat Oncol Biol Phys* 15:311-318, 1988.

Freifield A, Hathorn J, and Pizzo P: Infectious complications in the pediatric cancer patient. In Pizzo P and Poplack D, (editors): *Principles and practice of pediatric oncology,* Philadelphia, 1993, JB Lippincott, pp 987-1020.

Fricke SB et al: Chemotherapy-associated nausea and vomiting in pediatric oncology patients, *Cancer Nurs* 11:118-121, 1988.

Goede I, Betcher D: EMLA, *J Pediatr Oncol Nurs* 11:38-41, 1994.

Gootenberg J, Pizzo P: Optimal management of acute toxicities of therapy, *Pediatr Clin North Am* 38:269-297, 1991.

Gorelick M et al: Lack of association between neutropenia and the incidence of bacteremia associated with indwelling central venous catheters in febrile pediatric cancer patients, *Pediatr Infect Dis J* 10:506-510, 1991.

Harms D et al: Infectious risks of broviac catheters in children with neoplastic diseases: a matched pairs analysis, *Pediatr Infect Dis J* 11:1014-1018, 1992.

Hartman GE, Schochat SJ: Management of septic complications associated with silastic catheters in childhood malignancy, *Pediatr Infect Dis J* 6:1042-1047, 1987.

Hays DM et al: Educational, occupational, and insurance status of childhood cancer survivors in their fourth and fifth decades of life, *J Clin Oncol* 10:1397-1406, 1992.

Heyn R et al: Acute myeloid leukemia in patients treated for rhabdomyosarcoma with cyclophosphamide and low-dose etoposide on Intergroup Rhabdomyosarcoma study III: a preliminary report, *Med Pediatr Oncol* 23:99-106, 1994.

Hoffman B: Legal issues. In Schwartz C et al, (editors): *Survivors of childhood cancer: assessment and management,* St Louis, 1994, Mosby, pp 339-356.

Jaffe N: Osteosarcoma, *Pediatr Rev* 12:333-343, 1991.

Jones G et al: Risk factors for recurrent fever after the discontinuation of empiric antibiotic therapy for fever and neutropenia in pediatric patients with a malignancy or hematologic conditions, *J Pediatr* 124:703-708, 1994.

Katz J, Mustafa M: Management of fever in children with granulocytopenic cancer, *Pediatr Infect Dis J* 12:330-339, 1993.

Keegan-Wells D, Stewart J: The use of venous access devices in pediatric oncology nursing practice, *J Pediatr Oncol Nurs* 9:159-169, 1992.

Lawrence R et al: The risk of zoster after varicella vaccination in children with leukemia, *N Engl J Med* 318:543-548, 1988.

Leventhal B, Kato G: Childhood Hodgkin and non-Hodgkin lymphomas, *Pediatr Rev* 12:171-179, 1990.

Lunsford LD et al: Stereotactic radiosurgery of the brain using the first United States 210 cobalt-60 source gamma knife, *Neurosurgery* 24:151-159, 1989.

Marcoux C, Fisher S, and Wong D: Central venous access devices in children, *Pediatr Nurs* 16:123-133, 1990.

Marcus R et al: Long-term effects on the musculoskeletal and integumentary systems and the breast. In Schwartz C et al, (editors): *Survivors of childhood cancer: assessment and management,* St Louis, 1994, Mosby, pp 263-292.

Martinson I et al: Impact of childhood cancer on Korean families, *J Pediatr Oncol Nurs* 12:11-17, 1995.

McGuire P, Moore K: Recent advances in childhood cancer, *Nurs Clin North Am* 25:447-460, 1990.

Meadows A, Fenton G: Follow-up care of patients at risk for the development of second malignant neoplasms. In Schwartz C et al, (editors): *Survivors of childhood cancer: assessment and management,* St Louis, 1994, Mosby, pp 319-328.

Miser AW, Miser JS: The treatment of cancer pain in children, *Pediatr Clin North Am* 36:979-999, 1989.

Moore IM, Glasser ME, and Albin AR: The late psychosocial consequences of childhood cancer, *J Pediatr Nurs* 3:150-158, 1988.

Moore IM et al: Cognitive function in children with leukemia: effect of radiation dose and time since radiation, *Cancer* 68:1913-1917, 1991.

National Cancer Institute. Rie LA et al, (editors): *Cancer statistics review 1973-1988,* Bethesda, NIH Publication No 91-2789, 1991.

Ochs J, Mulhern RK: Late effects of antileukemic treatment, *Pediatr Clin North Am* 35:815-831, 1988.

Pack B, Maria B: Neurologic emergencies in pediatric oncology, *J Assoc Pediatr Oncol Nurses* 4:8-18, 1987.

Pedersen-Bjergaard J et al: Acute monocytic or myelomonocytic leukemia with balanced chromosome translocations to band 11q23 after therapy with 4-epi doxorubicin and cisplatin or cyclophosphamide for breast cancer, *J Clin Oncol* 10:1444-1451, 1992.

Perry M: Toxicity: 10 years later, *Semin Oncol* 19:453-457, 1992.

Pinkel D: Bone marrow transplantation in children, *J Pediatr* 122:331-341, 1993.

Pizzo P: Cancer and the pediatrician: an evolving partnership, *Pediatr in Rev* 12:5-6, 1990.

Pollock B, Krischner J, and Vietti T: Interval between symptom onset and diagnosis of pediatric solid tumors, *J Pediatr* 119:725-732, 1991.

Pui C, Crist W: Biology and treatment of acute lymphoblastic leukemia, *J Pediatr* 124:491-503, 1994.

Ramsay N: Bone marrow transplantation in pediatric oncology. In Pizzo P and Poplack D, (editors): *Principles and practice of pediatric oncology,* Philadelphia, 1993, JB Lippincott, pp 315-334.

Raney RB et al: Rhabdomyosarcoma and undifferentiated sarcoma. In Pizzo P and Poplack D, (editors): *Principles and practice of pediatric oncology,* Philadelphia, 1993, JB Lippincott, pp 769-794.

Renick-Ettinger A: Chemotherapy. In Foley G, Fochtman D, and Mooney K, (editors): *Nursing care of the child with cancer,* Philadelphia, 1993, WB Saunders, pp 81-116.

Riley-Lawless K: School reentry programs, *J Assoc Pediatr Oncol Nurses* 5:34-37, 1988.

Schwartz C et al: *Survivors of childhood cancer: assessment and management,* St Louis, 1994, Mosby.

Sherry D: Limb pain in childhood, *Pediatr Rev* 12:39-46, 1990.

Smith M, Rubinstein L, and Ungerleider R: Therapy-related acute myeloid leukemia following treatment with epipodophllotoxins: estimating the risks, *Med Pediatr Oncol* 23:86-89, 1994.

Strong L: Genetic implications for long-term survivors of childhood cancer. Facing the Challenge of the 90s. 14th Annual Conference Association of Pediatric Oncology Nursing, San Diego, 1991.

Tamaroff T et al: Therapeutic adherence to oral medication regimens by adolescents with cancer. II. Clinical and psychologic correlates, *J Pediatr* 120:812-817, 1992.

Thacker S et al: Infectious diseases and injuries in child day care: opportunities for healthier children, *JAMA* 268:1720-1725, 1992.

Thibaud E et al: Preservation of ovarian function by ovarian transposition performed before pelvic irradiation during childhood, *J Pediatr* 121:880-884, 1992.

Turner-Henson A et al: The experiences of discrimination: challenges for chronically ill children, *Pediatr Nurs* 20:571-577, 1994.

Voûte P, deKraker J: Ifosamide in pediatric oncology, *Semin Oncol* 19:2-6, 1992.

Walker C: Use of art and play therapy in pediatric oncology, *J Pediatr Oncol Nurs* 6:121-126, 1989.

Walker C et al: A delphi study of pediatric oncology nurses' facilitative behaviors, *J Pediatr Oncol Nurs* 10:126-132, 1993.

Wickham R, Purl S, and Welker D: Long-term central venous catheters: issues for care, *Semin Oncol Nurs* 8:133-147, 1992.

Wiley PM, House KU: Bone marrow transplant in children, *Semin Oncol Nurs* 4:31-40, 1988.

Woolery-Antil M, and Colter C: Biologic response modifiers. In Foley G, Fochtman D, and Mooney K, (editors): *Nursing care of the child with cancer,* Philadelphia, 1993, WB Saunders, pp 179-207.

Zeltzer L et al: A randomized controlled study of behavioral intervention for chemotherapy distress in children with cancer, *Pediatrics* 88:34-42, 1991.

Cerebral Palsy

Wendy M. Nehring and Shirley Steele

ETIOLOGY

Cerebral palsy, a condition first described in 1862 by Dr. George Little, is defined as a group of non-progressive disorders that cause aberrant movement and posture resulting from central nervous system damage or insult in the early periods of brain development, usually in the first 5 years of life (Galjaard, 1987). Cerebral palsy is described by both motor and anatomic groupings. Etiologically it is a set of disorders that is multifactorial and is diverse in clinical presentation.

The classification system developed by Minear (1956) remains the standard today. The four types of motor dysfunction seen in children with cerebral palsy are spastic, dyskinesia, ataxia, and mixed. Each of these types is then divided anatomically or by the number of extremities involved. Each category carries a different set of characteristics and prognoses (see box on classification system).

Spastic

Spasticity describes the presence of increased muscle tone, which is noted through the passive range of motion of a joint. Characteristics of spastic or pyramidal cerebral palsy include prolonged primitive reflexes, increased deep tendon reflexes (DTRs), rigidity of the extremities with movement, clonus, and later development of contractures and scoliosis. This form of cerebral palsy is most distinctly divided by the extremities involved. Damage occurs to the mo-tor cortex and pyramidal tracts in the brain (Geralis, 1991).

Spastic *diplegia* affects all of the extremities; however, the lower extremities are affected more than the upper extremities, with the presence of a positive Babinski reflex, tight heel cords, scissoring of the legs, and increased deep tendon reflexes (Avery and First, 1994; Behrman and Kliegman, 1992; Russman, 1992). Diplegia is frequently seen in low-birth-weight infants and is related to cerebral asphyxia with or without the presence of an intra-ventricular hemorrhage. The condition may not be recognized until the child is school age. Spastic diplegia cerebral palsy occurs in 10% to 33% of the cases (Behrman and Kliegman, 1992).

Spastic *quadriplegia* is characterized by a dysfunction of the four extremities (sometimes the legs are more affected) and often of the musculature surrounding the mouth and cheeks. In a few rare cases, three limbs can be affected which is called *triplegia* (Russman, 1992). Quadriplegia is the most common form associated with cerebral palsy and is diagnosed in low-birth-weight infants who have had severe asphyxial insults. Quadriplegia occurs in 9% to 43% of the cases (Avery and First, 1994; Behrman and Kliegman, 1992; Kurtz, 1992).

Spastic *hemiplegia* is characterized by a motor dysfunction on one side of the body with the upper extremity more affected than the lower. This form of cerebral palsy is seen in low-birth-weight infants

---

CLASSIFICATION SYSTEM FOR CEREBRAL PALSY

1. Spastic—described by the extremities involved. Characterized by prolonged primitive reflexes, increased DTRs, rigidity, clonus, contractures, and scoliosis.
   a. Diplegia—all extremities involved, lower > upper
   b. Quadriplegia—all extremities involved
   c. Hemiplegia—one side involved, upper > lower
   d. Double hemiplegia—both sides involved
2. Dyskinesia—characterized by abnormal voluntary movements.
   a. Hyperkinetic or choreoathetoid—large, jerky, and purposeless movements
   b. Dystonic—slow and twisting abnormal movements
3. Ataxia—described by the degree of muscle control, coordination of movements, and balance.
4. Mixed—spasticity and dyskinesias can be present together.

Data from Minear WL: A classification of cerebral palsy, *Pediatrics* 18:841-852, 1956.

with a past episode of asphyxiation, but also can be the result of a vascular malformation or embolism (Behrman and Kliegman, 1992).

Double hemiplegia occurs when each side of the body is affected and is caused by damage or insults to both hemispheres of the brain. The difference between this diagnosis and spastic quadriplegia is that the upper extremities are more affected than the lower (Behrman and Kliegman, 1992; Russman, 1992).

Dyskinesia

Dyskinesia represents the second motor dysfunction group and is characterized by abnormal involuntary movements after initiation of a voluntary movement. This aberrant positioning is a result of the coordination of muscle tone inadequately regu-

lated by the central nervous system, which is a result of insult to the basal ganglia or extrapyramidal tracts. The two forms of dyskinetic cerebral palsy are hyperkinetic, or choreoathetoid, and dystonic.

Hyperkinetic or *choreoathetoid* cerebral palsy has been classically associated with neonatal kernicterus. With prompt and aggressive management of hyperbilirubinemia in the first days of life, the incidence of cerebral palsy from this etiology has markedly decreased. Presently, low birth weight and perinatal asphyxia are more important risk factors (Behrman and Kliegman, 1992; Hagberg, Hagberg, and Olow, 1975; Yockochi et al, 1993). Choreoathetoid cerebral palsy is a result of damage to the basal ganglia (Geralis, 1991), and is characterized by dystonic and choreoathetoid movements. The dystonic movements often occur years after diagnosis. The choreoathetoid movements are grand in size, abrupt and slow, jerky, and purposeless. Hyperkinetic or choreoathetoid cerebral palsy occurs in 9% to 22% of the cases (Behrman and Kliegman, 1992; Geralis, 1991; Russman, 1992).

Dystonic cerebral palsy is characterized by slow and twisting abnormal movements of the child's trunk or extremities that may involve abnormal posturing. In other words, with a voluntary change in position, the extremity moved shifts into an abnormal position and stays in that position (Russman, 1992).

Ataxia

The third motor dysfunction group of cerebral palsy is *ataxia*. Neurologic damage is present in the cerebellum. Ataxia includes a range of conditions marked by the degree of muscle tone and coordination of movements and balance. These conditions can range from *ataxic* to *hypotonic* to *atonic*. Children with ataxia ambulate with an unstable, wide-based gait and have some mild tremors when attempting to move voluntarily. About one third of the children with ataxic cerebral palsy obtain this condition as a result of an autosomal recessive disorder (Geralis, 1991; Russman, 1992). Children with hypotonic cerebral palsy have increased deep tendon reflexes and may later develop ataxia, dysmetria, and, in rare cases, extrapyramidal movements (Avery and First, 1994). The children with atonic cerebral palsy have severe hypotonia and hyperreflexia. The range of incidence in this motor group is unknown (Behrman and Kliegman, 1992).

Mixed

The final motor dysfunction group of cerebral palsy is the *mixed* group, which is a result of many defects to various areas of the brain. Spasticity and dyskinesia can exist either alone or together. This mixed form occurs in 9% to 22% of the cases (Avery and First, 1994; Behrman and Kliegman, 1992).

Researchers generally believe that risk factors or causation of cerebral palsy can only be established in 35% to 40% of all cases (Russman, 1992). Others feel this number is as high as 75% (Eicher and Batshaw, 1993). Behrman and Kliegman (1992) divide the etiologic classification of cerebral palsy into four categories: (1) developmental anomalies, (2) perinatal trauma, (3) congenital infections, and (4) metabolic disorders in the perinatal period. Eicher and Batshaw (1993) separate their categories into prematurity, asphyxia, prenatal abnormalities, biochemical abnormalities (e.g., kernicterus), genetic causes, environmental toxins, congenital infections, and postnatal events (e.g., viral and bacterial infections and brain injury). They emphasize that in most cases where many of these risk factors are found, cerebral palsy does not occur (Eicher and Batshaw, 1993).

Finding the cause of each form of cerebral palsy is an area of ongoing research. The classic prospective National Collaborative Perinatal Project, completed in 1973, looked at 38,000 children who were followed through their seventh birthday. Researchers found that cerebral palsy occurred in 9% of the children weighing less than 1500 g at birth, compared to 0.3% of the children weighing more than 2500 g at birth (Nelson, 1988; Nelson and Ellenberg, 1978; Nelson and Ellenberg, 1986).

More recently, Pinto-Martin and her associates (1995) examined etiologic differences in disabling and nondisabling forms of cerebral palsy through ultrasound in 2-year-olds who were born at a low birth weight. The researchers found that perinatal brain injury is a more powerful risk factor in disabling cerebral palsy, especially in cases of parenchymal echodensities or lucencies and ventricular enlargement. A moderate risk factor was found with isolated germinal matrix/intraventricular hemorrhages (GM/IVH). Use of a mechanical ventilator in the neonatal period was also significant for later diagnosis of cerebral palsy. Pinto-Martin and associates believed that nondisabling forms of cerebral palsy, most often mild spastic diplegia, were a result of other perinatal variables. This 1995 study was a beginning effort to develop and validate a causal relationship between being born at a very low birth weight and developing cerebral palsy.

INCIDENCE

The incidence of cerebral palsy is approximately 7 per 1000 live births (Behrman and Kliegman, 1992). The prevalence rate in developed countries is 1.8 per 1000 children under 18 years of age. More specific findings from the 1988 National Health Interview Survey are found in Table 12-1 (Newacheck and Taylor, 1992). The incidence of cerebral palsy in the United States has remained steady or has slightly increased between 1970 and 1990 (see Table 12-1) mainly because of the decrease in incidences of kernicterus and the increase in very-low-birth-weight and premature infants who survive (Eicher and Batshaw, 1993; Kurtz, 1992). In contrast, the prevalence rates

Table 12-1.
PREVALENCE RATES OF CEREBRAL PALSY IN CHILDREN UNDER 18 YEARS OF AGE BASED UPON THE 1988 NATIONAL HEALTH INTERVIEW SURVEY

National prevalence	1.8/1000
Prevalence in children under 10 years of age	2.2/1000
Prevalence in children 10 to 17 years of age*	1.2/1000
Prevalence in boys	2.0/1000
Prevalence in girls*	1.5/1000
Prevalence in Caucasians	1.9/1000
Prevalence in African Americans*	0.5/1000*

Adapted from Newacheck PW, Taylor WR: Childhood chronic illness: prevalence, severity, and impact, *American Journal of Public Health* 82:364-371, 1992.
*Standard error exceeds 30% of the estimate value.

are higher in developing countries (Eicher and Batshaw, 1993). The specific prevalence of moderate and severe cerebral palsy is 1.2 per 1000 children at 3 years of age. Approximately 5000 children who will develop moderate and severe forms of cerebral palsy are born every year (Avery and First, 1994).

CLINICAL MANIFESTATIONS AT TIME OF DIAGNOSIS

Three elements leading to the diagnosis of cerebral palsy are: (1) the signs and symptoms of the motor deficit are nonprogressive; (2) the child is not reaching his or her normal motor milestones; and (3) there is a central nervous system abnormality(ies) (Russman, 1992). In severe cases, the diagnosis of cerebral palsy can be made early—43% of the cases within the first 6 months of life and 70% by the first year (Nelson and Ellenberg, 1978). For example, spastic hemiplegia usually is not medically diagnosed until the second year of life, although the parents note delays in the child's motor achievements in the first year. The spasticity does not begin early in the course of this condition. Instead, flaccidity and hemiparesis are present first (Avery and First, 1994; Behrman and Kliegman, 1992). On the other hand, some children who first present with risk factors of cerebral palsy no longer have these signs or symptoms after 24 months of age. This is especially true in cases of prematurity, although other communication and learning problems may persist (Piper et al, 1988).

Parents are often the first to discover their child's delayed or nonexistent attainment of motor milestones at the appropriate time and to bring this finding to the attention of their primary care provider. Specific signs include poor head control and clenched hands after 3 months of age, no presence of side protective reflexes after 5 months of age, extended moro and atonic neck reflexes past 6 months of age, no presence of the parachute reflex after 10 months of age, crossing of the midline to reach objects before 12 months of age, and hand preference before 18 months of age (sometimes as early as 6 months). These signs can appear in one or both sides (Taft and Barabas, 1982). The disappearance of the moro and atonic neck reflexes are more suspect in athetoid rather than spastic forms of cerebral palsy (Yockochi et al, 1993). An assessment of normal and abnormal muscle tone is outlined in the box below.

Other behavioral manifestations during the infancy period that may be indicative of cerebral palsy include: irritability, a weak cry, poor sucking ability with tongue thrust, excessive sleep patterns, and little interest in surroundings. The infant may also sleep in a ragdoll or floppy position or in an arched and extended position (opisthotonos). "Bunny hopping" (when crawling, the legs are brought forward together after the hands and arms are advanced) and "W sitting" may be signs indicative of this condition (Eicher and Batshaw, 1993; Kurtz, 1992). A summary of the clinical manifestations of cerebral palsy is found in the box on p. 236 with an example of scissoring in Figure 12-1.

ASSESSMENT OF TONE IN INFANTS

Normal tone

Infant moves well against gravity and lacks high or low tone characteristics

Low tone

Infant lacks tone to move against gravity; lacks resistance to passive movement; has low tone postures such as supine-lying with arm abducted, legs abducted in a frogged position; or has decreased movement

High tone

Infant becomes stiff when moving against gravity; the neck or extremities resist passive movement; infant has hypertonic head reactions such as hyperextension of the neck when rolling over, head pushing when supine or when pulled to sitting position; infant has high tone posturing such as increased extension of the head when supine-lying, retracted shoulder girdle, and lordosis of the back of extended lower extremities

CLINICAL MANIFESTATIONS OF CEREBRAL PALSY

Delayed or absent motor milestones
Poor head control
Clenched fists after 3 months
Absent protective reflexes after 5 months
Prolonged primitive reflexes after 6 months
No parachute reflex after 10 months
Crossing midline to reach before 12 months
Hand preference before 18 months
Irritability
Weak cry
Poor suck with possible tongue thrust
Prolonged sleeping patterns
Hypo- or hypertonia
Lack of interest in the environment
Scissoring of the legs
"Bunny hopping"
"W sitting"

Adapted from Eicher PS & Batshaw ML: Cerebral palsy, *Pediatric Clinics of North America* 40:537-551, 1993; Kurtz LA: Cerebral palsy. In Batshaw ML and Perret YM, eds: *Children with disabilities: a medical primer,* ed. 3, Baltimore, 1992, Brookes Publishing Co.; and Taft LT and Barabas G: Infants with delayed motor performance, *Pediatric Clinics of North America* 29:137-149, 1982.

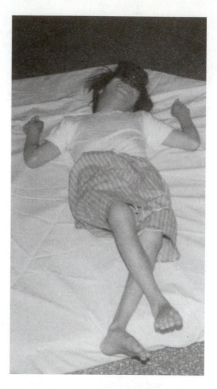

Fig. 12-1. An example of scissoring in a young girl. *(Photo courtesy of Matheny School, Inc., Peapack, NJ.)*

TREATMENT

The goals of treatment of children with cerebral palsy are designed to maintain mobility, maximal joint range of motion, optimal muscle control and balance, and the ability to communicate and to perform activities of daily living (Avery and First, 1994). The treatment always should be individualized and developmentally appropriate to the type and severity of the cerebral palsy (Russman, 1992). A summary of the forms of treatment used in cerebral palsy is included in the box on p. 237.

During infancy and toddlerhood when most diagnoses take place, the first line of treatment involves physical and occupational therapy. Several programs of physical therapy have been recommended to families, such as the Bobath method (a neurodevelopmental therapy program of sensori-motor positioning and handling techniques) (Bobath, 1980; Perin, 1989). The aim of these therapies is to enhance motor development and minimize the development of contractures, although the therapies' success has not been validated by replicated studies. In the majority of cases, parents are most helped emotionally from the support of other families facing similar issues (Russman, 1992).

More recently, physical therapists have used neuromuscular electrical stimulation to improve joint mobility, control muscle movement and strength, and reduce spasticity in tandem with standard active and passive therapies. This form of therapy has not been found useful for every muscle group, but has been used successfully in muscle groups responsible for achieving task-oriented activities (Carmick, 1993a; Carmick, 1993b).

From the preschool years through adolescence, the aim of a treatment program is to help the child with cerebral palsy function optimally in the class-

TREATMENTS FOR CEREBRAL PALSY

Therapies

Physical
    Method programs (e.g., Bobath)
    Neuromuscular electrical stimulation
Occupational
Speech

Orthotic devices

Braces
Splints
Casting

Adaptive equipment

For functional use (e.g., eating utensils)
Switches
Computers
Boards
Scooters and tricycles
Wheelchairs

Surgery

Orthopedic-corrective (e.g., tendon transfers,
    muscle lengthening)
Neurologic (e.g., neurectomies)
Selective dorsal rhizotomy

Medications (for)

Spasticity
Pain
Constipation
Urinary tract infections
Upper respiratory infections
Decubit:
Other secondary complications and conditions

Special education

Early intervention programs
Specialized learning programs and support
    services in school

room. Gross motor skills, muscle control, balance, and coordination are needed for sitting and moving. Fine motor skills, muscle control, and coordination are needed for writing and holding materials. Motor, cognitive, and language skills also are needed for self-care activities. Often the adolescent may decrease his or her amount of independent ambulation for the use of an orthotic device because of contractures, a lack of motivation, or weight gain (Russman, 1992).

Orthotic devices, which include braces and splints, usually accompany therapy when the therapy(ies) no longer assists, the child alone. Orthotic devices are used to provide stability to the joints, maintain optimal range of motion of the joints, prevent the occurrence or progression of contractures, and control involuntary movements. The most common types of orthoses are the short leg brace, the hand brace, and the molded ankle-foot orthosis (MAFO) which is worn inside the shoe. Other types of adaptive equipment include boards for positioning the child (sidelying, prone, and supine positions), scooters, tricycles, and wheelchairs. In severe cases, the wheelchairs are constructed and molded to the individual child (Nuzzo, 1980; Russman, 1992) (see Fig. 12-2). In each case, the orthosis is designed for the child and is altered as the child grows or the condition changes.

Surgery for cerebral palsy is not an early choice of intervention. Both orthopedic and neurologic forms of surgery have been performed; however, orthopedic surgery usually is not performed until after the child turns 7 or 8 years old. The child attains independent ambulation by this age if independence is at all possible. Orthopedic surgery is performed to achieve greater movements in the legs and better gait control, and to correct deformities in any extremity. Orthopedic surgeries are done to correct hip subluxation, hip dislocation, and spinal deformities such as scoliosis and to promote muscle balance, joint stabilization, and reduce spasticity through muscle lengthening and tendon transfers (Avery and First, 1994; Kurtz, 1992; Nuzzo, 1980; Russman, 1992).

Neurosurgery is used less frequently. Chronic cerebellar stimulation has shown mixed results, and stereotaxic thalamotomy and neurectomies have been performed on children with severe spasticity (Russman, 1992). Steinbok and his associates

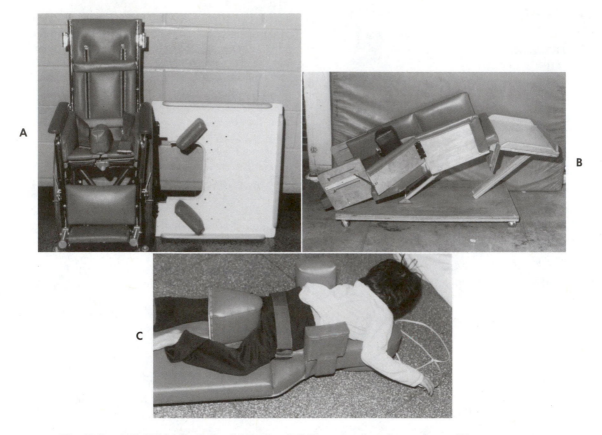

Fig. 12-2.   A, Individualized wheelchair. **B** and **C,** Two examples of prone lyers. *(Photos courtesy of Matheny School, Inc., Peapack, NJ.)*

(1992) in a study of 50 children who had received a selective rhizotomy found that in the postoperative period the children experienced a decrease in spasticity and an increase in range of motion; however, that function was not necessarily improved to a significant degree. It is also not known whether improvements after this surgery was more a result of the postoperative physical therapy or the actual procedure. Movement was not improved in children over 8 years of age who had received this operation.

Medications are usually unsuccessful, especially in children with ataxic and dyskinetic forms of cerebral palsy. Dantrolene sodium (Dantrium) occasionally helps spasticity (Ford et al, 1976), as well as baclofen (Lioresal) (Milla and Jackson, 1973) and diazepam (Valium) (Kurtz, 1992). In many children, the side effects of these medica-

tions have created further problems (Kurtz, 1992).

Along with a interdisciplinary health plan, which is mandatory for children with cerebral palsy, is the need for an individualized educational plan (IEP). Children also need special support services throughout their developing years. For more information on day care and school issues and needs, please refer to Chapter 5.

RECENT AND ANTICIPATED ADVANCES IN DIAGNOSIS AND MANAGEMENT

Selective dorsal rhizotomy has received recent attention for its use as a treatment to decrease severe spasticity in children with cerebral palsy. The long-

ASSOCIATED PROBLEMS WITH CEREBRAL PALSY

Cognitive

Learning disabilities
Mental retardation

Seizure disorders
Language and speech

Articulation
Vocal strength and quality
Language processing

Vision

Refractive errors
Strabismus
Amblyopia
Cataracts
Retinopathy of prematurity
Cortical blindness
Homonymous hemianopsia (Hemiplegia)

Hearing

Conductive
Sensorineural

Other sensory

Tactile hyper- or hyposensitivity
Dyspraxia
Balance and movement problems
Proprioception difficulties

Motor

Prolonged primitive reflexes
Absence of protective reflexes
Delayed motor milestones
Hip subluxation and dislocation
Scoliosis
Contractures

Feeding and eating problems

Chewing, sucking, and swallowing deficits
Drooling
Hypoxemia
Fatigue
Under- and overweight
Gastroesophageal reflux
Aspiration

Bowel

Constipation
Encopresis

Urinary

Bladder control
Urinary retention
Urinary tract infections

Dental

Malocclusions
Enamel defects and caries
Gum hyperplasia (with phenytoin)

Pulmonary

Respiratory infections
Pneumonia

Skin

Decubitus

Behavioral and emotional

Behavioral disorders
Attention deficit disorder with and without
    hyperactivity
Self-injurious behaviors

---

term effects have not been determined for any of these neurologic surgical treatments (Eicher and Batshaw, 1993). Other advances include further sophistication and refinement of the computer-assisted assessment programs for diagnosis and treatment used primarily by physical therapists.

ASSOCIATED PROBLEMS

Secondary conditions usually coexist and may include cognitive impairments (i.e., mental retardation or learning disabilities), seizures, sensory impairments (i.e., language and speech, vision, or hearing), motor problems, feeding issues, bowel and bladder problems, pulmonary infections, decubitus, dental problems, and behavioral and emotional problems (Russman, 1992). Plans for treatment, education, and habilitation must consider the child's individual presenting symptomatology and complaints. Secondary conditions may be acute, chronic, and transitory in nature.

Cognitive Impairments

Learning disabilities or mental retardation usually occur in children with cerebral palsy. Mental retardation is usually most profound in children with spastic quadriplegia and least profound with hemiplegia, where over 60% of these children have a normal intelligence quotient. Of the children with spastic quadriplegia, diplegia, and extrapyramidal and mixed type cerebral palsy, 50% to 70% also have mental retardation (Eicher and Batshaw, 1993; Kurtz, 1992; Russman, 1992). Even if the child's intelligence quotient is normal, often perceptual impairments and learning disabilities exist (Kurtz, 1992); however, any associated speech articulation problems should not be misconstrued as mental retardation.

Seizures

Approximately half of the children with cerebral palsy will also experience seizures (Aksu, 1990). Seizures are most commonly seen in children with spastic quadriplegia and hemiplegia and are less common in children with dyskinesias and ataxia. Generalized tonic-clonic and partial complex types of seizures are the most common (for a further discussion of seizure disorders, see Chapter 19).

Speech Impairments

The same muscle tone problems that make it difficult for children with cerebral palsy to move also create oral-motor problems. Limitations in trunk movements and positioning may limit lung capacity, which is needed for strength in speaking both clearly and loudly. Problems in articulation caused by muscle tone deficiencies are referred to as dysarthrias (Gersh, 1991a). In recent years, computers and adaptive equipment (e.g., switches) have allowed those persons with speech problems to dramatically improve their communication (see Fig. 12-3).

Impairments in communication, especially language processing, can be a major issue in children with hemiplegia (Behrman and Kliegman, 1992). Carlsson and his associates (1994) in a study involving 31 subjects of both genders with hemoplaque found that impairments of the left hemisphere result in greater speech disturbances. There is also a difference in the maximum amount of language abilities between boys and girls. Girls have less plasticity and greater verbal impairment with such deficits in the left hemisphere (Avery and First, 1994). Expressive and receptive speech problems are seen in children with quadriplegia, diplegia, and choreoathetoid cerebral palsy (Behrman and Kliegman, 1992).

Sensory Deficits

Children with cerebral palsy may develop a number of visual problems, including refractive error, strabismus, amblyopia, cataracts, and cortical blindness. About 75% of all children with cerebral palsy develop some form of refractive errors, most often farsightedness, approximately 50% develop strabismus (Gersh, 1991b), and approximately 25% develop homonymous hemianopsia (Russman, 1992).

A small percentage of children with cerebral palsy have hearing loss (5% to 15%). The hearing loss is either sensorineural (i.e., damage to the auditory nerve and/or the inner ear) or, more commonly, conductive (i.e., as a result of anatomic abnormalities and/or frequent otitis media). Hearing impairments further add to speech and communication delays (Gersh, 1991b).

As a result of damage to the parietal lobe of the brain, children with cerebral palsy have deficits in other sensory functions. These deficits may include tactile hypersensitivity or hyposensitivity, dyspraxia (i.e., difficulty in using one's senses to plan movements), balance difficulties, and problems with proprioception and movement (Gersh, 1991a).

Motor Impairments

Successful attainment of motor milestones is always delayed in children with cerebral palsy. Many children's primitive reflexes persist and protective reflexes never develop, thus permanently blocking their ability to ambulate. Often poor mus-

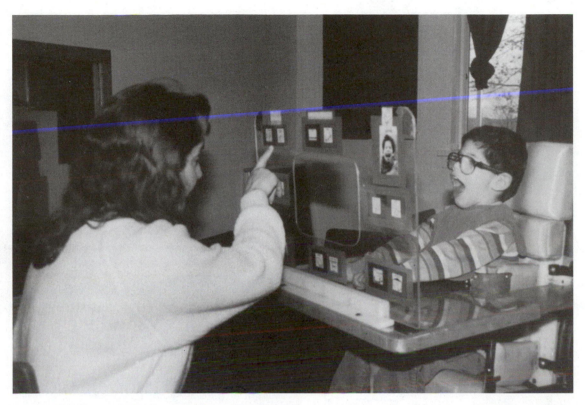

Fig. 12-3.   Child with communication board. *(Photo courtesy of Matheny School, Inc., Peapack, NJ.)*

cle tone and control lead to secondary physical problems, such as hip dislocations, scoliosis, and contractures, which create further motor impairment and other medical problems related to basic physiologic functioning. In the worst scenario, these impairments can be life-threatening (see Fig. 12-4).

Hip Dislocations, Scoliosis, and Contractures

Subluxation and dislocation of the hip are common in children with cerebral palsy. Subluxation occurs in 25% of children with spastic cerebral palsy (Gersh, 1991b) and dislocation occurs in 50% to 75% of bedridden spastic quadriplegics (Avery and First, 1994) (see Fig. 12-5). Complications can include further motor impairment, positioning difficulties, pain, chronic arthritis, scoliosis, and hygienic concerns (Gersh, 1991b).

Scoliosis can result from unequal muscle tension as a result of the cerebral palsy or because of poor posture or positioning in seating and recumbent positions. The degree of scoliosis directly coincides with the amount of spasticity and neurologic damage present. The prevalence of scoliosis varies from 5% to 65% (Avery and First, 1994; Gersh, 1991b).

Shortening and misalignment of the muscles can be created by a constant pull of tight muscles or spasticity, or diminished muscle use. This action creates contractures. Contractures in the lower extremities are most often seen in children with spastic quadriplegia and diplegia. Contractures in the upper extremities are most commonly found in children with spastic hemiplegia (Gersh, 1991b).

Feeding and Eating Problems

Feeding and eating difficulties are common in children with cerebral palsy primarily as a result of

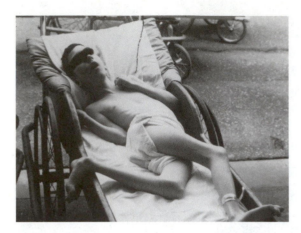

Fig. 12-4.   Boy with severe contractions. *(Photo courtesy of Matheny School, Inc., Peapack, N.J.)*

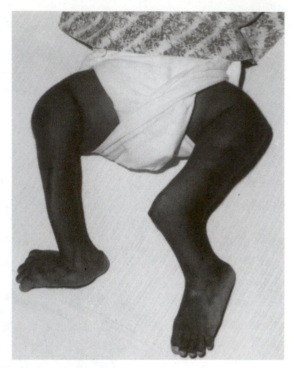

Fig. 12-5.   Hip dislocation in an infant. *(Photo courtesy of Matheny School, Inc., Peapack, N.J.)*

orofacial muscle impairments. Poor muscle tone (either hypertonic or hypotonic) in the neck, shoulders, and trunk can also impede the process of eating, as will compromise cardiopulmonary functioning. Specifically, these muscle tone and function deficits create problems with sucking, chewing, and swallowing. Increased drooling and gastroesophageal reflux may also occur. Feeding and eating disabilities are most often seen in children with choreoathetoid type cerebral palsy (Kurtz, 1992).

Bowel Problems

Constipation is a common and often chronic condition in children with cerebral palsy. Low muscle tone or spastic abdominal muscles can prohibit the ability to provide the contractility and pressure to adequately advance and empty the bowel contents. Further reasons for constipation include: lack of exercise, the inability to sense the signals of a bowel movement, painful defecations, inadequate fluid intake, a diet lacking in fruits, vegetables and fiber, medications, a fear of toileting, poor positioning on the toilet, and behavior problems (Gersh, 1991b). Bowel incontinence can also occur in cerebral palsy. Good dietary and bowel management is imperative.

Urinary Problems

Problems with bladder control and urinary retention that occur in cerebral palsy are often the result of neurologic insults (Mayo, 1992). Most children

with cerebral palsy do achieve bladder control between 3 and 10 years of age (Gersh, 1991b). Cognitive disabilities may lessen the child's ability to sense bladder fullness and the signals to urinate. A combination of incomplete bladder emptying, infrequent voiding, severe fluid restriction, and urinary reflux increase the likelihood of frequent urinary tract infections (Dorval, 1994), as do chronic constipation, improper perineal hygiene, and motor impairments. Overall there is a threefold increase of urinary tract infections in children with cerebral palsy compared to the general population (Gersh, 1991b). Prompt medical treatment of urinary tract infections is imperative.

Dental Problems

Malocclusions commonly occur in children with cerebral palsy as a result of orofacial muscle tone deficiencies. An over- or underbite can affect chewing and speech. Tooth enamel defects also occur frequently and if untreated, may lead to dental caries. Children who have seizures and take phenytoin may experience hyperplasia (i.e., excessive growth of the gums). Problems with gum disease and oral hygiene can occur (Gersh, 1991b). Other medications taken for spasticity such as sedatives or barbiturates can reduce the amount of saliva, increasing the propensity for dental caries (Leibold, 1994).

Pulmonary Effects

Alterations in positioning caused by abnormal muscle tone and spasticity, immobility, scoliosis, and contractures can affect pulmonary function and place the child with cerebral palsy at higher risk of respiratory infections such as pneumonia. When respiratory infections occur, they often linger beyond the usual period because many children have difficulty in coughing and in blowing their nose. Aspiration and gastroesophageal reflux can also cause pneumonia. Knowing the warning signs of respiratory infection and pneumonia is important for health professionals and families because pneumonia is the leading cause of death in children with cerebral palsy (78% of the cases reviewed in one study) (Evans and Alberman, 1990; Gersh, 1991b).

Children with severe dysphagia who show abnormal respiratory rates and fatigue during feeding likely are hypoxemic (Rogers et al, 1993). Choice of foods and especially textures can assist the child to oral feed for longer periods of time or identify life-threatening situations if oral feedings continue.

Skin Problems

Skin breakdown leading to raw and excoriated skin and decubitus is a common problem in children affected by cerebral palsy, especially in cases where mobility is most compromised. Good skin assessment and protection of bony prominences while seated or recumbent is necessary. Prompt and aggressive treatment of any evidence of skin breakdown is needed.

Behavioral and Emotional Problems

As a result of exaggerated and prolonged existence of primitive reflexes, especially the startle reflex, infants with cerebral palsy overreact to the mildest amounts of stimulation. As a result of the many associated problems with cerebral palsy, these chil-

dren become easily tired, frustrated, and sometimes demanding and uncooperative (Urbano, 1992). Approximately 20% of children with cerebral palsy may also develop attention deficit disorder and hyperactivity (Gersh, 1991a). In extreme cases, self-injurious behaviors can result (Kurtz, 1992).

PROGNOSIS

Prognosis, like treatment, depends on the type and severity of the cerebral palsy (Behrman and Kliegman, 1992). In general, the more extremities involved, the worse the prognosis (Eicher and Batshaw, 1993). In the 1988 National Health Interview Survey, 89.2% of the respondents with cerebral palsy indicated that their lives were limited in their ability to carry out everyday activities as a result of cerebral palsy. Yet approximately 75% of the same respondents to this survey indicated that they never or rarely were bothered by their conditions, suggesting that these individuals had adjusted well to their diagnosis (Newacheck and Taylor, 1992).

Although most children with cerebral palsy live to be adults, their projected lifespan is usually slightly less than the overall population (O'Grady et al, 1985). Children with spastic quadriplegia who are bedridden with many associated conditions may not survive beyond age 40 mainly because of complications of immobility (Kurtz, 1992). Prognosis is also specifically discussed in terms of independent ambulation. Generally if the primitive reflexes are still present at 12 months of age and the protective reflexes are not yet present, or the child has not walked by 6 to 7 years of age, the child will not ambulate independently. Children with severe dyskinesia also never walk (Russman, 1992). The locomotor prognoses based on attainment of selected motor milestones are located in Table 12-2 (dePaz, Burnett, and Braga, 1994).

Primary Care Management
HEALTH CARE MAINTENANCE
Growth and Development

Growth retardation does not occur in all cases of cerebral palsy. Children who have spastic quadriplegia, children who have seizures, and children who are nonambulatory are shorter in height than

Table 12-2.
PROGNOSIS FOR INDEPENDENT AMBULATION BASED ON SELECTED MOTOR MILESTONES

Prognosis and developmental milestone	Time in months
Head balance:	
Good	Less than 9 months
Guarded	9 to 20 months
Poor	Greater than 20 months
Sitting:	
Good	Less than 24 months
Guarded	24 to 36 months
Poor	Greater than 36 months
Crawling:	
Good	Less than 30 months
Guarded	30 to 61 months
Poor	Greater than 61 months

Adapted from dePaz AC Jr, Burnett SM, and Braga LW: Walking prognosis in cerebral palsy: a 22-year retrospective, *Developmental Medicine and Child Neurology* 36:130-134, 1994.

their same-aged peers (Stevenson et al, 1994). Children with spastic quadriplegia and children who are nonambulatory are generally thinner than their same-aged peers. A study of 171 infants and children from 10 months to 16 years of age found that all of the subjects' weights and heights were below the 5th percentile, and 30% had triceps skinfold measurements below the 3rd percentile for their age and sex. When nutritional factors were controlled, growth retardation continued across time. It appears that the etiology of cerebral palsy along with associated problems contribute largely to growth retardation (Stevenson et al, 1994).

Stallings and her associates examined nutritional status and growth in children with diplegic, hemiplegic, and quadriplegic cerebral palsy (Stallings et al, 1993a; Stallings et al, 1993b). In diplegic and hemiplegic children, these researchers discovered no differences in growth and nutrition patterns between these children and their same-aged peers, but they did find growth and nutritional

problems in younger children with cerebral palsy. Stallings and associates believe that in the subjects examined in the study, nutritional status improved over time probably as a result of improved oromotor, gross, and fine motor skills, general improvement in health status, and better nutritional intake (Stallings et al, 1993a).

Obtaining accurate measurements for height and weight can be challenging if the child experiences motor difficulty and has contractures. When a height cannot be taken in either a standing or recumbent position, the upper arm length (UAL) and lower leg length (LLL) measurements are adequate. Tricep and subscapular skinfold thicknesses are also obtained. A weight may be recorded from a standing position on a standardized scale or the child may have to be weighed sitting or supine on a chair or hammock scale (e.g., Hosey).

An interdisciplinary team is needed to longitudinally follow the development of the child with cerebral palsy. Periodic assessments of the child's mental, motor, language, self-care, and emotional development is warranted. There are many general and specific screening instruments that can be used by the primary care provider and should be an important part of the child's care (Urbano, 1992) (see Chapter 2). The most widely used general screening tool is the Denver Developmental Screening Test (DDST), but this tool is only used for screening and not practical after the child has been diagnosed with cerebral palsy (Meisels, 1989).

Motor assessment is most often completed by the physical or occupational therapist. Combining videotaping of the child's movements with computer analysis has greatly affected the ability of the physical therapist and physiatrist to plan and treat motor deficits and complications.

Speech and language problems can be screened with the use, for example, of the Preschool Language Scale or the Denver Articulation Screening Examination. There are also specific screening tools that assess receptive and expressive language ability (see Chapter 2). The primary care provider must accurately assess the parents' report of language skills, because mothers often overreport the number of spoken words, counting grunts and parts of words. The speech therapist is the best person for assessing language skills. Because of the many feeding and eating problems in infancy, a language assessment should be done in conjunction with a nutritional assessment around 6 months of age when solid foods are introduced.

Self-care skills should be assessed throughout childhood and adolescence during the history-taking at each primary health care visit. This can be done through an interview, a questionnaire, or a standardized test such as the American Association on Mental Retardation Adaptive Behavior Scales.

Emotional development is another important area for periodic assessment. Although there are a number of instruments available that measure self-concept and self-esteem, a good discussion with a trusted health professional is usually adequate for obtaining an understanding of how the child is coping at home, school, and other environments.

Diet

Undernutrition is most often seen in children with cerebral palsy during infancy. After any medical reasons for such difficulty are determined, further problems must be assessed. Exercises to improve facial muscle tone can be initiated. If the child has trouble controlling the jaw or keeping his or her mouth closed, external assistance or supports can be applied. The child may also have oral tactile defensiveness and require a program of desensitization to different textures and a food plan developed around the foods that the child will eat. Other children do not feel the food or drink in their mouths and the majority of the food or liquid falls out of the mouth creating skin problems. There may also be excessive drooling. Decreased independent mobility in late childhood and adolescence can lead to being overweight (Anderson, 1991).

Motor problems may also inhibit the child from being an independent feeder. Adaptive equipment can be designed for the growing child at each developmental stage. The infant may need to try different nipples until one is found that is preferred as a result of hypersensitivity. The size of the nipple hole may also need to be increased if thickened formula is prescribed. Most importantly, bottle feeding or baby foods should not be forced upon the infant because a high risk for aspiration exists. This risk is lifelong for the child with severe cerebral palsy (Anderson, 1991; Leibold, 1994).

The child's strengths and weaknesses for feeding should be assessed and recorded. An optimal environment should be provided to the child for successful feeding practices. Behavioral problems around feeding can also be minimized. A nutritionist and an occupational therapist can help in suggesting ways to assist the child who has oromotor difficulties and supplementing the diet to ensure adequate calories (Anderson, 1991).

Some children with severe cerebral palsy may eventually need a feeding tube surgically inserted in the stomach. Careful assessment of the child's oral feeding ability, degree of malnutrition, and health complications (i.e., respiratory distress) during feeding must be taken before a permanent tube is placed. A temporary nasogastric tube can be prescribed during an acute illness. In any event, careful lifelong monitoring of the child's feeding abilities and nutritional status is tantamount in cerebral palsy.

Safety

Children with motor impairments and seizure disorders are at increased risk for injury. Special concern should be taken for children with cerebral palsy in choosing physical activities, car seats, and environmental surroundings. Children with cerebral palsy may not be restricted in the type of physical activity, such as canoeing, but adult supervision is needed. Car seats should be appropriately padded and positioned for protection of the child's head (especially if head control is an issue), extremities, and skin. These precautions apply to any seating arrangement. The environment in which the child is in should be free of sharp edges in case of unexpected falls and roomy enough for the child to maneuver in it. If the child is in a wheelchair, the home environment should be accessible. Some engineers are specially trained to suggest adaptations to the home to make it more wheelchair accessible. Seizure precautions and helmets may be needed for the child with a seizure disorder. Home emergency plans should account for a child in a wheelchair and local police and fire departments should be alerted.

Immunizations

Diphtheria, tetanus, and pertussis. Children with seizure disorders are at increased risk of a seizure after receiving the pertussis vaccine. These seizures are usually fever related and show no evidence that neurologic disorders are aggravated. In infancy, the administration of the pertussis vaccine in the form of the DPT may hasten or parallel the diagnosis of a seizure disorder. Therefore the whole cell pertussis vaccination may be deferred when a child has a history of seizures. The risks and benefits for the administration of the pertussis vaccine when the child is at risk for seizures should be explained to the family (Committee on Infectious Diseases, American Academy of Pediatrics, 1994). Children with cerebral palsy who do not have seizures should maintain a regular schedule of immunizations.

Measles. Children with a seizure disorder are also at risk for a seizure after receiving the measles vaccine in the form of the MMR. However, because of the complications of measles, the high probability of contracting measles, and the unlikelihood of having a seizure after administration of the immunization, the standard schedule for measles vaccination should be followed (Committee on Infectious Diseases, 1994).

Chicken pox (varicella). Children with cerebral palsy need to follow the immunization schedule for varicella. For children with severe cerebral palsy where complications of the disease could be life threatening, prophylactic measures could be recommended (Committee on Infectious Diseases, 1994). Prophylactic treatment of varicella exposure with oral acyclovir has been used in lieu of the vaccine or varicella-zoster immunoglobulin to prevent the disease (Huang et al, 1995).

Haemophilus influenzae type B. The standard schedule for Haemophilus influenzae type B (Hib) vaccine should be followed for children with cerebral palsy. This schedule is especially pertinent for these children because of the increased risk for respiratory infections.

Influenza vaccine. Children with cerebral palsy are at risk for the complications of influenza. For those children with cerebral palsy living in institutions, influenza vaccines and chemophylaxis should be given during epidemics of influenza A (Committee on Infectious Diseases, 1994). Even though the Committee on Infectious Diseases from the American Academy of Pediatrics does not recommend influenza vaccine for all children with cerebral palsy, those children who are severely affected and who experience repeated respiratory infections would benefit from the yearly vaccine.

Other immunizations. Children with cerebral palsy should receive immunizations for mumps, rubella, hepatitis A, hepatitis B, and polio as recommended (Committee on Infectious Diseases, 1994).

Screening

Vision. A pediatric ophthalmologist should periodically assess vision in children with cerebral palsy because of the many types of visual impairments that may occur. Vision can also be screened each time the child comes for a primary care visit. When performing a visual acuity test, the child with motor problems may have difficulty showing which way the *E* points and the child with speech problems may have difficulty naming the letters. Allen cards may be useful for screening.

Glasses are often prescribed for refractive errors. Contact lenses are contraindicated in children with cerebral palsy because of their motor impairments which would inhibit placement and removal of the lenses. Glasses should be placed correctly on the child's face and adaptive equipment, such as velcro straps, may be recommended for comfortable and correct placement. Patching and surgery may be recommended for the other vision complications associated with cerebral palsy (e.g., strabismus and amblyopia) (Gersh, 1991b).

Hearing. A pediatric audiologist should regularly check the hearing of the child with cerebral palsy. For specific diagnostic information, the audiologist will use a tympanometer and an evoked response audiometry. An otolaryngologist may also be referred to assess hearing loss along with the audiologist. Infections can be treated with antibiotics, middle-ear fluid with decongestants, and if both conditions become chronic, surgical placement of myringotomy tubes can be performed (Gersh, 1991b).

Children with sensorineural hearing loss may be fitted with a hearing aid. A speech therapist may join the assessment team when a hearing aid is placed to facilitate language development through words or signs (Gersh, 1991b). Proper maintenance and use of the hearing aid(s) by the child and his or her family will assist in the child's optimal interaction with his or her environment.

Dental. Children with cerebral palsy need a dentist who has had some experience with children with movement and motor disorders. The environment of the dentist's office must be accessible, with a chair that allows for easy transfer from a wheelchair if the child uses one. The chair must also protect fragile skin and support spastic extremities (Leibold, 1994). Dental visits should occur at least every 6 months for the child with cerebral palsy, and more often if the child also has a seizure disorder and is taking phenytoin (Dilantin) so that gum hyperplasia can be prevented or treated early (Gersh, 1991b). Sedation may be needed for the child with severe spasticity.

Malocclusions can be prevented through a plan of oromotor exercises to improve tone in these muscles created by an interdisciplinary team consisting of the nutritionist, occupational therapist, and speech-language pathologist. Exercises can also be planned to reduce the oral reflexes that can lead to the development of over- or underbites. This team may also suggest adaptive equipment such as an altered toothbrush (Gersh, 1991b).

The interdisciplinary team can also address drooling problems and help the child to swallow his or her saliva and provide exercises to help the child keep his or her tongue in the mouth. If this problem persists, surgery may be warranted (Gersh, 1991b).

The dentist can place sealants on the teeth with enamel defects to prevent further tooth decay (Gersh, 1991b). The dentist can also suggest alternative positioning and ways to brush the child's teeth (i.e., using a wet washcloth and standing behind the child or having the child lay down) (Graff et al, 1990).

Blood pressure. Routine screening is recommended.

Urinalysis. Routine screening is recommended. If the child has frequent urinary tract infections, a referral to a pediatric urologist may be needed.

Hematocrit. Routine screening is recommended.

Tuberculosis. Routine screening is recommended.

Condition-specific screening

MOTOR AND MOVEMENT PROBLEMS. A motor assessment should be done at each primary care visit. Body alignment and positioning, passive and active range-of-motion, and signs of hip dislocation,

spinal deformities, contractures, and movement patterns (e.g., gait disturbances) should be assessed for and measured when appropriate. Dormans (1993) provides an excellent format for orthopedic assessment in his article on the orthopedic management of children with cerebral palsy. Use of x-rays and MRIs may be needed for further diagnosis. Correct management and follow-through by the child and his or her family are necessary to prevent the development of further complications.

COMMON ILLNESS MANAGEMENT

Differential Diagnosis

Fever. Children experience many febrile episodes in their lives as a result of the many viruses and bacteria that are present in their environment. Children with cerebral palsy are prone to respiratory and urinary tract infections. They may also get gastrointestinal infections. In each of these infections, fever is usually an accompanying symptom. The child with cerebral palsy needs to be seen by a primary care provider if the child is less than 6 months of age, has had a fever over 38.6°C for 3 or more days without symptoms, appears acutely ill with undefined symptoms, or has had a seizure(s) with a fever. A physical assessment and laboratory work need to be done at this time by the primary care provider for an accurate diagnosis and treatment.

Children with severe cerebral palsy may have impaired immune functions resulting from neurologic insult and thus a minor illness may manifest into a more severe condition if treatment is not begun promptly (Dorval, 1994). Regular follow-up by the primary care provider is essential.

Respiratory tract infections. Children with cerebral palsy are susceptible to upper and lower respiratory tract infections, namely otitis media, sore throats, rhinorrhea, sinusitis, and influenza. Routine management of these problems is warranted with careful monitoring of the resolution of the infection. Sometimes these infections are not resolved with one round of antibiotics, and a progressive condition is to be prevented, for example, additional hearing loss from a case of otitis media. Referral to a specialist may be recommended.

Pain with an infection is difficult to assess in children with severe cerebral palsy. The typical signs of pulling on the ear for an ear infection may not be present, for example. Often the parent is able to discern subtle signs in his or her child, such as increased irritability, decreased energy, less vocalizations, increased drooling, or the parent states, "My child is just not acting like him- or herself." The child can also be asked "yes" or "no" questions to identify the source of pain, or if the child uses a communication system, signs or symbols can be used to describe pain. Children's pain scales, such as the Wong Facial Scale, can be used by the primary care provider to further assess the child's pain.

It is important to stress the high probability of pneumonia occurring after an initial upper respiratory infection or bout of influenza in the child with severe cerebral palsy. Pneumonia can also be caused by aspiration and gastroesophageal reflux. Careful monitoring must be done to prevent a life-threatening situation. The child with cerebral palsy is unable to expectorate well and handle increased secretions. Dehydration can easily occur after a few days of fever. Hospitalization may be suggested as a preventive measure to ensure close observation of any changes in the child's health status. If the child is being cared for at home, the parents need to understand the importance of the treatment plan and be instructed to contact their primary care provider if the condition worsens.

Urinary tract infections. Urinary tract infections occur more frequently in children with cerebral palsy. The age of the child and any communication problems may impede getting detailed information on any pain or other symptoms experienced by the child. A urinalysis and urine cultures must be ordered if any suspicion exists of a urinary tract infection or the focus of the fever or other symptoms cannot be identified. After one or two urinary tract infections have been diagnosed and treated in a child with cerebral palsy, the parents and primary care provider should be able to identify the signs and symptoms that preceded the condition in *this* child. This information is especially important in the child who is nonverbal and should be recorded in the child's chart for further reference.

Standard antibiotic therapy for urinary tract infections is recommended when a diagnosis is made. Additional comfort measures such as increased fluid intake, perineal hygiene after voiding, increased rest, and taking acetaminophen based on body weight can be ordered. Follow-up after an urinary tract infection is imperative, including an urine culture 2 to 3 days after the initiation of the antibiotic to assess its effect. Follow-up urine cultures after the course of antibiotics is finished is also needed. If recurrent urinary tract infections occur, referral to a pediatric urologist is recommended.

Gastrointestinal problems. The parents may note that the child has abdominal pain, straining with hard stools, rectal bleeding, soiled underwear, and a distended, hard abdomen when constipated. Documenting the signs and symptoms of this problem in the infant or in the child who is nonverbal is especially important. Increased fluids, exercise, and a healthy diet with additional fiber is recommended. A bowel management program designed by an interdisciplinary team may be needed if constipation is a chronic problem. A program of stool softeners, laxatives, suppositories, and enemas can be prescribed, as well as suggestions for proper positioning and seating on the toilet. The effectiveness of this program should be closely monitored and recorded. A pattern for bowel elimination should be initiated and maintained. Complications of chronic constipation are urinary tract infections and impactions. Constipation is a very difficult chronic problem to deal with when the child is immobile and has a poor appetite. Bowel management programs must be individualized and evaluated periodically.

Drug Interactions

Children with cerebral palsy do not regularly receive prescription medications unless they also have a seizure disorder. A discussion of the drug interactions for seizure medications is included in Chapter 19. Medications are usually not prescribed for spasticity because they have no proven effectiveness and their side effects outweigh any benefit the child might receive (Gersh, 1991b).

DEVELOPMENTAL ISSUES

Sleep Patterns

A clinical manifestation of cerebral palsy in infancy is prolonged sleeping patterns. A variety of other sleeping problems also may exist with cerebral palsy. Kotagal and her associates (1994) found that obstructive and central sleep apnea can occur in children with severe cerebral palsy. Another problem may be severe hypoxemia during sleep, which may require a sleep apnea monitor. A neutral position of the body is encouraged during sleep with the neck and head slightly flexed. Bolsters or wedges can be used to facilitate appropriate positions. A side-lying position should be used for the child who drools so excessive fluid can drain out of the mouth instead of down the throat, which may cause choking.

Toileting

If children with cerebral palsy are able to be toilet trained, then, like any other children, they will give their parents clues of their physical and neurologic readiness. Importantly, the potty chair or toilet must offer adequate support for the child's body and minimize the risk of skin breakdown from extended sitting. The child's feet must be able to touch the floor so that the child can assist his or her abdominal muscles to push. Special potty chairs can be made or current chairs can be adapted. A physical or occupational therapist can inform the parents if their chair with the adaptations is acceptable. Diapers are now available for persons of all ages and sizes (Anderson, 1991).

Discipline

Children who have special health and developmental needs are disciplined by their parents differently than their siblings. As a result of their special needs and perhaps, past health care emergencies, parents are often reluctant to discipline their child with cerebral palsy. It is important that parents be consistent in their discipline with all of their children, that both parents are in agreement with the type of discipline, and that the discipline is developmentally appropriate for the child's mental age.

Child Care

Many child care programs today include children with and without chronic conditions and developmental disabilities. Parents of a child with cerebral palsy must be aware that the risk for infection is greater in settings where children are together, such as in day care (Committee on Infectious Diseases,

1994), and that issues of safety and accessibility are important to consider.

Schooling

The child with cerebral palsy may need to use different augmentative communication systems such as communication boards, computers, and keyboard voice synthesizers. Occupational, physical, and speech therapy as well as adaptive physical education are often needed and individually planned either for group or individual sessions. Adaptive equipment for seating, writing, and reading may be needed and should be obtained. For the child with severe cerebral palsy, an aide may be required to help with personal needs. Of the children with hemiplegic cerebral palsy, 25% develop a condition called *homonymous hemianopsia,* in which the child can see straight ahead but not to the affected side. Diagnosis of this condition is important for classroom seating arrangements (Russman, 1992). Transportation to and from school, transfer needs between classrooms, and emergency health and safety plans must also be arranged with school personnel.

Today most children with cerebral palsy participate in inclusive education. In this system, the child is integrated into the normal classroom for all subjects and receives specialized support systems within the classroom. Special attention must be paid to the child's cognitive ability and social integration into the regular classroom assisting the child with peer relationships and self-esteem. The primary care provider can assess the school situation and performance during well-child visits.

During the junior high and high school years, the child with cerebral palsy can be enrolled in vocational or college preparation programs depending on career interests and/or presence and degree of mental retardation. Adolescents with cerebral palsy may also experience renewed social problems during these years as they cope with adolescent self-esteem and contemplate life after school. Work and social opportunities are not as prevalent in the adult years as they are during childhood for persons with special health and developmental needs. Depression is often experienced as the adolescent is faced with the stigma of his or her condition and rejected in social situations. School performance also may decrease. Parents and professionals should look for signs that might alert them to these psychosocial issues during adolescence and offer support and professional counseling where needed.

Sexuality

The adolescent with cerebral palsy is a sexual being. Social isolation and chronic, low self-esteem and a poor body image can affect the development of intimate relationships. Sexuality education can be provided by an educator in the child's school or by a health care professional to aid the adolescent in developing both a positive self-esteem and body image. Role modeling and exposure to social situations can be planned and executed (Carmody, Brown, and Roth, 1991; Wadsworth and Harper, 1993). During the adolescent years, children often do not discuss sexuality and their feelings with parents. Therefore peers, other adults, and support groups should be available to assist the adolescent with cerebral palsy with these issues. In some cases, referral to a sexuality counselor may be needed.

Female adolescents should begin to receive gynecological care. Because of spasticity and poor muscle control, the woman's position for such an exam should be adapted. An annual pelvic ultrasound can be done by the physician for baseline data. Pregnancy is possible for the woman with cerebral palsy. Abnormal births can occur at an increased rate over the general population, but 90% of the births are normal (Winch et al, 1993).

Transition into Adulthood

Specific issues in the transition to adulthood in children with cerebral palsy relate to medical care, equipment, nutrition, vocational decisions, transportation, housing, and social needs. Throughout life, optimal independence should be encouraged and learned helplessness avoided. Independence and self-advocacy is stressed during the transitional period between adolescence and adulthood. The adolescent with cerebral palsy needs to take an active role in choosing a primary care provider and health care interdisciplinary team. Participation in decision making about dietary choices, medications, surgical interventions if needed, adaptive equipment, and chairs is important. Vocational decisions should also be discussed and plans for successful employment should be determined. When deciding upon a college or worksite, the physical layout, wheelchair accessibility, availability of personal aides, housing, and a repair shop for the wheelchair and any adaptive equipment must be considered and resources identified. Independence in the use of public transportation should be planned. In mild cases of cerebral palsy, driving may be possible. Independent living or assisted living arrangements need to be discussed and placement on waiting lists procured if living outside the home is desired. Social needs including activities, planned social programs, and time for successful relationships should be planned for and evaluated. The severity of the cerebral palsy will determine the amount of independence and decision making in which the individual can participate. Most importantly, the adolescent transitioning to adulthood must participate in decisions regarding his or her life to the extent possible.

SPECIAL FAMILY CONCERNS AND RESOURCES

In incidences of mild cerebral palsy, the effects on the family may be minimal or none at all. The needs of each individual family member must be attended and addressed. These needs will change across time and should be evaluated periodically.

In the case of a child who has severe cerebral palsy, parents usually experience chronic sorrow when their child does not achieve the developmental milestones that other children without this condition achieve. Hirose and Ueda (1994) found that the infancy period was most stressful for mothers and that the period from toddlerhood through adolescence was the most stressful for fathers.

Siblings are also affected. In a recent study of sibling interactions with children with cerebral palsy, researchers found that the children with cerebral palsy were unassertive and passive in their play behaviors. On the other hand, the unaffected siblings learned and exhibited more nurturant, directive, and extroverted behaviors (Dallas, Stevenson, and McGurk, 1993a; Dallas, Stevenson, and McGurk, 1993b).

Respite care is highly recommended to allow the family time away from the constant responsibilities of caring for a child with cerebral palsy. Respite care can be arranged for in the home or outside the home.

There are no specific cross-cultural or religious concerns for children with cerebral palsy, although a stigma, based on the diagnosis, is attached to all families. The visibility of this condition may create more of a stigma for some cultures than for others. For a discussion of these issues, see Chapter 4.

Community Resources

A variety of local, state, and regional services for children with cerebral palsy exist. "Social Services and Organizations" in the local yellow pages of the telephone directory usually list appropriate resources and organizations. Two books offer excellent resource lists for general and specific conditions at the state and federal levels (Geralis, 1991; Roth and Morse, 1994). *Children with Cerebral Palsy: A Parent's Guide* (Geralis, 1991) is an excellent guide for families and includes resources for adaptive equipment, wheelchairs, communication-technical equipment, toys, and clothing. *A Life-Span Approach to Nursing Care for Individuals with Developmental Disabilities* (Roth and Morse, 1994) is an excellent resource book for pediatric nurse practitioners and health care professionals. The national organization for cerebral palsy is:

United Cerebral Palsy Associations, Inc.
1522 K Street NW, Suite 1112
Washington, DC 20005
1-800-USA-5UCP (national office), 1-202-842-1266 (voice/tt), 1-202-842-3519 (fax), UCPA INC (American Online), and UCP.NAT (Applelink)

SUMMARY OF PRIMARY CARE NEEDS FOR THE CHILD WITH CEREBRAL PALSY

Health care maintenance

Growth and development

Undernutrition in infancy often leads to growth retardation.

Different techniques should be used to get height, arm length, leg length, and skinfold measurements.

Weights may be attained through standing scales, seating, or recumbent lifts.

Overweight conditions may occur in adolescence when mobility may decrease.

Delayed development in motor and communication skills is common.

Developmental strengths and weaknesses must be assessed and recorded.

Mental retardation and seizure disorders inhibit intellectual development.

Diet

Difficulty with sucking, swallowing, and chewing can be present in infancy. Assessment should be done early.

Drooling and aspiration can also be problems.

Nutritional concerns may be lifelong, and placement of a gastrostomy tube may be warranted in severe cases.

Referral to a nutritionist is needed.

Safety

The child is at risk for injury as a result of spasticity, muscle control problems, delayed protective reflexes, and potential seizures.

Positioning and adaptive equipment are often required.

Immunizations

If the etiology for seizure activity is unknown, the pertussis vaccine may be deferred or a cellular vaccine used when age appropriate.

The measles vaccine should be given as scheduled.

Fever management is necessary to decrease the possibility of febrile seizures.

Haemophilus influenzae type B (Hib) vaccine and other immunizations should be given as scheduled.

Children with cerebral palsy are at risk for the complications of influenza and varicella.

Continued.

SUMMARY OF PRIMARY CARE NEEDS FOR THE CHILD WITH CEREBRAL PALSY—cont'd

Screening

Vision

A pediatric ophthalmologist should be seen during the infancy period because of the likelihood of vision problems.

Vision should be checked for acuity, refractive errors, strasbismus, retinopathy of prematurity, and cataracts.

Hearing

Referral to a pediatric audiologist may be necessary during infancy to check for hearing problems and loss.

Both sensorineural and conductive hearing loss is possible.

Routine screening for conductive hearing problems and loss should be done.

Dental

Evaluation by a dentist experienced with children with motor problems should be done every 6 months.

Proper dental hygiene is needed.

Administration of phenytoin may cause hyperplasia of the gums and proper preventive care and early treatment of this condition is important.

Blood pressure

Routine screening is recommended.

Urinalysis

Routine screening is recommended.

A referral to a pediatric urologist may be needed if the child has chronic UTIs.

Hematocrit

Routine screening is recommended.

Tuberculosis

Routine screening is recommended.

Condition-specific screening

A motor assessment should be done at every well-child visit. This would include assessment for scoliosis, hip dislocation, and contractures.

Common illness management

Differential diagnosis

Fever

Management of fevers is routine.

Respiratory tract infections

Respiratory infections should be promptly treated. In the child with severe cerebral palsy, pneumonia may be life threatening. Follow-up is important.

Urinary tract infections

Treatment for urinary tract infections should be prompt and follow-up essential. Urinary tract abnormalities may also be present.

Gastrointestinal problems

Constipation is a chronic problem for many children. A bowel management program may be needed.

Drug interactions

No medications are routinely prescribed, except if a seizure disorder is also present.

Developmental issues

Sleep patterns

Correct positioning is needed during sleep because sleep apnea can occur.

Toileting

Often adaptive equipment is needed for correct positioning on the toilet. Bladder and bowel training may be delayed.

Discipline

It is important that consistent and age-appropriate discipline measures be taken.

Child care

Careful planning must be undertaken in choosing the best child care arrangements, especially regarding issues of safety, accessibility, health care needs, and increased rates of infection.

Schooling

Use IEPs and inclusive classrooms. Specialized services and therapies for the individual child must be procured. Adaptive equipment and computers have enhanced this child's ability to learn.

Behavioral and school problems can occur in adolescence as a result of poor esteem and body image.

Sexuality

Opportunities for social activities should be

Continued.

SUMMARY OF PRIMARY CARE NEEDS FOR THE CHILD WITH CEREBRAL PALSY—cont'd

arranged. Transportation needs are important to consider.

Opportunities for same sex and opposite sex relationships are needed. Classes in social interactions and sexuality may be needed.

Gynecological exams should begin for women with adaptations in the normal positioning.

Reproductive issues should be discussed.

Transition into adulthood

Promote independence and self-advocacy for the child.

Future residential and vocational plans need to be addressed.

Special family concerns

Respite care meets needs of family.

Effects on individual family members need to be assessed and addressed. Special support groups are available for fathers and siblings.

Family stigma may be perceived.

REFERENCES

Aksu F: Nature and prognosis of seizures in patients with cerebral palsy, *Dev Med Child Neurol* 32:661-668, 1990.

Anderson S: Daily care. In E Geralis, (editor): *Children with cerebral palsy: a parent's guide,* Bethesda, MD, 1991, Woodbine House, pp 91-132.

Avery ME, First LR: *Pediatric medicine,* ed 2, Baltimore, MD, 1994, Williams & Wilkins, pp 807-810, 1450-1451.

Behrman RE, Kliegman RM, (editors): *Nelson essentials of pediatrics,* ed 2, Philadelphia, PA, 1992, WB Saunders Co.

Bobath K: A neurophysiological basis for the treatment of cerebral palsy, *Br J Ophthamol* 66:46-52, 1980.

Carlsson G et al: Verbal and non-verbal function of children with right- vs left-hemiplegic cerebral palsy of pre- and perinatal origin, *Dev Med Child Neurol* 36:503-512, 1994.

Carmick J: Clinical use of neuromuscular electrical stimulation for children with cerebral palsy, part 1: lower extremity, *Phys Ther* 73:505-513, 1993a.

Carmick J: Clinical use of neuromuscular electrical stimulation for children with cerebral palsy, part 2: upper extremity, *Phys Ther* 73:514-522, 1993b.

Carmody MA, Brown M, and Roth SP: Perspectives: a case study, *Information Plus* 2:1-3, 1991.

Committee on Infectious Diseases, American Academy of Pediatrics. *1994 red book: report of the committee on infectious diseases,* ed 23, Elk Grove Village, IL, 1994, American Academy of Pediatrics.

Dallas E, Stevenson J, and McGurk H: Cerebral-palsied children's interactions with siblings - I. Influence of severity of disability, age, and birth order, *J Child Psychol Psychiat* 34:621-647, 1993a.

Dallas E, Stevenson J, and McGurk H: Cerebral-palsied children's interactions with siblings - II. Interactional structure, *J Child Psychol Psychiatr* 34:649-671, 1993b.

de Paz AC Jr, Burnett SM, and Braga LW: Walking prognosis in cerebral palsy: a 22-year retrospective analysis, *Dev Med Child Neurol* 36:130-134, 1994.

Dormans JP: Orthopedic management of children with cerebral palsy, *Pediatr Clin North Am* 40:645-657, 1993.

Dorval J: Achieving and maintaining body systems integrity and function: clinical issues. In DJ Lollar, (editor): *Preventing secondary conditions associated with spina bifida or cerebral palsy: proceedings and recommendations of a symposium,* Washington, DC, 1994, Spina Bifida Association of America, pp 65-77.

Eicher PS, Batshaw ML: Cerebral palsy, *Pediatr Clin North Am* 40:537-551, 1993.

Evans PM, Alberman E: Certified cause of death in children and young adults with cerebral palsy, *Arch Dis Child* 65:325-329, 1990.

Ford F et al: Efficacy of dantrolene sodium in the treatment of spastic cerebral palsy, *Dev Med Child Neurol* 18:770-783, 1976.

Galjaard H: *Early detection and management of cerebral palsy,* Netherlands, 1987, Martinus-Nijhoff Publisher.

Geralis E, (editor): *Children with cerebral palsy: a parent's guide,* Bethesda, MD, 1991, Woodbine House.

Gersh ES: What is cerebral palsy? In E Geralis, (editor): *Children with cerebral palsy: a parent's guide,* Bethesda, MD, 1991a, Woodbine House, pp 1-32.

Gersh ES: Medical concerns and treatment. In Geralis E, (editor): *Children with cerebral palsy: a parent's guide,* Bethesda, MD, 1991b, Woodbine House, pp 57-90.

Graff JC et al: *Health care for students with disabilities,* Baltimore, MD, 1990, Paul H Brookes Publishing Co.

Hagberg B, Hagberg G, and Olow I: The changing panorama of cerebral palsy in Sweden, 1954-1970. II: Analysis of the various syndromes, *Acta Paediatrics Scandinavia* 64:193-202, 1975.

Hirose T, Ueda R: Long-term follow-up study of children with cerebral palsy and coping behaviour of parents. In Smith JP, (editor): *Research and its application,* London, England, 1994, Blackwell Scientific Publications.

Huang Y-C et al: Acyclovir prophylaxis of varicella after household exposure, *The Pediatric Infectious Disease Journal* 14:152-154, 1995.

Kotagal S, Gibbons VP, and Stith JA: Sleep abnormalities in patients with severe cerebral palsy, *Dev Med Child Neurol* 36:304-311, 1994.

Kurtz LA: Cerebral palsy. In Batshaw ML and Perret YM, (editors): *Children with disabilities: a medical primer,* ed 3, Baltimore, MD, 1992, Brookes Publishing Company, pp 441-469.

Leibold S: Achieving and maintaining body systems integrity and function: personal care skills. In Lollar DJ, (editor): *Preventing secondary conditions associated with spina bifida or cerebral palsy: proceedings and recommendations of a symposium,* Washington, DC, 1994, Spina Bifida Association of America, pp 78-86.

Little WJ: On the influence of abnormal parturition, difficult labors, premature birth, and asphyxia neonatorum, on the mental and physical condition of the child, especially in relation to deformities, *Transactions of the Obstetric Society of London* 3:293-344, 1861-1862.

Mayo M: Lower urinary tract dysfunction in cerebral palsy, *J Urol* 147:419-420, 1992.

Meisels SJ: Can developmental screening tests identify children who are developmentally at risk? *Pediatrics* 83:578-584, 1989.

Milla JJ, Jackson ADM: A controlled trial of baclofen in children with cerebral palsy, *J Intern Med* 5:398-404, 1973.

Minear WL: A classification of cerebral palsy. *Pediatrics* 18:841-852, 1956.

Nelson KB: What proportion of cerebral palsy is related to birth asphyxia? *J Pediatr* 112:572-573, 1988.

Nelson KB, Ellenberg JH: Antecedents of cerebral palsy: multivariate analysis of risk, *New Engl J Med* 315:81-86, 1986.

Nelson KB, Ellenberg JH: Epidemiology of cerebral palsy. In Schoenberg BS, (editor): *Advances in neurology,* New York, 1978, Raven Press, pp 421-435.

Newacheck PW, Taylor WR: Childhood chronic illness: prevalence, severity, and impact, *Am J Public Health* 82:364-371, 1992.

Nuzzo RM: Dynamic bracing: elastics for patients with cerebral palsy, muscular dystrophy, and myelodysplasia, *Clin Orthop Related Res* 148:263-273, 1980.

O'Grady RS et al: Vocational predictions compared with present vocational status of 60 young adults with cerebral palsy, *Dev Med Child Neurol* 27:775-784, 1985.

Perin B: Physical therapy for the child with cerebral palsy. In Tecklin JS, (editor): *Pediatric physical therapy,* Philadelphia, PA, 1989, JB Lippincott, pp 68-105.

Pinto-Martin JA et al: Cranial ultrasound prediction of disabling and nondisabling cerebral palsy at age 2 in a low-birth-weight population, *Pediatrics* 95:249-254, 1995.

Piper MC et al: Resolution of neurologic signs in high-risk infants during the first 2 years of life, *Dev Med Child Neurol* 30:26-35, 1988.

Rogers BT et al: Hypoxemia during oral feeding of children with severe cerebral palsy, *Dev Med Child Neurol* 35:3-10, 1993.

Roth SP, Morse JS, (editors): *A life-span approach to nursing care for individuals with developmental disabilities,* Baltimore, MD, 1994, Paul H Brookes Publishing Co.

Russman BS: Disorders of motor execution I: Cerebral palsy. In David RB, (editor): *Pediatric neurology for the clinician,* Norwalk, CT, 1992, Appleton and Lange, pp 469-480.

Stallings VA et al: Nutritional status and growth of children with diplegic or hemiplegic cerebral palsy, *Dev Med Child Neurol* 35:997-1006, 1993a.

Stallings VA et al: Nutrition-related growth failure of children with quadriplegic cerebral palsy, *Dev Med Child Neurol* 35:126-138, 1993b.

Steinbok P et al: Selective functional posterior rhizotomy for treatment of spastic cerebral palsy in children, *Pediatric Neurosurgery* 18:34-42, 1992.

Stevenson RD et al: Clinical correlates of linear growth in children with cerebral palsy, *Dev Med Child Neurol* 36:135-142, 1994.

Taft LT, Barabas G: Infants with delayed motor performance, *Pediatr Clin North Am* 29:137-149, 1982.

Urbano MT: *Preschool children with special health care needs,* San Diego, CA, 1992, Singular Publishing Group, Inc.

Wadsworth JS, Harper DC: The social needs of adolescents with cerebral palsy, *Dev Med Child Neurol* 35:1015-1024, 1993.

Winch R et al: Women with cerebral palsy: obstetric experience and neonatal outcome, *Dev Med Child Neurol* 35:974-982, 1993.

Yockochi K et al: Motor function of infants with athetoid cerebral palsy, *Dev Med Child Neurol* 35:909-916, 1993.

Cleft Lip and Palate

13

Ginny Curtin

ETIOLOGY

Cleft lip and cleft palate result when there is a failure of the median maxillary, premaxillary, and palatine processes to fuse early in gestational age (Gorlin, Cohen, and Levin, 1990). The lip and alveolar ridge or primary palate is fully formed between 5 and 7 weeks' gestation and the secondary palate between 6 and 12 weeks' gestation (Gorlin, Cohen, and Levin, 1990). The specific etiology is usually unknown, although there is evidence to suggest maternal folic acid deficiency may play a role (Tolarova, 1993). Ingestion of teratogens such as alcohol and some prescriptive antiseizure medications such as phenytoin (Dilantin) as well as folic acid antagonists and retinoic acid have been implicated (Gorlin, Cohen, and Levin, 1990), although not definitively proven (Kelly, 1984). Occasionally a positive family history of clefting is noted.

All infants with cleft lip and cleft palate need to be examined by a dysmorphologist. There may be associated midline abnormalities and the clefting may be a component of a recognized syndrome (Gorlin, Cohen, and Levin, 1990; Parameters for Evaluation and Treatment of Patients with Cleft Lip and Palate or Other Craniofacial Anomalies, 1993). Isolated cleft palate, meaning without cleft lip, is more commonly accompanied by other findings than cleft lip and palate together (Gorlin, Cohen, and Levin, 1990). For example, cleft palate with micrognathia (small mandible) and glossoptosis (enlarged tongue) is known as Pierre Robin sequence and has important management implications. In this situation, researchers postulated that in fetal development the micrognathia is the primary problem and the cleft palate is a result of the tongue being placed superiorly, obstructing the movement of the maxillary shelves into the midline (Gorlin, Cohen, and Levin, 1990).

INCIDENCE

The generally accepted incidence rate of clefting is 1/700 births. Some ethnic differences exist with American Indians having an incidence of 3.6/1000 live births followed in descending order by Japanese, Chinese, Caucasian, Hispanic, and African Americans with the lowest reported incidence of 0.3/1000. Incidence rates are based on varied reporting mechanisms and problems occur with mixing together studies of live births, stillbirths, and spontaneous abortions. No registry or national database exists documenting clefting birth defects. Clefting may or may not be recorded when it is a component of a known syndrome. Submucous cleft palate is frequently undetected until the preschool years when the speech is unintelligible secondary to velopharyngeal insufficiency (Gorlin, Cohen, and Levin, 1990).

CLINICAL MANIFESTATIONS AT TIME OF DIAGNOSIS

Cleft lip is an obvious birth defect noted in the delivery room. It is described as unilateral or bilateral and incomplete or complete depending on whether the clefting extends into the nasal cavity (see Fig. 13-1). A microform cleft lip is characterized by very minor notching or the appearance of a well-healed surgical scar or "seam"; however, cleft lip is usually only described by a craniofacial team or plastic and reconstructive surgeon.

Cleft palate may involve the primary palate (lip and alveolus anterior to the incisive foramen) and the secondary palate (hard and soft palate) (see Fig. 13-2). A submucous cleft palate is characterized by a notch at the posterior spine of the hard palate and translucence at the midline. There is no standard classification system to describe cleft palate. Clinicians generally draw a diagram or use physical descriptors to define tissue deficiencies (see Fig. 13-3).

Infants with isolated cleft palate should be examined carefully for other anomalies, and as previously mentioned, all infants with clefting need a physical examination by a dysmorphologist (Hofstee, Kors, and Hennekam, 1993). Not all clefts of the palate are noted by the staff in the delivery room. Infants who are unable to breast feed successfully, who are unable to "latch on" or exhibit difficulties with bottle feedings such as prolonged (>30 to 45 minutes) feeding times should be reexamined carefully for the presence of clefting. Even

a small cleft of the soft palate usually produces ineffective sucking as a result of the infant's inability to create a seal to draw the milk out of the nipple (Curtin, 1990). Infants with cleft palate will present shortly after birth with feeding problems. The mother may report initially that the baby will wish to nurse for 45 minutes yet does not seem satisfied. The mother's breasts may still feel engorged at the end of a feeding and there is never a feeling that the breast is empty of milk. Frequent snacking usually results; however, urine output is inadequate and the baby continues to be fussy. After approximately 4 to 5 days of this feeding behavior, the infant becomes more sleepy, lethargic, and exhibits signs of dehydration including weight loss. For bottle-fed

CLINICAL MANIFESTATIONS AT TIME OF DIAGNOSIS

Cleft lip and palate—physical findings
Cleft palate—difficulty feeding because of infant's inability to create a seal around the nipple
Pierre Robin sequence—signs and symptoms of upper airway obstruction as a result of tongue repositioning in the airway, micrognathia
Submucous cleft palate—nasal sounding speech

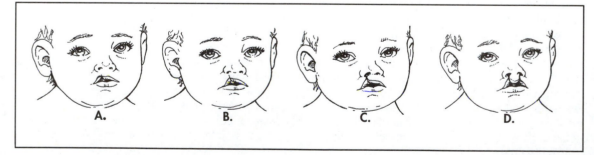

Fig. 13-1.   Varieties of lip clefts. **A, B,** and **C** show unilateral, or one-sided, clefts in the lip and gum ridge. A bilateral, or two-sided, cleft is seen in **D.** (*Redrawn from Moller KT, Starr CD, and Johnson SA: A parent's guide to cleft lip and palate, Minneapolis, 1990, University of Minnesota Press.*)

infants, the scenario is the same and parents report that it may take in excess of 1 hour for the infant to consume 1 oz of formula. It is at this time that a palatal cleft may be noted. Somnolent, dehydrated 4-day-old infants may be hard to examine because they are resistant to opening their mouth. Insertion of a water-moistened gloved finger may be useful in examining palatal integrity (Parameters for Evaluation and Treatment, 1993).

Pierre Robin sequence often has a rather benign presentation with the findings of cleft palate, glossoptosis, and micrognathia. (See box on page 258.) Discovery of airway obstruction may not be present until the infant is 2 weeks of age or until the first upper respiratory tract infection. It is therefore prudent to follow these infants closely during the first months of life and consider a baseline pediatric pulmonary evaluation within the first weeks of life. The infants are able to maintain adequate oxygen and carbon dioxide saturations initially after birth, but can tire over time with increased work of breathing. The tongue is retropositioned in the

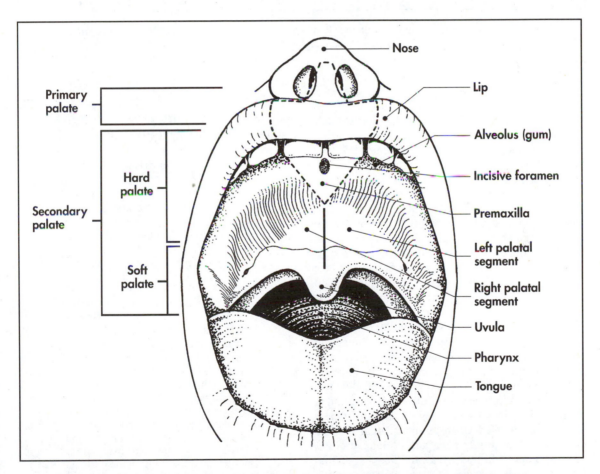

Fig. 13-2. The dashes outline the portion of the lip and the palate that develops separately from the hard and soft palate. *Unilateral clefts* of the lip occur on one side or the other along the dotted line through the lip and possibly the palate. *Bilateral clefts* of the lip occur on both sides of the incisive foramen and include the lip segment called the prolabium (the part of the lip attached to the premaxilla). (Redrawn from Berkowitz S: *The cleft palate story,* Chicago, 1994, Quintessence Publishing Co, Inc.)

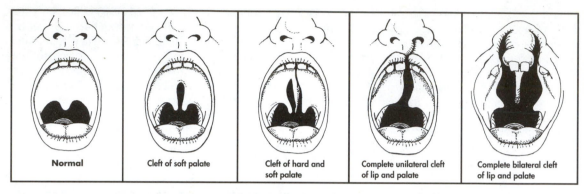

Fig. 13-3.   Types and examples of clefts. (Redrawn from Lynch JI, Brookshire BL, and Fox DR: *A curriculum for infants and toddlers with cleft palate,* Austin, 1993, Pro-Ed, Inc.)

mandible and the infant has great difficulty with expiration of carbon dioxide. This is particularly true when the baby is placed supine and also during sleep when the ventilatory effort is diminished (see Fig. 13-4).

The presentation of a child with a submucous cleft palate is more elusive. The observation of a posterior notch in the nasal spine at the juncture of the hard and soft palates along with a translucence of the soft palate are unusual unless there is clinical symptomatology to warrant closer physical examination of the soft palate. There may or may not be a bifid uvula, which can also be a normal variant, and a short soft palate with muscle separation in the midline.

Children who have nasal-sounding speech for all sounds should have a more detailed examination of their velopharyngeal mechanism. This nasal tone is oftentimes not noted until age 3 to 5 years. When the submucous cleft palate is found, then retrospectively a primary care provider may find a predictable history of nasal regurgitation of fluids, inability to breast feed in infancy, initial feeding problems, slow weight gain, and prolonged bottle feeding times. Additionally, a child may have a history of frequent episodes of serous and acute otitis media as a result of eustachian tube dysfunction associated with the cleft palate (Goldman, Martinez, and Ganzel, 1993; Muntz, 1993). Only submucous cleft palates that are symptomatic require intervention (McWilliams, 1991).

FINDINGS APPARENT IN THE INFANT WITH PIERRE ROBIN SEQUENCE

1. Increasing levels of carbon dioxide when measured serially as a result of carbon dioxide retention from intermittent upper airway obstruction with retropositioning of the tongue
2. Transient oxygen desaturations measured by pulse oximetry accompanied by increased work of breathing with chest wall retractions and gasping sounds as the tongue blocks the upper airway. These episodes usually self-correct within a short time as the infant repositions the tongue forward; however, the frequency may increase as the infant tires.
3. Difficulty during feedings especially when the nipple is removed from the mouth and the infant is still swallowing residual milk. The tongue becomes retropositioned easily without the stimulus of the nipple to move it forward. Gagging sounds may be heard and become worse with supine positioning.
4. Deceleration on the growth curve despite adequate intake of formula or expressed breast milk. This should signal a possible worsening respiratory status.

Sher 1992; Singer and Sidoti, 1992

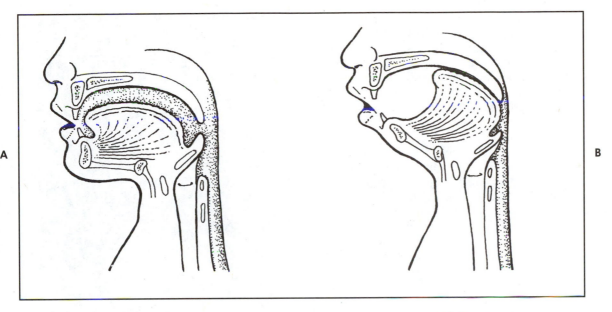

Fig. 13-4.   Pierre Robin sequence. Anatomical features of larynx. **A,** Normal. **B,** Mandibular hypoplasia. Note posterior placement of tongue makes larynx appear more anteriorly situated than normal.

TREATMENT

Goals of Treatment/Team Care

Goals of treatment are (1) to achieve optimum function in growth, speech, hearing, dental, and psychosocial development and (2) to achieve an optimal aesthetic repair. The American Cleft Palate-Craniofacial Association believes that every individual with cleft lip or cleft palate is best served by a multidisciplinary coordinated approach offered by a cleft palate or craniofacial team (see Appendix at the end of this chapter for listings). Parents may either contact the team independently or the contact can be facilitated by their primary health care provider.

Newborns should be referred to a team before discharge from the birthing hospital. Older children can and also should be referred for team consultation because management occurs over the first 18 years of life. The team must include a qualified speech pathologist, an orthodontist, and a plastic surgeon. Other specialties on a cleft palate team often include: audiology, otolaryngology, dental spe-

TREATMENT

- Establishment of adequate feeding
- Airway management for infants with Pierre Robin sequence
- Plastic surgery and oral-maxillofacial reconstruction
- Otolaryngology management
- Speech pathology treatment
- Dental/orthodontic care
- Psychosocial support

cialties (pediatric dentistry, prosthodontics, oral and maxillofacial surgery), genetics/dysmorphology, genetic counseling, nursing, social work, psychology, and pediatrics. Teams that care for children with more complex craniofacial deformities may also include members from anesthesia, neurosurgery, ophthalmology, radiology, and psychiatry.

Initial management of the newborn with a cleft involves diagnosis clarification (rule out associated syndromes), psychosocial support for the grieving family of the child with a congenital birth defect, feeding issues, and airway management for those infants with Pierre Robin sequence.

Establishment of Adequate Feeding

The goal of feeding is to maintain optimum nutrition utilizing a technique that is as normal as possible. Infants with an isolated cleft lip or a cleft lip and alveolus (gum) do not generally experience any feeding difficulties. Infants with cleft palate, on the other hand, require some minor adaptations to establish effective feeding. Establishment of negative intraoral pressure is necessary to draw milk out of a nipple and the infant with a cleft palate is unable to accomplish this aspect of the sucking process. There is generally no problem with the infant's ability to swallow and despite "noisy" feeding sounds there is not an increased incidence of aspiration pneumonia in infants with cleft palate. The feeding technique, therefore, must deliver the milk into the oral cavity so the baby can then swallow it normally.

Although infants with a cleft lip or cleft lip and alveolus may be able to breast feed with minor positioning modifications, infants with cleft palate are not able to breast feed owing to the inability to create a seal and develop adequate suction.

The most common feeding device utilized is the Mead Johnson Cleft Lip and Palate Nurser (see Fig. 13-5), which has a soft plastic compressible bottle and a cross-cut nipple that is slightly longer and narrower than regular nipples. The nipple, however, is not the crucial element of this device as evidenced by some infants' preference for an orthodontic type nipple that is also effective. The orthodontic nipple is useful in large clefts because it can serve to obturate the cleft. Its single hole provides a faster flow of milk and additionally the large nipple can provide some tongue stabilization during the sucking process. The soft plastic bottle allows the parent to control the rate of milk delivered, with rhythmic squeezing of the bottle timed to the infant's cues of swallowing. The nipple should be aimed at the parts of the palate that

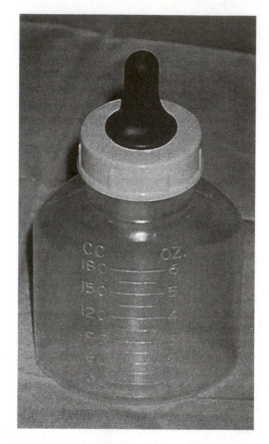

Fig. 13-5.   The Mead Johnson cleft palate nurser.

are intact to take advantage of any nipple compression that is possible between the tongue and the palate.

Alternatives to the Mead Johnson nurser are available, but are more costly and complicated without being more effective in establishing feeding. The Medula Company distributes a Haberman feeder which provides milk flow when the nipple is manually compressed by the feeder or when the infant's gums apply pressure to the plastic nipple. There are varying flow rates and also a one-way valve between nipple and bottle to decrease the chances of air ingestion with milk. The bottle has several plastic pieces and requires more training to utilize correctly than the Mead Johnson system. Additionally, the cost is $22.00 vs. approximately $1.00 per Mead Johnson bottle.

Another feeding device alternative is to cut the hole of a cross-cut nipple larger to ¼″ in length. A 2-oz bottle works well initially with the enlarged cross-cut nipple in order to provide jaw support more easily with a finger during the feeding. The Ross Cleft Palate nipple is intended for postoperative feeding and is not appropriate for newborns because the flow rate is too fast. Likewise, the Lamb's nipple is an outdated device that is bulky and causes gagging.

Whatever feeding method is chosen, there are principles or guidelines found to be most effective in achieving appropriate weight gain. The family needs personalized teaching within the first week of life regarding assessment, feeding methodology, and evaluation of response to feeding by a practitioner experienced in management of infants with clefts (American Cleft Palate-Craniofacial Association, 1993). Ideally this practitioner should be a member of a cleft palate or craniofacial team. Consistency with a chosen technique for a minimum of 24 hours is important to allow both parent and infant to adapt. Continuous switching of nipples is confusing. Feedings should last no longer than 30 to 45 minutes. Ideally the frequency should not be less than every 2½ to 3 hours. These guidelines promote conservation of energy and decreased caloric expenditure during the feeding process.

The infant who has Pierre Robin sequence requires a careful airway assessment, and effective management strategies must be in place before addressing feeding issues. This strategy may vary from placement of a tracheostomy for severe, obstructive, upper airway problems to prone positioning at rest and sitting upright during feedings for mild airway symptomatology (Sher, 1992; Singer and Sidoti, 1992).

The use of feeding appliances or acrylic prosthetic devices varies across the country. These devices assist the infant with a cleft in making a seal over the palatal cleft and creating negative intraoral pressure. Additionally, the appliance is utilized in maintaining or, in the case of an active appliance, manipulating the position of the dental arches and promotes the normal positioning of the tongue in the bottom of the oral cavity. The appliance is custom-made by a dental specialist (pedodontist, prosthodontist, or orthodontist) and is worn 24 hours a day, only to be removed for cleaning. It is larger than the airway and cannot be swallowed. Sometimes a thin coat of denture adhesive is required to maintain placement in the cleft area. This device may be useful in feeding; however, it does not enable an infant to successfully breast feed and bottle feeding can be established without it.

Surgical Reconstructive Management

There is a frequent misconception that cleft lip, palate, or both are merely surgical problems that are corrected in early childhood when the lip and palatal holes are closed. Parents who are very anxious to learn of the timing of surgical repairs, soon learn of the multidisciplinary rehabilitative services that must be coordinated with the surgeries. Specific timing of surgery is varied between different teams and individual primary care providers.

Surgical reconstruction of a cleft lip. In general, surgical repair of cleft lip is done between 3 and 5 months of age. Many surgeons utilize the rule of 10's—10 weeks of age, 10 g/dl hemoglobin level, and 10 pounds in body weight—in planning the repair. Occasionally if the cleft is very wide, especially in a unilateral defect, a surgical cleft lip adhesion is done at about 1 month of age in order to better approximate the lip tissue in preparation for the definitive procedure at the usual age.

The postoperative management for the infant with cleft lip has changed dramatically in recent years. Unrestricted breast or bottle feeding immediately after surgery has been demonstrated to decrease the length of hospital stay, increase oral intake, and improve parental satisfaction without negatively affecting suture line integrity (Boekelheide et al, 1992). Surgery is now performed on an outpatient basis with the infant discharged with elbow restraints. Parents are instructed to clean the suture line with normal saline for 1 to 2 weeks and pain management is usually adequate with oral acetaminophen.

Secondary lip revisions may be necessary before beginning school or during the school-age years. For children with bilateral clefts a nasal repair during the toddler years to lengthen the columella (soft tissue from nasal tip to nostril sill area) is frequently indicated.

Surgical reconstruction of a cleft palate. Surgical repair of a cleft palate is usually done between 9 and 18 months of age. This is timed in order to

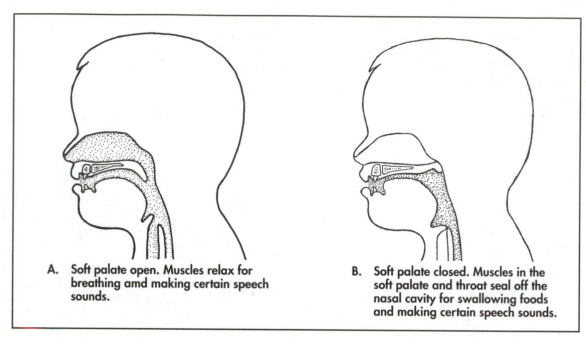

A. Soft palate open. Muscles relax for breathing amd making certain speech sounds.

B. Soft palate closed. Muscles in the soft palate and throat seal off the nasal cavity for swallowing foods and making certain speech sounds.

Fig. 13-6.   Anatomy of the roof of the mouth. The hard and soft palates separate the nasal cavity from the mouth. **A,** Soft palate open. Muscles relax for breathing and making certain speech sounds. **B,** Soft palate closed. Muscles in the soft palate and throat seal off the nasal cavity for swallowing foods and liquids and making certain speech sounds. (*Redrawn from Mead Johnson: Looking forward: a guide for parents of the child with cleft lip and palate.*)

provide a reconstructed palate needed for speech development (see Fig. 13-6). The repair most commonly is done at one time; however, a staged palatal reconstruction of the hard and soft palates is an option. The postoperative management usually dictates a 2-night hospital stay for airway monitoring and adequate enteral hydration. The use of elbow restraints and avoidance of straws and utensils for feeding for 2 weeks are routine. The use of bottles 24 to 48 hours after palatal surgery is variable depending on the center. Cup-feeding is taught for liquids and blenderized solid food. Some centers utilize mist tents for 1 night in order to provide humidification for dried bloody nasal and oral secretions. Good pain management usually requires a parenteral narcotic (morphine sulfate) on the day of surgery followed by an enteral narcotic analgesic (acetaminophen with codeine elixir) on the first postoperative day followed by an enteral analgesic (acetaminophen).

Secondary palatal surgery may be recom-

mended by the speech pathologist in order to address persistent nasal speech after a period of speech therapy. The procedures either create a smaller space in all dimensions (sphincter pharyngoplasty) or create a flap of tissue in the middle (pharyngeal flap) with two side ports to produce velopharyngeal sufficiency or closure during speech. This second surgery is most commonly done on children of preschool age in order to achieve clear speech before school entry (Witt and D'Antonio, 1993).

Repair of the bony defect along the gum or alveolar ridge is timed according to dental development and eruption of secondary teeth (Millard, 1980). Roots of the teeth need to be anchored on bone and generally iliac crest cancellous bone is harvested and packed into the alveolar cleft defect. This surgical procedure is usually done at 7 to 9 years of age. Dietary restrictions and the use of blenderized food for 2 weeks by cup are indicated.

Final nasal reconstruction surgical repair (rhinoplasty) is done when full growth has been attained. This is following menstruation in females and the growth spurt in males.

Some teens also require midface oral and maxillofacial surgery to address facial imbalances as a result of growth disturbance from the clefting that cannot be completely corrected by orthodontics.

Otolaryngology Treatment

Otolaryngology management involves monitoring persistent serous otitis media and aggressive management with placement of ventilation tubes in the tympanic membranes (Muntz, 1993). Ventilation tubes should be considered if there is fluid present in the middle ear space at the time of any other surgical procedures (i.e., cleft lip or palate repair). Because of the high incidence of middle ear problems, some centers favor placement of ventilation tubes at the time of surgical palate repair for all children.

Following placement of the tubes, parents are advised to utilize silicone ear plugs that work well in the pediatric population and are available in local pharmacies. Children with palate repair should use plugs while bathing and swimming to prevent water from entering the middle ear cleft.

A small percentage of children have chronic eustachian tube dysfunction after 5 years of age and may require multiple replacements of ventilating tubes to maintain normal hearing through the school-age years. The indication for tubes may be recurrent or persistent serous otitis media, or severe retraction of the tympanic membrane in which there is little air present in the middle ear space, resulting in an increased risk for cholesteatoma. The tympanic membranes may be very scarred and a persistent perforation of the tympanic membrane may be present following extrusion of the ventilating tube. This membrane does not need to be patched surgically if the perforation is functioning like a patent ventilating tube. Eventually when the child is a teenager it may be patched if the eustachian tube functioning improves with time (Muntz, 1993).

Dental/Orthodontic Treatment

A child with an isolated cleft palate requires regular pediatric dental care and orthodontic services. The palatal growth forward and laterally may be restricted especially if the cleft extends into the hard bony palate. The surgical palate procedure in infancy creates scarring along areas that normally experience significant growth during childhood. As a result, a palatal expansion appliance may be necessary in order to achieve adequate dental occlusion.

Children with Pierre Robin sequence who have micrognathia in infancy usually experience catch-up mandibular growth during the first year of life. Sometimes, however, children may need orthodontic management to deal with dental crowding as a result of the small mandible.

Children with clefts of the alveolar ridge, bilateral or unilateral, require considerable orthodontic management. Until the eruption of secondary dentition, these children should ideally be followed by a pediatric dentist.

RECENT AND ANTICIPATED ADVANCES IN DIAGNOSIS AND MANAGEMENT

There has been a recent focus on fetal surgery for cleft lip and palate repair (Oberg, Kirsch, and Hardesty, 1993). Proposed advantages of such surgical intervention include: decreased scar formation found in fetal wound healing; decreased potential costs as a result of less need for extensive postoperative care, orthodontia and speech therapy; and minimized psychologic trauma associated with facial deformity. This type of surgical repair has been done in the laboratory in fetal mice, rabbits, sheep, and monkeys.

Obvious limitations to this treatment modality include accurate prenatal diagnosis through ultrasound, which would capture some infants with cleft lip but would not include those with isolated cleft palate. The potential risks to the mother and the early fetus are considerable and at this point in time probably do not justify the intervention, because clefting is not considered a life-threatening problem. Nonetheless, the current research will be beneficial for an increased understanding of craniofacial development and early effects of management upon wound healing.

Potential advances in the management of children with cleft lip and palate include genetic testing to identify the genes that are transformed when an infant has a clefting disorder (Oberg, Kirsch, and

Hardesty, 1993). Further research regarding the effects of maternal vitamin deficiencies and environmental factors on gene transformation may provide clues into preventive measures that may be utilized during pregnancy (Tolarova, 1993).

ASSOCIATED PROBLEMS

Audiology/Otolaryngology

Infants and children with an isolated cleft lip or cleft lip and alveolus generally do not have abnormal audiologic findings at a rate above the general population. Infants and children with cleft palate, however, have significant audiologic and otolaryngology concerns. Audiologic testing is appropriate in children with cleft palate to monitor the degree of conductive hearing loss in order to guide the clinician in providing appropriate interventions and documenting the effectiveness of management. Newborns can be tested by audiologic screening known as algorithm auditory brain stem response screening, or ALGO (Amer CP-Cranf Assoc, 1993). If an infant does not pass the ALGO screening, the primary care provider may find it appropriate to proceed with more complex testing known as auditory brain stem response testing (ABR), which monitors the sensorineural auditory system.

Children who are 6 to 9 months of age and older may be tested by behavioral audiologic testing. This type of testing requires some degree of cooperation and is given when an infant can sit and respond to sounds. Ideally these findings should correlate with the physical examination by the otolaryngologist and a combined approach to management can then be devised.

The dynamic functioning of the eustachian tube, which serves as the communication link between the middle ear space and the back of the throat, is controlled by the palatal musculature. The child with cleft palate has abnormal placement and underdevelopment of palatal musculature. As a result, the functioning of the eustachian tube is suboptimal. When a child develops an upper respiratory tract infection, fluid normally accumulates in the middle ear space. Usually this fluid drains into the oral cavity when the infection and swelling of the eustachian tube subside. In the child with cleft

ASSOCIATED PROBLEMS

- Feeding difficulty
- Audiology/otolaryngology problems
- Speech pathology
- Dental/orthodontic problems
- Psychosocial adjustment to a physical deformity

palate, however, the eustachian tube may only rarely open and as a result the fluid remains behind the tympanic membrane on a chronic basis (Goldman, Martinez, and Ganzel, 1993). Infants and children with cleft palate have an 80% incidence of developing chronic serous otitis media associated with eustachian tube dysfunction.

Monitoring children with ear tubes in place is usually done every 6 months and more frequently as necessary for blocked, infected, or prematurely extruded tubes. It is especially important to monitor for the presence of middle ear fluid and resultant conductive hearing loss in the child who is rapidly acquiring speech and language skills and is already challenged by the cleft palate, which makes this acquisition more difficult.

Many parents query the primary care provider as to why the eustachian tube dysfunction continues after the surgical repair of the cleft palate. Even though palatal tissue is restored closer to normal, the dynamic mechanisms that control the palatal musculature influence on eustachian tube function are not normalized.

Speech Pathology

Children with isolated cleft lip usually do not have significant speech articulation problems. These children may only require short-term therapy that focuses on anterior sounds and bilabial sounds found in *m* and *b* and *p,* which require competent lip closure. Children with clefts of the alveolus have additional challenges with anterior sounds and also in managing air leakage from the front of the gums into the anterior nasal cavity before the cleft is surgically repaired with eruption of secondary dentition (Peterson-Falzone, 1986).

Children with clefts of the palate have problems with speech articulation (Witt and D'Antonio, 1993). Even before surgical repair of the palate at 9 to 18 months of age, children develop compensatory articulation errors to attempt to correct the nasal air escape caused by a cleft palate. The speech pathologist should meet with the family before the emergence of expressive speech and language development. Parents benefit from knowing how normal communication develops in their child. All families do not appreciate the fact that babies need to receive speech input directed at them and need to reciprocate in a turn-taking fashion with the use of body language and prespeech babbling behavior. Anticipatory guidance for this population is standard practice.

Following surgical closure of the cleft palate, parents can benefit from another visit with the speech pathologist who can provide information regarding speech sounds and communication styles such as turn-taking and expectations of oral communication. Formal speech therapy can begin with children who are as young as 2 years old. Without this intervention, it is common to see a toddler who has developed a complex jargoning system of partially articulated words and gestures to which the people in the child's environment respond. The child becomes frustrated in his or her inability to expand in expressive speech and language skills and may develop behavioral responses such as temper tantrums in order to communicate. Additionally, the child is unable to communicate even simple desires to strangers because the stranger is unfamiliar with the gestural system.

Ongoing monitoring and parental guidance on a 6-month basis with the speech pathologist is appropriate during the toddler and preschool years. At some point during this time, the speech pathologist usually determines that the child could benefit from regular speech therapy services. For children under 3 years of age, therapy may be provided by an infant development program that has specific speech therapy services or a speech pathologist that is community or hospital based. After 3 years of age, the child usually receives speech therapy that is provided by the local school district. An individual-

ized education plan (IEP) is necessary for this isolated service because it is a component of special education services. The speech pathologist at the craniofacial or cleft palate center should continue to monitor progress every 6 to 12 months and provide feedback and suggestions to the speech pathologist providing the therapy.

The desired outcome following cleft palate surgery and speech therapy is clear articulation by 4 years of age. Although many variables have been studied, including type of cleft, age of surgical repair, type of surgical technique utilized, initiation time and length of speech therapy services, no one factor has been determined to provide the desired outcome (Tatum and Senders, 1993; Witt and D'Antonio, 1993). Rather it is a combination of factors that produce the most optimal outcome.

Children who do not have clear speech development by 4 years of age may require secondary surgical palatal management ideally before school entry. This surgery is particularly helpful if the articulation of sounds is good but there is persistent nasal air emission as a result of a deficiency of palatal tissue or a palate that has inadequate motion. If secondary surgical or prosthetic management is done, follow-up speech therapy is usually needed to obtain maximum benefit from the intervention. It is not unusual for a school-age child to receive speech therapy during school, especially since they receive active orthodontic services which may further challenge speech articulation.

Dental/Orthodontic

Some children with a cleft alveolus have missing teeth or extra supernumerary teeth. Care should be taken not to remove these teeth because they maintain alveolar bone mass in a dental arch that is deficient in bone at the area of the cleft. Children often develop a crossbite in primary dentition because of the bony deficiency and alveolar and palatal collapse of the arches as a result of the cleft and the growth disturbance of the hard palate from surgical closure. The crossbite does not always need to be corrected in primary dentition; however, some pediatric dentists do offer early interceptive orthodontic treatment.

At 5 to 7 years of age, it is appropriate for the child with an alveolar cleft to have an orthodontic consultation, baseline records (photographs, dental study models, radiographs, examination), and a treatment plan. Initial management focuses on expansion of the maxillary arch with a removable or fixed active appliance in preparation for surgical grafting with iliac crest donor bone. The orthodontist usually indicates the appropriate time to perform the grafting surgery. Following the grafting procedure, the teeth adjacent to the cleft are mobilized and repositioned into the "new" alveolar bone mass.

Orthodontic management is usually done in phases and may have periods of rest when the teeth are held in place by a passive retention type of appliance. The timing and phase of intervention is dependent on maxillary and mandibular growth that occurs into the teen years. It is not uncommon for orthodontic management to span a period of 10 years. Compliance with the recommended regimen is crucial because active movement of teeth depends on keeping frequent appointments, maintaining appliances, and practicing good oral hygiene (Figueroa, Polley, and Cohen, 1993). Maintaining regular pediatric dental care services during the orthodontic treatment is also important.

Psychosocial Adjustment to a Physical Deformity

Parents of the infant with a cleft are the first clients for the long-term psychosocial management of the child. According to observations, families who positively accommodate to their child's chronic condition have children who appear to cope at a higher level than parents who exhibit negative adaptative behaviors. The degree of clefting is not predictive of the level of psychosocial functioning (Moller, Starr, and Johnson, 1990).

The birth of an infant with a facial deformity is a constant, daily reminder of the physical condition. Any bonding and attachment activities are related to the infant's face and it takes some time to adjust and positively regard an abnormal face (Moller, Starr, and Johnson, 1990). Most families learn over time to appreciate their infant's own personality and special way of expressing a "wide smile." Some families have a secondary grief reaction once the child's lip is repaired and express that they "miss the cleft" (Curtin, 1990). A second adjustment to the "new" face is necessary and may take 1 to 2 weeks after surgery. Parents do not regret deciding to have the lip repair done, but rather,

it is a normal adjustment. Parents are reassured when the team providers give them anticipatory guidance about their feelings. All parents initially experience grief reactions related to the loss of a perfect infant. These feelings can resurface at times of stress such as hospitalization, initiation of speech, dental eruption, and school entry.

Children in the preschool years gain an increased understanding of their clefting birth defect as they develop a sense of self-awareness and experience teasing from peers. Simple explanations about the cleft can be reviewed and strategies for deflecting the teasing can be suggested. School-age children may need support and strategies to cope with teasing and to promote a positive self-image. Teenagers are able to articulate their wishes and priorities in treatment planning and should participate in the decision-making process. Teenagers also have increased self-image concerns and may benefit from counseling services.

PROGNOSIS

The long-term prognosis for children with cleft lip and palate is excellent. The goals of team management are to achieve good speech articulation, functional dental occlusion, normal hearing acuity, an acceptable appearance, and a positive self-regard. Children with Pierre Robin sequence additionally have a goal of achieving adequate airway function. They are generally cared for in tertiary medical centers with cleft-craniofacial teams that work with pediatric pulmonary or pediatric otolaryngology specialists to achieve adequate airway function.

Primary Care Management
HEALTH CARE MAINTENANCE
Growth and Development

Growth and development in general is not known to be negatively affected in children with a clefting disorder. In the past, infant feeding devices used to provide nutrition for the neonate with a cleft palate were suboptimal. With the evolution of the squeeze bottle and also with the proliferation of team care and trained professionals to provide teaching, this aspect of management has been simplified. Additionally, current postoperative feeding routines are simpler and hospital stays are shorter, all contributing to a more normalized nutritional status.

Infants with cleft lip and palate are expected to grow along the same parameters as infants without clefting. Once the feeding methodology has been taught by a member of the cleft-craniofacial team, the primary care provider, will monitor the child's growth.

All children with craniofacial abnormalities should be referred to a pediatric endocrinologist if short stature (other than constitutional) is identified. A midline pituitary deficiency can result in depressed growth (Rudman et al, 1978). Children who have a known syndrome may have growth and developmental problems related to the syndrome. The primary care provider would need to refer to literature found in medical genetics-dysmorphology texts to determine the usual findings and prognoses for the specific disorder identified.

Diet

Mothers of infants with cleft palate can provide expressed breast milk for their children. Hospital-grade electric pumps work the best and can be rented from a lactation consultant who is trained to provide education and support regarding long-term pumping and storage of breast milk. Most mothers find it useful to use a double pumping system attachment to decrease the amount of time spent pumping milk. Mothers with a low income may be able to procure an electric pump from their local women, infants, and children (WIC) agency.

Mothers who are pumping breast milk 4 to 6 times a day in addition to then bottle-feeding the milk 6 to 8 times per day need support and assistance from others. It is important to balance the needs of the mother and the family with the needs of the infant with a cleft in such a way that the mother feels encouraged to continue, but also feels support if she decides to discontinue pumping. Mothers who are able to persevere with providing their infant expressed breast milk will be encouraged by a study that linked breast milk intake to a decreased incidence of otitis media specifically in infants with clefts (Paradise, Elster, and Tan, 1994).

Upright positioning of the infant during feeding will decrease the amount of nasal regurgitation. Parents should be reassured that a small amount of nasal regurgitation is expected and should be handled by simply wiping the nose of the infant with a cloth rather than interpreted as a signal of a problem. Cleansing of the nose and mouth with water or a cotton-tipped applicator or bulb syringe is not necessary because the mouth is self-cleaning and the nasal secretions and milk will drain by gravity. The parent may need to be reassured about the anatomy of the cleft palate. The oral and nasal cavity are combined and the parent may have an unspoken fear that the feeding will hurt the infant or that the nasal turbinates and the vomer represent brain tissue that can be injured with feeding.

The primary care provider can provide anticipatory guidance regarding discouraging the use of bottles in bed especially when filled with formula, milk, or juice. The supine position favors accumulation of the fluid into the middle ear space when the eustachian tube is open, in a population that is already at risk for recurrent otitis media.

Occasionally infants with clefting do not grow along the expected norms. There may be extenuating psychosocial factors that challenge the parent/caretaker in feeding the infant. Initially an observation and review of methodology of feeding should be pursued along with a 24- to 72-hour diet record. Serial weight checks can provide both parental and health care provider reassurance. For the infant with Pierre Robin sequence, deceleration on the growth curve should prompt a careful reassessment of ventilatory status and the probable finding of some degree of upper airway obstruction.

For the infant who is 4 to 6 months old, introduction of solid foods and progression to table foods is sequenced the same as for noncleft infants. There may be some nasal regurgitation as the infant learns this new skill. Varying textures can sometimes alleviate this issue. Some parents require extra encouragement to proceed with the introduction of solid foods by spoon. Delayed initiation of this normal developmental skill can create negative feeding behaviors and may interfere with normal oral motor development which is necessary in producing prespeech sounds. Utilization of bottle type infant feeders or enlarging nipple holes to accommodate solid foods also delay normal development. Messy spoon feedings are expected and nasal reflux of solids should be handled calmly similar to the milk intake. Infants and children have only minor dietary restrictions. Some tricky foods for the child with an unrepaired cleft palate include peanut butter, soft cheese, and sweets—all gummy in texture. Avoiding foods that are a "choking risk" such as peanuts, popcorn, and pellet candy is advised because these foods can get lodged in the nasal cavity. Parents are very concerned with future speech development in their infant with a cleft palate and therefore may respond to solid food progression as an aid toward a speech goal.

Safety

In addition to routine anticipatory guidance on safety issues, the child may have some restrictions during the first 2 to 4 weeks following reconstructive surgical procedures. Elbow restraints are generally used for 1 to 2 weeks after reconstructive surgery in the infant and toddler. Older preschool children may need these restraints, referred to as "reminders," especially at naptime and bedtime.

Dietary restrictions that are recommended postoperatively such as avoidance of utensils, straws, and textured foods are generally only necessary for about 2 weeks after surgery to allow for nontraumatic healing of the oral tissues. Some families may need to actually be encouraged and reassured to advance to soft foods 2 weeks after the surgery and an unrestricted diet 1 month after the surgery.

Youngsters need to avoid contact sports for 2 to 4 weeks following alveolar bone grafting procedures, nasal reconstruction, and midface jaw procedures to prevent disruption of the surgery before bone healing.

Infants with Pierre Robin sequence who require prone positioning for adequate ventilation may need a car safety bed rather than a car seat when traveling in an automobile. These are available commercially (see the Appendix at the end of this chapter).

Immunizations

Infants and children with cleft lip and palate should receive all routine immunizations at the ages recommended by the American Academy of Pediatrics. A planned surgical procedure is not a rationale for deferring routine immunizations; rather the child is better protected within the hospital setting when immunization status is current.

Administration of immunizations within 24 hours of a planned surgical procedure is not advisable for DPT because a low-grade fever following vaccine administration may preclude surgery. Administration of the MMR or varicella vaccine within a week before scheduled surgery is not recommended for similar reasons.

Screening

Vision. Routine vision screening is recommended. Children with isolated cleft palate should have a pediatric ophthalmology dilated examination at approximately 1 year of age and again before school entry at age 4 or 5 years to screen for Stickler syndrome, which is associated with myopia sometimes leading to retinal detachment.

Hearing. A high index of suspicion and prompt referral to an audiologist and otolaryngologist should be made if audiologic screening in the school-age years is not passed. Detailed audiologic testing (as previously described) is done by the specialty center in the early years of life.

Dental. Routine screening is recommended for the child with an isolated cleft lip. Dental and orthodontic care is indicated for children with clefts of the alveolar ridge or the secondary palate. A pediatric dental provider is strongly advised even if the family needs to travel some distance to obtain the service. The primary care provider should promote good oral hygiene practices, including initiation of tooth brushing or cleansing with a rough face cloth with eruption of the first tooth. Parents must be counseled on the hazards of baby-bottle tooth decay.

Dental eruption may be slightly delayed in a child with a cleft. Many families believe that once their child commences orthodontic care they no longer need to see the regular pediatric dentist. The dental cleanings and topical fluoride treatment are actually even more important during active orthodontic management.

Blood pressure. Routine screening is recommended.

Hematocrit. Routine screening is recommended.

Urinalysis. Routine screening is recommended.

Tuberculosis. Routine screening is recommended.

COMMON ILLNESS MANAGEMENT

Differential Diagnosis

Fever. The parents of a child with a cleft are alerted to the increased incidence of middle ear disease. The presence of a fever, increased irritability, tugging at the ears, and asking family members to repeat verbalizations should all signal the need to have the ears examined for acute or serous otitis media. Children with cleft palate are defined as an outlying population to the current AAP recommendations regarding middle ear disease favoring ongoing monitoring of serous otitis media rather than aggressive surgical management (Otitis Media Guideline Panel, 1994). Primary care providers are advised to refer these children to the otolaryngologist for a microscopic office examination if the child has persistent (i.e., longer than 1 to 2 months) middle ear fluid or recurrent (i.e., every 1 to 2 months) acute otitis media. Management of acute otitis media is with the usual oral antibiotics and possibly prophylactic antibiotics. If the fluid remains throughout the prophylaxis period of about 2 months or longer, or if there are breakthrough infections, more aggressive surgical management is usually indicated.

Drug Interactions

Medications are not required as part of the normal treatment regimen.

DEVELOPMENTAL ISSUES

Sleep Patterns

Infants and children with a unilateral cleft lip usually have a deviated nasal septum that causes noisy breathing during upper respiratory tract infections but does not negatively effect air exchange.

Children who have secondary palatal surgery to address nasal speech have a smaller upper airway space in the velopharyngeal area. These children are particularly at risk for sleep state upper airway obstruction during the first 6 weeks following surgery when local edema is present. Symptoms may include chest wall retractions with or without partial ventilation, irregular snoring with pauses greater than 15 to 20 seconds, diaphoresis, nighttime waking especially after an apneic episode, daytime somnolence, and enuresis (Sirois et al, 1994). The child's symptomatology should be reported to the specialty center physician, which may be a pediatric pulmonologist or otolaryngologist. The severity of the symptoms will be assessed and medical management such as steroid administration or inpatient observation may be warranted. Rarely does the surgical procedure need to be revised since the symptomatology is usually temporary and the desired outcome is to provide a decreased nasal airflow during speech without negatively affecting the ventilatory capabilities.

The infant with Pierre Robin sequence may have a disrupted sleep experience as a result of sleep state obstructive apnea. Careful history taking, evaluation, and management by the pediatric pulmonologist or otolaryngologist is appropriate.

Sleep patterns are usually disrupted following hospitalizations. Families should be told of this probable change in sleeping pattern both at the preoperative and postoperative visits. A required postoperative change in favored sleeping position from stomach to back to prevent rubbing of the incision site may also temporarily affect sleep.

Toileting

There is no physiologic effect on toileting. The psychologic impact of stressful surgeries and hospitalization experiences can delay acquisition of toileting skills temporarily or result in regression of recently acquired skills.

Discipline

Parents of children with a congenital birth defect often feel guilty that they "caused" the problem in some way. This can then translate into an altered perception of the child as being special and requiring extra attention to overcompensate for the guilt feelings. Additionally, parents are very saddened to learn of the long-term management, especially the initial surgeries that their child will require. Many parents report that they wish the treatment could be done on them rather than on the child. Because the initial surgeries are done in infancy, the psychologic burden is thrust on the parents.

Parents need to be encouraged to return to the infant's or child's normal routine following hospitalizations. A routine is reassuring for the child and promotes normalcy and a quicker return to normal behavior. Parents who focus exclusively on the needs of the infant or child who is sick and cater to every whim soon find that this is not functional or pleasant for the child or the family. Symptoms of this phenomenon include: no structured feeding or meal routine, irregular nap times, nighttime waking, nighttime feedings, co-sleeping in the parental bed (only if this is not the family's usual practice), excessive fussiness, irritability, or clinginess, loss of previously achieved developmental milestones, and inability to get along with others (Elmendorf, D'Antonio, and Hardesty, 1993). These are all normal reactions following a stressful experience such as a hospitalization; however, they usually do not persist beyond 2 to 6 weeks after a 24- to 48-hour hospital stay. Parents can benefit from anticipatory guidance and encouragement to promote normalcy which initially may appear harsh and unsympathetic. When it is presented as comforting for the child, however, most parents embrace the concept.

Issues regarding discipline arise again when the child with a cleft lip or palate enters school, especially if the child appears very different from his peers and is teased. Overprotectiveness and lack of appropriate limits actually can exacerbate these problems. The child and family can often benefit from short-term counseling regarding self-image concerns and development of skills to cope with teasing from others.

Child Care

Child care in a group day care setting can be stressful for the parent of a child who is at risk for frequent ear infections. For this reason, some parents elect to choose a setting with a more limited number of children especially during the winter months.

Once a child is old enough to attend a Head Start program or a structured preschool, it can be helpful as an adjunct to speech therapy because the child's peers will promote expressive language development. Peers will usually not understand the elaborate gesturing system and monosyllabic vocalizations that substitute for expressive language and may encourage the child to expand his or her repertoire by modeling.

Schooling

Children with cleft palate will be eligible for special education services, namely speech therapy, un-

der Public Law 94-142 and 99-457. Parents should be counseled to request in writing a speech evaluation focused on articulation when the child is 2 years 9 months of age. It is helpful if the parents provide medical information and any prior speech evaluations.

Peer teasing can occur as the child progresses through school. Some parents and children utilize the "class presentation" approach about clefting and teachers can incorporate this into their lesson plans about "differences" between people. Rarely a child reports teasing and ridicule so severe that school phobia and frequent absences become an issue. It is important to query the parents about these issues at primary care visits and offer supportive services and coordinated efforts between the primary care providers and the school system.

Children with cleft lip and palate do not have a predisposition to academic difficulties. Children who have an isolated cleft palate that is part of a syndrome may have a lower intellectual potential that is specifically associated with the syndrome (Strauss and Broder, 1993). These children should have an evaluation with the special education professionals as appropriate.

Sexuality

No special sexual problems are associated with cleft lip and palate. The obvious concerns regarding self-image may be exaggerated during adolescence.

When discussing reproductive issues, recurrence risks for clefting must be addressed. The rates quoted are between 2% and 7% (Gorlin, Cohen, and Levin, 1990; Hofstee, Kors, and Hennekam, 1993) depending on previous family history and the presence of a concurrent syndrome. Clefting is more common in males so females theoretically have a higher genetic component and therefore a slightly higher recurrence risk. A bilateral cleft lip is rare and more severe than a unilateral and likewise has a slightly higher recurrence risk. As a result, a male with a unilateral cleft lip would be at the low end (2%) and a female with a bilateral cleft lip would be at the high end (7%). A complete family history and physical examination of the affected individual by a geneticist and genetic counselor would be necessary to provide the most accurate information.

Women with increased risk for having a child with a cleft are eligible for a detailed ultrasound that has a better resolution of the facial features than a traditional ultrasound. Women of childbearing age are counseled to take a multivitamin that contains folic acid on a daily basis in the hope of preventing a clefting condition (Tolarova, 1993).

Transition into Adulthood

State funding for care of children with cleft lips and palates is available to financially eligible children up to age 21. Most individuals are able to complete the orthodontic and oral-maxillofacial surgical procedures by this age. Problems are encountered if there were treatment lapses or delays during crucial stages of dental development or orthodontic management that necessitated restarting the treatment. Additionally, orthodontic interventions are effective during active treatment and then the position of the teeth and the occlusion are often maintained with removable appliances; for example, a retainer worn at night. Adolescents and their families often do not appreciate the necessity for these appliances and then relapse occurs. If this happens before the insurance is terminated, some active management can be reinitiated. Otherwise the young adult will usually need to pay for these services as out-of-pocket expenses. Young adults who wish to have follow-up lip or nasal surgery have a very difficult experience in gaining third-party payment for what appears to be cosmetic procedures even if they relate to a congenital birth defect.

SPECIAL FAMILY CONCERNS AND RESOURCES

Parents of children with a cleft lip worry about their child's physical attractiveness to others, especially strangers. Parents are very sensitive to the reactions and comments of professionals and their family and look at others' facial and emotional reactions when viewing their baby with a facial deformity. Fears regarding feeding, fear of hurting the face and the mouth, and concern that the cleft extends into the brain are common. Demonstration of feeding techniques and promoting normal infant care routines provide opportunities for learning and alloying anxieties.

It is beneficial to recommend that parents take photographs of their infant with a facial cleft and to discuss with the parents the usefulness of retaining

a photograph that they will have available for their older child to view. If the parents are resistant, stating that they prefer to forget this time of sadness and wish to defer picture taking until after a cleft lip repair, it may be prudent for a professional working with the family to take a photograph and maintain it in the infant's chart.

Oral, auditory, and dental concerns may be verbalized as the family becomes more informed. These concerns and consequent stressors recur over time with rehospitalizations, tooth eruption, initial speech, school entry, and adolescent self-image concerns. Orthodontic services are a crucial component of the rehabilitation process and are covered by the local state CCS program if the family is financially eligible. Families who do not meet the financial eligibility often find this care very expensive.

Special cultural issues that affect families who have a child with a cleft lip and palate are mostly concerned with the etiology of the clefting condition. Superstitions exist regarding why clefting occurs that often originate in the family's country of origin. Hispanic and Filipino cultural folklore believe that clefting is related to the lunar cycle. A lunar eclipse or a crescent moon during a woman's pregnancy predisposes her unborn child to clefting. Some Asian cultural folklores relate construction, cutting, a fall, or moving the mother's bed during pregnancy, with birth defects, especially clefting. In Chinese culture the center of a person's face is very important and central to that person's being rather than the heart, which is common in Western culture. This has implications for a cleft lip and palate deformity in its central location.

Most young parents acknowledge that these beliefs are part of cultural folklores and are explanations that their parents and grandparents provided for the untoward events that happened during a pregnancy. Trying to disprove these theories is unnecessary especially since the etiology of clefting is unknown. It is more useful to focus on the common feeling of maternal guilt associated with a birth defect and to work through the grief process over time.

Some families bring with them extreme fears regarding surgery and hospitalization; however, fear usually seems to be experience related (i.e., relative who died after a surgical procedure) rather than related to a specific cultural framework. The concept of health care in general, especially preventive health care such as the routine dental care or anticipatory guidance needed to prevent speech articulation problems, is unfamiliar to some families. Particularly in families who originate from other countries outside the United States that do not have many health care resources, the very idea of seeking non-emergent health care services is unknown.

Resources

American Cleft Palate-Craniofacial Association Cleft Palate Foundation 1218 Grandview Ave Pittsburgh, PA 15211 (412) 481-1376 Fax (412) 481-0847 Internet NCS1 @ VMS.CIS.PITT.EDU CLEFTLINE 1-800-24-CLEFT— Referral to local cleft-craniofacial team—Written pamphlets and fact sheets in English and Spanish—Distribution of document—Parameters for Evaluation and Treatment 3/93.

About Face—USA PO Box 737 Warrington, PA 18976 1-800-225-FACE Internet ABTFACE @ AOL.COM—Newsletter, information, support.

Wide Smiles Newsletter PO Box 5153 Stockton, CA 95205-0153(209) 942-2812 Internet WIDESMILES @ AOL.COM

Mead, Johnson, & Co Nutritional Division Evansville, IN 47721-0001 (812) 429-5000 1-800-BABY123 Cleft lip and palate nursers—Free booklet—Your Cleft Lip and Palate Child: A Basic Guide for Parents. (For breast pump rentals and Haberman feeders)

Medela, Inc

4610 Prime Parkway

Mc Henry, IL 60050-7005

(800) 435-8316

(816) 362-1166

Dream Ride infant car bed/car seat

COSCO Columbus, IN 1-800-468-0174 Car safety bed for infants with Pierre Robin sequence who require prone positioning.

Books for parents

Moller KT, Starr CD, and Johnson SA: *A parent's guide to cleft lip and palate,* Minneapolis, 1990, University of Minnesota Press.

Berkowitz S: *The cleft palate story,* Chicago, 1994, Quintessence Publishing.

SUMMARY OF PRIMARY CARE NEEDS FOR THE CHILD WITH CLEFT LIP AND PALATE

Health care maintenance

Growth and development

Expectations for physical growth and development are the same as those for the noncleft population.

Diet

Use of cleft palate nurser enhances bottle feeding

Cleft palate—provision of expressed breast milk with use of an electric pump.

Introduction of solids by spoon at the same time as noncleft population.

Safety

Elbow restraints following surgical procedures.

Avoidance of utensils, straws, and textured foods approximately 2 weeks after surgical procedures to allow for nontraumatic oral healing.

Avoidance of contact sports for 2 to 4 weeks after surgeries.

Prone positioning for infants with Pierre Robin sequence; may need car safety bed vs. car seat.

Immunizations

All routine immunizations should be given on schedule.

May elect not to administer DPT within 24 hours of a surgical procedure and MMR/varicella 1 week before a surgery.

Screening

Vision:
Routine screening is recommended.

Children with isolated cleft palate or Pierre Robin sequence need a dilated eye examination by a pediatric ophthalmologist at 1 year of age and 4 to 5 years of age to rule out myopia which is found in Stickler syndrome.

Hearing:
Audiology screening for children with cleft lip and alveolus.

Ongoing close monitoring for conductive hearing loss in children with cleft palate.

Dental:
Screening for milk bottle caries.

Routine pediatric dental care for children with cleft lip. In addition to routine pediatric dental care children with cleft alveolus and palate need an orthodontic evaluation by age 5 to 7.

Blood pressure:
Routine screening is recommended.

Hematocrit:
Routine screening is recommended.

Urinalysis:
Routine screening is recommended.

Tuberculosis:
Routine screening is recommended.

Common illness management

Differential diagnosis

Fever
Rule out acute otitis media.

Developmental issues

Sleep patterns
Unilateral cleft lip and palate—deviated septum, noisy breathing especially with URI.

Increased risk of sleep state obstructive apnea following secondary palatal surgical procedures.

Disruption of sleep patterns following surgical procedures and hospitalization.

Signs of sleep state obstructive apnea requiring careful pulmonary evaluation and management in infants with Pierre Robin sequence.

Toileting
Temporary regression following surgical procedure and hospitalization.

Discipline
Expectations are normal, with allowances during hospitalizations and 1 to 2 weeks after surgery.

Overprotectiveness or lack of limit setting may result if family pities child.

Child care
May need to be in smaller group setting during winter months because of increased risk of otitis media.

Speech therapy sessions need to be coordinated with child care arrangements.

Continued.

SUMMARY OF PRIMARY CARE NEEDS FOR THE CHILD WITH CLEFT LIP AND PALATE—cont'd

Schooling

Speech therapy to begin at age 3 for children with cleft palate, requires an individualized education plan (IEP).

Peer teasing may negatively impact performance. Teasing may be because of lip, nose, and dentition appearance or speech articulation problems.

Sexuality

Genetic counseling recommended to discuss recurrence risks.

Women of childbearing age recommended to take folic acid to hopefully prevent clefting.

During pregnancy a detailed ultrasound is available to ascertain whether the fetus has a cleft lip.

Transition into adulthood

Treatment plan should be completed by age 21.

There is difficulty in procuring third-party payment for any orthodontic, oral-maxillofacial, or plastic surgical services in adulthood.

Special family concerns and resources

There is heightened awareness of physical appearance

Pre-surgical photographs are important.

Speech, audiology, and dental issues are challenging for families.

Cultural superstitions are common regarding the etiology of clefting.

Multiple surgical procedures during childhood is stressful for families.

REFERENCES

American Cleft Palate-Craniofacial Association. Parameters for evaluation and treatment of patients with cleft lip and palate or other craniofacial anomalies, *Cleft Palate-Cranf J* 30:(Suppl 1), 1993.

Boekelheide A et al: Comparison of postsurgical feeding techniques following cleft lip repair on suture line integrity, volume of oral fluid intake and length of hospital stay: a multicenter study. Presented at the *American Cleft Palate-Craniofacial Association Annual Meeting,* Portland, OR, 1992.

Curtin G: The infant with cleft lip or palate: more than a surgical problem, *J Perinat Neonatal Nurs* 3:80-89, 1990.

Elmendorf EN, D'Antonio LL, Hardesty RA: Assessment of the patient with cleft lip and palate—a developmental approach, *Clinics in Plastic Surgery* 20:607-621, 1993.

Figueroa AA, Polley JW, and Cohen M: Orthodontic management of the cleft lip and palate patient, *Clinics in Plastic Surgery* 20:733-753, 1993.

Goldman JL, Martinez SA, and Ganzel TM: Eustachian tube dysfunction and its sequelae in patients with cleft palate, *Southern Medical Journal* 86:1236-1237, 1993.

Gorlin RY, Cohen MM, and Levin LS: Orofacial clefting syndromes: general aspects. In Gorlin RY, Cohen MM, and Levin LS (editors): *Syndromes of the head and neck,* ed 3, New York, 1990, Oxford University Press, pp 693-714.

Hofstee Y, Kors N, Hennekam, RCM: Genetic survey of a group of children with clefting: implications for genetic counseling, *Cleft Palate-Cranf J* 30:447-451, 1993.

Kelly TE: Teratogenicity of anticonvulsant drugs. 1: Review of the literature, *Am J Med Genet* 19:413-434, 1984.

McWilliams BJ: Submucous clefts of the palate: how likely are they to be symptomatic?, *Cleft Palate-Cranf J* 28:247-249, 1991.

Millard DR: *Cleft craft: the evolution of its surgery,* vol 1: The unilateral deformity; vol 2: Bilateral and rare deformities; vol 3: Alveolar and palatal deformities, Boston, 1980, Little, Brown, & Co.

Millard DR: Introduction, clefts 1993, past, present and future, *Clinics in Plastic Surgery* 20:597-598, 1993.

Moller KT, Starr CD, and Johnson SA: *A parent's guide to cleft lip and palate,* Minneapolis, 1990, Univ. of Minnesota Press.

Muntz HR: An overview of middle ear disease in cleft palate children, *Facial Plastic Surgery* 9:177-180, 1993.

Oberg KC, Kirsch WM, and Hardesty RA: Prospectives in cleft lip and palate repair, *Clinics in Plastic Surgery* 20:815-821, 1993.

Otitis Media Guideline Panel. Quick reference guide for clinicians managing otitis media with effusion in young children, *J Am Acad Nurse Pract* 6(10):493-499, 1994.

Paradise JL, Elster BA, and Tan L: Evidence in infants with cleft palate that breast milk protects against otitis media, *Pediatrics* 94:853-860, 1994.

Peterson-Falzone S: Speech characteristics: Updating clinical Decisions, *Seminars in Speech & Language* 7(3):269-295, 1986.

Rudman D et al: Prevalence of growth hormone deficiency in children with cleft lip or palate, *J Pediatr* 93:378-382, 1978.

Sher AE: Mechanisms of airway obstruction in Pierre Robin sequence: implications for treatment, *Cleft Palate-Cranf J* 29:224-231, 1992.

Singer L, Sidoti EJ: Pediatric management of Pierre Robin sequence, *Cleft Palate-Cranf J* 29:220-223, 1992.

Sirois M et al: Sleep apnea following a pharyngeal flap: a feared complication, *Plastic & Reconstructive Surgery* 93(5):943-947, 1994.

Strauss RP, Broder H: Children with cleft lip and palate and mental retardation: a subpopulation of cleft-craniofacial team patients, *Cleft Palate-Cranf J* 30:548-556, 1993.

Tatum S, Senders C: Perspectives on palatoplasty, *Facial Plastic Surgery* 9:225-231, 1993.

Tolarova M: Primary prevention of cleft lip with or without cleft palate by vitamins and high folic acid. Presented at the *American Cleft Palate-Craniofacial Association Annual Meeting,* Pittsburgh, PA, 1993.

Witt PD, D'Antonio LL: Velopharyngeal insufficiency and secondary palatal management—a new look at an old problem, *Clinics in Plastic Surgery* 20:707-721, 1993.

Congenital Adrenal Hyperplasia

14

Judith A. Ruble

ETIOLOGY

The adrenal glands are small triangular organs located on the top of each kidney. They are divided into two major components: the adrenal medulla, which is in the center of the gland, and the adrenal cortex, which surrounds the medulla.

The adrenal cortex synthesizes glucocorticoids (primarily cortisol), mineralocorticoids (mainly aldosterone) and androgens through complex metabolic pathways. A simplified diagram of these pathways is shown in Fig. 14-1. Cortisol, aldosterone, and adrenal androgens play a crucial role in maintaining homeostasis by helping to regulate the body's blood pressure, glucose, sodium, and water levels, sexual development, and other metabolic processes (Bacon et al, 1990; New, 1995).

Congenital adrenal hyperplasia (CAH) is caused by a deficiency of one of the enzymes used by the adrenal cortex to produce cortisol and aldosterone. Although there are six possible enzyme defects, approximately 90% to 95% of CAH is caused by 21-hydroxylase deficiency (Bacon et al, 1990). The other five enzyme defects are quite rare and are not discussed here. Each of the enzyme defects causing CAH is inherited as a separate autosomal recessive genetic trait. The gene responsible for CAH has been identified and is located on the short arm of chromosome 6, linked to the human leukocyte antigen gene B (HLA-B) (New, 1995).

The adrenal production of glucocorticoids is regulated by a feedback system to the hypothala-mus and pituitary gland (see Fig. 14-2). Normally the hypothalamus secretes corticotropin-releasing factor (CRF), which causes the pituitary gland to produce adrenocorticotropic hormone (ACTH). In turn, ACTH stimulates the adrenal glands to synthesize glucocorticoids (primarily cortisol). The "switch" that controls this feedback system is cortisol. When blood levels of cortisol are low, the system turns on; the hypothalamus releases CRF, which signals the pituitary to release ACTH, which stimulates the adrenal glands to synthesize cortisol. When blood levels of cortisol rise, the system turns off; the hypothalamus stops releasing CRF, the pituitary gland stops releasing ACTH, and the adrenal glands stop synthesizing cortisol (Bacon et al, 1990). Because cortisol production is blocked in CAH, the hypothalamic-pituitary-adrenal system is not turned off, resulting in high ACTH levels that continuously stimulate the adrenal glands (Bacon et al, 1990; New, 1995). The continual stimulation by ACTH leads to hypertrophy of the adrenal glands and a buildup of precursors to cortisol and an overproduction of adrenal androgens, as described in Fig. 14-1.

Aldosterone synthesis is regulated primarily by the renin-angiotensin system of the kidney, so that a block in aldosterone synthesis will cause very high plasma renin activity levels, just as a block in cortisol synthesis will cause high ACTH levels (Bacon et al, 1990).

There are two forms of "classical" 21-hydroxylase deficiency: salt-losing CAH and non–

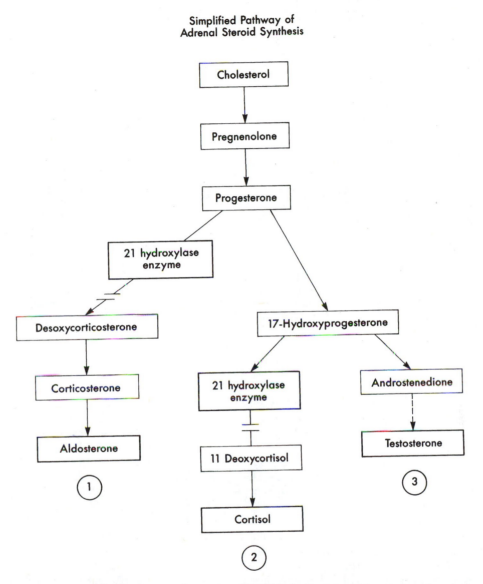

Simplified Pathway of Adrenal Steroid Synthesis

Fig. 14-1. In salt-losing CAH, pathways 1 and 2 are blocked, causing aldosterone and cortisol deficiencies. In non–salt-losing CAH, only pathway 2 is blocked, causing cortisol deficiency. In both forms of CAH there is a buildup of precursors and overproduction of adrenal androgens.

salt-losing (or simple virilizing) CAH. In the salt-losing form both cortisol and aldosterone production are blocked (see Fig. 14-1). The absence of aldosterone results in excessive sodium loss through the kidneys and the inability to maintain normal serum electrolyte balance. In the non–salt-losing form, only cortisol production is blocked and there is adequate aldosterone production to meet the body's normal needs. However, there may be a mild deficit, as indicated by elevated plasma renin activity levels or mild hyponatremia during stress (Bacon et al, 1990; New, 1995; Rosler et al, 1977).

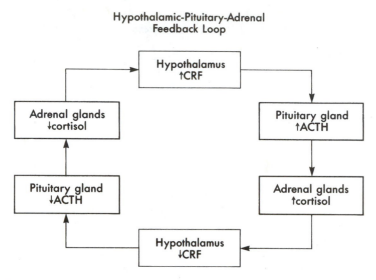

Fig. 14-2.   Blood levels of cortisol turn the hypothalamic-pituitary-adrenal system "on" and "off": low cortisol levels cause the hypothalamus to make CRF; CRF causes the pituitary to release ACTH; ACTH stimulates the adrenal cortex to synthesize cortisol; high cortisol levels cause the hypothalamus to stop making CRF; without CRF, the pituitary stops producing ACTH; without ACTH, the adrenal cortex stops synthesizing cortisol; the cycle repeats.

The alterations in adrenal steroid metabolism caused by 21-hydroxylase deficiency lead to the buildup of precursors of cortisol and aldosterone and overproduction of adrenal androgens, which do not require the 21-hydroxylase enzyme (see Fig. 14-1). Laboratory assays for these substances, such as serum 17-hydroxyprogesterone (17-OHP) or urine 17-ketosteroids and pregnanetriol, are used to monitor the adequacy of cortisol replacement therapy for CAH. Laboratory assay of plasma renin activity is used to monitor the mineralocorticoid replacement in the salt-losing form.

There is another type of 21-hydroxylase deficiency commonly called the "nonclassic" form, which is not apparent at birth by either physical findings or newborn screening tests. Its clinical features are similar to those of classical 21-hydroxylase deficiency but occur later in childhood and are much milder (many are asymptomatic) without salt-losing and acute adrenal insufficiency (New, 1995). Nonclassic 21-hydroxylase deficiency does not present the management difficulties and risks of the classical form.

INCIDENCE

A multinational neonatal screening study documented the overall incidence of classical 21-hydroxylase deficiency CAH in the United States, Italy, France, New Zealand, and Japan at approximately 1:5000 to 1:15,000 live births with males and females equally affected (Drucker and New, 1987; Pang et al, 1988). Some isolated populations have an extraordinarily high incidence of CAH, such as the Yu'pik-speaking Eskimos of Alaska (1:282) and the people of LaReunion, France (1:2141) (Pang et al, 1988). The incidence of CAH based on large-scale neonatal screening studies is significantly higher than that based on case reports, which suggests that many children with CAH go undiagnosed (Drucker and New, 1987; Pang et al, 1988).

The same neonatal screening study found that the salt-losing form of CAH is 2 to 3 times as frequent as the non-salt-losing form rather than the equal frequency previously described in case report studies (Pang et al, 1988). This discrepancy is believed to be the result of early deaths of infants with salt-losing CAH before the diagnosis was made. Methods for prenatal and neonatal screening of individuals known to have a blood relative with CAH are presently available. Screening could significantly reduce the number of deaths from undiagnosed CAH, as well as reduce the morbidity associated with nonfatal episodes of acute adrenal insufficiency and excessive virilization (New, 1995).

CLINICAL MANIFESTATIONS AT TIME OF DIAGNOSIS

Nearly all female infants with CAH will have virilization apparent on physical examination at birth (see Fig. 14-3). The findings range from a mildly enlarged clitoris to complete fusion and rugation of the labia, with the urethra opening through a urogenital sinus at the base of the phallus or even on the phallus (New, 1995).

Female infants with a mildly enlarged clitoris often go undetected, but the alert primary care provider can identify these infants by paying close attention to clitoral size. When measured at the base with redundant skin retracted, the normal clitoral breadth (not length) in a female infant is 2 to 6 mm; this range applies to all gestational ages of newborns and for infants up to 1 year of age (Riley and Rosenbloom, 1980).

The middle range virilization of a female infant looks abnormal enough to prompt an immediate search for the cause. Unfortunately, the severely virilized female infants may go undiagnosed, being mistaken for cryptorchid males with hypospadias or micropenis.

The label "ambiguous genitalia" should be applied to any infant with either hypospadias and no palpable gonads or a micropenis and no palpable gonads. Since the most common cause of ambiguous genitalia is CAH, it should be high in the clinician's index of suspicion and part of the diagnostic work-up (New, 1995).

Male newborns with CAH look normal and cannot be reliably identified by physical examination, although there may be slight enlargement of the penis and mildly increased genital pigmentation (New, 1995).

Newborns with salt-losing CAH will have elevated plasma renin activity levels at birth, although elevated serum potassium levels and decreased serum sodium levels may not be apparent for 1 week or more (Bacon et al, 1990). Newborns with either form of classical CAH will have significantly elevated 17-OHP levels by 24 to 36 hours of age (the infant's age should be noted on the specimen). However, there is a possibility of false positive results in premature infants or very sick term infants (Bacon et al, 1990). If salt-losing CAH is not diagnosed and replacement therapy is not begun at

---

CLINICAL MANIFESTATIONS AT TIME OF DIAGNOSIS

Ambiguous genitalia (females)
Elevated serum 17-OHP
Elevated plasma renin (salt-losing)
Acute adrenal insufficiency (see box on p. 282)
Accelerated growth and bone age

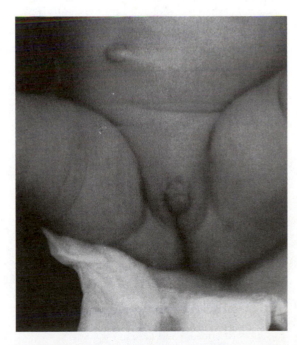

Fig. 14-3.   Infant girl with CAH-caused clitoromegaly.

birth, both male and female infants will have symptoms of acute adrenal insufficiency and a salt-losing crisis within the first few weeks of life. These symptoms include failure to thrive, weakness, vomiting, and dehydration. Unfortunately these symptoms are nonspecific and usually prompt a workup for sepsis, pyloric stenosis, or severe malabsorption. Because the routine evaluation of infants with these symptoms normally includes serum electrolyte values, hyponatremia and hyperkalemia should signal the clinician to suspect acute adrenal insufficiency.

The lack of specific symptoms combined with a low index of suspicion on the part of medical personnel can lead to a high mortality rate for undiagnosed infants, especially boys. The difference in the frequency of salt-losing CAH based on early case reports versus newborn screening reinforces the belief that many of these infants die because of a salt-losing crisis without being diagnosed (Fife and Rappaport, 1983; Pang et al, 1988).

Children with non–salt-losing CAH (who have only cortisol deficiency) may go undiagnosed for years. These children have impaired ability to withstand stress, so that minor illnesses such as acute otitis media, streptococcal pharyngitis, bronchitis, and febrile (temperature >38.4° C) illnesses may cause excessive weakness, pallor, hypotension, and prolonged convalescence (Burnett, 1980). Severe stress such as surgery or a fractured bone can trigger acute adrenal insufficiency with extreme weakness, abdominal pain, vomiting, dehydration, hypotension, and, if not adequately treated, vascular collapse and death (Bacon et al, 1990).

TREATMENT

It was not until the 1950s that an understanding of the metabolic defect in CAH led to the current concept of replacement therapy, and it was another decade before adequate therapy was routinely employed (Bartter, 1977). It is not yet possible to correct the genetic defect that blocks the adrenal metabolic pathways, but the clinical consequences of the defect can be prevented by replacing the blocked glucocorticoid and mineralocorticoid end products of cortisol and aldosterone.

TREATMENT

Glucocorticoids; dose increased for stress
Mineralocorticoids (salt-losing)
Sodium cloride supplement (salt-losing infants)
Injectable hydrocortisone for emergencies

In both salt-losing and non–salt-losing CAH, hydrocortisone tablets or liquid (Cortef) are given as a replacement for the glucocorticoid cortisol; in salt-losing CAH, fludrocortisone acetate (Florinef) is added as a replacement for the mineralocorticoid aldosterone.

The basal nonstress dose of hydrocortisone is designed to simulate normal cortisol serum levels and suppress ACTH production. A common regimen is 15 to 25 mg/m²/day divided into three doses and given orally every 8 hours, but there is still considerable disagreement on the optimal dosage regimen (Bacon et al, 1990; New, 1995; Sandrini, Jospe, and Migeon, 1993). Excessive hydrocortisone dosage can produce Cushing's syndrome, with stunted linear growth, truncal obesity, striae, bruising, hirsutism, muscle weakness, and hypertension (New, 1995). Inadequate dosage puts the child at risk for acute adrenal insufficiency and allows excessive androgen production, which causes virilization and accelerates growth and bone age advancement.

The basal hydrocortisone dose is doubled or tripled during the acute phase of an illness (e.g., temperature >38.4° C, significant malaise, or pain) or mild to moderate stress. Stress doses do not require prolonged tapering and should be returned to basal levels as soon as the acute stress is resolved (Bacon et al, 1990). Examples of stresses and dosage guidelines are provided in the accompanying box, page 281.

If the child vomits more than once, the stress is severe, or the child does not respond to oral treatment, injectable hydrocortisone (Solu-Cortef) must be given. The dose, typically 50 to 100 mg, is based

GUIDELINES ON STRESS DOSES OF HYDROCORTISONE*

1. For temperature 38.4° to 38.9° C (orally) or for mild illness, give double the basal dose orally
2. For temperature 38.9° C or higher (orally) or for moderate illness, give triple the basal dose orally
3. For minor injury (e.g., sprain), give double the basal dose orally
4. For vomiting only once and acting well, wait 20 minutes and give double the basal dose orally
5. For vomiting only once but acting ill, vomiting more than once, or acting ill in spite of increased oral dose, give hydrocortisone intramuscularly
6. For serious injury (e.g., fracture or concussion), give hydrocortisone intramuscularly
7. If the child looks severely ill or has symptoms of acute adrenal insufficiency, give hydrocortisone intramuscularly and go to the emergency room
8. If the child is unconscious for any reason, give injectable hydrocortisone intramuscularly and go to the emergency room
9. In general, emotional stress does not require increased hydrocortisone doses; for severe, prolonged emotional upheaval, consult with the endocrinologist for advice
10. Call the endocrinologist or primary care provider for all but mild illnesses
11. Before all surgical procedures consult with endocrinologist

NOTE: **When in doubt, give stress doses of hydrocortisone.** The stress dose should be reduced to basal levels after the acute phase of the illness, injury, or stress; it does not require a prolonged taper.

*From Children's Hospital, Oakland, California.

on the size and usual replacement dose of the child and should be prescribed in conjunction with the endocrinologist (Bacon et al, 1990). Parents should have injectable hydrocortisone on hand, know the indications for using it, and learn how to prepare and give an intramuscular (IM) injection. Parents who are unable to give injectable hydrocortisone must have rapid (5- to 10-minute) access to a hospital emergency room or health care provider who is equipped to administer hydrocortisone parenterally.

Whenever there is uncertainty about the necessity of giving emergency treatment, keep in mind that *there is no physical harm in treating for suspected acute adrenal insufficiency that is not present, and the consequence of not treating acute adrenal insufficiency can be the death of the child* (Bacon et al, 1990). In this type of situation it is always best to err on the side of prompt, aggressive treatment.

In a medical setting, acute adrenal insufficiency is treated with hydrocortisone (Solu-Cortef or hydrocortisone 21-phosphate) given intravenously in 5 to 10 times the basal dose, along with appropriate intravenous (IV) therapy to restore intravascular volume and electrolyte balance (see box page 282 for symptoms of acute adrenal insufficiency) (New, 1995). If IV access is not available, the hydrocortisone should be given intramuscularly rather than delaying until IV therapy can be started.

In addition to hydrocortisone therapy, salt-losing CAH also requires mineralocorticoid replacement with fludrocortisone (Florinef). The usual dose is 50 to 200 µg daily, given orally in a single dose. Newborns may temporarily need doses as high as 200 to 300 µg daily for stabilization, and adolescents may also require up to 250 to 300 µg daily during the rapid growth period (Bacon et al, 1990). Excessive amounts of mineralocorticoid will result in hypokalemia, weight gain, edema, hypertension, and headache. Inadequate dosage will impair growth and put the child at risk for a salt-losing crisis (Rosler et al, 1977).

The basal mineralocorticoid dose does not need to be increased during illnesses because the increased amount of hydrocortisone given during stress has enough mineralocorticoid activity to make additional fludrocortisone acetate unnecessary (Stern and Tuck, 1986).

**SIGNS AND SYMPTOMS
OF ACUTE ADRENAL
INSUFFICIENCY**

1. Nausea or vomiting
2. Pallor
3. Cold, moist skin
4. Weakness
5. Dizziness or confusion
6. Rapid heart rate
7. Rapid breathing
8. Abdominal, back, or leg pain
9. Dehydration
10. Hypotension

Sodium chloride supplementation may be required in infants if the salt loss continues to exceed the salt intake, in spite of mineralocorticoid therapy. The usual dose is 3 to 5 mEq/kg/day given divided into two to four doses and given dissolved in formula or other liquid (Bacon et al, 1990; Mullis, Hindmarsh, and Brook, 1990).

The majority of girls with CAH have severe enough virilization of their external genitalia to require surgical correction. The corrective surgery frequently requires more than one procedure (e.g., clitoral reduction, separation of the fused labia, correction of a urogenital sinus, and vaginoplasty), with the initial correction done before 2 years of age (Bailez et al, 1992). Although satisfactory cosmetic and functional results are usually achieved, additional surgery may be necessary during adolescence to enlarge the vagina to allow for intercourse and to avoid the need for repeated dilatation (New, 1995). All surgical procedures are a major stress to the child and require consultation with the endocrinologist for perioperative management.

RECENT AND ANTICIPATED ADVANCES IN DIAGNOSIS AND MANAGEMENT

Recent advances in diagnosis and treatment of CAH have been made in the areas of prenatal diagnosis and prenatal treatment. Prenatal testing has been done successfully by radioimmunoassay for adrenal steroids in amniotic fluid as early as 10 to 12 weeks' gestation, and by DNA probe of chorionic villus samples at 9 to 11 weeks' gestation (New, 1995). Early attempts to prevent virilization of female fetuses with CAH by administering glucocorticoids to the mother during pregnancy have produced promising results (New, 1990; Pang et al, 1990). Glucocorticoid therapy must be started before virilization begins at about 10 weeks' gestation. Because this may be before a prenatal diagnosis of CAH is available, a decision to treat will initially include nonaffected fetuses and their mothers.

Prenatal diagnosis and treatment for CAH are areas of intense interest and rapid progress; it is very likely that these procedures will be refined and become more readily available in the future. The procedures should be discussed with families who have a first-degree relative with CAH.

ASSOCIATED PROBLEMS

In children who are receiving appropriate therapy, the problems associated with CAH will be limited. However, the primary care provider must be aware of the potential for acute adrenal insufficiency, growth disorders, virilization, and problems surrounding issues of sexuality.

Acute Adrenal Insufficiency

Children with CAH may develop acute adrenal insufficiency with any significant illness or injury because they lack the ability to produce increased amounts of cortisol as part of the body's normal stress response.

Accelerated Growth and Bone Age

In children with undiagnosed or inadequately treated CAH, excessive androgen production will cause accelerated linear growth and muscle development so that a 5-year-old child could have the height and build of an 8- or 10-year-old. Another consequence of excessive androgen production is rapidly advancing bone age with early closure of the growth plates. The 5-year-old with the height and build of a 10-year-old may have the bone age of a 15-year-old. This means that a child who was unusually large for his or her age during the early

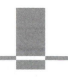

ASSOCIATED PROBLEMS

Acute adrenal insufficiency
Accelerated growth and bone age
Virilization
Precocious puberty
Fertility problems

years will stop growing early because of premature closure of the growth plates and end up as a significantly short adolescent and adult (New, 1995).

Virilization

Virilization of the fetus begins at approximately the tenth week of gestation, so virtually all newborn girls with CAH have virilized genitalia that will require surgical correction (Bacon et al, 1990; New, 1995).

By early school age, untreated boys may have an adult-sized penis (the testes remain normal size for age), and untreated girls will be severely virilized with fused labia and a markedly enlarged clitoris. Both sexes will have adult-appearing pubic and axillary hair. By adolescence, if the condition remains untreated, changes from prolonged exposure to very high testosterone levels may no longer be reversible. Boys may have benign testicular tumors, impaired testicular development or spermatogenesis, and girls will not have breast development or menarche (Srikanth et al, 1992).

Puberty

Most children with consistently well-controlled CAH can expect to have normal onset and progression of puberty. A few children with well-controlled CAH and many children who achieve good control of CAH after a prolonged period of poor control may enter puberty prematurely. The onset of precocious puberty shortly after improving control is believed to be caused by the "priming" of the pubertal timing system by the chronically high androgen levels which are characteristic of poorly controlled CAH. When these high androgen levels suddenly drop to normal ranges as a result of im-

proved control, the complex (and poorly understood) system which triggers pubertal development is activated.

This is a poor reward for a child and family who have put increased effort into achieving better control of CAH; however, children who do develop precocious puberty can be successfully treated with gonadotropin releasing hormone (GnRH) analogs (Dacou-Voutetakis and Karidis, 1993). GnRH analogs are presently available as SQ injections given daily, IM injections given every 4 weeks, and intranasal spray given QID.

Not only does the occurrence of precocious puberty increase the complexity, expense, and burden of the medical regimen for the family, it also increases the psychosocial stresses. Children with precocious puberty are faced with physical sexual development that they are not emotionally ready for, as well as teasing and sexual harassment. These children are also at increased risk for sexual abuse (Jackson and Ott, 1990).

Parents of a child with precocious puberty must meet with school and day care personnel to be sure that teasing and sexual harassment are not tolerated. The child must be taught how to maintain his or her "sexual boundaries," such as what kind of remarks, activities, or touching are "OK" and "not OK" and who to go to for help (Jackson and Ott, 1990; Ott and Jackson, 1989).

Fertility Problems

Menstrual irregularities are common in adolescent girls who are noncompliant with their replacement therapy, but the majority of girls who were diagnosed early and adequately treated can be expected to have normal pubertal development and fertility (Bacon et al, 1990).

Prolonged exposure to high levels of androgens in undiagnosed or inadequately treated children will eventually result in irreversible infertility and virilization in girls and may cause impaired fertility in boys (New, 1995; Mulaikal, Migeon, and Rock, 1987).

Congenital Anomalies

The incidence of congenital anomalies associated with CAH is not believed to be significantly increased over the general population. Although there have been reports of an increased incidence of upper urinary tract abnormalities, these have not been clearly established (Bacon et al, 1990).

PROGNOSIS

The major risk for children with CAH is death from an unrecognized salt-losing crisis early in infancy or from inadequately treated acute adrenal insufficiency during stress. Screening of individuals with a family history of CAH for the carrier state, prenatal screening, and routine neonatal screening have the potential for greatly reducing the number of children who die of CAH (New, 1995). Efforts are being made to include CAH in routine newborn screening programs in this country.

Currently nearly all female infants with CAH have morbidity associated with prenatal virilization and the surgical procedures necessary to correct it. If prenatal treatment of female fetuses to prevent virilization becomes available as a standard treatment, it should have a substantial effect on reducing the morbidity in girls with CAH (New, 1995).

Primary Care Management
HEALTH CARE MAINTENANCE

Growth and Development

Because abnormal linear growth is an indication of inappropriate treatment or noncompliance, careful monitoring of growth is an essential component of primary care. Linear growth should be measured every 1 to 4 months for infants and every 3 to 6 months for children more than 2 years of age. These measurements should be done carefully using an infantometer for lengths and a stadiometer for heights. The standard scale-mounted measuring device is not accurate enough to detect slight variations in growth. The measurements should be plotted on a standardized growth chart and assessed for changes in growth rate (e.g., increase or decrease in centile).

Poor growth. Linear growth is acutely sensitive to excessive levels of hydrocortisone; therefore any decrease in height centile on the growth chart should prompt a reassessment of the hydrocortisone dosage. Occasionally a child's hydrocortisone therapy will be increased based on a high laboratory 17-OHP result, when the result was high because of an acute illness, stress caused by an unusually traumatic venipuncture, or frequently missed hydrocortisone doses before sampling.

To avoid unnecessary and possibly harmful increases in hydrocortisone dosage, the clinician must rule out these other causes of high 17-OHP values with a careful history and comparison of the prescribed dose of hydrocortisone with established dosage ranges before making medication increases. The primary care provider may be in a position to identify these other causes and should contact the endocrinologist with this information.

Another cause of poor linear growth in children with CAH is chronically inadequate mineralocorticoid levels (Duck, 1980). A plasma renin activity level that is abnormally high indicates that the child needs additional mineralocorticoid or dietary sodium. A careful history and comparison with established dosage ranges will determine if the problem is one of compliance or inadequately prescribed dosage.

A child with poorly controlled CAH or one who was not diagnosed until preschool or school age may have early cessation of growth because of premature closure of the epiphyses. Bone-age x-ray studies should be done to assess skeletal maturity if this is suspected.

Excessive growth. Inadequate hydrocortisone replacement will cause excessive androgen synthesis by the adrenals and will result in accelerated linear growth. An elevated serum 17-OHP level or clinical findings of increased virilization (e.g., pubic and axillary hair, oily skin, acne, enlargement of the phallus) will confirm the cause of excessive growth. Again, the clinician must be careful to assess whether the inadequate hydrocortisone replacement is secondary to an inappropriately prescribed dose or poor adherence.

Development. Children with CAH that was diagnosed in infancy or very early in childhood and receive adequate, consistent treatment should develop normally.

If the diagnosis of CAH is not made until late childhood, the child will be much taller and more mature looking than his or her peers. Because of mature physical appearance, people may expect the child to have the emotional maturity and behavior of a much older child. This may lead to frustration for all concerned, inappropriate demands and punishment, and the possibility of creating or exacerbating behavior problems.

When these children stop growing early because of early epiphyseal closure, they will go from being the largest to the shortest child in their peer group. Short stature is known to have an impact on behavior and social relationships, and it is very likely to have an even greater impact on someone who spent early childhood as the largest person in any group of peers (Holmes, Karlsson, and Thompson, 1986; Young-Hyman, 1986).

Parents, school personnel, child care workers, and others who regularly interact with the child should be given clear, frequently reinforced guidelines on age-appropriate expectations to avoid demanding too much of the large but immature child or asking too little of the short adolescent.

Diet

The only required modification to a regular diet is to allow for adequate sodium intake. Although an appropriate dose of mineralocorticoid will prevent significant sodium depletion in children with salt-losing CAH the children should be offered salty foods and allowed to salt their food to taste. This recommendation also applies to children with non–salt-losing CAH because they may have a mild salt deficit compared with unaffected children (Rosler et al, 1977).

Safety

Children with CAH are not physically impaired and are not at increased risk for any of the usual physical hazards of childhood, but they are at risk for having their special needs neglected when they are away from home. Injuries, such as a broken bone, may not be recognized as a potentially life-threatening event.

Teachers, child care personnel, coaches, and others who are in regular contact with the child should have written information describing the condition and the need for prompt treatment in an emergency. The child should wear a Medic-Alert bracelet with similar information on it.

The decision of whether or not to keep injectable hydrocortisone at school or day care depends on the situation and must be made on a case-by-case basis. Factors to consider are: Can the primary care provider or emergency room be reached in 5 to 10 minutes? Is a parent always available at short notice? Are there personnel at the site who are trained and willing to give an IM injection? Does the child engage in activities with a high risk of serious injury?

If injectable hydrocortisone is kept at school or day care, the most convenient preparation is the 100-mg Solu-Cortef Mix-O-Vial, which is easy to use and store. Written indications for use and dosage should be provided by the endocrinologist.

Participation in sports is a normal part of childhood and should be encouraged; however, if at all possible the child with CAH should be directed toward activities with a low risk of serious injury, such as swimming, track, or tennis (bruises, mild or moderate sprains, abrasions, etc. are not cause for special concern). If the child is involved in high-risk sports such as football, the parents should meet with the coach to explain the child's special needs in an emergency and provide appropriate written materials, instructions, and authorization for treatment. Ideally someone such as a parent or team physician should be present and have hydrocortisone for IM injection on hand during competition. This should be mandatory if the activity takes place more than 15 minutes away from a source of emergency care.

Immunizations

Children with CAH are not immunosuppressed and should receive all of the standard immunizations at the usual ages. At present there is no recommendation for or against giving additional immunizations (e.g., pneumococcal, influenza); the benefits of immunity to these diseases must be weighed against the possibility of adverse reactions to the vaccine. In weighing these factors, many clinicians believe that giving additional immunizations is worthwhile to reduce the risk of acute adrenal insufficiency triggered by illness.

It is not necessary to increase the basal dose of hydrocortisone before immunizations are given unless there is a history of adverse reactions to previous immunizations with that vaccine. A common but discretionary recommendation is to give the child acetaminophen a few hours before giving an immunization that is likely to produce rapid-onset febrile reactions (e.g., pertussis) and continue it for 24 to 48 hours afterward.

For new vaccines or new combinations of vaccines, refer to the package insert for information on the type and timing of possible reactions and counsel the family to observe the child closely during the days when reactions are likely to occur (e.g., 5 to 12 days after measles vaccination).

Stress doses of hydrocortisone should be given if the child develops a temperature of more than 38.4° C or is very fussy or lethargic after an immunization. (See the box on p. 281 for stress dose guidelines.) Any immunization reaction should be documented so that stress doses of hydrocortisone can be given before subsequent immunizations with the same vaccine.

Screening

Vision. Routine screening is recommended.

Hearing. Routine screening is recommended.

Dental. Routine screening is recommended.

Blood pressure. Blood pressure should be checked at each primary care visit. This will require special equipment, such as a Dinamap, for infants. Every effort should be made to have the child relaxed and quiet so that the readings obtained are accurate.

Elevated blood pressure (in a quiet child) may indicate excessive mineralocorticoid or hydrocortisone dosage, whereas low blood pressure may indicate an inadequate mineralocorticoid or hydrocortisone dosage. Either situation should prompt an evaluation of the replacement therapy regimen and compliance.

Hematocrit. Routine screening is recommended.

Urinalysis. Routine screening is recommended.

Tuberculosis. Routine screening is recommended.

Condition-specific screening

SERUM 17-OHP. It may be desirable for the primary care provider to order additional screening tests to more closely monitor the adequacy of replacement therapy in children who have difficulty with compliance. The serum 17-OHP level has become widely accepted as a convenient measure of hydrocortisone therapy even though it has the disadvantage of being influenced by temporary stress (e.g., traumatic venipuncture), the length of time since the last hydrocortisone dose, and diurnal fluctuations. To help evaluate the significance of 17-OHP results, clinicians should note on the specimen the time of day (preferably morning) and the time of the last dose of hydrocortisone. Some clinicians continue to rely on 24-hour urinary 17-ketosteroid and pregnanetriol levels to monitor hydrocortisone therapy in spite of the difficulty in collecting a 24-hour specimen because of the lack of short-term fluctuations. Mineralocorticoid therapy is monitored by plasma renin activity level.

Serum 17-OHP levels should be no more than 3 times normal, preferably less than 200 ng/dl; urinary 17-ketosteroid and pregnanetriol levels should also be in the normal to near-normal range for age, as should plasma renin activity. Specimens ordered by the primary care provider should be coordinated with the endocrinologist and sent to the same laboratory to ensure consistency.

BONE AGE. The frequency of bone-age x-ray studies depends on the clinical course. Bone ages in newborns are not helpful. Initial bone age should be determined early in childhood at 2 to 3 years of age (or at the time of diagnosis if the diagnosis is delayed) and can be used as a baseline for future studies. If the child is growing normally and has consistently acceptable 17-OHP and plasma renin activity levels, routine screening should not be necessary more often than every few years.

If the child has growth acceleration, physical findings of increased virilization, or consistently high laboratory results, bone age should be determined to further assess the effects of androgen excess. If the bone age has accelerated, this finding can be used to help impress on the family the serious and permanent consequences of poor adherence. Ideally, all bone-age studies should be read by the same person to avoid inconsistencies in interpretation.

COMMON ILLNESS MANAGEMENT

Differential Diagnosis

Children with CAH are not immunosuppressed and are no different than their peers in their susceptibility to common childhood illnesses; it is their ability to withstand the stress of illness that is impaired. During periods of illness these children must be followed closely and consultation with the endocrinologist is necessary if the child shows any signs or symptoms of acute adrenal insufficiency.

The primary care provider should consider keeping injectable hydrocortisone in the office for emergencies. The most commonly used preparation is the 100-mg Solu-Cortef Mix-O-Vial because of its long shelf life and convenience. It does not require refrigeration. When reconstituted by rotating and depressing the plunger-stopper, it contains 100 mg of hydrocortisone in 2 ml and can be given intramuscularly or intravenously.

Upper respiratory infections and allergies. If the symptoms are mild and the child does not have fever or marked malaise, no specific treatment or increase in basal dose of hydrocortisone is necessary for upper respiratory infections or allergies. The parents should watch for worsening of the symptoms, fever, or unusual lethargy; a school-aged child should know to report these symptoms to the teacher and contact his or her parents.

If the symptoms worsen or complications develop, the child should be treated promptly with a stress dose of hydrocortisone and seen by the primary care provider for assessment and specific therapy for the illness.

Acute illnesses. Any known or suspected bacterial illness such as acute otitis media, urinary tract infection, streptococcal pharyngitis, and cellulitis should be treated aggressively with the appropriate antibiotic and stress doses of hydrocortisone during the acute phase of the illness if fever, pain, and malaise are present (see guidelines in the box on p. 281).

When the diagnosis is uncertain or has a significant risk of secondary infections or complications (e.g., a suspicious but not clearly inflamed tympanic membrane, viral pneumonia, or prolonged or marked nasal congestion in a child with a history of frequent acute otitis media or sinusitis), it is wise to treat with antibiotics rather than wait for the situation to worsen.

The child must be followed closely, with an initial office visit for diagnosis and assessment of the child's overall condition and daily telephone progress reports until the acute phase of the illness has passed. Follow-up office visits should be scheduled as for any other child.

Fever. Although fever is a physiologic response to illness, it is also a stress; for this reason fever in

DIFFERENTIAL DIAGNOSIS

Upper respiratory infections and allergies
Acute illness
Fever
Vomiting
Injury
Acute adrenal insufficiency

a child with CAH should be treated with acetaminophen in the usual recommended dose for age. Stress doses of hydrocortisone should be given using the guidelines in the box on p. 281. It is important to advise the family that reducing the fever does not cure the illness and that other treatments such as antibiotics and stress doses of hydrocortisone should continue to be given as directed.

The child must be followed closely, as described for bacterial and viral illnesses, until the illness has resolved.

Vomiting. If a child with CAH vomits once but appears well otherwise, wait about 20 minutes, give twice the usual oral dose of hydrocortisone, and observe the child closely. If the child appears weak or lethargic after vomiting only once or vomits more than once, the family should give injectable hydrocortisone intramuscularly and contact the endocrinologist immediately.

If family members are not able to give injectable hydrocortisone, they must immediately take the child to the nearest emergency room to receive parenteral hydrocortisone and appropriate fluid and electrolyte therapy. *This can be a life-threatening situation.* Emergency room personnel should contact the endocrinologist but should not delay hydrocortisone therapy while awaiting consultation.

Injury. The child with a significant injury such as a fracture or concussion or injury from an automobile accident should immediately be given hydrocortisone intramuscularly and evaluated further for acute adrenal insufficiency at an emergency room. Emergency room personnel should contact the endocrinologist but should not delay hydrocortisone therapy while awaiting consultation.

Acute adrenal insufficiency. *Acute adrenal insufficiency is a life-threatening situation.* Symptoms of acute adrenal insufficiency include weakness, nausea, abdominal discomfort, vomiting, dehydration, and hypotension. Any of these signs or symptoms in a child with CAH should be presumed to indicate acute adrenal insufficiency and be treated with hydrocortisone intravenously or intramuscularly in 3 to 5 times the basal dose; this should be done at home (or in the primary care setting if the child is there) rather than delaying initial treatment until the child arrives at an emergency room.

The diagnosis of acute adrenal insufficiency can be confirmed by laboratory values showing hyponatremia and hyperkalemia. Although consultation with an endocrinologist should be sought, treatment should not be delayed.

An IM injection of hydrocortisone or IV therapy in an emergency room are frightening experiences that no one wants to go through unnecessarily. However, as mentioned earlier, in this type of situation it is always best to err on the side of aggressive treatment.

Drug Interactions

Families often are afraid of giving their child steroids because of negative publicity in the popular press. It is important to stress to families that the Cortef and Florinef medications their child takes for CAH are replacing substances that are normally produced by their bodies and that the dosages recommended are calculated to match normal blood levels as closely as possible. This is an entirely different situation than taking a foreign substance such as an antibiotic. It is also very different from taking high doses of glucocorticoids to treat in-

flammatory diseases. Because the medications for CAH replace hormones that are normally present in the body, concern about using other medications is limited to their effect on absorption or rate of metabolism.

Barbiturates (phenobarbital, butalbital [Fiorinal, Fioricet], pentobarbital [Nembutal, Donnatal], secobarbital [Seconal, Tuinal], phenytoin [Dilantin], rifampin [Rifadin, Rifamate, Rimactane] increase the rate of metabolism of glucocorticoids; therefore children with CAH who are taking any of these medications for more than a few weeks may require a higher than usual dose of hydrocortisone for adequate cortisol replacement (Stern and Tuck, 1986).

A serum 17-OHP level done approximately 2 weeks after beginning any of the above medications will show if an adjustment in the hydrocortisone dose is necessary. The short-term use of barbiturates perioperatively or the prophylactic use of rifampin for *Haemophilus influenzae* meningitis should not require a change in hydrocortisone dose.

Antibiotics, decongestants, antihistamines, cough preparations, analgesics, antipyretics, and topical preparations have no unusual adverse effects.

DEVELOPMENTAL ISSUES

Sleep Patterns

Children with CAH do not differ from their peers in their sleep patterns or needs. Unusual fatigue may indicate an illness or inadequate cortisol replacement and should be evaluated.

Toileting

Children who have obvious virilization of their external genitalia should be allowed privacy when using the toilet to avoid being teased. Usually the initial corrective surgery for girls who are virilized is done at an early age to avoid problems related to looking different. Although boys who are excessively virilized may have some regression in pubic hair and penile size once they establish consistently adequate treatment, they will be noticeably different from their peers until adolescence.

These children are otherwise no different in toileting readiness or skills than their age group and are not unusually prone to constipation, inconti-

---

DRUG INTERACTIONS

Barbiturates
Phenytoin
Rifampin

nence, enuresis, polyuria, or other disorders related to toileting.

Discipline

Children with CAH should be expected to behave appropriately for their age. The only special consideration has to do with children who appear older than their actual age. Parents, teachers, and others must be given clear guidelines on appropriate expectations for the child's developmental stage if it differs from his or her appearance.

Another area that raises disciplinary issues is compliance with taking medication, especially during toddlerhood and adolescence when the child struggles with issues of dependency and autonomy. The parents should be advised from the beginning to use a matter-of-fact approach and avoid negotiating something that is not negotiable. During infancy and the early school years the parents have full responsibility for giving medications. As the child matures and is able to assume more responsibility, the parents should encourage more active participation by the child such as remembering when it is "pill time," marking off the calendar for each dose, or filling a pill box.

The adolescent should have the primary responsibility for taking the medication with the parents offering support. Using a watch with a beeper is helpful for adolescents, as is a pillbox, which coincidentally provides an unobtrusive way for a parent to see if the medication disappears on schedule.

Clinicians can help make older children and adolescents aware of the consequences of poor adherence by pointing out signs of virilization to the girls and slowed growth to both sexes and emphasizing that it is within their power to "get back to normal." The risks of acute adrenal insufficiency and impaired fertility associated with poor adherence should also be discussed with adolescents, again emphasizing that these things are avoidable.

Occasionally an adolescent will choose to make adherence with medications the focus of serious rebellion. Every effort should be made to explain the purpose and necessity of the medication, and counseling should be sought promptly if the problem is severe or chronic.

If the child's size differs from his or her peers, teachers may have inappropriate behavioral and academic expectations. This issue must be ad-

dressed in parent-teacher conferences and frequently reinforced.

The child with CAH may have more absences than usual because of the need for close observation at home during acute illnesses. Concerns about excessive absences should be brought to the attention of the primary care provider who can assess their appropriateness. Legitimate absences include any illness that would keep other children at home. In addition, symptoms such as a scratchy throat and malaise that might be ignored in other children should be initially observed at home.

Child Care

Parents should meet with child care personnel before enrollment to explain their child's special needs. Child care personnel do not require detailed knowledge of CAH, but they should be given a clear explanation that the child has a metabolic disorder that requires simple but very important treatment. Written information for the child care center should include written authorization to give hydrocortisone in oral form with instructions on the dose, time, and purpose, instructions on when to call the parents and telephone numbers where they can be reached, what symptoms or events require emergency care, where to take the child for care, authorization for treatment, and the name and telephone number of the primary care provider and endocrinologist.

It is neither necessary nor desirable to have special rules or restrictions on activities at school or child care for children with CAH. The usual policies on safety and appropriate play are sufficient to avoid serious injury.

Since hydrocortisone is usually given every 8 hours, many children will need at least one dose while in day care. Mineralocorticoid for children with salt-losing CAH is given once daily and can be administered at home. Although most child care providers are conscientious, occasionally they miss or delay doses of hydrocortisone because they do not understand its importance and are distracted by other demands on their attention. A routine that ties medication time to a regular activity, such as rest period or story time, can be established, or the child can wear a watch programmed to beep at the desired time. A letter from the primary care provider or the endocrinologist is very helpful in making this invisible condition real to people who care for these children.

Schooling

Children with well-controlled CAH should not have unusual learning disabilities or intellectual impairment related to their disorder (Galatzer and Laron, 1989; Ehrhardt and Baker, 1977). Not surprisingly however, children who have experienced episodes of acute adrenal insufficiency with severe hypoglycemia or convulsions do have significantly higher incidence of learning difficulties than children with or without CAH who did not suffer these events (Donaldson et al, 1994; Nass and Baker, 1991). Because hypoglycemia and convulsions are associated with learning difficulties, the findings may represent a complication of poor management rather than the biochemical abnormality of CAH. A child with CAH who has had severe hypoglycemia and convulsions should be assessed for learning difficulties and referred for special education intervention if indicated.

Sexuality

Virilization is nearly always present at birth in infant girls. Since multiple surgeries usually are needed, these girls learn that there is something "wrong" with them and that it has to do with their genitals. It is very important to reassure these girls that they have all the normal female organs, hormones, and chromosomes and that the surgeries are simply to correct a cosmetic mistake that happened before they were born (Mazur, 1983).

Although many observers have noted "tomboyish" behavior in girls with CAH, most of the early studies were difficult to interpret because of small sample size, lack of data on adequacy of treatment, and lack of control groups (Galatzer and Laron, 1989; Hochberg, Gardos, and Benderly, 1987; Money, Schwartz, and Lewis, 1984; Ehrhardt and Baker, 1977).

More recent research using better methodology has shown significant differences in gender-related and sexual behaviors between adolescent and adult women with CAH and their unaffected sisters; Dittmann and associates attribute these differences to prenatal exposure to high levels of adrenal androgens in the women with CAH (Dittmann et al,

1990a; Dittmann, Kappes, and Kappes, 1992). The data suggest that compared with their nonaffected sisters, more women with CAH have delays in establishing intimate relationships and more express a wish for or establish homosexual relationships (Dittmann, Kappes, and Kappes, 1992). Dittmann, Kappes, and Kappes believe prenatal androgen exposure is a predisposing rather than a causative factor in gender behavior, and they recommend that all aspects of psychosocial development be considered in the care of the girl with CAH (Dittmann, Kappes, and Kappes, 1992). The number of women with CAH in these studies was still rather small and the labeling of behaviors as "feminine" or "masculine" remains controversial; the primary care provider must use caution in interpreting these data and base discussions on the individualized assessment of each child and family.

Some studies have shown a high incidence of delayed menarche and menstrual irregularities in girls with CAH, but inadequate treatment or poor adherence with medications during puberty contributes to this (Mulaikal, Migeon, and Rock, 1987). Young women with CAH, particularly the salt-losing form, may have impaired fertility, and those who become pregnant may require cesarean delivery because of a small birth canal (Mulaikal, Migeon, and Rock, 1987). A significant number of women in one study had successful pregnancies in spite of late diagnosis, and treatment for CAH, inadequate reconstruction of the introitus, and poor compliance with replacement therapy all of which contribute to reduced fertility (Mulaikal, Migeon, and Rock, 1987).

Prolonged androgen excess can eventually result in infertility in men, but the majority are fertile (New, 1995).

When these children reach adolescence, the primary care provider or endocrinologist should discuss with them the availability and purpose of genetic counseling, screening for carriers, and prenatal and neonatal diagnosis. Because CAH is an autosomal recessive trait, children must receive an abnormal gene from each parent to have the disorder; if one parent has CAH and the other is not a carrier, their children will not have CAH. All unaffected children with a parent with CAH will be carriers of the trait.

Transition into Adulthood

As the child with CAH approaches adulthood, the primary care provider needs to help the family identify an internist or family practice provider to assume primary care responsibilities. If the child has had specialty care through a pediatric endocrinologist, the transition must also be made to adult endocrine care—usually the pediatric endocrinologist will have a list of names available.

Unfortunately, insurance may become a problem as the child reaches an age when he or she is no longer covered by CCS or the parents' insurance. Medicaid (for those who meet the criteria) and group insurance through employment (for those who have medical benefits) will cover care for CAH. Other possibilities to explore are coverage through the Genetically Handicapped Persons Program (GHPP) and purchasing pools. Information on these and other programs can be sought from county social services agencies, health departments, and state insurance commissions.

SPECIAL FAMILY CONCERNS AND RESOURCES

The parents of an infant girl with CAH must cope with the impact of ambiguous genitalia and possibly a delayed or even incorrect gender assignment. It is critical that the initial explanations and reassurances given to the family by health care personnel be both sensitive and accurate to prevent serious misperceptions of the child's condition and prognosis (Darland, 1986; Mazur, 1983). Discussions with parents should focus on listening to the parents' concerns and reinforcing the normality of their daughter's internal female organs and chromosomes and explaining that the appearance of the external genitals is correctable and the underlying condition treatable (Darland, 1986).

People tend to blame the occurrence of an abnormality in a baby on something the mother or father did. It is important to discuss this issue with the parents and the extended family, and to repeatedly reinforce the lack of fault. Even after the best of explanations and reassurances, these families continue to have a great deal of anxiety and guilt about their child's condition so that constant reinforcement and support are necessary.

The family must be taught to be assertive in communicating the urgency of their child's need for hydrocortisone to health care personnel who are not familiar with their child or with CAH. Unfortunately, it is common for treatment to be delayed because of lack of understanding of the implications of acute illness in a child with CAH. The primary care provider can help avoid delays in treatment by alerting other health care personnel (e.g., call group, emergency room staff) to the child's special needs. The endocrinologist should be consulted for any questions about treatment.

Parents initially have difficulty believing the seriousness of CAH unless the diagnosis was made during an episode of acute adrenal insufficiency. However, once they experience the rapidity with which their child can change from being robustly healthy to being deathly ill, they may become very fearful of future episodes. It is difficult for these parents to find a balance between protecting their child from serious harm and allowing them to have an active, normal life. This balance needs to be assessed at each primary care visit by asking about the child's social and academic progress, outside interests and activities, and special concerns. Any problem areas should then be discussed.

The child with CAH may experience emotional disturbances related to the multiple factors involved in having this chronic condition, including being concerned about sexuality and fertility, being perceived and treated as different by others (including their parents), receiving mixed or confusing messages from health care personnel, being overprotected by their parents, and dealing with their own fears related to life-threatening crises they may have experienced. Psychotherapy is indicated for significant emotional disturbance and behavioral problems and has proved to be helpful (Jones et al, 1970).

Newborn siblings should be screened for CAH. At birth their plasma renin activity and serum electrolyte levels should be evaluated, and at 24 to 36 hours of age their serum 17-OHP level should be checked (Hughes, Riad-Fahmy, and Griffiths, 1979). All older male and female siblings with virilization or accelerated growth should also be screened. Testing for the carrier state is available (although costly) and should be explained to unaffected siblings and other first-degree relatives (New, 1995).

The impact of CAH on a family will vary with their cultural beliefs regarding the causation of congenital disorders and with their attitudes toward sexuality. The primary care providers must determine what these beliefs are in order to provide sensitive and successful care to the child and family. Families will usually tell providers their beliefs if providers ask.

Individuals from cultures in which sexual topics are not openly discussed can be expected to have difficulty asking questions about CAH. The primary care provider and endocrinologist are faced with the challenge of presenting information on a sensitive subject without offending the family's values. It may be helpful to have a male health care provider speak to the men in the family and a female provider speak separately to the women in the family.

Resources

At present there is no national organization for CAH, but individual families can ask to be introduced to each other through their endocrinology clinic. Literature available on the subject of CAH is typically produced by individual medical centers and is available to patients and health professionals who request it (usually for a small charge).

Informational materials

Burnett J: A boy with CAH. *Am J Nurs* 80:1306-1308, 1980.
This article is easy to read, and families will identify with the description of life with a child with CAH. This is also a good article to give to school and child care personnel because it gives a simple explanation of the disorder and its management without overwhelming the reader with technical information.

From Department of Education, University of Wisconsin Hospital, 600 Highland Ave, Madison, WI 53792:

Guidelines for the Child Who is Cortisol Dependent, a leaflet for parents with information on cortisone replacement and illness management.
How to Mix and Inject Injectable Hydrocortisone, a small pamphlet for parents with a clear description of this procedure.
Congenital Adrenal Hyperplasia, an 8-page handout explaining CAH and its management. It is primarily for families but also is of interest to professionals unfamiliar with CAH.

From Patient/Parent Education Department, British Columbia's Children's Hospital, 4480 Oak St, Vancouver, British Columbia, V6H 3V4, Canada:

Congenital Adrenal Hyperplasia, a 28-page illustrated booklet describing the condition and treatment. It is primarily for families but also is of interest to professionals unfamiliar with CAH.
Hydrocortisone/Florinef Handout, a concise 2-page handout for parents that includes information on illness management.

From Pediatric Endocrinology, CB 7220, Burnett-Womack, University of North Carolina at Chapel Hill, Chapel Hill, NC 27599:

Medication Instructions for Patients with Congenital Adrenal Hyperplasia, instructions for families. It also describes dosages.

From Pediatric Endocrinology Nursing Society, PO Box 2933, Gaithersburg, MD, 20886-2933:

Cortisol Replacement Therapy, a booklet of instructions on cortisol replacement, primarily for families but also of interest to professionals unfamiliar with cortisol replacement.

Organizations

Pediatric Endocrinology Nursing Society (PENS): This organization has members in many regions who are willing to speak to parent, school, professional, or other groups. For information, write to PENS, PO Box 2933, Gaithersburg, MD, 20886-2933

Products

From Medic-Alert Foundation, PO Box 1009, Turlock, CA 95381-1009: Medic-Alert bracelets and necklaces, which are recommended for all children with CAH.

SUMMARY OF PRIMARY CARE NEEDS FOR THE CHILD WITH CONGENITAL ADRENAL HYPERPLASIA

Health care maintenance

Growth and development

If CAH is diagnosed in infancy and adequately and consistently treated, growth and development is normal.

Accelerated linear growth occurs if CAH is inadequately treated.

Accelerated bone age advancement and early closure of epiphyses with reduced final adult height will occur if CAH is inadequately treated.

Stunted linear growth will occur if CAH is overtreated with hydrocortisone.

Precocious puberty may occur with improved treatment.

Diet

Children should be allowed to salt to taste and eat salty foods.

Safety

These children have no increased susceptibility to injury.

There is a risk of acute adrenal insufficiency with a serious injury (e.g., fracture, concussion).

A Medic-Alert bracelet or necklace should be worn.

Immunizations

Give all routine immunizations according to usual guidelines.

Giving additional vaccines (pneumococcal, influenza, varicella when available) is discretionary.

Increased stress doses of hydrocortisone are not necessary prophylactically unless there is a history of previous adverse reaction to the vaccine.

Give increased stress dose of hydrocortisone for immunization reactions involving fever, unusual malaise, and lethargy.

Giving acetaminophen before immunization with likelihood of febrile reaction (e.g., pertussis) is discretionary.

Routine screening

Vision

Routine screening is recommended.

Hearing

Routine screening is recommended.

Dental

Routine screening is recommended.

Blood pressure

Blood pressure should be checked at each visit (including infants). Children with abnormal findings should be referred to an endocrinologist.

Hematocrit

Routine screening is recommended.

Urinalysis

Routine screening is recommended.

Tuberculosis

Routine screening is recommended.

Special screening

Screening serum 17-OHP levels or 24-hour urine pregnanetriol values may be indicated and should be coordinated with the endocrinologist.

Checking plasma renin activity levels may be indicated and should be coordinated with the endocrinologist.

Bone age should be checked every 2 to 3 years, more often if there are indications of androgen excess.

Common illness management

Differential diagnosis

If the child has nausea or vomiting, pallor, cold moist skin, weakness, dizziness or confusion, rapid heart rate, rapid breathing, abdominal, back or leg pain, dehydration, or hypotension, acute adrenal insufficiency should be ruled out.

Temperature greater than 38.4° C, significant malaise, pain, lethargy, or persistent vomiting (regardless of cause) should be covered by stress doses of hydrocortisone in addition to appropriate specific therapy.

Continued.

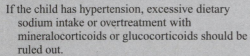

SUMMARY OF PRIMARY CARE NEEDS FOR THE CHILD WITH CONGENITAL ADRENAL HYPERPLASIA—cont'd

If the child has hypertension, excessive dietary sodium intake or overtreatment with mineralocorticoids or glucocorticoids should be ruled out.

If the child has hypotension, inadequate mineralocorticoid or glucocorticoid dosage should be ruled out.

Drug interactions

Long-term use of barbiturates, phenytoin, or rifampin increase the rate of metabolism of glucocorticoids. Adjustments in dosage may be required.

Developmental issues

Sleep patterns

Unusual fatigue or lethargy may indicate the need for increased doses of hydrocortisone.

Toileting

There is no impairment in readiness or functioning. Children with obvious virilization should be allowed privacy.

Discipline

Expectations are normal based on age and developmental level.

Physical appearance may differ from age and developmental level, leading to inappropriate expectations.

Child care

Child care providers must be aware of special needs with illness and injury and the importance of routine and stress medication.

Schooling

There are no special education needs.

School personnel should be aware of special needs regarding illness and injury.

Sexuality

Virilization of infant girls requires surgical correction.

Inadequate treatment results in continued virilization, menstrual irregularities, and infertility in girls and may impair fertility in boys.

Most will be fertile.

Transition into adulthood

Transition to providers of adult primary care and endocrine care.

Identify source of medical insurance.

Special family concerns

Rapid onset of acute adrenal insufficiency is possible.

Appropriate emergency treatment may be delayed because of lack of awareness or knowledge of CAH by health care providers.

The normality of girls should be stressed.

Others in the family may possibly be affected (siblings, children of affected child).

Family members may have difficulty speaking openly about sexuality and genitals.

REFERENCES

Bacon G et al: *A practical approach to pediatric endocrinology,* ed 3, Chicago, 1990, Year Book Medical Publishers, pp 157-182.

Bailez M et al: Vaginal reconstruction after initial construction of the external genitalia in girls with salt-wasting adrenal hyperplasia, *J Urology* 148:680-682, 1992.

Bartter F: Adrenogenital syndromes from physiology to chemistry (1950-1975). In Lee P, Plotnick L, Kowarski A, and Migeon C (editors): *Congenital adrenal hyperplasia,* Baltimore, 1977, University Park Press, pp 9-18.

Burnett J: A boy with CAH, *Am J Nurs* 80:1304-1305, 1980.

Dacou-Voutetakis C, Karidis N: Congenital adrenal hyperplasia complicated by central precocious puberty: treatment with

LHRH-agonist analog, *Ann N Y Acad Sciences* 687:250-254, 1993.

Darland N: Congenital adrenocortical hyperplasia: supportive nursing interventions, *J Pediatr Nurs* 1:117-123, 1986.

Dittmann R, Kappes M, and Kappes M: Sexual behavior in adolescent and adult females with congenital adrenal hyperplasia, *Psychoneuroendocrinology* 17:153-170, 1992.

Dittmann R et al: Congenital adrenal hyperplasia I: gender-related behavior and attitudes in female patients and sisters, *Psychoneuroendocrinology* 15:401-420, 1990a.

Dittmann R et al: Congenital adrenal hyperplasia II: gender-related behavior and attitudes in female salt-wasting and simple-virilizing patients, *Psychoneuroendocrinology* 15:421-434, 1990.

Donaldson M et al: Presentation, acute illness, and learning difficulties in salt-wasting 21-hydroxylase deficiency, *Arch Dis Child* 70:214-218, 1994.

Drucker S, New M: Nonclassic adrenal hyperplasia due to 21-hydroxylase deficiency. In Mahoney C (editor): *Pediatric clinics of North America: pediatric and adolescent endocrinology,* Philadelphia, 1987, WB Saunders, pp 1069-1081.

Duck S: Acceptable linear growth in congenital adrenal hyperplasia, *J Pediatr* 97:93-96, 1980.

Ehrhardt A, Baker S: Males and females with congenital adrenal hyperplasia: a family study of intelligence and gender-related behavior. In Lee P, Plotnick L, and Kowarski A (editors): *Congenital adrenal hyperplasia,* Baltimore, 1977, University Park Press, pp 447-461.

Fife D, Rappaport EB: Prevalence of salt-losing among congenital adrenal hyperplasia patients, *Clin Endocrinol* 18:259-264, 1983.

Galatzer A, Laron Z: The effects of prenatal androgens on behavior and cognitive functions. In M Forest (editor): *Androgens in childhood,* 1989, Karger, Basel, pp 98-103.

Hochberg Z, Gardos M, and Benderly A: Psychosexual outcome of assigned females and males with 46XX virilizing congenital adrenal hyperplasia, *Eur J Pediatr* 146:497-499, 1987.

Holmes C, Karlsson J, and Thompson R: Longitudinal evaluation of behavior patterns in children with short stature. In Stabler B and Underwood L, (editors): *Slow grows the child,* Hillsdale, NJ, 1986, Lawrence Erlbaum Assoc, pp 1-12.

Hughes IA, Riad-Fahmy D, and Griffiths K: Plasma 17 OH-progesterone concentrations in newborn infants, *Arch Dis Child* 54:347-349, 1979.

Jackson P, Ott M: Perceived self-esteem among children diagnosed with precocious puberty, *J Ped Nurs* 5:190-203, 1990.

Jones H, VerKauf B, Lewis V, et al: The relevance of surgical, psychologic, and endocrinologic factors to the long term end result of patient with congenital adrenal hyperplasia: A study of eighty-nine patients. *Int J. Gynaecol Obstet* 8: 398-401 1970.

Mazur T: Ambiguous genitalia: detection and counseling, *Pediatr Nurs* 9:417-422, 1983.

Money J, Schwartz M, and Lewis V: Adult erotosexual status and fetal hormonal masculinization and demasculization: 46XX congenital virilizing adrenal hyperplasia and 46XY androgen-insensitivity syndrome compared, *Psychoneuroendocrinology* 9:405-414, 1984.

Mulaikal R, Migeon C, and Rock J: Fertility rates in female patients with congenital adrenal hyperplasia as a result of 21-hydroxylase deficiency, *N Engl J Med* 316:178-182, 1987.

Mullis P, Hindmarsh P, and Brook C: Sodium chloride supplement at diagnosis and during infancy in children with salt-losing 21-hydroxylase deficiency, *Eur J Pediatr* 150:22-25, 1990.

Nass R, Baker S: Learning disabilities in children with congenital adrenal hyperplasia, *J Child Neurol* 6:306-312, 1991.

New M: Congenital adrenal hyperplasia. In DeGroot L et al, (editors): *Endocrinology,* ed 3, Philadelphia, 1995, WB Saunders, pp 1813-1835.

Ott M, Jackson P: Precocious puberty, *Nurse Practitioner* 14:21-30, 1989.

Pang S et al: Prenatal treatment of congenital adrenal hyperplasia due to 21-hydroxylase deficiency. (Review) *N Eng J. Med* 322(2):111-115, 1990.

Pang S et al: Worldwide experience in newborn screening for classical congenital adrenal hyperplasia as a result of 21-hydroxylase deficiency, *Pediatrics* 81:866-874, 1988.

Riley W, Rosenbloom A: Clitoral size in infancy, *J Pediatr* 96:918-919, 1980.

Rosler A et al: The interrelationship of sodium balance, plasma renin activity, and ACTH in congenital adrenal hyperplasia, *J Clin Endocrinol Metab* 45:500-512, 1977.

Sandrini R, Jospe N, and Migeon C: Temporal and individual variations in the dose of glucocorticoid used for the treatment of salt-losing congenital virilizing adrenal hyperplasia as a result of 21-hydroxylase deficiency, *Acta Paediatr Suppl* 388:56-60, 1993.

Srikanth M et al: Benign testicular tumors in children with congenital adrenal hyperplasia, *J Pediatr Surg* 27:639-641, 1992.

Stern N, Tuck M: The adrenal cortex and mineralocorticoid hypertension. In Lavin N, (editor): *Manual of endocrinology and metabolism,* Boston, 1986, Little, Brown, & Co, pp 107-130.

Young-Hyman D: Effects of short stature on social competence. In Stabler B and Underwood L (editors): *Slow grows the child,* Hillsdale, NJ, 1986, Lawrence Erlbaum Assoc, pp 27-45.

Congenital Heart Disease

15

Elizabeth H. Cook and Sarah S. Higgins

ETIOLOGY

Congenital heart disease (CHD) results from the abnormal development of structures within the heart or those leading to or from the heart. The condition is present, though not always manifested, at birth. Approximately one half of the infants born with congenital heart disease are symptomatic within the first year of life necessitating some form of intervention.

Congenital heart disease is commonly categorized as *acyanotic* or *cyanotic,* depending on the hemodynamic changes that occur as a result of the specific heart anomaly. In acyanotic heart disease, the systemic circulation is not exposed to unoxygenated blood; in cyanotic heart disease, unoxygenated blood mixes in the systemic circulation (see Fig. 15-1). A brief description of the intracardiac pressure-flow relationship may clarify this classification of CHD.

Blood returns to the heart from the venous system depleted of oxygen and enters the right atrium. From the right atrium, blood flows through the tricuspid valve into the right ventricle where it is pumped through the pulmonary arteries into the lungs to pick up oxygen. The oxygen saturation in the right side of the heart is therefore low (approximately 70%). Additionally, the pressure in the right-sided circulation is relatively low, ~$25/2$ mm Hg in the right ventricle and ~$25/10$ mm Hg in the pulmonary arteries.

The blood that enters the left atrium from the lungs is rich in oxygen, with the oxygen saturation reaching 95% to 100%. The blood flows through the mitral valve into the left ventricle where it is pumped into the systemic circulation via the aorta. Pressure in the left ventricle is under high pressure, ~$100/5$ mm Hg, and ~$100/60$ mm Hg in the aorta.

Because the pressure in the left side of the heart is greater than the pressure in the right side of the heart, blood will flow from the left to the right side of the heart if there is an abnormal connection between the two sides. This is called *left-to-right shunting.* Because of the significant difference in left- and right-sided pressure and oxygen saturations, heart defects that cause left-to-right shunting are acyanotic. Left-to-right shunts commonly cause overcirculation of the lungs and may result in congestive heart failure (CHF).

Cyanosis usually results from one or both of the following physiologic problems: (1) right-to-left shunting, which results from blood flow obstruction to the lungs plus an intracardiac communication, or (2) intracardiac mixing of oxygenated and deoxygenated blood. A summary and illustration of the most common defects, as created by Ross Laboratories (1970), can be found in Fig. 15-2. Additional information on cardiovascular disorders in children can be found in Hazinski (1992).

Most heart defects occur within the first 8 weeks of gestation (Nora, 1989). Approximately 90% of congenital heart defects have a multifactor-

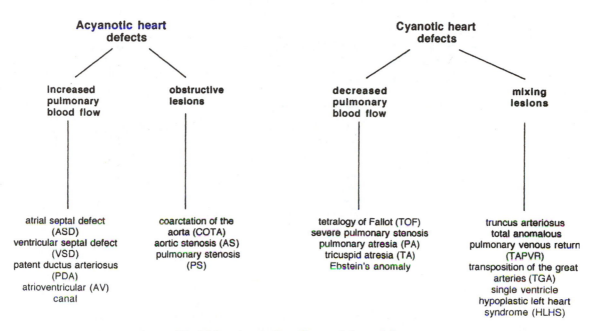

CLASSIFICATION OF CONGENITAL HEART DEFECTS

Acyanotic heart defects

- **Increased pulmonary blood flow**
  - atrial septal defect (ASD)
  - ventricular septal defect (VSD)
  - patent ductus arteriosus (PDA)
  - atrioventricular (AV) canal

- **obstructive lesions**
  - coarctation of the aorta (COTA)
  - aortic stenosis (AS)
  - pulmonary stenosis (PS)

Cyanotic heart defects

- **decreased pulmonary blood flow**
  - tetralogy of Fallot (TOF)
  - severe pulmonary stenosis
  - pulmonary atresia (PA)
  - tricuspid atresia (TA)
  - Ebstein's anomaly

- **mixing lesions**
  - truncus arteriosus
  - total anomalous pulmonary venous return (TAPVR)
  - transposition of the great arteries (TGA)
  - single ventricle
  - hypoplastic left heart syndrome (HLHS)

Fig. 15-1.   Acyanotic and cyanotic heart defects.

ial cause, in which there is an interplay of a genetic predisposition for cardiac maldevelopment with an environmental trigger (such as a virus or maternal ingestion of certain drugs) at the vulnerable time of cardiac development (Nora, 1989).

Genetic factors account for about 8% of CHD and are usually associated with a syndrome in which other systems are also affected (see Table 15-1). One of the most common genetic associations with CHD is Down syndrome; approximately 40% of these children have a heart defect (Ferencz et al, 1989). (See Chapter 18). Other syndromes, such as asplenia syndrome, DiGeorge syndrome, or VACTERL* syndrome, which do not have an identified chromosomal defect, frequently have CHD as one of many anomalies.

Maternal exposure to environmental effects during cardiac development of the fetus may also result in heart defects (see Table 15-1). A purely environmental cause for the development of CHD is estimated at 2% to 3% (Nora, 1989). The vulnerable period for exposure to a cardiac teratogen is during the first 8 weeks of gestation.

INCIDENCE

Congenital heart disease generally occurs in 0.8% to 1% of live births (Fyler, 1992a). The incidence of specific heart defects is presented in Table 15-2. Boys tend to have a higher overall incidence of CHD, and certain defects exhibit some sex preference.

The recurrence risk of CHD in the same family depends on several factors. If one child has a heart defect, the recurrence risk is about 1% to 4%, with the risk being higher in more common heart defects,

---

*VACTERL syndrome refers to abnormalities of vertebra, anus, cardiovascular tree, trachea, esophagus, renal system, and limb buds.

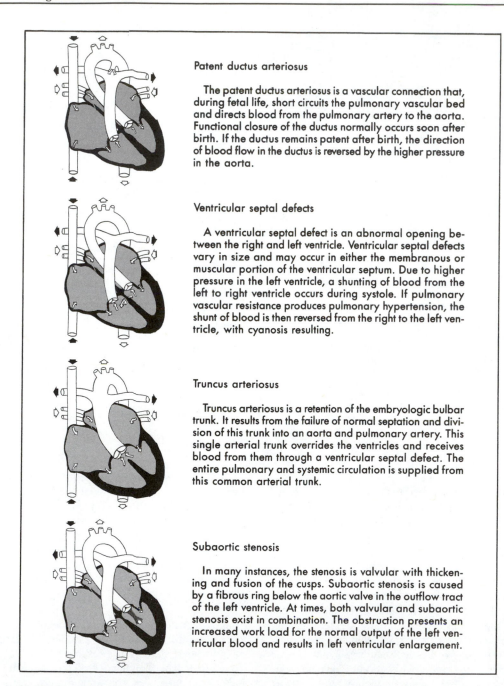

Patent ductus arteriosus

The patent ductus arteriosus is a vascular connection that, during fetal life, short circuits the pulmonary vascular bed and directs blood from the pulmonary artery to the aorta. Functional closure of the ductus normally occurs soon after birth. If the ductus remains patent after birth, the direction of blood flow in the ductus is reversed by the higher pressure in the aorta.

Ventricular septal defects

A ventricular septal defect is an abnormal opening between the right and left ventricle. Ventricular septal defects vary in size and may occur in either the membranous or muscular portion of the ventricular septum. Due to higher pressure in the left ventricle, a shunting of blood from the left to right ventricle occurs during systole. If pulmonary vascular resistance produces pulmonary hypertension, the shunt of blood is then reversed from the right to the left ventricle, with cyanosis resulting.

Truncus arteriosus

Truncus arteriosus is a retention of the embryologic bulbar trunk. It results from the failure of normal septation and division of this trunk into an aorta and pulmonary artery. This single arterial trunk overrides the ventricles and receives blood from them through a ventricular septal defect. The entire pulmonary and systemic circulation is supplied from this common arterial trunk.

Subaortic stenosis

In many instances, the stenosis is valvular with thickening and fusion of the cusps. Subaortic stenosis is caused by a fibrous ring below the aortic valve in the outflow tract of the left ventricle. At times, both valvular and subaortic stenosis exist in combination. The obstruction presents an increased work load for the normal output of the left ventricular blood and results in left ventricular enlargement.

Fig. 15-2.   Congenital heart abnormalities. Reprinted with permission of Ross Laboratories, Columbus, OH 43216, from Clinical Education Aid No. 7. Copyright 1970 Ross Laboratories.

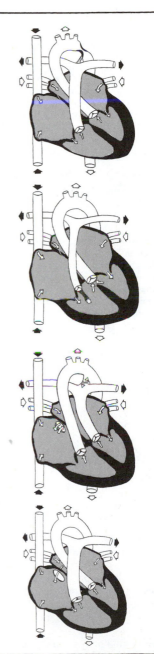

Coarctation of the aorta

Coarctation of the aorta is characterized by a narrowed aortic lumen. It exists as a preductal or postductal obstruction, depending on the position of the obstruction in relation to the ductus arteriosus. Coarctations exist with great variation in anatomic features. The lesion produces an obstruction to the flow of blood through the aorta causing an increased left ventricular pressure and work load.

Tetralogy of Fallot

Tetralogy of Fallot is characterized by the combination of four defects: (1) pulmonary stenosis, (2) ventricular septal defect, (3) overriding aorta, (4) hypertrophy of right ventricle. It is the most common defect causing cyanosis in patients surviving beyond two years of age. The severity of symptoms depends on the degree of pulmonary stenosis, the size of the ventricular septal defect, and the degree to which the aorta overrides the septal defect.

Complete transposition of great vessels

The anomaly is an embryologic defect caused by a straight division of the bulbar trunk without normal spiraling. As a result, the aorta originates from the right ventricle, and the pulmonary artery from the left ventricle. An abnormal communication between the two circulations must be present to sustain life.

Atrial septal defects

An atrial septal defect is an abnormal opening between the right and left atria. Basically, three types of abnormalities result from incorrect development of the atrial septum. An incompetent foramen ovale is the most common defect. The high ostium secundum defect results from abnormal development of the septum secundum. Improper development of the septum primum produces a basal opening known as an ostium primum defect, frequently involving the atrio-ventricular valves. In general, left to right shunting of blood occurs in all atrial septal defects.

Fig. 15-2. Congenital heart abnormalities.

Continued.

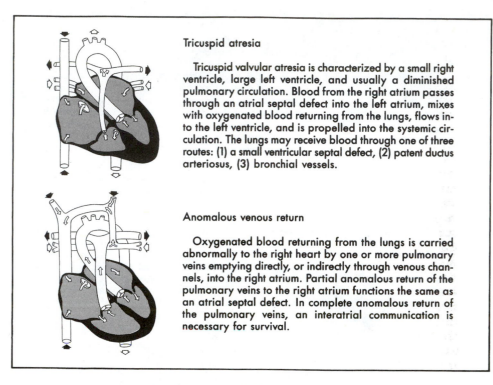

Tricuspid atresia

Tricuspid valvular atresia is characterized by a small right ventricle, large left ventricle, and usually a diminished pulmonary circulation. Blood from the right atrium passes through an atrial septal defect into the left atrium, mixes with oxygenated blood returning from the lungs, flows into the left ventricle, and is propelled into the systemic circulation. The lungs may receive blood through one of three routes: (1) a small ventricular septal defect, (2) patent ductus arteriosus, (3) bronchial vessels.

Anomalous venous return

Oxygenated blood returning from the lungs is carried abnormally to the right heart by one or more pulmonary veins emptying directly, or indirectly through venous channels, into the right atrium. Partial anomalous return of the pulmonary veins to the right atrium functions the same as an atrial septal defect. In complete anomalous return of the pulmonary veins, an interatrial communication is necessary for survival.

Fig. 15-2.   Congenital heart abnormalities.

than in defects with a lower incidence. If two first-degree relatives are affected, the recurrence risk is approximately tripled. If the defect is part of a syndrome or chromosomal abnormality the recurrence risk of the heart lesion is related to the recurrence risk of the syndrome. The recurrence risk if a mother has CHD may be from 2% to as high as 18%, whereas the risk to offspring if the father is affected is approximately 1% to 3% (Nora, 1989; Nora and Nora, 1987). Additional information indicates that certain left-sided cardiac lesions, most notably hypoplastic left heart syndrome, have a very high recurrence rate (Boughman et al, 1987).

CLINICAL MANIFESTATIONS AT TIME OF DIAGNOSIS

The clinical presentation of a child with CHD will vary depending on the specific defect. Symptoms usually relate to the degree of CHF or cyanosis.

CLINICAL MANIFESTATIONS OF CHD

- Congestive heart failure
  - -tachypnea
  - -tachycardia
  - -hepatomegaly
  - -dyspnea
  - -pale, cool skin
  - -diaphoresis
  - -periorbital edema
  - -persistent, dry cough
  - -poor feeding; failure to thrive
  - -easily fatigued
- Cyanosis
  - -blue coloration of lips, gums, nailbeds, around the eyes and mouth, skin and mucous membranes
  - -slowed growth
  - -decreased activity
  - -polycythemia

Table 15-1.   CONDITIONS COMMONLY ASSOCIATED WITH CARDIAC MALFORMATIONS

Condition	Associated defect
Infant syndrome	
Trisomy 13 syndrome	VSD, PDA, dextrocardia
Trisomy 18 syndrome	VSD, PDA, PS
Trisomy 21 syndrome	AV canal, VSD, ASD
Turner's syndrome	COTA, ASD, AS
Marfan syndrome	Great artery aneurysms, aortic insufficiency (AI), mitral regurgitation (MR)
Noonan's syndrome	PS, ASD, idiopathic hypertrophic subaortic stenosis (IHSS)
Cri du chat syndrome	VSD, PDA, ASD
Ellis-van Creveld syndrome	ASD, single atrium
Osteogenesis imperfecta	Aortic valve disease
DiGeorge syndrome	Interrupted aortic arch, TOF, truncus arteriosus, ASD
Holt-Oram syndrome	ASD, VSD, single atrium
Treacher Collins syndrome	VSD, PDA, ASD
Asplenia syndrome	VSD, single ventricle, common AV valve, TGA
VACTERL syndrome	TOF
Maternal condition	
Rubella	PDA, ASD, VSD, peripheral pulmonary stenosis
Diabetes	TGA, VSD, COTA, cardiomegaly
Lupus erythematosis	Heart block
Phenylketonuria	TOF, VSD, ASD
Maternal ingestion	
Alcohol	VSD, PDA, ASD
Trimethadione	TGA, TOF, HLHS
Lithium	Ebstein's anomaly, ASD, TA
Retinoic acid	VSD
Amphetamines	VSD, PDA, ASD, TGA
Hydantoin	PS, AS, COTA, PDA
Sex hormones	VSD, TGA, TOF
Thalidomide	TOF, truncus arteriosus, VSD, ASD

Adapted from Nora JJ: Etiologic aspects of heart disease. In Adams FH and Emmanouilides GC, eds: *Moss's Heart Disease in Infants, Children and Adolescents,* ed 4, Baltimore, 1989, Williams and Wilkins, pp 15-23.

Congestive Heart Failure

The majority of cases of CHF result from CHD, and most of these cases occur within the first year of life. Congestive heart failure occurs when there is a strain on the myocardium from pressure or volume overload that is severe enough to reduce cardiac output to a level insufficient to meet the body's metabolic demands (Freed, 1992). Symptoms of CHF result from the decreased cardiac output and the body's compensatory mechanisms. These include cardiac hypertrophy, cardiac dilatation, and stimulation of the sympathetic nervous system. The infant with CHF will be tachypneic, dyspneic, tachycardic, pale, cool, diaphoretic, and easily fatigued. Additional symptoms include periorbital edema, hepatomegaly, and a persistent cough. A history of difficult feeding and decreased food intake are classic signs of CHF. Failure to thrive is therefore common in the infant with CHF.

Table 15-2.
INCIDENCE OF SPECIFIC HEART DEFECTS

Defect	CHD (%)
Ventricular septal defect (VSD)	20-25
Patent ductus arteriosus (PDA)	10 (excluding premature)
Tetralogy of Fallot (TOF)	10
Coarctation of the aorta (COTA)	8
Atrial septal defect (ASD)	5-10
Pulmonary stenosis (PS)	5-8
Transposition of the great arteries (TGA)	5
Aortic stenosis (AS)	5
Atrioventricular (AV) canal	3-4
Hydroplastic left heart syndrome (HLHS)	1-2
Tricuspid atresia (TA)	1-2
Total anomalous pulmonary venous return (TAPVR)	1
Pulmonary atresia (PA)	<1
Ebstein's anomaly	<1
Truncus arteriosus	<1
Single ventricle	<1

From Park MK: *Pediatric cardiology for practitioners,* ed 2, Chicago, 1988, Year Book Publishers.

Congestive heart failure is manifested in the neonate with a severe cardiac defect such as transposition of the great arteries, hypoplastic left heart syndrome, or critical aortic stenosis. Infants with defects causing large left-to-right shunts such as PDA, AV canal defect, or VSD usually do not develop symptoms until 4 to 8 weeks of age, when the high pulmonary vascular resistance of the fetal period becomes low enough to cause increased pulmonary blood flow. The onset of symptoms is usually gradual, with tachypnea, changes in feeding patterns, and poor weight gain often being early clues. Premature infants with a left-to-right shunt may develop symptoms of CHF earlier than a term infant because pulmonary vascular resistance drops faster than in the term infant.

Hypoxemia and Cyanosis

Hypoxemia is defined as the presence of arterial oxygen saturation that is less than normal. *Cyanosis* is the blue coloration of the skin and mucous membranes caused by deoxygenated hemoglobin. The coloration is usually seen in the lips, gums, nail beds, and around the eyes and mouth. Cyanosis is more difficult to detect in children with dark skin pigmentation and is perceived best by observing mucous membranes and nail beds in natural light. The child with cyanosis often has slowed growth, although he or she is not usually a poor feeder. Polycythemia occurs in the child who is chronically hypoxemic as the body attempts to increase its oxygen-carrying capacity. Toddlers who are cyanotic usually limit their activity but will still become easily fatigued and breathless if running, climbing stairs, or playing for long periods of time. The child with symptomatic tetralogy of Fallot may assume a squatting position for relief of exertional dyspnea and fatigue. Increasing cyanosis may be subtle and difficult to discern; monitoring an increasing hemoglobin may help in the determination of progressive hypoxemia (O'Brien and Smith, 1994).

TREATMENT

Medical management of the child with CHD is aimed at allowing the infant to grow and the organs to mature so surgery can be performed at the optimal time. One goal of primary care management is

TREATMENT OF CHD

- Control CHF
- Support feeding
- Monitor for worsening cyanosis
- Cardiac catheterization—diagnostic or interventional
- Time surgery based on defect and symptoms

to control CHF, which is usually achieved with the use of digitalis and diuretics. Since failure to thrive is a common complication of CHF, support with feeding also becomes a priority in management. Support may include methods of decreasing fatigue during feeding, increasing the caloric concentration of formula, and occasionally providing gavage feeding.

The infant who is cyanotic additionally requires monitoring for progressive cyanosis, anemia, and dehydration. The parents of the child who is cyanotic must learn to identify increasing blueness and cyanotic spells. The parents can be taught the knee-chest position to alleviate cyanotic spells (Higgins and Kashani, 1986).

The decision for surgery depends on the severity of the lesion, associated defects, the child's age and size, concurrent medical or surgical problems, and family and cultural factors. The cardiologist follows the progress of the defect through cardiac ultrasound or echocardiography. For an increasing number of defects, this diagnostic technique provides all of the information needed to perform surgery (Sanders, 1992). For several cardiac defects, however, a cardiac catheterization or MRI may also be performed before surgery to determine the precise anatomy and physiology of the child's heart.

The natural history of some defects such as VSD, PDA, and ASD is such that spontaneous improvement may occur thus avoiding surgery. Most lesions, however, require surgery. The timing of surgical intervention varies among cardiac centers. As surgical techniques improve, the trend nationwide is toward earlier corrective surgery, often by early or middle infancy.

Crucial factors in determining the timing of surgery include the prevention of irreversible pulmonary hypertension, the prevention of the development of aortopulmonary collateral vessels, and the maintenance of adequate ventricular function. Large left-to-right shunts rarely cause irreversible changes in the pulmonary vasculature before 12 to 18 months of age. Once these irreversible changes occur however, surgery is contraindicated and the child will become progressively cyanotic.

Some neonates with complex defects require an initial palliative surgery at birth with definitive surgery occurring later. These infants have either inadequate pulmonary blood flow or uncontrolled CHF. They need close follow-up after surgery to ensure that pulmonary blood flow is maintained (when cyanotic) and excessive pulmonary blood flow is restricted (with CHF).

Infants who need surgery are followed closely by the cardiologist to manage CHF or cyanosis and to time surgery. Communication between the cardiologist and the primary care provider is important. Symptoms of increasing tachypnea, decreasing feeding, slowed weight gain, or increased cyanosis should be reported to the cardiologist.

Children whose cardiac defects warrant delaying surgery for several years include those who rarely develop early pulmonary hypertension or myocardial strain, such as small PDAs, ASDs, VSDs, and mild coarctation of the aorta. These children are usually asymptomatic. They may have more contact with their primary care provider than their cardiologist after initial diagnosis so communication with the cardiologist is again important.

For an increasing number of defects, interventional cardiac catheterization has replaced surgery as the treatment of choice. Some forms of aortic and pulmonary valvar or vascular stenosis can be repaired through balloon valvuloplasty and angioplasty. Vascular stents are being placed within the vessel to maintain patency of stenosed vessels after balloon angioplasty has been performed. Closure of PDAs, septal defects, and unnecessary collateral blood vessels is being performed through placement of various occlusion devices within the defect (Radtke, 1994; Callow, 1994). In addition, electrophysiologic studies in conjunction with cardiac catheterization are used to identify cardiac dysrhythmias, evaluate the effectiveness of certain drugs under controlled circumstances, and in some cases abolish or ablate the accessory pathway causing the dysrhythmia (Darling, 1994; Finkelmeier, 1994). As the field of interventional cardiac catheterization continues to develop, it is becoming a valuable therapy in managing many children with CHD.

RECENT AND ANTICIPATED ADVANCES IN DIAGNOSIS AND MANAGEMENT

The field of interventional cardiac catheterization is still in the early stages of development. Further advances in devices and techniques will continue to expand treatment options for the child with CHD. Simultaneously, the use of echocardiography as the primary diagnostic tool in CHD is decreasing the need for purely diagnostic cardiac catheterizations. Clinical electrophysiology is another growing field; rhythm control, whether it is accomplished through advanced antiarrhythmic drugs, ablative therapy, or implantable devices will continue to evolve as more clinical experience is gained and new technologies are refined. Several mechanical assist devices for children with cardiac failure are being used to provide circulatory support until myocardial function recovers. These interventions have met with varied success and will continue to evolve.

ASSOCIATED PROBLEMS

Hematologic Problems

Children with cyanotic heart disease develop polycythemia to increase the oxygen-carrying capacity of the blood. If the hematocrit reaches 70% or higher, there is a marked increase in the viscosity of the blood, an increase in the tendency for thrombus formation, and a possible decrease in oxygen delivery (Nadas, 1992). Bleeding disorders are also seen in the child with polycythemia, most commonly thrombocytopenia and defective platelet aggregation. These children may bruise easily or develop petechiae, gingival bleeding, or epistaxis (Park, 1996).

Anemia can be a special problem in the child with CHD. In the child with existing CHF, a decreased hemoglobin may exacerbate myocardial strain. In the infant who is cyanotic, iron deficiency anemia has been associated with cerebral vascular accidents and slowed growth (O'Brien and Smith, 1994). Children who are cyanotic with a low hematocrit may exhibit hypoxic spells more readily than if the oxygen-carrying capacity of the blood were normal. Cyanosis will not be as obvious in the child with anemia as in the child with a normal or elevated hemoglobin. Because of these problems associated with anemia, the child with an acyanotic heart defect should have a hemoglobin within normal range for their age; the child with a cyanotic heart defect should have a hemoglobin value of at

ASSOCIATED PROBLEMS IN CHD

- Hematologic
  - Polycythemia
  - Bleeding disorders
  - Anemia
- Recurrent respiratory infections
- Infective endocarditis
- CNS complications
  - Brain abscess in older children who are cyanotic
  - CVA
- Dysrhythmias
- Failure to thrive
- Slowed growth and development
- Vulnerable child syndrome

least 16 gm/dl (Gidding and Rosenthal, 1984). Although it is important for the child who is cyanotic with a low hematocrit to receive iron therapy, it is equally important to monitor the response to the therapy in order to prevent the hematocrit from rising to undesirably high levels thus increasing blood viscosity (Fyler and Nadas, 1992).

Adequate hydration must be maintained in children with cyanotic heart disease to avoid increased hemoconcentration. Problems associated with fever and exposure to hot weather can cause excessive perspiration; vomiting and diarrhea can cause dehydration (Miner and Canobbio, 1994).

Infectious Processes

Children with significant heart defects are at high risk for developing a variety of infections. Recurrent respiratory tract infections are especially common in children with lesions causing increased pulmonary blood flow. Other systemic infections such as sinusitis are common nonspecific infections seen in the older child who is cyanotic. Infections can significantly effect the child's health in the following ways: (1) severe respiratory tract infections can exacerbate hypoxemia in the cyanotic child; (2) fever can increase oxygen demands and precipitate myocardial decompensation; (3) dehydration in a child with polycythemia can lead to thrombus formation; and (4) electrolyte imbalances from vomiting, diarrhea, or fever in a child receiving digoxin can lead to digoxin toxicity.

The child with asplenia syndrome (a condition that includes absence of the spleen and complex cardiac defects) is extremely susceptible to bacteremia; *Streptococcus pneumonia, Haemophilus influenza type B,* and *Neisseria meningitidis* are the most common pathogens. Daily antimicrobial prophylaxis should be strongly considered for children under 5 years of age with asplenia syndrome. Some experts continue prophylaxis throughout childhood and into adulthood in particularly high-risk clients with asplenia. Recommended dosage is 125 mg of penicillin G or V twice daily, or 20 mg of amoxicillin/kg/day, or 4 mg/kg/day of trimethoprim and 20 mg/kg/day of sulfamethaxozole (Septra) for children less than 5 years of age. For children more than 5 years of age, 250 mg of penicillin twice daily is recommended (Committee on Infectious Diseases, 1994).

Infective Endocarditis

Endocarditis may occur because of blood-borne bacteria lodging on damaged or abnormal heart valves, on prosthetic material, or on the endocardium near congenital anatomic defects. Endocarditis may occur if prophylaxis precautions are not followed during all dental procedures, incision and drainage of infected tissue, and surgical or invasive procedures involving mucosal surfaces or contaminated tissues (Dajani et al, 1990) (see box on endocarditis prophylaxis, pg 306). The most common organisms are streptococci and staphylococci, which account for 80% to 90% of the cases (Park, 1994).

Central Nervous System Complications

In children who are cyanotic, bacteria normally filtered out of the blood in the pulmonary circulation may be shunted directly to the systemic circulation. As a result, these children are at increased risk for brain abscess, most commonly after 2 years of age. Infants who are cyanotic with iron deficiency anemia are prone to develop cerebral vascular accidents. A possible explanation for this finding is that relative anemia secondary to cyanosis leads to increased blood viscosity and increased coagulability, and thus venous thrombosis (Newberger, 1992a).

Dysrhythmias

Rhythm disturbances can occur in the child with CHD as a direct result of the cardiac defect or from the surgical repair. Atrial dysrhythmias are more common in children than ventricular rhythm disturbances. Infants with Ebstein's anomaly are predisposed to develop supraventricular tachycardia (SVT). Anatomically corrected transposition of the great arteries (L-TGA) is a rare congenital heart defect which may also lead to SVT or varying degrees of heart block.

Postoperatively, disturbances in atrial rhythms may be seen in children after surgical manipulation of the atrium, such as in the Fontan procedure, repair of total anomalous pulmonary venous return (TAPVR), ASD repair, or the Mustard procedure. Postoperative second- or third-degree heart block may occur in surgeries involving the ventricular septum, such as repair of VSD, atrioventricular (AV) canal repair, and TOF repair. In addition, children who have had a complete repair of TOF can develop ventricular dysrhythmias, which rarely leads to sudden death (Denfield and Garson, 1990).

Digoxin toxicity can cause a wide variety of dysrhythmias, including profound bradycardia, ventricular dysrhythmias, and varying degrees of heart block (Koren and Gorodischer, 1992). A low serum potassium concentration potentiates the effects of digoxin. A child receiving a non–potassium-sparing diuretic such as furosemide (Lasix) without potassium replacement may be at particular risk of digoxin toxicity. A therapeutic digoxin level is generally 0.5 to 2 ng/ml, although toxicity has been seen at lower levels and toxicity may not be seen at higher levels in some infants (Koren and Gorodischer, 1992). A sound rule is to assume that a dysrhythmia noted in a child on digoxin therapy is caused by digoxin until proved otherwise. If extra beats or an abnormal rhythm, including bradycardia and tachycardia, is identified by the primary care provider, an electrocardiogram should be obtained and the child should be referred to the cardiologist for further evaluation as soon as possible.

Failure to Thrive

Growth failure has been frequently observed in children with CHD (Barton et al, 1994; Gaedeke

INFECTIVE ENDOCARDITIS PROPHYLAXIS*

Cardiac conditions

Endocarditis prophylaxis recommended

Prosthetic cardiac valves
Most congenital cardiac malformations
Rheumatic and other acquired valvular dysfunction
Previous history of bacterial endocarditis
Mitral valve prolapse with valvular regurgitation
Hypertrophic cardiomyopathy

Endocarditis prophylaxis not recommended

Isolated secundum atrial septal defect
Surgical repair without residua beyond 6 months of
    secundum ASD, VSD, or PDA
Physiologic, functional, or innocent heart murmurs
Mitral valve prolapse without valvular
    regurgitation
Previous Kawasaki disease without valvular
    dysfunction
Previous rheumatic fever without valvular
    dysfunction
Indwelling cardiac pacemakers

Procedures for which endocarditis prophylaxis is recommended

Dental procedures known to induce gingival or
    mucosal bleeding, including professional
    cleaning
Tonsillectomy and/or adenoidectomy
Surgical procedures that involve intestinal or
    respiratory mucosa
Bronchoscopy with rigid bronchoscope, or with
    biopsy
Cystoscopy
Urethral dilatation
Urethral catheterization if urinary tract infection is
    present
Urinary tract surgery if urinary tract infection is
    present
Incision and drainage of infected tissue
Vaginal delivery in the presence of infection

Procedures for which endocarditis prophylaxis is not recommended

Dental procedures not likely to cause gingival
    bleeding, such as simple adjustment of
    orthodontic appliances or fillings above the gum
    line
Shedding of deciduous teeth
Insertion of tympanostomy tubes
Bronchoscopy with flexible bronchoscope, or
    without biopsy
Endotracheal intubation
Cardiac catheterization
Endoscopy with or without gastrointestinal biopsy
Cesarean section
In the absence of infection for urethral
    catheterization, dilatation and curettage,
    uncomplicated vaginal delivery, therapeutic
    abortion, sterilization procedures, or insertion or
    removal of intrauterine devices

From Dajani, AS et al.: Prevention of bacterial endocarditis, JAMA 264:2919-2922. Copyright 1990 by American Medical
Association. Adapted by permission.
*This table lists common pediatric conditions and procedures but is not meant to be all inclusive

Norris and Hill, 1994; Salzer et al, 1989). The decreased growth is usually more pronounced in weight than in height. Congestive heart failure is one of the most potent factors in the development of failure to thrive because of both inadequate caloric intake secondary to tachypnea and the relative hypermetabolism associated with CHF and pulmonary hypertension (Barton et al, 1994; Bougle et al, 1986; Salzer et al, 1989).

Growth failure is particularly important to recognize because it may suggest significant hemodynamic compromise necessitating an alteration in the drug regimen or surgery. Corrective surgery, particularly in infancy, generally restores a normal growth pattern. Weight usually improves more quickly than height. Palliative surgery generally improves growth, though not to the same degree as corrective surgery.

ENDOCARDITIS PROPHYLAXIS RECOMMENDATIONS*

For dental procedures and surgery of the upper respiratory tract

1. For most patients: amoxicillin 50 mg/kg (maximum 3.0 g) orally 1 hour before procedure; then half the dose 6 hours after the initial dose
2. For patients allergic to amoxicillin or penicillin: erythromycin ethylsuccinate 20 mg/kg (maximum 800 mg) or erythromycin stearate 20 mg/kg (maximum 1.0 g) orally 2 hours before procedure; then half the dose 6 hours after the initial dose;

or

clindamycin 10 mg/kg (maximum 300 mg) orally 1 hour before procedure; then half the dose 6 hours after the initial dose
3. For patients unable to take oral medications: ampicillin 50 mg/kg (maximum 2.0 g) IM or IV 30 minutes before the procedure; then half the dose 6 hours after the initial dose
4. For patients allergic to penicillin who are unable to take oral medications: clindamycin 10 mg/kg (maximum 300 mg) IV 30 minutes before the procedure; then half the dose 5 hours after the initial dose
5. For high-risk patients no candidates for standard regimen: ampicillin 50 mg/kg (maximum 2.0 g) IV, plus gentamicin 2.0 mg/kg (maximum 80 mg) IV, 30 minutes before procedure; then

amoxicillin 25 mg/kg (maximum 1.5 g) orally 6 hours after initial dose; alternatively, the IV dose may be repeated 8 hours after initial dose
6. For high-risk patients allergic to penicillin: vancomycin 20 mg/kg (maximum 1.0 g) IV starting 1 hour before procedure; no repeat dose necessary

For gastrointestinal and genitourinary tract procedures and surgery

1. For most patients: ampicillin, gentamicin, and amoxicillin. Ampicillin 50 mg/kg (maximum 2.0 g) IM or IV, plus gentamicin 2.0 mg/kg (maximum 80 mg) IM or IV 30 minutes before procedure; then amoxicillin 50 mg/kg (maximum 1.5 g) orally 6 hours after the initial dose; alternatively, the IV regimen may be repeated once 8 hours after initial dose
2. For patients allergic to penicillin: vancomycin and gentamicin. Vancomycin 20 mg/kg (maximum 1.0 g) IV, over 1 hour + gentamicin 2.0 mg/kg (maximum 80 mg) IV, 1 hour before procedure; may be repeated once 8 hours after initial dose
3. For low-risk patients: amoxicillin 50 mg/kg (maximum 3.0 g) orally 1 hour before procedure; then half the dose 6 hours after initial dose

From Dajani, AS et al.: Prevention of bacterial endocarditis, JAMA, 264:2919-2922. Copyright 1990 by American Medical Association. Adapted by permission.

*The American Heart Association recommends the standard oral prophylactic regimen to patients who have prosthetic heart valves and in other high-risk groups. Some practitioners may prefer to use parenteral prophylaxis in these high-risk group patients.

Development

The majority of children with CHD show development within the normal range (Wright and Nolan, 1994). However, studies of the effects of cyanosis on IQ have suggested that children who are cyanotic may have a lag in intellectual development (Linde, Rasof, and Dunn, 1970; Wright and Nolan, 1994). Generally, early correction of cyanotic lesions results in improved intellectual functioning (Newberger et al, 1984; Newberger, 1992a). CHF and cyanosis may significantly affect gross motor development. The child with CHD may sit, crawl, and walk much later than his or her peers. Parental overprotection and lack of activity may also contribute to delayed development (Linde, Rasof, and Dunn, 1966). Although delayed development has been identified, researchers have emphasized that both cyanotic and acyanotic groups have IQs well within the normal range, and the practical importance of the difference in IQ may be insignificant (O'Brien and Smith, 1994; Wright and Nolan, 1994).

Vulnerable Child Syndrome

Although overprotection may be a problem for the child with a chronic condition in general, the child with a heart defect is at high risk for overprotection and altered parent-infant attachment (Goldberg et al, 1991). Parental anxiety can occur as a result of the disturbing array of clinical symptoms of a child with CHF or cyanosis, feeding problems, and the fear of a sudden catastrophic event (D'Antonio, 1976; Goldberg et al, 1991; Higgins and Kashani, 1984; Stinson and McKeever, 1995). However, the mere presence of the defect unrelated to the severity of the heart disease can produce severe anxiety leading to overprotection and inappropriate limits being placed on the child (Linde, Rasof, and Dunn, 1966; Wright and Nolan, 1994). Because over-protection may delay the development in a child with existing physical impediments to development, the primary care provider should be aware of feelings of vulnerability in the parents and child and reinforce the importance of treating the child normally.

PROGNOSIS

The prognosis for children with CHD is good for the majority of lesions. Only the most complex defects require multiple surgeries. Therefore many children have had their definitive repair by their first or second year. The surgical mortality for the less complex defects is generally less than 5% (Park, 1994). Children with these defects usually are symptom-free postoperatively and do not require further surgery. The operative risk for some complex lesions may be as low as 5% to 10%, but can rise to 20% to 25% for the series of surgical procedures required with severe lesions (Park, 1994). The majority of children after surgery require long-term assessment of potential problems related to myocardial changes, ventricular failure, prosthetic materials, electrophysiologic sequelae, and infective endocarditis (Higgins, 1994).

Primary Care Management

HEALTH CARE MAINTENANCE

Growth and Development

Significant delays in both height and weight are seen in children with symptomatic CHD (Barton et al, 1994; Salzer et al, 1989). Generally height is not affected as much as weight, and head circumference is not affected at all by CHD. If growth is slowed to a point where the child's growth curve flattens, the child should be referred to the cardiologist for an evaluation of worsening CHF. A weight gain of approximately 1 pound a month is acceptable for the infant with controlled CHF (Higgins, 1987). Because the growth of a child whose CHF is well controlled may still be slow, it is important to look at trends of weight gain in addition to comparison with the norms.

In assessing the developmental and emotional status of the child with CHD, the primary care provider needs to take into account factors such as hypoxemia, CHF, parental overprotection, and physical incapacity. Preoperatively the infant with CHF is often too exhausted to pass all of the developmental tasks in screening tests. If a child is developing at a slower but progressive rate, referral for additional developmental testing is not immediately warranted. If there appear to be significant alterations in the level of alertness or if there is no progress in mastering developmental tasks, further screening is advised. If CHD is part of a syndrome which involves developmental delay, referral and enrollment in an infant stimulation program would be important.

Crying is a major developmental concern of most parents of children with CHD. They worry that crying will hurt the heart or precipitate a medical crisis. Parents need to be informed that short periods of crying will not harm the infant. They should treat crying as if the child did not have a heart defect. Parents can be counseled that prompt attention to crying will usually console the infant faster (Barnard, 1978) and reduce crying and irritability in subsequent months (Bell and Ainsworth, 1970). Parents should attend to the child who is crying for these reasons, not because crying is dangerous for the child. Discuss crying issues with both parents because there frequently are differences in philosophies and subsequent conflicts between parents regarding crying in children.

When discussing developmental concerns with parents, it is critical to help parents normalize responses to their child who has a chronic condition. The primary care provider can guide the parents in treating the child normally, reinforcing that children who are symptomatic will limit themselves naturally.

Diet

Feeding is often a major problem for children with CHD, particularly if they are in CHF. The infant in CHF often has difficulty coordinating the suck, swallow, and breath of feeding. The distribution of calories in these infants is similar to the recommended dietary allowances; however, caloric needs of infants in CHF with failure to thrive are about 150kcal/kg/day (Gaedeke Norris and Hill, 1994). If the infant is not gaining weight adequately, the caloric intake may need to be increased by concentrating formula. Concentrating the formula to 24 to 30 calories per ounce will improve total calories without increasing total volume. If formula is concentrated by decreasing the amount of water added to powder or concentrate, it is important to consider the increased renal solute load the infant receives. An alternative is to add low osmolarity glucose polymers or oils to standard formulas to increase the caloric density. A diet providing increased carbohydrates and fats may lead to increased retention of nitrogen for growth (Gaedeke Norris and Hill, 1994). Two common preparations used are Polycose, which delivers 23 calories per 15 cc, and medium chain triglycerides (or MCT oil), which delivers 120 calories per 15 cc. Consulting with a nutritionist and the cardiologist would be advised if nutritional manipulations are used.

Breast feeding the child with even a hemodynamically significant heart defect is not contraindicated if growth is adequate. Breast milk is the best source of nutrition for the child with CHD (Committee on Nutrition, American Academy of Pediatrics, 1985; Gidding and Rosenthal, 1984). The physiologic stress of breast feeding may actually be less than the stress related to bottle feeding (Meier and Anderson, 1987). Methods to decrease the work of feeding during breast or bottle feeding include holding the infant at a 45 degree angle to minimize

tachypnea, feeding for no more than 40 minutes at a time to minimize fatigue, allowing the infant to develop his or her own rhythm of feeding and resting, and following the infant's cues for hunger, satiety, and tiring (Higgins and Kashani, 1984).

Rarely, a child will not gain weight despite aggressive feeding and formula concentration. This child may need gavage feeding to minimize calories used with feeding. Using a pacifier during gavage feeding will help the infant develop a strong suck, facilitate the transition to oral feeding after surgery, and promote future language development (Bernbaum et al, 1983).

Parents often need a tremendous amount of support around feeding the child with CHD. The child with CHF and tachypnea has difficulty consuming adequate calories to satisfy hunger and may be irritable. Both the infant and mother may contribute to a less than optimal feeding situation. Infants with CHD give fewer feeding cues and respond less to caregivers, and mothers of infants with CHD may exhibit less fostering behavior such as eye contact, smiling, and cuddling the infant during feeding (Lobo, Barnard, and Coombs, 1992). Parents may also feel the pressure of getting the child to gain weight for surgery. In addition, a parent's self-esteem may be tied to feeding and growth of the child (D'Antonio, 1976). The primary care provider should stress to the parents that feeding can be a positive time for bonding and nurturing. Ongoing support includes teaching the parents to be sensitive to the infant's cues for hunger, satiety, and distress; pointing out the positive aspects of the child; and reinforcing their feeding skills. Through feeding, the parent and child are developing their relationship (Satter, 1986). The primary care provider who understands the potential problems with feeding can be instrumental in fostering a positive feeding relationship by providing support and counseling.

Safety

In addition to standard safety precautions, the child with CHD has unique safety needs. For example, digoxin elixir has a pleasant taste and attractive color, which increases the potential for accidental ingestion by the child or siblings. Therefore safe storage and administration of medications is essential. A surprising number of parents have inadequate knowledge for safely and wisely administering digoxin to their children (Jackson, 1979). Marking a syringe at the correct dose, giving written instructions on medication administration, and allowing the parent to practice drawing the medication will help ensure the safe use of digoxin, a valuable but potentially dangerous medication.

Electrical safety is critical for the child with a permanent pacemaker. An electric shock may irreparably damage the pacemaker requiring immediate surgical replacement. There is no risk of electromagnetic interference between a permanent pacemaker and common household items such as electrical appliances, radios, cellular phones, or electronic equipment. Microwave ovens and the pacemaker itself have filtering systems which prevent interference with the pacemaker's function. Large magnets placed directly over the pacemaker will temporarily change its function; magnetic resonance imaging (MRI) is therefore contraindicated for a child with a permanent pacemaker (Moses et al: 1987). Metal detectors should also be avoided because they have an electromagnetic field that may alter the pacemaker's function temporarily as well as set off the alarm as a result of the metal in the pacemaker. Small magnet toys, however, will not alter the pacemaker's function. A pacemaker identification card or letter from the primary care provider should be sufficient to avoid the metal detector. Older children with pacemakers and children on anticoagulants should wear Medic-Alert bracelets for emergencies.

Children with permanent pacemakers or on anticoagulants for prosthetic valves can maintain most normal activities. They should be counseled to avoid contact sports (such as football, boxing, or karate) which could damage the pacemaker or cause excessive bleeding (American College of Cardiology and American College of Sports Medicine, 1994; Shannon, 1986).

Travel may need to be altered for the child with CHD. Altitudes of 5000 feet or above are not recommended for children with moderate to severe pulmonary hypertension, severe CHF, or significant hypoxemia ($PO_2 < 50$ mm Hg) (Gidding and Rosenthal, 1984; Canobbio, 1987). Flying for these children may require precautions because cabin pressure is usually equivalent to an altitude of 5000 to 7500 feet. Supplemental oxygen can be supplied by the airlines to increase the inspired oxygen to 20%.

It has been reported that cardiopulmonary resuscitation (CPR) training for parents of children with CHD is effective and particularly warranted for certain problems (Higgins, Hardy, and Higashino, 1989). Suggesting CPR training to parents as a skill that is worthwhile for any parent to know can allay potential concerns about the importance of learning CPR. The American Red Cross or the American Heart Association may offer CPR training to families.

Immunizations

The standard immunization protocol, including varicella vaccine, is recommended for children with CHD. However, a significant percentage of infants with CHD either never receive immunizations or receive them well after the recommended dates (Gidding and Rosenthal, 1984; Uzark et al, 1983). Standard guidelines for immunization against hepatitis A and B should be followed for children with CHD. Immunizations should not be given before cardiac catheterization or surgery because a fever would delay the procedure. After surgery, immunizations should be delayed approximately 6 weeks so a fever from an immunization is not confused with a postoperative infection.

Children with hemodynamically significant CHD may be more susceptible to complications of influenza and should receive the influenza vaccine yearly beginning at 6 months of age (Committee on Infectious Diseases, 1994). Recommended dosage is 0.25 cc from 6 to 35 months and 0.5 cc thereafter. Polyvalent pneumococcal vaccine is recommended for all children who have asplenia and are 2 years old and older as a single intramuscular or subcutaneous 0.5 ml dose (Committee on Infectious Diseases, 1994).

Screening

Vision. Routine screening is recommended.

Hearing. Routine screening is recommended.

Dental. Routine dental care should be meticulously followed to prevent caries and gum disease that may predispose the child to bacteremia if left untreated. Endocarditis prophylaxis is recommended during all dental procedures except simple adjustment of braces and shedding of deciduous teeth (Dajani et al, 1990) (see boxes on pp 306).

Because oral procedures such as dental cleaning, drilling at the gum level, or pulling a permanent tooth all produce a higher inoculum of bacteria over a longer period of time than shedding of deciduous teeth, antibiotic coverage is recommended for these procedures (Danilowicz, 1995). Nearly all children with CHD need antibiotic prophylaxis both before and after dental procedures. The specific regimen depends on the type of defect, the procedure being performed, and the child's sensitivity to penicillin. This information should be communicated to the dentist by the child's cardiologist. Wallet size cards that outline specific prophylaxis regimens are available from the American Heart Association.

Blood pressure. Blood pressure should be obtained in upper and lower extremities for children with preoperative or postoperative repair of the aorta to identify discrepancies in pressure readings which may indicate progression of the heart defect. A child who has had a Blalock-Taussig shunt procedure to increase blood flow to the lungs will have a diminished or absent pulse in the upper extremity on the side of the surgical scar.

Hematocrit. A rise in hemoglobin and hematocrit may indicate progressive hypoxemia in the child with a cyanotic heart defect. Furthermore, because of the problems associated with anemia in the child with cyanosis or CHF, hemoglobin and hematocrit should be checked regularly. Iron supplementation should be prescribed if the hemoglobin is low for the child's specific condition. Since the child's cardiologist will be checking these values periodically, communication with the cardiologist may save the child the pain and expense of repeated laboratory tests.

Urinalysis. Routine screening is recommended.

Tuberculosis. Routine screening is recommended.

COMMON ILLNESS MANAGEMENT

Differential Diagnosis

Children with CHD may be susceptible to certain common pediatric problems which can be more severe than in the child with a structurally normal heart. It is important for the primary care provider

---

SCREENING

- Vision, hearing, tuberculosis, and urinalysis— routine recommended
- Dental—endocarditis precautions
- Blood pressure—check upper and lower
  extremities in child with
  COTA
  check contralateral arm of
  scar after Blalock-Taussig
  shunt
- Hematocrit—anemia problematic in CHF and
  cyanosis
  rising hct in cyanotic child may
  indicate progressive cyanosis

DIFFERENTIAL DIAGNOSIS

- Fever
    focus found: intercurrent illness unrelated to
      CHD postoperative:
    -wound infection: wound erythema, drainage
    -postpericardiotomy syndrome: pericardial
      friction rub, malaise, chest pain
    -infective endocarditis: malaise, anorexia,
      night sweats, new murmur
- Respiratory compromise
    URI or LRI: fever, productive cough, infil
      trates on CXR
    CHF: poor feeding, sweating, dry cough,
      cardiomegaly
- Gastrointestinal symptoms
    Acute gastroenteritis
    Digoxin toxicity
    Worsening CHF
- Neurologic symptoms
    CVA
    Brain abscess

to know these common problems which can lead to serious complications. It is equally important, however, to treat these children normally and look for the simple, uncomplicated problems. Families need reinforcement that the children are normal with special medical needs. Children who have had heart surgery are often scared or hesitant to allow an examination, particularly of their chest. Taking the time to gain the trust of the child before the examination will make visits less stressful for the child and more productive for the primary care provider.

Fever. Though febrile illnesses can have serious consequences in the child with CHD, an acute fever may also be caused by a common, uncomplicated childhood illness. The primary care provider should investigate and treat a fever the same way he or she would for any child the same age, keeping in mind the more serious possibilities. The chronic use of antibiotics without a diagnosis just because the child has CHD is not warranted and will put the child at risk of developing infections from resistant organisms (Lieberman, 1994; Woodin and Morrison, 1994).

A fever within a few weeks after heart surgery may be a sign of an operative infection or postpericardiotomy syndrome (an inflammatory reaction of the pericardial sac after heart surgery). A careful and complete examination is necessary to identify a source of infection. If no focus of infection such as otitis media or pharyngitis is found, the primary care provider should obtain a complete blood count (CBC) with differential and a blood culture and should consult with or refer the child to the cardiologist or surgeon. In addition, if there are any signs of a superficial wound infection, the child should be referred to the cardiologist or surgeon. Postpericardiotomy syndrome should be suspected by the presence of a fever soon after surgery with a pericardial friction rub, chest pain, malaise, or enlargement of the cardiac silhouette on a chest x-ray. It is rarely seen in children under 2 years of age. Generally it appears 7 days to 2 months after surgery (Fyler, 1992b). Referral to the cardiologist is necessary.

A fever will increase the metabolic demands thus the work of the heart. It is therefore important to evaluate the febrile child with symptomatic CHD for the development of or worsening CHF.

The infant or child with asplenia is at particular risk for infection. These children need to be seen by the primary care provider immediately on developing a fever for a complete work-up to identify the cause and initiate antibiotic therapy.

Infective endocarditis. The primary care provider should be alert to signs of endocarditis in a child with CHD who has a sustained, unexplained fever, because symptomatology may be nonspecific and insidious. Fever may be associated with decreased activity, anorexia, malaise, night sweats, petechiae, splenomegaly, or a new murmur. Children with an unexplained fever and these symptoms should be referred to their cardiologist for evaluation, including an echocardiogram, to look for vegetations within the heart. Blood cultures should be drawn before initiating antibiotics. Infective endocarditis rarely is seen in children under 2 years of age. Children at high risk are those who are cyanotic, have palliative systemic to pulmonary shunts, have prosthetic valves, and those with obstructive defects (Newberger, 1992b).

Parents' knowledge of measures to prevent endocarditis is limited (Cetta et al, 1993). It is therefore critical that the primary care provider reinforce endocarditis prophylaxis instructions at each visit.

Respiratory infection. The child with CHD, particularly the child with a defect causing left-to-right shunting, may have frequent or significant upper and lower respiratory infections. It is important to evaluate the degree of respiratory compromise compared to the child's baseline respiratory status. If there is an increase in respiratory effort or the presence of adventitious breath sounds, a chest x-ray should be obtained to rule out pneumonia or worsening CHF. Infiltrates by x-ray, fever, and productive cough could indicate a lower respiratory infection; cardiomegaly, poor feeding, sweating, and a dry cough would signal CHF. The primary care provider should have follow-up contact with the family 24 hours after initial contact to evaluate the child's progress.

Gastrointestinal symptoms. Vomiting or anorexia may occur secondary to gastroenteritis, worsening CHF, or digoxin toxicity. The child must be evaluated for other symptoms of CHF and a serum digoxin level obtained if the history and physical findings are not compatible with more common causes of gastrointestinal (GI) symptoms.

Excessive fluid losses from vomiting, diarrhea, or anorexia can lead to dehydration and thrombus formation in the child who is cyanotic and polycythemic. Replacement fluids or consultation with the cardiologist to hold diuretic therapy may be necessary until the GI disturbance is resolved.

Neurologic symptoms. The child with unexplained fever, headache, focal neurologic signs, or seizures requires immediate referral to a medical center because of the risk of a brain abscess or cerebrovascular accident (CVA).

Chest pain. Only a very small percentage of children complaining of chest pain have symptoms caused by significant cardiovascular abnormality (Hardy, 1994). The majority of these children have pain associated with musculoskeletal problems (such as costochondritis or trauma), pulmonary conditions (such as reactive airway disease, bronchitis, or pneumonia), hyperventilation, gastrointestinal reflux, or psychogenic chest pain (which is fairly common in adolescents). Cardiac etiologies of chest pain include coronary artery ischemia, tachydysrhythmias (particularly in toddlers who may be unable to differentiate pain from unusual sensations of dysrhythmias), myocarditis, or pericarditis.

Critical components in the child's history that may clarify the cause are: (1) Is the chest pain related to exercise, eating, or breathing? (2) Is there related lightheadedness or syncope? (3) Are there any other serious medical problems? (4) Is there unusual stress at home or school? (5) Is there a family history of sudden death or heart disease? (6) Did the child experience recent physical trauma or new physical activity? and (7) Is there a history of drug use? A careful history and physical examination can usually differentiate benign from dangerous conditions (Hardy, 1994). An electrocardiogram and referral to a cardiologist should occur if the primary care provider identifies chest pain in conjunction with syncope, dizziness, easy fatigue, palpitations, exertion, drug use, fever, or associated medical problems such as lupus erythematosis, diabetes, Marfan syndrome, or Kawasaki disease (Cohn, 1993; Hardy, 1994).

Syncope. *Syncope* is the transient loss of consciousness usually from decreased cerebral blood flow. Causes of syncope include autonomic nervous system abnormalities, cardiac dysrhythmias,

obstructive cardiac lesions, seizures, hyperventilation, vestibular diseases, drug use, or psychogenic causes. (Hardy, 1994; Heydemann, 1993). As with chest pain, a thorough history and physical examination are critical. Particular attention should be paid to the head, eyes, ears, nose, and throat for possible vestibular disease. A neurologic examination should be performed if symptoms suggest seizures, and cardiac auscultation to identify a murmur, click, or rub. Worrisome elements of the history include exercise-induced syncope or clonic-tonic movements suggesting seizures.

The most useful diagnostic test to evaluate for possible cardiac causes of syncope is the electrocardiogram (Hardy, 1994). Referral to a cardiologist for further evaluation including an exercise test and tilt-table test will be needed if the ECG is abnormal.

Drug Interactions

Children with CHF or dysrhythmias often receive combinations of digoxin, diuretics, and other medications. Several issues need to be considered when managing children on these medications: (1) coadministration of digoxin and quinidine (CinQuin), verapamil (Calan, Isoptin) or amiodarone (Cordarone) may elevate digoxin plasma concentrations (Koren and Gorodischer, 1992); (2) aminoglycosides can affect renal function and alter excretion of digoxin; (3) children with severe CHF may require medications such as captopril (Capoten) or enalapril (Vasotec) to decrease the resistance to left ventricular ejection (afterload) thus decrease the workload on the heart. These drugs may increase serum potassium. Therefore, if a child is on a potassium sparing diuretic such as spironolactone (Aldactone) and captopril, serum potassium should be checked periodically; (4) decongestants should be avoided in a child with a rapid heart dysrhythmia (e.g., supraventricular tachycardia or atrial fibrillation) or hypertension because they may exacerbate tachydysrhythmias or increase blood pressure; (5) aspirin should be avoided for 3 weeks before surgery because of its anticoagulant properties, and should be avoided altogether in children receiving coumadin. It is important for the primary care provider to counsel parents to read labels of over-the-counter medications since they may contain aspirin; (6) some antibiotics may alter the absorption of coumadin. Any time a child on coumadin requires antibiotics, the primary care provider should consult with the cardiologist before administering to prevent possible alteration of the prothrombin time.

The primary care provider may be monitoring certain drug levels (digoxin, antidysrhythmics) or response to drugs (prothrombin time in the child taking anticoagulants) in close association with the cardiologist.

DEVELOPMENTAL ISSUES

Sleep Patterns

Infants with CHF who are tachypneic may be unable to satisfy their hunger and have a difficult time sleeping through the night. Referral to the cardiologist is advised if the child's respiratory status is deteriorating to the point of interfering with feeding and sleeping. When discussing sleep with parents the primary care provider should ask the parents where the child sleeps. Because of the problem of parental anxiety and overprotection, some parents sleep with the child in the parents' bed for up to 2 years. The primary care provider should reinforce the stability of the child to help the parents deal with their anxiety. The transition to the child's bed should not occur when there has been a disruption in the child's routine or security, such as around hospitalization or surgery.

Toileting

The child on diuretic therapy may have difficulty with toilet training. If the child is receiving diuretics for a short period of time, the parents may want to delay toilet training until the medication has been discontinued. If the child is on chronic diuretic therapy, the timing of the diuretic may need to be adjusted to facilitate toilet training.

Discipline

Behavioral expectations of a child with CHD should be similar to those for a child without a heart defect. It is not uncommon for parents to overprotect and pamper children with CHD. Linde and associates (1966) observed that the mere label of congenital heart disease sets into motion complex changes in the family's approach and attitudes not only to the child with the disease but necessarily to his or her normal siblings. The primary care provider can play a key role in reinforcing the importance of setting limits and disciplining the child as if there were no heart disease and helping to normalize the family dynamics in light of the risk of overprotection.

On the other hand, the infant with CHF who is irritable, hard to console, and difficult to feed may present a very stressful situation for the parents. The primary care provider must be aware of the family stressors and infant characteristics that may lead to abuse in the child with a chronic condition.

Child Care

Some parents choose to stop work when they have a child with a chronic condition, but many do not have that option. Child care is necessary for most families. Several factors that need to be balanced when parents are deciding to return to work include: (1) the financial and emotional need to return to work, (2) parents' anxiety about leaving the child, (3) the increased incidence of infection for children in child care (Takala et al, 1995; Thacker et al, 1992) and the effect of infection on the child's cardiovascular status, and (4) parents' confidence in the child care provider's ability to recognize symptoms, give medications properly, and respond to emergencies appropriately.

Before surgery or cardiac catheterization, parents may be counseled to take their child out of child care to avoid exposure to infections which would cancel the procedure. Children with asplenia or DiGeorge syndrome are at the highest risk of infection. For these children who are prone to infection, home day care or small group day care would be advised. For 6 weeks after surgery, parents should limit the activities that stress the child's sternum, such as climbing, pulling, heavy lifting, rough playing, or lifting the child under the arms. The parents need to communicate these restrictions to the child care provider to see if it is realistic or safe to return the child to day care before normal activity is allowed. The primary care provider can play a key role in educating child care providers about the child's condition and reinforce activity limits, as well as lack of limits.

Schooling

Most school-aged children with CHD are able to attend school with their peers, though children with cyanotic heart disease are at risk of having difficulties in school (Wright and Nolan, 1994). Missed school is often related to hospitalizations, recuperation from surgery, and cardiology visits. The primary care provider can play an important role in assessing the need for home or in-hospital schooling for prolonged absences and facilitate services. Absenteeism may also be associated with the parents' perception of the child's vulnerability and lack of control over improving their child's health status (Fowler et al, 1987).

As children enter junior high and high school, they may have body image concerns related to their scar, their small stature, and their ability to keep up with peers. Parents frequently underestimate their child's activity tolerance (Casey et al, 1994) and adolescents with heart disease perceive their physical limitations as worse than medically indicated (Koster, 1994). In general, children should be encouraged to participate in physical activity to their tolerance based on discussions that include the child, primary care provider, cardiologist, parents, and school professionals (Committee on Sports Medicine and Fitness, 1994; Nelson, 1992). The American Heart Association has developed guidelines for activity for young clients with heart disease based on the particular defect and hemodynamic consequences (Gutgesell et al, 1986). Additionally, the Twenty-sixth Bethesda Conference in January, 1994, outlined in detail recommendations for determining the level of activity related to each congenital cardiac lesion, dysrhythmia, or acquired heart disease (American College of Cardiology, 1994).

A standard letter of recommendations for activity such as in Fig. 15-3 will clarify expectations and limits so the child can participate in physical activity to his or her highest potential. Stress testing may be performed by the cardiologist to develop an individualized activity plan. This information should be relayed to the primary care provider. An ongoing discussion with the parent and child will reinforce the realistic goals for activity and help to prevent overprotection.

Sexuality

Technologic and surgical advances have enabled the majority of young women with congenital heart disease to reach childbearing age. Many can successfully carry a pregnancy through delivery. A woman with complex congenital heart defects, however, warrants careful evaluation with respect to maternal and fetal risk (Canobbio, 1994). The increased risk of CHD in the offspring of persons with CHD should be discussed with a cardiologist or a genetic counselor before conception if possible.

The issues of contraception and the safety of pregnancy need to be discussed with the parents before their daughter becomes an adolescent and when the child is in early adolescence (Uzark, Von-Bargen-Mazza, and Messiter, 1989). Communication with the cardiologist will give the primary care provider critical information about the girl's risk factors for contraception and pregnancy given her particular physical status.

Oral contraceptives are not advised in women with pulmonary hypertension, cyanotic CHD, prosthetic valves, and those who smoke cigarettes because of the risks associated with increased coagulation and thrombus formation (Gleicher and Elkayam, 1990). Because of the potential for cervicitis and subsequent bacteremia, the intrauterine device (IUD) is contraindicated in women at risk for developing infective endocarditis (Canobbio, 1987; Gleicher and Elkayam, 1990). Barrier methods such as condoms and diaphragms with spermicidal cream are safe methods of birth control from a cardiac standpoint but are not as effective in preventing pregnancy. The condom represents the best method for preventing sexually transmitted diseases; with reliable use by her partner it is an acceptable form of contraception for the young woman with CHD (Gleicher and Elkayam, 1990).

For women at very high risk for cardiac compromise with pregnancy, surgical sterilization should be discussed. Tubal ligation in women with longstanding pulmonary hypertension leading to Eisenmenger's syndrome carries with it a high surgical risk and should not be performed unless absolutely necessary (Gleicher and Elkayam, 1990). If tubal ligation is recommended, it is best to wait, if possible, until young adulthood when the woman has gained maturity and can participate in the

---

RECOMMENDATIONS FOR PHYSICAL ACTIVITY IN SCHOOL
FOR CHILDREN WITH HEART DISEASE

DATE_____

To Whom it May Concern:

_____ is a patient of mine for a congenital heart condition. The
following recommendations are guidelines for physical activity in school. The child's cardiac diagnosis is
_____
_____.

_____(1) May participate in the entire physical education program, including varsity competitive sports
without any restriction.

_____(2) May participate in the entire physical education program EXCEPT for varsity competitive sports
where there is strenuous training and prolonged physical exertions, such as football, hockey, wrestling,
soccer, basketball, etc. Less strenuous sports such as baseball and golf are acceptable at varsity level. All
activities during the regular physical education program are acceptable.

_____(3) May participate in the physical education program except for restrictions from all varsity sports and
from excessively stressful activities such as rope climbing, weight lifting, sustained running (i.e., laps) and
fitness testing. MUST be allowed to stop and rest when tired.

_____(4) May participate only in mild physical activities such as walking, golf, and circle games.

_____(5) Restricted from the entire physical education program.

_____(6) Additional remarks: (see other side)

_____(7) Duration of recommendations: _____

If there are any additional questions about these recommendations, please contact me.

Sincerely,

_____ (cardiologist signature)

Fig. 15-3.   Sample letter of recommendation for activity.

---

decision (Canobbio, 1994). The preferred method of sterilization may therefore be vasectomy if there is one sexual partner.

Experts often look at the client's cardiovascular status based on the New York Heart Association (NYHA) Functional Classification to determine the relative risk of pregnancy. Adolescents with mild, unoperated heart disease or with well-repaired cardiac defects (NYHA Class I or II) are at no higher risk from pregnancy than the general population (Canobbio, 1987; Elkayam, Cobb, and Gleicher, 1990). The adolescent in class III will need special attention during pregnancy. The adolescent with pulmonary vascular disease or in CHF would be in

NYHA Functional Class IV. The young woman may not be able to safely carry a pregnancy to term and the pregnancy may need to be terminated for the safety of the mother (Gleicher and Elkayam, 1990). It is important for the primary care provider to discuss the risks of pregnancy with the cardiologist so the recommendation can be reinforced to the adolescent. A multidisciplinary approach involving the cardiologist, the high-risk obstetrician, and the primary care provider should be used for the adolescent with CHD who is pregnant.

Transition into Adulthood

There are approximately 600,000 adults with congenital heart disease in the United States, 400,000 of whom have had a surgical intervention (Perloff, 1991). Postoperative adolescents or adults are generally classified according to their clinical status: Category I—complete repair, asymptomatic; Category II—palliation/complete repair, asymptomatic; Category III—repair with residual defects, minimal; and Category IV—palliation/inoperable, moderate to severe symptoms (Canobbio, 1988). Problems requiring long-term follow-up include electrophysiologic sequelae, myocardial changes, prosthetic materials, ventricular failure, and infective endocarditis (Perloff, 1991).

The occurrence of dysrhythmias following intraatrial operations such as atrial septal defects is about 9%. Intraatrial baffling procedures (such as the Mustard procedure) for transposition of the great arteries has been essentially replaced by the arterial switch procedure because of the occurrence of dysrhythmias in over 50% of children and adolescents. The incidence of postoperative dysrhythmias in common intraventricular procedures is 30% in tetralogy of Fallot and 10% in ventricular septal defect repair (Vetter, 1991).

Additional long-term postoperative concerns include ventricular failure, which is particularly problematic after intraatrial baffling procedures and systemic to pulmonary shunts in functional single ventricles. Myocardial ischemia and fibrosis in open-heart repairs can effect the long-term performance of the myocardium (Somerville, 1991).

Synthetic valves can be associated with infective endocarditis and thromboembolism. These complications have been reduced with the use of human cadaver homograft valves which do not require anticoagulation and have a lower incidence of endocarditis (Tong, 1994).

Long-term surveillance of adolescents and adults with repaired or unrepaired congenital heart disease for infective endocarditis is of central importance. The individuals with the following conditions constitute the greatest risk: (1) rigid prosthetic valves, especially left-sided; (2) prosthetic conduits, such as the Fontan type operations; (3) cyanotic defects; (4) defects with high turbulence flow areas, such as VSDs; and (5) palliative shunts, such as the Blalock-Taussig anastamosis (Child and Perloff, 1991; Newberger, 1992b).

Evaluation for late postoperative concerns, as well as psychologic and social well-being is central as clients progress to adulthood. The goal for individuals who have survived congenital heart disease is to provide them with the best possible quality of life through their adulthood (Higgins and Reid, 1994).

SPECIAL FAMILY CONCERNS AND RESOURCES

The family of the child with CHD may have ongoing concerns about symptoms, feeding problems, sudden death, finances, and the long-term physical and emotional effects of multiple surgeries (Donovan, 1989). When parents are counseled about symptoms, it is important for the primary care provider to convey that the parents will be watching for trends over time rather than minute by minute. Reinforcing the fact that the parents become the expert in observing their child for changes decreases the parents' feelings that only health care providers can adequately monitor their child.

Young, Shyr, and Schork in a study (1994) found that a substantial number of parents of children with congenital heart disease believe that their primary care provider is unable to meet many of their children's illness needs. Parents' information needs related to caring for their infants following cardiac surgery are significant, and their level of understanding may be limited (Stinson and McKeever, 1995). Review of postoperative instructions by the primary care provider and ongoing, careful evaluation of the child will help solidify the parents' knowledge base and reinforce the health provider's position as a valuable asset to the child's care.

The insurability of a child with heart disease depends on the particular defect and repair. As children become older, they often lose their parents' coverage and have difficulty obtaining insurance as an adult (Canobbio, 1987; Hellstedt, 1994). Parents need to investigate the options for extended coverage of the child on their health insurance plan well in advance of the policy expiring for the child. Children with CHD may qualify for the supplemental insurance of Crippled Children's Services depending on their parents' income.

Parents may also be concerned about the occurence of CHD in subsequent children. Counseling a family about specific risks to future children should be performed by the cardiologist or genetic counselor; the primary care provider should then reinforce the information and support the family in their decision making. Early prenatal diagnosis of CHD is possible through ultrasound of the fetal heart (fetal echocardiogram).

Parent support groups are valuable resources and provide an important network for families coping with anxieties related to taking care of a child with CHD. Newsletters and special interest groups often develop from parent networking (see section on organizations at the end of this chapter). The primary care provider should contact the local American Heart Association (AHA) or the pediatric cardiology department to see if such groups exist. Written information covering many aspects of congenital heart disease is also available through the AHA. Public health or home health nursing may be an additional source of support, especially for the family learning to identify symptoms, give multiple medications, provide adequate nutrition to the newly diagnosed infant with CHD, or care for the child with complex home care needs.

Informational Materials

The following resource booklets and pamphlets are available for families through the local or national chapter of the AHA (this is not a complete listing of resources):
If Your Child Has a Heart Defect—A Guide for Parents
Feeding Infants with Heart Disease—A Guide for Parents
Dental Care for Children with Heart Disease
Abnormalities of Heart Rhythm—A Guide for Parents
Caring for a Child with a Heart Condition—A Guide for Parents [San Francisco Chapter]
Marfan's Syndrome
Kawasaki's Disease

Organizations
American Heart Association
   National Center
   7272 Greenville Ave
   Dallas, TX 75231
The Heartline Group, Inc.
   c/o Cindy & Harold Flocton
   229 Loving CT
   Sewell, NJ 08080-3005
   (609) 881-3734
This is a national newsletter for parents of children with complex CHD.
The Heart Connection
   415-666-6688 Sally Higgins RN, PhD consultant
This is a San Francisco Bay Area-based organization with monthly meetings for young adults with CHD.
Parents for Heart Support Group
Check with the local AHA for listings.

SUMMARY OF PRIMARY CARE NEEDS FOR THE CHILD WITH CONGENITAL HEART DISEASE

Health care maintenance

Growth and development

Significant delays in weight and height are common in children with symptomatic CHD preoperatively; corrective surgery improves growth.

Intellectual development is not significantly impaired by CHD; cyanosis, parental overprotection, and CHF may contribute to delayed development.

Infant crying is a major but unnecessary concern for parents.

Continued.

SUMMARY OF PRIMARY CARE NEEDS FOR THE CHILD WITH CONGENITAL HEART DISEASE—cont'd

Health care maintenance

Diet

Feeding is a major problem for the child with CHD, especially for the child in CHF; required daily allowances are normal, but formula may need to be concentrated for adequate caloric intake.

Breast feeding is encouraged if growth is adequate.

Teach methods to decrease work of breathing.

Feeding is a major source of stress for parents, who will need much support.

Safety

Safe storage of digoxin is critical.

For the child with a pacemaker, electrical safety is critical. There is no risk of damage with usual household appliances, including the microwave. Those with pacemakers should not have MRIs, should avoid metal detectors, and should wear a Medic-Alert bracelet.

Air travel and altitude may need to be limited depending on the defect.

Cardiopulmonary resuscitation training for parents is warranted for certain defects.

Immunizations

Standard immunization protocol is recommended; delay should occur only around cardiac catheterization or surgery.

With significant CHD, influenza vaccine is recommended.

With asplenia syndrome, daily antimicrobial prophylaxis and pneumococcal vaccine for children 2 years or older is recommended.

Screening

Vision

Routine screening is recommended.

Hearing

Routine screening is recommended.

Dental

Dental care is important to prevent caries, which predispose the child to bacteremia and endocarditis. Endocarditis prophylaxis is recommended for all dental procedures except routine adjustment of braces and shedding of deciduous teeth (see the boxes on pp. 306 and 307).

Blood pressure

Check blood pressure in all four extremities for children with coarctation of the aorta preoperatively and postoperatively. Child with a Blalock-Taussig shunt will have low or absent blood pressure values in the arm on the side of the shunt.

Hematocrit

A rise in hematocrit may indicate worsening cyanosis. Anemia is problematic in the child with CHF or cyanosis. Monitor hemoglobin levels closely in coordination with the cardiologist.

Urinalysis

Routine screening is recommended.

Tuberculosis

Routine screening is recommended.

Common illness management

Differential diagnosis

Fever

Postoperatively rule out (1) wound infection and (2) postpericardiotomy syndrome. If no focus is found, obtain CBC and blood culture. The child with asplenia with fever must be seen immediately.

Infective endocarditis

Symptoms are often vague; a high level of suspicion is needed to diagnose. It is rarely seen in children less than 2 years of age. Refer to the cardiologist if fever, malaise, anorexia, splenomegaly, or night sweats are present.

Respiratory infection

Frequent or significant upper and lower respiratory infections may occur; rule out CHF or pneumonia.

Gastrointestinal symptoms

Rule out digoxin toxicity and CHF; excessive fluid losses are dangerous in the child who is cyanotic or who is taking diuretics and digoxin.

Continued.

SUMMARY OF PRIMARY CARE NEEDS FOR THE CHILD WITH CONGENITAL HEART DISEASE—cont'd

Common illness management

Differential diagnosis

Neurologic symptoms

Cyanotic children are at increased risk of brain abscess (if >2 years) or CVA (if <2 years); unexplained fever, headaches, seizures, or focal neurologic signs need immediate referral to a medical center.

Chest pain

Most chest pain caused by noncardiac problems. Careful H&P usually differentiates benign from dangerous conditions.

Syncope

Many cardiac and noncardiac causes.

Close attention to HEENT to rule out vestibular disease.

ECG useful to rule out cardiac causes.

Drug interactions

Accurate administration of digoxin is critical.

Phenobarbital may lower the plasma level of digoxin.

Aminoglycosides may decrease renal function and increase the digoxin level.

Decongestants are not recommended for the child with rapid heart dysrhythmias or hypertension.

Digoxin or anticoagulant dosages may need to be monitored.

Developmental issues

Sleep patterns

Children may have difficulty sleeping through the night if they are tachypneic and unable to satisfy their hunger.

Toileting

Toilet training of the child receiving diuretics may be difficult.

Discipline

Normal behavior should be expected from children regardless of their CHD. Parents often overprotect and pamper children with CHD.

Child care

The provider must understand medications, must be able to recognize symptoms, and must know emergency procedures.

Infants with DiGeorge syndrome or asplenia syndrome are prone to infection; thus home day care or small group day care is recommended.

Vigorous activity is limited for 6 weeks after surgery.

Schooling

Children may need home tutoring around hospitalization and surgery time.

Self-image concerns about scar, keeping up with peers, and small stature may develop.

AHA publishes guidelines for activity limits based on each defect. Generally children limit themselves; the child who has a pacemaker or is taking anticoagulants should avoid rough contact sports.

Parents frequently underestimate their child's activity tolerance.

Sexuality

Oral contraceptives are not recommended for individuals with pulmonary hypertension, cyanotic CHD, or prosthetic valves.

An IUD is not recommended for individuals at risk for developing endocarditis.

Risks associated with pregnancy are determined by the individual's heart defect and functional ability as assessed by the cardiologist; teens need early and thorough counseling.

Transition into adulthood

Late postoperative concerns include dysrhythmias, ventricular failure, myocardial ischemia, prosthetic failure, thromboembolism, and infective endocarditis.

Special family concerns and resources

The family has ongoing concern about symptoms, multiple surgeries, and sudden death.

Insurability of the child is difficult.

Occurrence of CHD in subsequent children may be a concern; parents may want genetic counseling; prenatal diagnosis of CHD is possible through fetal echocardiography.

REFERENCES

American College of Cardiology and American College of Sports Medicine: 26th Bethesda conference. Recommendations for determining eligibility for competition in athletes with cardiovascular abnormalities. *J Am Coll Cardiol* 24:845-899, 1994.

Aram DM et al: Intelligence and hypoxemia in children with congenital heart disease: fact or artifact? *J Am Coll Cardiol* 6:889-893, 1985.

Barnard K: The nursing child assessment satellite training series. In *Learning resources manual,* Seattle, 1978, University of Washington School of Nursing Publications.

Barton JS et al: Energy expenditure in congenital heart disease. *Arch Dis Child* 70:5-9, 1994.

Bell SM and Ainsworth MDS: Infant crying and maternal responsiveness, *Child Dev* 43:1171-1190, 1970.

Bernbaum JC et al: Nonnutritive sucking during gavage feeding enhances growth and maturation in premature infants, *Pediatrics* 71:41-45, 1983.

Boughman JA et al: Familial risks of congenital heart defect assessed in a population-based epidemiologic study, *Am J Med Genet* 26:839-849, 1987.

Bougle D et al: Nutritional treatment of congenital heart disease, *Arch Dis Child* 61:799-801, 1986.

Callow LB: Nursing implications of interventional device placement in pediatric cardiology and pediatric cardiac surgery, *Crit Care Nurs Clin North Am* 6(1):133-151, 1994.

Canobbio MM: Counseling the adult with congenital heart disease. In WC Roberts, (editor): *Adult congenital heart disease,* Philadelphia, 1987, FA Davis.

Canobbio MM: Postoperative follow-up and counseling of adults with congenital heart disease. In CR Jillings, (editor): *Cardiac rehabilitation Nursing,* Baltimore, 1988, Aspen Publishers, pp 111-120.

Canobbio MM: Reproductive issues for the woman with congenital heart disease, *Nurs Clin North Am* 29(2):285-298, 1994.

Casey FA, Craig BG, and Mulholland HC: Quality of life in surgically palliated complex congenital heart disease, *Arch Dis Child* 70:382-386, 1994.

Cetta F et al: Parental knowledge of bacterial endocarditis prophylaxis, *Pediatr Cardiol* 14:220-222, 1993.

Child JS, Perloff JK: Infective endocarditis. In JK Perloff and JS Child, (editors): *Congenital heart disease in adults,* Philadelphia, 1991, WB Sanders, p 111.

Cohn HE: Chest pain. In RA Dershewitz, (editor): *Ambulatory pediatric care,* ed 2 Philadelphia, 1993, JB Lippincott Co, pp 228-231.

Committee on Infectious Diseases: *Report of the committee on infectious diseases,* ed 23, Elk Grove Village, Ill, 1994, The American Academy of Pediatrics, pp 57-61, 280-281, 372-375, 522, 525-532.

Committee on Nutrition: The American Academy of Pediatrics:

Pediatric nutrition handbook, ed 2, Elk Grove Village, Ill, 1985. The American Academy of Pediatrics, pp 1-15.

Committee on Sports Medicine and Fitness: Medical conditions affecting sports participation. *Pediatrics,* 94:757-760, 1994.

Dajani AS et al: Prevention of bacterial endocarditis: recommendations by the American Heart Association; *JAMA* 264:2919-2922, 1990.

Danilowicz D: Infective endocarditis, *Pediatrics in Review* 16:148-154, 1995.

D'Antonio IJ: Mothers' responses to the functioning and behavior of cardiac children in child-rearing situations, *Matern Child Nurs J* 5:207-256, 1976.

Darling EJ: Overview of cardiac electrophysiologic testing. *Crit Care Nurs Clin North Am* 6(1):1-14, 1994.

Denfield SW, Garson A Jr: Sudden death in children and young adults, *Pediatr Clin North Am* 37:215-231, 1990.

Donovan EF: Psychosocial considerations in congenital heart disease. In FH Adams and GC Emmanouilides, (editors): *Moss' heart disease in infants, children, and adolescents,* ed 4, Baltimore, 1989, Williams and Wilkins, pp 984-991.

Elkayam U, Cobb T, and Gleicher N: Congenital heart disease and pregnancy. In U Elkayam and N Gleicher, (editors): *Cardiac problems in pregnancy: diagnosis and management of maternal and fetal disease,* ed 2, New York, 1990, Alan R Liss, pp 73-98.

Ferencz C et al: Congenital cardiovascular malformations associated with chromosomal abnormalities: an epidemiologic study, *J Pediatri* 114:79-86, 1989.

Finkelmeier BA: Ablative therapy in the treatment of tachyarrhythmias, *Crit Care Nurs Clin North Am* 6(1):103-110, 1994.

Fowler MG et al: Factors related to school absence among children with cardiac conditions, *Am J Dis Child* 141:1317-1320, 1987.

Freed MD: Congestive heart failure. In DC Fyler, (editor): *Nadas' pediatric cardiology,* Philadelphia, 1992, Hanley and Belfus, Inc, pp 63-72.

Fyler DC: Trends. In DC Fyler, (editor): *Nadas' pediatric cardiology,* Philadelphia, 1992a, Hanley and Belfus, Inc, pp 273-280.

Fyler DC: Pericardial disease. In DC Fyler, (editor): *Nadas' pediatric cardiology,* Philadelphia, 1992b, Hanley and Belfus, Inc, pp 363-368.

Fyler DC, Nadas AS: History, physical examination, and laboratory tests. In DC Fyler, (editor): *Nadas' pediatric cardiology,* Philadelphia, 1992, Hanley and Belfus, Inc, pp 101-116.

Gaedeke Norris MK, Hill CS: Nutritional issues in infants and children with congenital heart disease, *Crit Care Nurs Clin North Am* 6(1):153-163, 1994.

Gidding SS, Rosenthal A: The interface between primary care and pediatric cardiology, *Pediatr Clin North Am* 31:1367-1388, 1984.

Gleicher N, Elkayam U: Fertility control in the cardiac patient. In U Elkayam and N Gleicher, (editors): *Cardiac problems in pregnancy: diagnosis and management of maternal and fetal disease,* ed 2, New York, 1990, Alan R Liss, pp 453-460.

Goldberg S et al: Congenital heart disease, parental stress, and infant-mother relationships, *J Pediatr* 119:661-666, 1991.

Gutgesell HP et al: Recreational and occupational recommendations for young patients with heart disease, *Circulation* 74:1195A-1198A, 1986.

Hardy CE: Syncope and chest pain: to worry, or not?, *Contemp Pediatr* 11:19-42, 1994.

Hazinski MF: Cardiovascular disorders. In MF Hazinsli, (editor): *Nursing care of the critically ill child,* ed 2, St Louis, 1992, Mosby, pp 117-394.

Hellstedt LF: Insurability issues facing the adolescent and adult with congenital heart disease, *Nurs Clin North Am* 29(2):331-343, 1994.

Heydemann PT: Syncope. In RA Dershewitz, (editor): *Ambulatory pediatric care,* ed 2, Philadelphia, 1993, JB Lippincott Co, pp 694-697.

Higgins SS: Long-term follow-up of the postoperative patient with congenital heart disease, *Nurs Clin North Am* 29(2):221-231, 1994.

Higgins SS: Patterns of impairment: congenital heart defects. In MH Rose and RB Thomas, (editors): *Children with chronic conditions: nursing in a family and community context,* Orlando, 1987, Grune and Stratton, pp 165-185.

Higgins SS, Hardy CE, and Higashino SM: Should parents of children with congenital heart disease and life-threatening dysrhythmias be taught cardiopulmonary resuscitation? *Pediatrics* 84:1102-1104, 1989.

Higgins SS, Kashani IA: Congestive heart failure: parent support and teaching, *Crit Care Nurse* 4(4):21-24, 1984.

Higgins SS, Kashani IA: The cyanotic child: heart defects and parental learning needs, *MCN* 11:259-262, 1986.

Higgins SS, Reid AR: Common congenital heart defects: long-term follow-up, *Nurs Clin North Am* 29(2):233-248, 1994.

Jackson PL: Digoxin therapy at home: keeping the child safe, *MCN* 4:106-109, 1979.

Koren G, Gorodischer R: Digoxin. In SJ Yaffe and JV Aranda, (editors): *Pediatric pharmacology: therapeutic principles in practice,* ed 2, Philadelphia, 1992, WB Saunders Co, pp 355-364.

Koster NK: Physical activity and congenital heart disease, *Nurs Clin North Am* 29(2):345-356, 1994.

Lieberman JM: Bacterial resistance in the '90s, *Contemp Pediatr* 11:72-99, 1994.

Linde LM et al: Attitudinal factors in congenital heart disease, *Pediatrics* 38:92-101, 1966.

Linde LM, Rasof B, and Dunn OJ: Longitudinal studies of intellectual and behavioral development in children with congenital heart disease, *Acta Paediatr Scand* 59:169-176, 1970.

Lobo ML, Barnard KE, and Coombs JB: Failure to thrive: a parent-infant interaction perspective, *J Pediatr Nurs* 7:252, 1992.

Meier P, Anderson GC: Responses of small preterm infants to bottle- and breast-feeding, *MCN* 12:97-105, 1987.

Miner PD, Canobbio MM: Care of the adult with cyanotic heart disease, *Nurs Clin North Am* 29(2):249-267, 1994.

Moses HW et al: *A practical guide to cardiac pacing,* ed 2, Boston, 1987, Little, Brown.

Nadas AS: Hypoxemia. In DC Fyler, (editor): *Nadas' pediatric cardiology,* Philadelphia, 1992, Hanley and Belfus, Inc, pp 73-76.

Nelson MA: Sports medicine. In SB Friedman, et al, (editors): *Comprehensive adolescent health care,* St Louis, 1992, Quality Medical Publishing, Inc, pp 1132-1151.

Newberger JW: Central nervous system sequelae of congenital heart disease. In DC Fyler, (editor): *Nadas' pediatric cardiology,* Philadelphia, 1992a, Hanley and Belfus, Inc, pp 77-82.

Newberger JW: Infective endocarditis. In DC Fyler, (editor): *Nadas' pediatric cardiology,* Philadelphia, 1992b, Hanley and Belfus, Inc, pp 369-376.

Newberger JW et al: Cognitive function and age at repair of transposition of the great arteries in children, *N Engl J Med* 310:1495-1499, 1984.

Nora JJ: Etiologic aspects of heart disease. In FH Adams and GC Emmanouilides, (editors): *Moss's heart disease in infants, children, and adolescents,* ed 4, Baltimore, 1989, Williams and Wilkins, pp 15-23.

Nora JJ, Nora AH: Maternal transmission of congenital heart diseases: new recurrence risk figures and questions of cytoplasmic inheritance and vulnerability to teratogens, *Am J Cardiol* 59:459-463, 1987.

O'Brien P, Smith PA: Chronic hypoxemia in children with cyanotic heart defects, *Crit Care Nurs Clin North Am* 6(1):215-226, 1994.

Park MK: *Pediatric cardiology for practitioners,* ed 3, St. Louis, 1996, Mosby.

Perloff SK: Congenital heart disease in adults: a new cardiovascular subspecialty, *Circulation,* 84:1881, 1991.

Radtke WAK: Interventional pediatric cardiology: state of the art and future perspective, *Eur J Pediatr* 153:542-547, 1994.

Salzer HR et al: Growth and nutritional intake of infants with congenital heart disease, *Pediatr Cardiol* 10:17-23, 1989.

Sanders SP: Echocardiography. In DC Fyler, (editor): *Nadas' pediatric cardiology,* Philadelphia, 1992, Hanley and Belfus, Inc, pp 159-186.

Satter EM: The feeding relationship, *J Am Diet Assoc* 86:352-356, 1986.

Shannon C: Care of the pediatric pacemaker patient. In Riegel B, (editor): *Dreifus' pacemaker therapy: an interprofessional approach,* ed 2, Philadelphia, 1986, FA Davis, pp 219-240.

Somerville J: The physician's responsibility. Residua and sequelae, *J Am Coll Cardiol* 18:325, 1991.

Stinson J, McKeever P: Mothers' information needs related to caring for infants at home following cardiac surgery, *J Pediatr Nurs* 10(1):48-57, 1995.

Takala AK et al: Risk factors for primary invasive pneumococcal disease among children in Finland, *JAMA* 273:859-864, 1995.

Thacker SB et al: Infectious diseases and injuries in child day care, *JAMA* 268:1720-1726, 1992.

Tony, E and Sparacino, P.S.:Special management issues for adolescents and young adults with congenital heart defects, Critical Care Nursing Clinics of North America, 6:199-214, 1994.

Uzark K et al: Primary preventive health care in children with heart disease, *Pediatr Cardiol* 4:259-264, 1983.

Uzark K, VonBargen-Mazza P, and Messiter E: Health education needs of adolescents with congenital heart disease, *J Pediatr Health Care* 3:137-143, 1989.

Vetter VL: Electrophysiologic residua and sequelae, *J Am Coll Cardiol* 18:331, 1991.

Woodin KA, Morrison SH: Antibiotics: mechanisms of action, *Pediatrics in Review* 15:440-447, 1994.

Wright M, Nolan T: Impact of cyanotic heart disease on school performance, *Arch Dis Child* 71:64-70, 1994.

Young PC, Shyr Y, and Schork A: The role of the primary care physician in the care of children with serious heart disease, *Pediatrics,* 94(3):284-290, 1994.

Cystic Fibrosis

16

Ann Hix McMullen

ETIOLOGY

Cystic fibrosis (CF), a condition characterized by complex multisystem involvement, is the most common lethal genetic illness among white children, adolescents and young adults. Significant advances in genetic and biomedical research have been made over the past 15 years that have influenced health professionals' understanding of the condition, its etiology, clinical management, and approaches to detection.

In 1989, following a succession of scientific breakthroughs in genetics, the CF gene was isolated on the long arm of chromosome 7 which encodes a protein product, cystic fibrosis transmembrane conductance regulator (CFTR) (Rommens et al, 1989). More than 300 mutations in the CFTR gene have been reported, the most common of which is the delta F508 mutation accounting for 70% of CF alleles (Beaudet et al, 1989; Fernbach and Thomson, 1992). Scientists initially hoped that a relationship could be identified between specific mutations, defects in CFTR functioning, and subsequent clinical manifestations of the disease. Those genotype-phenotype relationships have proven to be more complex and are probably complicated by such factors as multiple person environment interactions and other gene products (Cutting, 1994). This area of scientific study should be closely followed by primary care providers because findings will have specific implications for genetic counseling of carriers and of parents con-

sidering prenatal diagnosis, as well as for counseling of individuals with the illness.

Breakthroughs in genetics have been accompanied by advances in biomedical research which are leading to improved understanding of the pathophysiology of CF. At least one function of CFTR appears to be as a chloride ion channel regulated by cyclic AMP. Scientists have demonstrated defective chloride ion transport across secretory epithelial cells in affected tissue (Quinton, 1989). This impermeability to chloride ions leads to decreased water movement across cell membranes causing secretions to become less well-hydrated, viscous, and cause obstruction of the lumen of airways and ducts (Cutting, 1994). The pathogenesis of an ion transport defect leads to pathologic sequelae of mucus obstructing ducts in various body organs. Progressive pathologic changes are produced in nearly every organ of the body. The most consistent changes occur in the exocrine glands (e.g., pancreatic acini, bile ducts and gallbladder, prostatic glands, salivary and lacrimal glands, mucous glands of the tracheobronchial tree, upper respiratory tract and intestinal wall, and the sweat glands) (Lloyd-Still, 1983; Abrons, 1993). Table 16-1, an overview of cystic fibrosis, delineates organ system pathogenesis, clinical manifestations, and treatment.

INCIDENCE

The transmission of CF follows an autosomal recessive mode of inheritance and occurs in

Table 16-1.   OVERVIEW OF CYSTIC FIBROSIS

System	Pathogenesis	Clinical manifestations	Complications	Management
Sweat glands	Abnormal electrolytes	High rate of salt loss; salt depletion	Heat prostration	Dietary salt replacement, sweat test (see p. 328)
Lungs	Thick, tenacious mucus	Cough, decreased exercise tolerance	Infection	Chest physiotherapy: postural drainage, cupping/vibration; alternative methods
	Mucus plugging	Air trapping: increased anteroposterior chest diameter	Fibrosis, bronchiectasis	Antibiotics: oral, intravenous (IV), aerosolized
	Obstruction	Hyperresonance	Atelectasis	Bronchodilators
	Decreased mucociliary clearance	Wheezing, fine and coarse crackles, clubbing	Hypoxia, respiratory failure	DNase
			Pneumothorax, hemoptysis	Antiinflammatories
			Cor pulmonale	Ibuprophen
			Allergies	Cromolyn sodium
			bronchopulmonary aspergillosis	Inhaled corticosteroids
			Failure to thrive (increased energy expenditure)	Oral corticosteroids
			Hypertrophic osteoarthropathy	
Upper airway	Viscous mucus	Chronic sinusitis	Obstruction, mouth breathing	Decongestants; intermittent use
		Nasal polyposis		Nasal cromolyn sodium or corticosteroids
				Antibiotics
				Surgery

Continued.

Table 16-1.   OVERVIEW OF CYSTIC FIBROSIS—cont'd

System	Pathogenesis	Clinical manifestations	Complications	Management
Gastrointestinal (GI tract)	Inspissated tenacious meconium Maldigested food and viscous mucus in gut	No passage of meconium Abdominal distension Crampy abdominal pain Fecal mass in colon	Obstruction: meconium ileus Distal ileal obstruction syndrome (DIOS) Volvulus, intussusception	Enema; surgery Pancreatic enzyme replacement Dietary changes to avoid constipation Laxatives Gastrografin with Tween 80 enema or Go-LYTELY
Pancreas	Viscous secretions obstructions, fibrosis Abnormal electrolytes Suboptimal enzyme function	Maldigestion; bulky, greasy, foul-smelling stools Fat malabsorption, including fat-soluble vitamins	Pancreatitis Fibrosis Failure to thrive Delayed maturation Vitamin deficiency Rectal prolapse Insulin or oral hypoglycemics Glucose intolerance Portal hypertension Cholelithiasis	Enzyme replacement Antacids H_2 antonists High-energy diet; normal fat intake Concentrated dietary supplements Vitamin supplements Aggressive nutritional supplementation Actigal Cholecystectomy
Biliary	Obstruction Fibrosis	Subclinical cirrhosis		
Salivary glands	Abnormal electrolyte concentrations	Probably not clinically significant		
Reproductive tract	Abnormally viscous secretions	Male: obliteration of vas deferens Sterility Female: thick vaginal and cervical secretions, decreased fertility		Counseling Genetic and birth control counseling

approximately 1 in 2000 to 2500 live births. The incidence in blacks is lower, about 1 in 17,000; Asians and American Indians are rarely affected, though its occurrence in any race is possible. With a gene frequency of 1 in 25 in the white population, it is estimated that 1 in 400 to 500 couples are both carriers of this recessive trait, with a subsequent 1 in 4 risk with each pregnancy of bearing an affected child (Schwartz, 1987; Stern, 1986).

CLINICAL MANIFESTATIONS AT TIME OF DIAGNOSIS

The pathophysiologic hallmarks of CF are: (1) pancreatic enzyme deficiency from duct blockage by viscous mucus, (2) progressive chronic obstructive lung disease associated with viscous infected mucus and subsequent interstitial destruction, and (3) sweat gland dysfunction resulting in abnormally high sodium and chloride concentrations in the sweat (Schwartz, 1987).

There are three common clinical presentations. The first is *meconium ileus in the neonate,* occurring in 7% to 10% of newly diagnosed infants. Occurrence of meconium ileus should be presumed to be CF until testing confirms or rules out the diagnosis. Meconium plug syndrome, although less frequently associated with the diagnosis of CF, should also raise the primary care provider's suspicion.

Second is *malabsorption with failure to thrive* as a result of lost or diminished exocrine pancreatic function. This occurs in 80% to 90% of children with CF. These children exhibit varying degrees of weight loss or poor growth patterns usually in the presence of a normal to voracious appetite; fre-quent foul-smelling, greasy, bulky stools; rectal prolapse (seen in 25% of children), and a protuberant belly with decreased subcutaneous tissue of the extremities.

Third, *chronic or recurrent upper and lower respiratory infections* occur. Manifestations include: nasal polyps, chronic sinusitis, recurrent pneumonia and bronchitis, bronchiectasis, or atelectasis. These children have a chronic cough that persists after a respiratory infection and may become paroxysmal and productive, provoking choking and vomiting. Auscultatory findings may include fine crackles and expiratory wheezes, particularly in the upper lobes and right middle lobe; however, some children have no findings on auscultation. Infants may have recurrent episodes of wheezing and tachypnea. *Staphylococcus aureus,* often seen initially, and subsequently *Pseudomonas aeruginosa* as well as *Haemophilus influenzae* are frequent isolates in a respiratory tract culture. Fungi, including *Candida albicans* and *Aspergillus* are also often cultured from the respiratory tract (Colin and Wohl, 1994). Early roentgenographic changes include air trapping and peribronchial thickening, followed by atelectasis, infiltrates, and hilar adenopathy (Rosenstein and Langbaum, 1984; Schwartz, 1987). Without treatment, these early signs and symptoms progress and complications occur. The box on progressive changes and Fig. 16-1 summarize the clinical picture of CF lung disease.

Although these presentations are most common, CF's multisystem involvement (see Table 16-1) may lead to a presentation of symptoms that are variable and sometimes subtle, leading to diagnostic delays and creating an anxious and difficult period for both the family and the primary care provider. Manifestations may be minimal or absent during childhood. Of the children with CF, 8% to 10% are diagnosed after 9 years of age (Fitzpatrick, Rosenstein, and Langbaum, 1986, Cystic Fibrosis Foundation, 1992). Diagnostic delays may be decreased if the primary care provider maintains a high level of suspicion of the wide variety of symptoms associated with cystic fibrosis. See the box on page (330) for indications for sweat testing, the gold standard laboratory test for diagnosing CF.

Diagnosis of CF requires a positive sweat test in the presence of either (1) clinical symptoms

CLINICAL MANIFESTATIONS AT TIME OF DIAGNOSIS

Meconium ileus in the neonate
Malabsorption with failure to thrive
Chronic/recurrent upper and/or lower respiratory
  infections

PROGRESSIVE CHANGES IN THE CLINICAL PICTURE OF CYSTIC FIBROSIS

I. Early
   A. Dry, hacking, nonproductive cough
   B. Increased respiratory rate
   C. Decreased activity
II. Moderate
   A. Increased cough, increased sputum production
   B. Rales, musical rhonchi, scattered or localized wheezes
   C. Repeated episodes of respiratory tract infection
   D. Signs of obstructive lung disease
      1. Increased anteroposterior diameter
      2. Depressed diaphragm
      3. Palpable liver border
   E. Decreased appetite
   F. Failure to gain weight or grow, or weight loss
   G. Decreased exercise tolerance
III. Advanced
   A. Chronic, paroxysmal, productive cough
   B. Increased respiratory rate, shortness of breath on exertion, orthopnea, dyspnea
   C. Diffuse and localized fine and coarse crackles

   D. Signs of severe obstructive lung disease
      1. Marked increase in anteroposterior diameter (barrel chest, pigeon breast)
      2. Limited respiratory excursion of thoracic cage
      3. Depressed diaphragm
      4. Hyperresonance over entire chest
      5. Decreased ventilation, persistent hypoxemia
   E. Noisy respirations
   F. Marked decrease in appetite
   G. Muscular weakness
   H. Cyanosis
   I. Digital clubbing
   J. Rounded shoulders
   K. Fever, tachycardia, toxicity
   L. Hemoptysis
   M. Pneumothorax
   N. Lung abscess
   O. Signs of cardiac failure (cor pulmonale, edema, enlarged tender liver)
   P. Bone pain and osteoarthropathy

consistent with CF or (2) a family history of CF. Sweat testing is done by pilocarpine iontophoresis with quantitative analysis of sweat sodium and chloride. Collection and assay of sweat should be done only through a qualified laboratory. All of the 115 regional CF centers certified by the CF Foundation have clinical chemistry laboratories that meet specifications for accuracy and reliability of sweat tests. Sweat sodium and chloride concentrations of greater than 60 mEq/L are consistent with the diagnosis of CF. A value of 40 to 60 mEq/L is considered borderline and should be repeated. These values should be considered reliable only if an adequate quantity of sweat, minimally 75 mgm, has been collected (National Academy of Sciences, 1976; National Committee for Clinical Laboratory

Standards, 1993). Adequate quantities of sweat may be difficult to obtain on infants less than 4 weeks of age, and CF centers may elect to obtain DNA analysis to facilitate early diagnosis in these children. Once the diagnosis has been established in a child, all siblings should also be sweat tested.

Neonatal screening of immunoreactive trypsinogen (IRT), although possible, remains controversial because of the high number of false positives and because it is unclear whether the potential benefits of early diagnosis outweigh the cost of testing the newborn. Pilot programs currently underway in Colorado and Wisconsin are anticipated to address these questions (Shapiro and Seilheimer, 1994).

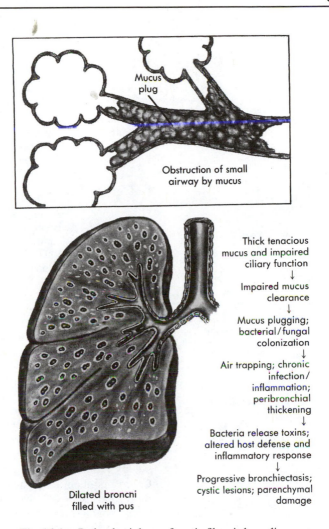

Fig. 16-1. Pathophysiology of cystic fibrosis lung disease.

TREATMENT

Pancreatic Enzyme Deficiency

The principal treatment for the resulting malabsorption in cystic fibrosis is oral pancreatic enzyme replacement. Enteric coating of enzyme preparations decreases the likelihood of inactivation by gastric acid and dosing may be adjusted to achieve weight gain and one to two formed stools per day. Recently, concerns have been raised by reports of colonic strictures in children with CF. These strictures have occurred in children receiving high doses of enzymes. As this problem continues to be investigated, current recommendations are that pancreatic enzyme doses should be reduced to the lowest effective dose while not altering the child's diet. Dosing guidelines of 1000 to 2000 units of lipase per kilogram per meal have been adopted by many CF centers (Grand, 1994).

Neutralization of gastric acid with antacids or inhibition of its production with H_2 antagonists may improve the efficacy of the enzyme preparation. Because fat malabsorption is particularly problematic in CF, and deficiencies in fat-soluble

INDICATIONS FOR SWEAT TESTING

Pulmonary

Chronic cough
Recurrent or chronic pneumonia
Staphylococcal pneumonia
Recurrent bronchiolitis
Atelectasis
Hemoptysis
Mucoid *Pseudomonas* infection

Gastrointestinal

Meconium ileus, steatorrhea, malabsorption
Rectal prolapse
Childhood cirrhosis (portal hypertension or
    bleeding esophageal varices)
Hypoprothrombinemia beyond newborn period

Other

Family history of CF
Failure to thrive
Salty sweat, salty taste when kissed, salt frosting
    of skin
Nasal polyps
Heat prostration, hyponatremia, and
    hypochloremia, especially in infants
Pansinusitis
Aspermatism
Digital clubbing

From Schwartz RH: Cystic fibrosis. In Hoekelman RH, ed:
Primary pediatric care, 1205, St Louis, 1987, CV Mosby Co.

TREATMENT

Nutrition: Enzyme and vitamin
                  supplementation
             Salt replacement
             High-calorie diet
Respiratory: Chest physical therapy
             Antibiotics
             Antiinflammatory therapy
             Bronchodilators
             Antifungal therapy
             RhDNase
             Lung transplantation

vitamins have been reported, CF centers recommend doubling the recommended daily allowance of multivitamins and adding a water-miscible form of vitamin E supplementation. Vitamin K may also be supplemented during infancy, and in the presence of hemoptysis, or when clotting studies are prolonged (Hubbard, 1985). Newer water-miscible preparations combining the fat-soluble vitamins A, D, E, and K have recently been marketed, providing the convenience of supplementation with a single vitamin preparation for most children.

Caloric and protein requirements may be increased in children with CF by malabsorption related to inadequate enzyme supplementation and by progressive pulmonary disease. Most authorities agree that these children have a basal energy requirement 25% to 50% greater than the usual recommended daily allowance for energy intake (Hubbard, 1985). With pulmonary disease progression, children usually have chronic weight and nutrition problems as a result of their increased pulmonary energy requirements. The goal is for children with CF to maintain a weight-height index equal to or more than 90% of ideal weight (Nutrition in CF Consensus Report, 1992).

Calories are encouraged in both complex carbohydrates and fats. Dietary fat is the highest density source of calories. Dietary fat improves palatability of foods and maintains normal essential fatty acid status. Whenever possible, children with CF should follow a normal diet pattern with no specific restrictions (Nutrition in CF Consensus Report, 1992). Energy boosting tips are found in the box on page 331. An individual may have difficulty with certain high-fat foods and these may be limited; however, children generally should be encouraged to cover high-fat intake with additional enzymes. Aggressive nutritional supplementation (oral, enteral, and parenteral) has been used for children with weight loss problems and growth delay de-

TIPS TO BOOST ENERGY INTAKE

- Include snacks regularly, especially before bedtime. Serve snacks at least 2 hours before the next meal.
- Serve vegetables with cheese or cream sauces
- Serve meats, potatoes, and other foods with sauces and gravies
- When preparing fruit juice from concentrate, reduce water added by one fourth
- Use whole milk fortified with powdered milk as a beverage, in cooking, and on food such as cereal

Make the following additions to foods served:

Amount	Food	Adds (calories)	Use in or on
1 tsp	Butter or margarine	40	On hot cereal, vegetables, sandwiches, soups, casseroles, breads
1 T	Sour cream	26	Add to vegetables, salads
1 T	Mayonnaise	100	Use in salads, sandwiches, vegetables, deviled eggs
1 oz	Light cream	60	Cereal, hot chocolate, in cooking
1 oz	Evaporated milk*	50	Substitute for water or milk in cooking; add to hot cereal, hot chocolate
1 T	Powdered milk*	23	Add to whole milk, milkshakes, mashed potatoes, scrambled eggs, meatloaf, or hamburgers
1	Hard boiled egg*	80	Add to casseroles, meatloaf
1	Egg yolk, chopped*	60	Sandwich spreads
1 T	Peanut butter*	100	On bread, crackers, toast, apples or celery, in hot cereal, baked goods, milk shakes
1 oz	Cheese*	100	On vegetables, casseroles, meats, in sandwiches, salads, pasta, soup, dips
1 oz	Cream cheese	100	On toast, sandwiches, raw vegetables; add to scrambled eggs, jello salads
1 T	Chopped nuts*	49	Top puddings, ice cream; add to salads, casseroles, cereal, baked goods, fruit cup

From Adams EA: Nutrition care in cystic fibrosis. *Nutrition news,* Seattle, WA 1988, University of Washington Child Development and Mental Retardation Center.

*These foods add protein as well as calories

spite a reasonable intake. In the short term, improved weight gain and stabilization of pulmonary function has been achieved with this approach (Soutter et al, 1986; Levy et al, 1985). Long-term studies have documented decreased mortality and improved growth; however, a demonstrated rate of pulmonary decline, however, has not been as clearly demonstrated (Dalzell et al, 1992).

Pulmonary Disease

Progressive lung disease is the major cause of morbidity and mortality in CF. The pathophysiologic basis of CF lung disease is impaired mucociliary clearance of dehydrated mucus followed by endobronchial infection. Children with CF become chronically colonized with Gram negative organisms, which may be quantitatively decreased with antimicrobial therapy but cannot be eradicated long term. The child's susceptibility to this bacterial growth is not fully understood and controversies are widespread concerning the optimal approach to its long-term treatment. General agreement exists, however, that bacterial infection, particularly *Pseudomonas aeruginosa* with its virulence factors, and the host inflammatory response to infection (i.e., antibody response and neutrophil influx) lead to chronic bronchiectasis and progressive damage to lung tissue (Fig. 16-1). CF centers recognize that antimicrobial therapy plays a significant role in decreasing the rate of this deterioration (Marshall, 1994).

Pulmonary exacerbations often follow mild viral illnesses, particularly upper respiratory infections. Although the mechanism has not been clearly defined, it has been hypothesized that viruses may cause suppression of host defenses (Mischler, 1985; Wang et al, 1984; Prober, 1991). Early use of oral antibiotic therapy with viral illness symptoms can be argued on the basis of its use to prevent exacerbation of the bacterial pulmonary infection during the viral illness. Traditional concerns regarding development of resistant organisms with overuse of antibiotics must be balanced against the greater concern for progressive deteriorative bronchiectasis (Stern, 1989). Initial choice of an antibiotic and its dosage should include consideration for broad spectrum coverage, specifically for *Staphylococcus aureus, Streptococcus pneumoniae,* and *Hemophilus influenza.* Further considerations in children whose pulmonary infections have not responded to initial therapy include antibiotic sus-ceptibility or resistance, lack of compliance, or abnormal pharmacokinetics (Taussig, Landau, and Marks, 1984; MacLuskey, 1993).

Other ongoing pulmonary therapeutic interventions are aimed at relief of bronchial obstruction. Chest physical therapy (postural drainage and cupping/clapping/vibration done two to four times a day) has demonstrated efficacy and has been standard therapy (Desmond et al, 1983). More recently, other techniques of airway clearance have been developed for school-age children and adolescents, including active cycle of breathing (ACB) and forced expiration technique (FET), autogenic drainage (AD), positive expiratory pressure (PEP), the Flutter valve, and mechanical percussors. The common advantage of these techniques is that they allow independence in performing airway clearance of mucus. Although more definitive studies are needed, the efficacy of these techniques has been demonstrated.

Routine chest therapy is recommended for all children with pulmonary involvement; the specific regimen recommended for an individual with CF should be made by the CF center's physician and respiratory or physical therapist (Davidson and McIlwaine, 1995). Exercise, particularly an aerobic conditioning program, is also encouraged as it positively influences general health, cardiopulmonary and musculoskeletal function, and airway clearance (Orenstein, Henke, and Cerney, 1983; deJong et al, 1994). Reactive airways disease (RAD) may result from chronic inflammation and infection; bronchodilators are often used if a clinical response can be observed or if a beneficial response can be demonstrated by pulmonary function testing (Rosenstein, 1990). Many children with CF use an aerosolized bronchodilator before chest physical therapy and some may also be on a theophylline preparation.

Children with CF mount a significant inflammatory response to chronic bronchial infection, contributing to parenchymal destruction and disease progression. Konstan and associates (1994) reported that adolescents and adults with mild CF lung disease who appeared clinically healthy were found on bronchoalveolar lavage to have evidence of bacterial infection and significant local inflammatory response. Even lavage fluid from infants has been shown to have increased DNA levels (Kirchner et al, 1993). Clinicians have long recognized the clinical efficacy of antiinflammatory therapy and have used short courses of oral and inhaled corticosteroids as well as cromolyn sodium in reactive airway disease associated with CF. However, initial enthusiasm for chronic use of systemic corticosteroids is now being more closely scrutinized because of the development of significant side effects (i.e., cataracts, growth retardation, and glucose abnormalities) (Rosenstein and Eigen, 1991).

More recently, long-term use of high-dose ibuprofen by preadolescents with mild lung disease has been reported to decrease progression of lung disease over a 4-year study period (Konstan et al, 1995). Use of ibuprofen is expected to increase in the future; it requires monitoring of serum drug levels to establish therapeutic doses and careful selection of individuals most likely to benefit.

In 1994, the FDA released aerosolized recombinant human DNase, a breakthrough in new CF pharmacotherapy. rhDNase cleaves extracellular DNA, which is present in high concentrations in purulent CF airway mucus, and reduces its viscosity to a more liquid form (Hubbard et al, 1992). Studies have demonstrated its efficacy in improving pulmonary function as well as decreasing frequency of hospitalizations, school or work absenteeism, and CF-related symptoms in individuals with mild to moderate pulmonary disease (FVC ≥40% predicted). Side effects were limited to upper airway irritation resulting in hoarseness, rash, chest pain and conjunctivitis, and were usually mild and transient. (Accurso, 1995; Hodson, 1995). Children started on DNase should be monitored by serial pulmonary function testing and clinical markers of morbidity. Selection of children to be started on DNase should be based on efficacy data, which continues to emerge. Initial studies document that ongoing efficacy is based on daily use (Ramsey, 1993) and clinicians should continue to follow emerging data on the cost-effectiveness of this expensive drug. The mucolytic agent, acetylcysteine (Mucomist) and expectorants have no clear efficacy; acetylcysteine may irritate the respiratory tract (Rosenstein, 1990).

Aerosolized aminoglycosides have demonstrated increasing efficacy by delivering antibiotics at high concentrations to the site of infection while decreasing the risk of systemic absorption and toxicity. Aerosolized aminoglycosides may reduce the frequency of intravenous antibiotic therapy; however, the potential for developing resistant strains of *Pseudomonas* may concern clinicians (Marshall and Ramsey, 1994). Clinical expertise in CF management is therefore helpful in selecting appropriate individuals, the specific drug and dosage to be used, and the length of therapy.

When pulmonary exacerbations are not controlled by oral and aerosolized antibiotics, intravenous antibiotics may be necessary. A pulmonary and nutritional "tune-up" or "clean-out" may be initiated in the hospital or at home. These 2-week (or longer) courses of therapy allow the CF center team to employ more aggressive strategies to contain infection and supplement nutrition. Strategies include use of intravenous antibiotics, often an aminoglycoside with either a synthetic penicillin or third generation cephalosporin; increased pulmonary toilet; and nutritional support measures. Intravenous antibiotics are chosen for their efficacy in treating *Pseudomonas aeruginosa,* which is less responsive to oral therapy. Quinolone antibiotics, specifically ciprofloxacin (Cipro), are currently the only oral preparations available that effectively treat *Pseudomonas* species. Because of lack of data about side effects in children, Cipro has not been approved by the FDA for use in individuals under 18 years of age. However, in clinical trials, children with CF have generally tolerated Cipro well and many CF centers make judicious use of it (Hooper and Wolfson, 1991).

RECENT AND ANTICIPATED ADVANCES IN DIAGNOSIS AND MANAGEMENT

Genetic Testing

The impact of genetic discoveries on understanding etiology and pathophysiology is only beginning to unfold. At the same time, approaches to detection are changing and reflect the new technologic advances. Carrier screening is available and reliable for siblings and family members of a child with CF whose deletions have been identified (Beaudet et al, 1989). Appropriate DNA deletion and linkage analysis studies are highly complex and any family member contemplating such screening should be referred to a regional CF center or pediatric genetics center for counseling.

Prenatal diagnosis is now available to parents with a child affected with CF and to other at-risk couples. As a result, increasing numbers of at-risk families are utilizing these diagnostic resources and confronting the ethical dilemmas of therapeutic abortion versus continuation of the pregnancy. At present, their decision making occurs in a milieu of rapidly advancing science of treatment and the variability of phenotypic expression of CF illness severity in an individual child. Chorionic villus sampling (CVS) at 8 to 10 weeks' gestation or amniocentesis at 12 to 16 weeks' gestation may be utilized for information regarding CF mutations in the fetus. Wertz and associates (1992) surveyed childbearing-age parents who had a child with CF regarding the parents' attitudes about prenatal diagnosis. Almost half of the couples surveyed desired more children and intended to use prenatal diagnosis. Of those expected users of prenatal diagnosis, 44% would carry a fetus found to have CF to term, 28% would abort, and 28% were undecided. Prenatal diagnosis services and related counseling is clearly an area of specialization and should be coordinated by the regional CF center (Beaudet & Buffone, 1989; Fernbach and Thomson, 1992; Shapiro and Seilheimer, 1994).

Heterozygote (carrier) detection of the general population is at present technically possible. Specialized genetic laboratories now offer screening for up to 32 of the most common CF mutations which account for about 85% of mutant CF genes in ethnically diverse North America. In 1990, a National Institutes of Health (NIH) workshop report recommended that carrier screening in the general population should only be offered if a 90% to 95% level of carrier detection could be achieved. The report also noted that a number of mass population screening issues remain unstudied (i.e., public and professional education, the system's ability to provide genetic counseling services, and effects of information on legislative and health insurance systems). Before mass screening would be a feasible and responsible endeavor, pilot screening programs were suggested and are currently underway in several areas of the country (Wilfond and Fost, 1990; National Institutes of Health (NIH) Workshop on Population Screening for the CF Gene, 1990).

Pharmacological and other Advances

New breakthroughs in pharmacologic interventions that focus on the treatment of CF lung disease, the major determinant of morbidity and mortality in CF, should be expected in the future. Interventions are designed to interrupt the cascade of pathophysiologic phenomena by either (1) preventing the development of abnormal airway secretions and lung infections, or (2) treating the existing infection and inflammation. (See Fig. 16-2.) Four of the most promising areas of research include:

1. Modulation of salt and water transport in CF airway epithelium. Initial studies of aerosolized amiloride and uridine triphosphate (UTP) demonstrated success in stimulating chloride secretion and inhibiting sodium absorption in CF airway epithelium, leading to better hydrated airway mucus. Multicenter trials are underway (Knowles et al, 1995).

2. Interruption of the neutrophil-mediated inflammatory cascade with such agents as antiproteases, pentoxifylline, and intravenous immune globulin (Davis, 1994, Moss et al, 1994).

3. Gene therapy. The first human trial of gene therapy for CF was initiated at NIH in April,

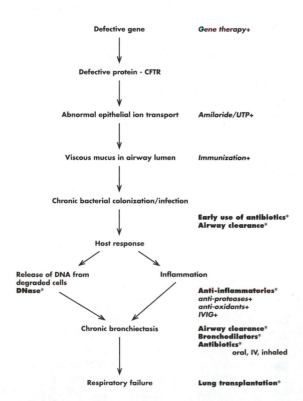

Fig. 16-2. Pathologic sequence of CF lung disease and therapies used.

1993. (Wilson, 1994). The goal is to insert coding for normal CFTR protein in airway epithelial cells. Clinical studies of safety, efficacy, and methodology are in progress in a number of research centers across North America. Ultimately, all individuals with CF, their families, and their health care providers hope that researchers of gene therapy will eventually realize the therapy's potential as a cure for CF (Drumm et al, 1992; Wilson, 1994).

4. Bilateral lung transplantation has emerged as a viable therapeutic option for individuals with end-stage CF lung disease. As of 1993, anticipated actuarial 1-year survival in North America was 70% and was as high as 80% at some transplant centers. Long-term survival statistics are accumulating and are projected to be at 50% in 3 to 5 years. Improved surgical techniques and antirejection drugs have had, and will continue to have, a marked impact on survival statistics. The most difficult impediment to more widespread use of this intervention is the critical shortage of suitable organ donors (Egan and Detterbeck, 1993; Ramirez, et al., 1992). Although this procedure offers hope to individuals with end-stage disease and their families, it presents them with significant psychosocial and financial challenges as well. Consideration of transplantation, individual and family counseling, and referral for evaluation should be coordinated through the CF center.

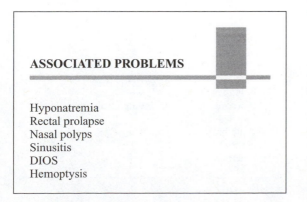

ASSOCIATED PROBLEMS

Hyponatremia
Rectal prolapse
Nasal polyps
Sinusitis
DIOS
Hemoptysis

ASSOCIATED PROBLEMS

Salt Depletion—Hyponatremia and Dehydration

Children with CF have abnormal sodium and chloride loss in their sweat and therefore are at risk for dehydration secondary to electrolyte imbalance. Risk factors include hot weather, febrile illnesses with or without vomiting and diarrhea, and strenuous physical activity. Excessive salt loss may lead to listlessness, vomiting, heat prostration, and dehydration. Infants are at particular risk because of the low salt content of breast milk, commercial infant formulas, and infant foods. Prevention includes supplementation of salt in infant formulas (¼ tsp/day) and adding salt to the older child's diet (Adams, 1988).

Rectal Prolapse

Rectal prolapse was present in about 3% of individuals with CF who were reported in the National Patient Registry in 1991 (Cystic Fibrosis Foundation, 1992). It may be the presenting symptom and may occur only once, or be a recurrent problem. Often, initiation of appropriate enzyme replacement or adjustment of enzyme dosage prevents its reoccurrence. Rarely, persistent or recurrent prolapse requires surgical intervention; (Borowitz, 1994). The first episode of rectal prolapse is frightening to both parents and child, and its reduction usually requires both immediate phone guidance and assistance in the primary care provider's office or an emergency room.

If a child experiences recurrent episodes of rectal prolapse, parents may learn to manually reduce a prolapse. With the child side-lying and using a glove and KY jelly, the parent is usually able to gently invert the mucosa through the rectal opening.

Nasal Polyps and Pansinusitis

Nasal polyps occur in 10% of children with CF and their finding on physical examination of a child should raise the suspicion of CF if not already diagnosed. The upper respiratory tract, including sinuses, is lined with respiratory epithelial cells similar to the lining in the lungs, and is therefore also affected by CF pathology. Sinuses are frequently chronically infected, producing symptoms of frontal headaches, tenderness on palpation, purulent nasal discharge, and postnasal discharge which further contributes to the chronic cough. Treatment includes extended use of antibiotics, nasal cromolyn sodium and steroids, and intermittent use of nasal decongestants. Children may also find warm mist and saline nasal rinses to be helpful comfort measures; some CF clinicians and otolaryngologists recommend sinus irrigations with saline. Surgical interventions for polyposis and sinusitis are occasionally necessary with variable degrees of success (King, 1991).

Distal Ileal Obstruction Syndrome/Constipation

Although the prevalence of distal ileal obstruction syndrome (DIOS) is higher in adolescents and young adults, even young children with CF are at risk for developing total or partial intestinal obstruction. Constipation is often the result of a combination of malabsorption, either from inadequate pancreatic enzyme dosage or failure to take enzymes, decreased intestinal motility, and abnormally viscous intestinal secretions. DIOS is seen when there is sludging of intestinal contents at the ileocecum. Abdominal cramping with either diarrhea or absence of stool and anorexia occurs. A stool mass may be palpable in the right lower quadrant. If the obstruction becomes complete, vomiting and increased pain and distention occur. Appendicitis, intussusception, and volvulus occur with increased frequency in children with CF and must be considered. A plain abdominal film may help to confirm the diagnosis of DIOS. Contrast enemas (gastrograffin with Tween 80) may be both diagnostic and therapeutic; these enemas are the treatment of choice for children with complete obstruction. Children with partial obstruction may be treated with polyethylene-glycol solutions (Golytely, Colyte) or gastrograffin given orally or by nasogastric tube (Borowitz, 1994). Follow-up should include long-term use of some combination of a stool softener, mild stimulant, and bulk laxative, as well as the addition of bulk to the diet, consistent enzyme use, and exercise (Rubinstein, Moss, and Lewiston, 1986; MacLusky, 1993).

Hemoptysis

The appearance of blood-streaked mucus and small quantities of bright red blood is not uncommon in CF. Though initially alarming to the child and family, the bleeding is usually self-limiting. Bleeding reflects increased bronchial infection, inflammation, and irritation, which require more aggressive treatment. Initiation or change of antibiotic therapy should be considered in addition to increasing routine pulmonary toilet. Massive hemoptysis (usually defined as ≥240 ml/24 hours), on the other hand, requires immediate referral to the CF center team for management.

Other Associated Problems

CF is a multisystem condition with an increased rate of complications and morbidity with disease progression. Complications listed in the box below are more serious and usually require the expertise of the CF center team in their management. The primary care provider must recognize early signs and symptoms of these complications so that timely referral for evaluation and treatment can be implemented.

Of note, colonization with *Pseudomonas cepacia* has emerged as a perplexing problem in a number of CF centers. The organism is highly resistant to antibiotic therapy and has been implicated in rapid progression of lung disease. The

SERIOUS COMPLICATIONS OF CYSTIC FIBROSIS

Cor pulmonale
Massive hemoptysis
Pneumothorax
Hypertrophic pulmonary osteoarthropathy
Liver disease including portal hypertension
Gallbladder disease
Glucose intolerance, including insulin dependent diabetes
Allergic bronchopulmonary aspergillosis (ABPA)
Pancreatitis

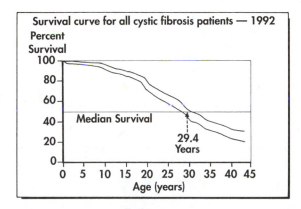

Fig. 16-3. Survival curve for all cystic fibrosis patients for the year 1992. *(Courtesy of the Cystic Fibrosis Foundation, National CF Patient Registry, 1992.)*

organism is also known to be transmitted between children with CF; however, its true significance is the subject of ongoing debate (MacLusky, 1993).

PROGNOSIS

Despite 40 years of remarkable progress in treatment and a recent surge of new approaches to treatment, CF remains a progressive disease without cure. The median survival age is 28 to 30 years (see Figs. 16-3 and 16-4), which has markedly increased over the past 20 years. This change is likely a result of both improved treatment and appreciation and detection of the milder phenotypic expressions of the disease (Schwartz, 1987). With continued improvement in survival, CF has become an illness of children, adolescents, and young adults.

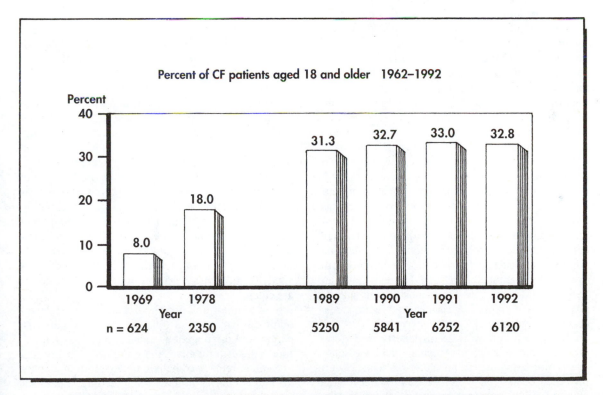

Fig. 16-4. Percentage of patients aged 18 years and older for the years 1969 through 1992. *(Courtesy of the Cystic Fibrosis Foundation, National CF Patient Registry.)*

Primary Care Management
HEALTH CARE MAINTENANCE

Growth and Development

Growth delay and difficulty maintaining adequate weight for height are common problems in CF. Weight loss and linear growth retardation may be presenting clinical signs both in infancy and in early adolescence. Following diagnosis and initiation of pulmonary and nutritional therapy, catch-up growth is frequently observed.

Growth and developmental failure may be observed in children with CF who have significant progression of pulmonary disease; it may be more observable as they approach puberty and during adolescence when a growth spurt is normally expected. These delays involve not only height and weight but also skeletal and sexual maturation and are explained by a complex interrelationship of degree of severity of pulmonary disease, maturational delay, and caloric intake (Shepherd, Cooksley, and Cooke, 1980; Levy et al, 1985; Mahaney and McCoy, 1986; Pencharz and Durie, 1993). Aggressive nutritional supplementation has been associated with short-term improvement in growth velocity and well being in addition to slowed decline in pulmonary function (Levy et al, 1985; Shepherd et al, 1986; Wooten et al, 1991). Primary care providers should be alert to weight loss or a flattened growth curve associated with loss of appetite since these may be indicators of a pulmonary exacerbation; their presence should prompt further investigation with the child and family about an increase in pulmonary symptoms. Growth retardation also should prompt review of gastrointestinal status, specifically stool pattern and consistency, as well as symptoms of abdominal cramping or gastric "burning." The primary care provider may adjust the enzyme dosage if stools are frequent and greasy; however, consultation with the CF center team regarding further interventions may become necessary.

The mean age of onset of puberty in children with CF is 14.5 years (Moshang and Holsclaw, 1980); this delay may be an acute source of concern for adolescents. The primary care provider may be able to help the teenager understand that this delay is neither unusual nor unexpected and that sexual development, though delayed, will occur. Menar-

chal age has been associated with severity of illness and adolescent girls who are underweight because of advancing disease, despite rigorous efforts in nutritional supplementation, need support and reassurance.

Cystic fibrosis is not associated with intellectual deficits or delays in cognitive development. Problems in school performance are more likely to be related to either absenteeism as a result of physical illness or fatigue at school associated with an impending exacerbation.

Diet

Children with CF require high-calorie, high-protein diets. In infancy, breast feeding should be continued whenever possible with enzyme supplementation and, when necessary, supplementation of higher calorie per ounce formula. Formula-fed infants are often given a hydrolysate formula with medium chain triglycerides (e.g., Pregestimil, Alimentum). Even though these formulas are predigested, enzyme supplementation may also be necessary. Enzymes are given to infants by mixing the beads contained in the capsule into pureed fruit, usually applesauce, and feeding these by mouth.

Parents often have questions about enzyme supplementation dosage. Requirements depend on the degree of pancreatic insufficiency, the fat content of the food ingested, the quantity eaten, and the type of enzymes used. Dosage is adjusted by trial until the stool pattern is acceptable (e.g., one to two stools per day in older children with more in infancy) and the child demonstrates reasonable growth. Enzymes should be taken within 30 minutes of eating, and the beads should not be chewed or crushed—destroying the enteric coating causes inactivation of the enzymes and excoriation of oral mucosa. Children should be encouraged to add extra enzymes when high-fat foods are eaten.

As toddlers and preschoolers experience developmentally appropriate changes in eating patterns, parents are often anxious about providing adequate food intake to maintain the child's well-being and growth. Parents need help in understanding that abnormal emphasis on food, force feeding, and mealtime battles should be avoided. Instead, parents should provide appropriate foods, set limits for mealtimes, and suggest trying some of each food offered. Multiple, small serving portions and nutritious snacks may also boost intake.

In preschool-age and older children, oral high-calorie, high-protein supplementation may be achieved using commonly purchased foods (see box on page 331). The CF center nutritionist can provide many suggestions for fortifying the child's diet, and printed educational material is also available to families (see pages 334-335).

Taking enzymes in front of classmates may be difficult for school-age children. Parents, the teacher, the school nurse, and the child can devise the best plan for enzyme administration. As children grow older and have more control in selecting their diets, parents need to pay particular attention to the quality of snack foods available in the home. Parents often find that an adolescent's intake is better if a structured mealtime is maintained, despite individual schedules.

Safety

In addition to routine anticipatory guidance about safety issues, the primary care provider should emphasize safe storage and handling of the large quantities of medications frequently used by children with CF. Issues of accidental ingestion of pancreatic enzymes by another child may arise because these are routinely in ample supply at mealtimes in the home and carried by the child for use. Medications are not likely to be harmful if small quantities are ingested; they are activated in the small intestine and excreted in stool without major absorption in the blood stream.

Immunizations

Infants and children with CF should receive all routine immunizations at the ages recommended by the American Academy of Pediatrics (AAP). In a few instances, the CF team may recommend a brief delay in order to stabilize an acute pulmonary or nutritional problem; however, there is no evidence to support delay of routine immunizations.

The FDA approved varicella vaccine in April, 1995. Following AAP guidelines, a single dose should be given to children with CF between 12 and 18 months of age who do not have a history of chicken pox. Older children with CF, especially those who are steroid dependent, may be immunized at the earliest opportunity. Two doses of

vaccine 4 to 8 weeks apart are recommended for adolescents (American Academy of Pediatrics (AAP), Committee of Infectious Diseases, 1995).

Annual influenza vaccine is also recommended, following Centers for Disease Control guidelines which include use of split virus vaccine in children under 13 years of age. Pneumococcal vaccine is not routinely recommended because pneumococcal infections are rarely reported in children with CF (Stern, 1989; AAP, 1994).

Screening

Vision. Routine screening is recommended. If steroid dependent, the child should be monitored annually by a pediatric ophthalmologist for early detection of cataracts or glaucoma.

Hearing. Routine screening is recommended, the child should be monitored by an audiologist for occurrence of high frequency hearing loss with each course of intravenous aminoglycoside therapy.

Dental. Routine screening is advised. Precautions regarding use of tetracyclines before permanent tooth formation is advised.

Hematocrit. Routine screening is advised. The role of pancreatic insufficiency and pancreatic enzyme replacement therapy in iron absorption in CF is unclear. Iron status should be evaluated periodically and appropriate supplementation provided if anemia is present (Nutrition Assessment and Management in Cystic Fibrosis: A Consensus Report, 1992).

Tuberculosis. Skin tests with PPD are routinely performed at CF centers. Although active disease caused by *Mycobacterium tuberculosis* in individuals with CF is probably no more prevalent than in the general population, recent reports have documented the presence of atypical mycobacteria in individuals with CF. The general prevalence and clinical pathogenesis remain to be determined (Kilby et al, 1992).

Condition-specific screening

PULMONARY FUNCTION TESTING. Pulmonary function testing (PFT) is routinely performed in children over 6 years of age during CF center visits at least annually and more often as indicated. PFTs and chest roentgenography monitor pulmonary disease progression and identify acute problems.

MULTISYSTEM SCREENS. Other screening routinely performed at CF center visits include sputum cultures with antibiotic sensitivities, blood and urine assay of liver function, renal function, cell counts and differential, glucose, and serum and anthropometric measures of nutrition status.

COMMON ILLNESS MANAGEMENT

Differential Diagnosis

Symptoms associated with common pediatric illnesses may also be symptoms specific to CF and questions often arise regarding their etiology and management. Parents may need to hear often that their child will develop common minor childhood illnesses and will usually respond to routine management. Parents may be reassured to know that the CF center team is readily available to the primary care provider whenever questions arise regarding etiology and treatment of an acute illness. Thorough history taking and examination are not only essential to the primary care provider in making a differential diagnosis, but reassuring to parents and the child.

Gastrointestinal symptoms. Diarrhea, constipation, and abdominal cramping may be presenting complaints of a partial or complete intestinal obstruction. A history of cramping pain and changes in stool pattern in the absence of other acute gastrointestinal and systemic symptoms is suggestive

of distal ileal obstruction syndrome (DIOS). Abdominal pain may also be suggestive of gallstones or pancreatitis (Borowitz, 1994).

Fever and viral illness. Fever associated with a CF pulmonary exacerbation is a relatively uncommon presentation, and evaluation of fever in children with CF should elicit the same broad-based approach used with other children. A brief initial febrile period with a viral illness should be anticipated in children with CF and symptomatically treated per usual practice protocols. When a viral illness exacerbates lower respiratory tract symptoms, as frequently occurs with upper respiratory tract infections, an increase in chest physical therapy as well as prompt and sustained (2 to 3 weeks) oral antibiotic coverage are usually recommended. Prevention of hyponatremia and dehydration during febrile illness includes adding salt to the child's intake and reviewing warning signs of dehydration with parents. When a rehydration solution is indicated, electrolyte-balanced clear liquids such as Pedialyte may be used.

Chest pain. Children with CF frequently have complaints of chest pain. These should always be evaluated because of the potential occurrence of pneumothorax. Complaints associated with pneumothorax are typically a sudden onset of sharp pain unilaterally followed by dull aching, and accompanied by profound shortness of breath and activity intolerance. This complication, confirmed by physical examination and chest roentgenogram, is best managed at the regional CF center following local emergency stabilization as indicated.

Bilateral musculoskeletal pain from coughing paroxysms is usually diffuse and occurs with a pulmonary exacerbation. It may also be localized and the child will have pain on palpation at the site. Both usually respond to use of nonsteroidal antiinflammatory and pain therapy. Some children and adolescents with CF experience midline chest and epigastric burning related to gastroesophageal reflux (GER) and esophagitis (Schidlow, Taussig, and Knowles, 1993). If antacids are not effective, the CF center team should be consulted, specifically regarding use of H_2 antagonists.

Varicella. There has been no report in the CF literature of higher rates of complications from chicken pox in children with CF; however, there have been reports of exacerbation of pulmonary

---

DIFFERENTIAL DIAGNOSIS

Constipation:	common vs DIOS
Abdominal pain:	rule out appendicitis, volvulus, intussuception, gallstones, pancreatitis
Fever:	viral illness with exacerbation of chronic infection
Chest pain:	pneumothorax vs muscle pull vs GER
Cough:	sinusitis vs lower respiratory tract exacerbation
Wheezing:	heightened bronchial activity due to chronic infection and inflammation

symptoms (MacDonald, Morris, and Beaudry, 1987). Management of coryzal symptoms is no different from other children. The same approach to antibiotic use with increased pulmonary symptoms should also apply to this viral illness. Use of antipruritic medications is not contraindicated; but the child's cough may be suppressed by their use and parents should increase chest physical therapy as soon as lesions permit. In some children with severe CF lung disease, the CF center may recommend varicella-zoster globulin (VZIG) with exposure to chicken pox; if recommended. It should be administered within 48 hours of exposure. Acyclovir given within 24 hours of onset of the rash of chicken pox may be recommended by the CF center to attenuate the clinical course in children with moderate to severe lung disease (AAP, 1994).

Cough. A chronic cough which may vary in intensity is a hallmark of CF lung disease. At baseline, it may be present in the early morning and with exercise. An increase in cough is always of significance and requires intervention. Nighttime coughing may develop and may be associated with reactive airway disease, increased pulmonary infection and inflammation, or postnasal discharge from sinusitis or rhinitis. Delineating a clear etiology can be challenging. Both antibiotic therapy and initiation or increase in the use of aerosolized bronchodilators and antiinflammatory agents may be helpful. Cough suppressants are generally contraindicated and should only be used after consultation with the CF center team. A trial of decongestants may be useful. Antihistamines may be used when allergy is playing a role in symptomatology; however, the primary care provider should be aware that antihistamines potentially may increase the viscosity of mucus and inhibit its mobilization.

Wheezing. Wheezing is a common manifestation of CF, particularly in infancy. It is most often attributed to heightened bronchial reactivity from chronic infection and inflammation (Taussig, 1993). Aerosolized bronchodilators and antiinflammatory agents may be effective, as will a course of an antibiotic. Wheezing in infancy may be difficult to alleviate, but often diminishes with age (Stern, 1989).

Drug Interactions

Primary care providers routinely include anticipatory guidance about substance abuse with children,

adolescents, and parents. The effect of tobacco smoke, both active and passive, is an obvious burden for children with CF. The growing evidence of an increased incidence of viral respiratory illness in all children exposed to passive smoke makes caregiver smoking an added risk to the child with cystic fibrosis (Wall, 1987). More alarming are Campbell and associates' (1992) findings of a significant association between heavy exposure to tobacco smoke and lower clinical scores, poorer pulmonary function results, and higher rates of hospitalization in children with CF. Smoke is also known to increase airway reactivity (Stern et al, 1987).

In addition to the overall impact of alcohol, smoke, and psychoactive drugs on organ systems of the child and adolescent with CF, specific interactions have been reported. Alcohol use in individuals on chloramphenicol or cephalosporins has been associated with episodes of nausea, vomiting, and headache. Alcohol has also been reported to be associated with increased pulmonary symptoms, perhaps from suppression of the cough reflex, and with episodes of hemoptysis.

The primary care provider should also be cognizant of certain interactions of drugs commonly used in the management of CF lung disease. Both erythromycin and ciprofloxacin alter the metabolism and excretion of theophylline, requiring a reduction in the theophylline dose during use of these drugs. With use of these antibiotics, the primary care provider should review signs of theophylline toxicity with children and parents and discuss a plan for dosage reduction if indications arise. Increased ultraviolet light sensitivity may occur in some children on tetracyclines and sulfonamides and their use should be avoided when sun exposure is anticipated.

DEVELOPMENTAL ISSUES

Sleep Patterns

Children with CF have a busy early morning routine, requiring early rising for school-age children and adolescents. At the same time, they are often more vulnerable to fatigue because of their increased basal metabolic rate. Sleep requirements, though not necessarily greater, should not be shortened.

Onset of nighttime coughing may also interfere with rest and contribute to general fatigue. Prompt attention to these symptoms is important to overall well-being.

Toileting

As in other children, toilet training should proceed as cues of developmental readiness are noted in the child. However, many children with CF continue to have stools more frequently than once a day, and may have some abdominal cramping before stooling even on adequate enzyme therapy. These problems may impede the child's interest in toileting and allowances should be made by parents for this delay.

Even though enzymes improve digestion of nutrients, some maldigested food passes through the intestine. As a result, stools may be malodorous and an embarrassment to children and adolescents. Parents, teachers, and friend's parents should be aware of the need for privacy during toileting and assist the child with managing bathroom odor.

Discipline

From the time of diagnosis, parents of children with CF not only grieve their loss of a healthy child, but also experience feelings of guilt associated with their genetic contribution. Parents struggle to redefine a future for their child and their family. The primary care provider can provide ongoing support and counseling during this difficult adjustment period. Setting limits and encouraging similar responsibilities for the child with CF and his or her siblings will help maintain consistency in family life.

The time commitment of daily therapy may not only create periodic conflict between parent and child but may also be seen by siblings as an inequity in parental attention. Conscious efforts by parents to give individual attention to each child may prevent feelings of jealousy and guilt. Extended family and community support are important ingredients in daily therapy, for parents need respite and the opportunity to develop individual interests (Venters, 1981; Quittner et al, 1992).

Parents of adolescents with CF are frequently frustrated and anxious about disease progression when they experience difficulty in maintaining their child's adherence to the treatment program. Factors influencing compliance with chronic illness regimens are numerous and complex (Pidgeon, 1989). Normal adolescent behavior of testing limits, perceived invincibility, and taking risks is com-

plicated by the chronicity and morbidity of CF. Experimentation with medications, both overuse and underuse, and refusal of chest physical therapy frequently occurs. Teenagers with CF often experience no immediate consequences of these experimentations, further reinforcing their behaviors. Although the relative risk of not doing therapy is difficult to quantify, documentation of the efficacy of chest physical therapy cannot be ignored. Parents who begin during early school years to transfer responsibility for illness management to their child often report fewer problems in adolescence. Even children 5 to 6 years of age are old enough to understand the need for such treatments as enzymes and vitamins. Adolescents with CF may also be more compliant if allowed to take control of parts of their illness management (e.g., using a mechanical percussor, Flutter valve, or one of the independent drainage techniques, or substituting an exercise program for a therapy session). Encouraging school-age children and adolescents to actively participate in clinic visits and involving them in decision making is essential to the child's development of accountability. Behavioral contracts may be useful tools for families and health care providers who are experiencing more problems with the adolescent (Sinnema et al, 1988).

Child Care

Parents of children with CF often struggle with day care issues. Parents need reassurance that a child with CF is not immunocompromised and will mount an adequate response to communicable diseases. However, choosing a day care setting with fewer children, and therefore potentially lower viral illness exposure, may be a more appropriate decision for parents of an infant or toddler. When a day care program has been selected, day care providers will need specific education regarding issues such as: (1) the child's individual nutritional and pulmonary treatment program, (2) the child's chronic cough and lack of contagion, and (3) methods to prevent the spread of viral illness in the setting. (See listing of educational materials at the end of this chapter.)

Schooling

A number of issues may surface for the child with CF in the school environment, and it may be helpful for a CF center provider to make a school visit, and meet with the school nurse, classroom teacher(s), physical education teacher, principal, and when appropriate, the director of special education. Commonly, school personnel have questions about the child's cough, bowel and pulmonary toilet needs, exercise tolerance, nutrition and medication needs during the school day, and school absenteeism for illness and hospitalization. Advice in handling these issues is greatly dependent on the individual child's severity of illness. Specific educational materials for school personnel are also available (see pages 344-345).

The degree to which short stature, difficulty in gaining and maintaining weight, and delayed pubertal development are present is variable. When significant, they effect the development of a positive body image and associated self-esteem, particularly in adolescence. These delays are often associated with increasing pulmonary involvement, and both alter the child's ability to fully participate in academics, social life, and sports and exercise programs. The primary care provider may be able to suggest choices of recreational activities and skills which are more likely to be tolerated and in which the child may have an opportunity to excel (e.g., swimming, diving, baseball, archery, gymnastics, certain track and field events, playing a musical instrument, and art) (AAP Committee on Sports Medicine and Fitness, 1994).

Sexuality

Of the men with cystic fibrosis, 98% are sterile because of blockage of the vas deferens; a sperm count is recommended to confirm the expected aspermia (Kotloff, 1994). Male adolescents need reassurance that this condition does not indicate impotency and will not diminish their ability to have normal sexual relations. Women with CF may have more difficulty becoming pregnant because of thick cervical mucus. Women also should be carefully evaluated and counseled about the degree of risk of pregnancy in their individual condition. This counseling is complex and includes such considerations as the woman's level of pulmonary function and overall health status, the statistical genetic risk of having a child with CF, and the woman's shortened life expectancy.

Contraception alternatives for adolescent and young adult women with CF have been controversial. Oral contraceptives have been reported to in-

crease the viscosity of cervical mucus and therefore carry the theoretical increased risk of having a similar effect on pulmonary mucus viscosity, although this has not been documented. Because of the comparative risk of pregnancy, many CF center providers recommend oral contraceptives after full discussion of these issues with the young woman. Reproductive issues in CF should be managed in consultation with the CF center team and the team's high-risk obstetrician/gynecologist consultant.

Transition Into Adulthood

Today, adolescents, whose parents were given a less than optimistic picture on survival at diagnosis, are being challenged to set goals for a future which may include college and vocational education, a career, and social relationships including marriage. At the same time, adolescents with CF struggle with increasing morbidity and higher rates of CF complications as they grow older.

Primary care providers, as well, are faced with meeting the needs of a growing population of young adults. In most regional CF centers, about 35% of the client population is over 18 years of age. Transition programs which move the adolescent into care by adult providers have been developed in a number of these centers. These programs feature a committed team of adult providers who have developed CF care expertise and who become jointly involved with pediatric providers in care delivery during adolescence. Implementation of these programs has not been without problems; but they have innovatively addressed client's developmental needs for independence and identity (Cappelli, MacDonald, and McGrath, 1989).

SPECIAL FAMILY CONCERNS AND RESOURCES

Families who deal with CF have a myriad of special concerns including the stress of its prognosis, the added financial burden of medical care, and maintaining family life despite the uncertainty of exacerbations, hospitalizations, and disease progression. It has been demonstrated that families, though stressed, generally cope successfully (Phillips et al, 1985; Buchanan and Morrison, 1992). McCubbin (1984) has identified circumstances which place a family dealing with CF at high risk for dysfunction and maladaptation. These include single-parent families, families with an adult with CF, and families with limited income.

Parents often need guidance in presenting information and answering questions about CF with their child and with other family members. In addition to the CF center team's help, written material is available, including books for school-age children (see pages 344-345). By age 10 to 12 years, most children's cognitive development is reaching formal operational thinking. Information regarding morbidity and mortality should be presented honestly, and within a framework of hope for continued breakthroughs in treatment research.

The financial burden of this condition is formidable and families often need additional assistance with health care costs. CF is a diagnosis covered in most states by programs for physically handicapped children or children with special needs. Eligibility requirements as well as benefits are highly variable; the CF center staff can be helpful in coordinating these efforts for a family.

CF is commonly seen in Caucasians of European origin. In a CF center population, it is not unusual to find few, if any, Black, Asian, or Indian children. When these children are diagnosed, the children and their families face the additional problem of limited support networks within their community. One-to-one contact between families may be helpful and can be facilitated by the CF center.

In families who are Amish and Mennonite, use of herbal medicine (e.g., garlic and pleurisy root) to treat the pulmonary and nutritional problems of CF is common. Remedies are often shared among families by mail. Coverage of health care costs can be a significant issue for families in many of the Anabaptist communities. Often, neither private insurance nor government programs are acceptable to them because of their religious beliefs. In addition, homes may not have electricity. Providers of health care to these children are well served by both sensitivity and creativity as they address issues in care delivery with these families.

When considering genetic testing of cultural, ethnic, and racial subpopulations, it is important to identify differences in prevalence of various CF mutations and their potential phenotypic expressions within and between these groups (e.g., Amish, Mennonite, Hutterite communities; Blacks,

Ashkenazi Jews). In addition, cultural differences in beliefs, attitudes, and feelings, and behavior regarding testing and intervention should be identified and understood by the counselor (Miller and Schwartz, 1992).

Community Resources

The CF Foundation is a national organization committed to supporting research for the treatment and cure of CF. Local chapters are found in many of the larger cities in the United States. The CF Foundation also develops and distributes excellent informational material for the lay public as well as the professional community (see list of informational materials). The 115 regional CF care centers in the United States offer expertise in the care and management of CF-related issues. Parents should be encouraged to keep in regular contact with the center; this ongoing and regular specialist care has been demonstrated to correlate with improved survival statistics (Wood, 1984). The CF center also offers a specialty team approach with physicians, nurse or nurse practitioner, nutritionist, social worker, respiratory or physical therapist, and clinical psychologist. The centers have a family focus in programming which often includes parent, adolescent, and young adult support groups, education programs, education and support for newly diagnosed families, genetic counseling and testing services, and medical specialty consultation for multiple organ systems involvement in CF.

Educational Materials

Cystic Fibrosis Foundation
6931 Arlington Rd
Bethesda, MD 20814.
1-800-FIGHT CF
  Chest Physical Therapy: Segmental Bronchial Drainage
  An Introduction to Cystic Fibrosis
  The Genetics of Cystic Fibrosis
  A Teacher's Guide to CF
  Living with Cystic Fibrosis: A Guide for Adolescents

Farmer G, Wilcox S: *Fat and loving it,* 1990.
  This is a book on nutrition written for individuals with CF and is available from Gail Farmer, PO Box 5127, Belmont, CA 94002.

Orenstein DM: *Cystic fibrosis: a guide for patient and family,* New York, 1989, Raven Press.

Ribando C, Langbaum T: *I have cystic fibrosis,* The Johns Hopkins Medical Institutes, 1985. *A story for school-aged children.*

Nakielna B, O'Loane M, and Durbach E: *For adults with cystic fibrosis.* Vancouver, BC V6H3N1, 1986, Shaughnessy Hospital CF Clinic.

Sondel S, Hartman L: *A way of life: cystic fibrosis nutrition handbook and cookbook,* 1988. Available for $5.00/copy from Karen Luther, F4/120 Food and Nutrition Services, University of Wisconsin Hospital and Clinics, Madison, WI 53792

Storey M, Adams E: *Snacks and more,* 1988, Pediatric Pulmonary Center, University of Rochester Medical Center, Rochester, New York 14642.

Available through pharmaceutical representatives

Luder E: *Living with cystic fibrosis: family guide to nutrition,* 1987, McNeil Pharmaceuticals, Spring House, PA 19477.

Mandolfo A: *Cystic fibrosis,* 1988, Solvay Pharmaceuticals, Marietta, Ga. *A booklet for young children.*

Stanzone A, Godwin SL: *Lets look at me,* 1989, Solvay Pharmaceuticals, Marietta, Ga. *A workbook for young children.*

A guide to cystic fibrosis for parents and children, a manual and video through McNeil Pharmaceuticals.

Cystic fibrosis in the classroom, available from Solvay Pharmaceuticals.

Available through the CF Center

Cystic fibrosis family education program: a comprehensive program developed by DK Seilheimer, et al at Baylor College of Medicine/Texas Children's Hospital. Distribution underwritten by Genentech.

This is a partial listing of helpful information for children and families. Contact a regional CF center for help with additional resources, particularly in specific content areas.

SUMMARY OF SPECIAL PRIMARY CARE NEEDS OF CHILDREN WITH CYSTIC FIBROSIS

Health care maintenance

Growth and development

Growth and developmental delay reported and variable; associated with pulmonary disease severity and maturational delay.

Degree of malabsorption and presence of pulmonary exacerbation are also factors affecting growth delay.

Pubertal delay may be anticipated in most adolescents.

Diet

High calorie, high protein diet recommended.

Fat intake not restricted; target of 35% to 40% daily intake in fat sources.

Pancreatic enzyme replacement and vitamin supplementation necessary in children with malabsorption.

Safety

Safe storage of multiple medications emphasized.

Immunizations

Generally, all routine immunizations should be given on schedule.

Influenza vaccine should be given annually per CDC guidelines.

Pneumococcal vaccine is not currently recommended.

Screening

Vision: routine screening is recommended.

Hearing: routine screening recommended; audiology screen for high-frequency hearing loss with aminoglycoside therapy.

Continued.

SUMMARY OF SPECIAL PRIMARY CARE NEEDS OF CHILDREN WITH CYSTIC FIBROSIS—cont'd

Dental: routine care

Hematocrit: routine screening recommended with full review of iron status as indicated.

Tuberculosis: routine testing with PPD at CF center.

Condition-specific screening: PFTs, chest roentgenography, sputum culture with drug sensitivities and blood and urine assays of liver function, renal function, cell counts and differential, glucose and nutrition status usually monitored at routine CF center visits.

Drug interactions

Erythromycin and ciprofloxacin may increase serum theophylline levels.

Alcohol use with cephalosporins or chloramphenicol may cause headaches, nausea, and vomiting.

Common illness management

Differential diagnosis

Constipation or diarrhea. rule out DIOS

Abdominal pain: rule out DIOS, appendicitis, volvulus, intusseption

Chest pain: rule out pneumothorax

Cough: further differentiation of component of RAD, lower respiratory tract infection/ inflammation, rhinitis/sinusitis may be helpful in selecting treatment choices.

Developmental issues

Sleep patterns:

Early morning routines require adjustment of bedtime. Nighttime cough may interfere with rest and require prompt attention.

Toileting:

Delayed bowel training may occur secondary to increased frequency of stools and associated abdominal cramping.

Discipline:

Normal expectations with allowances during periods of illness exacerbation.

Lack of compliance with treatment programs may effect disease progression in adolescence.

Child care:

Home care and small day care programs recommended during first year of life to reduce viral exposure. Day care workers need information on CF.

Schooling

Multiple school questions may be best addressed in a school visit.

Possible adjustment problems during adolescence related to altered body image and self-esteem.

School performance may be affected by fatigue and lethargy with an impending pulmonary exacerbation.

School absenteeism for hospitalizations requires coordination for ongoing academic services.

Sexuality

Male sterility should be confirmed.

Female reproductive issues are complex and require specialty consultation and counseling.

Transition to Adulthood:

Developmentally appropriate specialty health care should begin in adolescence.

Special family concerns

Uncertainty of illness progression and predicted lethality.

Family functioning during illness exacerbations requiring hospitalizations.

Impact of treatment program, particularly chest physical therapy on family life.

Cultural issues of minority and subpopulations include isolation, use of alternative therapies, sensitive counseling for genetic screening, and insurance coverage for health care.

REFERENCES

Abrons HL: Cystic fibrosis: current concepts, *West Virginia Medical Journal* 89(6):236-240, 1993.

Accurso FJ: Aerosolized dornase alfa in cystic fibrosis patients with clinically mild lung disease, *Dornase Alfa Clinical Series* 2(1):1-6, 1995.

Adams EA: Nutrition care in cystic fibrosis, *Nutrition news,* Seattle, WA, 1988, University of Washington Child Development and Mental Retardation Center.

American Academy of Pediatrics Committee on Sports Medicine and Fitness, Medical conditions affecting sports participation, *Pediatrics* 94(5):757-760, 1994.

American Academy of Pediatrics, *Report of the committee on infectious diseases,* American Academy of Pediatrics, IL, 1994.

American Academy of Pediatrics, AAPCom: AAP alert re varicella vaccine. American Academy of Pediatrics, IL, 1995.

Beaudet AL, Buffone GJ: Prenatal diagnosis of cystic fibrosis, *J Pediatr* 111:630-633, 1989.

Beaudet AL et al: Linkage disequilibrium, cystic fibrosis, and genetic counseling, *American Journal of Human Genetics* 44:319-326, 1989.

Borowitz D: Pathophysiology of gastrointestinal complications of cystic fibrosis, *Semin Respir Crit Care Med* 15(5):391-401, 1994.

Buchanan E, Morrison LM: Cystic fibrosis: a full-time occupation or more of a way of life? *European Journal of Clinical Nutrition* 46, suppl 1:S41-S46, 1992.

Campbell PW et al: Association of poor clinical status and heavy exposure to tobacco smoke in patients with cystic fibrosis who are homozygous for the delta F 508 deletion, *J Pediatr* 120(2):261-264, 1992.

Cappelli M, MacDonald N, and McGrath P: Assessment of readiness to transfer to adult care for adolescents with cystic fibrosis, *Child Health Care* 18:218-224, 1989.

Colin AA, Wohl MEB: Cystic fibrosis, *Pediatrics in Review* 15(5):192-200, 1994.

Cutting GR: Genotype defect: its effect on cellular function and phenotypic expression, *Semin Respir Crit Care Med* 15(5):356-363, 1994.

Cystic Fibrosis Foundation, *Patient registry 1991 annual data report,* Bethesda, MD, October 1992.

Dalzell AM et al: Nutritional rehabilitation in cystic fibrosis: a 5-year follow-up study, *J Pediatr Gastroenterology and Nutrition* 15(2):141-145, 1992.

Davidson AGF, McIlwaine M: Airway clearance techniques in cystic fibrosis, *New Insights into Cystic Fibrosis* 3(1):6-11, 1995.

Davis PB: Advances in treatment of cystic fibrosis. Plenary session presented at the 8th Annual North American Cystic Fibrosis Conference, *Pediatric pulmonology supplement 10,* 69-70, 1994.

deJong W et al: Effect of a home exercise training program in patients with cystic fibrosis, *Chest* 105(2):463-468, 1994.

Desmond KJ et al: Immediate and long-term effects of chest physiotherapy in patients with cystic fibrosis, *J Pediatr* 103:538-542, 1983.

Drumm MT et al: Correction of the cystic fibrosis defect in vitro by retrovirus-mediated gene transfer, *Cell* 62:1227-1233, 1992.

Egan TM, Detterbeck, FC: Techniques and results of double lung transplantation, *Chest Surg Clin North Am* 3:89-111, 1993.

Fernbach SD, Thomson EJ: Molecular genetic technology in cystic fibrosis: implications for nursing practice, *J Pediatr Nurs* 7(1):20-25, 1992.

Fitzpatrick SB, Rosenstein BJ, and Langbaum TS: Diagnosis of cystic fibrosis during adolescence, *J Adolesc Health* 7:38-43, 1986.

Grand RJ: Gastrointestinal and nutritional issues. *Highlights: Selected Proceedings from the 8th Annual North American Cystic Fibrosis Conference,* Orlando Florida, October 1994.

Hodson ME: Aerosolized dornase alfa (rhDNase) for therapy of cystic fibrosis, *Am J Respir Crit Care Med* 151:S70-S74, 1995.

Hooper DC, Wolfson JS: Floroquinolone antimicrobial agents, *New Engl J Med* 324(6):384-394, 1991.

Hubbard RC et al: A preliminary study of aerosolized recombinant human deoxyribonuclease I in the treatment of cystic fibrosis, *New Engl J Med* 326(12):812-815, 1992.

Hubbard VS: Nutritional considerations in cystic fibrosis, *Semin Respir Med* 6(4):308-313, 1985.

Kilby JM et al: Nontuberculous mycobacteria in adult patients with cystic fibrosis, *Chest* 201(1):70-75, 1992.

King VV: Upper respiratory disease, sinusitis, and polyposis, *Clinical Review of Allergy* 9(1-2):143-157, 1991.

Kirchner KK et al: Increased DNA levels in bronchoalveolar lavage fluid obtained from infants with cystic fibrosis, *Pediatr Pulmonol,* suppl 9:288, 1993.

Knowles MR et al: Pharmacologic modulation of salt and water in the airway epithelium in cystic fibrosis, *Am J Respir Crit Care Med* 151:S65-S69, 1995.

Konstan MW et al: Bronchoalveolar lavage findings in cystic fibrosis patients with stable, clinically mild lung disease suggest ongoing infection and inflammation, *Am J Respir Crit Care Med* 150:448-454, 1994.

Konstan MW et al: Effect of high dose ibuprofen in patients with cystic fibrosis, *New Engl J Med* 332(13):848-854, 1995.

Kotloff RM: Reproductive issues in patients with cystic fibrosis, *Semin Respir Crit Care Med* 15(5):402-413, 1994.

Levy LD et al: Effects of long-term nutritional rehabilitation on body composition and clinical status in malnourished children and adolescents with cystic fibrosis, *J Pediatr* 107:225-230, 1985.

Lloyd-Still JD: Pathology. In JD Lloyd-Still, (editor): *Textbook of cystic fibrosis,* Boston, 1983, John Wright-PSG Inc, pp 19-31.

MacDonald N, Morris R, and Beaudrey P: Varicella in children with cystic fibrosis, *Pediatric Infectious Disease Journal* 6:414-416, 1987.

MacLusky I: Cystic fibrosis for the primary care pediatrician, *Pediatr Ann* 22(9):541-549, 1993.

Mahaney MC, McCoy KS: Developmental delays and pulmonary disease severity in cystic fibrosis, *Human Biology* 58(3):445-460, 1986.

Marshall BC: Pathophysiology of pulmonary disease in cystic fibrosis, *Semin Respir Crit Care Med* 15(5):364-374, 1994.

Marshall SG, Ramsey BW: Aerosol therapy in cystic fibrosis: DNase, tobramycin, *Semin Respir Crit Care Med* 15(5):434-438, 1994.

McCubbin M: Nursing assessment of parental coping with cystic fibrosis, *West J Nurs Res* 6:407-422, 1984.

Miller SR, Schwartz RH: Attitudes toward genetic testing of Amish, Mennonite, and Hutterite families with cystic fibrosis, *Am J Public Health* 82(2):236-242, 1992.

Mischler EH: Treatment of pulmonary disease in cystic fibrosis, *Semin Respir Med* 6:271-284, 1985.

Moshang T, Holsclaw DS: Menarchal determinants in cystic fibrosis, *Am J Dis Child* 134:1139-1142, 1980.

Moss R et al: Safety and pharmacokinetics of a mucoid *Pseudomonas aeruginosa* immune globulin, intravenous (human) in patients with cystic fibrosis. Preliminary results of a phase I/II trial. Abstract presented at the 8th Annual North American Cystic Fibrosis Conference, Orlando, FL, October 1994.

National Academy of Sciences: Report of the committee for a study for evaluation of testing for cystic fibrosis, *J Pediatr* 88(4):711-750, 1976.

National Committee for Clinical Laboratory Standards: *Sweat testing: sample collection and quantitative analysis, proposed guideline.* NCCLS document C34-P (ISBN 1-56238-188-1). NCCLS, 771 East Lancaster Ave, Villanova, PA 19085, 1993.

National Institutes of Health Workshop on Population Screening for the CF Gene: *New Engl J Med* 323:70-71, 1990.

Nutrition assessment and management in cystic fibrosis: a consensus report, *Am J Clin Nutr* 55:108-116, 1992.

Orenstein DM, Henke KG, and Cerney FJ: Exercise and cystic fibrosis, *Phys Sports Med* 11:57-62, 1983.

Pencharz PP, Durie PR: Nutrition management of cystic fibrosis, *Ann Rev Nutr* 13:111-136, 1993.

Phillips S et al: Parent interview findings regarding impact of cystic fibrosis on families, *Dev Behav Pediatr* 6(3):122-127, 1985.

Pidgeon V: Compliance with chronic illness regimens: school-aged children and adolescents. *J Pediatr Nurs* 4(1):36-47, 1989.

Prober CG: The impact of respiratory viral infections in patients with cystic fibrosis. *Clin Review of Allergy* 9(1):87-102, 1991.

Quinton PM: Defective epithelial ion transport in cystic fibrosis, *Clin Chem* 35(5):726-730, 1989.

Quittner AL et al: *J Pediatr Psychol* 17(6)m:683-704, 1992.

Ramirez JC et al: Bilateral lung transplantation for cystic fibrosis, *Journal of Thoracic Cardiovascular Surgery* 103:287-294, 1992.

Ramsey B: A summary of the results of the phase III multicenter clinical trial: aerosol administration of recombinant human DNase reduces the risk of respiratory tract infection and improves pulmonary function in patients with cystic fibrosis, *Pediatr Pulmonol Suppl* 9:152-153, 1993.

Rommens JM et al: Identification of the cystic fibrosis gene: chromosome walking and jumping, *Science* 245:1059-1065, 1989.

Rosenstein B: Cystic fibrosis. In FA Oski, (editor): *Principles and practice of pediatrics,* Philadelphia, 1990, JB Lippincott, pp 1362-1372.

Rosenstein BJ, Eigen H: Risks of alternate-day prednisone in patients with cystic fibrosis, *Pediatrics* 87:245-246, 1991.

Rosenstein BJ, Langbaum TS: Diagnosis. In LM Taussig, (editor): *Cystic fibrosis,* New York, 1984, Theime Stratton Inc, pp 85-114.

Rubenstein S, Moss R, and Lewiston N: Constipation and meconium ileus equivalent in patients with cystic fibrosis, *Pediatrics* 78(3):473-479, 1986.

Schidlow DV, Taussig LM, and Knowles MR: Cystic fibrosis foundation consensus conference report on pulmonary complications of cystic fibrosis. *Pediatr Pulmonol* 15(3):187-198, 1993.

Schwartz RH: Cystic fibrosis. In RH Hoekelman, (editor): *Primary pediatric care,* St Louis, 1987, Mosby.

Shapiro SK, Seilheimer DK: Screening for cystic fibrosis: clinical issues and genetic counseling implications, *New Insights into CF* 2(1):6-11, 1994.

Shepherd R, Cooksley WGE, and Cooke WDD: Improved growth and clinical nutritional and respiratory changes in response to nutritional therapy in cystic fibrosis, *J Pediatr* 97:351-357, 1980.

Shepherd RW et al: Nutritional rehabilitation in cystic fibrosis: controlled studies of effects on nutritional growth retardation, body protein turnover, and course of pulmonary disease, *J Pediatr* 109:788-794, 1986.

Sinnema G et al: The development of independence in adolescents with cystic fibrosis, *J Adol Health* 9:61-66, 1988.

Soutter VL et al: Chronic undernutrition/growth retardation in cystic fibrosis, *Clin Gastroenterol* 15(1):137-155, 1986.

Stern RC: Cystic fibrosis: recent developments in diagnosis and treatment, *Pediatr in Rev* 7(9):276-286, 1986.

Stern RC: The primary care physician and the patient with cystic fibrosis, *J Pediatr* 114(1):31-36, 1989.

Stern RC et al: Recreational use of psychoactive drugs by patients with cystic fibrosis, *J Pediatr* 111:293-299, 1987.

Taussig LM: Desired outcomes in cystic fibrosis airway disease: opportunities for pharmacologic intervention, *New Insights into Cystic Fibrosis* 1(1):5-8, 1993.

Taussig LM, Landau LI, and Marks MI: Respiratory system. In LM Taussig, (editor): *Cystic fibrosis,* New York, 1984, Thieme-Stratton, Inc, pp 115-174.

Venters M: Familial coping with chronic and severe illness: the case of cystic fibrosis, *Soc Sci Med* 15A:289-297, 1981.

Wall M: Update on the effects of passive smoking in children, *J Respir Dis* 8(7):31-36, 1987.

Wang EEL et al: Association of respiratory viral infections with pulmonary deterioration in patients with cystic fibrosis, *New Engl J Med* 311:1653-1658, 1984.

Wertz DC et al: Attitudes toward abortion among parents of children with cystic fibrosis, *Am J Public Health* 81:992-996, 1992.

Wilfond BS, Fost N: The cystic fibrosis gene: medical and social implications for heterozygote detection. *JAMA* 263(20):2777-2783, 1990.

Wilson JM: Cystic fibrosis: strategies for gene therapy, *Semin Respir Crit Care Med* 15(5):439-445, 1994.

Wood RE: Prognosis. In LM Taussig, (editor): *Cystic fibrosis,* New York, 1984, Thieme-Stratton, Inc, pp 434-460.

Wooten SA et al: Energy balance and growth in cystic fibrosis, *J Rehab Social Med* 84, suppl 18:22-27, 1991.

Diabetes Mellitus (Type I)

17

Margaret Grey and Elizabeth A. Boland

ETIOLOGY

Diabetes mellitus was first described in the Egyptian *Ebers Papyrus* in 1500 BC. Type I, or insulin-dependent diabetes mellitus (IDDM), occurs most commonly in young people, and it is characterized by β-cell failure. In type II, or non–insulin-dependent diabetes mellitus (NIDDM), clients are often overweight, are usually more than 30 years of age, overproduce insulin, and have a receptor site defect. Thus those with NIDDM can often be treated orally with hypoglycemic agents, whereas those with IDDM must be treated with insulin.

The etiology of IDDM is unknown, but many factors have been hypothesized to contribute to the cause of the disease. Genetic susceptibility is a necessary precursor to the development of IDDM (Drash, 1987). Certain histocompatibility leukocyte antigen (HLA) genes are believed to play a role in the genetic inheritance of the tendency to develop IDDM. Individuals with IDDM have an increased frequency of HLA genes B8, B15, DR3, and DR4 (Lernmark, 1991). The HLA-DR genes are known to be associated with autoimmunity. Evidence of autoimmunity is necessary but not sufficient for the development of IDDM. It is hypothesized that without genetic susceptibility, other factors will not initiate the autoimmune process. In autoimmunity, "self" antigens are no longer recognized as such, and a self-destructive process occurs. Islet cell antibodies can be detected in a majority of newly diagnosed individuals with IDDM (Lendrum, Walker, and Gamble, 1975; Skyler and Marks, 1993), and evidence of an autoimmune response may be present up to 9 years before the onset of clinical symptoms (Srikanto et al, 1983).

Other factors such as host and environmental factors may influence the development of the illness, because the concordance rate is only 50% in identical twins. Such factors include age, race, stress, and infectious agents (Vialettes et al, 1989). Recent studies have also suggested that the early introduction of dairy products is associated with an increased risk of IDDM, and that breast feeding may be protective (Virtanen et al, 1993).

INCIDENCE

Insulin-dependent diabetes mellitus is the most common metabolic disorder of childhood and it affects 1.7 cases per 1000 people, and approximately 123,000 children (American Diabetes Association, 1993a). Overall, the annual incidence of IDDM in the United States is approximately 18 new cases per 100,000 people under the age of 20, with a peak incidence at about 10 to 12 years of age in girls and 12 to 14 in boys (ADA, 1993a).

CLINICAL MANIFESTATIONS AT TIME OF DIAGNOSIS

Despite the fact that the autoimmune process may be long standing before the diagnosis of diabetes is made, the signs and symptoms of IDDM are usually present for a short period of time. Once the autoimmune process has destroyed enough of the pancreatic β, or islet cells to produce clinical evidence of illness, the classic symptoms (polydipsia, polyuria, polyphagia) of diabetes occur. As can be seen in Fig. 17-1, the lack of insulin production leads to disturbances in carbohydrate, protein, and fat metabolism.

The hormone insulin, produced by the pancreatic β cells, or islets of Langerhans, is responsible for the utilization of glucose in the cell. In its absence, there are three general alterations: (1) reduced entry of glucose into the cell; (2) unavailability of carbohydrate as a substrate for energy needs; and (3) utilization by the cell of alternate substrates, namely, fatty acids derived from adipose stores and amino acids from body protein. Thus when there is lack of insulin, glucose cannot be used in the cell for energy, and hyperglycemia results. The extraordinary concentration of glucose in the blood serves to promote an osmotic diuresis, so that large amounts of urine are produced. This osmotic diuresis is responsible for the symptom of polyuria, and as the body struggles to maintain homeostasis, polydipsia ensues.

If glucose is not available as a source of energy, alternative sources must be used. There is a reliance on lipolysis, as well as proteolysis. When this occurs, polyphagia becomes prominent as the body attempts to avoid starvation. Should these symptoms go uncorrected, the hyperglycemia and ketonemia secondary to increased lipolysis will progress to severe levels, and diabetic ketoacidosis will occur.

The diagnosis of diabetes is easily established. Any child with the classic symptoms should have levels of blood glucose and urinary glucose and ketones determined. If the blood glucose level is more than 200 mg/dl and glucose, ketones, or both are present in the urine, the diagnosis is established (ADA, 1995).

TREATMENT

Management of the illness has two major objectives: to return the blood glucose levels to near normal and to prevent complications (ADA, 1995). Controversy exists about the relative roles of primary care providers and specialists in the care of children with diabetes. Current recommendations are that most children should be followed by the primary caregiver for routine ongoing care but that the specialist team approach is best for education and ongoing oversight of the diabetes. This arrangement, of course, depends on many factors, including the proximity of the specialist and the expertise of the primary care provider.

Replacement of insulin results in dramatic reversal of the symptoms of the disease. At diagnosis, the majority of children are hospitalized, in part for correction of the metabolic derangement but also for education in the management of the condition. Once any acidosis is corrected, subcutaneous treatment with insulin is the mainstay of therapy.

Table 17-1 shows the actions of the most common types of insulin. Insulin may be derived from pork or it may be genetically engineered as human insulin. In general, the action of human insulins is more rapid in onset and peak than pork insulins. In the past, animal insulins were associated with

---

CLINICAL MANIFESTATIONS

- Hyperglycemia
- Polydipsia
- Polyuria
- Polyphagia

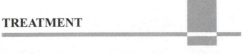

TREATMENT

- Insulin to achieve near-normal blood glucose
- Diet sufficient for growth
- Monitoring of blood sugars several times daily
- Glycosylated hemoglobin to assess overall control

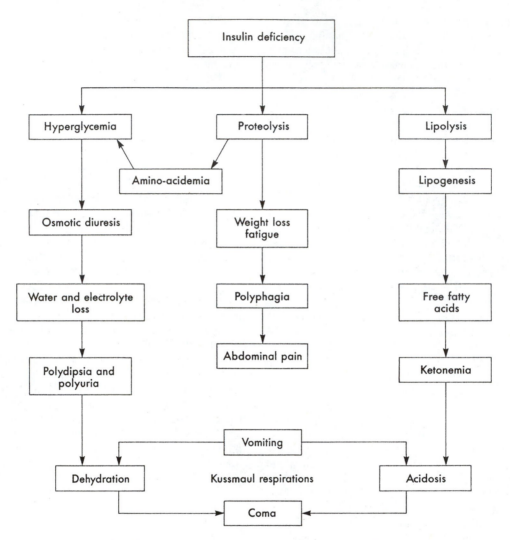

Fig. 17-1.   Signs and symptoms of type I diabetes mellitus.

various local reactions, including reddening, itching and inflammation, which eventually led to the development of lipoatrophy at injection sites. Human insulins are thought to be less immunogenic. Although the incidence of these local reactions decreased dramatically with the introduction of more highly purified pork insulins in the late 70s, most newly-diagnosed children with diabetes are now started on human insulins (Santiago, 1993a).

Most children are given two injections daily, one before breakfast and one before the evening meal. Although doses must be individually titrated, often two thirds of the daily dose is given in the morning as one-third short-acting insulin and two-thirds intermediate-acting insulin. The remaining one third is given in the evening, similarly divided between short- and intermediate-acting insulin. Based on the blood glucose response, the dose is al-

Table 17-1.
TYPES AND ACTIONS OF INSULIN PREPARATIONS

	Approximate action curves (hr)		
Class/name	Onset	Peak	Duration
Rapid acting			
Regular	0.5-1	2-4	4-6
Intermediate acting			
NPH	1.5-2	6-12	18-24
Lente	1.5-2	6-12	16-24
Long acting			
Ultralente	4-8	10-20	16-24

tered as necessary for maintenance of blood glucose levels as close to normal as possible. Children on intensive therapy regimens, which are currently recommended for individuals over the age of 13, may receive multiple injections of insulin daily or continuous subcutaneous insulin infusion to more closely mimic the body's normal insulin response (see Tamborlane et al, 1994).

Shortly after the diagnosis is made, many children experience a sharp reduction in the insulin requirement. In some cases no insulin is necessary for a period of time, which may last up to 6 months, but some health care providers will continue a small dose to maintain the injection schedule. However, the insulin requirement will return, and children should be cautioned that this honeymoon period does not indicate that the diabetes has gone away. Once destruction of the β cells is complete, usually within 2 years of diagnosis, most children will require insulin replacement of approximately 1 U/kg of body weight (Travis, Brouhard, & Schreiner, 1987), although the total may reach 1.5 to 2.0 U/kg (Plotnick, 1994; Santiago, 1993a).

Because exogenous insulin cannot mimic the normal moment-to-moment response of the β cells to changes in blood glucose levels, regulation of both diet and exercise help to minimize the variation in blood glucose levels. The child with diabetes, unlike the individual with NIDDM, is often slender. Therefore, the goal of dietary therapy is to

provide sufficient calories for normal growth and development distributed in three meals and two or three snacks. Such a meal plan, when concentrated sugars are limited or avoided, serves to help avoid hyperglycemia, prevent hypoglycemia, and maintain metabolic balance (Brink, 1988). Consistent with the current recommendations of the American Academy of Pediatrics, American and Canadian Diabetes Associations, and the American Dietetic Association, the composition of the diet should be 55% to 60% carbohydrate, 10% to 20% protein, and 10% to 20% fats, with less than 10% saturated fats (Franz et al, 1994).

Daily caloric needs can be estimated to be 1000 calories for the first year of life with approximately 100 calories added per year of age until age 10 to 12 years. Thereafter, females may need a reduction in total calories to the common adult level of 1400 to 1600 calories daily unless they are exceptionally active on a regular basis, whereas males will continue to need approximately 2000 calories daily. Shortly after diagnosis, children may need an additional 200 to 700 kcal per day to make up the negative energy balance at diagnosis (Connell and Thomas-Doberson, 1991).

Maintenance of near-normal or normal blood glucose levels requires constant self-monitoring. Self-monitored blood glucose (SMBG) levels allow people with diabetes to have more precision in monitoring than is permitted with urine testing. Glucose is not found in the urine until the blood glucose level rises above the renal threshold, usually about 180 mg/dl. Because the goal of therapy is to maintain blood glucose levels between 80 to 120 mg/dl before meals and 100 to 140 mg/dl at bedtime (ADA, 1995), self-monitoring blood glucose levels allows the individual to know exactly what the blood glucose level is at any moment in time and allows the child to adjust the dose of insulin in response to his or her actual blood glucose level. Several methods can determine SMBG levels, all of which are similar. A droplet of capillary blood is obtained from a fingerstick and placed on a small glucose reagent strip. After the required period of time, the degree of color change on the strip is measured by inserting it in a meter or, rarely, comparing it with a standardized color chart.

The pattern of testing varies with providers. Most children are advised to test three to four times daily, at various times throughout the day, and when symptoms are present. However, some health care providers prefer that tests be done at times of peak insulin action (e.g., 3 PM to 5 PM, bedtime), whereas others prefer to see tests at varying times. In any case, the results of SMBG testing are used to identify asymptomatic hypoglycemia, to determine patterns in insulin action, and to make appropriate alterations in the insulin dose. For example, if a child consistently has high blood glucose levels before the evening meal, the morning intermediate-acting insulin (NPH or Lente) would be increased to prevent this effect.

Children and adolescents with diabetes are routinely seen approximately every 3 months. Quarterly visits correspond to the rate at which the glycosylated hemoglobin levels can be expected to change. Glycosylated hemoglobin (Plotnik, 1994) or hemoglobin A_{1c} is a measure of the attachment of glucose to the circulating hemoglobin molecule. In nondiabetic individuals, glycosylated hemoglobin will comprise 3% to 6% of the total hemoglobin, whereas those with diabetes have levels in excess of 6%, varying in proportion to the blood glucose levels. The glycosylated hemoglobin level reflects the average blood glucose level over the most recent 3 months, because the life span of the hemoglobin molecule is approximately 120 days. It is not affected by short-term fluctuations and is considered to be an objective and accurate measure of long-term diabetes control (Gabbay et al, 1977; ADA, 1993b).

Because diabetes is an autoimmune disease, it is associated with other autoimmune diseases, especially Hashimoto's thyroiditis (Eisenbarth, 1986). Children and adolescents who demonstrate any change in growth pattern or who develop signs and symptoms of either hypothyroidism or hyperthyroidism should be tested with thyroid function studies (triiodothyronine, thyroxine, and thyroid-stimulating hormone levels).

RECENT AND ANTICIPATED ADVANCES IN DIAGNOSIS AND MANAGEMENT

Primary care providers should be aware of several recent advances in the treatment of IDDM. These include the seminal findings of the Diabetes Control and Complications Trial (DCCT) (DCCT Research Group, 1993b; 1994), and the Diabetes Prevention Trial.

Before publication of the results of the Diabetes Control and Complications Trial (DCCT) in 1993, a convincing benefit of intensive therapy had not been demonstrated, despite suggestions from animal and epidemiologic studies (DCCT Research Group, 1986). The DCCT was a multicenter, randomized clinical trial designed to compare intensive with conventional diabetes therapy to determine its effects on the development and progression of early vascular and neurologic complications of IDDM (DCCT Research Group, 1993b). A total of 1441 people (age 13 to 39) with IDDM, 726 of whom had no retinopathy at baseline and 715 who had mild retinopathy, were randomly assigned to intensive therapy or to conventional therapy. Intensive therapy consisted of three or more injections per day of insulin with frequent blood glucose monitoring, whereas conventional therapy consisted of one or two insulin injections per day. Goals of intensive therapy were reduction of glucose to normal range, with glycosylated hemoglobin in the normal range. Subjects in the intensive therapy group had monthly visits and were followed frequently by telephone (Santiago, 1993b). After 6.5 years, the study was terminated because the results were so impressive—in the cohort without retinopathy, the risk for developing it decreased 76% with intensive therapy, and in the secondary prevention cohort, the progression of retinopathy was slowed by 54%. Further, microalbuminuria was reduced by 39%, albuminuria by 54%, and clinical neuropathy by 60%. Intensive therapy, however, was associated with a two- to three-fold increase in severe hypoglycemia and clinically significant weight gain. There were no differences between those in the intensive treatment group and those in the conventional group in mean total scores on a quality of life (DQOL) measure as well. On the basis of these findings, the researchers and the American Diabetes Association recommended in individuals with IDDM, "a primary treatment goal should be blood glucose control at least equal to that achieved in the intensively treated cohort" (ADA, 1993b, p 1555).

Among the 1441 clients in the DCCT were 195 adolescents (13 to 17 years of age at entry), 125 with no retinopathy and 70 with mild retinopathy. Since adolescents face unique issues with regard to diabetes compared with adult subjects, data on these subjects were analyzed separately (DCCT Research Group, 1994). In contrast with the larger study cohort, the adolescents took longer to attain near normal glycosylated hemoglobin (6 to 12 months versus 6 months at nadir). Nevertheless, similar positive results of intensive treatment were also found with this cohort; decreased risk of retinopathy, retinopathy progression, microalbuminuria, and clinical neuropathy by 53% to 70%. In terms of quality of life, none of the subjects voluntarily withdrew from the study, and adolescents in the intensively treated group did not differ from the conventional treatment group on a measure of quality of life. Thus the DCCT Research Group (1994) recommend that "the same recommendations [as in the full DCCT] should be made for most subjects in the 13- to 17-year-old age group." Further, they note that the adolescents in the DCCT were the most difficult to manage and required the most time of the treatment team, but that the potential savings to young people with IDDM in suffering and long-term costs are worth the investment of treatment resources.

Given the results of the DCCT and the recommendation that all individuals over the age of 13 be urged to achieve control equal to that in the DCCT, more diabetes providers are implementing intensive therapy regimens. Intensive therapy involves three or more insulin injections per day or insulin delivered by continuous subcutaneous insulin infusion (CSII). Dosage of insulin is adjusted frequently according to frequent blood glucose monitoring (at least four times per day, and once per week at 3 AM), strict dietary intake, and anticipated exercise. These regimens require frequent and careful monitoring by the diabetes team (physician, nurse, dietician, behavioralist), and are difficult to accomplish in a primary care setting (Drash, 1993).

Children younger than adolescence can be taught the principles behind intensive therapy, but care must be taken to avoid severe hypoglycemia which may complicate intensive therapy regimens. The concern with severe hypoglycemia in young children is the effect of lowered blood sugar on brain development and functioning. Some health care providers believe that frequent monitoring and careful adjustment of insulin therapy can help to prevent severe hypoglycemia in younger children attempting intensive therapy.

The Diabetes Prevention Trial-Type 1 (DPT-1) is currently being conducted in the United States. All consenting first-degree relatives of IDDM are being screened to see if they are at risk for developing the disease in the next 5 years. If the relatives are positive, they will be asked to have more specific testing, including glucose tolerance testing and HLA typing. If these tests show the relative to be at significant risk, the relative will be asked to participate in a randomized clinical trial to determine if small doses of insulin will prevent the onset of the disease. The trial is based on animal and human studies with small samples (Keller, Eisenbarth, and Jackson, 1993) that suggest that small doses of insulin may protect the pancreatic β cells from the destruction associated with IDDM by preventing the autoimmune process from proceeding.

In addition, researchers are developing artificial insulin delivery systems (Clark and Plotnick, 1990) and transplantation of β cells (Lacy, 1994) as new methods of treatment. The artificial insulin delivery systems will improve on the CSII by incorporating a feedback loop that will alter the insulin delivered according to the blood glucose level. Transplantation of β cells results in a cure for people with diabetes who are already on immunosuppression for previous organ transplants. The challenge remaining is to prevent autoimmune destruction of these cells in those who are not immunosuppressed. Techniques have been developed to encapsulate the islets, and studies are underway to determine if these techniques will be effective early in the course of the disease.

Research advances are also being made in home blood glucose monitoring. Future technology has the potential to monitor blood glucose levels on an almost continuous basis. Near-infrared and implantable continuous monitoring devices may either decrease or eliminate the pain and inconvenience of home blood glucose monitoring; therefore, individuals will be able to test more frequently. This increased monitoring is likely to improve metabolic control and decrease the risk of hypoglycemic episodes (ADA, 1995).

ASSOCIATED PROBLEMS

Diabetic Ketoacidosis and Hypoglycemia

Fig. 17-1 shows the physiologic process that results in diabetic ketoacidosis (DKA) when there is a lack of insulin. Any potential stressor, such as illness, fever, injury, and psychosocial stress, can increase the risk of metabolic derangement caused by disturbances in counterregulatory hormones and lead to DKA. Thus any stressor in a child with diabetes must be managed with care. Management of intercurrent illness is discussed later.

Children with well-controlled diabetes will occasionally experience mild to moderate hypoglycemia. Because the symptoms of DKA and hypoglycemia can sometimes be confused, they are compared in the box below. Hypoglycemia may be caused by too much insulin, too little food, too much exercise, or any combination of these factors. Although it is easily treated, prevention is the best approach. Again, SMBG determination is helpful. Using SMBG testing, children can identify patterns of lower blood glucose levels that may indicate periods of increased risk. During these periods, the insulin dose can be altered to prevent the hypoglycemia. If the child anticipates unusual physical activity, both insulin and diet can be adjusted to prevent low glucose levels.

Hypoglycemia presents particular problems at different ages. Infants are unable to express the feelings associated with hypoglycemia, and they must be observed for listlessness, sleepiness, or irritability (Charron-Prochownik and Schwartz, 1984; Lipman, et al, 1989a). Parents should be instructed that any unusual behavior at any time is an indication for blood glucose levels to be measured. If the result is less than 80 mg/dl, the conscious infant should be given 2 to 4 oz of sweet liquids or a small amount of cake frosting; the unconscious or convulsing infant should be given glucagon by injection (Lipman et al, 1989a). Older children can be taught the symptoms of hypoglycemia and how to prevent its occurrence. They should also be instructed to carry high-sugar foods with them at all times. All children with IDDM should wear medical identification so that they can be diagnosed and treated appropriately should they lose consciousness while away from home.

Some substances have the potential to increase the likelihood of hypoglycemia. Adolescents need to know that alcohol augments the glucose-lowering effects of insulin and that the symptoms of alcohol intoxication and hypoglycemia are similar. Low blood glucose levels can increase the body's sensitivity to alcohol. Many experimenting teenagers have found themselves in the emergency room with profound hypoglycemia. Stimulants such as amphetamines and cocaine may increase metabolism and decrease appetite, with a potential for hypoglycemia to occur (Lipman et al, 1989b).

Monilial Infections

Once healthy girls are toilet trained, monilial infections of the perineum are rare until adolescence, when the estrogenation of the vagina provides a potential environment for monilial growth. Hyperglycemia also leads to increased glucose levels in vaginal secretions, which provides an ideal medium for monilia. Thus girls with diabetes have an increased risk for monilial vaginitis, and any complaint of vaginal discharge and itching should be investigated with a potassium hydroxide preparation and treated appropriately.

ASSOCIATED SYMPTOMS

•Hyperglycemia	•Hypoglycemia
Slow onset	Rapid onset
Increased thirst and urination	Excessive sweating
High blood and urine glucose levels	Fainting
Urinary ketones	Headache
Weakness and abdominal pain	Trembling and shaking
Heavy, labored breathing	Hunger
Anorexia	Inability to waken
Nausea and vomiting	Irritability
Monilial infections	Personality change

PROGNOSIS

Diabetes is the seventh leading cause of death in the United States (National Center for Health Statistics, 1994). The life expectancy of a child with diabetes at the age of 10 is 44 years, whereas his or her peers can be expected to live 62 more years (Raskin and Rosenstock, 1987). For the most part, this early mortality is a result of the long-term complications of the illness.

Diabetic complications appear to be a function of the years of diabetes after puberty rather than the absolute number of years of diabetes (Rogers et al, 1986). Complications can range from asymptomatic mild proteinuria to blindness, renal failure, and painful neuropathies. Raskin and Rosenstock (1987) suggest that hyperglycemia is a necessary but not sufficient factor for the development of complications. In addition to hyperglycemia, genetic factors appear to influence the development of complications. Epidemiologic evidence suggests that in the general diabetic population prevalence of microvascular complications is relatively high, with approximately 40% of affected individuals experiencing renal failure and 50% of affected individuals having diabetic retinopathy after 15 years. Although the DCCT showed that improvement in metabolic control to near normal levels delays the onset or progression of complications, complications were not eliminated. It is clear, however, that the better the metabolic control, the better the chance of avoiding complications.

Primary Care Management
HEALTH CARE MAINTENANCE
Growth and Development

Because IDDM is a metabolic disorder affecting carbohydrate metabolism, growth and sexual development may be slowed. Children and adolescents in poor control may fail to grow normally. Therefore, accurate measurement of height and weight and comparison with growth norms are imperative.

Even when children have normal linear growth, there may be delays in the onset and progression of puberty if glycemic control is not adequate. At each visit, Tanner stages of secondary sexual development should be assessed and recorded. Any deviation from the normal pattern should be investigated. In girls, menarche may be delayed. Loss of regular menses once cycling has been established may indicate a further degeneration in diabetic control and should be investigated.

Obesity can occur in children and adolescents with IDDM, especially those on intensive regimens. Rapid weight gain in the presence of high SMBG levels may suggest that a child is having undetected hypoglycemia with rebound of the blood glucose to high levels. This phenomenon is known as the "Somogyi phenomenon" and is frequently a cause of overtreatment with insulin. Management of the obesity should be done carefully, with attention to the need to maintain self-monitoring, because glucose levels may change dramatically when a weight loss diet is followed.

Another concern is the adolescent who manipulates overeating by reducing or omitting insulin. Some adolescent girls with IDDM engage in insulin withholding to maintain body shape or to lose weight (Rodin and Daneman, 1992). Researchers have studied the incidence of eating disorders in adolescents with IDDM with conflicting results. Some have found that adolescents with diabetes are at higher risk for eating disorders than those without diabetes (Steel et al, 1989), while others have not found differences (Peveler et al, 1992; Striegel-Moore, Nicholson, and Tamborlane, 1992). Nonetheless, alterations in insulin dosage may affect the adolescent's ability to grow and develop normally and should be considered in the evaluation of children with growth difficulties.

Diet

Although insulin therapy is the cornerstone of treatment, a dietary plan is important in maintaining near-normoglycemia without wide swings in blood glucose levels. Long-term adherence to the dietary plan is probably the most difficult aspect of management for families (Hodges and Parker, 1987).

Many meal plans are based on the exchange system. Current exchange lists can be obtained from the ADA (see the resources listed at the end of this chapter), but the basic components are listed in Table 17-2. There are six food groups, including a "free" group. Within the groups, the nutritional

Table 17-2.   DIETARY EXCHANGE SYSTEM

Food exchange	Calories	Approximate content gm/serving		
		Carbohydrate	Protein	Fat
Fruit	60	12	0	0
Starch	68	15	2	0
Milk				
Whole	170	12	8	10
Skim	90	12	8	Trace
Meat				
Lean	55	0	7	3
Medium fat	75	0	7	5
High fat	95	0	7	8
Fat	45	0	0	5
Free	0	Negligible	0	0

composition of a serving of different foods is relatively constant. In the starch category, for example, one exchange is one slice of bread, ½ cup of white rice, or one medium, baked potato. The system helps families learn portion sizes and healthy childhood nutrition.

All dietary management plans have the goal of providing adequate calories and nutrients for normal growth and maintenance of near-normal blood glucose as possible. Daily consistency of intake with regular meals and snacks is important. The selection of the appropriate meal plan should be made by the family in consultation with the diabetes team. The family is in the best position to judge the approach that will work for them. The imposition of a rigid approach on a nonwilling family will only lead to problems of nonadherence to the diet. In addition, for any child to adhere without question to a diet perceived as different from that of peers is clearly unrealistic. Thus primary care providers need to be understanding in their approach and work with families to ensure as much dietary consistency as possible.

Two approaches to dietary management most commonly used with children are the ADA Exchange Lists (see Table 17-2) and carbohydrate counting. With the ADA Exchange Lists, the goal is for the child to have adequate calories for growth,

distributed appropriately through the day and through the food groups. The dietary plan should be developed with the child and the parents so that usual routines and favorite foods can be incorporated.

Carbohydrate counting is used most frequently by those on intensive regimens (DCCT Research Group, 1993a). This method provides more flexibility in the diet by providing for varying amounts of carbohydrates at meals and snacks with appropriate coverage with regular insulin. Protein and fat intake is not controlled, but efforts to remain within low-fat guidelines are encouraged. For example, adolescents who choose to eat a second sandwich at lunch (30 g extra carbohydrate in the bread) may need to take 5 to 10 units of regular insulin before the meal depending on their regimen.

The wide availability of artificially sweetened foods and drinks has eased some of the difficulties children with diabetes faced in following the meal plan. Parents sometimes express concern, however, that extensive use of artificial sweeteners will be problematic for their children.

Currently there are three nonnutritive sweeteners approved for use by the FDA in the United States—saccharine, aspartame, and acesulfame K. For these and all other additives, the FDA determines an acceptable daily intake (ADI), or the amount that can be safely consumed on a daily basis over a person's lifetime without any adverse effects. This includes a 100-fold safety factor. In reality, average intake is much less than the ADI. For example, the average aspartame consumption in the general population (including children) is 2 to 3 mg/kg per day or approximately 4% of the US ADI of 50 mg/kg (Franz et al, 1994).

Safety

The safety issues faced by families with a child or adolescent with diabetes are twofold. As discussed earlier, hypoglycemia is a significant risk for all affected children, and families and others in the child's social sphere should be prepared to respond appropriately. Older children need to know how to prevent severe hypoglycemia, especially when exercising. Children should be taught to eat a snack composed of complex carbohydrate and protein before exercise, not to inject insulin into an exercising muscle, and to carry glucose with them at all times. When traveling, children or their parents should carry their supplies with them, not in checked baggage, and always have food available should a meal be delayed. Some airlines require a letter from a health provider explaining the need for syringes to be carried on board an airplane.

Parents or caretakers must learn to treat episodes of severe hypoglycemia with glucagon. Glucagon is the antagonist hormone to insulin and serves to release glycogen from the liver. When a child or adolescent is unable to take sugar by mouth, glucagon is administered by intramuscular injection to rapidly raise the blood glucose. The dose for an infant or toddler is 0.5 mg, and the dose for older children is 1 mg.

The other important safety issue is the proper disposal of syringes. Children and parents need to be taught the importance of proper disposal of syringes to reduce the risk of injury to themselves and others.

Immunizations

Children and adolescents with diabetes should follow the immunization schedule recommended by the American Academy of Pediatrics including vaccines for hepatitis and chicken pox. Children with diabetes are considered to be potentially at an increased risk for developing complicated influenza

SCREENING

• Vision	Visual acuity yearly or if complaints
	Cataracts at diagnosis
	Retinopathy within 5 years, then yearly thereafter (after puberty)
• Hearing	Routine
• Dental	Routine
• Blood pressure	Each visit
• Urinalysis	Routine
	After 5 years, screen for microalbuminuria
• Tuberculosis	Routine
• Lipids	Yearly

illness; therefore, they may benefit from yearly influenza vaccination after the age of 6 months (American Academy of Pediatrics, 1994).

Screening

Vision. Vision screening is of particular importance in children with diabetes as visual problems are not uncommon. A small number of children will develop cataracts early in the course of the illness, therefore observing the normalcy of the red reflex during the ophthalmic examination is very important. Fluctuations in blood glucose levels can also affect visual acuity. Children experiencing hypoglycemia may complain of visual disturbances, and those with hyperglycemia may also complain of blurred vision. Thus it is important to relate the results of routine visual screening to the level of diabetic control, because improvement in metabolic control may improve the results of the visual testing.

Parents and children are often most concerned about the risk of diabetic retinopathy. Retinopathy of diabetes is the leading cause of blindness. Therefore, the ADA (1995) recommends that fundoscopic examination be performed at each primary care visit in all individuals with diabetes. Further, in those children who are more than 12 years of age and who have had diabetes for at least 5 years, annual examination with dilation by a pediatric ophthalmologist is recommended.

Hearing. Routine screening is recommended.

Dental. Routine screening is recommended.

Blood pressure. Screening should be performed at each visit. Hypertension has been reported in up to 45% of all individuals with diabetes. Thus the ADA (1995) recommends that orthostatic measurements be performed and recorded routinely.

Hematocrit. Routine screening is recommended.

Urinalysis. Screening is performed yearly, with examination for levels of ketones, glucose, and protein. After 5 years of diabetes or after puberty, total urinary protein excretion should be measured yearly by the microalbuminuria method to screen for renal complications. If proteinuria is detected, serum creatinine clearance or blood urea nitrogen concentration should be measured and glomerular filtration assessed.

Tuberculosis. Routine screening is recommended.

Condition-specific screening

LIPIDS. Individuals with IDDM are at risk for disorders of lipid metabolism, and these disorders may increase the risk of macrovascular complications. Children with IDDM should be screened yearly after puberty with blood lipid profiles. If the child has other risk factors, lipid screening should begin earlier, as is true for children without diabetes.

COMMON ILLNESS MANAGEMENT

Differential Diagnosis

When the classic symptoms of diabetes are present, there are few other diagnoses to consider. Polydipsia and polyuria may be caused by diabetes insipidus, but urinary and serum glucose levels will be normal. Urinary tract infections may also cause urinary frequency, but, again, glucose levels will be normal. Renal glycosuria is possible but unusual, and it will not be characterized by ketosis. (See box on diagnostic criteria.)

Illness management and prevention of diabetic ketoacidosis. Children and adolescents with

DIFFERENTIAL DIAGNOSIS

- Diabetes insipidus—urinary & serum glucose will be normal
- Urinary tract infection—urinary frequency, without glycosuria
- Renal glycosuria—not associated with ketosis
- Stressors, including illness, can lead to DKA
- Illness requires "sick day" management
- Important to maintain hydration during illness

DIAGNOSTIC CRITERIA FOR DIABETES MELLITUS IN CHILDREN

- Classic symptoms of diabetes, including polydipsia, polyuria, polyphagia, and weight loss, with random plasma glucose ≥200 mg/dl
- Fasting plasma glucose level ≥140 mg/dl on two occasions and two oral glucose tolerance tests (OGTT) with the 2 hour plasma glucose and one intervening value ≥200 mg/dl, using 1.75 g/kg to maximum of 75 g glucose load

Data from American Diabetes Association: Clinical practice recommendations 1995, *Diabetes Care* 18(suppl 1):entire issue, 1995.

diabetes are at no higher risk for most common infectious diseases of childhood than their peers, provided that the diabetes is under reasonable metabolic control. Because any stressor may lead to DKA in a child with diabetes, infections and other stressors must be managed with care.

Regardless of the insult, there are several important principles for management. Of utmost importance is the need to continue to take insulin even when the child is unable to eat the normal diet, because the excess of counterregulatory hormones released in response to the stressor will more than offset the decreased oral intake. Thus even though dietary intake may be decreased, insulin requirement may be increased.

The principles of management include monitoring parameters of control, maintaining hydration, preventing hypoglycemia, and preventing DKA. For these principles to work effectively, it is imperative that the child and family know that any illness or insult involving fever, gastrointestinal symptoms, congestion in the head or chest, or urinary symptoms should be managed as a sick day (Ley and Goldman, 1990). Once a day is identified as a sick day, the usual rules for self-monitoring are altered to reflect the need for closer monitoring. Blood glucose levels should be tested every 1 to 4 hours, and those with blood glucose levels greater than 200 mg/dl should test urine for ketones. Blood glucose levels of more than 400 mg/dl on two determinations and moderate or high ketone levels in the urine that do not decrease with additional insulin should be viewed as an indication that the child should be seen and evaluated by either the primary care provider or the specialist.

Maintaining hydration is important in helping clear extra glucose and ketones. If children are unable to eat their usual diet, a large fluid intake should be maintained. In adolescents this amount should be more than 8 oz of fluid hourly. Such fluids should contain adequate amounts of carbohydrate (50 to 75 gm/6 to 8 hr) to maintain their usual caloric intake. Children will often drink nondiet sodas, flavored gelatin water, or suck on ice pops when ill. If the child is vomiting or has diarrhea, broths or electrolyte solutions may be helpful with replacing sodium losses.

To prevent DKA, the child may need additional insulin. In general, the family should administer the usual dose of insulin and add up to 20% of the total daily dose as regular insulin every 4 hours if the blood glucose level is greater than 300 mg/dl. Such management should be done in careful consultation with the child's diabetes team.

The box above lists those indications for which a child or adolescent should be seen and evaluated. Most important is the need for the child with any alteration in mental status to be evaluated. The primary care provider should never assume that sleepiness in a child with diabetes is merely the result of the fatigue associated with an illness.

INDICATIONS FOR EVALUATION BY A HEALTH CARE PROVIDER

Vomiting for more than 6 hours or more than five diarrheal stools in 1 day
Any change in mental status
Syncope
Temperature greater than 38.9° C for 12 hours
Blood glucose levels more than 400 mg/dl twice
Moderate or high ketone levels that do not decrease with extra insulin intake
Dysuria or other symptoms of urinary tract infection
Decrease in urinary output

Drug Interactions

Many over-the-counter medications and antibiotics contain glucose, and some contain alcohol or traces of gluconeogenic substances such as sorbitol or glycerine (Kumar, Weatherly, and Beaman, 1991). In amounts usually ingested, these compounds may raise blood glucose levels slightly, but they should not markedly impair diabetic control. Pseudoephedrine has the potential to increase blood glucose levels because of its stimulant effect. This effect is minimal at usual doses, but all such products contain warnings that individuals with diabetes should consult their provider before taking the product, so primary care providers should be aware of the potential effect.

DEVELOPMENTAL ISSUES

Sleep Patterns

Children with diabetes who are in good control should have no problems sleeping. However, those who are hyperglycemic overnight will have difficulty sleeping because of the recurrent need to urinate. This problem can be managed by improving metabolic control.

Hypoglycemia at night is a concern of parents. The child may not awaken with the usual early signs and symptoms, and the first sign may be a severe reaction with nightmares or seizures. Thus, prevention of nighttime hypoglycemia by adjusting the evening insulin dose appropriately and offering a bedtime snack with carbohydrate and protein or fat is important. Parents should also be instructed in the use of the counterregulatory hormone glucagon in the event the child is not arousable.

Nightmares are common in young children and may be caused by hypoglycemia. Parents should determine the blood glucose level before assuming the cause of a nightmare. If the cause is hypoglycemia, treatment would include administration of glucose; if the nightmares are not related to hypoglycemia, appropriate comfort measures should be instituted. Prevention is the key, though, and significant nighttime hypoglycemia is to be avoided as much as possible by careful adjustment of diet and insulin.

Toileting

Several issues related to toileting are important in the management of diabetes in children. Many children have secondary enuresis at the time of diagnosis. It is important to tell children who were previously dry that diabetes is the cause of their enuresis and that when the diabetes is adequately controlled, the enuresis should remit. It is also true that enuresis can occur with well-controlled diabetes. Other methods of diagnostic confirmation and treatment should be explored with these families.

Although testing urine for glucose is not as critical to management as it was before SMBG testing became available, urinary ketone levels are important indicators of status when a child is ill. Parents should know how to obtain such samples from infants and toddlers. Cotton balls tucked into a diaper can provide an adequate sample for use on a dipstick to determine ketone levels in pretoilet-trained children. During toilet training when a child uses a potty chair, urine is readily obtainable. When the child moves onto the bathroom commode, the parent needs to teach the child to urinate into a paper cup so that the urine can be tested. Taught at a time when the child is feeling well, this task can be made into a game so that, when necessary, the behavior has been learned.

Discipline

Although the issues related to discipline of a child with diabetes are not different from those of all children with a chronic condition, parents of chil-

dren with diabetes report that their second most common concern in raising the child is discipline (Hodges and Parker, 1987). Parents most often worry that a hypoglycemic episode will be missed by attributing the unruly behavior to lack of discipline. It is appropriate for parents to test the blood glucose level at any time hypoglycemia is suspected. Then, if the result is within the normal range, the child can be disciplined appropriately. Some parents also worry that the stress of imposed discipline will raise the blood glucose level because of the presence of counterregulatory hormones. Although severe stressors may increase blood glucose levels (Aikens et al, 1992), no evidence suggests that usual disciplinary measures increase blood glucose levels or worsen diabetic control. Indeed, some authors (Betschart, 1993; Lipman et al, 1989a) have suggested that parents who set reasonable limits for their children are more likely to have children in good metabolic control.

Child Care

Toddlers and preschoolers with diabetes benefit from the socialization of preschool programs. They do not need specialized medical day care. Preschool teachers should be informed of parents' expectations such as blood glucose testing. Snack and lunch intake is very important, so preschool teachers need to be aware of the child's need to eat and what should be served at each mealtime. They should be aware of appropriate food substitutions when food is refused. All caregivers should be told how to manage symptoms of hypoglycemia. Emergency telephone numbers should always be available and should include telephone numbers of the parents, another emergency contact, the primary care provider, and the diabetes specialists.

Parents of children with diabetes often express concerns about the abilities of baby-sitters or day care workers to manage a young child's diabetes (Hodges and Parker, 1987). Parents of young children can begin by leaving the child for only short periods of time, thus reassuring themselves that the sitter can successfully care for the child. Clear instructions regarding the child's diet and management of hypoglycemia should be provided in writing. Parents should be encouraged to train sitters in blood glucose monitoring and in recognition of hypoglycemic symptoms. Emergency telephone numbers should always be available.

Schooling

Children and adolescents with diabetes should participate fully in school activities. Children whose diabetes is adequately controlled should attend school regularly and participate in any activity for which they are otherwise suited. Parents should be encouraged to inform the school nurse and the child's teachers when the diabetes is diagnosed. It is important that someone in the school be knowledgeable about the child's care so that hypoglycemia or illness can be managed appropriately. The need for other involvement, such as SMBG testing or injections, will depend on the child's usual regimen.

With older children, providers need to work with the child, family, and school personnel to arrange a school schedule that fits the child's diabetes regimen (Balik, Haig, and Moynihan, 1986). For example, a child who has had regular and NPH insulin at 7 AM should probably have a snack before a gym class which precedes a late lunch period. Arrangements need to be made so that the child can always have access to glucose-containing foods or tablets in the event of a hypoglycemic episode. For field trips the child should always have food available. A sack lunch with all food groups serves nicely as a substitute should a meal be unexpectedly delayed.

Sports are also encouraged. Coaches should be aware of the diabetes and keep glucose-containing foods on hand. Depending on the degree of exercise, insulin dose may be lowered on extraactivity days, diet may be increased, or both in an attempt to prevent hypoglycemia. Hypoglycemia following exercise may occur up to 12 hours after the event, so children should be carefully monitored when any new activity is undertaken. Children should be advised that insulin is absorbed more rapidly from exercising muscle; therefore, if a muscle is to be exercised, insulin should be injected in another site. For example, if a child will run track, the insulin could be administered in the arm or the abdomen rather than the leg.

Children whose diabetes is in poor control may experience difficulties in school performance. Because hypoglycemia can cause a child to lose the ability to concentrate when the blood glucose level is low, learning can be a problem. When the blood glucose level is consistently too high, many children experience difficulties in concentration and grades may suffer. Thus any child with diabetes whose school performance changes should be carefully assessed for alterations in metabolic control.

As with all children who have a chronic condition, emphasis should be on the normality of the child, not the diabetes. Such an approach helps to minimize the sense of being different that is experienced by all affected children.

Sexuality

The achievement of normal growth and development is a goal of therapy. If the diabetes is adequately controlled, sexual development should be normal. If, on the other hand, sexual development is delayed, normal concerns about self and physical adequacy may be amplified. Primary care providers need to monitor secondary sexual development carefully in children with diabetes, and any deviation from normal should be investigated. Often, tightening the metabolic control will improve growth. If not, the cause should be investigated.

All sexually active teenagers need information about birth control. Such information is especially important for those with diabetes because the risks of complications of pregnancy are at least 5 times greater than the already high risk for adolescents. Because of the risk of acquired immunodeficiency syndrome (AIDS), many providers are encouraging condoms for birth control over all other methods. Unfortunately, as with all teenagers, proper and consistent use of condoms is variable. Other barrier methods, such as diaphragms, foams, and creams, may also be used by those with diabetes, but these methods share the same disadvantages as condoms and do not prevent sexually transmitted diseases.

Teenagers who are willing to use contraceptives often find the use of the birth control pill acceptable. The combination pill, containing both estrogen and progesterone, may have considerable risks for adolescents with diabetes. Side effects include cerebral ischemia, myocardial infarction, and rapid progression of retinopathy, so the combination pill is not recommended. The low dose estrogen combination pill, appears to be reasonably well tolerated and is the oral contraceptive of choice.

Although the avoidance of adolescent pregnancy is clearly preferred, some teenagers will express the desire to become pregnant. It has been clearly demonstrated (Aucott et al, 1994) that pregnancy outcomes can be dramatically improved if euglycemia is maintained both in the months preceding conception and throughout the pregnancy. Therefore, female adolescents who are at risk for pregnancy or who are contemplating pregnancy should be counseled regarding pregnancy outcomes and helped to achieve better metabolic control.

Male adolescents will often express concern about the well-known complication of impotence in adult men. This problem is thought to be a result of both vascular and neurologic compromise in those with long-standing diabetes. Fortunately, impotence caused by diabetes is very rare in adolescence, and most can be reassured.

Transition into Adulthood

The challenges of transitioning into adulthood may be more complex for adolescents with IDDM as a result of the extraordinary demands of disease self-management on the client and the family. Wysocki and colleagues (1992) found that older adolescents had poorer adjustment to diabetes and poorer metabolic control than younger children, and that difficulties in adjustment in early adolescence tended to persist into young adulthood.

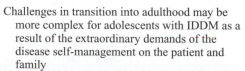

TRANSITION INTO ADULTHOOD

Challenges in transition into adulthood may be more complex for adolescents with IDDM as a result of the extraordinary demands of the disease self-management on the patient and family

Some young adults with IDDM may have more difficulty with vocational adjustment and marital relationships than other adults

If adjustment is better in early adolescence, the young adult is more likely to have better adjustment and metabolic control

Further, some studies have suggested that young adults with IDDM have more difficulty with vocational adjustment (Gutezeit and Gilde, 1983) and marital relationships (Karlsson, Holmes, and Lang, 1988) than other young adults. Thus the care provided during this crucial time may be important for long-term quality of life.

Wysocki and colleagues (1992) also found that if adjustment was better in early adolescence, the young adult is more likely to have better adjustment and metabolic control. This finding suggests that the care provided in early adolescence with attention to improving psychosocial adjustment is just as important as providing quality transitional care. Little empirical work on the provision of care in the transition from adolescence to adulthood has been accomplished, but Court (1993) surveyed adolescents to elicit their views on the process of transfer from pediatric to adult care. Court found that adolescents value continuity of care by a provider they trust; adolescents expect confidentiality and privacy, informality and waiting rooms tailored to their needs. In addition, young adults and late adolescents may be less capable of insulin self-regulation than is assumed by providers (Pless et al, 1988). Therefore, transition to adult care needs to be designed to respect the wishes of these young people and to support their assumption of self-care and development in their vocational and social roles.

Another concern of young adults is the increasing risk of complications. A recent study (Dunning, 1995) found that concerns about complications were common among young adults with IDDM and included concerns about eye disease, pregnancy and childbirth, hypoglycemia, and loss of independence. It is clear that these young people need help in implementing intensive insulin regimens and self-care management styles that will help to delay complications.

SPECIAL FAMILY CONCERNS AND RESOURCES

Diabetes is a disease that requires ongoing active involvement of the child and the family in its management. Some children will neglect all aspects of care, even insulin injections, and be repeatedly hospitalized with DKA, whereas others will take their insulin but never perform SMBG testing or follow their dietary plan. Compliance is a behavioral coping strategy (Grey and Thurber, 1991) that is an issue in many chronic conditions and therefore is not discussed in depth here. However, any child or adolescent with repeated problems in management (poor control with or without repeated hospitalization) should be carefully questioned about adherence to the diabetic regimen.

Families worry about the appropriate assumption of self-care because of its importance in preventing long-term complications. Recommendations for understanding the levels at which children should assume various self-care activities are available (Daneman, 1991). There is, however, broad disagreement among professionals as to the appropriate age for management of skills (Wysocki et al, 1990), and some authors (Ingersoll et al, 1986) have suggested that the too-early assumption of self-management is associated with poorer psychologic and metabolic outcomes. Therefore, decisions about assumption of self-care activities should be made with the family, the child, and the providers working together. Until more data on the impact of assuming self-care at different ages are available, the strict regulation by providers of such activities may be unwarranted.

In addition to the family issues that are common to many chronic conditions, families with a child with diabetes face some unique problems. In studies of parents' concerns (Hauenstein et al, 1989; Hodges and Parker, 1987), several issues appear to be prominent. First is the adherence to the diabetes regimen, especially diet and the assumption of self-care. Second is the question of genetics and inheritance. In addition, psychosomatic issues may be of particular importance to families dealing with diabetes, because poorly functioning families have been shown to be associated with poorer diabetic control (Baker, 1970; Kovacs et al, 1989). Parents frequently also express concerns about long-term complications and the risk of hypoglycemia. As noted earlier, the risk of severe hypoglycemia is 3 to 4 times greater in children on intensive treatment regimens; par-

ents may be more concerned about the child participating in sports on these regimens than on conventional regimens.

Guilt is often of concern to parents of children with diabetes, particularly because the disease is inherited. Families need to be provided with appropriate genetic counseling so that they are aware of the risks to other family members and the risks to offspring of the individual with diabetes. Such information will often help to assuage the guilt present at diagnosis, because the risk for first-degree relatives is low. The sibling of a child with IDDM has about a 5% to 10% risk, and the risk in an offspring of a single parent with diabetes is about 1% to 2%.

Considerable attention has been paid to family problems and their impact on metabolic control in children with diabetes. It is hypothesized that the well-functioning family facilitates a child's well-being by providing emotional support, advice, and practical help (Anderson and Auslander, 1980) and that poor family functioning interferes with self-care or causes stress-related metabolic deterioration (Baker, 1970). Results of studies of the influence of family life on diabetes control have been inconclusive (Kovacs et al, 1989). However, some families exhibit psychosomatic characteristics that have a clear adverse effect on the child with diabetes. Such families should be referred for family therapy.

Multiple factors may influence adjustment in children and adolescents with IDDM. Burns, Green, and Chase (1986) studied the association of age with a number of psychosocial variables in three age groups of 15 to 22 subjects each. The researchers' results suggest that parental and family factors have less importance in predicting metabolic control in adolescents than in younger children.

There also may be social issues which influence adaptation to diabetes in youth, such as cultural differences, but little work on these questions has been accomplished with adolescents with IDDM. Auslander and colleagues (1990) demonstrated that African American children and children from single-parent families were at higher risk for poor control. Hanson, Henggeler, and Burghen (1987) and Delamater and colleagues (1991) all found that black children and adolescents had

CULTURAL IMPLICATIONS

African American children and children from
single-parent homes are at highest risk for poor
metabolic control

Black children and adolescents tend to have
worse metabolic control than white children

Differences in metabolic control may be from
cultural dietary factors, or participation in less
exercise, both which may be influenced by
cultural values

worse metabolic control than white children. Hanson and colleagues (1987) did not find differences in psychosocial status and family functioning between white and black families. Differences in metabolic control may be because of cultural dietary factors, such as eating more foods that affect blood glucose swings or participating in less exercise. Since eating behaviors and participation in sports may be influenced by cultural values, families should be assessed for their beliefs and values about food and exercise.

Resources

Two national organizations provide help for families coping with diabetes in a child: the ADA and the Juvenile Diabetes Association (see the list of organizations that follows). The ADA is the largest such organization, composed of both lay individuals and professionals. They support research, education, fund raising, and camps, as well as provide lobbying efforts related to diabetes. They publish several pamphlets and books for families to use in understanding diabetes. At the local level, many affiliates provide support and educational programs for families and children. The ADA deals with all types of diabetes, not only IDDM.

The primary focus of the Juvenile Diabetes Foundation, on the other hand, is research toward a cure for IDDM. The organization does provide some support for families, but its major effort is devoted toward fund raising for research to find a cure for IDDM. Some families find that working toward the cure is helpful.

Organizations
American Diabetes Association
1660 Duke St
Alexandria, VA 22314
(800) ADA-DISC
Juvenile Diabetes Foundation
23 E 26th St
New York, NY 10010
(212) 689-7868

SUMMARY OF PRIMARY CARE NEEDS FOR THE CHILD WITH DIABETES MELLITUS (TYPE I)

Health care maintenance

Growth and development

Height and weight are normal unless control is less than adequate.

Secondary sexual development may be delayed.

Rapid weight gain may signal overtreatment with insulin.

Weight loss usually indicates poor control.

Diet

Maintenance of normoglycemia is critical.

Stress the importance of regular distribution of meals and snacks.

Of the various approaches to diet, all emphasize consistency and low concentrated sweets.

Safety

Prevent hypoglycemia with careful monitoring; be sure a glucose source is always available.

Dispose of syringes properly.

Use glucagon for severe hypoglycemic episodes.

Immunizations

Routine immunizations are recommended.

Yearly influenza vaccine recommended.

Screening

Vision

Check red reflex and perform fundoscopic examination at each visit.

Thorough pediatric ophthalmologic examination is advised every 5 years.

Cataracts at diagnosis

Hearing

Routine screening is recommended.

Dental

Routine screening is recommended.

Blood pressure

Check blood pressure each visit and orthostatic variation.

Hematocrit

Routine screening is recommended.

Urinalysis

Perform urinalysis yearly for ketones, glucose, and protein determinations; after 5 years screen for microalbuminuria yearly.

Tuberculosis

Routine screening is recommended.

Condition-specific screening

Check hemoglobin A_{1c} every 3 months.

Perform thyroid function studies if a change in growth patterns occurs.

Perform other studies as indicated.

Common illness management

Differential diagnosis

Diabetes insipidus—urinary & serum glucose will be normal

Urinary tract infection—urinary frequency without glycosuria

Renal glycosuria—not associated with ketosis

Stressors— including illness, can lead to DKA

Illness requires "sick day" management

Important to maintain hydration during illness

Drug interactions

Beware that many OTC medications and antibiotics contain glucogenic substances or alcohol.

Pseudoephedrine may increase blood glucose as a result of stimulant effect.

Developmental issues

Sleep patterns

Prevention of nighttime hypoglycemia is important.

Nightmares may be the result of hypoglycemia.

Toileting

Enuresis may be present when control is poor.

Measurement of urinary ketones is important when blood glucose levels are high or when the child is ill.

Discipline

Unruly behavior may be caused by hypoglycemia.

The potential for conflict over diet, blood testing, and insulin administration should be recognized.

Continued.

SUMMARY OF PRIMARY CARE NEEDS FOR THE CHILD WITH DIABETES MELLITUS (TYPE I)—cont'd

Child care

Teachers and baby-sitters need training in management of dietary needs and hypoglycemia.

Schooling

Full attendance and participation are expected.
School personnel must be aware of the child's special needs.
If control is poor, performance may be affected.

Sexuality

If diabetes is adequately controlled, sexual development should be normal.
Pregnancy prevention is very important because of combined risks of diabetes and adolescent pregnancy.
Low dose estrogen combination OCs are recommended as a result of risk of complications with estrogen-containing OCs or oral contraceptives.
Pregnancy outcomes are dramatically improved if euglycemia is maintained preceding and during pregnancy.
Impotency caused by long-term vascular and neurologic compromise is a rare problem during adolescence.

Transition into adulthood

Challenges in transition to adulthood may be more complex for adolescents with IDDM as a result of the extraordinary demands of the disease self-management on the patient and family.
Some young adults with IDDM may have more difficulty with vocational adjustment and marital relationships than other adults.
If adjustment is better in early adolescence, the young adult is more likely to have better adjustment and metabolic control.

Special family concerns

Assumption of self-care activities and adherence to the regimen are of prime concern.
Parents often experience guilt concerning the inheritance of IDDM.
Psychosomatic families may have more problems with diabetic management.
African American children and children from single-parent homes are at highest risk for poor metabolic control.
Black children and adolescents tend to have worse metabolic control than white children and adolescents.
Differences in metabolic control may be from cultural dietary factors, or participation in less exercise, both which may be influenced by cultural values.

REFERENCES

Aikens JE et al: Daily stress variability, learned resourcefulness, regimen adherence, and metabolic control in type I diabetes mellitus: evaluation of a path model, *J Consult Clin Psychol* 60:113-118, 1992.

American Academy of Pediatrics: Summaries of infectious diseases. In G Peter, (editor): *1994 red book: report of the committee on infectious diseases,* ed 23, Elk Grove Village, IL, 1994, Author.

American Diabetes Association: *Diabetes: 1993 vital statistics,* Alexandria, VA, 1993a, Author.

American Diabetes Association: Position statement: implications of the Diabetes Control and Complications Trial, *Diabetes* 42:1555-1558, 1993b.

American Diabetes Association: Clinical practice recommendations 1995, *Diabetes Care* 18, suppl 1, entire issue, 1995.

Anderson BJ, Auslander WF: Research on diabetes management and the family: a critique, *Diabetes Care* 3:696-702, 1980.

Aucott SW et al: Rigorous management of insulin-dependent diabetes mellitus during pregnancy, *Acta Diabetologica* 31:126-129, 1994.

Auslander W et al: Risk factors to health in diabetic children: a prospective study from diagnosis, *Health Soc Work* 15:133-142, 1990.

Baker L: Psychosomatic aspects of diabetes mellitus. In OW Hill, (editor): *Modern trends in psychosomatic medicine,* ed 2, Stone Ram, MA, 1970, Butterworth, pp 105-124.

Balik B, Haig B, and Moynihan PM: Diabetes and the school-aged child, *MCN* 11:324-330, 1986.

Betschart J: Children and adolescents with diabetes, *Nurs Clin North Am* 28:35-44, 1993.

Brink SJ, (1988). Pediatric, adolescent, and young-adult nutritional issues in IDDM. *Diabetes Care, II.* 192-200.

Burns KL, Green P, and Chase HP: Psychosocial correlates of glycemic control as a function of age in youth with insulin-dependent diabetes mellitus, *J Adolesc Health* 7:311-319, 1986.

Charron-Prochownik D, Schwartz S: Care of the infant with type I diabetes mellitus, *Diabetes Educ* 10:46-50, 1984.

Clark LM, Plotnick LP: Insulin pumps in children with diabetes, *J Pediatr Health* 4:3-10, 1990.

Connell JE, Thomas-Doberson D: Nutritional management of children and adolescents with insulin-dependent diabetes mellitus: a review by the Diabetes Care and Education Dietetic Practice Group, *J Am Diet Assoc* 91:1556-1564, 1991.

Court JM: Issues of transition to adult care. *J Pediatr Child Health* 29, suppl 1:S53-S55, 1993.

Daneman D: When should your child take charge? . . . diabetes care, *Diabetes Forecast* 44:60-66, 1991.

Delameter AM et al: Racial differences in metabolic control of children and adolescents with type I diabetes mellitus, *Diabetes Care* 14:20-25, 1991.

DCCT Research Group. The Diabetes Control and Complications Trial (DCCT): Design and methodologic implications for the feasibility phase, *Diabetes* 35:530-545, 1986.

DCCT Research Group. Expanded role of the dietician in the DCCT: implications for clinical practice, *J Am Diet Assoc* 93:758-767, 1993a.

DCCT Research Group. The effect of intensive treatment of diabetes on the development and progression of long-term complications in Insulin-Dependent Diabetes Mellitus, *New Engl J Med* 329:435-459, 1993b.

DCCT Research Group. Effect of intensive diabetes treatment on the development and progression of long-term complications in adolescents with Insulin-Dependent Diabetes Mellitus: DCCT, *J Pediatr* 125:177-188, 1994.

Drash AL: The child, the adolescent, and the DCCT, *Diabetes Care* 16:1515-1516, 1993.

Drash AL: The epidemiology of insulin-dependent diabetes mellitus, *Clin Invest Med* 10:432-436, 1987.

Dunning PL: Young-adult perspectives of insulin-dependent diabetes, *Diabetes Educ* 21:58-65, 1995.

Eisenbarth GS: Type I diabetes mellitus: a chronic autoimmune disease, *N Engl J Med* 314:1360-1368, 1986.

Franz MJ et al: Nutritional principles for the management of diabetes and related complications, *Diabetes Care* 17:490-518, 1994.

Gabbay KH et al: Glycosylated hemoglobins and long-term blood glucose control in diabetes mellitus, *J Clin Endocrinol Metab* 44:859-864, 1977.

Grey M, Thurber FW: Adaptation to chronic illness in childhood: diabetes mellitus, *J Pediatr Nurs,* 1991.

Gutezeit G, Gilde HP: Vocational integration of diabetic adolescents. In Z Laron and A Galatzer, (editors): *Pediatric and adolescent endocrinology, vol 11,* Basel, Switzerland, 1983, S Karger, pp 45-49.

Hanson CL, Henggeler SW, and Burghen GA: Race and sex differences in metabolic control of adolescents with IDDM: a function of psychosocial variables, *Diabetes Care* 10:313-318, 1987.

Hauenstein EJ et al: Stress in parents of children with diabetes mellitus, *Diabetes Care* 12:18-23, 1989.

Hodges LC, Parker J: Concerns of parents with diabetic children, *Pediatr Nurs* 13:22-24, 1987.

Ingersoll GM et al: Cognitive maturity and self-management among adolescents with insulin-dependent diabetes mellitus, *J Pediatr* 108:620-623, 1986.

Karlsson JA, Holmes CS, and Lang R: Psychosocial aspects of disease duration and control in young adults with type I diabetes, *J Clin Epidemiol* 41:435-440, 1988.

Keller RJ, Eisenbarth GS, and Jackson RA: Insulin prophylaxis in individuals at high risk of type I diabetes, *Lancet* 341:927-928, 1993.

Kovacs M et al: Family functioning and metabolic control of school-aged children with IDDM, *Diabetes Care* 12:409-414, 1989.

Kumar A, Weatherly M, and Beaman DC: Sweeteners, flavorings, and dyes in antibiotic preparations. *Pediatrics* 87:352-360, 1991.

Lacy PE: Pancreatic islet cell transplant. *Mt Sinai J Med* 61:23-31, 1994.

Lendrum R, Walker SG, and Gamble DR: Islet cell antibodies in juvenile diabetes mellitus of recent onset, *Lancet* 1:880-882, 1975.

Lernmark A: Insulin dependent diabetes mellitus. In JK Davidson, (editor): *Clinical diabetes mellitus—a problem-oriented approach,* New York, 1991, Thieme, pp 35-49.

Ley B, Goldman D: Sick-day management: a partnership in preparation for the expected, *Clin Diabetes* 8:25-30, 1990.

Lipman TH et al: A developmental approach to diabetes in children: birth through preschool, *MCN* 14:225-259, 1989a.

Lipman TH et al: A developmental approach to diabetes in children: school age-adolescence, *MCN* 14:330-332, 1989b.

National Center for Health Statistics: Advance report of final mortality statistics, *Monthly Vital Stat Rep* [MVSR], 43(6), suppl 1-76, 1994.

Peveler RC et al: Eating disorders in adolescents with IDDM. *Diabetes Care* 15:1356-1360, 1992.

Pless IB et al: Expected diabetic control in childhood and psychosocial functioning in early adult life, *Diabetes Care* 11:387-392, 1988.

Plotnick L: Insulin-dependent diabetes mellitus, *Pediatr Rev* 15:137-148, 1994.

Raskin P, Rosenstock J: Hyperglycemia, genetic susceptibility, and diabetic complications, *Clin Diabetes* 5:135-141, 1987.

Rodin GM, Daneman D: Eating disorders and IDDM: a problematic association, *Diabetes Care* 15:1402-1412, 1992.

Rogers DG et al: Glycemic control and bone age are independently associated with muscle capillary basement membrane width in diabetic children after puberty, *Diabetes Care* 9:453-459, 1986.

Santiago JV: Insulin therapy in the last decade: a pediatric perspective, *Diabetes Care* 16(suppl 3):143-154, 1993a.

Santiago JV: Lessons from the Diabetes Control and Complications Trial. *Diabetes* 42:1549-1554, 1993b.

Skyler JS, Marks JB: Immune intervention in type I diabetes mellitus, *Diabetes Reviews* 1:15-42, 1993.

Srikanto S et al: Islet cell antibodies and beta cell function in monozygotic triplets and twins initially discordant for type I diabetes mellitus, *N Engl J Med* 308:322-325, 1983.

Steel JM et al: Abnormal eating attitudes in young insulin-dependent diabetics, *Br J Psychiatr* 155:515-521, 1989.

Striegel-Moore RH, Nicholson TJ, and Tamborlane WV: Prevalence of eating disorder symptoms in preadolescent and adolescent girls with IDDM. *Diabetes Care* 15:1361-1368, 1992.

Tamborlane WV et al: Implications of the DCCT in treating children and adolescents with diabetes, *Clin Diabetes,* 115-116, 1994.

Travis LB, Brouhard BH, and Schreiner BJ: *Diabetes mellitus in children and adolescents,* Philadelphia, 1987, WB Saunders.

Vialettes B et al: Stress antecedents and immune status in recently diagnosed type I (insulin-dependent) diabetes mellitus, *Diabete Metab* 15:45-50, 1989.

Virtanen SM et al: Early introduction of dairy products associated with increased risk of IDDM in Finnish children, *Diabetes Care* 42:1786-1790, 1993.

Wysocki T et al: Survey of diabetes professionals regarding developmental changes in diabetes self-care, *Diabetes Care* 13:65-68, 1990.

Wysocki T et al: Diabetes mellitus in the transition to adulthood: adjustment, self-care, and health status. *Dev Behavior Pediatr* 13:194-201, 1992.

18

Down Syndrome

Judith A. Vessey

ETIOLOGY

Down syndrome, first described by Esquirol in 1838 and promulgated by John Langdon Down in 1866, is a condition associated with a recognizable phenotype and limited intellectual endowment because of extra chromosome 21 material. It is the most frequent autosomal chromosomal anomaly. The exact band of chromosomal material implicated in Down syndrome has been isolated, indicating that an entire replication of chromosome 21 is not needed for expression.

Nondisjunction

Nondisjunction of chromosome 21 is responsible for the majority of cases of Down syndrome and is not inherited. Nondisjunction, or the uneven division of chromosomes, can occur during anaphase 1 or 2 in meiosis (reduction division of germ cells) or in anaphase of mitosis (somatic cell division). Although the exact mechanism remains unconfirmed, the pair of chromosomes fail to separate and migrate properly during cell division. When this occurs in meiosis, the haploid number for the respective daughter cells is unequal. If the cell receiving 24 rather than 23 chromosomes is fertilized, a trisomic zygote will result (see Fig. 18-1).

Nondisjunction may also occur early in mitosis. The resulting zygote will possess two or more cell lines with varying chromosomal constitutions. The earlier nondisjunction occurs, the greater the percentage of affected cells. This inheritance pattern, referred to as mosaicism, is associated with fewer phenotypic features (see Fig. 18-2).

Translocation

In Down syndrome caused by translocation, there are also three copies of chromosome 21. The third copy does not occur independently, however, but is attached to another chromosome, usually to one of the D or G group. Robertsonian translocations, where the long arms of chromosome 21 attach to the long arms of chromosome 14, 21, or 22, are the most common although other forms of translocation can occur (Pueschel, 1992).

The total chromosome count is 46 despite the fact that the material for 47 chromosomes is present. Although the phenotype for Down syndrome caused by translocation is the same as in nondisjunction, the inheritance pattern is quite different. In this form the disorder may reoccur in future pregnancies. If one parent has 45 chromosomes that include a translocation of chromosome 21, the gametes produced could result in a trisomic zygote. Although theoretically six combinations are possible, three of these are nonviable. Of the three that are viable, one is normal (N = 46), one results in a balanced translocation (N = 45), and one is an unbalanced translocation resulting in Down syndrome (N = 46) (see Fig. 18-3). Although this would translate to a 33% chance of having a child with Down syndrome with each pregnancy, in clinical practice the actual distribution is different than the theoretical distribution. Risk of recurrence is 10%

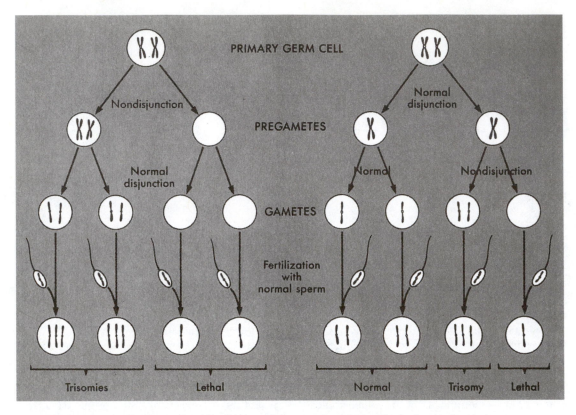

Fig. 18-1.   Mechanisms of maldistribution of chromosomes during first and second meiotic divisions caused by nondisjunction.

to 15% if the mother is the carrier and 5% to 8% if the father is the carrier.

A variety of hypotheses have been offered over the years as to the cause of Down syndrome, including: (1) a genetic predisposition to nondisjunction, (2) autoimmunity, (3) hormonal alterations in aging women, (4) viral disease, (5) environmental factors such as abdominal radiation before conception and drug exposure, and (6) frequency of coitus (Pueschel, 1992). No one factor has been confirmed although new genetic findings suggest that the cause is probably multifactorial.

INCIDENCE

The prevalence rate for Down syndrome is approximately 1 in 1000 live births with the incidence rate dropping to approximately 1 in 700 live births. Prenatal diagnosis in women of advance maternal age explains this difference (Hagerman, 1992). Prevalence rates vary by inheritance pattern. Nondisjunction is found in 92% to 95% of cases, mosaicism in 2% to 3% of cases, and translocation in 5% to 6% of cases (Pueschel, 1992). Because the overwhelming percentage of cases of Down syndrome are caused by nondisjunction, parental age directly affects the overall incidence (see Fig. 18-4).

Down syndrome caused by translocation is independent of parental age, and the incidence remains stable across age cohorts. Advanced parental age, however, is implicated in nondisjunction. For women in their early 20s, the incidence is approximately 1 in every 1500 births. The incidence rises gradually until maternal age surpasses 35, with the incidence then climbing to approximately 1 in 32 for 45-year-old women. Advanced paternal age has also been shown to correlate slightly with the inci-

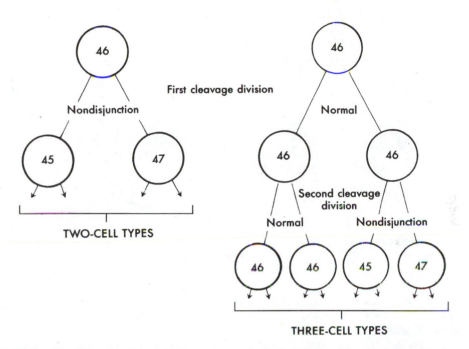

Fig. 18-2.   Nondisjunction during the first and second mitotic division of the zygote, resulting in a mosaic phenotype. *(From Whaley L and Wong D: Nursing care of infants and children, ed 4, St Louis, 1991, Mosby.)*

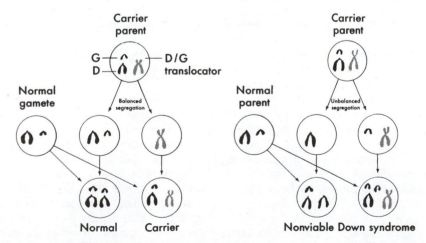

Fig. 18-3.   Possible zygotes from the union of a somatically normal carrier of D/G translocation and with a genetically and somatically normal individual. *(From Whaley L and Wong D: Nursing care of infants and children, ed 4, St Louis, 1991, Mosby.)*

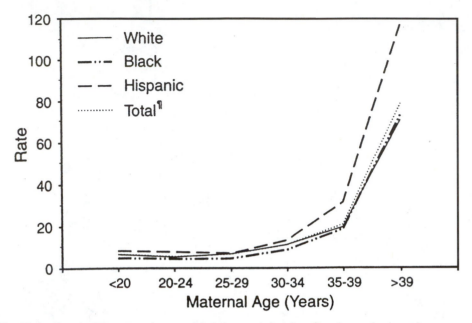

Fig. 18-4.   Rate* of Down syndrome at birth, by race/ethnicity of mother and maternal age group—17 state-based birth defects surveillance programs†, United States, 1983–1990§.
*Per 10,000 live-born infants. US Department of Health and Human Services: Down syndrome prevalence at birth —United States, 1983-1990, *Morbidity and Mortality Weekly Report* 43:617-622, 1994.
†Arizona, Arkansas, California, Colorado, Georgia, Hawaii, Illinois, Iowa, Kansas, Maryland, Missouri, Nebraska, New Jersey, New York, North Carolina, Virginia, and Washington.
§Because of the variability in surveillance periods (e.g., 1983–1987 or 1986–1989) and the low number of annual cases in some states, rates are presented as period prevalence rates.
¶Includes infants from all racial/ethnic groups and infants for whom race/ethnicity was unknown.

dence of Down syndrome in approximately 20% to 30% of the cases. Although the extra chromosome is paternal in origin, nondisjunction still occurs after fertilization. Because the overwhelming percentage of cases of Down syndrome are caused by nondisjunction, parental age directly affects the overall incidence.

Down syndrome occurs more frequently in males than females (Sharav, 1991) and is found in all races and ethnic groups. Although the incidence rates of Down syndrome vary little among whites, blacks, and Hispanic infants born to mothers under 35 years of age, significantly higher rates are seen in Hispanic infants born to mothers over 35 years of age. Differences in these rates may be a reflection of differences in early prenatal care, prenatal diagnosis, and views on abortion (Centers for Disease Control [CDC], 1994).

CLINICAL MANIFESTATIONS AT TIME OF DIAGNOSIS

Down syndrome is most frequently diagnosed immediately following birth as a result of its distinctive phenotype. In infants of color or those born very prematurely, diagnosis may be delayed because the clinical features may not be as clearly recognized. Although more than 50 physical characteristics can be identified at birth (see box on common findings), no one feature is considered diagnostic. Features vary in their expression and are not always present. Some of the most commonly associated features, however, include generalized hypotonia, epicanthal folds, single transverse palmar creases, and diminished vigor.

A variety of congenital anomalies commonly occur in association with Down syndrome. Con-

CLINICAL MANIFESTATIONS IN DOWN SYNDROME

Skull

False fontanel
Flat occipital area
Brachycephaly
Separated sagittal suture
Hypoplasia of midfacial bones
Reduced interorbital distance
Underdeveloped maxilla
Obtuse mandibular angle

Eyes

Oblique narrow palpebral fissures
Epicanthical folds
Brushfield spots
Strabismus
Nystagmus
Myopia
Hypoplasia of the iris

Ears

Small, shortened ears
Low and oblique implantation
Overlapping helices
Prominent antihelix
Absent or attached earlobes
Narrow ear canals
External auditory meatus
Structural aberrations of the ossicles
Stenotic external auditory meatus

Nose

Hypoplastic
Flat nasal bridge
Anteverted, narrow nares
Deviated nasal septum

Mouth

Prominent, thickened and fissured lips
Corners of the mouth turned downward
High arched, narrow palate
Shortened palatal length
Protruding enlarged tongue
Papillary hypertrophy (early preschool)
Fissured tongue (later school years)

Periodontal disease
Partial anodontia
Microdontia
Abnormally aligned teeth
Anterior open bite
Mouth held open

Neck

Short broad neck
Loose skin at nape

Chest

Shortened rib cage
Twelfth rib anomalies
Pectus excavation or carinatum
Congenital heart disease

Abdomen

Distended and enlarged abdomen
Diastasis recti
Umbilical hernia

Muscle tone and musculature

Hyperflexibility
Muscular hypotonia
Generalized weakness

Integument

Skin appears large for the skeleton
Dry and rough
Fine, poorly pigmented hair

Extremities

Short extremities
Partial or complete syndactyly
Clinodactyly
Brachyclinodactyly

Upper extremities

Short, broad hands
Brachyoclinodactyly
Single palmar transverse crease
Incurved short fifth finger
Abnormal dermatoglyphics

Continued.

CLINICAL MANIFESTATIONS IN DOWN SYNDROME—cont'd

Lower extremities

Short and stubby feet
Gap between first and second toes
Plantar crease between first and second toe
Second and third toes grouped in a forklike
    position
Radial deviation of the third to the fifth toe

Physical growth and development

Short stature
Increased weight in later life

Other findings seen in the newborn

Enlarged anterior fontanel
Delayed closing of sutures and fontanels
Open sagittal suture
Nasal bone not ossified, underdeveloped
Reduced birth weight

---

genital cardiac disease is seen in approximately 40% of children, with endocardial cushion defects accounting for about 60% and septal defects comprising another 28% of cardiac malformations (Ferencz et al, 1989). Gastrointestinal (GI) malformations are seen, with duodenal atresia, congenital megacolon (Hirschsprung's disease), imperforate anus, annular pancreas, and pyloric stenosis among the most common problems. In male individuals an increase in urogenital conditions such as micropenis, hypospadias, and cryptorchidism has also been documented, although no rise in the incidence of anatomic abnormalities of the kidneys or ureters was noted (Lang et al, 1987). Surgical correction of anomalies can usually be undertaken in the neonatal period. Although many children experience total correction of the anomaly, others will suffer from untoward sequelae throughout their lives.

TREATMENT

No treatment can eliminate the chromosomal defect that causes Down syndrome. Extensive interdisciplinary services and research over the last 20 years has, however, transformed society's view of children with Down syndrome and accepted treatment protocols. Current accepted approaches include (1) genetic counseling, (2) prompt referral for surgical correction of congenital anomalies, and (3) enrollment in an early intervention program.

TREATMENT

- Genetic counseling
- Surgical correction of abnormalities
- Early intervention programs

Genetic Counseling

Validation of Down syndrome and its genotype by chromosomal analysis should be considered for all affected children. Although this will not affect the child's treatment or prognosis, it has significant implications for genetic counseling of family members. Because translocation is the cause in 4% to 6% of cases, parents and siblings will need to be tested to determine their carrier status and the risk of recurrence in future pregnancies carefully explained.

Surgery

Today, surgical corrections of most major cardiac, GI, and genitourinary anomalies are performed routinely. Historically this was not the standard practice in some settings. Amidst moral and ethical controversy, however, the federal judiciary decreed in 1984 that treatment of life-threatening congenital anomalies could not be refused only because a child was developmentally disabled (Mahon, 1990) (see Chapter 3).

In addition to life-saving surgeries, some children with Down syndrome are also undergoing plastic procedures to alter their phenotypic appearance. As these children continue to become more integrally mainstreamed into society, they are frequently stigmatized because of their physiognomy. Some parents, concerned about their child's social acceptance, will seek plastic surgery. Procedures include partial glossectomies, neck resections, Silastic implants for the chin and nose, and reconstruction of dysplastic helices. Better articulation of speech, less mouth breathing, fewer and less severe upper respiratory tract infections, and improved mastication and swallowing may be realized. However, the degree of success may be small (Katz and Kravetz, 1989; Klaiman and Arndt, 1989; Strauss et al, 1988). Plastic surgery is not indicated for all children. If after counseling it is still deemed appropriate, initial revisions begin when the child is approximately 3 years old.

Early Intervention

Infant stimulation programs and continued early childhood education are designed to optimize a child's rate of development and minimize the amount of developmental lag that will occur between the child with Down syndrome and developmentally normal peers. Specific therapeutic exercises are devised to stimulate the infant's cognitive, social, motor, and language domains. Parents are usually taught these skills by special education teachers, physical therapists, occupational therapists, and speech pathologists so that therapy may be conducted at home. The child will later be referred to a specialized program designed to continue these intervention strategies and then mainstreamed into generic child care or school.

The research as to the results of early intervention programs has been extensive but as yet not conclusive. Short-term gains on children's developmental outcomes are often substantial. Although the long-term cognitive effects remain questionable (Gibson and Harris, 1988), improved family functioning and better social integration of the child are

seen. It does appear that timing is a critical factor, with earlier interventions being correlated with greater developmental gains.

Numerous other approaches designed to improve these children's developmental outcomes such as patterning, megavitamin therapy, and the administration of butoctamide hydrogen succinate have also been tried. Unfortunately, the results of all of these interventions have been disappointing.

RECENT AND ANTICIPATED ADVANCES IN DIAGNOSIS AND MANAGEMENT

Because no effective treatment for Down syndrome is on the horizon, increased attention is being given to prenatal diagnosis. Antenatal screening for Down syndrome using three serum markers (alpha-fetoprotein, unconjugated oestriol, and human chorionic gonadotrophin) has been shown to be more efficacious than using only alpha-fetoprotein or amniocentesis when screening is initiated based solely on maternal age (Haddow et al, 1992; Wald et al, 1992).

Growth hormone therapy has been effective in increasing height, occipital-frontal circumference, and muscle strength in children with Down syndrome (Hurwitz, 1992). However, this therapy is investigational and controversial (Giordano, 1992, Underwood, 1992). Many ethical issues around its usage exist such as: How will the child benefit from being taller? Is the discomfort associated with the therapy warranted? Who will pay for the therapy? (Binder, 1992). Moreover, growth hormone therapy has been associated with leukemia. The risks versus the benefits of this therapy have not been clearly evaluated as of yet.

ASSOCIATED PROBLEMS

Mental Retardation

Intellectual capabilities of children with Down syndrome vary dramatically. Most are moderately retarded (IQ 40 to 55, SD = 15), but a small percentage are either mildly affected (IQ 56 to 69, SD = 15) or severely impaired (IQ $\leq$39, SD = 15). For a few children, their intelligence quotients are not

---

ASSOCIATED PROBLEMS

- Mental retardation
- Cardiac defects
- Gastrointestinal tract anomalies
- Growth retardation
- Musculoskeletal and motor abilities
- Vision
- Hearing
- Immune system
- Dental changes
- Respiratory functioning
- Thyroid function
- Leukemia
- Seizure disorders

consistent with a diagnosis of mental retardation (Pueschel, 1992). Known correlates to children's intelligence and adaptive behavior skills are their physical condition, home environment, and individualized early intervention (Gibson and Harris, 1988). Unfortunately, cognitive function often deteriorates with aging, and significant losses in intelligence and social skills are seen earlier (frequently by age 40) than in persons who do not have Down syndrome (Brown et al, 1990).

Mental retardation may or may not be accompanied with behavior disorders. Depression, autisticlike behavior, and psychotic episodes have been reported. Neurologic deterioration, institutionalization, disturbed family life, stress associated with mainstreaming, and normal childhood stressors may have an effect on the mental health of children with Down syndrome.

Cardiac Defects

Approximately 40% of children with Down syndrome have congenital heart defects. In order of decreasing frequency, anomalies include: atrioventricular canal, ventricular septal defect, tetralogy of Fallot, patent ductus arteriosus, atrial septal defect, and others (Pueschel, 1990). (See Chapter 15). Many of these conditions are associated with a

greater degree of elevation of pulmonary vascular obstructive disease than would normally be expected (Clapp et al, 1990). In addition, children with Down syndrome who do not have congenital heart disease are at risk for developing mitral valve prolapse as they age; by the end of adolescence, mitral valve prolapse has been detected in over 50% of tested individuals (Geggel, O'Brien, and Feingold, 1993).

Gastrointestinal Tract Anomalies

Common congenital gastrointestinal tract anomalies include tracheoesophageal fistula, pyloric stenosis, duodenal atresia, annular pancreas, aganglionic megacolon, and imperforate anus (Pueschel, 1990). Most of these require immediate surgical correction and careful follow-up throughout the individual's life.

Growth Retardation

Infants with Down syndrome weigh less, are typically shorter, and have smaller occipital-frontal circumferences than unaffected children at birth (Palmer et al, 1992). The velocity of linear growth is also reduced, with the most marked reductions seen between 6 and 24 months of age. This reoccurs during adolescence, when the growth spurt is less vigorous than what would normally be expected (Cronk et al, 1988). This reduction in linear growth is not unexpected as children with Down syndrome have hypothalmic dysfunctions that affect the secretion of growth hormone (Pueschel, 1993).

Children with Down syndrome have a tendency toward being overweight. Beginning around 2 years of age (Chumlea and Cronk, 1981), untoward weight gain persists throughout the child's lifetime. For virtually every age, more than 30% of children with Down syndrome are above the 85th percentile for weight/height ratios (Cronk et al, 1988). Those of school age show the greatest propensity for weight/height percentile gain.

Differences by sex are noted, with boys being heavier and taller than girls from 3 to 24 months and again during the teenage years (Cronk et al, 1988). No meaningful differences in weight, stature, or head circumference, however, have been seen between white and black children with Down syndrome (Ershow, 1986). Environment also plays a role, with a greater number of children raised by their families showing increased weight/height ratios than for those children raised in institutions (Cronk, Chumlea, and Roche, 1985). Significant differences have been seen between growth parameters of children with Down syndrome with and without congenital heart defects, with the severity of growth delay being correlated to the severity of disease (Cronk et al, 1988).

Musculoskeletal and Motor Abilities

Orthopedic problems are second only to cardiac defects as a cause of morbidity in Down syndrome. Flaccid muscle tone and ligamentous laxity occur to some extent in all affected children, possibly because of an intrinsic defect in their connective tissue. Among these conditions are pes planus, patellar subluxation, scoliosis, dislocated hips, atlantoaxial subluxation, joint and muscle pain, and rapid muscle fatigue. These problems may occur throughout the child's lifetime and should be carefully screened for by the primary care provider at each visit.

Surgical correction may be indicated for patellar hypermobility with subluxation, scoliosis, or dislocated hips. It should be noted that although the incidence of congenital dislocated hip in children with Down syndrome is similar to that of unaffected peers, approximately 1 in 20 will acquire dislocated hips between learning to walk and the end of the school-aged period.

Another significant disorder is atlantoaxial instability. Atlantoaxial instability results from a "loose joint" between C1 and C2 and increased space between the atlas and odontoid process. It affects 9% to 30% of children with Down syndrome (Goldberg, 1993). At least 85% of affected children are asymptomatic. Subluxation or dislocation may result. Early manifestations may include head tilt, torticollis, deteriorating gait, or changes in bowel or bladder function. If left untreated, symptoms may progress to frank neurologic findings associated with spinal cord compression. Those at greatest risk are children under the age of 10 years and girls with very lax ligaments. The atlantodens interval may change over time in a small percentage of children, generally narrowing but occasionally widening (Pueschel, Scola, and Pezzullo, 1992). Secondary to the numerous studies done on atlantoaxial instability, other cervical spinal abnormalities such as occiput-C1 instability, odontoid dysplasia, and premature arthritis have been noted (Goldberg, 1993; Pueschel, et al, 1990).

Vision

Increased prevalence of numerous ocular deviations is associated with Down syndrome. In order of decreasing frequency the most commonly occurring abnormalities are slanted palpebral fissures, spotted irises, refractive errors, strabismus, nystagmus, cataracts, blepharitis, pseudopapilledema, and keratoconus (Roizen, Mets, and Blondis, 1994). A significant loss in visual acuity will result if many of these conditions are not diagnosed and treated in early childhood. Moreover, visual problems increase with age.

Hearing

Structural deviations of the skull, foreface, external auditory canal, and middle and inner ears accompanied by eustacian tube dysfunction are associated with congenital and acquired hearing loss (Brown et al, 1989). The incidence of hearing loss in children with Down syndrome is estimated to range from 50% to 76% (Davies, 1988). Children with stenotic auditory canals are at particular risk for problems.

Immune System

It is well documented that children with Down syndrome have altered immune function, although the evidence is conflicting as to the exact nature of the changes (Levin, 1987). All areas of immune function appear to be altered in part because of changes in the thymus. Responsible for controlling many immunologic mechanisms, the thymus is histologically and functionally abnormal. Documented alterations include depressed neutrophil chemotaxis, numerous variations in phagocytosis, and a somewhat diminished complement system. The ability of B cells to produce immunoglobins to selected antigens is also impaired despite the relative normality in the number of cells. This is possibly the result of the influence of T-cell regulation, because qualitative and quantitative differences have been shown to exist in their number and function (Levin, 1987; Wysocki, Wysocki, and Wierusz-Wysocka, 1987). Immune system deficits contribute directly to an increased incidence and severity of numerous other conditions. These include but are not limited to periodontal disease, respiratory problems, lymphocytic thyroiditis, leukemia, diabetes mellitus, alopecia areata, adrenal dysfunction, gluten enteropathy, and vitiligo.

Dental Changes

Children with Down syndrome seem to develop fewer caries than unaffected children. Numerous other dental problems, however, including bruxism, malocclusion, defective dentition, and periodontal disease, are more prevalent in this population because of a combination of anatomic anomalies of the oral cavity and immunologic dysfunction. Of particular significance is juvenile periodontitis, which is present in approximately 100% of children with Down syndrome. The disease progresses rapidly and may be noted even in deciduous dentition (Reuland-Bosma and van Dijk, 1986). Not accounted for merely by poor dental care, it is suspected that the altered immune function in conjunction with the extensive gingival inflammation seen in children with Down syndrome are responsible (Reuland-Bosma, van Dijk, and van der Weele, 1986). Mouth breathing and consumption of a diet high in soft foods, two common occurrences in children with Down syndrome, also contribute to their dental problems.

Respiratory Functioning

Pulmonary hypertension and pulmonary hyperplasia, fewer alveoli, a decreased alveolar blood capillary surface area, and associated upper airway obstruction (lymphatic hypertrophy in the Waldeyer ring), combined with a compromised immune system, predispose children with Down syndrome to respiratory tract infections. If recurrent severe respiratory tract infections occur, they will have a significant effect on the child's development.

Thyroid Dysfunction

Thyroid dysfunction in Down syndrome is commonly associated with autoimmune dysfunction (Pueschel, 1990). Usually it is an acquired rather than a congenital condition, and the prevalence may reach 40% in adults. Graves' disease, goiter, chronic lymphocytic thyroiditis, and hypothyroidism occur most frequently. Although thyroid dysfunction may remain subclinical for an extended period, alter-

ations in thyroid-stimulating hormone, thyroid-binding globulin, iodine-131 uptake, and the presence of antithyroglobulin and antimicrosomal antibodies may be seen (Pueschel et al, 1991).

Sleep Disordered Breathing

Anatomic and physiologic differences (e.g., midfacial hypoplasia, glossoptosis) predispose the child with Down syndrome to obstructive sleep apnea and other sleep disordered breathing problems. A recent study by Marcus and colleagues (1991) demonstrated that overnight polysomnograms were abnormal in 100% of the children tested. Frequent problems diagnosed included hypoventilation (81%), obstructive sleep apnea (63%), desaturation (56%), and multiple abnormalities (63%). Age, obesity, and cardiac disease did not affect the incidence of these problems.

Seizure Disorders

An increased frequency of seizure disorders is seen in children with Down syndrome, with approximately 8% of children being affected. Structural differences and biochemical changes associated with Down syndrome have been implicated although not confirmed. The distribution of the onset of seizures is bimodal. Of the affected children, 40% will begin to have seizures before 1 year of age; generally these seizures are infantile spasms and tonic-clonic seizures (Stafstrom and Konkol, 1994). The onset of seizures again peaked in adults in their 30s, with tonic-clonic seizures and partial simple and partial complex seizures being the most common (Pueschel, Louis, and McKnight, 1991). (See Chapter 19.)

Leukemia

Children with Down syndrome have approximately a fifteenfold risk of developing leukemia compared with other children. Neither acute lymphoblastic leukemia (ALL) nor acute nonlymphoblastic leukemia (ANL) predominate. Children with Down syndrome have the same prognosis as children without Down syndrome if they are able to achieve an initial remission. Unfortunately, remission is more difficult to achieve from both ALL and ANL, because children with Down syndrome often have a poor tolerance to antineoplastic drugs (Robison, 1992).

PROGNOSIS

Because of the association of Down syndrome with numerous anatomic and physiologic aberrations, life expectancy is reduced, with approximately a 10% mortality in the first year of life, rising to 14% by 10 years of age (Carr, 1994). The number and severity of congenital anomalies significantly decrease life expectancy for some of these children. Premature aging and a high incidence of Alzheimer's disease are also seen in Down syndrome and reduce life expectancy for adults. With correct medical, educational, and social interventions, the majority of individuals live well into adulthood and have satisfying, productive lives (Carr, 1994). Successful outcomes appear to depend heavily on the early interventions children and their families receive. Aggressive, interdisciplinary management is paramount if a child with Down syndrome is to reach his or her full potential.

Primary Care Management
HEALTH CARE MAINTENANCE
Growth and Development

Evaluating the growth of children with Down syndrome is a detailed process. When linear growth is assessed, the variations in velocity must be taken into account by the primary care provider. Whereas growth adequacy is often determined by maintaining a particular percentile rank, variations in growth velocity affect these children's growth curves during early childhood. Growth velocities for children with and without Down syndrome are similar during the school-aged period, however, and stability will then be seen in percentile curves.

Measurements should be plotted on both the National Center for Health Statistics (NCHS) growth charts and growth charts specifically normed for children with Down syndrome (see Figs. 18-5 to 18-10). The NCHS growth charts allow comparisons of children with Down syndrome to their chronologic-age peers and provide a frame of reference for parents. Weight/height percentiles found on the NCHS growth charts are independent of the child's age and are also useful in determining appropriate weight in children before adolescence. The specialty charts, where all percentiles for

stature are less than their analogous percentiles on the NCHS charts, provide an excellent reference point for comparing growth among children with Down syndrome and in determining those at risk for failure to thrive or obesity. Because inappropriate growth and excessive weight gain have ramifications for motor performance and social acceptance for children with Down syndrome, yearly assessments are required. Interventions for weight management may be introduced as necessary. Caloric reduction and increased exercise incorporated into a behavior management program is the approach most likely to be effective.

Development. Because Down syndrome is associated with global development delay, virtually all children with Down syndrome will have intelligence quotients below the second standard deviation on standardized tests such as the Weschler Intelligence Scale for Children—Revised or the Stanford-Binet Intelligence Test. Performance on other language, motor, and social aptitude tests will also be less than age norms for almost all children.

Children with Down syndrome will pass through the normal developmental milestones but at a much slower rate than expected. The primary care provider can assist in the child's development by referring the family to an early intervention program as soon as possible after the child's birth. As the child grows older, a variety of activities such as Special Olympics and summer camp that are known to assist in development can be encouraged. In the presence of significant congenital anomalies, program personnel will need guidance as to the intensity of activity the child is allowed. The child's progress should be carefully documented on standardized developmental schedules (see Fig. 18-11) at each primary care visit. Sharing the results of the child's developmental gains with the parents will objectively demonstrate the child's improvement, reinforcing the parents' efforts.

Diet

Among the most significant concerns are feeding difficulties in young children and obesity in older children. Feeding problems may be encountered because of the children's disproportionately large tongues, muscle flaccidity, poor coordination, significantly delayed social maturation, and congenital heart disease.

Text continued on p. 386

Boys with Down Syndrome:
Physical Growth: 1 to 36 Months

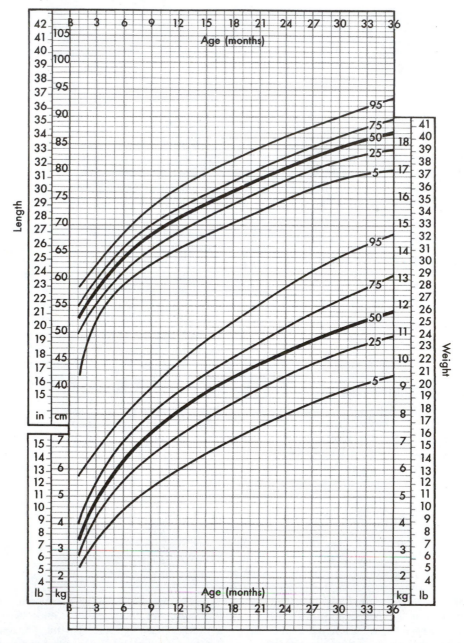

Fig. 18-5.   Based on data from the Developmental Evaluation Clinic of the Children's Hospital, Boston, The Child Development Center of Rhode Island Hospital, and the Clinical Genetics Service of the Children's Hospital of Philadelphia. Supported by March of Dimes grant 6-449.

Girls with Down Syndrome:
Physical Growth: 1 to 36 Months

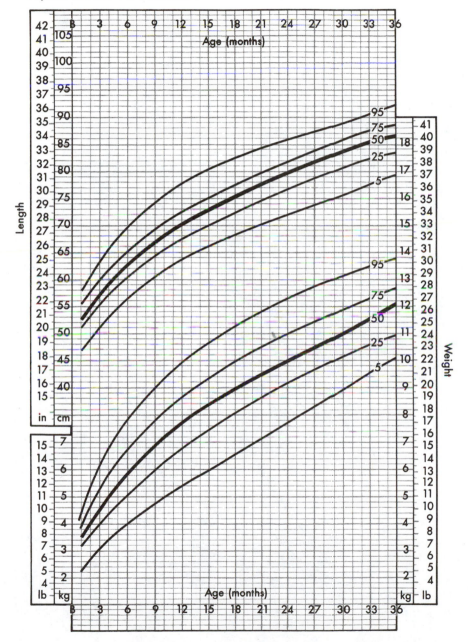

Fig. 18-6.   Based on data from the Developmental Evaluation Clinic of the Children's Hospital, Boston, The Child Development Center of Rhode Island Hospital, and the Clinical Genetics Service of the Children's Hospital of Philadelphia. Supported by March of Dimes grant 6-449.

Boys with Down Syndrome:
Physical Growth: 2 to 18 Years

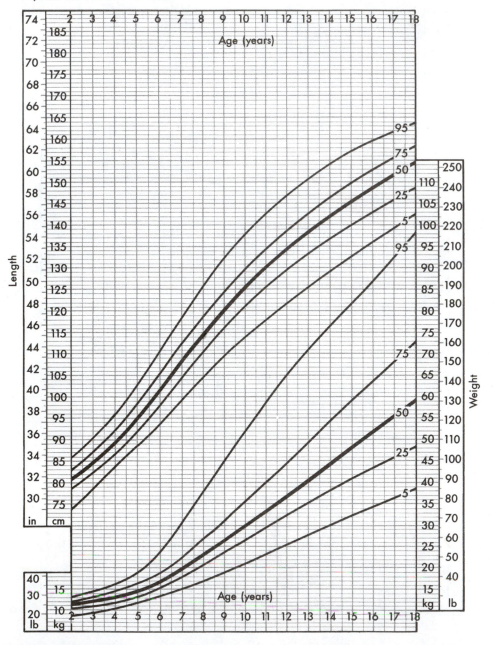

Fig. 18-7.   Based on data from the Developmental Evaluation Clinic of the Children's Hospital, Boston, The Child Development Center of Rhode Island Hospital, and the Clinical Genetics Service of the Children's Hospital of Philadelphia. Supported by March of Dimes grant 6-449.

Girls with Down Syndrome:
Physical Growth: 2 to 18 Years

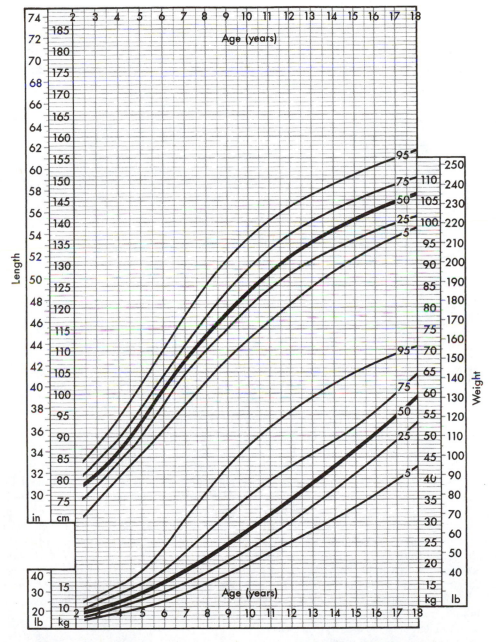

Fig. 18-8.   Based on data from the Developmental Evaluation Clinic of the Children's Hospital, Boston, The Child Development Center of Rhode Island Hospital, and the Clinical Genetics Service of the Children's Hospital of Philadelphia. Supported by March of Dimes grant 6-449.

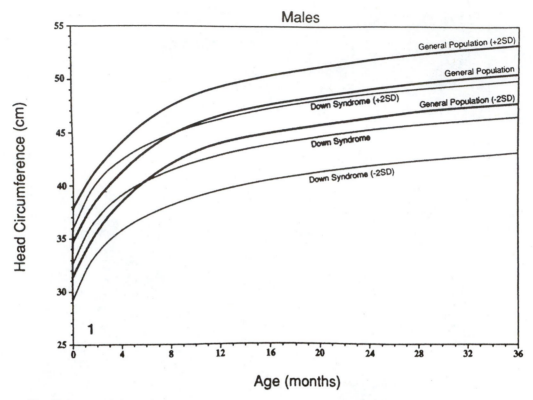

Fig. 18-9.   Head circumference growth curves for male individuals with Down syndrome (shaded) compared with male individuals from a general population. *(From Palmer CGS et al: Head circumference of children with Down syndrome (0 to 36 months), Am J Med Genetics 42:61-67, 1992.)*

For infants, breast feeding should be encouraged. The immunogenic qualities offer additional protection against upper respiratory tract infections and other illnesses. The extra effort required of the child who is breast feeding also helps develop the baby's orofacial muscles and tongue control and promotes greater jaw stability. Breast feeding will take longer at first, and mothers will need to be encouraged in their efforts. In addition to standard guidance concerning breast feeding, the primary care provider may also suggest other helpful tips such as (1) awaking the infant for feeding as necessary; (2) initially expressing some milk to encourage the infant to latch onto the breast; (3) ensuring that the infant's nose and mouth are free of mucus; (4) checking that the infant's lip is turned out during feeding; and (5) holding the infant in an upright position during feeding (Danner and Cerutti,

1984). For infants who are not breast feeding, using soft, large-hole nipples may be helpful.

Blended and chopped foods and shallow-bowl, latex-covered spoons may be of some help in children who are learning to eat solids. If significant problems occur, consultation with an occupational therapist or other developmental therapist in designing an individualized feeding program is suggested.

For older children there are no routine dietary restrictions. Care should be taken to avoid excessive caloric intake if inappropriate weight gain is a problem.

Safety

Safety issues for children with Down syndrome are the same as for their developmental, not chronologic, peers. Primary care providers must adjust

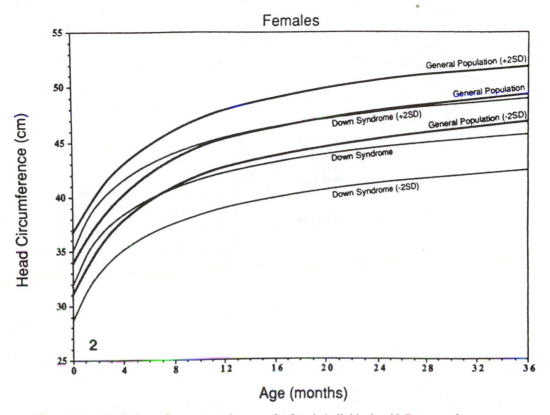

Fig. 18-10.   Head circumference growth curves for female individuals with Down syndrome (shaded) compared with female individuals from a general population. *(From Palmer CGS et al: Head circumference of children with Down syndrome (0 to 36 months), Am J Med Genetics 42: 61-67, 1992.)*

their normal schedule for providing anticipatory guidance to the development of the child with Down syndrome. If information is given too far in advance of the child's developmental progression, parents may forget or find it a painful reminder that their child is progressing more slowly than unaffected children.

Children with Down syndrome are more likely to sustain joint injuries as a result of their musculoskeletal problems. For children with atlantoaxial instability or those who have not yet been adequately evaluated, contact sports, somersaults, or other activities that may result in cervical injury should be restricted. Documentation that the child is not in danger of subluxation may be required for children participating in the Special Olympics.

Immunizations

Vaccination does not necessarily confer immunity in individuals with compromised secondary immune responses such as those seen in children with Down syndrome. Research that has investigated antibody response to immunization in children with Down syndrome is conflicting (Stiehm, 1989), and immunity should not be assumed by the primary care provider. Additional immunizations may be necessary because this group of children is considered high risk for infection. In areas endemic for specific diseases, antibody titer levels may be assessed to determine a child's immune status. There are, however, no contraindications for immunizations for children with Down syndrome, and the national immunization schedule should be followed including the immunizations for varicella and

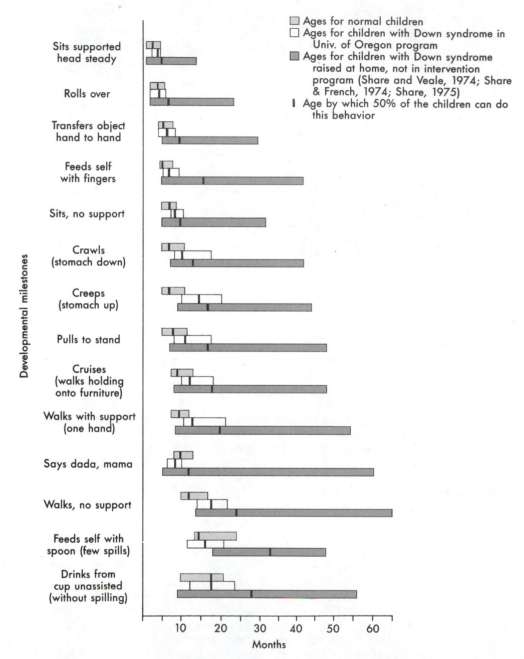

Fig. 18-11. Developmental milestones for children with Down syndrome. A new parents' guide. *(Kensington, MD, 1986, Woodbine House.)*

hepatitis A. (Committee on Infectious Diseases, 1994).

Other immunizations. Pneumococcal polysaccharide vaccine (Pneumovax) is indicated for this population and is given at 2 years of age (Immunization Practices Advisory Committee, 1984). Yearly immunoprophylaxis for influenza should also be considered for all children more than 6 months of age. Current recommended dosages are two doses of 0.25 ml of split-virus vaccine for children 6 to 35 months of age and 0.50 ml of split-virus vaccine for children aged 3 to 12 years. Only split-virus vaccines should be given to children because they lessen the risk of postimmunization febrile episodes. Adolescents need only one 0.50-ml dose of either whole or split-virus vaccine (Immunization Practices Advisory Committee, 1989).

Although immunization for hepatitis B is universally recommended for children, the status of children who are or have been cared for in an institutional setting should be assessed because there is an increase in the prevalence of hepatitis B carriers among individuals with a history of institutionalization and they may not have been immunized. For those children who are surface antibody negative, immunization with hepatitis B vaccine is highly recommended. Family members, respite care providers, teachers, or other individuals working closely with children with Down syndrome may also be at increased risk of hepatitis B infection, depending on the child's status and the individual's situation. Even though hepatitis B is not spread through casual contact, immunization for others is also recommended if circumstances warrant it.

Screening

Vision. Because of the large number of ocular defects associated with Down syndrome, all children should be evaluated by an ophthalmologist during infancy. Early referral is critical considering the synergistic effects that diminished vision and hearing have on development. Significant visual impairment is usually preventable because those conditions common in Down syndrome such as strabismus and myopia are treatable (Courage et al, 1994). Future screening recommendations should be determined in conjunction with the ophthalmologist according to the status of the child's eyes. At the minimum, the primary care provider should screen for visual problems at each well child visit. Screening should include testing acuity, examining the red reflex and optic fundi, and checking alignment and oculomotor functions. Because children with Down syndrome may have difficulty using a Snellen or lazy E chart, acuity screening performed with the Titmus picture test, Teller Acuity cards, or Allen picture cards will yield more valid results. The primary care provider should note that some visual disorders, including cataracts and keratoconus, frequently do not develop until adolescence.

Many children with Down syndrome have difficulty keeping their glasses in place; therefore, parents should be counseled that purchasing glasses with lightweight plastic lenses and using an elastic strap around the child's occiput to secure them will help correct this problem. Contact lenses are not routinely recommended but may be appropriate for children with keratoconus.

Hearing. Because good hearing is a requisite for cognitive, social, and language development and because these children are at high risk for conductive hearing losses, careful assessment is needed. It is recommended that all infants be evaluated for auditory brain stem responses during the first 6 months of life (Roizen et al, 1993). If the external ear orifice is so stenotic or other difficulties occur as to preclude adequate pneumootoscopic examination, alternate methods of evaluation must be used. Tympanometry provides one useful adjunct to assessment but is not reliable in children less than 1 year of age. Because of the importance of early intervention, infants should be referred for microotoscopy between 9 and 12 months of age if examination is difficult. Accumulation of cerumen leading to impacted canals is common; removal of cerumen every 6 months is recommended for children who have this problem. When middle ear disease occurs, it deserves aggressive intervention and close follow-up if further developmental insult is to be prevented.

If hearing aids are required, those that fasten onto the earpiece of eyeglasses may be better than ear molds. Hearing aids dependent on ear molds are difficult to fit for children who are just beginning to wear them. Frequently these children do not like the increased sound. Parents may need to be helped to find methods, such as behavior management, that will help improve their child's compliance for leaving the hearing aid in place. Parents must also be cautioned to devise mnemonic cues for remembering to change the batteries on a routine basis because it is unlikely that their child will be able to identify that their hearing aid is malfunctioning.

Dental. Because of the extremely high prevalence of dental problems in young children, aggressive dental care is necessary. The primary health care provider needs to document and carefully follow these children's dental problems. All children with Down syndrome should be evaluated before the age of 2 years by a dentist or pediodontist skilled in the care of children with developmental disabilities. Locating such dentists is often difficult for parents, and specific referrals to such professionals may be warranted.

Good dental hygiene, including frequent brushing and flossing, is indicated to reduce the amount of periodontal disease. If this is difficult, using a Water Pik should be considered. Effective toothbrushing techniques may be difficult to achieve because of the child's limited manual dexterity, enlarged tongue, and small mouth. Close supervision is required, and independent toothbrushing and mouth care may not be feasible until the child is of school age or older.

Weaning children from the bottle by 18 months and diets that contain low-sugar crunchy foods, such as fresh vegetables, will also help deter dental deterioration and should be encouraged. In areas where the water supply is nonfluoridated, fluoride supplementation should be initiated (Randell, Harth, and Seow, 1992). If periodontal disease is severe, chemical plaque control may be necessary. For children with congenital heart disease, prophylactic antibiotics should accompany all dental interventions (Dajani et al, 1990) (see Chapter 15).

Blood pressure. Routine screening is recommended. If there is a history of cardiac disease or a positive family history of cardiac disease or a positive family history of hypertension, more careful assessment is required.

Hematocrit. Routine screening is recommended.

Urinalysis. Routine screening is recommended.

Tuberculosis. Routine screening is recommended. No special precautions need to be taken unless the child is or has been institutionalized.

Condition-specific screening

THYROID DYSFUNCTION. As the abnormalities seen in Down syndrome are similar to some seen in thyroid dysfunction, a diagnosis of thyroid problems by clinical examination is difficult. Thyroid-stimulating hormone levels should be assessed yearly from birth. In the presence of any signs or symptoms suggestive of thyroid dysfunction, a complete thyroid panel should be drawn.

ATLANTOAXIAL INSTABILITY. The risk of atlantoaxial subluxation must be appraised by the primary care provider for all children with Down syndrome who are planning on engaging in physically active exercise, participating in Special Olympics, or are to undergo surgical or rehabilitative procedures (Morton et al, 1995). In general, cervical spine x-ray studies should be considered after age 2½ years. Reevaluation at around age 8 years may be appropriate depending on the child's initial findings and activity levels (Pueschel, Scola, and Pezzullo, 1992).

HIP DISLOCATION. Assessing hip stability through age 10 years is indicated because early detection before the dislocation is fixed and acetabular dysplasia occurs will allow for optimal surgical correction. Early presenting signs of habitual dislocation are an increasing limp, decreasing activity, and an audible click. Pain does not usually occur unless the dislocation is acute. In older children, x-ray studies may be necessary for assessment.

MITRAL VALVE PROLAPSE. Screening should begin in adolescence. Echocardiographic evaluations are recommended before surgical or dental procedures (Geggel, O'Brien, & Feingold, 1993).

SCREENING

- Thyroid dysfunction
- Atlantoaxial instability
- Hip dislocations
- Mitral valve prolapse

COMMON ILLNESS MANAGEMENT

Differential Diagnosis

Immune dysfunction. The significant changes in the immune systems of children with Down syndrome have significant implications for the primary care provider. Specifically, all infections need to be treated aggressively because negative sequelae are more likely to develop. The incidence of many autoimmune diseases, including diabetes mellitus and juvenile rheumatoid arthritis, are also much greater in this population. Should a child exhibit signs and symptoms compatible with a diagnosis of any of these, thorough evaluation is indicated. Parents need to be educated about the signs and symptoms of conditions and the need to seek medical advice promptly (see Chapters 17 and 25).

Upper respiratory tract infections. Children with Down syndrome are prone to upper respiratory tract infections. These should be managed aggressively because untoward sequelae, including otitis media and pneumonia, are more apt to develop. Children with congenital heart disease should be examined at the first signs of illness; children are more likely to develop secondary problems, and parents may confuse an upper respiratory tract infection with early congestive heart failure. These children may also need to be given subacute bacterial endocarditis prophylaxis (see Chapter 15).

Behavioral changes. Behavioral changes may be caused by a variety of physiologic and psycho-logic problems, including (1) thyroid dysfunction, (2) obstructive sleep apnea, (3) neurodegeneration (primarily in older individuals), (4) declining physical competence (e.g., congestive heart failure), (5) disturbed home environment, and (6) overstimulation. Interventions must be cause specific. Trials with antidepressants or antipsychotic drugs may be indicated in some cases after thorough evaluation.

Gastrointestinal symptoms. Because pyloric stenosis and Hirschsprung's disease are more common, the primary care provider should carefully pursue complaints of persistent vomiting, constipation, or chronic diarrhea in infants. Constipation, a common problem, may also be related to inadequate peristalsis, poor diet, lack of exercise, or thyroid dysfunction. The cause of constipation must clearly be assessed so that the correct interventions are initiated.

Leukemia. Children with Down syndrome are at 15 to 20 times the risk for developing leukemia than other children. Easy bruising, unusual pallor, or listlessness need to be fully evaluated. Parents must be alerted to seek health care immediately for their child if any of these signs or symptoms develop.

Drug Interactions

Down syndrome is associated with functional abnormalities in the neurotransmitter enzyme systems, with the cholinergic and noradrenergic systems particularly vulnerable (Coyle, Oster-Granite, and Gearhart, 1986). This may predispose children with Down syndrome to a hypersensitivity to cholinergic drugs, although the evidence is conflicting. Caution is advised if atropine, pilocarpine, or other related medications are to be given.

DEVELOPMENTAL ISSUES

Sleep Patterns

Sleep disorders are uncommon in children with Down syndrome, with the exception of obstructive sleep apnea and related conditions. Anatomic and immunologic differences predispose school-aged children in particular to this condition. The primary care provider should have a high index of suspicion if a history of snoring, restless sleep, night terrors, or daytime somnolence is given or failure to thrive, pulmonary hypertension, or behavioral

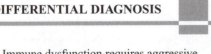

DIFFERENTIAL DIAGNOSIS

- Immune dysfunction requires aggressive treatment
- Upper respiratory tract infections common
- Behavioral changes may have physical cause
- Gastrointestinal symptoms in infants may be due to congenital anomalies
- Leukemia, 15 to 20% more common

problems are present. Referral to a sleep laboratory for an overnight polysomnography is warranted (Carskadon, Pueschel, and Millman, 1993).

Toileting

The median age for toilet training children with Down syndrome is approximately 36 months. Parents need to be advised of this to reduce frustrations associated with unrealistic expectations. Routine toilet training techniques are effective. It will take longer, however, to train a child with Down syndrome, and additional positive reinforcement will be necessary.

Children with Down syndrome may suffer from constipation secondary to their generalized muscle flaccidity and low activity levels. Dietary corrections, occasional use of bulk laxatives, and increases in exercise can alleviate this problem.

Discipline

Children with Down syndrome are more likely to display disruptive behavior and repetitive actions than their nonaffected peers (Myers and Pueschel, 1991). They are, however, not usually more difficult to discipline than other children. Parents must be encouraged to remember that discipline needs to be appropriate for the child's developmental age, however, and not their chronologic age. Consistency in parental expectations and limit setting help prevent aberrant behavioral patterns from developing. Behavior management programs can be developed for specific discipline problems when the child has not been responsive to the parents' usual methods.

Child Care

Day care should provide appropriate social, cognitive, and physical stimulation for the child with Down syndrome. When selecting the type of day care setting, parents should be encouraged to consider the child's personality and medical needs as well as their own philosophy about mainstreaming. Many generic day care centers willingly mainstream children with Down syndrome into their programs and are sufficiently staffed to provide an excellent experience for the child. If the child has significant medical problems, specialized day care, often available through the school system, may be a better option. Primary care providers should be aware of resources in their community to which

parents may be referred to assist with day care placement. The local affiliates of the Association of Retarded Citizens, the Association for the Care of Children's Health, or other specialty agencies may be helpful with this task.

All young children who attend group day care are more likely to experience a greater number of illnesses (Thacker et al, 1992), have more frequent hospitalizations (Bell et al, 1989), and have a greater need for myringotomies (Wald et al, 1988) than children in home care.

If the individual child has proven to be highly susceptible to infections, a home care setting (less than six children) is recommended. As with all individuals who are immunocompromised, immunizations are an important component in prevention.

Schooling

A variety of options for academic placement ranging from mainstreaming to residential placement exist. If circumstances permit, children with Down syndrome do best in a fully integrated environment with nondisabled peers. Children with Down syndrome, however, do need support from their families as they deal with being exceptional and with social pressures from peers. Parents and teachers working together to create a supportive environment can ensure that the child has some social and academic successes. Failing to accomplish this will result in the child becoming frustrated and demoralized leading to disruptive behaviors and poor self-esteem.

Families may need assistance in choosing the school setting they think is most appropriate for their child. The primary care provider can be instrumental in helping the family locate the appropriate community services (e.g., mental health–mental retardation base service units) that will assist in educational placement. All children with Down syndrome are eligible for educational provisions under Public Law 101-476 (see Chapter 5). Parents should be encouraged to contact their social worker or local office of mental retardation shortly after the child's birth so they can receive those educational, vocational, and supportive services for which the child is eligible.

Sexuality

Pubertal changes in adolescents with Down syndrome occur at approximately the same time as in their unaffected peers (Scola and Pueschel, 1992). Accompanying these physical changes, adolescents will have similar social interests and biologic drives to their chronologic-age peers (Pueschel and Scola, 1988) and will need to be provided with the opportunity to participate in social activities with their peers. For parents who are highly protective, the social and sexual education that must accompany their children's increasing independence are often difficult and sensitive issues (Smith et al, 1995). The primary care provider needs to help parents recognize their responsibility in ensuring that their child can handle himself or herself in a socially and sexually appropriate manner.

Individualized instruction about self-care skills, biologic changes, social implications, and contraception is paramount so that both appearance of sexual impropriety and the risk of being sexually exploited may be minimized. Genetic counseling for both parents and child is necessary, because although men virtually always will be sterile, women are capable of reproducing. Planned Parenthood, the Association of Retarded Citizens, and parent support groups offer printed and audiovisual materials specifically designed for use with these families.

For some female adolescents, handling pubertal changes will be difficult. Family members need to be helped to recognize the behavior changes that may be related to normal hormonal cycles. For those who are menstruating and are unable to manage their own hygienic care, parents and other caregivers must also take precautions in assisting if the young woman is positive for hepatitis B.

Some parents may request sterilization of a daughter with Down syndrome. The right to procreative choice is protected by law, and statutes regarding sterilization vary dramatically from state to state. The primary care provider is strongly suggested to consult with the state office of mental retardation for current guidelines, because in some jurisdictions sterilization is illegal. Professional practice standards from the American College of Obstetricians and Gynecologists and the American Academy of Pediatrics provide ethical guidelines for this difficult issue (Committee on Bioethics, 1990). If sterilization is to be pursued, the adolescent must participate in the decision to the extent possible and state and local laws strictly followed.

Transition into Adulthood

The life expectancy for individuals with Down syndrome has increased dramatically and most individuals are now reaching adulthood, raising many specific issues that until now remained unaddressed. Some of these issues are: independent living, sexuality, vocational choices, and health maintenance.

Individuals with Down syndrome range in their abilities to live independently from requiring ongoing, consistent supervision to minimal guidance with complex tasks. Most individuals remain at home until a crisis forces different arrangements. Because individuals with Down syndrome often have aged parents, families can help plan for a smooth transition to a different living situation within the context of normal development. For example, some parents may help their son or daughter move to a group home at about the age as their other children left for college. Recreation activities such as bowling, swimming, and dancing are encouraged because these activities promote social relationships and physical fitness.

Vocational choices are directed by the individual's cognitive abilities, social skills, and adaptive abilities. Many will be able to seek competitive employment in custodial work, offices, housekeeping, restaurants, landscaping, or other occupations where the required skills are not too difficult, fairly repetitive, and there is ongoing supervision. Skills necessary to survive in the work force such as basic money management, telling time, or using public transportation need to be mastered before seeking such positions. For others, working in sheltered workshops is a better option because this type of job requires fewer adaptive abilities.

Generally, most individuals' overall health is good, although premature aging occurs as early as age 20 with dental changes. Dermatologic, thyroid, cardiac, and sensory problems are the most troublesome and worsen with aging. Changes in mental health are also a concern after the child completes formal schooling at 21 years of age. The overall prevalence of psychiatric disorders is 22% with depression and dementia being the most common (Carr, 1994). This may be a result of decreased social opportunities and lack of readily available transportation. Perhaps of greatest concern is Alzheimer's disease, which may occur as early as age 20. IQ levels also decline over time. These changes do not bode well for maintaining the self-help skills and independence that individuals with Down syndrome worked so hard to achieve during their childhood. Further longitudinal study of the adult with Down syndrome, especially documentation of health status changes, is warranted.

SPECIAL FAMILY CONCERNS AND RESOURCES

Parenting a child with Down syndrome can be difficult. Although Down syndrome is associated with numerous health and developmental needs, most parents meet these challenges with resilience and adaptive functioning (Van Riper, Ryff, and Pridham, 1992). Yet for some parents, raising these children can become overwhelming. Locating and coordinating acceptable medical, educational, and ancillary personnel may be highly stress producing. The primary care provider may be of tremendous assistance to the family in identifying appropriate resources and helping the parents become their child's lifelong case manager. Mothers in particular may find it difficult to balance their time and responsibilities among their children and spouse. Although many concerns are similar for all families with a child who has special needs, one notable issue for families of children with Down syndrome is the need for long-range planning. Some children with Down syndrome may never become totally self-sufficient, and families will need to plan for the child's lifetime. Others may marry and live semiindependent lives. The severity of the child's difficulty, internal family strengths, and the support offered from extended family and community networks all affect a family's adjustment.

Parents of children with Down syndrome will experience joy and pride in the child. They may also experience chronic sorrow. A natural response to an abnormal event, chronic sorrow is the prolonged sadness that parents may periodically experience at points throughout their child's lifetime (Olshansky, 1962). This occurs most commonly when developmental milestones, such as graduating from high school, are missed (Wikler, Wascow, and Hatfield, 1981). For some parents this continued grief work is discomfiting, particularly if it is misinterpreted by professionals as pathologic

grieving. Primary care providers have the unique opportunity to assist families in recognizing that chronic sorrow is a normal extension of the grieving process and that their reactions are normal and healthy.

Resources

Caring for a child with Down syndrome is a complex task because of the numerous physical, cognitive, and social concerns that must be addressed. Lists of additional resources for professionals and parents of children with Down syndrome follow.

Informational materials

Cunningham C: *Down syndrome: an introduction for parents,* ed 2, Cambridge, MA, 1988, Brookline Books. It is available from Brookline Books, PO Box 1047, Cambridge, MA 02238.

Hanson M: *Teaching the infant with Down syndrome: A guide for parents and professionals,* ed 2, Austin, TX, 1988, Pro-Ed. It is available from Pro-Ed, 8700 Shoal Creek Blvd, Austin, TX 78757.

Brill MT: *Keys to parenting a child with Down syndrome,* Hauppauge, NY, 1993 Barron's Educational Series. It is available from Barron's Educational Series, Inc, 250 Wireless Blvd, Hauppauge, NY 11788.

Pueschel S, ed: *The young person with Down syndrome: transition from adolescence to adulthood,* Baltimore, 1988, Brookes Publishing. It is available from Paul H. Brookes Publishing Co, Box 10624, Baltimore, MD 21285-0624.

Stray-Gundersen K, ed: *Babies with Down syndrome: a new parents guide,* Kensington, MD, 1986, Woodbine House. It is available from Woodbine House, Inc, 10400 Connecticut Ave, Kensington, MD 20895.

Tingey C: *Down syndrome: a resource handbook,* Waltham, MA, 1988, College-Hill Press. It is available from College-Hill Press/Little, Brown, & Co, Order Dept, 200 West St, Waltham, MA 02254-9931.

Trainer M: *Differences in common: straight talk on mental retardation, Down syndrome, and life,* Kensington, MD, 1991, Woodbine House. It is available from Woodbine House, Inc, 10400 Connecticut Ave, Kensington, MD 20895.

Van Dyke DC et al, eds: *Medical and surgical care for children with Down syndrome: a guide for parents,* Kensington, MD, 1995, Woodbine House. It is available from Woodbine House, Inc, 10400 Connecticut Ave, Kensington, MD 20895.

Teaching aids

Dollydowns (teaching doll)
    Camp Venture, Inc
    100 Convent Rd

Box 402
Nanuet, NY 10954

Organizations

The ARC (formerly: Association for Retarded Citizens of the United States)
500 E Border St
Suite 300
Arlington, TX 76010
(800) 433-5255
(817) 261-6003

Canadian Down Syndrome Society
12837 76th Ave, Suite 206
Surrey, BC V3W 2V3, CANADA
(604) 599-6009
(604) 599-6165 FAX

The Commission on Mental and Physical Disability Law
American Bar Association
740 15th St NW
Washington, DC 20005-1009
(202) 662-1570
(202) 662-1032 FAX

National Down Syndrome Congress
1605 Chantilly Dr, Suite 250
Atlanta, GA 30324
(800) 232-6372
(404) 833-2817 FAX

National Down Syndrome Society
666 Broadway, Suite 810
New York, NY 10012
(800) 221-4602
(212) 974-2873 FAX

SUMMARY OF PRIMARY CARE NEEDS FOR THE CHILD WITH DOWN SYNDROME

Health care maintenance

Growth and development

Children usually have shorter stature and increased weight (after infancy).

Occipitofrontal circumference may be decreased.

Children should have height and weight measured at each visit and plotted on NCHS growth charts and growth charts for children with Down syndrome.

Virtually all children will be mentally retarded and have global developmental delay.

Virtually all children will have hypotonia and joint laxity. Obesity compounds complications.

Cognitive function often deteriorates with age. High incidence of early Alzheimer's disease.

Diet

Diets may need to be tailored to help correct constipation or obesity.

Safety

Anticipatory guidance needs to be based on the child's developmental level, not chronologic age.

Increased incidence of musculoskeletal injuries from laxity.

Atlantoaxial instability a hazard. Must be ruled out before active sports program or surgery. Spine x-rays usually done after 2½ years of age.

Immunizations

Immunity may not be conferred from immunizations because of a compromised immune system. Titer analysis during outbreaks of communicable diseases is recommended.

Pneumococcal polysaccharide and influenza immunoprophylaxis should be considered.

Screening

Vision

High incidence of ocular defects. All infants should be evaluated by ophthalmologist.

Acuity and alignment testing and examination of the red reflex and optic fundi should be done at each visit.

Hearing

Anatomical abnormalities of ears common. Evaluation by specialist recommended during infancy.

Otoscopy and tympanometry should be performed at each visit.

Continued.

SUMMARY OF PRIMARY CARE NEEDS FOR THE CHILD WITH DOWN SYNDROME—cont'd

50% to 76% have hearing loss. Many will require hearing aids.

Dental

Dental screening should be done a minimum of every 6 months from age 18 months because of the high incidence of periodontal disease.

Children with CHD may require antibiotic prophylaxis to prevent endocarditis.

Blood pressure

Routine screening is recommended.

Hematocrit

Routine screening is recommended.

Urinalysis

Routine screening is recommended.

Tuberculosis

Routine screening is recommended.

Condition-specific screening

Thyroid-stimulating hormone levels should be checked yearly if dysfunction is suggested.

Cervical spine x-ray studies to determine atlantoaxial stability should be done after age 2 years or before first surgery or athletic involvement.

Screening for hip dislocation is necessary through age 10 years.

Screening for mitral valve prolapse beginning in adolescents.

Common illness management

Differential diagnosis

Immune dysfunction

Children with Down syndrome are more susceptible to infections and autoimmune disorders.

Upper respiratory tract infections

Upper respiratory tract infections are often associated with otitis media and pneumonia and should be managed aggressively, especially when child has CHD.

Behavioral changes

Thyroid dysfunction, obstructive sleep apnea, neurodegeneration, declining physical competence, disturbed home environment, and overstimulation should be ruled out.

Gastrointestinal symptoms

Pyloric stenosis, megacolon, inadequate peristalsis, and thyroid dysfunction should be ruled out.

Leukemia

Unusual pallor, easy bruising, and listlessness should be fully evaluated.

Drug interactions

Hypersensitivity to cholinergic drugs (e.g., atropine) is possible.

Developmental issues

Sleep patterns

Obstructive sleep apnea may occur; it is a problem of primarily school-aged children. Surgical intervention may be necessary.

Toileting

Delayed bowel and bladder training may occur as a result of developmental lag; constipation is common because of low activity level, decreased peristalsis, poor diet.

Discipline

Discipline must be developmentally appropriate; behavior management programs are often successful.

Child care

Small group day care lessens the risk of repeated infections.

Eligible for special programs through Public Law 99-457 and 94-142.

Schooling

Associated problems are covered by Public Law 101-476; it assists families with school planning and mainstreaming.

Sexuality

Sex education must be taught so that children with Down syndrome are not abused and do not display inappropriate sexual behaviors.

Girls may need assistance with menstrual hygiene.

Continued.

**SUMMARY OF PRIMARY CARE NEEDS FOR THE CHILD
WITH DOWN SYNDROME**—cont'd

Hepatitis B precaution advised.
Boys are usually infertile but girls may be fertile.

Transition into adulthood

Emphasis on independent living, vocational skills,
and health maintenance.

Mental health problems including Alzheimer's
disease may be problematic.

Special family concerns

Special family concerns include long-term care and
chronic sorrow.

REFERENCES

Bell DM et al: Illness associated with child day care: a study of incidence and cost, *Am J Public Health* 79:479-484, 1989.

Binder ND: Growth hormone therapy in children with Down syndrome (letter), *J Pediatr* 120:832, 1992.

Brown FR et al: Intellectual and adaptive functioning in individuals with Down syndrome in relation to age and environmental placement, *Pediatrics* 85(suppl 3):450-452, 1990.

Brown PM et al: The skull base and nasopharynx in Down's syndrome in relation to hearing impairment, *Clin Otolaryngol* 14:241-246, 1989.

Carr J: Annotation: long-term outcome for people with Down's syndrome, *J Child Psychol Psychiatr* 35:425-439, 1994.

Carskadon MA, Pueschel SM, and Millman RP: Sleep-disordered breathing and behavior in three risk groups: preliminary findings from parental reports, *Child's Nervous System* 9:452-457, 1993.

Centers for Disease Control: Down syndrome prevalence at birth—United States, 1983–1990, *Morbidity and Mortality Weekly Review* 43:617-622, 1994.

Chumlea WC, Cronk CE: Overweight among children with trisomy 21, *J Ment Defic Res* 25:275-280, 1981.

Clapp S et al: Down's syndrome, complete atrioventricular canal, and pulmonary vascular obstructive disease, *J Cardiovasc Surg* 100:115-121, 1990.

Committee on Bioethics: Sterilization of women who are mentally handicapped, *Pediatrics* 85:868-871, 1990.

Committee on Infectious Diseases: *1994 red book: report of the Committee on Infectious Diseases,* ed 23, Elk Grove Village, IL, 1994, American Academy of Pediatrics.

Courage ML et al: Visual acuity in infants and children with Down syndrome, *Dev Med Child Neurol* 36:586-593, 1994.

Coyle JT, Oster-Granite ML, and Gearhart JD: The neurobio-logic consequences of Down syndrome, *Brain Res Bull* 16:773-787, 1986.

Cronk CE, Chumlea WC, and Roche AF: Assessment of overweight children with trisomy 21, *Am J Ment Defic* 89:433-436, 1985.

Cronk C et al: Growth charts for children with Down syndrome: 1 month to 18 years of age, *Pediatrics* 81:102-110, 1988.

Dajani RS et al: Prevention of bacterial endocarditis: recommendations by the American Heart Association, *JAMA* 264:2919-2922, 1990.

Danner SC, Cerutti ER: *Nursing your baby with Down's syndrome,* Rochester, NY, 1984, Childbirth Graphics.

Davies B: Auditory disorders in Down's syndrome, *Scand Audiol* 30 (suppl):65-68, 1988.

Ershow AG: Growth in black and white children with Down syndrome, *Am J Ment Defic* 90:507-512, 1986.

Ferencz C et al: Congenital cardiovascular malformations associated with chromosome abnormalities: an epidemiologic study, *J Pediatr* 114:79-86, 1989.

Geggel RL, O'Brien JE, and Feingold M: Development of valve dysfunction in adolescents and young adults with Down syndrome and no known congenital heart disease, *J Pediatr* 122:821-823, 1993.

Gibson D, Harris A: Aggregated early intervention effects for Down's syndrome persons: patterning and longevity of benefits, *J Ment Defic Res* 32:1-17, 1988.

Giordano BP: The impact of genetic syndromes on children's growth, *J Pediatr Health Care* 6:309-315, 1992.

Goldberg MJ: Spine instability and the special olympics, *Clin Sports Med* 12:507-515, 1993.

Haddow JE et al: Prenatal screening for Down's syndrome with use of maternal serum markers, *New Engl J Med* 327:588-593, 1992.

Hagerman RJ: Chromosomal conditions. In MD Levine, Carey WB, and Crocker AC, (editors): *Developmental-behavioral pediatrics,* ed 2, Philadelphia, 1992, WB Saunders, pp 213-220.

Hurwitz A: Helping Down syndrome children to reach new heights: the role of the pediatric nurse, *Pediatr Nurs* 18:485-489, 1992.

Immunization Practices Advisory Committee: Update: Pneumococcal polysaccharide vaccine usage—United States, *MMWR* 33:273-281, 1984.

Katz S, Kravetz S: Facial plastic surgery for persons with Down syndrome: research findings and their professional and social implications, *Am J Ment Retard* 94:101-110, 1989.

Klaiman P, Arndt E: Facial reconstruction in Down syndrome: perceptions of the results by parents and normal adolescents, *Cleft Palate J* 26:186-192, 1989.

Lang DJ et al: Hypospadias and urethral abnormalities in Down syndrome, *Clin Pediatr* 26:40-42, 1987.

Levin S: The immune system and susceptibility to infections in Down's syndrome. In McCoy EE, Epstein CJ, (editors): *Oncology and immunology of Down syndrome,* New York, 1987, Alan R Liss, pp 143-162.

Mahon M: The nurse's role in treatment decision making for the child with disabilities, *Issues in Law and Medicine* 6:247-268, 1990.

Marcus CL et al: Obstructive sleep apnea in children with Down syndrome, *Pediatrics* 88:132-139, 1991.

Morton RE et al: Atlantoaxial instability in Down's syndrome: a 5-year follow up study, *Arch Dis Child* 72:115-119, 1995.

Myers BA, Pueschel SM: Psychiatric disorders in persons with Down syndrome, *J Nerv Ment Dis* 179:609-613, 1991.

Olshansky S: Chronic sorrow: a response to having a mentally defective child, *Soc Casework* 43:190-193, 1962.

Palmer CGS et al: Head circumference of children with Down syndrome (0 to 36 months), *Am J Med Genetics* 42:61-67, 1992.

Pueschel SM: Growth hormone response after administration of L-dopa, clonidine, and growth hormone releasing hormone in children with Down syndrome, *Res Devel Disabil* 14:291-298, 1993.

Pueschel SM: The child with Down syndrome. In MD Levine, WB Carey, and AC Crocker, (editors): *Developmental-behavioral pediatrics,* ed 2, Philadelphia, 1992, WB Saunders, pp 221-228.

Pueschel SM: Clinical aspects of Down syndrome from infancy to adulthood, *Am J Med Genetics* 7(suppl.):52-56, 1990.

Pueschel SM: Growth, thyroid function, and sexual maturation in Down syndrome, *Growth Genet Horm* 6:1-5, 1990.

Pueschel SM et al: Thyroid function in Down syndrome, *Res Devel Disabil* 12:287-296, 1991.

Pueschel SM, Louis S, and McKnight P: Seizure disorders in Down syndrome, *Arch Neurol* 48:318-320, 1991.

Pueschel SM, Scola FH, Pezzullo JC: A longitudinal study of atlanto-dens relationships in asymptomatic individuals with Down syndrome, *Pediatrics* 89:1194-1198, 1992.

Pueschel SM et al: Skeletal anomalies of the upper cervical spine in children with Down syndrome, *J Pediatr Orthop* 10:607-611, 1990.

Pueschel SM, Scola PS: Parents' perception of social and sexual functions in adolescents with Down's syndrome, *J Ment Defic Res* 32:215-220, 1988.

Randell DM, Harth S, and Seow WK: Preventive dental health practices of noninstitutionalized Down syndrome children: a controlled study, *J Clin Pediatr Dent* 16:225-229, 1992.

Reuland-Bosma W, van Dijk LJ: Periodontal disease in Down's syndrome: a review, *J Clin Periodontol* 13:64-73, 1986.

Reuland-Bosma W, van Dijk LJ, and van der Weele L: Experimental gingivitis around deciduous teeth in children with Down's syndrome, *J Clin Periodontol* 13:294-300, 1986.

Robison LL: Down syndrome and leukemia, *Leukemia* 6(suppl 1):5-7, 1992.

Roizen NJ, Mets MB, and Blondis TA: Ophthalmic disorders in children with Down syndrome, *Dev Med Child Neurol* 36:594-600, 1994.

Roizen NJ et al: Hearing loss in children with Down syndrome, *J Pediatr* 123:S9-S12, 1993.

Scola PS, Pueschel SM: Menstrual cycles and basal body temperature curves in women with Down syndrome, *Obstet Gynecol* 79:91-94, 1992.

Sharav T: Aging gametes in relation to incidence, gender, and twinning in Down syndrome, *Am J Med Genetics* 39:116-118, 1991.

Smith K et al: The role of the pediatric nurse practitioner in educating teens with mental retardation about sex, *J Pediatr Health* 9:59-66, 1995.

Stafstrom CE, Konkol RJ: Infantile spasms in children with Down syndrome, *Dev Med Child Neurol* 36:576-585, 1994.

Stiehm ER: *Immunologic disorders in infants and children,* Philadelphia, 1989, WB Saunders.

Strauss RP et al: Social perceptions of the effects of Down syndrome facial surgery: a school-based study of ratings by normal adolescents, *Plast Reconstruct Surg* 81:841-846, 1988.

Thacker SB et al: Infectious diseases and injuries in child day care, *JAMA* 268:1720-1726, 1992.

Underwood LE: Growth hormone therapy in children with Down syndrome (letter), *J Pediatr* 120:833, 1992.

US Department of Health and Human Services: Down syndrome prevalence at birth—United States, 1983–1990, *Morbidity and Mortality Weekly Report* 43:617-622, 1994.

Van Riper M, Ryff C, and Pridham K: Parental and family well-being in families of children with Down syndrome: a comparative study, *Res Nurs Health* 15:227-235, 1992.

Wald NJ et al: Frequency and severity of infections in day care, *J Pediatr* 112:540-546, 1988.

Wald NJ et al: Antenatal maternal serum screening for Down's syndrome: results of a demonstration project, *Br Med J* 305:391-393, 1992.

Wikler L, Wascow M, and Hatfield E: Chronic sorrow revisited: parent and professional depiction of adjustment of parents of mentally retarded children, *Am J Orthopsychiatry* 51:63-67, 1981.

Wysocki H, Wysocki J, and Wierusz-Wysocka B: The influence of thymus extract on the phagocytosis and the bactericidal capacity of polymorphonuclear neutrophils from children with Down's syndrome, *Ann NY Acad Sci* 496:740-742, 1987.

Epilepsy

Judith A. Farley

ETIOLOGY

Epilepsy is a chronic condition defined by *repeated* occurrence of seizure activity. Seizures are the abnormal discharge of electric activity within the brain. When a sufficient number of neurons become overexcited, they discharge abnormally. This activity may or may not display clinical manifestations. If clinical manifestations do occur, the specific physical activity displayed will depend on the origin of the electric activity and its expanse within the brain. Epilepsy may be the result of either an underlying disorder of the central nervous system or a disorder that directly or indirectly affects the normal function of the central nervous system. Often, the true cause of epilepsy remains unknown (Dreifuss, 1994).

Certain types of epilepsy have a familial predisposition and/or a genetic component. Congenital structural anomalies of the central nervous system may also cause epilepsy. In the prenatal period, fetal infections, trauma, and maternal diseases have also been identified as precipitating factors of epilepsy (American Association of Neuroscience Nurses, [AANN], 1990; Pellock 1993b; Dreifuss, 1994).

During the first month of life, asphyxia, intracranial hemorrhage, trauma, electrolyte imbalances, and inborn metabolic errors are all thought to be potential causes of epilepsy (Pellock 1993b; Dreifuss, 1994; O'Donohoe, 1994). Primary infections of the central nervous system, including encephalitis and meningitis, or systemic infections resulting in persistent high fever, also have been implicated as causative factors. Infants born to drug addicted mothers may withdraw during the neonatal period resulting in frequent reoccurring seizure activity (AANN, 1990; Holmes, 1986; Pellock 1993a; Dreifuss, 1994; O'Donohoe, 1994).

The etiology of epilepsy in children over a year old is generally the same as in infants during the first month of life. In addition to the conditions already discussed, this population may present with acute neurologic disorders or chronic conditions that have continued from earlier in life. These conditions may include infections, trauma, intracranial neoplasms, and degenerative disorders, all of which are associated with epilepsy (AANN, 1990; O'Donohoe, 1994; Annegers, 1993).

INCIDENCE

The incidence of epilepsy varies greatly with age. The incidence is greatest in children 0 to 1 year of age, averaging approximately 1 per 1000 in the United States (Epilepsy Foundation of America, 1994). Infants are particularly susceptible to developing epilepsy during the first 12 months of life. This incidence decreases with age. Of all epilepsy cases, 50% initially occur before 25 years of age with 20% of the cases initially occurring within the first 5 years of life. Approximately 125,000 individuals in the United States are newly affected each year (Epilepsy Foundation of America, 1994; Penry, 1986; Holmes, 1986).

CLINICAL MANIFESTATIONS AT TIME OF DIAGNOSIS

Clinical manifestations at diagnosis depend on primary cause and the extent and involvement of abnormal electric discharges within neuronal tissue. (See accompanying box.) Because of the diversities and complexities displayed in seizure activity, the International Seizure Classification System was adopted in 1970 and later revised in 1981 (see Table 19-1). This classification system groups seizures that have similar clinical presentations. The general purposes of the classification system are to assist the health care provider with the assessment of the clinical course, to institute appropriate treatment, and to evaluate the individual's response to therapy (Gastaut, 1970; Bancaud et al, 1981).

Three major classifications within the international system of epilepsy are: (1) partial seizures, (2) generalized seizures, and (3) unclassified epileptic seizures. Each major grouping is divided into subsets based on clinical manifestations and electroencephalographic (EEG) findings.

Partial seizures are characterized by seizure activity that begins in and is usually limited to one part of either the left or right cerebral hemisphere. A *simple partial seizure* refers to seizure activity that occurs without loss of consciousness. A *complex partial seizure* refers to seizure activity that occurs with impairment or alteration in level of consciousness. The clinical activity is contingent on which part of the cortex generates the activity. For example, partial seizures may result in either abnormal activity such as focal muscle-twitching and loss of tone, or sensory changes such as tingling and numbness (Dreifuss, 1984; Holmes, 1986; Penry, 1986).

In general, a simple partial seizure is confined to one cerebral hemisphere, whereas a complex partial seizure involves both hemispheres. A partial seizure (either simple or complex) may evolve into a generalized tonic-clonic, tonic, or clonic convulsion (see Table 19-1) (Dreifuss, 1994; Holmes, 1986; Penry, 1986, Pellock, 1993a).

Generalized seizures are those in which the first clinical manifestations indicate that the seizure activity starts or involves both cerebral hemispheres. In this grouping of seizures, consciousness is impaired. The clinical manifestations may present as convulsive activity, although others such as absence seizures which are typically characterized by staring, have nonconvulsive activity. Because both hemispheres are involved, the clinical manifestations are almost always bilateral (see Table 19-1) (Dreifuss, 1994; Holmes, 1986; Penry, 1986; Pellock, 1993a; O'Donohoe, 1994).

Not all seizure disorders fit neatly into a classified grouping. These seizures are referred to as **unclassified epileptic seizures** and characteristically have a wide variety of abnormal clinical activity. Examples may include rhythmic eye movements, chewing, and swimming movements. These activities are commonly seen in neonatal seizures (Dreifuss, 1994; Holmes, 1986; Penry, 1986, Pellock, 1993a; O'Donohoe, 1994)

Status epilepticus is defined as the state of continuing or recurring seizure activity in which recovery between seizures is incomplete. The seizure activity is unrelenting and usually lasts for 30 minutes or more. Any classified seizure activity can evolve into status epilepticus. The state of status epilepticus is considered a medical emergency and requires immediate intervention (AANN, 1990; O'Donohoe, 1994; Pellock, 1993b).

In addition to the seizures classified by the international system, several types of **epileptic syndromes** also exist. These are seizure disorders that display a *group* of signs and symptoms that collectively characterize or indicate a particular

---

CLINICAL MANIFESTATIONS

- International Seizure Classification System
  - Partial seizures
    - Simple partial seizures
    - Complex partial seizures
  - Generalized seizures
  - Unclassified epileptic seizures
  - Status epilepticus

- Epileptic Syndromes
  - Infantile spasms
  - Lennox-Gestaut syndrome
  - Juvenile myoclonic epilepsy

Table 19-1.   INTERNATIONAL CLASSIFICATION SYSTEM

I. Partial (focal, local) seizures

Partial seizures are those in which, in general, the first clinical and electroencephalographic (EEG) changes indicate initial activation of a system of neurons limited to part of one cerebral hemisphere. A partial seizure is classified primarily on the basis of whether or not consciousness is impaired during the attack. When consciousness is not impaired, the seizure is classified as a simple partial seizure. When consciousness is impaired, the seizure is classified as a complex partial seizure. Impairment of consciousness may be the first clinical sign, or simple partial seizures may evolve into complex partial seizures. In patients with impaired consciousness, aberrations of behavior (automatisms) may occur. A partial seizure may not terminate but instead progress to a generalized motor seizure. Impaired consciousness is defined as the inability to respond normally to exogenous stimuli by virtue of altered awareness and/or responsiveness.

There is considerable evidence that simple partial seizures usually have unilateral hemispheric involvement and only rarely have bilateral hemispheric involvement; complex partial seizures, however, frequently have bilateral hemispheric involvement.

Partial seizures can be classified into one of the following three fundamental groups:

- Simple partial seizures
- Complex partial seizures:
    With impairment of consciousness at onset
    Simple partial onset followed by impairment of consciousness
- Partial seizures evolving to generalized tonic-clonic convulsions:
    Simple evolving to generalized tonic-clonic convulsions
    Complex evolving to generalized tonic-clonic convulsions (including those with simple partial onset)

Clinical seizure type	EEG seizure type

A. Simple partial seizures (consciousness not impaired)
  1. With motor signs
    (a) Focal motor without march
    (b) Focal motor with march (jacksonian)
    (c) Versive
    (d) Postural
    (e) Phonatory (vocalization or arrest of speech)
  2. With somatosensory or special-sensory symptoms (simple hallucinations, e.g., tingling, light flashes, buzzing)
    (a) Somatosensory
    (b) Visual
    (c) Auditory
    (d) Olfactory
    (e) Gustatory
    (f) Vertiginous
  3. With autonomic symptoms or signs (including epigastric sensation, pallor, sweating, flushing, piloerection and pupillary dilation)
  4. With psychic symptoms (disturbance of higher cerebral function); these symptoms rarely occur without impairment of consciousness and are much more commonly experienced as complex partial seizures
    (a) Dysphasic
    (b) Dysmnesic (e.g., dé-jà vu)
	Local contralateral discharge starting over the corresponding area of cortical representation (not always recorded on the scalp)

Continued.

Table 19-1.   INTERNATIONAL CLASSIFICATION SYSTEM—cont'd

Clinical seizure type	EEG seizure type
(c) Cognitive (e.g., dreamy states, distortions of time sense)	
(d) Affective (fear, anger, etc.)	
(e) Illusions (e.g., macropsia)	
(f) Structured hallucinations (e.g., music, scenes)	
B. Complex partial seizures (with impairment of consciousness; may sometimes begin with simple symptoms)	Unilateral or, frequently, bilateral discharge; diffuse or focal in temporal or frontotemporal regions
1. Simple partial onset followed by impairment of consciousness	
(a) With simple partial features, followed by impaired consciousness	
(b) With automatisms	
2. With impairment of consciousness at onset	
(a) With impairment of consciousness only	
(b) With automatisms	
C. Partial seizures evolving to secondarily generalized seizures (may be generalized tonic-clonic, tonic, or clonic)	Discharges listed earlier become secondarily and rapidly generalized
1. Simple partial seizures (A) evolving to generalized seizures	
2. Complex partial seizures (B) evolving to generalized seizures	
3. Simple partial seizures evolving to complex seizures evolving to generalized seizures	

II. Generalized seizures (convulsive or nonconvulsive)

Generalized seizures are those in which the first clinical changes indicate initial involvement of both hemispheres. Consciousness may be impaired, and this impairment may be the initial manifestation. Motor manifestations are bilateral. The ictal EEG patterns initially are bilateral and presumably reflect neuronal discharge that is widespread in both hemispheres.

Clinical seizure type	EEG seizure type
A. Absence seizures	
1. Typical absence seizures	Usually regular and symmetric 3-Hz, but may be 2 to 4-Hz, spike-and-slow-wave complexes; may have multiple spike-and-slow-wave complexes; abnormalities bilateral
(a) Impairment of consciousness only	
(b) With mild clonic components	
(c) With atonic components	
(d) With tonic components	
(e) With automatisms	
(f) With autonomic components (b-f may be used alone or in combination)	
2. Atypical absence seizures, which may have:	EEG more heterogeneous; may include irregular spike-and-slow-wave complexes, fast activity or other paroxysmal activity; abnormalities bilateral but often irregular and asymmetric
(a) Changes in tone that are more pronounced	
(b) Onset and/or cessation that is not abrupt	
B. Myoclonic seizures (single or multiple myoclonic jerks)	Polyspike and wave or sometimes spike and wave or sharp and slow waves

Continued.

Table 19-1.   INTERNATIONAL CLASSIFICATION SYSTEM—cont'd

Clinical seizure type	EEG seizure type
C. Clonic seizures	Fast activity (≥10 c/sec) and slow waves; occasional spike-and-wave patterns
D. Tonic seizures	Low voltage fast activity, a fast rhythm of 9 to 10 c/sec, or more decreasing in frequency and increasing in amplitude
E. Tonic-clonic seizures	Rhythm at ≥10 c/sec, decreasing in frequency and increasing in amplitude during tonic phase, interrupted by slow waves during clonic phase
F. Atonic seizures (astatic) (combinations of the above may occur, e.g., B and F, B and D)	Polyspikes and waves or flattening or low-voltage fast activity

III. Unclassified epileptic seizures

These include all seizures that cannot be classified because of inadequate or incomplete data and some that defy classification in hitherto described categories. They include some neonatal seizures (e.g., rhythmic eye movements, chewing, and swimming movements).

IV. Addendum

Repeated epileptic seizures occur under a variety of circumstances:
1. As fortuitous attacks, coming unexpectedly and without any apparent provocation.
2. As cyclic attacks, at more or less regular intervals (e.g., in relation to the menstrual cycle, or the sleep-waking cycle).
3. As attacks provoked by (a) nonsensory factors (fatigue, alcohol, emotion, etc.) or (b) sensory factors, sometimes referred to as "reflex seizures."

The term "status epilepticus" is used whenever a seizure persists for a sufficient length of time or is repeated frequently enough that recovery between attacks does not occur. Status epilepticus may be divided into partial (e.g., jacksonian), or generalized (e.g., absence status or tonic-clonic status). When very localized motor status occurs, it is referred to as "epilepsia partialis continua."

Adapted from *Epilepsia* 22:489-501, 1981.

condition. An additional classification system of these syndromes has been proposed by the International League Against Epilepsy. This classification system was revised in 1989 (see box page) (Dreifuss et al, 1985; International League Against Epilepsy, 1989). Several syndromes that are associated with epilepsy occur in infants and children. Three syndromes that occur most often are infantile spasms, Lennox-Gastaut syndrome, and juvenile myoclonic epilepsy.

Infantile spasms are a form of epilepsy characterized by a variety of clinical manifestations. The infant may present with episodes of sudden flexion or extension movements involving the neck, trunk, and extremities. The resulting spasms may range in presentation from subtle head nods to violent body contractions, commonly referred to as "jackknife seizures." Onset of infantile spasms is usually between 3 and 12 months of age. They may be idiopathic or occur in response to a central nervous system insult. An EEG will display a classic hypsarrythmia pattern of epileptic spike and wave discharges on a slow, disorganized background (Lombroso, 1983; Dreifuss, 1994). Infantile spasms manifest a typical clinical course. The spasms usually occur in clusters as frequent as 5 to 150 times a day and are usually worse when waking or falling asleep. Once the spasms begin, the seizure activity

INTERNATIONAL LEAGUE AGAINST EPILEPSY
CLASSIFICATION OF EPILEPSIES AND EPILEPTIC SYNDROMES

1.   Localization-related (focal, local, partial) epilepsies and syndromes
1.1 Idiopathic (with age-related onset)
At present the following syndromes are established, but more may be identified in the future:
Benign childhood epilepsy with centrotemporal spike
Childhood epilepsy with occipital paroxysms
Primary reading epilepsy
1.2 Symptomatic
Chronic progressive epilepsia partialis continua of childhood (Kojewnikow's syndrome)
Syndromes characterized by seizures with specific modes of precipitation
1.3 Cryptogenic
Presumed to be symptomatic; etiology unknown
2.   Generalized epilepsies and syndromes
2.1 Idiopathic (with age-related onset; listed in order of age)
Benign neonatal familial convulsions
Benign neonatal convulsions
Benign myoclonic epilepsy in infancy
Childhood absence epilepsy (pyknolepsy)
Juvenile absence epilepsy
Juvenile myoclonic epilepsy (impulsive petit mal)
Epilepsy with grand mal seizures on wakening
Other generalized idiopathic epilepsies not already defined
Epilepsies with seizures precipitated by specific modes of activation
2.2 Cryptogenic or symptomatic (in order of age)
West's syndrome (infantile spasms, Blitz-Nick-Salaam Krämpfe)
Lennox-Gastaut syndrome
Epilepsy with myoclonic-astatic seizures
Epilepsy with myoclonic absences
2.3 Symptomatic

2.3.1 Nonspecific etiology
Early myoclonic encephalopathy
Early infantile epileptic encephalopathy with suppression burst
Other symptomatic generalized epilepsies not already defined
2.3.2 Specific syndromes
Epileptic seizures may complicate many disease states; under this heading are diseases in which seizures are the presenting or predominant feature
3.   Epilepsies and syndromes undetermined whether focal or generalized
3.1 With both generalized and focal seizures
Neonatal seizures
Severe myoclonic epilepsy in infancy
Epilepsy with continuous spike-waves during slow-wave sleep
Acquired epileptic aphasia (Landau-Kleffner syndrome)
Other undetermined epilepsies not already defined
3.2 Without unequivocal generalized or focal features; all cases with generalized tonic-clonic seizures in which clinical EEG findings do not permit classification as clearly generalized or localization related (e.g., in many cases of sleep-grand mal) are considered not to have unequivocal generalized or focal features
4.   Special syndromes
4.1 Situations-related seizures (Gelegenheitsanfälle)
Febrile convulsions
Isolated seizures or isolated status epilepticus
Seizures occurring only when there is an acute metabolic or toxic event caused by such factors as alcohol, drugs, eclampsia, nonketotic, hyperglycemic

Adapted from Commission on Classification and Terminology of the International League Against Epilepsy: *Epilepsia* 30:389-399, 1989.

increases in intensity and severity over time. Invariably there is a loss of developmental milestones with infantile spasms (Lombroso, 1983; Pellock, 1993a; Dreifuss, 1994; O'Donohoe, 1994).

Lennox-Gastaut syndrome is characterized by an onset of seizures early in childhood, usually around 1 to 5 years of age. This epileptic syndrome presents with a variety of generalized seizures, in which predominantly tonic-clonic, atonic (drop attacks), akinetic, absence, and myoclonic activity are seen. Mental retardation and delayed psychomotor development are often associated with Lennox-Gastaut syndrome (Holmes, 1986; Dreifuss, 1994; Pellock, 1993a; O'Donohoe, 1994).

Juvenile myoclonic epilepsy is a primary generalized epilepsy that usually affects adolescents and young adults. This is a relatively benign form of epilepsy involving myoclonic jerks of neck, shoulders, and arms. The seizures may occur singularly or repetitively. Juvenile myoclonic epilepsy is usually associated with a normal neurologic exam, normal intelligence, and a positive family history of seizures (Dreifuss, 1989; Pellock, 1993a; Dreifuss, 1994; O'Donohoe, 1994).

TREATMENT

Specific treatment for epilepsy is directed at particular clinical manifestations or the syndrome of seizure activity and its underlying causes. Several other factors must be considered in addition to the clinical manifestations presented at time of diagnosis. The history and examination, which covers the child's physical and developmental activities, provides invalu-able information necessary to combine the multitude of pieces that contribute to the diagnosis. The child's birth history and record of milestone achievements must be explored, along with family history for seizures. Report of presenting signs and symptoms—associated factors such as fever or head trauma—are important considerations for the primary care provider. Evaluation and testing includes an EEG to isolate the focus or origin and involvement of seizure activity in the brain, and a computerized tomography (CT) scan and a magnetic resonance imaging (MRI) of the brain to investigate the presence of a lesion or abnormal tissue. Finally, a complete metabolic workup must be reviewed to explore the possibility of a deficiency or malabsorp-

---

TREATMENT

- Need for thorough assessment
  - Complete data base
  - Evaluation may include:
    - EEG
    - CT scan
    - MRI scan
    - PET scan
    - SPECT scan
    - Metabolic workup
- Therapies
  - Pharmacologic therapy (see table 19-2)
    - Focal resective surgery
    - Hemispherectomy
      - Considered for intractable hemispheric disease
    - Corpus collosotomy
  - Ketogenic diet

---

tion (Pellock, 1993a; Dreifuss, 1994; O'Donohoe, 1994; Holmes, 1986; Penry, 1986).

Treatment usually begins with anticonvulsant medications (see Table 19-2). Often the epileptic pattern and clinical course require more than one drug to control the abnormal discharges. The child's age, classification of seizures, medication side effects, and compliance must all be considered when deciding on a medication regimen (Holmes, 1986; Penry, 1986; Pellock, 1993a; Dreifuss, 1994; O'Donohoe, 1994).

Surgery is also a treatment for some forms of epilepsy. As with medical interventions, surgery for epilepsy is directed at the particular clinical manifestations of seizure activity, the EEG findings, and underlying causes. If a site of origin or a seizure focus is identified, it may be possible to remove this area of the brain, eliminating seizure activity with little or no neurologic impairment. Certain forms of partial seizure disorders can be treated successfully with focal resective surgery (Spencer, 1986; Santilli and Sierzant, 1987; Brewer and Sperling, 1988; Holmes, 1993).

The surgical removal or disconnection of a cerebral hemisphere is a treatment for children with unilateral hemispheric disease and medically intractable epilepsy. Total or partial hemispherec-

Table 19-2.   COMMONLY USED ANTIEPILEPTIC DRUGS*

Drug	Dosage/internal	Therapeutic plasma level	Seizure type	Common side effects	Adverse side effects
ACTH	Begin 40 units IM qd (taper gradually) Treatment course 2-4 mo		Infantile spasm	Hypertension Gastrointestinal distress Weight gain Electrolyte disturbance	Infection Gastrointestinal bleeding Sodium retention
Clonazapam (Clonopin)	0.1-0.2 mg/kg tid	0.01-0.08	Absence Generalized tonic-clonic Myoclonic Simple partial Complex partial	Drowsiness Ataxia Gastrointestinal distress	Behavioral changes Hyperactivity Cognitive dysfunction
Valproic acid (Depakote)	30-60 mg/kg qid	40-150	Absence Generalized tonic-clonic Myoclonic Simple partial Complex partial	Nausea-vomiting Fatigue with initiation Hair loss	Thrombocytopenia Pancreatitis Hepatic dysfunction Liver toxicity
Primidone (Mysoline)	10-25 mg/kg/day 3-4 times/day	5-12†	Tonic-clonic Complex partial Simple partial	Drowsiness Hyperactivity Ataxia Behavior changes	Oversedation Behavioral disturbances Gastrointestinal dysfunction
Phenytoin (Dilantin)	4-8 mg/kg bid	10-20	Generalized tonic-clonic Simple partial Complex partial	Gingival hyperplasia	Lethargy; ataxia; dizziness Skin reaction (rash) Hepatic dysfunction
Phenobarbitol	2-4 mg/kg qd; bid	15-40	Generalized tonic-clonic Myoclonic Simple partial Complex partial	Fatigue with initiation of treatment Hyperactivity Mood changes Irritability	Rash Lethargy Learning difficulties Behavioral changes Hepatic dysfunction
Carbamazepine (Tegretol)	10-30 mg/kg tid; qid	6-12	Generalized tonic-clonic Simple partial Complex partial	Drowsiness Ataxia; dizziness Gastrointestinal distress Irritability	Leukopenia Movement disorders Rashes Hepatic dysfunction Bone marrow suppression

Modified from *Physicians' Desk Reference*, ed 44, Oradell, NJ, 1994, Edward R Barnhart.

*ACTH, adrenocorticotropic hormone; IM, intramuscular; qd, every day; tid, 3 times daily; qid, 4 times daily; bid, twice daily.

†When testing mysoline levels, always check phenobarbital levels as well.

tomy may be performed to control localized epileptic conditions that are extremely complex and have a profound impact on the child's activities and life span (Bare, 1989; Spencer, 1986; Holmes, 1993).

Corpus collosotomy is another neurosurgical treatment used to help control generalized seizures (involving both hemispheres) that are medically intractable. Basically the corpus callosum is the connecting bridge between the right and left hemisphere. In this classification of epilepsy, the abnormal electric discharge begins in one hemisphere then crosses over the corpus callosum to the opposite hemisphere, thereby creating a generalized response. Corpus collosotomy partially or completely severs this connecting bridge. The main objective of this treatment is to stop or decrease generalization of seizure activity. A palliative procedure, it is done in effort to minimize physical injury that may occur during seizure activity and decrease the need for anticonvulsant medications (Spencer and Spencer, 1989).

The ketogenic diet is a form of treatment for certain types of medically intractable epilepsies. This diet consists of foods high in fat and low in carbohydrate and protein. The exact therapeutic mechanism is not completely known. It is thought, however, the ketone bodies produced by this diet may have an antiepileptic effect (Huttenlocher, 1976; Schwartz et al, 1989; Kinsmen et al, 1992). Both surgical and nutritional interventions almost always require concurrent medical treatment with antiepileptic drugs.

RECENT AND ANTICIPATED ADVANCES IN DIAGNOSIS AND MANAGEMENT

There have been significant advances in the diagnosis and subsequent management of pediatric epilepsy. In general, diagnosis and treatment is directed at the underlying cause. Recent advances in medical technology with EEG studies and neuroimaging have served to support this primary objective (Jackson, 1994). Surgical placement of electrodes directly on the cortex helps obtain diagnostic information to localize the seizure origin. The continued development and refinement of high-resolution magnetic resonance imagery (MRI), positron emission tomography (PET), and single photon emission computed tomography (SPECT) have led to the early identification of underlying pathologies that may have previously gone undetected. Major advances in genetics have allowed researchers to examine the genetic basis for several epilepsies (Kotagal and Luders, 1994; Dreifuss, 1994; Jackson, 1994).

Results from diagnostic studies and data all lead to enhancement of treatment options and opportunities for individuals with epilepsy. Genetic counseling, advances in surgical procedures and interventions, and development and introduction of new and challenging antiepileptic medications are all additional considerations for future developments and outcomes.

ASSOCIATED PROBLEMS

The etiology, age of onset, type of seizures, frequency of occurrence, and success of treatment all influence problems related to epilepsy.

Injury During Seizures

Injury during seizure activity is always possible. A child may sustain direct trauma, or fall or aspirate during a seizure. It is therefore vital for parents, primary care providers, and teachers to be knowledgeable about appropriate first aid to minimize injury during a seizure (see box on first aid for seizure management, pg 409).

Cognitive Dysfunction

Children with epilepsy may also present with various cognitive dysfunctions. In general, the intelligence quotients of children with epilepsy are

ASSOCIATED PROBLEMS

- Vary according to etiology
- Injury secondary to seizures
- Cognitive dysfunction
- Psychiatric problems

FIRST AID FOR SEIZURE MANAGEMENT

The following is a guide for first aid in the event of a generalized seizure. Parents, teachers, and caretakers must know these steps to follow in the event of such an occurrence:

- It is important to lower the child to the floor, or leave the child where he or she is when the seizure begins
- Be careful to move any objects in the area away from the child to prevent injury. Cushion the child's head from the floor with a pillow or soft barrier.
- Turn and keep the child on his or her side to prevent aspiration. It is very important NOT to attempt to put anything in the child's mouth. This can actually cause injury or further damage, such as a broken tooth or a bite to the individual providing aid.
- Loosen tight, restrictive clothing on the child that may be too confining and cause further injury such as a buttoned shirt collar or tie. Clear the location of objects that may cause further injury to flailing extremities.
- Stay with the child and do not restrain the movements
- Try to remain calm
- When the seizure clears, the child may be sleepy or confused. Allow for adequate rest after the seizure finishes.
- If there are breathing difficulties or the seizure does not stop for an extended period of time, the local Emergency Medical Services (EMS) should be called for further assistance
- Never hesitate to call EMS for help if concern is present

slightly lower than average (Holmes, 1986; Wossum, 1994). Children with seizures that emanate from the temporal lobe region may have difficulty with language and memory functions (Wossum, 1994). Children with partial seizures manifested as staring spells may have an impaired attention span.

Specific antiepileptic drugs may further alter or impair selected facets of cognition, including memory and attention span (Holmes, 1986; Dreifuss, 1984; O'Donohoe, 1994; Trimble, 1993).

Psychiatric Problems

A greater incidence of psychiatric problems, emotional disturbances, psychosocial and behavioral problems exist in children with epilepsy than in children with other chronic conditions or in the general population (Hermann and Austin, 1993; Kim, 1991).

PROGNOSIS

Prognosis for epilepsy depends primarily on the type and severity of the disorder, the age of onset, coexisting disorders, and the type and success of medical, surgical, and nutritional therapy. Clearly, if a child's brain is active with abnormal electric activity, the opportunity for normal growth, development, and learning is limited. The convulsive disorders do not in themselves cause irreversible brain damage, rather they detract from the potential of normal brain and intellectual development.

As with the classification of epilepsy and clinical manifestations and treatment, the prognosis of epilepsy is dependent on many factors (Dreifuss, 1994). Some seizure disorders cease or improve with age, some persist at the same level, and some seizures worsen. The type of seizure and the age of onset help to determine treatment responsiveness and, therefore, the impact on the child's general prognosis. Prognosis depends primarily on etiology (Dreifuss, 1994).

Impaired neurologic functioning and altered growth and development occur more frequently in the forms of epilepsies that are more difficult to treat. The functional outcomes in these seizure disorders are more difficult to predict and in general have a poorer prognosis (Dreifuss, 1994; Holmes, 1986; Penry, 1986).

Primary Care Management
HEALTH CARE MAINTENANCE

Growth and Development

A primary care provider must monitor body growth and total development in all children. Obtaining body heights and weights regularly on children with epilepsy is particularly important, especially if there has been significant losses, gains, or dramatic growth spurts such as occurs with adolescents. This information must be kept current because anti-epileptic drug dosages are calculated and usually prescribed for the child according to his or her body weight and maintenance of therapeutic levels.

Primary care management and interventions related to the child's social, cognitive, and motor development depend greatly on the severity of the seizure disorder and the underlying neurologic complications. Screening and assessment tools such as the Denver Developmental Screening Tool and Wechsler Intelligence Scale for Children, accompanied by regular neuropsychologic evaluations, help to identify the particular strengths and weaknesses (or potential for weaknesses) as the child matures.

If developmental delays are detected, these infants, children, and families may benefit from early intervention programs or infant stimulation programs. These programs are usually community based and provide therapy for the child and education for the parents, focusing on developmental needs and appropriate child-centered interventions.

Diet

Infants with epilepsy may have difficulty with feeding because of the frequency of their seizure activity or increased lethargy from anticonvulsant therapy or the post-ictal state. In addition, seizure activity may produce a temporary state of increased metabolism. This increase, in combination with poor intake, may result in an inadequate nutritional balance for growth and development. Assessment of growth curves over time in combination with the parents' reports of intake help to determine if interventions such as increased calories per feeding and supplemental feedings are necessary. Temporary assistance and supplementation can be supported with use of a nasogastric tube. Children with persistent weight loss, poor oral feeding abilities, and failure to thrive may require a gastric tube for caloric, fluid, and medication intake.

Conversely, excessive weight gain may occur in infants and children with epilepsy. Neurologic impairments that accompany epilepsy may result in poor motor function leading to decreased physical activity, which requires less caloric intake for nor-

mal body growth. Again, assessment of growth curves over time in addition to the parents' reports of intake help to determine if interventions such as decreased calories per feeding are necessary.

Weight gain is a significant issue in infants with infantile spasms. Infants with this epileptic syndrome commonly present with *extreme* irritability. This irritability is frequently quieted with feeding, and therefore in an effort to soothe their distressed baby, parents may overfeed their infant. In addition, the treatment of choice for this seizure disorder is administration of adrenocorticotropic hormone (ACTH). A major side effect of this drug is weight gain. The child's weight and growth must be monitored closely while on this medication. It will usually return to normal after the ACTH treatment is discontinued.

The ketogenic diet is an accepted form of therapy to control intractable seizures in children with certain forms of epilepsy with the objective of producing ketosis. An extremely difficult diet for a child to maintain, the ketogenic diet is often associated with weight loss and hypoglycemia. Careful monitoring of these children's nutritional status is necessary.

Safety

Being aware of the many issues regarding safety that are particular to the infant and child with epilepsy is important. Parents must be educated on any changes that occur and that threaten their child's safety, including instruction on how to intervene safely and appropriately during frequent or prolonged seizure activity. In the event of such an occurrence, parents, teachers, and caretakers must know the following steps: (1) maintain an adequate airway, (2) lower the child to the ground, (3) turn and keep the child on his or her side to prevent aspiration, (4) protect the child from injury to the head and limbs by loosening tight, restrictive clothing and clearing away objects, and (5) remain with the child and call for help. (Emergency Medical Services (EMS) should be called in situations of prolonged seizure activity, such as when dramatically different seizures occur other than baseline or when there is respiratory distress; however, never hesitate to call if concern is present.) The primary care provider should emphasize to the parents that *never* should anything be placed in the child's mouth. In addition, a child's tonic-clonic movements should not be restrained during the seizure activity, unless the child is in danger of greater injury. Parents and child care providers of children with life-threatening seizures should also be certified to perform cardiopulmonary resuscitation (CPR) in the event of a respiratory and cardiac arrest. After a seizure episode, the child may experience a post-ictal period of confusion, disorientation, or sleepiness. The child should be allowed to rest during this time of recovery following a seizure.

Certain seizure types, including complex partial seizures, atonic seizures, and Lennox-Gastaut syndrome, often result in a sudden loss of consciousness and a change in body muscle tone. These seizure types may exhibit loss of muscle tone (atonia) or extreme tension of muscle groups (tonic). These changes may occur independently, or just before a generalized body convulsion. Because the onset of this seizure activity is unpredictable, the actual clinical manifestation is a sudden body drop to the floor resulting in a great potential for injury, especially to the head. If the child has ever had these symptoms, the primary care provider should advise the parents to have their child wear a helmet in effort to protect the child's head in the event of such seizure activity. A hockey or bicycle helmet provides adequate protection to the areas (forehead, back of head) most commonly hit during these drop attacks. These helmets are lightweight, come in various colors and sizes, and are available wherever sports equipment is sold. The child's individuality and cooperation may be fostered by placing creative designs, stickers, and labels on the helmet.

For similar reasons, consideration must be given to the child's participation in certain activities that may increase the risk of injury should a seizure occur. Participation in activities such as swimming and gymnastics is commonly questioned by parents and school teachers. Restricting the child from taking part in these exercises, however, is not necessary provided there is adequate supervision by a responsible adult who is able to intervene appropriately should an emergency arise.

A tremendous amount of safety issues exist for the adolescent with epilepsy related to the use of various machinery (i.e., lawn mowers, equipment in machine shop classes). If adequate adult supervision is possible, participation in such activities supports the child's normal growth and development and peer relationships. Each state has laws pertaining to an individual with epilepsy securing a license to operate a motor vehicle.

Compliance with antiepileptic drugs presents another safety issue for the adolescent. Adolescence is a time of tremendous peer pressure and personal challenges. Alcohol use and experimentation with other drugs are common occurrences in today's society. Intake of these substances often lowers the anticonvulsant's therapeutic effects and therefore lowers the seizure threshold. Education on the individual's personal responsibility for health maintenance may minimize these complications.

As discussed in the previous section, a potential for limited cognitive ability and altered judgment exists in children with epilepsy. This is an important concept to discuss with parents when they are considering independence issues.

Immunizations

Much has been written regarding the controversial opinions and data surrounding immunizations, such as with the immunization schedule and the potential interaction in children with neurologic disorders. Infants and children with underlying seizure disorders or a family history of seizures are at increased risk of having a seizure after receiving either the DTP (diphtheria, tetanus, and pertussis) or the measles vaccine (American Academy of Pediatrics [AAP], 1994). These seizures are usually brief, generalized, and associated with a fever. Such characteristics typically classify this seizure type as a febrile convulsion (AAP, 1994). No evidence suggests that these seizures (1) cause permanent brain damage or epilepsy, (2) increase or advance underlying neurologic disorders, or (3) affect the prognosis of children with underlying disorders (AAP, 1994).

The present recommendations from the AAP regarding the DTP immunization in infants and children with neurologic disorders are as follows: (1) administration of the pertussis vaccine may be, and in many cases should be, deferred in children with a progressive neurologic disorder (i.e., infantile spasm, uncontrolled epilepsy); (2) infants and children with a history of seizures should have the pertussis vaccine deferred until the progress of the neurologic condition is determined. Children with well-controlled seizures and who are neurologically stable should receive the pertussis vaccine, (3) children who are suspected or predisposed to developing a progressive neurologic condition with seizures should have the pertussis vaccine deferred until the diagnosis can be determined; and (4) a family history of seizures is not a contraindication for the child to receive the pertussis vaccine (AAP, 1994).

If deferment of the pertussis vaccine is necessary, the AAP recommends the DTP vaccine be held completely until the child is 1 year of age. At this time a decision to administer either the complete DTP or just the DT vaccine can be made based on the above criteria. Receipt of the DTP immunization frequently results in fever; therefore, the AAP also recommends that children who are predisposed to seizures *and receive the DTP vaccine* be given acetaminophen 15mg/kg/dose) every 4 to 6 hours after the vaccine for as long as 24 hours after vaccination to prevent a fever that may lower the child's seizure threshold (AAP, 1994). As with all difficult health care questions, the primary care provider must view each infant and child in question individually and involve the family in the decision-making process.

Receipt of the measles vaccine frequently results in fever approximately 1 week after the vaccine is given. The AAP recommends the measles vaccine be administered to children who are predisposed to *develop* seizures or who have a positive history of seizures. Therefore, the same prophylactic therapy of acetaminophen (15mg/kg/dose) for 24 hours after receipt of the vaccine is advised (AAP, 1994).

All other immunizations should be given according to routine schedule.

Screening

Vision. Routine vision screening is recommended.

Hearing. Routine screening is recommended.

Dental care. Routine dental care is recommended. In severe seizure disorders, routine dental care may be difficult with resulting dental caries or gum disease. Gingival hyperplasia is a common occurrence in children on phenytoin (Dilantin) (Physicians' Desk Reference, 1994), therefore children on phenytoin require more frequent brushing and flossing with particular attention given to gums. The dentist should be informed if the individual is taking phenytoin and more frequent dental cleaning should be scheduled.

Blood pressure. Infants treated with ACTH therapy require daily blood pressure monitoring for potential hypertension. Parents should be taught how to take and monitor the infant's blood pressure while the infant is on ACTH therapy. If the parents are unable to do this, the visiting nurse or health care provider should check the blood pressure at least twice a week during therapy.

Hematocrit. Routine screening is recommended.

Urinalysis. Routine screening is recommended.

Tuberculosis. Routine screening is recommended.

Condition-specific screening

DRUG TOXICITY SCREENING. Decreased hematocrit with increased bruising or bleeding in a child taking valproic acid (Depakene), carbamozepine (Tegretol), and phenytoin (Dilantin) may indicate thrombocytopenia, blood dyscrasia, and liver dysfunction. Complete blood counts with platelets, SGOT, and SGPT should be obtained every 2 weeks when Depakene or Tegretol is initiated, and then monthly for at least the first 6 months of treatment (Physicians' Desk Reference, 1994).

COMMON ILLNESS MANAGEMENT

Differential Diagnosis

Seizurelike episodes. The primary care provider will evaluate children with epilepsy who present with common childhood illnesses that may or may not be related to this underlying disorder. The following presenting signs and symptoms must be evaluated in order to provide appropriate treatment for the illness or to change the treatment regimen for the diagnosed seizure disorder.

Gastroesophageal reflux is a condition that produces vomiting. In this condition, the reflux of the stomach contents may enter only the lower esophagus which produces pain and symptoms of

DIFFERENTIAL DIAGNOSIS

- Seizurelike episodes
  - Gastroesophageal reflex
  - Breath-holding spells
  - Migraine headaches
  - Cardiac dysfunction
  - Pseudoseizures
  - Unusual body movements
- Fever

choking, laryngospasm, apnea, arching, and occasionally loss of body tone (Pellock, 1993c). This event is dramatic and frightening for the parents to witness. Parents commonly report that the child has had a seizure or convulsion. Pathophysiologic cause and response may be more common when infants are laid supine after feeding. Diagnosis of gastro-esophageal reflux can be confirmed through a barium swallow and esophagram, an esophageal manometry, or a nuclear medicine test called a "scintiscan." Treatment may include thickening feedings, maintaining the child in an upright position for approximately 30 minutes after feeds, using agents to alter sphincter tone, and performing surgery for fundoplication (Pellock, 1993c).

Breath-holding spells are common occurrences in infants and young children that present much like seizure activity. Such events usually begin with and are provoked by the child crying; the crying worsens and the child may hold his or her breath and actually stop breathing. This breath holding leads to cyanosis, the child loses consciousness, and becomes limp. Once the child loses consciousness, normal breathing returns. If persistent apnea occurs, the child may actually have seizure activity (Holmes, 1986; Pellock, 1993c). The key to accurate diagnosis of breath-holding spells versus seizure activity depends greatly on meticulous history taking on the part of the primary care provider. Reliable reporting of a witnessed event by the parents is essential. These attacks are

always associated with crying, and the apnea and cyanosis occur *before* loss of consciousness (Holmes, 1986; Pellock, 1993c). EEG findings demonstrate no abnormal electric activity. Treatment of breath-holding spells may include use of behavior modification (Pellock, 1993c).

Migraine headaches are often difficult to differentiate from seizure activity. Migraine headaches are frequently associated with clinical manifestations similar to those seen with simple partial seizures such as visual changes, weaknesses, nausea, and flushing. A complete history of presenting signs and symptoms, family history, and EEG findings may help to confirm the differential diagnosis (Holmes, 1986; Wilson, 1992).

Treatment of migraine headaches may include use of antiepileptic drugs—60% of children with migraine headaches report relief with antiepileptic medications (Pellock, 1993c).

Cardiac dysfunction such as arrhythmias and syncopal episodes may be mistaken for seizure activity. The child may have a loss of consciousness, presenting much like drop attacks or an atonic seizure. Cardiac dysfunction is different from seizure activity because it usually presents with a gradual change in consciousness accompanied by dizziness, decreased or irregular pulse, pale clammy appearance, and mild neurologic impairment after the event (confusion, lethargy). An EEG performed during an event is usually normal. In addition, there may be a positive family history of cardiac anomalies and syncopal attacks (Holmes, 1986; O'Donohoe, 1994).

Pseudoseizures are behavioral manifestations that closely resemble seizures but do not correlate with epileptic activity on an EEG. Pseudoseizures may occur in children and adolescents with a diagnosed seizure disorder. These spells are sometimes quite convincing and are not necessarily intentional. A psychiatric referral in combination with medical therapy is appropriate to evaluate, differentiate, and treat this diagnosis separate from electrically discharged seizures (Taylor, 1989; Kim, 1991).

Unusual body movements in infants and children such as a hyperstartle response to stimuli, muscle tics, muscle spasticity, and altered gait pattern are conditions that may be confused with epileptic patterns. Diagnosis can usually be differentiated by careful testing, assessment, precise history taking, and accurate reporting of signs and symptoms experienced by the child and witnessed by the parents (Pellock, 1993c).

Differential diagnosis of common pediatric problems are sometimes very difficult and may require additional testing to rule out seizure activity. Referral to other specialists such as a pediatric neurologist, cardiologist, gastroenterologist, and psychologist may also be necessary for supportive consultation and diagnostic confirmation.

Fever. The presence of infection and fever in a child with epilepsy may alter the serum levels and therapeutic effects of antiepileptic drugs. Moreover, the fever may lower a child's seizure threshold. Parents should be advised by the primary care provider of methods of fever management including increasing fluid intake, controlling environmental factors, and using antipyretics appropriately. Parents should be advised not to increase antiepileptic drugs without consulting the primary care provider.

Drug Interactions

Many antiepileptic drugs are available for use today. Control of seizure activity is often enhanced with the use of more than one antiepileptic drug. The primary care provider must know the particular regimen and combination of drug therapy, serum levels, and common side effects (Table 19-

---

DRUG INTERACTIONS

- Combination drug therapy for epilepsy
- Altered seizure threshold may occur with:
  - Antihistamines
  - Antidepressants
- Aspirin
  - Decreases Dilantin's effectiveness
  - Increases plasma levels of valproic acid
- Anticonvulsants may lessen therapeutic effect of oral contraceptives
- Erythromycin increases plasma level of Tegretol

---

2). Several of these antiepileptic drugs have altered therapeutic effects when combined with common drugs used in pediatric care. Caution should be used in recommending or prescribing antihistamines, antidepressants, aspirin, oral contraceptives, and erythromycin.

Drugs such as antidepressants and antihistamines may alter the threshold of seizure activity and may interact with the therapeutic effects of antiepileptic medications. Because of the wide variety of antihistamines and antidepressants available it is beyond the scope of this chapter to address each of the interactions specifically. The primary care provider should explore further the individual medication regimen and the potential complications that may arise from combining these drugs.

The use of aspirin may decrease therapeutic plasma levels of Dilantin by displacing the Dilantin from binding sites. This displacement causes an increase level of free Dilantin which may result in toxic effects despite a decreased plasma level. The use of aspirin may increase therapeutic plasma levels of valproic acid by displacing the Valproate from the protein-binding sites. This would potentiate the drug's toxic side effect (Physicians' Desk Reference, 1994; Kutt and Pippenger, 1993; Holmes, 1986).

The therapeutic effect of oral contraceptives may be altered when used in combination with antiepileptics. Failure rates have been reported to be higher in women taking certain antiepileptic drugs. As a result, a higher dose of oral contraceptive may be necessary in some women to achieve a full contraceptive effect (Kutt and Pippenger, 1993).

The use of the erythromycin results in an increased plasma level of Tegretol. Erythromycin decreases the metabolism or breakdown of Tegretol, potentiating toxic effects (Physicians' Desk Reference, 1994; Kutt and Pippenger, 1993).

DEVELOPMENTAL ISSUES

Sleep Patterns

Sleep patterns may be altered if seizure activity occurs at night. Infants and children with seizures are at increased risk for apnea or respiratory difficulties because the seizure activity may be unwitnessed. It is recommended that these children wear a cardiac-apnea monitor during sleep. If the child does not have a history of respiratory difficulties during sleep, a room intercom monitor may be used to alert the parents to seizure activity. Early recognition of seizure activity helps to limit complications. Pillows should also be used with caution. A firm pillow and mattress are advised.

Seizure activity during the day may result in prolonged post-ictal states interfering with the child's sleep pattern at night. Parents should be instructed not to allow their child to sleep for extended periods during the daytime hours. The post-ictal state often cannot be interrupted however, and even the greatest effort to keep a child awake may not be successful.

Toileting

There are usually no particular concerns related to toileting the child with epilepsy. Toilet training should be appropriate for the child's developmental level.

Discipline

Children with epilepsy have an increased risk of psychosocial adjustment problems (Kim, 1991). In fact, these children have a greater incidence of psychiatric problems, emotional disturbances, and psychosocial and behavioral problems than children with other chronic conditions or children in the general population (Kim, 1991). This invariably influences the parents' and family members' response to discipline. Parents may be hesitant to set limits for their child for fear that this would upset the child and cause a seizure. Parental guidance on discipline should be provided early in the child's life and should always reflect the child's cognitive ability. Need for discipline, direction, and encouragement toward the child's independence should be ongoing. Referral for parent counseling may be necessary to assist with the particular needs and challenges that may arise (Austin and McDermott, 1988; Kim, 1991).

Child Care

Finding appropriate day care often presents a challenge for parents. This challenge is even greater for parents of children with a chronic condition such as epilepsy. The primary care provider can assist the family in this endeavor by helping to identify local agencies familiar with the care involved with a child with epilepsy, or by providing the education needed about epilepsy to the child care agencies willing to support these children's special needs.

Specific needs of the child in day care are dependent on the individual seizure disorder. The child care providers must be educated in the same manner as the parents regarding emergency aid and interventions during seizures (see box on p. 409). They must have an understanding of the clinical manifestations and what type of seizure activity to expect and monitor.

Frequently medications must be administered to a child while he or she is at day care. It is therefore necessary for the day care providers to have information regarding (1) the rationale for the anticonvulsant, (2) potential side effects, and (3) proper administration of the prescribed drugs. All medications should be stored in a safe, locked location to prevent accidental ingestion.

Schooling

Children with epilepsy may have social, intellectual, and cognitive difficulties. These difficulties need to be assessed and identified so that interventions for the child's particular learning needs can be individualized and addressed. Staff from early intervention or infant stimulation programs should be consulted if the seizure disorder begins during infancy or early childhood. These children are at risk for developmental delay. Early assessment allows for appropriate interventions to begin, which maximizes learning potentials.

If needed, this pre-school plan can be carried into the formal educational program as a child ages. Core evaluations by the individual school systems are necessary and appropriate for children at risk (see Schooling in Chapter 5).

Establishing a supportive, well-informed environment for the child is important. School staff should be informed of the child's medical diagnosis, even if the child progresses well and does not require special educational classes. This information allows the teachers to be helpful in assessing behavioral side effects of anticonvulsant therapy. A teacher who is informed of the potential for seizure occurrence and who has been instructed by the parents and the primary care provider on proper interventions is more apt to be calm and intervene appropriately if needed (Bannon, Wildig, and Jones, 1992).

A tremendous social stigma accompanies the diagnosis of epilepsy. The primary care provider must recognize the stress this diagnosis places on the child and its impact on the child's self-concept, his or her relationships with peers, and the educational system. The unpredictability and lack of control of seizure activity are part of this stress. Misconceptions, fears, apprehensions, and judgments of the peer group commonly have a negative effect on the child's self-esteem (O'Donohoe, 1994; Kim, 1991). The primary care provider should explore opportunities to educate the community and increase knowledge and understanding concerning this condition. Greater understanding of epilepsy may yield compassion and acceptance rather than ridicule and fear of children with epilepsy (Bannon, Wildig, and Jones, 1992).

The primary care provider should inquire about school performance and peer interactions at each well-child visit. It may be appropriate to refer the child for additional counseling and professional support to help manage with these ongoing stresses (Kim, 1991).

Sexuality

In the female adolescent with epilepsy, the seizure threshold may fall with cyclic changes induced by the menstrual cycle. This decline is presumably related to water retention, electrolyte imbalances, and decreased levels of progesterone. Cyclic adjustments of the antiepileptic medications should be considered (Cramer and Mattson, 1993). Regulation of the menstrual cycle may also help in the control of seizure activity (Uthman and Wilder, 1993).

As with all women, oral contraceptives should be considered on an individual basis. The therapeutic effect of oral contraceptives may be altered when used in combination with antiepileptics. Therefore, a higher dose of oral contraceptive may be necessary in some women to achieve a full contraceptive effect (Kutt and Pippenger, 1993). Caution should be taken if the woman with epilepsy becomes pregnant because certain antiepileptic drugs are potentially teratogenic. Antiepileptic drugs such as valproic acid, carbamazeopine, primidone, and phenobarbital have been associated with birth defects and fetal loss. The use of particular antiepileptic drugs, especially in combinations,

may need to be altered during pregnancy (Yerby, 1993; Tanganelli and Regesta, 1992).

Transition into Adulthood

The etiology and neurologic status of the individual with epilepsy is a significant issue when considering the concept of transition into adulthood. Young adults who have epilepsy that develops as a result of inborn metabolic disease such as congenital malformations, brain trauma, or brain tumors are less likely to achieve complete seizure control than those with idiopathic epilepsy (Gross-Tsur and Shinnar, 1993). As such, the diagnosis of epilepsy and associated complications follow them into adulthood and through the life span. Primary care and clinical management of specific issues should be directed by internists in consultation with epileptologists. Consultation and advisement on educational training programs and careers must take into account both the individual's cognitive and physical abilities and the safety concerns regarding environments with significant hazards (in case of a seizure) such as construction work or fire fighting.

SPECIAL FAMILY CONCERNS AND RESOURCES

Families of children with epilepsy all experience some sense of grief as parents mourn for the "loss of the normal" child they once had (Ferrari, 1989). Societal stigma and misconceptions concerning epilepsy are particularly stressful to the family. The diagnosis has implications through all aspects of growth and development such as child care, health care, recreation, education, transportation, employment, and insurance coverage (life and health).

Epilepsy presents a chronic and intense stress on the family system. This, in addition to the unpredictability of seizure occurrence, often results in overprotective parents and dependent children (Austin and McDermott, 1988; Ferrari, 1989).

Community Resources

The health care system must be empathic to the multitude of needs of these children and their families. Health care workers provide the physical, emotional, and social care that individuals with epilepsy very much need. Nevertheless, no person understands or feels the problems these children and families face during their day-to-day lives as well as another child or family with the same disorder. For this reason, parent support groups and peer support groups are available to provide this network of support within the community. These resources are not only necessary, but have proven to be a major factor in coping and adaptation for these families (Wallander and Varni, 1989).

Epilepsy Foundation of America
National Epilepsy Library and Resource Center
4351 Garden City Dr
Landover, MD 20785-2267
(301) 459-3700
(800) EFA-4050

National Easter Seal Society
2030 W Monroe St Suite 1800
Chicago, IL 60606-4802
(312)726-6200

SUMMARY OF SPECIAL PRIMARY NEEDS FOR CHILDREN WITH EPILEPSY

Health care maintenance

Growth and development

Obtain heights and weights at each visit. Medications must be based on current accurate measurements.
Provide regular screening and assessment of cognitive and motor skills.
Provide regular neuropsychologic screening.
If developmental delays present, recommend early intervention with infant stimulation program.

Diet: Diets may be tailored to meet child's caloric needs.

Ketogenic diet is difficult to maintain.

Safety: Provide instructions regarding emergency interventions for seizure activity.

Use helmet for certain seizure types.
Use caution with certain sports and activities.
Use caution with use of machinery, including motor vehicles.

Immunizations

Increased risk for children with underlying seizure disorders of having a seizure after DTP or measles vaccine. May defer pertussis and use DT. Measles vaccine continues to be recommended.

Screening

Vision: Routine screening is recommended.
Hearing: Routine screening is recommended.

Dental: Routine screening is recommended. Dilantin (phenytoin) may cause gingival hyperplasia. Children on Dilantin require more frequent cleaning by the dental hygienist.
Blood pressure: Routine screening is recommended. Infants on ACTH therapy may require daily monitoring of blood pressure.
Hematocrit: Routine screening is recommended.
Urinalysis: Routine screening is recommended.
Tuberculosis: Routine screening is recommended.

Condition-specific screening

Drug toxicity screening: Necessary first 6 months of therapy for Depakene, Tegretol, and Dilantin.

Common illness management

Differential diagnosis

Need to rule out seizurelike symptoms.
Gastrointestinal symptoms: Rule out gastroesophageal reflux.
Respiratory symptoms: Rule out breath-holding spells and apnea.
Severe headaches and migraines may occur.
Cardiac symptoms: arrhythmias, syncopal episodes may occur.
Pseudoseizures may occur.
Movement disorders, hyperstartle, muscle tics, muscle spasticity, altered gait patterns may occur.

Continued.

SUMMARY OF SPECIAL PRIMARY NEEDS FOR CHILDREN WITH EPILEPSY—cont'd

Management of illness with fever: increased risk of seizures. Close observation needed and antipyretic therapy.

Drug interactions

Several antiepileptic drugs have altered therapeutic effects when combined with antihistamines, aspirin, antidepressants, oral contraceptives, and certain antibiotics. Careful monitoring is required.

Developmental issues

Sleep patterns

May require use of cardiac-apnea monitor.
May be altered with prolonged or frequent seizure activity.

Toileting

Reflective of child's cognitive and developmental ability.

Discipline

Developmentally appropriate.

Child care

Instructions to agency regarding emergency interventions for seizure activity. Instructions on medication given at day care.

Schooling

Learning needs must be individualized and addressed.
Teachers should be informed of seizure history and instructions regarding emergency interventions for seizure activity should be given.
Social stigma of epilepsy may adversely affect child's self-concept.

Sexuality

Cyclic changes induced by menstrual cycle may alter antiepileptic effects. Some antiepileptic drugs are teratogenic. Counseling may be necessary.

Transition into adulthood

Issues are dependent on complexity of disorder.
Career counseling, recognizing potential safety concerns with seizures are of particular importance.

Special family concerns

Chronic sorrow and stress are present.
Social stigma is present.
Unpredictability of seizure activity is a major concern.

REFERENCES

American Academy of Pediatrics: *Report on the Committee on Infectious Diseases,* ed 23, Illinois, 1994, American Academy of Pediatrics.

American Association of Neuroscience Nurses: *Core curriculum for neuroscience nursing,* ed 3, Park Ridge, 1990, AANN.

Annegers JF: Epidemiology of childhood onset seizures. In WE Dodson and JM Pellock, (editors): *Pediatric epilepsy. Diagnosis and treatment,* New York, 1993, Demos, pp 57-63.

Austin JK, McDermott N: Parental attitude and coping behaviors in families of children with epilepsy, *J Neurosci Nurs* 20:174-179, 1988.

Bancaud J et al: Proposal for revising clinical electroencephalographic classification of epileptic seizures, *Epilepsia* 22:489-501, 1981.

Bannon MJ, Wildig C, and Jones PW: Teachers' perception of epilepsy, *Arch Dis Child* 67:1467-1471, 1992.

Bare MA: Hemispherectomy for seizures, *J Neurosci Nurs* 21:18-23, 1989.

Brewer K, Sperling MR: Neurosurgical treatment of intractable epilepsy, *J Neurosci Nurs* 20:366-372, 1988.

Cramer JA, Mattson RH: Hormones and epilepsy. In E Wyllie, (editor): *The treatment of epilepsy. Principles and practice,* Philadelphia, 1993, Lea & Febiger, pp 686-692.

Dreifuss FE: *Pediatric epileptology,* Boston, 1984, Wright.

Dreifuss FE: Prognosis of childhood seizure disorders: present and future, *Epilepsia* 35(suppl 2):S30-S34, 1994.

Dreifuss FE et al: Proposal for classification of epilepsies and epileptic syndromes, *Epilepsia* 26:268-278, 1985.

Dreifuss FR: Juvenile myoclonic epilepsy: characteristics of a primary generalized epilepsy, *Epilepsia* 30:S1-S7, 1989.

Epilepsy Foundation of America: *Basic statistics on the epilepsies,* Philadelphia, 1994, Davis.

Ferrari M: Epilepsy and its effects on the family. In BP Hermann and M Seidenberg, (editors): *Childhood epilepsies: neuropsychological, psychosocial and intervention aspects,* New York, 1989 Wiley, pp 159-173.

Gastaut H: Clinical and electroencephalographic classification of epileptic seizures, *Epilepsia* 11:102, 1970.

Gross-Tsur V, Shinnar S: Discontinuing antiepileptic drug treatment. In E Wyllie, (editor): *The treatment of epilepsy. Principles and practice,* Philadelphia, 1993, Lea & Febiger, pp 858-867.

Hermann BP, Austin J: Psychosocial status of children with epilepsy and the effects of epilepsy surgery. In E Wyllie, (editor): *The treatment of epilepsy. Principles and practice,* Philadelphia, 1993, Lea & Febiger, pp 1149-1163.

Holmes GL: *Diagnosis and management of seizures in children,* Philadelphia, 1986, Saunders.

Holmes GL: Surgery for intractable seizures in infancy and early childhood, *Neurology* 43(suppl 5):S28-S37, 1993.

Huttenlocher PR: Ketonemia and seizures: metabolic and anticonvulsant effects of two ketogenic diets in childhood epilepsy, *Pediatr Res* 10:536-540, 1976.

International League Against Epilepsy: Proposal for revised classification of epilepsies and epileptic syndromes, *Epilepsia* 30:389-399, 1989.

Jackson GD: New techniques in magnetic resonance and epilepsy, *Epilepsia* 35(suppl 6):S2-S13, 1994.

Kim WJ: Psychiatric aspects of epileptic children and adolescents, *J Am Acad Child Adolesc Psychiatr* 30(6):874-886, 1991.

Kinsman SL et al: Efficacy of the ketogenic diet for intractable seizure disorders: review of 58 cases, *Epilepsia* 33(6):1132-1136, 1992.

Kotagal P, Luders HO: Recent advances in childhood epilepsy, *Brain and Development* 16:1-15, 1994.

Kutt H, Pippenger C: Drug interactions. In WE Dodson and JM Pellock (editors): *Pediatric epilepsy. Diagnosis and treatment,* New York, 1993, Demos, pp 357-367.

Lombroso CT: A prospective study of infantile spasms: clinical and therapeutic correlations, *Epilepsia* 24:135, 1983.

O'Donohoe NV: *Epilepsies of childhood,* ed 3, Oxford, 1994, Butterworth-Heinemann, LTD.

Pellock JM: Seizures and epilepsy in infancy and childhood, *Neurol Clin* 11(4):755-775, 1993a.

Pellock JM: Status epilepticus. In WE Dodson and JM Pellock, (editors): *Pediatric epilepsy. Diagnosis and treatment,* New York, 1993b, Demos, pp 197-207.

Pellock JM: The differential diagnosis of epilepsy: nonepileptic paroxysmal disorders. In E Wyllie, (editor): *The treatment of epilepsy. Principles and practice,* Philadelphia, 1993c, Lea & Febiger, pp 697-709.

Penry JK: *Epilepsy. Diagnosis, management, quality of life,* ed 2, New York, 1986, Raven Press.

Physician's Desk Reference, ed 44, Oradell, New Jersey, 1994, Barnhart.

Santilli N, Sierzant TL: Advances in the treatment of epilepsy, *J Neurosci Nurs* 19:141-157, 1987.

Schwartz RH et al: Ketogenic diets in the treatment of epilepsy: short-term clinical effects, *Dev Med Child Neurol* 31:145-151, 1989.

Spencer DD, Spencer SS: Corpus callosotomy in the treatment of medically intractable secondarily generalized seizures of children, *Cleveland Clin J Med* 56:69-78, 1989.

Spencer SS: Surgical options for uncontrolled epilepsy. *Neurol Clin* 4:669-695, 1986.

Tanganelli P, Regesta G: Epilepsy, pregnancy, and major birth anomalies: an Italian prospective, controlled study, *Neurology* 42(suppl 5):89-93, 1992.

Taylor DC: Psychosocial components of childhood epilepsy. In BP Hermann and M Seidenberg, (editors): *Childhood epilepsies: neuropsychological, psychosocial and intervention aspects,* New York, 1989, Wiley, pp 119-143.

Trimble MR: Behavioral and cognitive issues in childhood epilepsy. In WE Dodson and JM Pellock (editors): *Pediatric epilepsy. Diagnosis and treatment,* New York, 1993, Demos, pp 387-409.

Uthman BM, Wilder BJ: Less commonly used antiepileptic drugs. In E Wyllie, (editor): *The treatment of epilepsy. Principles and practice,* Philadelphia, 1993, Lea & Febiger, pp 959-974.

Wallander JL, Varni JW: Social support and adjustment in chronically ill and handicapped children, *Am J Commun Psychol* 17:185-201, 1989.

Wilson J: Migraine and epilepsy, *Dev Med Child Neurol* 44:645-647, 1992.

Wossum DJ: Neuropsychologic issues in children with disabilities, *Compr Ther* 20(2):79-83, 1994.

Yerby MS: Treatment of epilepsy during pregnancy. In E Wyllie, (editor): *The treatment of epilepsy. Principles and practice,* Philadelphia, 1993, Lea & Febiger, pp 844-858.

Fragile X Syndrome

20

Randi J. Hagerman and Amy Cronister

ETIOLOGY

Fragile X syndrome is a relatively newly recognized condition that causes cognitive impairment ranging from mild learning disabilities to severe mental retardation. This condition derives its name from the presence of a fragile site or break in the X chromosome at Xq27.3 (see Fig. 20-1) which is identifiable by chromosome analysis. Because of the phenotypic variability among children with fragile X syndrome and because this condition was only recently discovered, the majority of individuals with fragile X syndrome remain undiagnosed.

Fragile X syndrome is caused by a mutation in the gene called the Fragile X Mental Retardation 1 gene (FMR1) which is located at Xq27.3. The FMR1 gene was discovered and sequenced in 1991 by an international collaborative effort (Verkerk et al, 1991; Oberle et al, 1991; Yu et al, 1991). The FMR1 gene has a unique trinucleotide expansion located within the gene. This expansion is the source of the mutation that causes the fragile X syndrome. All individuals have the FMR1 gene but when the trinucleotide repeat expansion $(CGG)_n$ increases in size dramatically, this expansion causes dysfunction and lack of protein production from the FMR1 gene. Normal individuals in the general population have between 6 and 50 CGG repeats within their FMR1 gene. Individuals who are carriers for the fragile X syndrome have an expansion of the CGG repetitive sequence that goes beyond 50 repeats up to 200. This change in the DNA is called a "premutation" and it causes an increase in the instability of this region so that further expansion can take place when this mutation is passed on to the next generation through a female carrier. Individuals who are significantly affected by fragile X syndrome have greater than 200 repeats, called "full mutation." This full mutation is usually associated with methylation, which is a process of silencing the gene so that no FMR1 protein is produced from a full mutation. The absence of protein production actually causes the physical, behavioral, and cognitive problems that comprise the fragile X syndrome.

INCIDENCE

Fragile X syndrome is the most common cause of inherited mental retardation known. Down syndrome, which rarely is inherited, has an incidence of approximately 1 per 700. In comparison, fragile X syndrome affects approximately 1 per 1250 males and 1 per 2500 females in the general population (Herbst and Miller, 1980; Webb, Thake, and Todd, 1986). Studies by Rousseau et al (1995) have shown that approximately 1 in 259 females in the general population is a carrier of the premutation. Screening of individuals with mental retardation in institutional and other residential settings has shown that 2% to 10% (Hagerman et al, 1988) of this high-risk population have fragile X syndrome as the cause of their mental impairment.

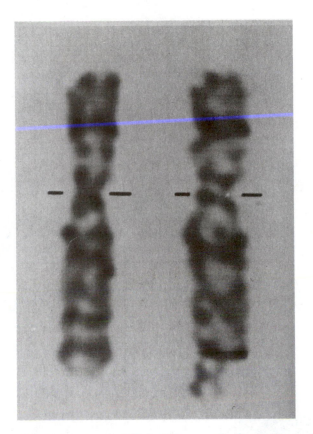

Fig. 20-1. A normal X chromosome and a fragile X chromosome demonstrating the fragile X site at Xq27.3.

Population studies of such diverse groups as the Aborigines in Australia, the Zulus of Africa, and individuals screened in Sweden, Finland, New South Wales, England, and France suggest that fragile X is equally common among all racial and ethnic groups (Sherman, 1991). As mentioned earlier, however, the majority of families affected by this syndrome are still undiagnosed and therefore remain unaware of available treatment and intervention.

CLINICAL MANIFESTATIONS AT TIME OF DIAGNOSIS

When most health care providers hear the word syndrome, they think of an individual who appears phenotypically abnormal. Similarly, most syndromes have consistent cognitive and physical fea-tures that succinctly describe the clinical manifestations. Although the majority of individuals with fragile X syndrome share certain clinical findings, there is much variability. The health care provider should note that children with this syndrome may not be immediately recognizable by their phenotype.

Males

The majority of males with fragile X syndrome have IQs in the mild to moderate range of mental retardation. A significantly smaller percentage are severely to profoundly retarded. Hagerman, Kemper, and Hudson (1985) have described learning disabled boys with fragile X who have IQs in the normal range. This may not be a rare occurrence but instead a continuum of the cognitive spectrum of involvement (Chudley, de von Flint, and Hagerman, 1987). The cognitive profile of males with fragile X includes difficulty with abstract reasoning, math, and attention.

Delayed onset of language is present in nearly all males with fragile X syndrome. In some children difficulties are evidenced by only language problems related to weaknesses in abstract reasoning. Other children as young as 18 months of age have delayed speech and significant deficits in receptive and expressive language. Perseveration and echolalia, or repetitive speech, are common speech characteristics of the individual with fragile X. A fast rate of speech, cluttering, mumbling, rambling, and poor topic maintenance are also frequent findings (Madison, George, and Moeschler, 1986; Newell, Sanborn, and Hagerman, 1983; Scharfenaker and Schreiner, 1989).

The three classic physical features associated with the fragile X syndrome phenotype are a long narrow face, prominent or large ears, and, in males,

enlarged testicles. Approximately 80% of all males with fragile X will exhibit one or more of these features (Hagerman, 1987; Sutherland and Hecht, 1985). A long, narrow face is a more subjective measurement, although Butler and colleagues (1991) and Loesch, Lafranchi, and Scott (1988) have described anthropometric methods that may lead to better characterization of facial features.

Large ears (>2 SD above the norm) are seen in 50% of boys with fragile X (see Fig. 20-2). Prominent or cupped ears are often a more useful discriminating feature among this younger group. This finding is observed in 60% to 70% of boys and is frequently the only obvious physical feature associated with fragile X syndrome (Simko et al, 1989; Hagerman, 1991a).

Enlarged testicles are frequently observed in the mentally retarded population; 70% to 90% of

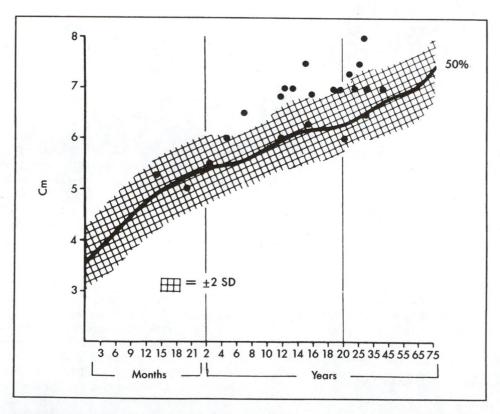

Fig. 20-2. Mean ear length. *(From Hagerman R, Smith ACM, Manner R: Clinical features of the fragile X syndrome. In Hagerman R, McBogg P, editors:* The fragile X syndrome: diagnosis, biochemistry and intervention, *Dillon, CO, 1983, Spectra.)*

men with fragile X have a testicular volume greater than 30 ml (Sutherland and Hecht, 1985). An orchidometer (see Fig. 20-3) consisting of ellipsoid shapes of varying size is a useful instrument to measure testicular volume, especially in prepubescent boys in whom testicular volume may be less obvious (4 ml or greater in approximately 30% of boys with fragile X compared with a normal testicular volume of 2 ml in those up to age 8 years).

Other more subtle physical features noted among the fragile X population include a prominent jaw, prominent forehead, and long palpebral fissures (Brondum-Nielsen et al, 1983; Butler et al, 1991; Hagerman, 1991a). A high-arched palate, mitral valve prolapse, hypotonia, hyperextensible finger joints, and flat feet suggest these individuals may have an underlying connective tissue disorder (Opitz, Westphal, and Daniel, 1984; Hagerman et al, 1984).

It is very important to recognize that the majority of males with fragile X, especially the younger boys, appear quite normal (see Fig. 20-4). Often what is more concerning to the parents are the behavioral characteristics. Hyperactivity is observed in more than 70% of boys with fragile X syndrome yet frequently disappears after puberty. Poor attention span, often combined with impulsivity, is also problematic for all boys with fragile X regardless of their level of cognitive functioning (Hagerman, Kemper, and Hudson, 1985; Fryns et al, 1984). Approximately 90% have poor eye contact (Hagerman,

1991a; Pueschel and Finelli, 1984), and 60% to 70% display unusual hand mannerisms, including hand flapping and hand biting (Hagerman, 1987).

Females

Overall, females who are affected by fragile X syndrome display milder phenotypic features than males, although some have been described with moderate and severe retardation (see Fig. 20-5).

Females who carry the premutation (CGG repeat number between 50 and 200) are usually unaffected intellectually by fragile X. However, females who carry the full mutation are often affected to a mild or severe degree. Approximately 25% of females with the full mutation have mental retardation, 25% have borderline intellectual abilities, and 50% have normal intellectual abilities; however, learning difficulties are common within girls with

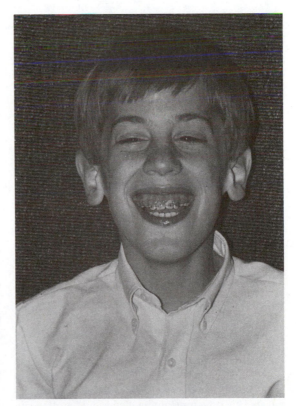

Fig. 20-4.   Prepubertal fragile X male.

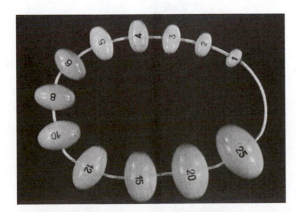

Fig. 20-3.   Prader orchidometer used to measure testicular volume.

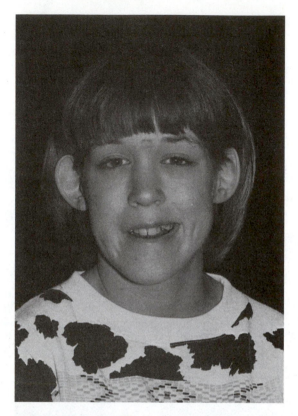

Fig. 20-5. Young heterozygous fragile X female who is affected physically and cognitively by fragile X syndrome.

the normal IQ range in full mutation (Hagerman et al, 1992; Rousseau et al, 1991 and 1994; Reiss et al, 1993). Executive function deficits including attention and organizational difficulties are common in the majority of females with the full mutation but with an overall normal IQ. In addition, math difficulties, shyness, and poor eye contact are also common to females with the full mutation (Mazzocco, Pennington, and Hagerman, 1993; Sobesky et al, 1994; Freund, Reiss, and Abrams, 1993).

Speech and language difficulties are noted in children with a heterozygote gene pattern. Although more work is needed in this area, receptive and expressive language deficits, including difficulties with auditory processing, inappropriate and tangential speech, poor topic maintenance, and written language difficulties, have been reported (Hagerman,

1987; Madison, George, and Moeschler, 1986; Scharfenaker and Schreiner, 1989).

The physical characteristics are less obvious than those described in males with fragile X. Prominent ears, a long narrow face, a prominent forehead and jaw, and hyperextensible finger joints have been described by several authors (Cronister et al, 1991, Fryns, 1986). Phenotypic expression is more frequently observed in the mentally impaired population; however, penetrance of the fragile X gene or genes is seen in normal functioning heterozygous females also (Cronister and Schreiner, 1991; Loesch and Hay, 1988).

To improve diagnosis in fragile X syndrome, the primary care provider must be familiar with the characteristic gestalt that defines this very common condition. It is important to recognize that none of the physical, behavioral, or psychologic characteristics looked at individually is diagnostic of fragile X syndrome. However, the finding of one or more of these features in combination with developmental delay or mental retardation of unknown cause should alert the clinician to order chromosome studies. The fragile X checklist (see box page 425) was designed to assist the primary care provider with screening children who are developmentally delayed or mentally retarded. A child receives a zero for each feature not present, one point for those present in the past or questionably present, and two points for those definitely present. The higher the score, the greater the risk for fragile X syndrome (Hagerman, Amiri, and Cronister, 1991).

TREATMENT

To date few health care professionals are knowledgeable about the diagnosis and treatment of individuals with fragile X syndrome. It is not uncommon, however, for an undiagnosed child with fragile X to be seen by the primary care provider with one of several associated medical problems including repeated ear infections, strabismus, hyperactivity, delayed language, tantrums, violent outbursts, seizures, or hypotonia. Although much of the medical intervention is approached as it would be with any child, certain treatment options specific to the fragile X diagnosis can significantly improve the developmental outcome of these children.

FRAGILE X CHECKLIST

	Score		
	0 (Not present)	1 (Borderline or present in the past)	2 (Definitely present)
Mental retardation	————	————	————
Perseverative speech	————	————	————
Hyperactivity	————	————	————
Short attention span	————	————	————
Tactile defensiveness	————	————	————
Hand flapping	————	————	————
Hand biting	————	————	————
Poor eye contact	————	————	————
Hyperextensible finger joints	————	————	————
Large or prominent ears	————	————	————
Large testicles	————	————	————
Simian crease or Sydney line	————	————	————
Family history of mental retardation	————	————	————
TOTAL SCORE: ————			

Adapted from Hagerman RJ: Fragile X syndrome, *Curr Probl Pediatr* 17:621-674, 1987.

Any signs that indicate developmental delay, sensory integration dysfunction, or language delays deserve immediate and aggressive treatment in a child with fragile X. All areas of a child's presenting signs and symptoms should be addressed, and thus a multidisciplinary approach to evaluation and therapy is essential.

Medication

Medical management of hyperactivity and attentional problems can augment learning and behavioral management at home and in the school. Central nervous system stimulant medication has proved the most reliable, with improvements in as many as two thirds of affected children (Hagerman, Murphy, Wittenberger, 1988). No one drug is effective for all children. Most commonly children will be prescribed methylphenidate (Ritalin), but pemoline (Cylert) and dextroamphetamine (Dexedrine) have also proved beneficial (Hagerman, 1991b) (see Chapter 26).

TREATMENT

Genetic counseling for all extended family
   members at risk
Medications for hyperactivity
   Ritalin, Dexedrine, or Cylert
   Folic acid
   Catapres (clonidine)
Medications for aggression or severe mood
   lability
   Serotonin agents Tegretol or depakote
Counseling for behavioral problems including
   aggression
Special education support including
   speech/language therapy and occupational
   therapy
Genetic counseling

Folic acid therapy appears to be helpful for approximately 50% of prepubertal boys with fragile X (Hagerman, 1991b). Its use is controversial, and several studies have shown a lack of efficacy. Other studies have shown noticeable improvements in activity level, attention span, unusual mannerisms, and coping skills. The mechanism of action of folate is unclear, but it does not appear to be specific to fragile X syndrome. Because harmful side effects are rare, many families request that their child be given folic acid as a trial. A prepubescent child can be placed on a regimen of 10 mg/day (divided twice daily) for 3 to 6 months. Regardless of the dosage, careful follow-up is warranted to monitor vitamin B_6 and zinc serum levels, which may become deficient. If, however, improvements are not noticeable within the trial period, the clinician should consider an alternative treatment.

Clonidine (Catapres) has been shown to be beneficial in approximately 80% of children with fragile X syndrome who have significant hyperactivity. Clonidine is a high blood pressure medication which lowers plasma and CNS norepinephine levels. It is particularly helpful for children with severe hyperactivity, overexcitability, and aggression. It has an overall calming effect on hyperactivity and it can be used in conjunction with stimulants (Hagerman et al, 1995).

Individuals who suffer from significant mood lability, mood instability, or aggression may benefit significantly from the use of carbamezapine (Tegretol). Although carbamezapine is an anticonvulsant medication, it has beneficial behavioral effects in many disorders, including fragile X syndrome (Hagerman, 1991b).

In adolescence, aggression can be a significant difficulty and recently serotonin agents such as Prozac have been helpful in fragile X syndrome (Hagerman et al, 1994a). A survey of fluoxetine's efficacy in fragile X reported that 70% had a beneficial response, including a decrease in aggression, improvement in anxiety, and improvement in moodiness or outburst behavior. Fluoxetine is widely known as an antidepressant medication but it may also be helpful in decreasing obsessive or compulsive behavior. The side effects of fluoxetine can include gastrointestinal upset or nausea and an activation effect which can sometimes exacerbate hyperactivity. A rare child may experience an increase in obsessive or compulsive behavior or suicidal ideation while taking fluoxetine. For this reason, it is recommended that children be followed in therapy on a weekly basis while taking this medication.

Educational Intervention

Several studies have indicated that IQ declines with age (Borghgraef et al, 1987; Dykens et al, 1989; Lachiewicz et al, 1987). Some males, however, whose IQs have remained stable over time have been followed (Hagerman et al, 1989), and an occasional individual may maintain an IQ within the normal range (Hagerman et al, 1994b). This finding has been associated with a novel pattern on DNA testing, an unmethylated full mutation (CGG expansion >200). This is unusual because the full mutation is typically completely methylated. The lack of methylation in these high-functioning males has been associated with a limited level of FMR1 protein production, leading to a less severe degree of involvement intellectually and behaviorally than typical fragile X males (Hagerman et al, 1994b; Merenstein et al, 1994). There is a tendency for the individual with fragile X to perform better on some academic tests than the IQ score would predict. Children with fragile X syndrome typically are better visual learners than auditory learners. Significant memory abilities and well-developed skills in recognizing visual gestalts make reading, spelling, and vocabulary obvious areas of strength for many (Kemper, Hagerman, and Altshul-Stark, 1987; Scharfenaker and Schreiner, 1989; Wilson et al, 1994).

When developing an educational program, one must consider the child's overall intellectual abilities. Mainstreaming is a realistic goal for some children, whereas others may need a more structured and specialized program. The child with fragile X will improve most significantly if he or she is shown appropriate role models. Educational intervention strategies should emphasize a child's strengths, such as imitating abilities, memory, visual skills, and vocabulary. The curriculum should also be focused on areas of interest (Scharfenaker and Schreiner, 1989; Scharfenaker, Hickman, and Braden, 1991). Logo reading is an example of a learning tool developed to capitalize on the child's interesting sense of incidentally acquired knowledge (Braden, 1988). The idea is to use logos from popular television commercials and advertisements as the basis for a sight word vocabulary. The logos are gradually faded away such that only the word, phrase, or number remains.

Another learning tool that has proved successful is the use of computers for learning enhancement. This medium may be used to enhance language ability and academic progress in reading, spelling, and math. It can utilize visual matching skills and can help focus attention with colorful programs.

Speech and language and occupational therapy intervention are critical components of the education program and are recommended for all children with fragile X syndrome. Therapy is most effective when it incorporates a child's primary areas of interest. When possible, speech and language therapy sessions should include one or two other children who function at a higher level. Again, early intervention and vigorous treatment can optimize a child's speech and language abilities (Scharfenaker and Schreiner, 1989; Scharfenaker, Hickman, and Braden, 1991). Occupational therapy can be combined with speech and language therapy so that attention is maintained and the child is provided with an experiential approach to language (Windeck and Laurel, 1989).

Because the child with fragile X is easily overstimulated, occupational therapy should be geared toward helping a child reorganize, interpret, and adjust to sensory stimulation. For this reason, sensory integration therapy is the method of choice when working with these children. With this form of treatment, improvements should be noticeable in motor skills, balance, coordination, movement, sequencing, and attention (Scharfenaker, Hickman, and Braden, 1991).

Genetic Counseling

Fragile X syndrome is known to affect generation after generation, and many families have two or more children affected by this condition. Early diagnosis can provide relatives with important information regarding fragile X inheritance, recurrence risks, carrier testing, and family planning options (Silverman, 1991).

Fragile X syndrome is inherited in an X-linked fashion. Males are typically affected by any deleterious gene they carry on the X chromosome. Females, on the other hand, are usually normal because the abnormal gene on one X chromosome is compensated for by the normal gene on the other X chromosome. Heterozygous females have a 50% chance to pass the abnormal gene to their children. Males who carry the fragile X gene, on the other hand, will pass the premutation to all of their daughters but none of their sons.

Males who are carriers have the premutation, which is a CGG repeat between 50 and 200. When males pass on this premutation to all of their daughters, only minimal changes occur in the CGG repeat number and it never increases to the full mutation. However, when the premutation is passed on by a female, there is a high probability that the premutation will increase to a full mutation in the offspring who inherit the fragile X chromosome. The larger the size of the premutation in the carrier mother the greater the chance that expansion will occur to a full mutation. In women with a premutation of 100 CGG repeats the expansion to the full mutation will occur 100% of the time when the fragile X chromosome is passed on to the next generation. All family members who are at risk to carry either the premutation or the full mutation should be studied by DNA testing, which is done on a blood sample. DNA testing is available throughout the United States and at large genetic centers internationally. For a list of laboratories that can carry out DNA testing for fragile X syndrome, contact the National Fragile X Foundation (see pg 343).

Because fragile X syndrome is inherited, it is essential that a thorough family history or pedigree be taken. Questions regarding intellectual deficits, learning disabilities emotional problems, and physical features associated with fragile X syndrome should be asked. Any relative with positive findings should be suspected as either a carrier or an affected individual.

Prenatal diagnosis is available to all families with a confirmed diagnosis of fragile X syndrome or in families with a history of mental retardation. This testing includes amniocentesis (performed at 14 to 18 weeks' gestation), chorionic villi sampling (performed at 9½ to 12 weeks' gestation) and percutaneous umbilical blood sampling (18 to 22 weeks' gestation). Each procedure has specific benefits and drawbacks that should be carefully discussed with a genetic counselor before a pregnancy or testing is pursued. The accuracy of prenatal diagnostic testing has improved significantly (>98% accurate) with DNA-FMR1 studies.

RECENT AND ANTICIPATED ADVANCES IN DIAGNOSIS AND MANAGEMENT

The most significant advance in the future will be the utilization of antibodies to the FMR1 protein to identify individuals who have fragile X syndrome. Since normal individuals produce a normal level of FMR1 protein, the fluorescent antibody test will light up the protein within the lymphocytes of individuals who are normal. However, a fluorescent antibody test will not detect antibody production in males who are affected by fragile X syndrome because they do not produce FMR1 protein. Females, on the other hand, produce some level of FMR1 protein because their other normal X chromosome is producing FMR1 protein to a level dependent on the pattern of X-inactivation in the female. Therefore, this diagnostic test will not clearly differentiate females with the full mutation compared to controls because of the variable FMR1 protein expression in females. However, this advance will be helpful for diagnosing the fragile X syndrome in males. A fluorescent antibody test should be much less expensive than the DNA testing. Such an antibody test should be considered as a screening for individuals who may be affected by fragile X syndrome and then the diagnosis would be confirmed by DNA testing.

In the future, new medications will be developed that will no doubt help with the behavior problems in children with fragile X syndrome including hyperactivity and aggression. Probably within the next 10 years the technology either to replace the FMR1 protein or to replace a normal FMR1 gene in individuals who are affected by this syndrome will be developed. This very important advance could mean a cure or significant alleviation of this disorder. Extensive animal studies will be needed over the next decade to improve methods for inserting a gene or normal FMR1 protein inside of neurons. It is unclear at this time how significant the improvements will be in children or adults who receive a new gene or normal levels of FMR1 protein, (RaHazzi and Ioannou, 1996).

ASSOCIATED PROBLEMS

Otitis Media

Recurrent otitis media has been reported in 45% to 60% of all children with fragile X syndrome. Approximately 40% of these children will require myringotomy tube insertions (Hagerman, Altshul-Stark, and McBogg, 1987; Simko et al, 1989). There has been some speculation that this may be caused by an unusual angle or collapsibility of the eustachian tube (Hagerman, 1991a). Appropriate intervention is critical to avoid conductive hearing loss and a compounding of language deficits typical for fragile X (Rapin, 1979).

Connective Tissue Problems

Of all individuals with fragile X syndrome, 50% will have pes planus (Davids, Hagerman, and Eilert, 1990). Clubfoot has also been reported and may be related to hypotonia in utero. In the study by Davids and associates (1990), joint laxity was documented in approximately 70% of children 10 years or younger. For reasons not clearly understood, hypotonia tends to disappear with age. Scoliosis may be present, and hernias appear to be more common in children with fragile X than in the general population. These problems may also be related to an underlying connective tissue disorder. Routine intervention is recommended.

ASSOCIATED PROBLEMS

Otitis media
Pesplanus
Scoliosis
Mitral valve prolapse
Strabismus
Nystagmus
Seizures
Dental malocclusions
Autisticlike features (hand flapping, hand biting)
Psychiatric manifestations
Surgery integration difficulties

Cardiac problems have also been noted in persons with fragile X syndrome. These may be secondary to a connective tissue disorder. Mitral valve prolapse has been diagnosed in 22% to 55% of individuals affected (Loehr et al, 1986; Sreeran et al, 1989). Although usually benign, mitral valve prolapse can predispose a person to arrhythmias. Thus far this has not been noted in males with fragile X, but 30% of heterozygous females complain of heart palpitations (Cronister et al, 1991). Mild dilation of the base of the aorta has also been observed with ultrasound studies in as many as 50% of this population. It does not appear to be progressive (Loehr et al, 1986; Sreeran et al, 1989).

Vision Problems

Strabismus (either esotropia or exotropia) appears to be present in approximately 30% to 56% of those with fragile X syndrome (Maino et al, 1990; King, Hagerman, and Houghton, 1995). Other eye problems such as myopia, nystagmus, and ptosis have been observed with and without strabismus (Schnizel and Largo, 1985; Storm, DeBenito, and Ferretti, 1987).

Seizures

Seizures have been documented in approximately 20% of all individuals with fragile X. Generalized seizures and partial complex seizures have been reported (Musumeci et al, 1988a, b; Wisniewski et al, 1991). A careful history should be taken and if clinical seizures are present, treatment with an anticonvulsant such as carbamazepine (Tegretol) is warranted (Hagerman, 1991b).

Oral Problems

A high-arched palate is seen with greater frequency among the fragile X population and can explain the increased incidence of dental malocclusion (Partington, 1984). Several reports have also noted of Pierre Robin syndrome (micrognathia and cleft palate) in combination with the fragile X syndrome.

Autisticlike Tendencies

Much has been written in the literature to suggest an association between autism and fragile X syndrome. Studies have estimated that 5% to 53% of all individuals with fragile X meet *Diagnostic and Statistical Manual of Mental Disorders DSM-IV*

criteria for autism (Benezech and Noel, 1985; Brown et al, 1982, 1986; Partington, 1984). The majority of individuals, however, are more appropriately described as autisticlike. In addition to poor eye contact and unusual hand mannerisms, many children have fascinations with certain objects such as vacuum cleaners and record players. What differentiates the majority of individuals with fragile X from those with autism is that individuals who are autistic characteristically lack an ability to relate. Although social anxiety is obvious at times, many children with fragile X can be intermittently quite sociable, demonstrating a spontaneous and natural sense of humor (Hagerman, 1987; Scharfenaker, Hickman, and Braden, 1991).

Psychiatric Manifestations

Researchers have only recently investigated the psychiatric manifestations of the fragile X gene in females. As with males with fragile X, social anxiety is a common complaint. Many of the affected girls appear shy, are withdrawn, and have poor eye contact (Freund, Reiss, and Abrams, 1993; Hagerman et al, 1992). Occasional cognitively normal women recall their childhood burdened by similar types of problems. Poor self-image and depression have also been described (Hagerman and Sobesky, 1989; Reiss et al, 1988). Reiss and colleagues (1988) have reported an increased incidence of schizotypal features, including emotional withdrawal and odd communication patterns. The schizotypal features appear to be related to the executive function or frontal deficits which are seen in the majority of females with the full mutation (Mazzocco, Pennington, and Hagerman, 1993; Sobesky et al, 1994).

Sensory Integration Difficulties

Other behavioral concerns include an inability to calm when the child is overstimulated or overwhelmed. New stimuli or novel situations can be frightening. Many parents describe their child as being hypersensitive to touch or tactilely defensive. Sensory integration difficulties are evidenced by an inability to screen out noises, lights, or confusion. Common responses to this overloading can include tantrums or outburst behavior, aggressive behavior, emotional instability, and, rarely, psychotic behavior (Scharfenaker and Schreiner, 1989; Scharfenaker, Hickman, and Braden, 1991; Hagerman, 1991b).

PROGNOSIS

Individuals with fragile X syndrome are expected to live a normal life span regardless of intellectual functioning.

Primary Care Management
HEALTH CARE MAINTENANCE

Growth and Development

Increased head circumference (greater than the 75th percentile) at birth and throughout childhood has been reported by several authors (Borghgraef, Fryns, and Van den Berghe, 1990; Turner, Daniel, and Frost, 1980; Turner et al, 1986). This may lead to a possible misdiagnosis of Sotos' syndrome (cerebral gigantism). Others, however, have concluded that this deviance of head circumference into the upper range of normal occurs only occasionally and therefore is not a consistent finding (Partington, 1984). No special intervention is necessary for a large head circumference.

Controversy also exists regarding birth weights and growth. Prouty and others (1988) found growth to be normal and noted only a mild increase in growth percentiles from childhood into adult life. Partington (1984) reported similar findings. Sutherland and Hecht (1985), on the other hand, reported that 9 of 29 (31%) boys studied were above the 95th percentile.

In addition to deficits in cognitive functioning and speech, children with fragile X may be delayed in meeting other age-appropriate developmental milestones. Developmental delay will be evident with early developmental testing, such as the Bayley Scales of Infant Development (see Chapter 2). Other early warning signs are clumsiness and poor balance. Toe walking, unusual gait, lack of flow of movement, and trouble with motor planning may also occur secondary to hypotonia, joint laxity, and sensory integration difficulties (Scharfenaker, Hickman, and Braden, 1991).

Diet

Obsessive-compulsive behavior can be seen in children with fragile X syndrome, and this may involve food cravings. Obesity has been a problem for a small subgroup of children with fragile X (Fryns et al, 1987). This may, in fact, be secondary to perseverative eating or hypothalamic dysfunction (Fryns et al, 1987). Parents of obese children should be encouraged to place their children on appropriate diets. Exercise programs for older children may also be beneficial, as well as exercise videos, which encourage children to use their visual and mimicking abilities. Failure to thrive is not uncommon in infants with fragile X syndrome. On the other hand, this may be the result of aversion to some food textures, frequent infections, or problematic mothering skills if the mother herself is affected by the syndrome.

Safety

Families and educators should not expect every child with fragile X to be able to learn age-appropriate safety. It will depend on each child's individual strengths and weaknesses. With strong visual and mimicking abilities and through the use of repetition, many children can be taught to follow safety tips.

Hyperactivity may lead to more accidents, so these children should be monitored closely. Because children with fragile X can be overstimulated by their environment, the home setting and particularly the child's playroom and bedroom should be a calm and uncluttered environment. The use of bean bag chairs, vibrating pillows, musical tapes, and appropriate environmental changes can be discussed with an occupational therapist.

Parents also may be concerned about their child's safety if they display self-injurious behavior. Head banging is rare but can be harmful to the child. Hand biting, despite its frequency, does not commonly cause scarring. Nevertheless, parents may wish to pursue behavior management therapies to decrease the frequency of these behaviors. Parents and professionals should also be advised of possible seizure activity and taught appropriate intervention.

Immunizations

Vaccination regimen is the same as it would be for any infant or child. Should a child have a seizure disorder, the American Academy of Pediatrics guidelines for administering pertussis and measles vaccinations to those with seizures should be followed (see Chapter 19) (Committee on Infectious Diseases, 1994).

Screening

Vision. An eye examination is recommended as early as possible after the fragile X diagnosis is made to rule out strabismus and the less frequent findings of myopia, hyperopia, astigmatism, nystagmus, and ptosis. The evaluation should include a complete case history, visual acuity evaluation, refractive error determination, oculomotor assessment, and fundoscopy. Other testing may include an assessment of focusing function and visual developmental-perceptual skills. Yearly screening is sufficient unless visual difficulty is suspected. Early intervention is encouraged to avoid the development of blurred vision, amblyopia, or diplopia as a result of an uncorrected refractive error or strabismus. Treatment for many of the ophthalmologic problems includes corrective lenses, patching, or both—treatment that is relatively inexpensive and noninvasive. For some cases of strabismus, however, surgery may be the treatment of choice. Although early intervention may not dramatically influence cognitive functioning, corrected vision will maximize a child's learning potential.

Hearing. Because of the increased risk for recurrent ear infections, hearing evaluations are strongly recommended in the newly diagnosed child. Audiometry testing is usually sufficient to assess hearing. Any child who has a history of recurrent ear infections is best referred to an ear, nose, and throat (ENT) specialist to determine whether pressure equalizing (PE) tubes are warranted.

Dental. A routine dental screening by the practitioner may reveal a high-arched palate, cleft palate, or dental malocclusion, all of which compound speech problems. Any child requiring dental work should be evaluated for mitral valve prolapse. If it is present, prophylactic antibiotic treatment to avoid subacute bacterial endocarditis is warranted (see Chapter 15). Although it is not always possible, families should be referred to a pedodontist experienced in working with developmentally delayed and hyperactive children.

Blood pressure. Routine screening is recommended.

Hematocrit. Routine screening is recommended.

Urinalysis. Routine screening is recommended.

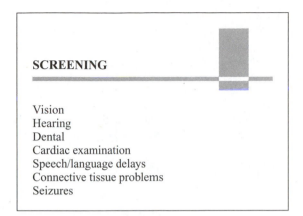

SCREENING

Vision
Hearing
Dental
Cardiac examination
Speech/language delays
Connective tissue problems
Seizures

Tuberculosis. Routine screening is recommended.

Condition-specific screening

MITRAL VALVE PROLAPSE. Children with fragile X syndrome are at increased risk of mitral valve prolapse. Careful screening to detect a click or murmur is essential to detect this problem or any other cardiac involvement. Any child with an abnormal cardiac examination should be referred to a cardiologist for formal evaluation.

SPEECH AND LANGUAGE. Some children will have early speech delays that may be so subtle that they go undetected by the parents or teachers. An early and annual speech and language evaluation should be performed to detect any speech or language deficits that can be improved through early intervention. Because of the diversity of speech and language difficulties in children with fragile X, no one screening tool is recommended, and thus each child should be approached on an individual basis. Routine screening tools such as the Denver II will identify developmental delays but subsequent DNA testing is necessary to identify fragile X syndrome as the cause of the delays. Children identified with fragile X syndrome should have a formal evaluation by a licensed speech and language pathologist preferably experienced with fragile X syndrome.

CONNECTIVE TISSUE PROBLEMS. Early detection of scoliosis can often prevent further sequelae. Screening should also include a careful examination for excessive joint laxity and other complications of loose connective tissue, such as hernias.

SEIZURES. When the clinical history suggests seizures, an electroencephalogram (EEG) is indicated. Unusual findings can include a slow background rhythm and spike-wave discharges that are often similar to rolandic spikes (Musumeci et al, 1988a, 1988b). Any child who appears to be having seizures should be treated with anticonvulsant medication and should be followed closely by a pediatric neurologist. If a child is taking medication to control seizures, anticonvulsant serum levels should be followed (see Chapter 19).

COMMON ILLNESS MANAGEMENT

Differential Diagnosis

Recurrent otitis media. As mentioned earlier, a frequent pediatric health problem in the child with fragile X is ear infections. It is imperative that these children be vigorously monitored and treated for recurrent otitis media to avoid sequelae that could further compromise language development and learning. In young children parents may not recognize otitis as the cause of their child's irritability. It may be helpful to inform parents of children with fragile X that recurrent otitis media is a common problem and review for them which signs or symptoms are indicators of infection.

To best determine a child's individualized medical management, newly diagnosed families should be referred to a health care team with expertise in fragile X syndrome for a thorough evaluation and consultation.

Drug Interactions

Carbamazepine is a commonly prescribed anticonvulsant and is also used to control behavior problems such as violent outbursts, aggression, and self-injurious behavior. Concurrent treatment with macrolide antibiotics, cimetidine (Tagamet), propoxyphene (Darvon), and isoniazid (INH) can interfere with the breakdown of carbamazepine, causing nausea, vomiting, and lethargy. Folic acid therapy may worsen the seizure frequency in the child with epilepsy.

DEVELOPMENTAL ISSUES

Sleep Patterns

Frequent wakefulness in early childhood is a common problem in children with fragile X. Overstim-ulation can often interfere with sleeping, and calming techniques such as music are useful in quieting the child in preparation for bedtime.

Toileting

Parents of children with fragile X often need help in setting realistic expectations regarding toilet training. Some children achieve this milestone on time, but delayed training is more common. Parents should not be discouraged if a child takes longer to learn. The establishment of a predictable routine and consistent positive reinforcement are general principles that are helpful for children with fragile X. As with parents of any child having toilet-training difficulties, parents are discouraged from being overly critical or reprimanding.

Discipline

Children with fragile X syndrome are especially noncompliant in response to an unexpected event or change in routine and therefore need a highly structured environment. Sending the child to school the same way each day, having meals on a scheduled basis, and using the same nightly routines are encouraged. Behavior problems should be anticipated if the child is faced with an unexpected event. The prevention of unpredictable events in the home or at school is obviously an unrealistic expectation and should not be overemphasized. On the other hand, change and transitions should be gradually programmed into the child's learning and home environment. Setting limits, giving the child timeouts, and being consistent are appropriate responses when disciplinary action is required.

Child Care

Issues related to child care are common concerns for parents of a child with fragile X. Because of the short attention span and hyperactivity, child care providers should be knowledgeable about behavior modification techniques. The environment in which the child is placed is also important. Colors, noise level, and the amount of light can be altered to avoid overstimulation. Slowly but gradually new events can be programmed into the child's day. Setting a common time each week to introduce a new game, playing in a new space, or meeting a new day care provider can help a child anticipate and deal more effectively with change. If these aspects of day care are well managed, there is no reason why a child with fragile X cannot be placed in full-day or half-day programs. Placement with nonaffected children is very helpful for modeling appropriate behavior.

Schooling

Most children with fragile X syndrome identified thus far are receiving special education. Mainstreaming is a potential goal as described under the treatment section. Children can be mainstreamed in preschool programs as well, but child care providers should be experienced in specialized education. A program that provides for individualized attention and a high teacher/student ratio is best. The success of any approach will depend on a number of factors specific to each child, including the child's level of cognitive functioning, distractibility, impulsivity, the structure of the class, classroom environment, and appropriate role models.

Because few educators are knowledgeable about fragile X syndrome, the health care professional can play an active role in helping families educate the teachers and therapists about the specialized needs of their child and why an integrative approach that emphasizes a child's overall strengths and weaknesses is essential for effective learning.

Parents should be encouraged to become actively involved in their child's program. Frequent visits to the classroom and observing therapy sessions helps establish open communication among parents, teachers, and support personnel.

Sexuality

Masturbation and other forms of self-stimulatory behavior are common among the mentally retarded population and are occasionally problematic for the adolescent with fragile X. Families can be supportive by providing appropriate sex education and by talking openly about sexuality issues. This need can also be met through family or individual counseling (Brown, Braden, and Sobesky, 1991). Counseling or therapy can also train new behaviors that can replace socially inappropriate behavior, such as masturbation in public. Most important, counseling can provide an environment in which the adolescent can discuss and deal with issues of sexuality in a supportive environment.

Fertility is usually normal in men with fragile X, although reproduction is rare because of cognitive deficits (Cantú et al, 1976). Ovarian problems and premature menopause have been reported in heterozygous women (Cronister et al, 1991). Fryns (1986) has reported increased fertility and twinning in heterozygous fragile X women. Mildly retarded individuals will require support in parenting. Sex education and genetic counseling should therefore be available to them.

Transition into Adulthood

The transition into adulthood is usually difficult for adolescents affected by fragile X syndrome because living independently is a problem as a result of mental retardation. It is important for adolescents to have adequate vocational training. Most individuals affected by fragile X syndrome can carry out jobs in the community consistent with their level of mental functioning. Many individuals require a job trainer who can work with them for the first several days, or the first few weeks, when a new job is started. A focus on daily living skills is also critical for young adults with fragile X syndrome if they are to be successful in living independently or semi-independently. Individuals with mild or moderate mental retardation can learn how to use public transportation and can carry out activities in the home, including laundry, self-care, and cooking. Most adults who are affected by fragile X syndrome will do well with limited supervision in an apartment living situation. Females affected with fragile X syndrome have their greatest difficulty when trying to raise their children who are affected by fragile X syndrome. This can be extremely stressful and may overwhelm their limited resources, particularly if the mother is mildly retarded. Additional help from family or from social services agencies is usually necessary.

The connective tissue problems usually improve in adulthood and medical complications are uncommon. Hernia and mitral valve prolapse are more common in adulthood than childhood. Follow-up with a cardiologist and the use of antibiotic prophylaxis for subacute bacterial endocarditis (SBE) prevention is necessary for mitral valve prolapse.

Approximately 30% of young adults, particularly males, with fragile X syndrome may have difficulty with episodic outburst behavior. This should be treated with medications such as the serotonin agents, fluoxetine or sertraline, in addition to counseling. Counseling can help with development of calming techniques and recognition of environmental situations that can lead to outburst behavior.

SPECIAL FAMILY CONCERNS AND RESOURCES

Perhaps the most frustrating aspect of having a child diagnosed with fragile X syndrome is realizing that so few professionals have a good understanding of this disorder and how it can affect a child and other family members. As a consequence many parents become the main advocate for their child in both the educational and medical settings. Health care professionals who are unfamiliar with fragile X syndrome should make every effort to listen carefully to families. It is also the parents' responsibility to (1) educate themselves about this unique disorder so that they too appreciate these children's specialized needs and (2) recognize their own needs if they require additional support because they themselves may be affected by the syndrome.

Fragile X syndrome occurs in all ethnic and racial groups that have been studied. There is no evidence of increased prevalence in any individual group. In some cultural groups, such as certain Asian populations, it is sometimes difficult to do genetic counseling in extended family members because of the negative cultural implications of knowing about a genetic disorder that affects large numbers within the family tree. When these cultural concerns exist, often permission will not be given to inform extended family members about this genetic disorder. In these cases it is helpful to write an explanatory letter regarding fragile X syndrome that the immediate family can pass out to other family members who may be affected or may be carriers for fragile X syndrome.

The National Fragile X Foundation was established to educate parents, professionals, and the lay public regarding the diagnosis and treatment of fragile X syndrome and other forms of X-linked mental retardation. In addition, the National Fragile X Foundation promotes research pertaining to fragile X syndrome in the areas of biochemistry, genetics, and clinical applications. All parents who have a child diagnosed with fragile X syndrome and interested professionals working with the developmentally delayed population are encouraged to write or call the foundation so they may receive the newsletter and other services available to them.

Organizations

National Fragile X Foundation
  1441 York St, Suite 303
  Denver, CO 80231
  (800) 688-8756
  (303) 333-6155

SUMMARY OF PRIMARY CARE NEEDS FOR THE CHILD WITH FRAGILE X SYNDROME

Health care maintenance

Growth and development

Physical growth is usually within normal limits.
Some children are reported to have large heads for body size.
Deficits in cognitive function and speech are common.
Developmental delays in gross motor skills are common.

Diet

Obsessive eating may result in obesity in older children.
Infants may have failure to thrive.

Safety

Cognitive dysfunction may limit the child's awareness of safety issues.
Hyperactivity may make the child more accident prone.
Self-injurious behavior may occur, and parents can be taught behavior management therapies.
If seizures are present, seizure precautions are necessary.

Immunizations

Routine immunizations are recommended.
AAP guidelines for immunizations in children with seizures should be followed where indicated.

Screening

Vision
Eye examination for strabismus, refractive errors, and visual perceptual skills is recommended at the time of diagnosis. If no problems are found, annual vision screening is recommended.
Hearing
An increased risk of otitis media warrants audiometric testing. The child may need referral to an ENT specialist for PE tubes.
Dental
Screening for palate and dental abnormalities is recommended. If mitral valve prolapse is present, prophylactic antibiotics will be needed for dental work.

Blood pressure
Routine screening is recommended.
Hematocrit
Routine screening is recommended.
Urinalysis
Routine screening is recommended.
Tuberculosis
Routine screening is recommended.
Condition-specific screening
MITRAL VALVE PROLAPSE
In the presence of an abnormal cardiac examination, mitral valve prolapse must be evaluated by a cardiologist.
SPEECH AND LANGUAGE
Speech and language evaluation should be done annually, with early intervention if a problem is detected.
CONNECTIVE TISSUE PROBLEMS
The child should be screened for flat feet, scoliosis, and excessive joint laxity.
SEIZURES
A clinical history suggestive of seizures should be evaluated by electroencephalography. If the child is taking anticonvulsants, blood levels must be monitored.

Common illness management

Differential diagnosis

Recurrent otitis media is common.

Drug interactions

Carbamazepine is altered by macrolide antibiotics, cimetidine, propoxyphene, and isoniazid.
See Chapter 19 for drug interactions with seizure medications.

Developmental issues

Sleep patterns

Frequent wakefulness in early childhood is not uncommon.
Overstimulation should be avoided.

Toileting

Delayed continence is not uncommon.

Continued.

SUMMARY OF PRIMARY CARE NEEDS FOR THE CHILD WITH FRAGILE X SYNDROME—cont'd

Discipline

Children behave better in highly structured environments.
Consistent limit setting is beneficial.
Positive reinforcement is essential.

Child care

Short attention span and hyperactivity may be modified by subdued environments.
New activities must be introduced slowly.

Schooling

Most children receive special education services. The provider can help educate the school system personnel on condition and treatment.

Sexuality

Self-stimulatory behaviors are common. Counseling may help decrease inappropriate behavior.

Fertility is normal in men; carrier females may experience premature menopause.
Sex education, birth control, and genetic counseling are necessary.

Transition into adulthood

Living independently is difficult, individuals will likely need support from others.
Connective tissue problems improve.
Outburst behavior may be a problem.

Special family concerns

The family may have difficulty adjusting to the diagnosis; parents may also be affected.
Genetic counseling is warranted.
Because the condition is not well known, care may be nonspecific.

REFERENCES

Benezech M and Noel B: Fra(X) syndrome and autism, *Clin Genet* 28:93, 1985.

Borghgraef M et al: Fragile X syndrome: a study of the psychological profile in 23 patients, *Clin Genet* 32:179-186, 1987.

Borghgraef M, Fryns JP, and Van den Berghe H: The female and the fragile X syndrome: data on clinical and psychological findings in fragile X carriers, *Clin Genet* 37:341-346, 1990.

Braden M: *Optimal educational strategies to maximize learning potential in the fragile X patient,* Unpublished manuscript, 1988.

Brondum-Nielsen K et al: Diagnosis of the fragile X syndrome (Martin-Bell syndrome): clinical findings in 27 males with the fragile site at Xq28, *J Ment Defic Res* 27:211-226, 1983.

Brown J, Braden M, and Sobesky W: Treatment of behavioral and emotional problems. In RJ Hagerman and AC Silverman, (editors):*The fragile X syndrome: diagnosis, treatment, and research,* Baltimore, 1991, Johns Hopkins University Press.

Brown WT et al: Fragile X and autism, *Am J Med Genet* 23:341-352, 1986.

Brown WT et al: Autism is associated with the fragile X syndrome, *J Autism Dev Disord* 12:303-307, 1982.

Butler MG et al: Anthropomorphic comparisons in mentally retarded males with and without the fragile X syndrome, *Am J Med Genet* 38:260-268, 1991.

Cantú JM et al: Inherited congenital normofunctional testicular hyperplasia and mental deficiency, *Hum Genet* 33:23-33, 1976.

Chudley AE, de von Flindt R, and Hagerman RJ: Cognitive variability in the fragile X syndrome, *Am J Med Genet* 28:13-15, 1987 (invited editorial comment).

Committee on Infectious Diseases: *Report of the Committee on Infectious Diseases,* ed 23, Elk Grove Village, IL, The American Academy of Pediatrics, 1994.

Cronister A et al: The heterozygous fragile X female: historical, physical, cognitive, and cytogenetic features, *Am J Med Genet* 38:269-274, 1991.

Davids JR, Hagerman RJ, and Eilert RE: The orthopaedic aspects of the fragile X syndrome, *J Bone Joint Surg BR* 72:889-896, 1990.

Dykens E et al: The trajectory of cognitive development in males with the fragile X syndrome, *J Am Acad Child Adolesc Psychiatry* 28:422-426, 1989.

Freund LS, Reiss AL, and Abrams M, Psychiatric disorders associated with fragile X in the young female, *Pediatrics* 91:321-329, 1993.

Fryns JP: The female and the fragile X: a study of 144 obligate female carriers, *Am J Med Genet* 23:157-169, 1986.

Fryns JP et al: A peculiar subphenotype in the fragile X syndrome: extreme obesity, short stature, stubby hands and feet, diffuse hyperpigmentation. Further evidence of disturbed hypothalamic function in the fragile X syndrome? *Clin Genet* 32:388-392, 1987.

Fryns JP et al: The psychological profile of the fragile X syndrome, *Clin Genet* 25:131-134, 1984.

Hagerman RJ: Fragile X syndrome, *Curr Probl Pediatr* 17:621-674, 1987.

Hagerman RJ: Physical and behavioral phenotype. In RJ Hagerman and AC Silverman, (editors): *The fragile X syndrome: diagnosis, treatment, and research,* Baltimore, 1991a, Johns Hopkins University Press.

Hagerman RJ: Medical follow-up and pharmacotherapy. In RJ Hagerman and AC Silverman, editor: *The fragile X syndrome: diagnosis, treatment, and research,* Baltimore, 1991b, Johns Hopkins University Press.

Hagerman RJ, Amiri K, and Cronister A: The fragile X checklist, *Am J Med Genet* 38:283-287, 1991.

Hagerman RJ et al: Institutional screening for the fragile X syndrome, *Am J Dis Child* 142:1216-1221, 1988.

Hagerman RJ et al: Fragile X girls: physical and neurocognitive status and outcome, *Pediatrics* 89:395-400, 1992.

Hagerman RJ et al: Fluoxetine therapy in fragile X syndrome, *Developmental Brain Dysfunction* 7:155-164, 1994a.

Hagerman RJ et al: High functioning fragile X males: demonstration of an unmethylated fully expanded FMR1 mutation associated with protein expression, *Am J Med Genet* 51:298-308, 1994b.

Hagerman RJ, Kemper M, and Hudson M: Learning disabilities and attentional problems in boys with the fragile X syndrome, *Am J Dis Child* 139:674-678, 1985.

Hagerman RJ et al: A survey of the efficacy of clonidine in fragile X syndrome. *Developmental Brain Dysfunction,* 8:336-344, 1995.

Hagerman RJ, Murphy M, and Wittenberger M: A controlled trial of stimulant medication in children with fragile X syndrome, *Am J Med Genet* 30:377-392, 1988.

Hagerman RJ et al: Longitudinal IQ changes in fragile X males. *Am J Med Genet* 33:513-518, 1989.

Hagerman RJ, Altshul-Stark D, and McBogg P: Recurrent otitis media in boys with the fragile X syndrome, *Am J Dis Child* 142:1216-1221, 1987.

Hagerman RJ, Smith ACM, and Mariner R: Clinical features of the fragile X syndrome. In RJ Hagerman and PM McBogg, editors): *The fragile X syndrome: diagnosis, biochemistry and intervention,* Dillon, CO, 1983, Spectra Publishing, pp 83-94.

Hagerman RJ, Sobesky WE: Psychopathology in fragile X syndrome, *Am J Orthopsychiatry* 59:142-152, 1989.

Hagerman RJ et al: Consideration of connective tissue dysfunc-

tion in the fragile X syndrome, *Am J Med Genet* 17:111-121, 1984.

Jenkins EC et al: Recent experience in prenatal fra(X) detection, *Am J Med Genet* 30:329-336, 1988.

Kemper MB, Hagerman RJ, and Altshul-Stark D: Cognitive profiles of boys with the fragile X syndrome, *Am J Med Genet* 30:191-200, 1987.

King RA, Hagerman RJ, and Houghton M: Ocular findings in fragile X syndrome. In press *Developmental Brain Dysfunction,* 1995.

Lachiewicz AM et al: Declining IQ scores of young males with fragile X syndrome, *Am J Med Genet* 30:272-278, 1987.

Loehr JP et al: Aortic root dilatation and mitral valve prolapse in the fragile X syndrome, *Am J Med Genet* 23:189-194, 1986.

Loesch DZ, Hay DA: Clinical features and reproductive patterns in fragile X female heterozygotes, *J Med Genet* 25:407-414, 1988.

Loesch DZ, Lafranchi M, and Scott D: Anthropometry in Martin-Bell syndrome, *Am J Med Genetics* 30:149-164, 1988.

Madison LS, George C, and Moeschler JB: Cognitive functioning in the fragile X syndrome: a study of intellectual, memory and communication skills, *J Ment Defic Res* 30:129-148, 1986.

Maino DM et al: Ocular anomalies in fragile X syndrome. *J Am Optom Assoc* 61:316-323, 1990.

Mazzocco MM, Pennington BF, and Hagerman RJ: The neurocognitive phenotype of female carriers of fragile X: additional evidence for specificity, *J Dev Beh Ped* 14:328-335, 1993.

Merenstein SA et al: Fragile X syndrome in a normal IQ male with learning and emotional problems, *J Am Acad Child Adoles Psychiat* 33:1316-1321, 1994.

Musumeci SA et al: Prevalence of a novel epileptogenic EEG pattern in the Martin-Bell syndrome, *Am J Med Genet* 30:207-212, 1988a.

Musumeci SA et al: Fragile X syndrome: a particular epileptogenic EEG pattern, *Epilepsia* 29:41-47, 1988b.

Newell K, Sanborn B, and Hagerman RJ: Speech and language dysfunction in the fragile X syndrome. In RJ Hagerman and P McBogg, (editors): *The fragile X syndrome: diagnosis, biochemistry and intervention,* Dillon, CO, 1983, Spectra Publishing, pp 175-200.

Oberle I et al: Instability of a 550-base pair DNA segment and abnormal methylation in fragile X syndrome, *Science* 252:1097-1102, 1991.

Opitz JM, Westphal JM, and Daniel A: Discovery of a connective tissue dysplasia in the Martin-Bell syndrome, *Am J Med Genet* 17:101-109, 1984.

Partington MW: The fragile X syndrome: preliminary data on growth and development in males, *Am J Med Genet* 17:175-194, 1984.

Prouty LA et al: Fragile X syndrome: growth development and intellectual function, *Am J Med Genet* 30:123-142, 1988.

Pueschel SM, Finelli PV: Neurologic investigations in patients with fragile X syndrome. Proceedings of the American Academy of Cerebral Palsy and Developmental Medicine, Washington, DC, April 1984 (abstract).

Rapin I: Conductive hearing loss effects on children's language and scholastic skills: a review of the literature, *Ann Otol Rhinol Laryngol* 88:3-12, 1979.

Rattazzi, MC and Ioannou, YA. Molecular approaches to therapy. In Hagerman RJ and Cronisten A. (eds.) Fragile X syndrome. Diagnosis, treatment, and research. 2nd ed. Johns Hopkins University Press, Baltimore, 1996.

Reiss AL et al: Neurobehavioral effects of the fragile X premutation in adult women; a controlled study. *Am J Hum Genet* 52:884-894 1993.

Reiss AL et al: Psychiatric disability in female carriers of fragile X chromosome, *Arch Gen Psychiatry* 45:25-30, 1988.

Rousseau F et al: Direct diagnosis by DNA analysis of the fragile X syndrome of mental retardation, *New Engl J Med* 325:1673-1681, 1991.

Rousseau F et al: Mal prevalence carriers of premutation—size alleles of the FMRI gene—and implications for the population genetics of the fragile X syndrome, *Am J Hum Genet* 57:1006-1018:1995.

Rousseau F et al: A multicenter study on genotype-phenotype correlations in the fragile X syndrome using direct diagnosis with probe StB12.3: the first 2253 cases, *Am J Human Genet* 55:225-237, 1994.

Scharfenaker S, Hickman L, and Braden M: An integrated approach to intervention with fragile X individuals. In RJ Hagerman and AC Silverman, (editors): *Fragile X syndrome: diagnosis, treatment, and research,* Baltimore, 1991, Johns Hopkins University Press.

Scharfenaker S, Schreiner R: Cognitive and speech language characteristics of the fragile X syndrome, *Rocky Mountain J Commun Disorders,* 1989.

Schnizel A, Largo RH: The fragile X syndrome (Martin-Bell syndrome) clinical and cytogenetic findings in 16 prepubertal boys and in 4 of their 5 families, *Helv Paediatr Acta* 40:133-152, 1985.

Sherman SL: Introduction and epidemiology of the fragile X syndrome. In RJ Hagerman and AC Silverman (editors): *Fragile X syndrome: diagnosis, treatment and research,* Baltimore, 1991, Johns Hopkins University Press.

Silverman AC: Genetic counseling. In RJ Hagerman and AC Silverman, (editors): *Fragile X syndrome: diagnosis, treatment, and research,* Baltimore, 1991, Johns Hopkins University Press.

Simko A et al: Fragile X syndrome: recognition in young children, *Pediatrics* 83:547-552, 1989.

Sobesky WE et al: Emotional and neurocognitive deficits in fragile X, *Am J Med Genet* 51:378-384, 1994.

Sreeran N et al: Cardiac abnormalities in the fragile X syndrome, *Br Heart J* 61:289-291, 1989.

Storm RL, De Benito R, and Ferretti C: Ophthalmologic findings in the fragile syndrome, *Arch Ophthalmol* 105:1099-1102, 1987.

Sutherland GR, Hecht F: *Fragile sites on human chromosomes,* New York, 1985, Oxford University Press.

Turner G, Daniel A, and Frost M: X-linked mental retardation, macroorchidism, and the Xq27 fragile site, *J Pediatr* 96:837-841, 1980.

Turner G et al: Conference report: second international workshop on the fragile X and on X-linked mental retardation, *Am J Med Genet* 23:11-67, 1986.

Verkerk AJMH et al: Identification of a gene (FMR-1) containing a CGG repeat coincident with a breakpoint cluster region exhibiting length variation in fragile X syndrome, *Cell* 65(5):905-914, 1991.

Webb TD, Thake A, and Todd J: Twelve families with fragile Xq27, *J Med Genet* 23:400-406, 1986.

Wilson P, et al: Issues and strategies for educating children with fragile X syndrome: a monograph, Dillon, CO, 1994, Spectra Publishing Co, Inc.

Windeck SL, Laurel M: A theoretical framework combining speech-language therapy with sensory integration treatment, *Am Occup Ther Assoc Sensory Integration Spec Interest Sect Newslett* 12:1-5, 1989.

Wisniewski KE et al: The fragile X syndrome: neurological, electrophysiological, and neuropathological abnormalities, *Am J Med Genet* 38:476-480, 1991.

Yu S et al: Fragile X genotype characterized by an unstable region of DNA, *Science* 252:1179-1181, 1991.

Head Injury

Carole Low

21

ETIOLOGY

Traumatic brain injury (TBI) is defined as physical damage to, or functional impairment of, the cranial contents from acute mechanical energy exchange (exclusive of birth trauma) (Michaud, Duhaime, and Batshaw, 1993). As defined by the National Head Injury Foundation, it is a traumatic insult to the brain capable of producing physical, intellectual, emotional, social, and vocational changes (Walleck and Mooney, 1994). The *primary injury* is that which results from the impact or initial insult. The causes of *secondary injury* include hypoxia, hypercapnia, hypotension, and intracranial hypertension (Altimier, 1992).

Craniocerebral trauma is the most common cause of acquired disability in the pediatric population, with nearly one fourth of those head injuries being inflicted in the child younger than 2 years of age (Reynolds, 1992; Michaud, Duhaime, and Batshaw, 1993). The majority of these injuries are preventable.

The cost of care for the child who experiences a TBI is overwhelming. The scope of this issue and increasing technologic development in the child's treatment have lead to an increased recognition of the unique challenges the child with a head injury presents. As a result, the 1990s have been declared by Congress and the Office of the President as the Decade of the Brain. During this decade the National Institute of Neurologic Disorders and Stroke (NINDS) has targeted programs which improve the long-term outcome of individuals with a traumatic brain injury (Coburn, 1992).

Mechanisms of Injury

The mechanisms of injury associated with TBI involve the effect of forces on the skull and brain. These injuries result from either primary or secondary injury to the head. Primary injury occurs as the result of direct traumatic forces. These include the forces of penetrating injuries, deceleration, acceleration, and rotation. Secondary injuries occur as a result of effects from the primary injury and include shearing forces and tension strains from extreme stretching of the neck or torsion within the cranium. In addition, the development of sustained intracranial hypertension, persistent cerebral edema, cerebral hemorrhage, seizures, systemic hypotension, hypercapnia, infection, or hypoxemia, increase the morbidity and mortality in children with TBI.

Deceleration forces occur when the head strikes an immovable object, such as the ground or the dashboard of a car. *Acceleration* forces occur when the head is struck by an object, such as from a bar or forceful hand slap. *Coup-contrecoup,* or acceleration-deceleration injuries, occur in combination (see Fig. 21-1). A decelerating force causing compression trauma to the head frequently produces a double injury to the brain: the first injury occurs when the brain strikes the cranium on the side of impact; the second occurs when the brain rebounds and strikes the cranium on the contralateral side

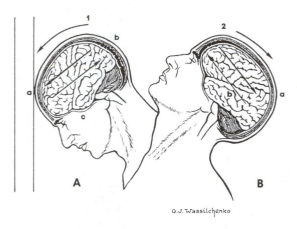

G.J. Wassilchenko

Fig. 21-1.   Coup and contrecoup head injury following blunt trauma. **A,** Coup injury: impact against object. a, Site of impact and direct trauma to brain. b, Shearing of subdural veins. c, Trauma to base of brain. **B,** Contrecoup injury: impact within skull. a, Site of impact from brain hitting opposite side of skull. b, Shearing forces through brain. These injuries occur in one continuous motion—the head strikes the wall (coup), then rebounds (contrecoup). (From Rudy E: *Advanced neurological and neurosurgical nursing,* St Louis, 1984, Mosby.)

(Chipps, Clanin, and Campbell, 1992). Contrecoup injuries are considered more severe and the size of the impact area also affects the injury severity; the smaller the area of impact the greater the severity of the injury as a result of the concentration of force in the smaller area (Walleck and Mooney, 1994).

Rotational trauma is characterized by a twisting type of deceleration which frequently occurs in combination with coup-contrecoup injuries, resulting in tension and shearing of the tissues. Blunt trauma or gunshot wounds to the brain are examples of *deformation* injuries which are the result of direct blows to the head that change the skull contour and symmetry; the higher the velocity of impact the greater the explosive effect within the cranium (Chipps, Clanin, and Campbell, 1992).

Open Versus Closed Head Injuries

Head injuries are classified as either open or closed. Open head injuries are the result of penetrating wounds or skull fractures (linear, depressed, comminuted, or perforated). Closed or blunt head

trauma can result in cerebral concussion, contusion, or laceration.

Concussion

The least serious type of traumatic brain injury is a *concussion,* which is a transient neurologic dysfunction involving immediate and transitory alterations in consciousness, equilibrium, and vision. Although the injuries may be considered minor, this can be deceiving and may lead to complications and a prolonged course of recovery. The duration of unconsciousness can be an indicator of the severity of the concussion (i.e., the longer the coma, the worse the injury). Long-term sequelae or postconcussive syndrome can include fatigue, dizziness, headache, irritability, poor concentration, memory difficulties, emotional lability, decreased attention span, and cognitive changes occurring from a week to a year after injury (Walleck and Mooney, 1994).

Contusion

Cerebral contusions result in bruising of neuronal tissue and can be accompanied by hemorrhage of surface blood vessels. Contusions are the most frequently seen lesion after a head injury. Common locations for contusions include the frontal and temporal lobes, orbital area, and, less frequently, in the occipital and parietal areas. Lacerations are also commonly seen in these areas and are more serious than contusions. Lacerations involve tearing of the cortical surface with damage to the surrounding tissues. As a result, lacerations tend to bleed profusely because of the poor vasoconstrictive ability of the cortical vasculature (Walleck and Mooney, 1994).

Diffuse Axonal Injury

Diffuse axonal injury (DAI) is more serious than a concussion and carries with it a poorer prognosis. This lesion is the most common cause of prolonged coma following a traumatic brain injury (Michaud, Duhaime, and Batshaw, 1993). The symptoms of DAI range from a mild confusion to prolonged unresponsiveness and occurs during the primary traumatic event (Slazinski and Johnson, 1994). DAI results from damage to nerve fibers produced by linear and rotational sheer strains following high-speed deceleration injuries (Coburn, 1992; Walleck

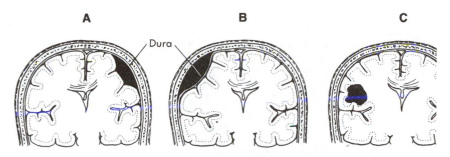

Fig. 21-2.   Different types of hematomas. **A,** Subdural. **B,** Epidural. **C,** Intracerebral. (From Thelan LA, Davie JK, Urden LD, and Lough ME: *Critical care nursing: diagnosis and management,* ed 2, St Louis, 1994, Mosby.)

and Mooney, 1994). MRI neuroimaging demonstrates small hemorrhagic lesions. Function may be lost as a result of physiologic blockage at the neuronal cell body, synapse, axons, dendrites, or any combination thereof (Slazinski and Johnson, 1994). The severity corresponds with the amount of shearing force applied. The resulting injury to the brain tissue leads to widespread cerebral edema and neuronal dysfunction. The prognosis ranges from severe disabilities to remaining in a persistent vegetative state to even death.

Secondary Head Injuries

Secondary head injuries, also known as delayed responses, are those which are preceded by the primary injury. Cerebral hemorrhage, or hematoma, results in a mass lesion effect that causes elevated intracranial pressure (see Fig. 21-2). Epidural and subdural hematomas occur outside the brain parenchyma, whereas intracerebral hematomas occur within the brain parenchyma (Coburn, 1992; Chipps, Clanin, and Campbell, 1992). Of individuals with skull fractures, 25% develop a surgically significant hematoma. Subdural hematomas are the most common type and have the highest mortality rate. They occur in approximately 10% to 20% of all traumatic brain injuries (Walleck and Mooney, 1994).

Expanding lesions, such as hematomas, and cerebral edema are major causes of increased intracranial pressure after craniocerebral trauma. This cerebral edema, either focal or generalized, is the result of an increase in tissue fluid content from intracellular or extracellular sources. It may be caused from either the initial injury to the neuronal tissue or secondarily in response to hypoxia, hypercapnia, and cerebral ischemia.

Cerebral edema following a traumatic brain injury occurs in one of two types: cytotoxic or vasogenic. *Cytotoxic* edema is intracellular and believed to be caused by an alteration in metabolic responses following hypoxia (Walleck and Mooney, 1994). It results from failure or impairment of the cation pump, allowing sodium to infiltrate into the intracellular space. Water follows into the cell because of the osmotic gradient. *Vasogenic* edema is extracellular. It is the most common type of edema and is caused damage to the cerebral vasculature. The blood-brain barrier helps to keep the normal brain water volume constant by osmotically stopping the escape of active substances to the vascular system. Vasogenic edema is believed to be a result of an alteration in the blood-brain barrier (Walleck and Mooney, 1994).

Cerebral edema peak response usually occurs up to 72 hours after the neurologic insult, and gradually resolves over a 2- to 3-week period (Walleck and Mooney, 1994). If left untreated or poorly controlled, cerebral edema can have a devastating effect resulting in intracranial hypertension and altered cerebral perfusion. This can lead to neuronal tissue hypoxia and cerebral herniation.

Brain herniation, or a shift of tissue from a compartment of high pressure to a compartment of low pressure, can occur after a traumatic brain injury if the effects of increased intracranial pressure fail to adequately respond to aggressive management. Downward displacement of the cerebellar tonsils of the lower brainstem through the foramen magnum can lead to irreversible loss of brain function. The prognosis associated with brainstem injuries is poor as a result of the brainstem's control of vital functions (Chipps, Clanin, and Campbell, 1992).

INCIDENCE

Trauma is the major cause of death in the pediatric population, with children between the ages of 1 and 19 years more likely to die from trauma than any other cause (Dandrinos-Smith, 1991). The incidence of traumatic brain injury is approximately 200 per 100,000 children annually in the United States. Head injuries are the most common injuries in the pediatric population, accounting for 4000 deaths annually (Dandrinos-Smith, 1991). Most commonly these result from falls, motor vehicle accidents, sports, and assaults. Of traumatic head injuries in children, 82% are considered mild, 14% are moderate or severe, and 5% are fatal. Approximately 20% of those children who survive will have a significant residual disability (Michaud, Duhaime, and Batshaw, 1993). Factors influencing traumatic head injury in children include gender and time of the year (increased incidence in spring and summer). Boys incur injuries twice as often as girls (Reynolds, 1992; Vernon-Levett, 1991). Peak occurrence is during evenings, nights, weekends, and holidays when children are outside playing, swimming, riding bicycles, traveling in cars, or victims of gunshot wounds.

CLINICAL MANIFESTATIONS AT TIME OF DIAGNOSIS

The clinical manifestations at the time of diagnosis will vary depending on the primary cause of head injury and the extent and involvement of associated secondary injuries.

The Glasgow Coma Scale (GCS) has become the most widely used tool to assess a child's level of consciousness (Vernon-Levett, 1991; Altimier, 1992). The GCS objectively scores the child's best responses to motor, verbal, and eye opening stimulation (see Table 21-1). The highest combined score is 15 and the lowest is 3. Any score less than a maximum of 15 is considered an alteration in the level of consciousness. GCS scores of 13 to 15 reflect a

CLINICAL MANIFESTATIONS

Assessment tools for TBI
  Glascow Coma Scale (GCS)
  Children's Coma Scale (CCS)
  Rancho Los Amigos Scale of Cognitive
    Functioning
Physical findings determined by severity and type
  of injury

minor injury, scores of 9 to 12 reflect moderate brain injury, and scores of 8 or less are considered a severe brain injury.

Despite its limitations for use in infants and young children, for other individuals with a focal deficit (such as hemiparesis) or for individuals who are intubated, this scoring method is routinely used as an assessment tool because it is universally understood and provides for a rapid assessment of the child's level of consciousness. The modified GCS has proven to be more useful for assessing the child with a head injury who is less than 2 years of age, is nonverbal, or is developmentally delayed. The GCS along with the clinician's physical assessment should be utilized in the evaluation of the child with a head injury.

A Children's Coma Score (CCS) was developed as a method of assessing infants and toddlers who are unable to speak or follow commands appropriately (see Table 21-2) (Ghajar and Hariri, 1992). The maximum score of the CCS is 11 compared with 15 on the adult GCS. Although gaining in popularity, many clinicians continue to use the GCS.

The Rancho Los Amigos Scale of Cognitive Functioning is useful in assessing the level of dysfunction (see Rancho Los Amigos Table 21-3). This table categorizes in more descriptive terms the cognitive functioning and behaviors of individuals with brain injuries. The scale is divided into eight levels that range from purposeful and appropriate responses to no response from any stimulus. It is useful in tracking the sequence of recovery from coma (Walleck and Mooney, 1994).

Table 21-1.   GLASGOW COMA SCALE

	Child >2 years old or adult		Child <2 years old or developmentally delayed	
Best eye-opening response	Spontaneously	4	Spontaneously	4
	To verbal command	3	To verbal command	3
	To pain	2	To pain	2
	No response	1	No response	1
Best verbal response	Oriented, converses	5	Coos, babbles	5
	Disoriented, converses	4	Irritable cry	4
	Inappropriate words	3	Cries to pain	3
	Incomprehensible sounds	2	Moans to pain	2
	No response	1	None	1
Best motor response				
To verbal command	Obeys	6	Spontaneous	6
To painful stimulus	Localizes pain	5	Withdraws to touch	5
	Flexion-withdrawal	4	Withdraws to pain	4
	Flexion-decorticate	3	Abnormal flexion	3
	Extension-decerebrate	2	Abnormal extension	2
	No response	1	None	1
Total		(3-15)		(3-15)

Adapted from Chipps EM, Clanin NJ, and Campbell VG: Neurologic disorders, St. Louis, 1992, Mosby, and Hazinski MF: Neurologic disorders. In Hazinski MF (editor): Nursing care of the critically ill child, St. Louis, 1992, Mosby.

Alterations in level of consciousness can range from irritability, agitation, restlessness, and confusion to coma. Acute pain can be manifested by verbalization of a headache, irritability, and crying. Skull fractures may or may not show bony displacement. Unilateral swelling may present from a possible hematoma. Asymmetry, focal neurologic deficits, cranial nerve injuries, CSF rhinorrhea or otorrhea, ecchymosis, and hearing impairments may also be evident with skull fractures.

The child with a closed head injury may have a transient period of unconsciousness with recovery in minutes to hours afterwards, along with residual amnesia and memory loss. Hemorrhage from a hematoma may first present with a transient loss of consciousness followed by a lucid period and then suddenly deteriorate with signs of rapidly increasing intracranial pressure. Seizures, unilateral pupillary changes, and hemiplegia may be present. As cerebral edema and increased intracranial pressure rise, the following may be evident: changes in level of consciousness, abnormal respiratory patterns, loss of protective reflexes (e.g., cough, gag, or corneal), changes in blood pressure and pulse pressure with bradycardia (a late sign), pupillary dysfunction, papilledema (a late sign), changes in motor function or posturing, nausea and projectile vomiting, positive Babinski's sign, and visual disturbances (Chipps, Clanin, and Campbell, 1992).

TREATMENT

Medical management begins in the prehospital setting where the goal is rapid, accurate assessment of the primary injury and the prevention or management of associated secondary injuries (Altimier, 1992). These children should be treated for cervical spine injuries until definitive neurodiagnostic studies demonstrate otherwise (Cox, 1994). Those children who are considered to be high risk for hypoxia or aspiration and are who unable to protect their airway need assistance from an artificial airway.

Table 21-2.
CHILDREN'S COMA SCALE

Maximum score = 11
Minimum score = 3
Motor response: maximum score = 4
    4   flexes and extends
    3   withdraws from painful stimulus
    2   hypertonic
    1   flaccid
Verbal response: maximum score = 3
    3   cries
    2   spontaneous respirations
    1   apneic
Ocular response: maximum score = 4
    4   pursuit
    3   extraocular muscles (EOM) intact, reactive
       pupils
    2   fixed pupils of EOM impaired
    1   fixed pupil and EOM paralyzed

Adapted from Ghajar J and Hariri R: Management of pediatric head injury, *Pediatric Clinics of North America* 39:1093-1125, 1992.

TREATMENT

- Prehospital stabilization
- Early treatment determined by severity of TBI
- Need to control for hypoxia, increased cerebral CO_2, and brain edema
- Surgical intervention for bleeding, trauma, or cerebral edema may be necessary
- Recovery from coma follows predictable patterns but with varied time sequence
- Rehabilitation program key to long-term recovery

Children with a GCS of 8 or less should be provided with intubation and hyperventilation immediately. Hypoxia before intubation exacerbates secondary injury by producing vasodilation and subsequently an increase in intracranial pressure (Walleck and Mooney, 1994).

Hyperventilation is used to control intracranial pressure by lowering the $PaCO_2$ to between 25 and 30 mm Hg, leading to vasoconstriction of cerebral vasculature (Cox, 1994). The goal with regard to circulation is to stabilize and maintain cerebral perfusion pressure above 50 mm Hg. Because neuronal tissue lacks metabolic reserves, it depends on arterial blood flow to meet its metabolic needs (Walleck and Mooney, 1994). Injuries to the cerebral contents cause edema and loss of autoregulation, increase intracranial pressure, decrease cerebral perfusion pressure, and ultimately decrease cerebral blood flow. Short-term management of hypotension with vasopressors is the favored approach to maintain adequate cerebral perfusion pressure.

To manage the excess fluid in brain tissue, fluid restriction and osmotic diuresis have been com-monly used. Maximizing oxygenation of cerebral tissues by maintaining PaO_2 at greater than 100 mm Hg is also recommended. In addition, decreasing the cerebral metabolic rate by use of sedation, paralytic agents, and barbiturate coma can be effective in lowering metabolism and cerebral blood flow, ultimately leading to further decreases in intracranial pressure (Reynolds, 1992).

Surgical management for mass lesions include craniotomies, craniectomies, cranioplasties, ventriculostomies with placement of an intracranial measuring device, and burr holes.

Recovery from Coma

Despite variations as a result of injury type and severity of traumatic brain injury, there are certain patterns of behavior commonly seen in children recovering from a head injury (Michaud, Duhaime, and Batshaw, 1993). Initially the child is either unresponsive to external stimuli or unable to localize after a painful stimulus. The child could also display a generalized, purposeless motor response. Autonomic dysfunction such as central fever, hypertension, agitation, restlessness, or diffuse intermittent diaphoresis may be seen, as well as teeth grinding. There may be spontaneous eye opening; however, there is no tracking or fixation on objects.

Emergence from a coma typically follows a variable course of waxing and waning levels of

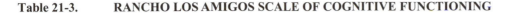

Table 21-3.   **RANCHO LOS AMIGOS SCALE OF COGNITIVE FUNCTIONING**

Level	Response	Description
1	None	Completely unresponsive to any stimulus
2	Generalized	Reacts inconsistently and nonpurposefully to stimuli; may respond with physiologic changes, gross body movements, or utterances
3	Localized	Reacts specifically but inconsistently to stimuli; responds directly to a stimulus; shows vague awareness of self and body; may pull at tubes and react to discomfort
4	Confused Agitated	Heightened state of activity but unable to process information correctly; reacts to internal confusion; nonpurposeful behavior with confabulation present; cries, screams, and manifests aggressive behavior; cannot discriminate among people; performs gross motor activities but not self-care activities
5	Confused Inappropriate	Follows simple commands; may show agitated behavior from inability to cope with external demands; gross inattention to environment, easily distracted; impaired memory and inappropriate verbalization; cannot initiate tasks; often uses things incorrectly
6	Confused Appropriate	Displays goal-directed behavior but requires direction from others; follows simple commands; shows carryover of information from previously learned tasks; memory problems persist; inconsistently oriented to time and place; increased awareness of self and others
7	Automatic Appropriate	Oriented in hospital and home settings but performs tasks in robotlike manner; superficial awareness of own condition but lacks good problem-solving abilities; carryover for new learning; independent in self-care activities; needs structure but can initiate tasks of interest
8	Purposeful Appropriate	Alert and oriented; few memory problems; can begin vocational rehabilitation; carryover for new learning; social, emotional, and intellectual capacities may be decreased from pretrauma level

Modified from original scale developed by Los Amigos Research and Education Institute, Inc. of Rancho Los Amigos Medical Center, Downey, California.
From Walleck CA and Mooney KF: Neurotrauma: head injury. In Barkin E, ed: *Neuroscience Nursing,* St. Louis, 1994, Mosby.

consciousness. Rarely is it a sudden or smooth rise to being alert and oriented. The first to notice a heightened response to external stimulation are family members or health care providers who assist in the daily activities of the child. There may be a period of intermittent agitation including behaviors such as pulling at restraints, entanglement in bed linens or equipment attached to the child, flailing or contortion of extremities, crying or moaning, and repetitive movements. There may be spontaneous eye opening; however, little recognition of familiar objects or family members will be evident. This "nightmare state" can be difficult for family members. Reassurance that posttraumatic amnesia will lessen the memories of these events can be helpful (Michaud, Duhaime, and Batshaw, 1993).

The child will begin to show increasing awareness of his or her surroundings as this agitation period begins to subside. The child may utter a familiar phrase or word, follow a simple command, show a common gesture, or visually focus on a familiar face or object. This heightened level of awareness may come and go and be initially brief in duration.

The return of consciousness can be functionally defined as the child's ability to reliably and consistently follow commands (Michaud, Duhaime, and

Batshaw, 1993). However, in aphasic or preverbal children, a more general assessment must be used in observing the child's behaviors or purposeful actions. Passive interventions such as range-of-motion exercises can then be modified to include those movements that encourage more active participation by the child. During this period of rehabilitation, assessment of the child's abnormal physical, behavioral, and cognitive problems is necessary in order to establish long-term goals (Michaud, Duhaime, and Batshaw, 1993). Behavioral problems for the child with a head injury can include altered attention span and memory, poor impulse control and emotional outbursts, and frustration at the lengthy process of rehabilitation and adaptation.

Long-Term Management and Rehabilitation

Most children who lapse into a coma as a result of a traumatic brain injury eventually regain consciousness—only a small number of children remain in a persistent vegetative state (Michaud, Duhaime, and Batshaw, 1993).

The goals of rehabilitation in the child with a head injury are to maximize abilities and functions in physical, cognitive, communicative, emotional, and social areas (Michaud, Duhaime, and Batshaw, 1993). Rehabilitation can hasten and maximize restoration of lost functions, promote adaptation to disabilities, and aid age-appropriate independence and reintegration into family and school life. Rehabilitation can enhance the quality of life of these children and can greatly reduce future health care expenditures (Osberg, DiScala, and Gans, 1990).

A child's cognitive development is incomplete at the time of injury. During the course of rehabilitation, the child undergoes whatever recovery processes occur after the injury, in addition to the naturally occurring processes of his or her development itself (Goldberg and Sachs, 1992).

Methods to accomplish rehabilitative goals include limiting problems which are secondary in nature, retraining of skills which were lost, and facilitating compensatory skills. Use of passive range-of-motion exercises, limb splinting, and proper support and positioning are methods aimed at prevention of physical deformities (e.g., extremity contractures) that result from prolonged immobilization and increased tone.

Rehabilitation must start early in the acute care phase and, for some children and their families, continue throughout life (Ylvisaker, Hartwick, and Stevens, 1991). These child survivors recover better and at a lower level of cost if they are appropriately assessed and evaluated during their acute care hospitalization and then matched with appropriate rehabilitation programs. Not all children with a serious head injury need intensive inpatient rehabilitation programs; some children do quite well at home with their families and specific supportive rehabilitation services.

A good rehabilitation plan for the management of the child with a head injury includes a coordinated, multidisciplinary team approach. It should consist of children and their families, primary care providers, specialist clinicians, nurses (during acute care, rehabilitation, and home health care), psychiatrists/psychologists, social workers, dietitians, child life therapists, physical and occupational therapists, speech and language pathologists, special educators, school counselors, and clergy who are all participants in setting realistic goals and making treatment decisions. The acute care hospital or rehabilitation center phase should include a coordinator or case manager. Once back in the home setting, the primary care provider can assume that role.

The process of rehabilitation does not stop when the child is discharged from the hospital or rehabilitation center. There needs to be continued support in the home until the quality of life obtained is maximal and acceptable to the child, family, and care providers. Respite opportunities for the family and the health care providers are important. Such opportunities should be planned for and utilized.

Regular weekly evaluation of progress and adjustment of treatment regimens should be made during the initial acute care phase. Following this, progress evaluations should be done at biweekly periods followed by monthly intervals, then as needed to justify continued rehabilitation efforts. Discharge from a rehabilitation program should be considered when reasonable treatment goals have been achieved or no further progress is demonstrated.

Reliable predictions of outcome in the child who has suffered a severe head injury should be addressed between 6 and 12 months after injury, at which point the child has regained 90% of his or her previous neurologic function (Ghajar and Hariri, 1992).

RECENT AND ANTICIPATED ADVANCES IN DIAGNOSIS AND MANAGEMENT

The question still remains: Why do some very young children respond to craniotrauma better than others? Technologic advances have aided the clinician's understanding of recovery after severe neurologic injury. These advances include recent developments in improved diagnostic technology, neurosurgical techniques, and neurologic interventions (Coburn, 1992). Recent technology has provided important information about normal human brain development and the young child's immature brain response to neurologic insult; however, clinical assessment and imaging studies are not completely reliable. A child can have a neuroimaging study that is interpreted as severely pathologic but clinically have a good outcome, and vice versa.

Advances in the areas of neurologic surgery techniques and sophisticated surgical equipment have enabled many children with a craniotrauma to live who would have otherwise died. Current research is attempting to assist the clinician in identifying those individuals who will not survive. Neurodiagnostic imaging tools including magnetic resonance images (MRI), computerized tomography (CT), positron emission tomography (PET), and cranial ultrasonography continue to be evaluated for their accuracy in initial diagnosis and sequential evaluation. In addition, their potential as long-term outcome predictors is being explored (Walker, 1993). Recently developed tools such as the Innsbruck Coma Scale and the Leeds Scale attempt to predict mortality based on admission assessments (Walleck and Mooney, 1994). These scales should be used, however, in conjunction with other assessment data in the management of children with a traumatic brain injury.

Another area of research involves the use of pharmaceutical agents to neutralize the complication that can occur during reperfusion of injured brain tissue (Reynolds, 1992). These processes include alterations in the calcium channel system, formation of oxygen-derived free radicals, and cell membrane phospholipid hydrolysis. The extent and significance of these areas and the effects of induced hypothermia in the management of pediatric head trauma are yet to be established.

ASSOCIATED PROBLEMS

Neurologic Dysfunction

Neurologic assessment protocols have been developed and may provide some insight into the child's likely course of management and outcome (see Table 21-4) (Ghajar and Hariri, 1992). Children in a coma will either meet the preestablished criteria for brain death or will respond to external stimulation within the first 2 weeks post injury. A child's eventual outcome after eye opening can range from a persistent vegetative state to the preinjury state. It should be recognized that in even the best of situations, other behavioral and personality changes may occur.

Posttraumatic hydrocephalus occurs in a small number of individuals after head trauma, most commonly in those who have suffered a subarachnoid hemorrhage. Cerebral ventriculomegaly may arise weeks or months after the craniotrauma (Humphreys, 1991). Surgical management via

ASSOCIATED PROBLEMS

- Neurologic dysfunction
    Posttraumatic hydrocephalus
    Posttraumatic meningitis
    Seizures
- Abnormal motor and sensory function
- Altered cognitive and neuropsychologic functions
- Psychosocial and psychiatric deficits
- Additional physiologic problems (See box p. 449)

Table 21-4.
STAGING PROGNOSIS
IN THE CHILD WITH A
NEUROTRAUMA INJURY

Time	Examination	Prognosis
Within 24 hours following resuscitation	Absent ocular brainstem reflexes	Poor
	GCS ≤8	Significant probability of death or major neurologic deficits
	GSC ≥8	Low probability of death but with high risk of temporary or permanent neurologic deficits
Within first week after neurotrauma with GCS <8	Patient meets brain death criteria	Follow institutional protocol
	Intracranial pressure (ICP) consistently >40 mm Hg	Significant probability of death or major neurologic deficit including persistent vegetative state
	ICP generally <20 mm Hg	Low probability of death; high probability of long-term neurologic deficits

Adapted from Walker C: The young pediatric patient: Predicting outcome after cerebral insult, *Headlines* 4:4-11, 1993.

a shunt relieves the acute symptoms (see Chapter 23).

Posttraumatic meningitis may be associated with a basilar skull fracture. Indications of cerebrospinal fluid (CSF) leakage from the nares or ear canal, periorbital ecchymosis, Battle's sign, scleral hemorrhage, fever, irritability, or an altered level of consciousness indicate the need for further assessment and CSF sampling (Humphreys, 1991).

Seizure reports vary from 2% to as high as 50% in individuals requiring hospitalization for TBI. Children who experience an open head injury have a much higher incidence as opposed to children with a closed head injury (Altimier, 1992; Walleck and Mooney, 1994). Posttraumatic seizures show no correlation with respect to age, location of skull fracture, parenchymal injury, fixed neurologic deficits, or type of cranial operation (Humphreys, 1991). Both focal and generalized seizures can occur, which increases oxygen requirements, increases the metabolic rate of neuronal tissues, and worsens ischemic injury. Seizures are usually well controlled with antiepileptic medications. The onset of these seizures varies greatly, from soon after the initial injury to 2 years following the injury. (See Chapter 19 on epilepsy).

Abnormal Motor and Sensory Function

Common motor disabilities for children following a head injury include: incoordination, quadriparesis, hemiparesis, spasticity, rigidity, tremors, decreased motor speed, and ataxia (Carney and Gerring, 1990; Michaud, Duhaime, and Batshaw, 1993). For children with any impairment at all after craniotrauma, difficulty in walking was identified as the single most frequently impaired function (DiScala et al, 1991). Tics have also been shown to occur following a central nervous system insult (e.g., anoxia secondary to trauma). As much as 10% of new onset tic disorders arise following head trauma (Moskowitz, 1994). In addition, audiologic problems and visual deficits may develop. Occupational and physical therapies are provided at regular intervals in order to maximize balance, coordination, and strength as well as to retrain in assisted (followed by independent) ambulation and other functional activities leading to developmentally appropriate self-care. Adaptive equipment may be utilized as needed, including crutches, walkers, wheelchairs, lifts, and mechanical seats. Pharmacologic management of spasticity with baclofen, dantrolene, or benzodiazepines may have variable levels of success (Michaud, Duhaime, and Batshaw, 1993).

Altered Cognitive and Neuropsychologic Function

In children who have developed verbal skills, alterations in speech and language capability can be either expressive, receptive, or mixed. In the preverbal child, delays in expressive and receptive language can be present. Deficits may be noted in the areas of memory, word retrieval, naming, verbal organization, comprehension of verbal information, comprehension of verbal abstractions, efficient verbal learning, and effective conversation and discourse. Difficulties in attention and concentration, poor judgment, and impulsivity may persist (Michaud, Duhaime, and Batshaw, 1993). There may also be perceptual impairment, poor motor planning, tactile sensory dysfunction, and spatial disorientation (Carney and Gerring, 1990). Improvement of speech is consistent with gains in motor function. Improvement in language ability (predominantly a cognitive function) may lag in severe cases despite aggressive therapy by speech and language specialists.

Psychosocial and Psychiatric Deficits

Post concussion syndrome may potentially be seen following a mild head injury or after any form of head trauma. Personality changes (which can be the most difficult to manage), mood lability, loss of self-confidence, impaired short-term memory, headaches, and subtle cognitive impairments can be present (Walker, 1993; Walleck and Mooney, 1994). There is no specific treatment. Reassurance and support for the child and family are key factors in management.

Deficits noted include: lack of goal direction and initiative, social withdrawal, depression, denial of disabilities, immature behavior, apathy, reduced self-image, self-centeredness, disinhibition, aggression, and family dysfunction (Miller, 1991; Carney and Gerring, 1990). Peer acceptance is extremely important, without which social isolation may persevere. Assistance leading to self-motivation will improve self-worth.

Additional Problems Associated with Traumatic Brain Injury

The following box lists additional physiologic problems found in children with TBI.

TRAUMATIC BRAIN INJURY SEQUELAE AND COMPLICATIONS

Focal neurologic deficits
Neurogenic pulmonary edema
Pneumonia
Gastrointestinal hemorrhage
Cardiac dysrhythmias
Syndrome of inappropriate secretion of antidiuretic hormone (SIADH)
Diabetes insipidus
Disseminated intravascular coagulation
Pulmonary emboli
Heterotopic ossifications
Increased muscle tone
Contractures
Aspiration
Hypertension
Disturbances of respiratory control
Hypopituitarism
Impaired nutritional status
Bladder incontinence
Bowel incontinence
Hyperphagia

Adapted from Chipps EM, Clanin NJ, and Campbell VG: Neurologic Disorders, St. Louis, 1992, Mosby.

PROGNOSIS

The key factor associated with overall outcome is the severity and type of traumatic brain injury. Of the children who sustain traumatic brain injury, 95% survive; however, for those children who sustain a severe head injury, there is only a 65% survival rate (Michaud, Duhaime, and Batshaw, 1993). Children with diffuse injury have better outcomes than those with focal lesions in addition to a diffuse injury. Secondary brain injuries have a significant impact on both survival and quality of cognitive and physical outcome. In addition, significant extracranial injuries, most notably involving the chest or abdomen and related problems of hypoxia and hypotension, are also associated with a poorer survival rate and outcome (Michaud, Duhaime, and Batshaw, 1993).

Despite improvements in imaging techniques and aggressive management for infants, toddlers, and young children with traumatic brain injuries, initial appearance, level of consciousness, and recovery time are still the best tools for primary care providers to determine long-term prognosis (Walker, 1993). Potential outcomes range from coma and permanent neurologic damage to a brief loss of consciousness followed by the resumption of full neurologic functioning. Of survivors with traumatic brain injury, 20% have a residual disability; 10% in mild injuries and 90% to 100% for moderate to severe injuries (Michaud, Duhaime, and Batshaw, 1993) (see box on Glasgow Outcome Scale and see Table 21-5).

The highest mortality rate occurs in children less than 2 years of age, reflecting the increased risk of physical abuse and resultant subdural hematomas. A second rise in mortality occurs during midadolescence, likely related to increased motor vehicle accidents and resultant diffuse axonal injury (Michaud, Duhaime, and Batshaw, 1993). The duration of coma is also an important factor associated with severity of the underlying brain injury— longer duration is associated with a less favorable outcome (Michaud, Duhaime, and Batshaw, 1993). The speed at which the child recovers provides a good predictive scale of how well the child will recover over the long term (Walker, 1993).

The initial Glasgow Coma Scale scores can be helpful in providing a gross predictor of outcome. In addition, other factors such as pupillary response to light and intracranial pressure measurements can improve the accuracy in predicting mortality and morbidity (Walker, 1993).

The effect of age at the time of injury on neurologic outcome is a complex factor. Cerebral water content, extent of normal myelination, level of brain development, developmental stage and amount of cortical function, and neurochemical content vary in children at different ages. Each of these factors may have an impact on brain plasticity and the potential level of functional recovery (Michaud, Duhaime, and Batshaw, 1993).

Long-term prognosis is far more difficult to evaluate. Of the large proportion of children who are survivors of severe head trauma, many will remain comatose or have permanent disabling neuro-

GLASGOW OUTCOME SCALE

Vegetative state:	No cerebral cortical function that can be judged by behavior
Severe disability:	Conscious but dependent
Moderate disability:	Independent but disabled
Good recovery:	Able to participate in normal social life and can return to daily activities

From Chipps EM, Clanin NJ, and Campbell VG: Neurologic disorders, St. Louis, 1992, Mosby.

Table 21-5.
GLASGOW COMA SCALE SCORES VS GLASGOW OUTCOMES SCALE

GCS at 24 hrs	Good recovery or moderate disability %	Vegetative or dead %
11-15	91	6
8-10	59	27
5-7	28	54
3-4	13	80

From Chipps EM, Clanin NJ, and Campbell VG: Neurologic disorders, St. Louis, 1992, Mosby.

logic damage. Although being realistic is important, the primary care provider should not convey an overly pessimistic outlook in counseling families because there have been many stories of children who have defied the odds and made remarkable recoveries. The reasons for higher percentages of good neurologic outcome in the pediatric population are unclear, although it could be attributed to the resilient properties of the immature brain.

Primary Care Management
HEALTH CARE MAINTENANCE

Growth and Development

Body growth and total development must be monitored in the child with a head injury. Head circumference measurements should be taken at each visit and recorded on a head circumference chart which plots this information versus the 50% mean value from birth to late adolescence (see Chapter 23 on hydrocephalus). For children with seizures, antiepileptic drug dosages are calculated based on body weight for therapeutic effectiveness. Alterations in growth for weight as well as height may be present because of altered nutritional intake (see diet), therefore weight and height measurements should be taken and plotted on each visit.

Precocious puberty may occur in association with central nervous system lesions including head trauma. As a result of this insult and potential disruption of the normal hypothalamus and pituitary function, children with a traumatic brain injury are at risk and should be monitored for clinical features of puberty before age 8 years in girls or age 9 years in boys. Premature sexual characteristics can take the form of isolated breast or pubic hair development. The most significant long-term complication is early epiphyseal fusion and resulting short stature as an adult. Should these sexual changes arise, referral to a pediatric endocrinologist is recommended for more in-depth management (Pescovitz, 1990).

Children who have suffered a severe head injury frequently demonstrate signs of regression and may take on infantlike behavior. Often the child is completely dependent on supportive nursing care by health professionals and family members (Appleton, 1994). In the young infant, major motor milestones are often delayed. Developmental progress should be monitored as well as progress in therapy programs. Contractures and impaired motor function may persist as a result of alterations in muscle tone, decreased range of motion, and immobility.

Diet

Feeding difficulties frequently affect children who have sustained a traumatic brain injury. These include poor manual dexterity in handling utensils, dysphagia and inability to communicate when hungry, vomiting, insufficient caloric intake to meet metabolic demands, and gastroesophageal reflux. A decreased level of arousal interferes with adequate nutrition and a negative nitrogen balance develops. Difficulty with immobility may lead to increased bone calcium loss as a result of inadequate weight bearing (Boss, 1994). Management of these nutritional difficulties usually begins with hyperalimentation during the acute phase and then transition to high-calorie, gastric tube feedings when bowel function is stabilized. At this point, tube feedings may continue for an indefinite period of time. Placement of a gastrostomy tube and fundoplication may be considered for long-term management. Potential aspiration or gastroesophageal reflux concerns may be addressed by placing the child in a side-lying position during and after meals.

Once the level of consciousness has improved along with an intact cough and gag reflex, occupational and speech therapy can assist in optimizing feeding positions, evaluating swallowing function, facilitate coordinated tongue-lip-jaw control, and promote oral desensitization. Alterations in smell and taste also may be associated with feeding difficulties (Michaud, Duhaime, and Batshaw, 1993). Disability in the dominant hand will require new spatial and motor learning for effective self feeding.

Oral hygiene, mucosal and tongue lesions, and poor dentition may affect appetite, as well as depression, overstimulation, fatigue, and frustration with trying to relearn how to self-feed. Cognitive or behavioral deficits can cause poor intake through problems with confusion, inability to concentrate, attentional deficits, and distractibility.

Children who need to learn new eating skills may be unable to eat without repeated cueing and supervision (Whitney, 1994). Soft foods that are easy to swallow should be offered with assistance in feeding. Inadequate oral intake of a high-calorie, balanced diet consisting of three small meals with three snacks during the daytime may be supplemented by tube feedings at nighttime. Weight should be monitored at regular intervals, more frequently if there is evidence of inadequate weight gain or the presence of excessive weight gain as a result of poor motor function and decreased physical activity. In addition, supplementation of vitamins and minerals may be considered to address the amount of calcium loss.

Safety

Safety practices and injury prevention are important in children who have previously sustained a traumatic brain injury. These children are at an increased risk for future injury as a result of neuropsychologic and neurobehavioral deficits resulting in overactivity, poor judgment, impulsivity, and perceptual deficits (Michaud, Duhaime, and Batshaw, 1993). Keeping an environment free of clutter, sharp angled objects, steps, or uneven surfaces is recommended along with adequate anticipatory supervision as independence increases (see Chapter 26 on learning disabilities). Assistive devices (e.g., wheelchairs and walkers) should be assessed for safety and kept in repair (Whitney, 1994). Consideration of appropriate emergency exit routes from the home and other locations should be evaluated. Family members and care providers should be knowledgeable in regard to seizure precautions and seizure first aid (see Chapter 19 on epilepsy).

Use of appropriate motor vehicle passenger seat restraints, helmets, and home child-proofing should be reinforced. Normal childhood activities such as bike riding, swimming, gymnastics, and softball should be considered for each individual child with regard to the benefits gained from active participation versus the possible risks. The adolescent with post TBI may have increased safety risks as a result of neuropsychiatric sequelae impairing judgment and motor-coordination. Parents may need assistance in determining appropriate adolescent responsibilities and activities.

Immunization

Infants and children with head injuries and posttraumatic seizures are at a slightly increased risk of having a seizure after receiving either the diphtheria, tetanus, and pertussis (DTP) vaccine or the measles vaccine (Committee on Infectious Diseases, 1994). Withholding these immunizations during the acute phase should be considered. The immunizations can be given when the neurologic situation is stabilized. Postimmunization fever management with acetaminophen is recommended for children with seizures.

Discussion of the risk of contracting these diseases versus the risk of the vaccine's side effects should be discussed with the family. Consultation with the child's neurologist is recommended during the acute and rehabilitation period. Known exposure to a vaccine-preventable illness can be managed with disease-specific immunoglobulin therapy.

Screening

Vision and hearing. A thorough evaluation is recommended 6 to 8 weeks post injury during the recovery period (Humphreys, 1991). Both vision and hearing can be adversely affected in the child following a traumatic brain injury. Formal evaluation including brainstem auditory or visual evoked potentials should be considered in assessing function. Mild deficits of either disorder should be corrected if possible in order to facilitate recovery (Michaud, Duhaime, and Batshaw, 1993). Continued routine periodic screening is recommended if deficits are not determined in the immediate postinjury period.

Dental. Routine dental care is recommended. The child with a head injury may have fractured or missing teeth secondary to facial trauma. Use of sedation may be necessary for dental work if voluntary cooperation is difficult as a result of spasticity. Assessment of gingival hyperplasia is recommended with more frequent dental examinations at 3-month intervals for children on phenytoin (Dilantin) therapy. For persistent bruxism, a mouth guard should be considered.

Blood pressure. Routine screening as well as evaluation during episodic visits are recommended. Persistently elevated blood pressure should be evaluated, including assessment of the blood pressure on all four extremities, particularly in the presence of an intracranial shunt.

Hematocrit. Routine screening is recommended.

Urinalysis. Bi-monthly screening is recommended for the first 6 months post head injury to rule out indication of trauma or diabetes insipidus. Afterwards, routine screening is recommended.

Tuberculosis. Routine screening is recommended. If prophylactic medications are needed, evaluate potential drug interactions in children on anticonvulsant therapy. Consultation with the child's neurologist and pharmacist are recommended.

Condition-specific screening

POSTTRAUMATIC SEIZURE THERAPY. Complete blood cell counts and chemistry panels to assess for blood dyscrasias and liver dysfunction are recommended. This screening should be done biweekly then monthly for 6 months post injury, then periodically thereafter. Anticonvulsant medications must be titrated for therapeutic effect and management of adverse side effects. Repeat drug levels should be done within 2 weeks of adjustments in dosage (see Chapter 19 on epilepsy).

COMMON ILLNESS MANAGEMENT

Differential Diagnosis

Alterations in cognition or level of consciousness. As the primary care provider, a thorough

---

DIFFERENTIAL DIAGNOSIS

- Need to know child's current baseline neurologic status
- Respiratory tract infections—children with severe neurologic or motor deficits are more prone to complications such as pneumonia or aspiration
- Nausea and vomiting—may be indicative of shunt malfunction in child with posttraumatic hydrocephalus. Prolonged or severe vomiting may require aggressive rehydration in child with poor nutritional intake.
- Skin rashes—evaluate for possible allergic reaction to medication, especially anticonvulsant drugs
- Headaches—post TBI often associated with frequent headaches. Headache diaries may help determine frequency, intensity, and effectiveness of mild analgesics.

---

knowledge of the child's baseline health and neurological status, level of consciousness, and behavior is the key to accurate assessment. Children with impairment to their neurologic system are more at risk for developing an acute illness. A significant change in cognitive functions should be viewed as pathologic and assessed (Boss, 1994). Many different etiologies may produce decreases in arousal or cognition. Various types of trauma, infections, tumors, and metabolic imbalances may cause such alterations. The severity of the pathology as well as the site of the pathology can often determine whether this is an acute exacerbation of the child's chronic condition or a new focus. The onset may be sudden, subacute over a period of several days, or progressive over several weeks to months. Fevers should be assessed early, especially in children with seizures (see Chapter 19).

Respiratory tract infections. Upper respiratory tract illnesses are common in children and adolescents. Acute illnesses such as fever, otitis media, and other respiratory infections may exacerbate the manifestations of post TBI (e.g., worsening posttraumatic seizure pattern or level of consciousness) and should be appropriately monitored and treated (Martinez, Schreiber, and Hartman, 1991). Children with severe motor or neurologic sequelae will need to be evaluated closely for respiratory complications such as pneumonia and aspiration. Any adjustments to antiepileptic medications should be withheld until after the acute phase of the respiratory illness has passed.

Common infectious diseases such as varicella, rubella, or rubeola can cause potentially serious complications such as pneumonia or worsening encephalopathy in the child with a serious head injury. Any signs of acute deterioration should be urgently evaluated and further treatment initiated.

Nausea and vomiting. Symptoms of nausea and vomiting are of concern, particularly in the child with an intracranial shunt. Mild gastrointestinal symptoms should be evaluated and then reevaluated in 24 to 48 hours by telephone or a return appointment with close follow-up by the family or primary care provider. Fluid rehydration either orally or via gastroesophageal or gastrostomy tube may be necessary in the child with severe vomiting or difficulty feeding. Persistent vomiting or developing lethargy should be evaluated urgently.

Skin rashes. The onset of skin rashes should be evaluated for early signs of a possible allergic reaction, particularly in cases where a new anticonvulsant has been initiated for seizure management. Potentially serious complications may require consideration of alternate anticonvulsant therapies.

Headaches. Posttraumatic headaches can be a frequent concern, especially in the older child. Use of a 2-week log by the family or primary care provider can be extremely valuable in recording patterns of onset, frequency, and relief-producing actions. Symptom management with mild analgesics is usually adequate. If the headaches persist in frequency to a chronic pattern, as indicated by continuation of the headache log book, further evaluation is recommended.

Drug Interactions

Drug interactions between multiple medications, in particular multiple anticonvulsants, should be evaluated. The use of antihistamines with anticonvulsants should be done with caution. The use of erythromycin-based antibiotics should be avoided with carbamazepine (Tegretol). Aspirin can alter therapeutic effects of anticonvulsants and should be used with caution. Acetaminophen is recommended instead of aspirin (see Chapter 19 on epilepsy). The use of stimulant medications (e.g., Ritalin, Dexedrine, Cylert) can result in a prolonged half-life of many anticonvulsants (e.g., Dilantin, Mysoline, Phenobarbitol) (see Chapter 26 on learning disabilities). Consultation with a pharmacist and the child's neurologist may be indicated.

DEVELOPMENTAL ISSUES

Sleep Patterns

Alterations in the child's sleep-wake cycle may result from the irregular pattern experienced during the acute phase of management. The child may experience excessive wakefulness or insomnia and irregular sleep patterns, or he or she may be fearful and experience nightmares as a result of the recent head injury. Alterations in the child's sleep routine may lead to difficulties in the family's or care provider's sleeping routine because of the need for adequate supervision. A 2-week sleep log may be helpful in identifying specific patterns.

Irregular sleep-wake patterns are generally managed with behavioral therapy. A schedule of daily activities may be necessary to develop a consistent pattern. A regular bedtime that allows a sleep period of 8 to 10 hours should be established with a short daytime nap if needed. A regular arousal time in the morning can strengthen circadian rhythms and can lead to regular times of sleep onset. Regular daily exercise can deepen existing sleep patterns. A soothing evening bath or shower can offer increased relaxation. A light snack may enhance sleep. Caffeinated beverages (e.g., tea, soda, cocoa) may need to be withheld. The number and duration of any daytime naps may need to be limited (Boss, 1994). Timing of medication doses may need to be adjusted if a correlation with sleep patterns is identified. Encouraging verbalization of fears and concerns and the use of relaxation techniques may be helpful. Appropriate pain management also should be addressed.

Transient insomnia is treated symptomatically with short-term use of antihistimines (for their sedative effect) or intermediate-acting hypnotics (e.g., chloral hydrate). Long-acting hypnotics are contraindicated because of impairment in daytime functioning (Boss, 1994).

Toileting

Bowel and bladder continence may be disrupted in the older child who had voluntary control before the head injury. Establishment of a progressive training program with positive reinforcement as cognition increases will assist in regaining control (Kersenbrock, Kirchner, and Sammons, 1983). This routine may also be helpful for younger children as they are ready for toilet training.

Routine toileting every 2 hours can reduce the incidence of incontinence. Longer interval periods are introduced as continence is achieved. The goal should be to obtain bowel and bladder control during the waking hours and then progress to nighttime hours. The child should be monitored for an adequate fluid intake during the daytime hours with limitation of fluid intake near bedtime. Caffeinated beverages (e.g., tea, soda) may need to be withheld during the training schedule (Whitney, 1994). Appropriately sized disposable diapers, easy to manipulate clothing, and adaptive equipment can assist in the training program. In addition, labeling bathroom doors with large pictures and use of a night light in the room at night may be helpful (Bunting and Fitzsimmons, 1994).

Children with a head injury who are immobile can be prone to constipation as well. They may require the use of natural or medicated stool softeners, glycerin suppositories, additional fluid intake, dietary bulk expanders, or manual rectal stimulation for assisted elimination (Coffman, 1992).

Discipline

Alterations in behavior and personality should be anticipated, even following mild brain injury. The most common behavioral changes noted are social withdrawal, decreased attention span, hyperactivity, aggression, and poor anger control. If deficits secondary to traumatic brain injury persist, they may lead to future behavior and learning problems. The child may have changes in temperament including apathy, poor motivation, and being socially withdrawn, or the child may be hyperactive, irritable, impulsive, aggressive, or inattentive (Michaud, Duhaime, and Batshaw, 1993).

Parents and primary care providers need to be encouraged to remain consistent with discipline and reinforce normal household rules as much as possible (Diamond, 1994). Persistent behavior difficulties in the home environment, altered family and peer relationships, disruption in the school setting, or issues in the use of leisure time can lead to interruption in learning situations.

Difficulties with behavior and discipline are generally managed with behavioral therapy. Clear, simple expectations explained at an appropriate cognitive level for the child should be established. Consistency between care providers in their style of discipline and behavior management is important in order to avoid giving mixed messages of what is appropriate and acceptable behavior. Regular periods of unrestricted physical activity can be helpful in allowing for release of excessive energy. Role modeling of acceptable behavior should be done by the parents, care providers, and other family members. Acceptable behaviors should be positively reinforced. Unacceptable behaviors should have an appropriate consequence.

Referral and evaluation by a behavior specialist should be considered for persistent behavior suggestive of attention deficit disorder syndrome.

These problems are often more easily recognized in the school setting, where the group situation may provide distractions that intensify the child's attentional difficulties (Cantwell and Baker, 1987). The primary care provider will be able to assist in coordination and collection of the data for a comprehensive evaluation from the parents, school teachers, the child, and from significant others in the child's life. Several standardized behavior rating scales can be utilized for assessment (Kelly and Aylward, 1992).

Appropriate assessment and management in a multidimensional, interdisciplinary, and adaptive behavior modification program should: (1) reflect a developmental base, (2) survey multiple developmental and behavioral dimensions, (3) use several norm-based, curriculum-based, and clinical judgment scales, (4) blend the assessments of several team members and parents or care providers, (5) link assessment and curriculum goals, (6) adapt tasks for various disabilities, and (7) monitor the child's program (Bagnato et al, 1988).

Pharmacologic management with the use of stimulants (e.g., Ritalin, Dexedrine, Cylert) or other psychotropic medications (e.g., Clonidine) may be considered (see Chapter 26). These medications should never be used as an isolated treatment program and should be initiated on a trial basis (Kelly and Aylward, 1992; Campbell and Cohen, 1990).

Child Care

Short-term child care or longer periods of respite care have frequently been identified by families as priority needs (Coffman, 1992). The majority of care to meet the needs of these children's activities of daily living is provided by household members (Folden and Coffman, 1993). Mildly disabled children may be appropriately cared for in a day care or home care setting. Severely disabled children often required assisted nursing care in the home.

Respite care is the temporary care of a disabled child for the purpose of providing relief to the primary caregiver (Folden and Coffman, 1993). Respite care can provide an important gift of time and potential peace of mind. This time can be used to go on errands, provide a needed vacation from the day-to-day activities of providing care, spend extra time with other family members, or become involved in new activities. Respite providers must be aware that while their assistance is very supportive, their presence can also be disruptive to the family dynamics and relationships (Coffman, 1992). Federal funds from Title XX of the Social Security Act are available for respite services, homemaker services, and foster home care (Folden and Coffman, 1993).

For children in a day care or preschool setting, an Individualized Health Plan (IHP) can be useful in communicating medical information with early childhood educators and individual curriculum goals (Donlin-Shore, 1993.)

Schooling

Discharge from an acute care or rehabilitation facility marks a return to normalcy for the child and his or her family. However, it can also be a time of confrontation with the realities of the physical, cognitive, psychiatric, or neuropsychologic impairments as a result of the brain injury.

A critical phase in recovery for the child with a head injury is the return to school. Successful school reentry is determined by intellect and cognitive ability, social skills, and peer relationships. Initially, home schooling, tutoring, or part-time attendance may be appropriate on return to a school program, especially if limited endurance or fatigue problems are present.

Cognitive recovery ranges from a return to preinjury ability to severely impaired intellectual function and is often not as complete as motor function recovery (Michaud, Duhaime, and Batshaw, 1993). Unlike other special education students who have a stable neurologic status, children who have experienced a traumatic brain injury continue to change neurologically for weeks, months, and even years following resumption of their school program (Ylvisaker, Hartwick, and Stevens, 1991). In the young child with a head injury, particularly in the preschool age, many of the school difficulties may not occur until 2 or 3 years later when the child is expected to develop math and reading skills.

Post head injury behavior and cognitive difficulties may be sufficient to interfere with learning in a mainstream classroom setting and referral for special education evaluation and services is war-

ranted. Public Law 101-476, the Individuals with Disabilities Education Act of 1990, identifies traumatic brain injury as a specific disability category within special education (Michaud, Duhaime, and Batshaw, 1993). Parents and family members should be introduced early to advocacy skills that will assist in developing an IEP.

Neuropsychologic deficits can include information processing, impaired attention and memory, problem-solving skills, processing of abstract information, judgment, and organizational skills. Performance IQ can be more adversely affected than verbal IQ (Michaud, Duhaime, and Batshaw, 1993). Neurobehavioral and neuropsychologic problems may not be recognized as resulting from a previous traumatic brain injury, especially if there has been a long interval of time between the injury and detection of deficits. Formal neuropsychologic and school performance testing can be helpful in identification of problems and development of an IEP.

Depending on the depth of persistent deficits, children with traumatic brain injury can receive services ranging from regular classes with help in a resource room to special education classes, speech-language therapy, occupational or physical therapies, special services for hearing or visual impairments, behavior management, and counseling as components of the child's IEP (Carney and Gerring, 1990; Michaud, Duhaime, and Batshaw, 1993). Flexibility in educational programming is of utmost importance as the children's changing profile may at no point resemble that of other children who are classified under existing special education categories (Ylvisaker, Hartwick, and Stevens, 1991). The child's strengths and weaknesses should be identified and utilized in the IEP assessment and planning process. Family counseling in regard to realistic performance expectations and anticipatory guidance for the parents and primary care providers in their role as the child's advocate in the school reentry process are important and should be emphasized.

Sexuality

Individuals who have sustained a head injury may have altered inhibitions or may make socially inappropriate sexual comments and gestures. Impairment in motor and sensory function or impaired communication may alter sexual functioning. Concerns regarding sexuality expressed by the child or adolescent, family, and significant others should be addressed early (Miller, 1991; Chipps, Clanin, and Campbell, 1992). For adolescents, educational programs or counseling sessions should include the topics of sexuality, substance abuse, and other risk-taking behaviors. For female adolescents on long-term antiepileptic medication, consideration of teratogenic effects should be made when prescribing or altering medications (see Chapter 19).

Transition into Adulthood

Traumatic brain injury may have a major impact on the subsequent education, vocational development, independent living skills, and future productivity of the affected adolescent. Supported living programs, supervised housing, shared services, or foster care should be evaluated with respect to level of assistance provided for the activities of daily living (Jackson, 1994). School guidance and vocational counselors should be aware of the importance of appropriate work experiences for children and adolescents with a head injury such as is offered in adult rehabilitation programs (Goldberg and Sachs, 1992). Supervised work experiences may be necessary to develop appropriate skills, work habits, and attitudes in order to succeed in gainful employment and contribute to the community (Ylvisaker, Hartwick, and Stevens, 1991). In addition, health care insurance coverage and financial assistance programs should be addressed as the adolescent enters adulthood.

SPECIAL FAMILY CONCERNS AND RESOURCES

Severe stresses on the family unit arise following the sudden occurrence of a head injury. Although difficult to predict, families want to know exactly how their child is going to be at the end of the recovery period. They want to know whether their child will have the same intelligence, personality, and sensory motor functions that were present before the head injury. The need of the parents to deal with the physical, social, cognitive, and communicative changes is emotionally draining, especially if there is a likelihood of permanent disability (Miller, 1991; Michaud, Duhaime, and Batshaw,

1993). An uncertain outcome followed by numerous weeks and months of medical treatment further contributes to the family's stress. Parents, family members, and primary care providers should be encouraged to become actively involved in the day-to-day care of the child. This will reduce their sense of helplessness and result in confidence building (Appleton, 1994). They should be actively involved in any recommendations or decision. Support groups or family counseling for both parents and siblings may be of assistance during the rehabilitation and recovery period in order to express and discuss any concerns or anxieties (Miller, 1991; Appleton, 1994).

The primary caretaker, usually the mother, may have difficulty meeting the care needs of the injured child and the needs of the spouse and siblings. The noncaretaker parent, usually the father, may feel neglected by the exhausted mother who is coping with the child for the majority of the daytime hours. Often, there are unresolved feelings of denial, guilt, and remorse. It is not uncommon for marriages to dissolve within 1 to 2 years following the onset of a significant brain impairment in a child (Miller, 1991).

Siblings of the child who had the head injury also suffer from a loss of parental attention and may demonstrate guilt feelings. Many siblings may initially experience a sense of relief that the injury happened to their brother or sister and not to them, followed by a sense of guilt over having been spared. Younger siblings may fear that the same thing or worse may happen to them (Miller, 1991).

Significant financial issues and conflict related to the parents' return to work may arise, further adding to the family's stress. Long-term family support and counseling should be advocated.

Use of a home health record would assist parents and primary care providers in organizing health care information about the child's disabilities and ongoing health condition. As an adjunct to formal medical records, this health summary could be used during periods of respite care or travel. Components of a home health record include: emergency medical information, birth history, hospitalizations, medications used, information about primary health care, growth and nutrition, use of special equipment or supportive devices, daily schedule and special care routines, therapy and communication needs, and toileting regimen (Smigielski and Parton, 1992).

Head trauma in the pediatric population does not discriminate and can occur in all walks of life. Despite the tremendous benefits of family centered care, cultural differences may become a barrier to adequate services. Differences in English-speaking capability, level of literacy, knowledge of the sophisticated level of care required, coordination of health services, compliance in the treatment regimen, and adequacy of health care resources based on legal residency status are all issues to be addressed by these families. Primary health care providers are in a key position to assist in providing comprehensive care services that are congruent with and respectful toward the child's and family's cultural background (Folden and Coffman, 1993).

Caring for a child with a head injury is a complex task because of the numerous physical, cognitive, and psychosocial concerns that must be addressed. The following is a list of additional resources for professionals as well as for parents and primary care providers of these children:

Neurologic Organizations

American Speech, Language, Hearing Association
    10801 Rockville Pike
    Rockville, MD 20852
    (301) 897-5700

Brain Injury Association
    1776 Massachusetts Ave NW, Suite 100
    Washington, DC 20036-1904
    (800) 444-6443 or 202/296-6443
National Rehabilitation Information Center
    8455 Colesville Rd, Suite 935
    Silver Spring, MD 20910
    (301) 588-9284
Rehabilitation Services Administration
    Department of Human Services, Rm 101M
    605 G Street NW
    Washington, DC 20001
    (202) 727-3211

Neurologic Organizations for Professionals

American Association of Neuroscience Nurses
    224 N Des Plaines, Suite 601
    Chicago, IL 60661
    (312) 993-0043
American Congress of Rehabilitative Medicine
    5700 Old Orchard Rd
    Skokie, IL 60077
    (708) 966-0095
Association of Rehabilitation Nurses
    5700 Old Orchard Rd, 1st Floor
    Skokie, IL 60077-1024
    (708) 966-3433

SUMMARY OF THE PRIMARY CARE NEEDS FOR THE CHILD WITH A HEAD INJURY

Health care maintenance

Growth and development

Height, weight, and head circumference should be assessed to monitor growth. Medications (e.g., anticonvulsants) are based on current accurate weight measurements for therapeutic effectiveness.

Delayed development may be present. Regularly screen and assess cognitive and motor skills. Interventional therapy programs are recommended.

Monitor for early signs of precocious puberty and short stature.

Diet

Eating and feeding problems contribute to poor growth patterns. Decreased physical activity and immobility may lead to excessive weight gain. Tailor dietary intake to meet the child's caloric needs.

Regularly monitor protective reflexes to prevent potential of aspiration and determine need for fundoplication with feeding tube placement.

Occupational and speech therapy can assist with optimal feeding programs.

Safety

Increased risk of injury is present as a result of instability, incoordination, potential seizures, and delays in motor skill acquisition.

Provide ongoing anticipatory guidance in general safety precautions.

Review emergency seizure procedures, helmet use for certain seizure types.

Use caution with risk-taking sports and activities, evaluate emergency exit routines.

Immunization

Avoid routine immunizations until child is well into postinjury recovery stage.

Children with posttraumatic seizures are at increased risk of having a seizure following a DPT or measles vaccine. Pertussis vaccine may be deferred and DT used instead. Benefit of measles immunization should be evaluated versus risk of contracting disease with potentially serious complications in endemic areas.

Fever prophylaxis with acetaminophen is recommended.

Other immunizations are given as recommended.

Screening

Vision

A complete evaluation is recommended 6 to 8 weeks post injury during the recovery period, with correction of minor deficits.

Hearing

A complete evaluation is recommended 6 to 8 weeks post injury during the recovery period, with correction of minor deficits.

Dental

Routine screening is recommended.

Evaluate for dental trauma post head injury.

More frequent evaluations may be necessary for children on phenytoin.

Blood pressure

Monitor blood pressure with each visit. Assess elevations from baseline.

Hematocrit

Routine screening is recommended.

Hematologic monitoring for chronic medication therapy may be warranted.

Urinalysis

Monitor periodically for the first 6 months post head injury. Afterward, routine screening is recommended.

Tuberculosis

Routine screening is recommended. If prophylactic medications are needed, evaluate potential drug interactions in children on anticonvulsant therapy.

Condition-specific screening

POST TRAUMATIC SEIZURE THERAPY

Monitor complete blood cell counts and chemistry panels along with anticonvulsant levels for the first 6 months postinjury and periodically thereafter.

Continued.

SUMMARY OF THE PRIMARY CARE NEEDS FOR THE CHILD WITH A HEAD INJURY—cont'd

Common illness management

Differential diagnosis

A thorough knowledge of the baseline level of health and neurologic status, level of consciousness, and behavior is key in assessing significant pathologic deviations.

Risk of seizures is increased with acute illness and fever. Closely observe, maintain hydration, and provide antipyretic therapy. Children with severe motor or neurologic sequelae must be monitored for respiratory complications.

Common communicable diseases may result in high incidence of pulmonary or neurologic complications.

Evaluate potential for increased intracranial pressure in the presence of an intracranial shunt with signs of nausea and vomiting.

Skin rashes must be evaluated for possible indication of allergic reactions to chronic medication therapy.

Evaluation of headaches will require careful history and symptom management.

Drug interactions

Altered therapeutic effects have been seen between several antiepileptic medications and certain antibiotics, antihistamines, behavior stimulants, and aspirin. Careful monitoring is required.

Developmental issues

Sleep patterns

Disruption in sleep patterns may be evident. A structured behavioral program is recommended.

Toileting

Bowel and bladder continence may be delayed in the younger child or disrupted in the older child who previously had voluntary control. Establishment of a progressive training program with positive reinforcement as cognition increases will assist in regaining control.

Discipline

Alterations in behavior and personality should be anticipated with early guidance counseling instituted. Standard developmentally appropriate discipline is recommended with reinforcement of normal household rules.

Persistent difficulties with behavior and discipline are managed with behavioral therapy. Referral and evaluation by a behavior specialist may be warranted.

Child care

Child care and respite care have been identified as priority needs by the primary caretakers. Assistance in this area is priority.

Schooling

Cognitive changes continue to occur from weeks to months following the recovery from head trauma.

Assessment of learning needs must be fully individualized and addressed as soon as feasible post injury. Public Law 94-142 and 99-457 outline mandated educational programs.

Families may require assistance with IEP process.

Toddlers and preschoolers need close monitoring because of increasing cognitive demands with age.

Formal neuropsychologic and school performance testing may be necessary.

Sexuality

Impairment in the motor and sensory function or impaired communication may alter sexual functioning. Anticipatory guidance in counseling is advised.

Transition in adulthood

Traumatic brain injury can have a major impact on the future education, vocational development, and independent living skills of the affected adolescent. School guidance and vocational counseling are recommended.

Continued.

SUMMARY OF THE PRIMARY CARE NEEDS FOR THE CHILD WITH A HEAD INJURY—cont'd

Special family concerns

Severe stresses on the family unit arise following the sudden occurrence of a head injury. Support groups or family counseling for parents and siblings may be helpful.

Cultural differences can be considered a barrier to adequate services despite the benefits of family centered care. Comprehensive care that is congruent with and respectful toward the child's and family's cultural background is a key element.

REFERENCES

Altimier LB: Pediatric central neurologic trauma: issues for special patients, *AACN Clin Issues* 3:31-41, 1992.

Appleton R: Head injury rehabilitation for children, *Nurs Times* 90:29-31, 1994.

Bagnato SJ et al: An interdisciplinary neurodevelopmental assessment model for brain-injured infants and preschool children, *J Head Trauma Rehabil* 3:75-86, 1988.

Boss BJ: Coma and cognitive deficits. In E Barker, (editor): *Neuroscience nursing,* St Louis, 1994, Mosby, pp 175-202.

Bunting L, Fitzsimmons F: Degenerative disorders. In E Barker, (editor): *Neuroscience nursing,* St Louis, 1994, Mosby, pp 517-535.

Campbell LR, Cohen M: Management of attention deficit hyperactivity disorder: a continuing dilemma for physicians and educators, *Clin Pediatr* 29:191-193, 1990.

Cantwell DP, Baker L: Attention-deficit disorder in children: the role of the nurse practitioner, *Nurse Pract* 12:38, 43-44, 46-48, 50-51, 54, 1987.

Carney J, Gerring J: Return to school following severe closed head injury: a critical phase in pediatric rehabilitation, *Pediatrician* 17:222-229, 1990.

Chipps EM, Clanin NJ, and Campbell VG: *Neurologic disorders,* St Louis, 1992, Mosby.

Coburn D: Traumatic brain injury: the silent epidemic, *AACN Clin Issues* 3:9-18, 1992.

Coffman SP: Home care of the child and family after near drowning, *J of Pediatr Health Care* 6:18-24, 1992.

Committee on Infectious Diseases: *Report of the committee on infectious diseases,* ed 23, Elk Grove Village, IL, 1994, The American Academy of Pediatrics.

Cox SA: Pediatric trauma: special patients/special needs, *Crit Care Nurs Q* 17:51-61, 1994.

Dandrinos-Smith S: The epidemiology of pediatric trauma, *Crit Care Nurs Clin North Am* 3:387-389, 1991.

Diamond J: Family-centered care for children with chronic illness, *J of Pediatr Health Care* 8:196-197, 1994.

DiScala C et al: Children with traumatic head injury: morbidity and postacute treatment, *Arch Phys Med Rehabil* 72:662-666, 1991.

Donlin-Shore K: The hospital to preschool transition: new guidelines for clinicians, *Headlines* 4:25-28, 1993.

Folden SL, Coffman S: Respite care for families of children with disabilities, *J Pediatr Health Care* 7:103-110, 1993.

Ghajar J, Hariri R: Management of pediatric head injury, *Pediatr Clin North Am* 39:1093-1125, 1992.

Goldberg AL, Sachs PR: A guide to evaluating residential postacute programs for children and adolescents with brain injury, *J Cognit Rehabil* 10:28-32, 1992.

Hazinski MF: Neurologic disorders. In MF Hazinski, (editor): *Nursing care of the critically ill child,* St Louis, 1992, Mosby, pp 521-528.

Humphreys RP: Complications of pediatric head injury, *Pediatr Neurosurg* 17:274-278, 1991.

Jackson JD: After rehabilitation: meeting the long-term needs of persons with traumatic brain injury, *Am J Occup Ther* 48:251-255, 1994.

Kelly DP, Aylward GP: Attention deficits in school-aged children and adolescents: current issues and practice, *Pediatr Clin North Am* 39:487-512, 1992.

Kersenbrock P, Kirchner KM, and Sammons J: Transdisciplinary approach to a brain injured child, *Rehabil Nurs* 8:22-23, 26-27, 1983.

Martinez NH, Schreiber ML, and Hartman EW: Pediatric nurse practitioners: primary care providers and case managers for chronically ill children at home, *J Pediatr Health Care* 5:291-298, 1991.

Michaud LJ, Duhaime AC, and Batshaw ML: Traumatic brain injury in children, *Pediatr Clin North Am* 40:553-565, 1993.

Miller L: Significant others: treating brain injury in the family context, *J Cognit Rehabil* 9:16-25, 1991.

Moskowitz C: Movement disorders. In E Barker, (editor): *Neuroscience nursing,* St Louis, 1994, Mosby, pp 536-558.

Osberg JS, DiScala C, and Gans BM: Utilization of inpatient rehabilitation services among traumatically injured children discharged from pediatric trauma centers, *Am J of Phys Med Rehabil* 69:67-72, 1990.

Pescovitz OH: Precocious puberty, *Pediatrics in Review* 11:229-237, 1990.

Reynolds EA: Controversies in caring for the child with a head injury, *MCN* 17:246-251, 1992.

Slazinski T, Johnson MC: Severe diffuse axonal injury in adults and children, *J Neurosci Nurs* 26:151-154, 1994.

Smigielski PA, Parton E: A home health record for children with chronic health conditions, *J Pediatr Health Care* 6:121-126, 1992.

Vernon-Levett P: Head injuries in children, *Crit Care Nurs Clin North Am* 3:411-421, 1991.

Walker C: The young pediatric patient: predicting outcome after cerebral insult, *Headlines* 4:4-11, 1993.

Walleck CA, Mooney KF: Neurotrauma: head injury. In Barker E (editor): *Neuroscience nursing,* St Louis, 1994, Mosby, pp 324-351.

Whitney F: Stroke. In E Barker, (editor): *Neuroscience nursing,* St Louis, 1994, Mosby, pp 469-515.

Ylvisaker M, Hartwick P, and Stevens M: School reentry following head injury: managing the transition from hospital to school, *J Head Trauma Rehabil* 6:10-22, 1991.

HIV Infection and AIDS

22

Rita Fahrner and Mindy Benson

ETIOLOGY

The human immunodeficiency virus (HIV) causes a continuum of infection to occur, and the end stage of that infectious process is called acquired immune deficiency syndrome (AIDS). The HIV type 1 (HIV-1) belongs to the family of retroviruses, which means that its viral RNA is copied into DNA using the enzyme reverse transcriptase. This virus selectively infects the T-helper (T4 or CD4) subset of T-cell lymphocytes. Other cells that express CD4, such as monocytes, macrophages, and glial cells, are capable of becoming infected, as are some cells without detectable cell surface CD4. Through a process of replication, HIV perpetuates and integrates itself into the genetic material of the organism it infects (Demmler and Taber, 1990). The primary pathologic condition of HIV causes specific immunodeficiency that destroys the host's ability to withstand infection. In addition, the HIV directly invades other major organ systems, including the peripheral and central nervous system (CNS), lungs, heart, kidneys, and gastrointestinal (GI) tract.

Although HIV infection in children and adults share common pathologic conditions, an infant with HIV infection, particularly one who is infected perinatally, represents a distinctive immunologic host with a developing, immature immune system. The fetus and neonate have a well-developed T-cell or cell-mediated immune system, whereas their B-cell, or humoral, immune system is

physiologically immature (Kamani and Douglas, 1991). Although the function of both B and T cells is altered in HIV-infected children, the consequences of B-cell dysfunction, including hypergammaglobulinemia and failure to form functional antibodies, often become problematic early in the course of disease. For this reason children with HIV disease are more susceptible to bacterial infections than their adult counterparts. T-cell defects, allowing for opportunistic infections (OIs) such as *Pneumocystis carinii* pneumonia (PCP), are also frequently seen in young infants. In addition, the degree of lymphopenia, percentage of T4 (CD4) cells, absolute T4 (CD4) count, and degree of reversal of the helper/suppressor (T4/T8) ratio are more variable in infants. In general, depletion of T-cell numbers and inversion of the helper/suppressor ratio occurs at a later stage of disease than in adults (Koup and Wilson, 1994). Another major difference between adults and children with HIV infection is that the time period from infection to development of signs and symptoms appears to be shorter in children (Pizzo, 1990).

HIV is transmitted to children by a variety of modes (see Table 22-1). Perinatal transmission is the most common (89%) mode of transmission. Perinatal transmission is believed to occur transplacentally in utero (vertical), during delivery by exposure to infected maternal blood and vaginal secretions, and by postpartum ingestion of infected breast milk. Current prospective studies estimate the risk of perinatal transmission to be around 20%

463

Table 22-1.
U.S. PEDIATRIC AIDS CASES BY
ROUTE OF TRANSMISSION*

Mode of transmission	%
Mother has or is at risk for HIV infection	89
Recipient of blood, blood product, or tissue	6
Hemophilia or coagulation disorder	4
Undetermined	1
TOTAL	100

Adapted from Centers for Disease Control: HIV/AIDS surveillance report, June, 1994.
*N = 5734.

RESULTS OF ACTG 076:

A randomized, double-blind, placebo-controlled clinical trial of the efficacy and safety of zidovudine (AZT) in reducing the risk of maternal-infant HIV transmission

Mothers and infants	Risk of transmission
Those who took zidovudine	8.3%
Those who took placebo	25.5%

Data from Connor EM, et al: Reduction of maternal-infant transmission of human immunodeficiency virus type I with zidovudine treatment, *N Engl J Med* 331:1173-80, 1994.

to 30% (Oxtoby, 1994). It is becoming clear that many factors seem to influence mother-to-infant transmission of virus including maternal factors, fetal factors, viral factors, placental factors, obstetrical factors, and neonatal factors (Mofenson, 1994).

Children have become infected with HIV from contaminated blood and blood products, tissues, and factor concentrates received between the years of 1978 and 1985. The risk of infection through this route was extremely high, with infection estimated to occur in up to 95% of those receiving contaminated products. Because of safeguards instituted during the mid-1980s in blood and tissue collection and heat treatment of factor concentrates, few new cases of infection by this route have been reported.

A small number of children have become HIV infected as a result of sexual abuse. Practitioners caring for children who have experienced abuse must include HIV infection in their differential diagnosis of sexually transmitted diseases.

Approximately 25% of the AIDS cases in the United States are among young adults age 20 to 29 years (Centers for Disease Control [CDC], HIV/AIDS Surveillance Report, 1994). Because the average period from HIV infection to the development of AIDS is about 11 years (Brookmeyer, 1991), most of these young adults were infected as teenagers. Teenagers are especially at risk for HIV because many behaviors that put a person at risk for HIV begin during adolescence (i.e., sexuality, drug use). In addition, as the management and therapeu-

tic treatments for children with perinatally acquired HIV infection improve, more of these children will reach adolescence.

INCIDENCE

Although pediatric and adolescent AIDS is a reportable condition, the actual incidence/prevalence is unknown because of significant underreporting of AIDS cases both in the United States and worldwide. However, the actual incidence/prevalence of HIV infection in children is becoming better known as national confidential HIV infection reporting has recently begun in 27 of the 50 states. The occurrence of AIDS in children was established as early as 1982; 20 children less than 13 years of age had been diagnosed by the end of 1981. By mid-1994, more than 5700 cases of AIDS in children had been reported to the Centers for Disease Control (CDC), comprising 1.4% of the total number of reported AIDS cases in the United States (CDC, 1994). Estimates from the CDC suggest that currently there are 18,000 to 23,000 infants and children in this country who are infected with HIV. The incidence of pediatric HIV disease is

Table 22-2.   **PEDIATRIC AIDS CASES ($N = 5095$) BY MATERNAL EXPOSURE CATEGORY AND RACE OR ETHNICITY***

Exposure	White (%)	Black (%)	Asian/ Latino (%)	Am Ind/ Pac Is (%)	Alaskan (%)	Total (%)
Injection drug use (IDU)	44	43	44	22	50	43
Sex with IDU	19	15	28	11	12	19
Sex with other at-risk person	16	11	11	34	13	12
Recipient of blood, blood products, or tissue	5	2	2	0	0	2
Risk unspecified	16	29	15	33	25	24
TOTAL						100

Adapted from Centers for Disease Control: HIV/AIDS surveillance report, June, 1994.
*Pac Is, Pacific Islander; Am Ind, American Indian; IDU, injection drug user.

rapidly increasing as HIV infection continues to increase in the injection drug-using and heterosexual communities. All states in the United States have now reported at least one case of pediatric AIDS.

Because most children with AIDS have been perinatally infected, the demographics of this group closely parallel that of women with AIDS (see Table 22-2). In this population HIV is a disease primarily associated with poverty and drug use and is clustered in inner cities and ethnic minority communities. The parenteral cases, on the other hand, represent a broader geographic distribution and a wider ethnic apportionment.

Early diagnosis and treatment of HIV-infected infants is believed to enrich and prolong their lives. Currently there are no accurate methods of prenatal diagnosis of HIV infection. However, in February 1994 the results of a major national study were released showing that AZT (Zidovudine, Retrovir, ZDV) may reduce perinatal transmission from 25% to about 8% (Connor et al, 1994). (See box on p. 469.) The study included only relatively healthy women with CD4 counts above 200 and who had never taken AZT before.

CLINICAL MANIFESTATIONS AT TIME OF DIAGNOSIS

Developing a clinical definition of HIV infection and AIDS in children has proved to be a complex task. The initial pediatric AIDS definition provided direction for surveillance but did not describe the spectrum of infection. In 1987 the CDC therefore developed a classification system for HIV infection in children; however, as more information about pediatric HIV became available the 1987 classification system proved to be inadequate. In 1994 the CDC once again revised the classification system for children under 13 years of age. The current classification system places perinatally exposed and infected children into mutually exclusive categories according to infection and clinical and immunologic status (see box on p. 466). Although HIV infection is most accurately identified by viral culture from blood or tissue, in adults it is generally diagnosed by the presence of specific antibodies to the virus. The presence of passively acquired maternal antibodies, however, limits the use of HIV antibody testing in infants suspected of perinatal infection up to the age of 18 months. For this reason two definitions of infection in children are necessary: one for infants up to 18 months of age and one for older children (see box on p. 466).

For those children meeting the definition of HIV exposure or infection, they may be further grouped into one of six mutually exclusive classes based on clinical signs and symptoms and immunologic status (see Table 22-3). This classification system is helpful for health care planning and for epidemiologic purposes.

DIAGNOSIS OF HUMAN IMMUNODEFICIENCY VIRUS INFECTION IN CHILDREN*

Diagnosis: HIV infected

A. A child <18 months of age who is known to be HIV seropositive or born to an HIV-infected mother **and:**
  • Has positive results on two separate specimens (excluding cord blood) from any of the following HIV detection tests:
    —HIV culture
    —HIV polymerase chain reaction
    —HIV antigen (p24)
      or
  • Meets criteria for acquired immunodeficiency syndrome (AIDS) diagnosis based on the 1987 AIDS surveillance case definition
B. A child >18 months of age born to an HIV-infected mother or any child infected by blood, blood products, or other known modes of transmission (e.g., sexual contact) who:
  • Is HIV-antibody positive by confirmatory Western blot or immunofluorescence assay (IFA);
      or
  • Meets any of the criteria in A above

Diagnosis: perinatally exposed (prefix E)

A child who does not meet the criteria above who:
  • Is HIV seropositive by ELISA and confirmatory Western blot or IFA and is ≤18 months of age at the time of test;
      or
  • Has unknown antibody status, but was born to a mother known to be infected with HIV

Diagnosis: seroreverter (SR)

A child who is born to an HIV-infected mother and who:
  • Has been documented as HIV-antibody negative (i.e., two or more negative ELISA tests performed at 6 to 18 months of age or one negative ELISA test after 18 months of age);
      and
  • Has had no other laboratory evidence of infection (has not had two positive viral detection tests, if performed);
      and
  • Has not had an AIDS-defining condition

*Adapted from Centers for Disease Control MMWR 43: 2-3, 1994.

Many pediatric HIV-AIDS centers now use more specific laboratory tests to determine infectivity in perinatally exposed infants. HIV blood culturing has been considered the gold standard in virology testing of infants for many years. Unfortunately it is very expensive and labor intensive, and results are not usually available for 4 to 6 weeks after specimen processing. The p24 antigen assay is another virologic test which is very inexpensive and has been available for many years. Unfortunately, in the presence of HIV antibodies, an immune complex is formed with the p24 antigen, thereby making it impossible to detect the antigen itself. This test becomes more accurate in children at 6 months of age, when maternal antibody titers

in the infant begin to drop. A third test, which is proving to be superior to viral culture and p24 antigen assay, is the polymerase chain reaction (PCR). PCR is a method of gene amplification that directly detects proviral sequences of HIV within DNA using small amounts of blood (Rogers et al, 1989). PCR is somewhat less expensive than viral culture and more sensitive than p24 antigen assays. In addition, PCR results are usually available within 1 week of processing the specimen.

Using HIV cultures, PCRs, or a combination of both, the infection status of an infant can be determined with 90% to 100% certainty by 3 to 6 months of age (Rogers, Schochetman, and Hoff, 1994). Because these tests are not yet widely available, com-

Table 22-3.   **PEDIATRIC HUMAN IMMUNODEFICIENCY VIRUS (HIV) CLASSIFICATION***

	Clinical categories			
Immunologic categories	**N: no signs/ symptoms**	**A: mild signs/ symptoms**	**B: moderate signs/symptoms**	**C: severe signs/symptoms**
1: No evidence of immune suppression	N1	A1	B1	C1
2: Evidence of moderate immune suppression	N2	A2	B2	C2
3: Severe immune suppression	N3	A3	B3	C3

*Children whose HIV infection status is not confirmed are classified by using the above grid with a letter E (for perinatally exposed) placed before the appropriate classification code (e.g., EN2).
*Adapted from Centers for Disease Control MMWR 43: 2-3, 1994.

munity clinicians caring for these children may not have direct access to them but will need to refer to the closest pediatric HIV specialty center or contact the National Institute of Allergy and Infectious Diseases or the Maternal-Child Health Bureau for the nearest participating research group.

Because HIV infection is clearly a multisystem disease process, infants and children who are infected may have a wide range of signs and symptoms. Often the clinical manifestations that occur early in infection are nonspecific and may be seen in healthy children and children with other conditions. However, children with HIV infection generally experience more chronic and severe signs and symptoms and often fail to respond to appropriate therapy. Some children have acute opportunistic infections (OIs) with the same protozoal, viral, fungal, and bacterial pathogens as do adults, which are indicator diseases for an AIDS diagnosis. Others may have nephropathy, hepatitis, cardiomyopathy, and hematologic abnormalities.

Most children are diagnosed with HIV infection before they exhibit any signs or symptoms of illness. Infants and children born to mothers known to be HIV infected should be tested to determine if

---

CLINICAL MANIFESTATIONS ASSOCIATED WITH EARLY HIV INFECTION IN INFANCY AND CHILDHOOD

Failure to thrive
Diarrhea, chronic or recurrent
Fever of unknown origin
Atopic dermatitis
Persistent or recurrent fungal infections such as thrush or diaper dermatitis
Thrombocytopenia
Hepatosplenomegaly
Parotitis
Frequent infections
Developmental delay; loss of milestones

---

they are also infected. Retrospective transfusion programs have identified many children who are infected. Children with hemophilia or other hematologic conditions who received factor concentrates or other blood products before 1985 should be counseled about HIV testing (see Chapter 9).

TREATMENT

HIV infection is gradually becoming a chronic, treatable, life-threatening disease. The most significant treatments are those aimed at killing HIV in an attempt to eradicate the virus. Currently the only antiretroviral agents approved for use in children by the Food and Drug Administration are zidovudine (AZT, Retrovir) and didenosine (ddI). Unfortunately neither of these drugs alone is capable of completely eradicating the virus or keeping it suppressed over the long term.

Many questions regarding the use of antiretrovirals in children have yet to be completely answered, but there are a growing number of investigational treatment protocols for children concerning such issues as when to start treatment, how long to continue, and when and how to modify dosage. Rather than having to prove efficacy in adults before allowing children access to them, new drugs are now simultaneously tested in adults and children. This process parallels the approval process for new chemotherapeutic agents used in cancer therapy.

Much controversy exists over the use of intravenous immune globulin (IVIG) to reconstitute the immune system of a child with HIV infection. IVIG has been shown to reduce serious bacterial infections in children with HIV (Marwick 1991; Spector et al, 1994). This benefit did not hold true in children receiving zidovudine who were also receiving trimethoprim-sulfamethoxazole as *Pneumocystis carinii* pneumonia (PCP) prophylaxis. In addition, IVIG has never been shown to have an effect on survival time.

In the absence of a definitive cure, the treatment for children with HIV infection is comprehensive, multidisciplinary care with prompt diagnosis and aggressive therapy of concurrent infections and other clinical manifestations of disease. One of the most frequent problems in children with HIV infection is recurrent and severe systemic bacterial infection, which can progress to pneumonia, meningitis, and sepsis. Although this type of infection contributes greatly to morbidity, it is potentially preventable and treatable. The major bacterial pathogens encountered are those seen in pediatric practice with children who are immunocompetent. Reducing the frequency and intensity of bacterial infection may potentially modify HIV replication and primary disease progression (Krasinski, 1994).

TREATMENT

- Antiviral drugs
- Intravenous immune globulin
- Therapies for concurrent infectious and other clinical manifestations

Most children with HIV infection, even those with symptomatic disease, are active, playful, functional children who see themselves as healthy. They may take medications and spend time in the hospital, but they also attend day care and school. It is important for the primary care provider to remember that these children will develop common childhood illnesses and that all symptoms are not related to their underlying immunodeficiency. However, children with HIV disease need to be quickly assessed and aggressively managed when the possibility of intercurrent illness occurs. A wait-and-see attitude is rarely appropriate. These children and their families need to develop a strong partnership with their primary care provider so that prompt evaluation and treatment is assured. Children with HIV infection need to be linked with a comprehensive pediatric HIV-AIDS treatment center whenever possible. Centers ensure access to clinical trials, the most up-to-date information and expertise, and other children and families who are living with this disease. Clear lines of access to and responsibility of the primary care provider and the center team need to be developed for each family.

RECENT AND ANTICIPATED ADVANCES IN DIAGNOSIS AND MANAGEMENT

Prevention and early diagnosis have been at the forefront of pediatric HIV research for many years. In the early 1980s before blood banks began screening blood products for HIV, large numbers of children were infected by transfusion. Today transfusion is rarely cited as a route of transmission for pediatric HIV. In the late 1980s research began fo-

AZT TO REDUCE VERTICAL TRANSMISSION (FROM ACTG 076 PROTOCOL)

Maternal:

Antepartum	Begin after 14 weeks' gestation Zidovudine 100 mg PO 5×/day
Intrapartum	Zidovudine loading dose 2 mg/kg IV over 1 hr then 1 mg/kg/hr IV infusion
Diluent:	D$_5$W
Preparation:	Zidovudine 1000 mg in 250 ml D$_5$W
Final Concentration:	4 mg/ml

Infant:

Begin as soon as possible within the first 12 hours of life

For PO infant:

Zidovudine 2 mg/kg PO q6h × 6 weeks plus extra week supply

For NPO infant:

Zidovudine 1.5 mg/kg IV q6h infuse over 30 to 60 minutes

Diluent:	D$_5$W
Final Concentration:	0.5 mg/ml

ers who had been randomized to the treatment arm of the study transmitted virus to their infants only 8% of the time compared to women who had been on the placebo arm of the trial who transmitted to their infants 25% of the time. The study included only relatively healthy women who had CD4 counts above 200 and who had never taken AZT before. There were no congenital anomalies that could be attributed to AZT. The only adverse reaction in the infants receiving AZT was short-term transient anemia which resolved after completion of the treatment as specified by the protocol. It is unclear if there will be any long-term consequences for the infants or mothers who received AZT, but all women in the study are being monitored for up to 3 years following delivery, and infants may be followed in a long-term follow-up protocol until they are 21 years of age.

The CDC has published guidelines in the *Morbidity and Mortality Weekly Report (MMWR)* for the use of zidovudine to reduce perinatal transmission of HIV (Center for Disease Control RR-11, 1994). These guidelines are based on the ACTG 076 protocol and are not meant to be interpreted as required treatment regimens. There may be many reasons why a pregnant, HIV-infected woman might choose not to take AZT therapy or her primary care provider may deem it inappropriate for her. The decision as to whether or not a pregnant woman should take AZT should be made by the woman herself in consultation with her primary care provider.

Advances in early diagnosis of infants at risk for HIV have been dramatic over the past 5 years. One of the reasons that the ACTG 076 efficacy results were available earlier than anticipated is because when the study was first drafted in 1990, it was thought that infection could only be ruled out at 15 to 18 months of age when maternal antibody levels in the infant dissipate. However, more recently, the use of HIV culture and PCR has made diagnosis of HIV possible by 3 to 6 months of age. Unfortunately these tests are not ideal because of their high cost and labor intensity. A new antigen assay, the immune-complex dissociated p24 antigen assay (ICDp24), has been recently developed which applies an acidification process to the sample in an effort to dissociate the antibody from the antigen. This dissociation then allows the antigen to be detected. The ICDp24 is showing much

cusing on preventing vertical transmission as a means to reducing pediatric HIV. In 1991 the National Institutes of Health (NIH) through its newly established AIDS Clinical Trials Groups (ACTG) began a study using AZT in an attempt to reduce perinatal transmission of HIV (CDC, 1994). ACTG 076 was a double-blind, placebo-controlled study of the efficacy of zidovudine in preventing perinatal transmission of HIV. The box above outlines these treatment protocols. The study was abruptly stopped by the Data and Safety Monitoring Board (DSMB) after only half of the expected 800 mother-infant pairs had enrolled. In a routine analysis of the data the DSMB found that the moth-

ASSOCIATED PROBLEMS

Failure to thrive
  Chronic diarrhea
  Candida esophagitis
  Malnutrition
Neurologic manifestations
  HIV encephalopathy
    Developmental delay
    Deterioriation of motor skills
    and/or cognitive functions
  Acquired microcephaly
    Impaired brain growth
    Cortical atrophy
    Calcifications
  Gait disturbances
  Deficits in expressive language
Pancytopenia
  Thrombocytopenia
  Anemias
  Leukopenia
    Neutropenia
    Lymphopenia

Opportunistic infections
  Major cause of death
  PCP most common OI
Pulmonary disease
  Noninfections
    LIP
    Nonspecific pulmonary fibrosis
    Pulmonary hyptertension
    Aspiration pneumonia
  Infectious
    PCP
    CMV
    RSV
    MTB
Fungal infections
  Candidiasis
Drug exposure
  Delayed development
  Learning/behavioral difficulties

promise and is much less expensive than either culture or PCR. This assay has been shown to be highly sensitive and specific for diagnosing HIV infection in infants, but more refinement is needed to improve sensitivity and specificity in infants during the first week of life.

ASSOCIATED PROBLEMS

Failure to Thrive

Nutrition can be a significant problem in children with HIV disease, particularly those with chronic diarrhea and *Candida* esophagitis. Many infants and children with symptomatic disease demonstrate poor weight gain and frequently fall below the 5th percentile for weight on the National Center for Health Statistics growth curves.

Specific etiologies of chronic diarrheas such as *Cryptosporidium, Giardia,* and *Mycobacterium avium-intracellular* (MAI) are rarely found even after exhaustive gastrointestinal (GI) and stool examinations. Some children thrive better on lactose-free diets, whereas others experience cyclical diarrhea unresponsive to dietary manipulations. Many clinicians believe that these problems are caused by changes in the GI tract secondary to direct invasion by HIV (Winter and Miller, 1994).

HIV-associated malnutrition is no different than malnutrition from other etiologies. Children with chronic conditions who are experiencing malabsorption may also have malnutrition-induced immuno-deficiency. This creates an atmosphere where enteric pathogens are likely to thrive. In this way, there appears to be an interrelatedness between malabsorption, malnutrition, immunodeficiency, and enteric infections (Winter and Miller, 1994). Fig. 22-1 shows the obvious necessity of good nutrition in supporting the immune system of children with HIV infection.

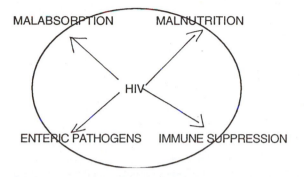

Fig. 22-1.   Link between malabsorption, malnutrition, and HIV infection. *(From Winter HS and Miller TL: Gastrointestinal and nutritional problems in HIV disease. In PA Pizzo and CM Wilfert, eds: Pediatric AIDS: the challenge of HIV infection in infants, children, and adolescents, ed 2, Baltimore, 1994, Williams and Wilkins.)*

Neurologic Manifestations

The brain is a target site for HIV infection in infants and children, and a variety of clinical patterns of neurodevelopmental involvement emerge (Browers, Belman, and Epstein, 1994). HIV encephalopathy may result in developmental delay, deterioration of motor skills and cognitive functioning, and behavioral abnormalities. This course may be static, progressive, or episodic with plateaus of relative stability lasting months alternating with intervals of marked deterioration occurring over weeks. The degree of neurologic deficit is influenced by both the extent of immunodeficiency and the age of the child. Usually some degree of neurologic impairment is found in all symptomatic children; however, CNS involvement may be the first and only sign of HIV disease in a child (Tovo et al, 1992).

Acquired microcephaly is frequently observed in infants and young children with HIV disease. Computerized tomographic scanning and magnetic resonance imaging often demonstrate impaired brain growth with diffuse cortical atrophy and basal ganglia calcifications in severely affected infants (Falloon et al, 1989). Cerebrospinal fluid (CSF), even if HIV culture positive, usually shows normal glucose, protein levels and cell count.

These children may demonstrate gradual apathy, progressive motor deficits resulting in general-ized weakness and gait disturbances, and difficulties with expressive language. It is often perplexing to differentiate the impact of HIV infection from the effects of prenatal and perinatal drug exposure, prematurity, chronic disease, and chaotic social environments (Browers, Belman, and Epstein, 1994).

Opportunistic Infections

Opportunistic infections (OIs) are the major cause of death for children with HIV infection. In comparison to adults, OIs in children usually develop from primary infections. *Pneumocystis carinii* pneumonia (PCP) is the most frequent OI diagnosed in children who are HIV infected, and occurs in about 50% of children with an AIDS diagnosis (Hughes, 1994). The initial episode of PCP is most often fatal, even with appropriate treatment (Cvetkovich and Frenkel, 1993). The high rate of recurrence makes prophylaxis imperative.

Pulmonary Disease

Pulmonary disease and resultant respiratory failure contribute profoundly to the morbidity and mortality of pediatric HIV infection. Pulmonary complications of pediatric HIV infection may be divided into noninfectious and infectious etiologies. Lymphoid interstitial pneumonitis (LIP), the most common noninfectious pulmonary disease, is characterized by a chronic interstitial process of diffuse bilateral infiltration of the alveolar and small airway walls with lymphocytes and plasma cells and is often combined with hypertrophy of the bronchial-associated lymphoid tissue (Church, 1993). Symptoms may be subtle and include tachypnea, dyspnea, cough and exercise intolerance. Treatment is generally symptomatic and supportive, but it is now believed that antiretroviral therapy aimed at the underlying HIV infection may help to ameliorate LIP (Connor and Andiman, 1994).

Other noninfectious pulmonary manifestations of pediatric HIV infection include nonspecific pulmonary fibrosis and pulmonary hypertension, as well as recurrent and severe aspiration pneumonia as a complication of encephalopathy (Church, 1993).

Pneumocystis carinii pneumonia, a diffuse, desquamative alveolopathy that results in hypoxia, is the most frequent OI seen in pediatric AIDS. The clinical manifestations of the child with PCP are age and immune status-dependence. Symptoms are likely to be acute with fever, dyspnea, dry cough, cyanosis, and hypoxemia. Treatment of acute infection is usually begun with trimethoprim-sulfamethoxazole (Bactrim, Septra) and corticoste-roids. Prophylaxis, both primary and secondary, with oral Bactrim or Septra is extremely effective (Church, 1993).

Other pathogens causing pulmonary infection include cytomegalovirus (CMV), respiratory syncytial virus (RSV), *Mycobacterium tuberculosis,* Mycobacterium Avium Intracellulare, rubeola, varicella, and a variety of other viral, fungal, and bacterial sources. Reactive airway disease is common, and considered to be chronic airway inflammation associated with frequent and persistent infection (Church, 1993).

Pancytopenia

Hematologic abnormalities are common in children with HIV infection, occurring as a result of HIV infection itself or as an adverse effect of treatment. Some children have thrombocytopenia, which is usually an immune response to circulating platelets, because their bone marrow produces megakaryocytes, which break down into platelets in the peripheral blood. Intravenous immunoglobulin (IVIG) is sometimes effective in raising the platelet count, and platelet transfusions are rarely required. Anemias of chronic disease or iron deficiency are common among this population and often require iron supplementation. Red blood cell (RBC) transfusions are sometimes indicated, particularly in AZT-induced anemia. Cytomegalovirus-negative, washed, irradiated RBCs and irradiated platelets are used to avoid introducing new infection and to protect against graft-versus-host disease. Abnormalities of the white blood cell (WBC) line including neutropenia, lymphopenia, and leukopenia are also frequently observed.

Fungal Infections

Candidiasis occurs frequently and may be manifested as either oral thrush or diaper dermatitis. The usual first-line treatments for oral thrush include topical nystatin (Mycostatin) and clotrimazole (Mycelex) oral troches. However, clotrimazole vaginal suppositories (100 mg) used orally are often more efficacious because they are 10 times more potent than the oral suspensions or troches. Infants can be treated either by placing the suppository into the nipple of a bottle, allowing the infant to suck formula through it, or by dissolving the

suppository in warm water and swabbing the mouth. Older children can suck the suppositories. Both nystatin and clotrimazole creams are available for skin infections. Refractory cases of mucous membrane and dermatologic infections may be treated systemically with oral ketaconazole (Nizoral) or the newer fluconazole (Difucan).

Prenatal and Perinatal Drug Exposure

Children with HIV who have been born to drug-using and alcohol-using HIV-infected mothers are frequently premature, small for gestational age, and have very immature immune systems. Their development is often delayed, and learning and behavioral difficulties are common (see Chapter 26).

PROGNOSIS

Acquired immune deficiency syndrome is among the 10 leading causes of death in children, and is the seventh leading cause of death in 1 to 4 year olds in the United States (Oxtoby, 1994). More than 50% of the children diagnosed with AIDS have died, but the actual mortality rate may be changing as treatment advances are made. Two distinct disease courses of perinatally infected children seem to exist: those infants who have a shorter medial survival time appear to develop symptoms by 4 to 6 months of age, qualify for an AIDS diagnosis by 1 year of age, and often die by the age of 2 years; and those infants with a longer median survival time usually develop mild symptoms during the first year which resolve over the second and third years, may not have an AIDS diagnosis for many years, and may live to be teenagers (European Collaborative Study [ECS], 1991).

Data now exist to support the well-accepted hypothesis that those children who have a rapidly progressive HIV course were infected early in gestation and those with a more indolent course were infected late in gestation or during the delivery process (Dickover et al, 1994).

Primary Care Management
HEALTH CARE MAINTENANCE

Growth and Development

The poor growth of children with symptomatic HIV disease appears to be more related to the general failure to thrive associated with the underlying HIV infection rather than to specific problems with caloric intake or GI losses (Church, 1993). Height and weight should be measured carefully by a practitioner or a skilled assistant and plotted on the child's individual National Center for Health Statistics growth chart at least monthly. The same scale should be used at each visit if at all possible. Nutritionists need to be part of the multidisciplinary primary care team, taking dietary histories and performing nutritional assessments to guide clinical decisions.

As previously noted, cortical atrophy and acquired microcephaly are common findings in the more severely affected infants. All children up to age 3 years require serial head circumference measurements at least every 3 months, with results plotted on the child's growth chart and carefully evaluated. Symptomatic children need careful measurements by the practitioner.

Standard developmental screening tests used by primary care providers, such as the Denver Developmental Screening Test, are of little value in assessing the child with HIV disease. Developmental delay is a hallmark of pediatric HIV infection, and early intervention appears to produce significant results; therefore, it is imperative that these children be assessed regularly by a skilled clinical psychologist as part of the comprehensive team approach. It is important for the primary care provider and the psychologist to discuss their developmental assessments and to formulate a plan of action together.

Intervention strategies must begin as early as possible in an attempt to maximize the child's capabilities. Infant stimulation programs that focus on motor and language skills and add specialties such as physical, occupational, and speech therapy can be provided at home, in the hospital, or in clinic or group settings. Preschool and school-aged children who have the physical stamina necessary can best be mainstreamed into regular programs, with special services added.

Diet

Children with HIV infection need a well-balanced diet with emphasis on adequate calories to maintain and increase weight with growth. There are no special dietary recommendations or restrictions based on HIV infection. Because failure to thrive is common in this population, early nutritional intervention before wasting occurs is important. Dietary supplementation and special formulas (e.g., Instant Breakfast for those who can tolerate dairy products and Pediasure for infants and younger children and Ensure for older children and adolescents who are lactose intolerant) are often beneficial for weight stabilization and potential weight gain. Enteral feedings and IV alimentation may be used acutely, intermittently, or chronically for children with severe anorexia, vomiting, diarrhea, and other GI problems. Consultation between the family and primary care provider regarding the child's particular needs should take place on a regular basis.

Safety

The primary care provider must teach the family safety precautions for children with neutropenia and thrombocytopenia and how to evaluate the neutropenic child for signs and symptoms of infection (see Chapter 11).

Caretakers may benefit from education on infectious disease transmission and control, such as the need for frequent handwashing and avoiding crowds. Children with HIV infection and their household contacts need to learn universal blood and body substance precautions. Because there is such concern in the community regarding casual contagion, families need to be well educated and able to withstand the apprehension of others. Several prospective studies of family and school contacts have found no evidence of HIV infection spread within these settings (Rogers et al, 1990). Although HIV has been isolated in a variety of body fluids, including blood, CSF, pleural fluid, breast milk, semen, cervical secretions, saliva, and urine, only blood, semen, cervical secretions, and human milk have been implicated in its transmission (Hollander, 1990).

It is important to counsel the child's caretaker concerning safe storage of medications and equipment in the home. Parents who are HIV infected also may have many potentially hazardous medications at home. Children with HIV infection may be developmentally delayed or exhibit neurologic regression as the infection progresses. Safety precautions must be adjusted accordingly. If the child is cared for by a parent with HIV infection, the parent's ability to safely care for the child must be frequently assessed because of the symptom of dementia often associated with adult HIV infection.

Immunizations

Much controversy exists regarding immunization practices in children with HIV infection. Historically, live-virus vaccines have not been recommended for children with congenital or drug-induced immunodeficiencies because of the concern that administration of live, attenuated vaccine viruses have the potential to produce infection in an immunocompromised host. Prospective studies, however, have failed to reveal such problems.

In addition, the dysfunction of the B-cell system typical of infants with HIV disease, which includes markedly elevated immunoglobulins, reflects nonspecific stimulation suggestive of poor immune response to antigens and therefore to vaccines. Because of this immunologic dysfunction, immunogenicity and vaccine efficacy may be lower than in children who are immunocompetent. In general, children with symptomatic HIV infection have poor immunologic responses to vaccines, and therefore, when exposed to a vaccine-preventable disease such as measles or tetanus, these children should be considered susceptible regardless of history of vaccination and should receive passive immunoprophylaxis if indicated (Committee on Infectious Disease, 1994).

Because live-virus, attenuated immunizations may be ineffective if given to children who have received IVIG during the previous 3 months, the general practice is to administer these vaccinations at the midpoint between monthly IVIG infusions.

Hepatitis B virus (HBV). Hepatitis B vaccine is now recommended as part of the regular schedule of immunizations for children who are asymptomatic and HIV infected; generally, symptomatic children do not receive this live-virus vaccine (Committee on Infectious Disease, 1994).

Tetanus. Children who are HIV infected should receive tetanus immune globulin (human) (TIG) regardless of vaccine status following an injury that places the child at risk for acquiring tetanus infection (Committee on Infectious Disease, 1994).

Polio. Although oral polio vaccine (OPV) has been administered to children who are HIV infected without adverse effects, the injectable enhanced, inactivated poliomyelitis vaccine (EIPV) is generally recommended because both the child and the HIV-infected family members may be immunosuppressed as a result of HIV infection and hence, may be at risk for vaccine-associated paralytic poliomyelitis caused by vaccine virus infection (Committee on Infectious Disease, 1994).

Measles, mumps, and rubella. The measles, mumps, and rubella (MMR) vaccination should be administered at the standard age of 12 to 15 months unless there is an increased risk of measles or rubeola exposure. Monovalent measles vaccine can be used for infants 6 to 11 months old, with revaccination with MMR at 12 months of age or older.

Regardless of vaccination status, children with both asymptomatic and symptomatic HIV infection should be prophylaxed with immune globulin (IG) after an exposure (Committee on Infectious Disease, 1994). Immune globulin may be helpful in preventing or minimizing measles if it is administered within 6 days of exposure. It is also indicated for measles-susceptible household contacts of children with asymptomatic HIV disease, especially for infants less than 12 months of age. Immune globulin may be unnecessary if the child is receiving regular IVIG infusions, and the last dose was within 3 weeks of exposure (Committee on Infectious Diseases, 1994).

Haemophilus influenzae type b. Conjugated polysaccharide-diphtheria *Haemophilus influenzae* type b vaccine is recommended for all children starting at 2 months of age (Committee on Infectious Diseases, 1994). As previously noted, *H. influenzae* is a common and serious pathogen in children with HIV infection, increasing the importance of immunization. Even children who have had one or more episodes of documented infection with *H. influenzae* before the age of 2 years may not produce enough antibody to prevent subsequent infections, making vaccination imperative. Prophylaxis with rifampin (Rifadin) is required even after vaccination if there is a known contact with HIB (Committee on Infectious Diseases, 1994).

Pneumococcus. Polyvalent pneumococcal vaccine (Pneumovax) should be administered to children with HIV disease at 2 years of age because of their underlying immunosuppression and the fact that pneumococcus is a prevalent pathogen in this population (Committee on Infectious Diseases, 1994).

Influenza. Yearly influenza vaccination with the subvirion (split-virus) bivalent vaccine is recommended for children more than 6 months of age with HIV exposure or infection and their household contacts (Committee on Infectious Diseases, 1994).

Varicella. Varicella (HZV) poses significant risks for dissemination, encephalitis, and pneumonia in children who are immunosuppressed. Although the vaccine is now approved and released for use in healthy children, the efficacy of the vaccine in children with HIV infection is unknown and may vary depending on the child's degree of immune suppression. A study of the use of the varicella vaccine in children who are HIV infected has begun.

Children with HIV infection who are susceptible to varicella need to receive varicella-zoster immune globulin (VZIG) IM within 72 hours of exposure if they have not received IVIG within the past 3 weeks.

Screening

Vision. Because of the incidence of CMV retinitis in adults with HIV disease and therefore the theoretical risk of a similar process affecting children, the primary care provider must elicit a thorough visual history and provide a careful visual and fundoscopic examination. Comprehensive pediatric HIV centers may recommend that all children with HIV infection be referred to a knowledgeable pediatric ophthalmologist for baseline screening. If the findings are normal, the primary care provider can then continue to provide regular follow-up.

Hearing. Because of the frequent acute suppurative otitis media (OM) in children with HIV infection and the possibility of hearing loss, periodic audiometry and tympanometry should be performed. Children who require myringotomy tube placement require special precautions for swimming and showers, such as regular use of well-fitting earplugs.

Children with severe neurologic disease, some children with chronic OM, and those on maintenance aminoglycoside therapy need baseline brainstem auditory evoked response hearing testing if routine acuity testing cannot be done or is abnormal.

Dental. Early screening beginning at 2 to 3 years of age is strongly recommended because dental caries can create a focus of infection. Fluoride treatments are recommended if the community water supply does not contain adequate amounts to protect enamel. Severe dental caries and gingivitis, as well as dental abscesses, are being reported in some infected children. The clinician must educate families regarding appropriate oral hygiene and encourage regular dental care.

Blood pressure. Blood pressure measurements should be taken every 3 to 6 months unless changes warrant more frequent measurements. Increased blood pressure can indicate renal disease.

Hematocrit. Screening is deferred because of the need for frequent CBC assessment.

Urinalysis. Children with HIV disease require urinalysis with microscopic examination at least every 3 months because urine abnormalities can be the first sign of illness. Findings can include hematuria and proteinuria and can result in azotemia and nephrotic syndrome (Falloon et al, 1989).

Tuberculosis. Yearly screening is strongly advised. As more tuberculosis is being diagnosed in adults with HIV infection, more children in infected households are at risk. Because many individuals infected with HIV demonstrate anergy to skin testing, close surveillance of families may include regular chest x-ray studies. *Mycobacterium avium-intracellulare* (MAI) is a common bacterium of the same family as *M. tuberculosis* that is prevalent in the population of persons infected with HIV. Unlike *M. tuberculosis,* MAI is not contagious by the respiratory route but may be transmitted through infected GI secretions. Because it can invade many organ systems, including the bone marrow and the GI system, MAI may be responsible for much morbidity.

Condition-specific screening

VITAL SIGNS. Vital signs should be assessed and documented at each visit. Children can be asymptomatic yet febrile, needing a work-up. Elevations in heart and respiratory rate can indicate pulmonary or cardiac dysfunction.

COMPLETE BLOOD COUNT. Because of bone marrow suppression caused by HIV and some OIs, as well as by many of the drugs used in treatment, children with HIV disease require regular determinations of CBCs with differential and platelet counts. Asymptomatic children should have a CBC done every 3 to 6 months; symptomatic children usually need them done at least monthly. This blood work can be performed by the primary care provider or at the pediatric HIV center.

Anemia should be investigated as to the cause, because children with iron deficiency anemia will usually benefit from oral iron supplementation. Often no specific cause is discovered. Children taking AZT need CBC and reticulocyte counts assessed frequently because anemia is a common adverse effect. Complete blood counts with reticulocyte counts are usually completed every 2 weeks for the first 2 months and then done monthly as long as the counts are stable. Dosage is modified based on the degrees of anemia. Some children taking AZT require RBC transfusions. Neutropenia and thrombocytopenia are also common side effects of AZT, and dose reductions may be indicated.

IMMUNOLOGIC MARKERS. Baseline T-cell and B-cell counts and quantitative immunoglobulin (QUIG) determinations are necessary to assess immunologic status. T-cell subset values and T4/T8 ratios are usually checked every 3 to 6 months. T4 counts less than $500/mm^3$ are generally an indication for prescribing antivirals, such as AZT. Children receiving monthly IVIG infusions do not have serial QUIG assessments because they would reflect the infused rather than endogenous immunoglobulins.

CHEMISTRY PANEL. Routine serum chemistry panels should be obtained every 3 to 6 months and more frequently for symptomatic children or those taking medications (i.e., AZT, ddI) that might affect liver or kidney function. Children taking ddI also need to be monitored for pancreatitis by checking amylase levels. Many children who are HIV-infected have elevated baseline liver function test results, with both aspartate aminotransferase (AST) and alanine aminotransferase (ALT) enzyme levels frequently 2 to 3 times normal.

PULMONARY FUNCTION. Children with chronic lung disease need baseline pulmonary function testing with oxygen saturation and regular serial testing based on disease severity. Pulse oximetry, a noninvasive technique, is used in place of arterial blood gas sampling when available. A baseline radiograph is useful as a comparison study for pulmonary complaints. Often the child with either acute infection or chronic pneumonitis has no adventitial sounds. Pulmonary consultation is a useful adjunct for the primary care provider in following these children.

COMMON ILLNESS MANAGEMENT

Differential Diagnosis

Fever. Fever is a frequent sign in children with HIV disease. It can be caused by HIV disease itself or can indicate a separate infectious process. Practitioners must ensure that families have a thermometer, are able to use it accurately, and have clear guidelines about when to contact their primary care provider. Generally, whenever a child's temperature measures 38.5°C or greater, the child needs to be examined and a treatment plan initiated based on the objective and subjective findings.

DIFFERENTIAL DIAGNOSIS

Fever

HIV infection vs other infectious process
Cultures essential

Respiratory distress

LIP vs PCP
Cardiomyopathy
Reactive airway disease

Otitis media

Very common
Refer to ENT for tube placement

Sinusitis

Common following UTI
Untreated can lead to meningitis

Varicella

Risk of dissemination high

A thorough interval history and complete physical examination are the most important part of the work-up of a febrile child with HIV infection. Some of these children will have otitis media, sinusitis, pneumonia, or sepsis; others will have common colds and other viral infections that can be traced to school or household contacts.

In consultation with the infectious disease specialist or the HIV center, the primary care provider can order cultures of blood and other body fluid as indicated for aerobic, anaerobic, and fungal organisms. Cultures are essential in an attempt to identify the infectious process. Frequently the cultures are negative, even in seriously ill children, but positive cultures will determine specific antibiotic therapy. Chest x-ray studies may be an important part of the work-up of a febrile child with HIV infection.

Respiratory distress. A variety of respiratory complaints may plague children with HIV disease. Again, the history and physical examination are of paramount importance in the differential diagnosis. A dry, hacking cough is a common complaint of children with LIP but can also be a sign of PCP. Children with acute onset of respiratory distress need speedy evaluation, because the condition can progress extremely rapidly, sometimes over hours. Pulmonary consultation is often necessary. Occasionally children with cardiac disease have respiratory complaints. These children need cardiology consultation and diagnosis.

Children with known reactive airway disease may benefit from having equipment and medications for aerosol delivery at home. The primary care provider must evaluate the family's ability to provide such sophisticated assessment and treatment, and if parents are capable, they can be taught the necessary skills.

Otitis media. Otitis media (OM) is one of the most common infectious diseases seen in children with HIV disease. Frequently it is diagnosed on routine physical examination when no pain or fever is present, even at times when the tympanic membrane may be ruptured with pus filling the external canal. Follow-up must be done after treatment is completed because the OM may not resolve and complications may occur. Children who have persistent and refractory OM should be referred to an ear, nose, and throat (ENT) specialist for evaluation for myringotomy tube placement.

Sinusitis. Although sinusitis is rare in children, it is seen commonly in children with HIV disease, often occurring after a viral respiratory tract infection. The primary care provider can teach the family to report changes in the color of nasal mucus from clear or white to yellow or green, which may indicate infection. Sinusitis, if not appropriately treated, can lead to mastoiditis and can directly extend into the brain, causing meningitis.

Varicella. Because of the risk of dissemination as a result of immunocompromise, varicella in the child with HIV disease is potentially life threatening. Because these children may not respond adequately to vaccines and the general herd immunity to varicella will not be high until the vaccine has been distributed on a wide basis for many years, herpes zoster virus (HZV) will continue to cause chickenpox as a primary manifestation and zoster as a secondary manifestation of infection in most children who are HIV infected. If primary prevention with VZIG fails, or if the child was not known to be exposed until the rash occurs, the usual practice at most centers is to hospitalize and treat with acyclovir IV as soon as the disease is diagnosed. With this treatment few children progress to disseminated disease, and most go home within 5 days of starting therapy, continuing with oral therapy to complete a 7-day to 10-day course.

Drug Interactions

AZT. Zidovudine interferes with reverse transcriptase and inhibits replication of HIV. The main toxicity of AZT in children is bone marrow suppression—anemia and neutropenia. There are no specific drug interactions known for ddI. This nucleoside analog is similar to AZT, but rather than hematologic toxicity, its major toxicity is pancreatitis. ddI is often used in conjunction with AZT.

TMP-SMX. One of the major toxicities of this sulfa combination is hematologic—neutropenia and thrombocytopenia. Children on PCP prophylaxis or treatment regimens who develop persistent neutropenia secondary to TMP-SMX either alone or in combination with AZT often need to discontinue the drug. Pentamidine administered intravenously or by aerosol in older children can be used as an alternative. Allergic reactions to sulfa are not uncommon, and primary care providers need to teach families how to recognize the

symptoms of skin rash and hives as part of the reaction complex. The child who shows allergy to
one form of sulfa should not be prescribed other
antibiotics containing sulfa.

IVIG. There are no specific drug interactions
noted with IVIG. Allergic reactions have been documented but appear to be rare.

DEVELOPMENTAL ISSUES

Sleep Patterns

Children taking AZT or other medications that interrupt normal sleeping hours may experience difficulty in returning to sleep. Parents may need to try
a variety of schedules to find one that works best
for them and their child. The primary care provider
must ensure that the family has access to a reliable
alarm clock so that doses are not missed.

Toileting

Nontoilet-trained children with HIV infection may
experience profound diaper dermatitis. This is frequently associated with candidiasis, as well as with
chronic and cyclical diarrhea. Impeccable perineal
care including frequent diaper changes, exposure
of the perineum to air, and the use of topical medications can significantly reduce morbidity. When
the perineum is bloody or the child has hematuria
or diarrhea, the caretakers should wear gloves to
protect themselves during diapering.

Discipline

Discipline is often difficult for the family of a child
with a life-threatening illness. Some parents are unable to set developmentally appropriate and necessary limits and need guidance and information from
their provider. Discipline needs and appropriate expectations will vary as the illness progresses and
neurologic and motor deterioration occur. Caretakers must be provided with anticipatory guidance in
these areas. Other factors such as homelessness,
chaotic lifestyle, and parental illness can make consistent discipline difficult. Practitioners may be
helpful in assisting families and caregivers to understand the child's needs for safety and limits.

Child Care

Child care, respite care, and preschool placement
are difficult issues for families of children with

HIV infection. The primary care provider must advise parents that children who are in group settings
have an increased risk of exposure to infectious diseases and common childhood illnesses compared
with children who remain at home (Takala et al,
1995). The particular setting for each child must be
individualized, based on the child and family's
needs and resources. Practitioners can provide education regarding universal infection control and infectious disease guidelines for these agencies.

Child care and respite care are important resources for families who are caring for children
with chronic conditions. Some foster families have
access to respite hours through their social services
division, whereas others have none. In some areas
there are few, if any, child care or respite workers
who are willing to care for infants and children
with HIV infection. This is an enormous problem
for infected families who need time to care for their
own HIV disease, as well as for their infected and
noninfected children. The regular availability of
respite care and other support services may allow
many infected mothers to continue to care for their
children.

Public Laws 101-476 and 99-457 may offer
valuable services for children with HIV (see Chapter 5). Head Start, a federal preschool program
that provides preschool for economically deprived
children, is specifically mandated to enroll children
with HIV infection.

Because day care and preschool are not a legal
requirement for children, individual day-care providers may develop their own policies in accordance with local, state, and federal regulations.
Many private day care centers and preschools
refuse to accept children with HIV infection, probably because of their fears of casual contagion, litigation, and disenrollment if other families discover
the diagnosis. Some areas of the country with high
prevalence of pediatric HIV disease have developed day care programs specifically for these children. Such services are directed toward children
who are too ill to attend regular day care programs.

It is optimal to educate day care and preschool
personnel and families before a child with HIV disease is enrolled. It may be useful for the primary
care provider to call the preschool, stating that a
family is interested in enrolling their child who is
HIV infected. The school is notified that there is no

"duty to inform" and that the child will not be identified. Feelings regarding children with HIV infection are explored, and an offer is made to provide in-service training about pediatric HIV disease and general infection control.

Some families choose to conceal the fact of HIV in their family; other families discuss it openly. As more children take antiviral medications such as AZT that need to be administered frequently, it is becoming harder to conceal HIV infection from day care providers. However, many families schedule dosing around school hours and create unusual stories about why they need to know immediately about chickenpox or other contagious illnesses in the classroom. The clinician has an important role to play in helping families to decide how, when, and to whom information about HIV disease should be disclosed.

Schooling

The major school issues faced by young children with HIV infection have little to do with their educational needs and much to do with concerns regarding confidentiality, information sharing, and infection control. This issue has created strife in many communities nationwide. As these children age, however, their needs for special education programs will undoubtedly increase. The primary care provider can help the family secure the appropriate services (see Chapter 5).

Because AIDS is recognized as a handicap, attendance in public schools is supported by Public Law 101-476. In some areas of the country, public school attendance is decided by committees composed of educators, public health officials, and the child's primary care provider. If the decision is made to ban the child from attending school, the school district then must provide home teaching. Children benefit greatly from attending school, and this option should be strongly encouraged. When children are too ill to attend, home teaching is a viable alternative for that time period only. As the child's condition progresses, particularly with neurologic deterioration, there will be increasing needs for frequent meetings of school resource personnel, health care providers, and family members to ensure that appropriate services are provided.

There is no legal duty to inform school officials about a child's diagnosis, although this will vary from state to state. However, as more children become aware of their own HIV infection, there will be more discussion among the children themselves. This will lead to greater awareness in the school and larger community that a child with HIV infection is in attendance. It is important for the provider to be available to the school—students, faculty, and parents—for educational discussion sessions.

Teenagers with HIV infection often have difficulty in school. Rumors that circulate about HIV infection and students who are believed to be infected can cause tremendous anxiety for an infected adolescent regardless of the route of infection. Primary care providers can support their teenaged clients, helping them gain more knowledge and differentiate whom they might trust with this sensitive information. Referral to the school nurse or counselor may be appropriate.

Sexuality

Children and adolescents with HIV disease need to learn about sexual and perinatal transmission of this condition. Adolescence is the time for sexual experimentation and the emergence of sexual identity. Sexual activity increases steadily throughout these years. Teens who are infected with HIV face much difficulty in attaining a healthy, integrated sexual identity because of the risks of oral and genital sexual transmission. Some teens deny the reality of their HIV infection, refusing to practice safer sex. The primary care provider needs to be comfortable discussing transmission and sexual risk reduction strategies, as well as demonstrating the proper use of condoms and dental dams.

Transition into Adulthood

The advent of new and more effective HIV therapies is likely to transform HIV infection from a terminal illness to a chronic but manageable condition. Survival times will likely continue to increase. As these children with perinatally-acquired HIV infection get older, there may be more teen and possibly even young adult survivors. These individuals will doubtless continue to need a vast array of medical and psychosocial services throughout their childhood and transition into adulthood. Because this group of children was born to HIV-infected mothers, most often there are many infected family members that are at risk of death from HIV disease while the children are young. As these children reach sexual maturity, they need to be educated about and helped to deal with the fact that they are capable of transmitting HIV to their sexual partners.

Children and teenagers who have been infected as a result of nonperinatal transmission (i.e., sexual activity, injection drug use, transfusion or transplantation) have an abundance of other concerns to face. Some of these issues include risk of sexual transmission, intimacy, and stigma. As HIV infection becomes a more chronic, life-threatening disease integrated into the mainstream of health care, these special issues may gradually decline.

SPECIAL FAMILY CONCERNS AND RESOURCES

Human immunodeficiency virus infection is a family disease, and when a child is diagnosed, a family crisis results. The majority of children with HIV disease have infected mothers who are ill, dying, or deceased; there may be an infected father and siblings in the family as well. Most infected mothers who transmit HIV to their children experience tremendous guilt. The physical and emotional burden of caring for a child who requires frequent medical and supportive treatments, who may have developmental delay, and who will probably die as a result of the illness is enormous.

The most significant psychosocial issue facing children with HIV infection and their families is the social stigmatization associated with the disease. Initially many families feel isolated and unable to call on their normal support systems for fear of rejection and retaliation. In addition, these families may lack other resources; they are primarily poor, of minority heritage, undereducated, and burdened by the social ills of inner-city life. With support the family may reach out to utilize extended family, friends, and community agencies.

The vast majority of children who were perinatally infected with the HIV disease are children of color. Some children are placed in foster or adoptive care after birth if the mother is unable to care for the infant. Others are placed out of the home at a later date when resources are insufficient to support the parents' ability to care for the child. Foster

and adoptive parents need considerable support to provide optimal care for these children. They need ongoing education, financial support, respite care, emotional support and counseling, and social and legal counseling. Because children in foster care are wards of the juvenile court, decisions regarding consent for investigational drugs and experimental protocols, as well as do-not-resuscitate orders, must be court ordered. Working relationships need to be developed between the primary care provider, HIV center, and social services to ensure that children with HIV disease in the child welfare system receive optimal care.

Helping a child and family face a chronic, life-threatening illness that ultimately leads to death is a pivotal role for the primary care provider. Counseling about the physical and emotional issues of the death and dying process, options for hospital or home death, hospice services, funeral plans, and bereavement is imperative as an integral part of the clinician's role. Support groups are invaluable resources for networking, keeping current, and decreasing social isolation. Most pediatric HIV-AIDS comprehensive treatment centers offer such groups on an ongoing basis. The primary care provider should become familiar with the local, national, and international organizations (see the list that follows).

Organizations

AIDS Resource Foundation for Children
182 Roseville Ave
Newark, NJ 07107
(201) 483-4250

Camp Sunburst National AIDS Project
PO Box 2824
Petaluma, CA 94953
(707) 769-0169

Northern Lights Alternatives
Children's Care Program
601 W 50th St, 5th Floor
New York, NY 10019
(212) 765-3202

National AIDS Hotline
(800) 342-AIDS

CDC National AIDS Clearinghouse
PO Box 6003
Rockville, MD 20849-6003
(800) 458-5231

National Center for Youth Law
  114 Sansome St, Suite 900
  San Francisco, CA 94104-3820
  (415) 543-3307
National Pediatric HIV Resource Center
  15 S 9th St
  Newark, NJ 07107
  (800) 362-0071
NIAID Intramural Trials for HIV Infection and AIDS
  (800) AIDS-NIH (800-243-7644)
Pediatric AIDS Foundation
  1311 Colorado Ave

Santa Monica, CA 90404
(310) 395-9051
Foundation for Children with AIDS, Inc
  1800 Columbus Ave
  Roxbury, MA 02119
  (617) 442-7442

Local and State Resources

County health department
State health department
AIDS task forces
AIDS hotlines

SUMMARY OF PRIMARY CARE NEEDS FOR THE CHILD WITH HIV INFECTION

Health care maintenance

Growth and development

Growth in both weight and height may be poor; measure and plot monthly.
Cortical atrophy and acquired microcephaly are common in severely affected infants.
Measure and plot head circumference monthly until the child is 3 years of age.
Standard developmental screening tests are not useful; serial screening by a psychologist if available is recommended.
Early intervention programs are recommended.
  Diet
Emphasize a balanced, high-calorie diet.
Use nutritional supplements.
  Safety
The risk of infection because of immunocompromise is increased.
The risk of bleeding because of thrombocytopenia is increased.
Universal blood and body substance precautions should be taught to the family and community.
Safe storage of medication in the home is important.
Developmental delay or regression may alter safety requirements.
Parents with HIV infection must be evaluated for

safe care practices because of symptoms of dementia.

Immunizations

Hepatitis B Vaccine given to asymptomic children with HIV.
Tetanus immunglobulin (TIG) should be given to child at risk of infection due to injury.
Use EIPV for exposed or infected child, all household members, and close contacts.
Give immune globulin within 6 days of measles exposure to prevent or modify course unless child received IVIG within previous 3 weeks.
Haemophilus influenzae type b and polyvalent pneumococcal vaccines are recommended.
Pneumovac should be given to children with HIV > 2 years of age
Yearly influenza vaccine is recommended.
Varicella-zoster immune globulin is recommended within 72 hours of varicella exposure.

Screening

  Vision
Ophthalmologist should do baseline fundoscopic examination; practitioner follow-up every 3 to 6 months.
  Hearing
Periodic audiometry and tympanometry screening is recommended.

Continued.

SUMMARY OF PRIMARY CARE NEEDS FOR THE CHILD WITH HIV INFECTION—cont'd

A BSER hearing test should be given to those with chronic OM or abnormal screening.

Dental

Early screening is recommended to prevent dental infections.

Blood pressure

Measurements should be taken every 3 to 6 months.

Hematocrit

Routine screening is deferred because of the need for frequent CBC tests.

Urinalysis

Urinalysis with microscopic examination should be done at least every 3 months.

Tuberculosis

Yearly screening is recommended. Chest x-ray studies may be needed if the child is anergic.

Condition-specific screening

VITAL SIGNS

Temperature, heart rate, and respiratory rate should be checked at each visit.

COMPLETE BLOOD COUNT

The CBC should be assessed every 3 to 6 months if the child is asymptomatic; every 2 to 4 weeks if the child is taking AZT or another myelosuppressive agent.

IMMUNOLOGIC MARKERS

Baseline T-cell and B-cell counts, QUIG values, repeat T-cell subset levels, and T4/T8 ratios should be checked every 3 to 6 months.

CHEMISTRY PANEL

Serum chemistry panels should be obtained every 3 to 6 months if the child is asymptomatic; more frequently if the child is symptomatic or is taking liver or kidney toxic agents.

PULMONARY FUNCTION

Baseline pulmonary function testing, including pulse oximetry if available, is recommended for children with lung disease.

Common illness management

Differential diagnosis

Fever

Rule out bacterial infection and OI.

Respiratory distress

Rule out LIP, PCP, and cardiac disease.

Otitis media

Rule out tympanic membrane perforation.

Sinusitis

Rule out bacterial sinusitis, mastoiditis, and meningitis.

Varicella

Use VZIG as primary prevention and acyclovir as secondary prevention.

Drug interactions

Zidovudine

Bone marrow suppression may occur.

ddI—check amylase for pancreatitis.

Trimethoprim-sulfamethoxazole

Bone marrow suppression (neutropenia, thrombocytopenia) and allergic reactions may occur.

Developmental issues

Sleep patterns

Sleep patterns may be disturbed because of medications needed around the clock.

Toileting

Impeccable perineal care needed to reduce morbidity of diaper dermatitis. Caretaker to use gloves for blood or diarrhea.

Discipline

Discipline is often difficult for the family; lifestyle issues can exacerbate problems.

Child care

The child care program should be individualized to meet the child's and family's needs.

Public Laws 99-457 and 101-476 cover early intervention services.

Schooling

Public school attendance is aided by Public Law 101-476.

There is no duty to inform school officials of a child's HIV status.

The school community may benefit from education.

Teens may need extra support from the school nurse or counselor.

Continued.

SUMMARY OF PRIMARY CARE NEEDS FOR THE CHILD
WITH HIV INFECTION—cont'd

Sexuality

Discuss sexual and perinatal transmission.
Demonstrate safer sex techniques and the use of condoms and dental dams.

Transition into adulthood

With improved treatment HIV may become a chronic condition.
Parents may have died from condition years before.
Must be educated about possible transmission of HIV to others.

Special family concerns

Human immunodeficiency virus is a family disease.

Many families lack resources.
The disease is an enormous physical and emotional burden.
Stigmatization is a major issue.
Many of these children are placed in foster or adoptive homes.
Counseling on death and dying, and during bereavement is helpful.
Many of these children are of color. Primary care provider must have sensitivity to specific cultural issues.

REFERENCES

Benson MS: Management of infants born to women infected with the human immunodeficiency virus, *J Perinat Neonatal Nurs* 7:79-89, 1994.

Brookmeyer R: Reconstruction and future trends of the HIV epidemic in the United States, *Science* 253:37-42, 1991.

Browers P, Belman AL, and Epstein L: Central nervous system involvement: manifestations, evaluation and pathogenesis. In PA Pizzo and CM Wilfert, (editors): *Pediatric AIDS: the challenge of HIV infection in infants, children and adolescents,* ed 2, Baltimore, 1994, Williams and Wilkins, pp 433-455.

Centers for Disease Control: *HIV/AIDS surveillance report,* June, 1994.

Centers for Disease Control: 1994 revised classification system for human immunodeficiency virus infection in children less than 13 years of age, *MMWR* 43(RR-12):1-10, 1994.

Centers for Disease Control: Recommendations of the U.S. Public Health Service task force on the use of zidovudine to reduce perinatal transmission of human immunodeficiency virus, *MMWR* 43(RR-11):1-19, 1994.

Church JA: Clinical aspects of HIV infection in children, *Pediatr Ann* 22:417-427, 1993.

Committee on Infectious Disease: Report of the Committee on Infectious Disease, ed 23, Elk Grove Village, IL, 1994, The American Academy of Pediatrics.

Connor EM, Andiman WA: Lymphoid interstitial pneumonitis. In PA Pizzo and CM Wilfert, (editors): *Pediatric AIDS: the challenge of HIV infection in infants, children and adoles-*

cents, ed 2, Baltimore, 1994, Williams and Wilkins, pp 467-481.

Connor EM et al: Reduction of maternal-infant transmission of human immunodeficiency virus type 1 with zidovudine treatment, *N Engl J Med* 331:1173-1180, 1994.

Cvetkovich TA, Frenkel LM: Current management of HIV infection in children, *Pediatr Ann* 22:428-434, 1993.

Demmler GJ, Taber LH: Virology of HIV-1, *Semin Pediatr Infect Dis,* 1:17-20, 1990.

Dickover RE et al: Rapid increases in load of human immunodeficiency virus correlate with early disease progression and loss of CD4 cells in vertically infected infants, *J Infect Dis* 170:1279-1284, 1994.

European Collaborative Study: Children born to women with HIV-1 infection. Natural history and risk of transmission, *Lancet* 337:253-260, 1991.

Falloon J et al: Human immunodeficiency virus infection in children, *J Pediatr* 114:1-30, 1989.

Hollander H: Transmission of HIV in body fluids. In PT Cohen, MA Sande, and PA Volberding, (editors): *The AIDS knowledge Base,* Waltham, MA, 1990, The Medical Publishing Group, pp 2-1.2.1.

Hughes WT: Pneumocystis carinii pneumonia. In PA Pizzo and CM Wilfert, (editors): *Pediatric AIDS: the challenge of HIV infection in infants, children and adolescents,* ed 2, Baltimore, 1994, Williams and Wilkins, pp 405-418.

Kamani NR, Douglas SD: Structure and development of the immune system. In DP Sites and AF Terr, (editors): *Basic and clinical immunology,* ed 7, Norfolk, CT, 1991, Appleton and Lange, pp 9-33.

Koup RA, Wilson CB: Clinical immunology of HIV-infected children. In PA Pizzo and CM Wilfert, (editors): *Pediatric AIDS: the challenge of HIV infection in infants, children and adolescents,* ed 2, Baltimore, 1994, Williams and Wilkins, pp 405-418.

Krasinski K: Bacterial infections. In PA Pizzo and CM Wilfert, (editors): *Pediatric AIDS: the challenge of HIV infection in infants, children and adolescents,* ed 2, Baltimore, 1994, Williams and Wilkins, pp 241-253.

Marwick C: Example of prepublication data release: Immunoglobulin for concomitant infections, *JAMA* 265:953, 1991.

Oxtoby MS: Vertically acquired HIV infection in the United States. In PA Pizzo and CM Wilfert, (editors): *Pediatric AIDS: the challenge of HIV infection in infants, children and adolescents,* ed 2, Baltimore, 1994, Williams and Wilkins, pp 3-20.

Pizzo PA: Pediatric AIDS: problems within problems, *J Infect Dis* 161:316-325, 1990.

Rogers MF et al: Lack of transmission of human immunodeficiency virus from infected children to their household contacts, *Pediatrics* 85:210-214, 1990.

Rogers MF et al: Use of polymerase chain reaction for early detection of the proviral sequences of human immunodeficiency virus in infants born to seropositive mothers, *N Engl J Med* 320:1649-1654, 1989.

Rogers MF, Schochetman G, and Hoff R: Advances in diagnosis of HIV infection in infants. In PA Pizzo and CM Wilfert, (editors): *Pediatric AIDS: the challenge of HIV infection in infants, children and adolescents,* ed 2, Baltimore, 1994, Williams and Wilkins, pp 219-238.

Spector SA et al: A controlled trial of intravenous immune globulin for the prevention of serious bacterial infections in children receiving zidovudine for advanced human immunodeficiency virus infection, *N Engl J Med* 331:1181-1187, 1994.

Takala AK et al: Risk factors for primary invasive pneumococcal disease among children in Finland, *JAMA* 273(11):859-864, 1995.

Tovo PA et al: Prognostic factors and survival in children with HIV-I infection, *Lancet* 339:1249-1253, 1992.

Winter HS, Miller TL: Gastrointestinal and nutritional problems in HIV disease. In PA Pizzo and CM Wilfert, (editors): *Pediatric AIDS: the challenge of HIV infection in infants, children and adolescents,* ed 2, Baltimore, 1994, Williams and Wilkins, pp 513-533.

23

Hydrocephalus

Patricia Ludder Jackson and Joyce Harvey

ETIOLOGY

Hydrocephalus is a condition that results from an imbalance between the production and the absorption of cerebrospinal fluid (CSF), leading to the enlargement of the ventricular system and increased intracranial pressure. It is most frequently caused by an intraventricular or extraventricular blockage in the normal circulation and absorption of CSF (see Fig. 23-1). Hydrocephalus may be categorized as communicating hydrocephalus, in which there is extraventricular obstruction to CSF flow or diminished absorption of CSF, and noncommunicating hydrocephalus, caused by intraventricular obstruction of CSF flow (Barkovich, 1995). (See box p. 486.) In some cases, CSF flow and absorption may be obstructed at multiple sites causing both communicating and noncommunicating hydrocephalus (Barkovich, 1995; Carey, Tullous, and Walker, 1994; Rekate, McCormick, and Yamada, 1991).

Noncommunicating hydrocephalus can result from obstruction of any portion of the ventricular system—from the foramina of Monro, the posterior third ventricle, the aqueduct of Sylvius, the fourth ventricle, and the fourth ventricular outflow foramina (Barkovich, 1995). In *congenital noncommunicating hydrocephalus,* the flow of CSF to the arachnoid spaces is blocked resulting in enlargement of the ventricular system proximal to the site of obstruction. The most common obstruction is congenital aqueductal stenosis or gliosis usually

at the aqueduct of Sylvius. This may occur as the result of a perinatal infection (toxoplasmosis, cytomegalovirus, mumps, syphilis, meningitis) or as a result of compression and obstruction of the aqueduct by a lesion (congenital aneurysm, arachnoid cyst, subdural hematoma caused by birth injury, intraventricular or subarachnoid hemorrhage or early neonatal brain tumors) (Barkovich, 1995; Carey, Tullous, and Walker, 1994). Congenital malformations of the brain, such as Chiari II malformations, which are commonly associated with myelomeningocele, and Dandy-Walker malformations also result in hydrocephalus, with both intraventricular and extraventricular blockage of CSF.

After the neonatal period, noncommunicating hydrocephalus may occur as a result of CNS infections, tumors, trauma, arteriovenous malformations or systemic bleeding disorders (Barkovich, 1995; Carey, Tullous, and Walker, 1994).

Communicating hydrocephalus occurs when CSF flow is blocked in the subarachnoid spaces, basilar cisterns, and finally the arachnoid villi. It may be the result of CNS infection (bacterial or viral), subarachnoid hemorrhage, or as the result of congenital malformation of the subarachnoid spaces. In communicating hydrocephalus the lateral third and fourth ventricles enlarge (Barkovich, 1995). Hydrocephalus may also be a component of numerous syndromes (Carey, Tullous, and Walker, 1994). The etiology of hydrocephalus associated with achondroplasia and various cranial facial

485

CLASSIFICATION OF HYDROCEPHALUS

I. Noncommunicating
   A. Congenital
      1. Chiari malformation (usually associated with myelomeningocele)
      2. Aqueductal stenosis
      3. Aqueductal gliosis (postperinatal hemorrhage or infection)
      4. Obstruction from congenital lesions (neoplasms, vascular malformation, vein of Galen)
      5. Arachnoid cyst, benign intracranial cyst
   B. Acquired
      1. Infectious ventriculitis
      2. Obstruction from lesions (neoplasms, vascular malformation)
      3. Chemical ventriculitis
      4. Intraventricular hemorrhage

II. Communicating
   A. Congenital
      1. Arachnoid cyst
      2. Encephalocele
      3. Associated with congenital malformation: craniofacial syndromes, achondroplasia
      4. Dandy-Walker malformation
   B. Acquired
      1. Chemical arachnoiditis
      2. Infections (postmeningitis)
      3. Posthemorrhagic (postsubarachnoid hemorrhage, intraventricular hemorrhage)
      4. Associated with spinal tumors and seeding from CNS tumors

Adapted from Carey CM, Tullous MW, and Walker ML: Hydrocephalus: Etiology, pathologic effects, diagnosis, and natural history. In Cheek WR, (editor): *Pediatric neurosurgery: surgery of the developing nervous system,* ed 3, Philadelphia, 1994, WB Saunders, and Barkovich AJ: *Hydrocephalus.* In Barkovich AJ: *Pediatric neurosurgery,* New York 1995, Raven Press.

syndromes is thought to be a result of venous hypertension, leading to a decreased pressure gradient across the arachnoid villi and decreased CSF absorption (Barkovich, 1995).

INCIDENCE

The overall incidence of hydrocephalus is unknown. The incidence of infantile hydrocephalus is approximately 3 to 4 per 1000 live births (Carey, Tullous, and Walker, 1994), with aqueductal stenosis responsible for approximately one third of the cases. The incidence of myelomeningocele varies dramatically from region to region. In the United States the incidence is approximately 1 per 1000 births (Carey, Tullous, and Walker, 1994). Of these children, 80% will develop hydrocephalus during the first year of life as a result of either a Chiari II malformation or associated aqueductal stenosis.

CLINICAL MANIFESTATIONS AT TIME OF DIAGNOSIS

Although the signs and symptoms of hydrocephalus may be somewhat varied as a result of the specific cause of the condition, there are common clinical manifestations associated with the increased intracranial pressure. The rate of CSF production, the degree of flow obstruction, and the amount of absorption will determine the degree of hydrocephalus; the presence or absence of an expandable cranium and the volume and compliance of the cerebral tissue will determine the degree of symptoms (Carey, Tullous, and Walker, 1994). If the accumulation of excessive CSF occurs slowly, the infant or young child may be asymptomatic until the hydrocephalus is quite advanced. Significant dilation of the ventricle may occur before abnormal head growth is apparent. Full or distended fontanels, frontal bossing, prom-

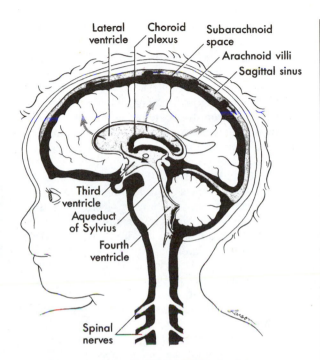

Fig. 23-1.   Cerebrospinal fluid (CSF) circulatory pathway. Drawing shows a view of the center of the brain. *Solid arrows* show major pathway of CSF flow; *broken arrows* show additional pathways. (From Edwards MS and Derechin M, eds: *About hydrocephalus: a book for parents.* Drawings by Lynne Larson. San Francisco, 1986, University of California. Reprinted with permission.)

CLINICAL MANIFESTATIONS

Manifestations determined by degree of hydrocephalus, degree of increased intracranial pressure, and etiology.

Associated symptoms

Associated symptoms in infants:

Abnormal head growth
Distended fontanels
Frontal bossing
Vomiting
Irritability or lethargy
Opisthotonic posturing

Associated symptoms in child >18 months:

Headache
Nausea
Vomiting
Irritability/lethargy
Alterations in motor development
Eye changes

inent scalp veins, poor feeding, vomiting, irritability, lethargy, and even opisthotonic posturing may be observed by the primary care provider before dramatic changes are noted in head circumference.

In the child more than 18 to 24 months of age with fused cranial sutures, the development of hydrocephalus may result in the nonspecific symptoms of headache, nausea, vomiting, and personality changes, including irritability, lethargy, and loss of interest in normal daily activities. Depending on the cause of the hydrocephalus and the degree of increased intracranial pressure, these symptoms can be either acute in onset or chronic (Carey, Tullous, and Walker, 1994). Spasticity or ataxia of the lower extremities, as well as urinary incontinence, may occur. These children frequently complain of vision problems because increased intracranial pressures on the second, third, or sixth cranial nerves result in extraocular muscular paresis and papilledema (Gaston, 1991). Alterations in growth, sexual development, and fluid and electrolyte imbalance may occur if there is increased pressure at the site of the hypothalamus.

TREATMENT

Surgical treatment for hydrocephalus is directed at restoring CSF flow either by removing the obstruction or creating a new CSF pathway. The latter usually involves the placement of a ventricular catheter or shunt to divert the flow of CSF to another internal site for absorption (Rekate, 1994). Ventriculoperitoneal shunts are most common; however, ventriculoatrial or ventriculopleural shunts are used when the peritoneal cavity is inaccessible (Piatt, 1994;

TREATMENT

Treatment determined by etiology. Goal is to restore CSF flow by removing obstruction or creating new pathway

Shunting pathways

Ventriculo peritoneal
Ventriculo atrial
Ventriculo pleural

Management of shunt malfunction, shunt infection

Neuroendoscopy

Drug therapy

Punt, 1993). The ventricular portion of the shunt is inserted into the lateral ventricle via a frontal or occipital burr hole (Scott, 1990). The distal portion is tunneled under the child's skin to the designated location where a small incision is made and the shunt is either inserted through the peritoneum into the peritoneal cavity (VP shunt), or through the neck into the superior vena cava and into the right atrium (VA shunt) (see Fig. 23-2). The distal end of the ventriculopleural shunt is guided subcutaneously to an area just below the nipple where an incision is made and the tube is inserted into the pleural space (Rekate, 1994).

A variety of shunt designs exist, with most consisting of a soft silastic tube ⅛ inch in diameter, a dome-shaped reservoir, and a one-way valve (Shiminski-Maher and Disabato, 1994). The reservoir and tubing are palpable from the burr hole in the skull to the tube's insertion at either the abdomen or chest. Identification of and access to the shunt reservoir is important in evaluating shunt infection and malfunction. The reservoir should be easy to depress and should rebound readily when released. A small 25-gauge needle can be inserted into the reservoir to collect CSF for culture, to obtain intracranial pressure readings, or to inject radioisotopes for shunt flow studies (Piatt, 1994; Rekate, 1994).

Although CSF shunting has dramatically improved the prognosis for children with hydrocephalus, shunts continue to have inherent problems (Rekate, 1991). Shunt malfunction may occur because of chronic or acute inflammation, accumulation of cellular debris or blood, or occlusion of either the distal or proximal end of the shunt as a result of growth (Kast et al, 1994; Rekate, 1991; Sainte-Rose, 1993; Scott, 1990). Shunts in children with cranial neoplasms were found to have the highest rate of complications in a previous study (Serlo et al, 1990). Shunt revisions are necessary at some point in almost all children who have been treated for hydrocephalus. Most individuals require two to five revisions during childhood and adolescence (Kokkonen et al, 1994; Lumenta and Skotarczak, 1995; Vernet, Campiche, and de Tribolet, 1995). Although shunt revisions are traumatic for the child and family and pose physical risk because of surgery and increased intracranial pressure, the number of revisions has not been correlated with poor neurodevelopmental outcome (Lumenta and Skotarczak, 1995; Riva et al, 1994).

The incidence of shunt infection has decreased significantly in the past decade, but continues to be a major source of shunt malfunction and potential morbidity. Shunts create a medium in the host where normal phagocytosis is impaired, allowing the child to be more susceptible to CNS infection (Klein, 1990; Marlin and Gaskill, 1994). Reported rates of infection range from 2% to 17.8% (Andretta, 1987; Klein, 1990; Piatt and Carlson, 1993; Serlo et al, 1990), with infants less than 1 year of age having a higher incidence than older children. Children with hydrocephalus as a result of perinatal intracranial hemorrhage have the highest rate of infection. Staphylococcus aureus and Staphylococcus epidermidis are responsible for 60% to 75% of infections, and gram negative bacilli is the third most common organism associated with peritoneal shunt infection (Shapiro et al, 1988). More than 50% of staphylococcal infections occur within 2 weeks of a shunt operation, and 70% of all infections occur within 2 months of surgery, probably from a slow-growing contaminate such as Staphylococcus epidermidis (Scott, 1990). Haemophilus influenzae meningitis is also believed to be more

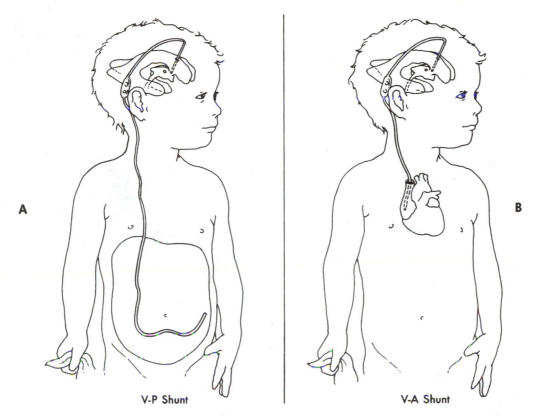

V-P Shunt   V-A Shunt

Fig. 23-2.   Pathway used for **A,** ventriculoperitoneal shunt and **B,** ventriculoatrial shunt. *(From Edwards MS and Derechin M, (editors):* About hydrocephalus: a book for parents. *Drawings by Lynne Larson. San Francisco, 1986, University of California. Reprinted with permission.)*

common in children with shunts (Patriarca and Lauer, 1980; Rennels and Wald, 1980). Although shunt malfunction has not been associated with cognitive deficits, shunt infections especially resulting from gram negative organisms have a significant detrimental effect (Hendrick, 1993).

The incidence of shunt infections following dental or surgical procedures other than shunt placement is relatively low (Pittman et al, 1992). Although some authors propose that antibiotic prophylaxis are unnecessary (Pittman et al, 1992), most neurosurgeons recommend that children with shunts receive antibiotic prophylaxis before dental work with anticipated bleeding, oral and upper respiratory tract procedures, and genitourinary and gastrointestinal procedures (Graham et al, 1993; Pittman et al, 1992). The recommended prophy-

laxis is the same for prevention of bacterial endocarditis in children with congenital heart disease (see box on p. 306, Chapter 15) (Dajani et al, 1990). In children with ventriculoatrial shunts, the possibility of bacterial endocarditis as a complication must not be overlooked. Peritoneal shunts are preferred over atrial shunts because the latter often result in cardiac complications.

In view of the multiple problems with ventricular shunts, surgeons continue to look for ways to restore CSF flow without placement of a permanent shunt. The removal of intracranial mass lesions may restore normal CSF flow and cure the associated hydrocephalus. Unfortunately, as many as 25% to 30% of children with brain tumors and hydrocephalus will require shunting subsequent to tumor resection (Rekate, McCormick, and Yamada,

1991; Warnick and Edwards, 1991). Clinical and experimental data suggest the etiology of hydrocephalus in these children is more complex than simply obstruction of flow by the lesion (Rekate, McCormick, and Yamada, 1991).

These children, as well as others with obstructive hydrocephalus, may benefit from recent advances in neuroendoscopy (Walker, Petronio, and Carey, 1994). Using a fiber optic ventriculoscope, neurosurgeons can navigate through the ventricular system and create a new pathway or communication for CSF between the third ventricle and prepontine subarachnoid cistern. This enables the CSF to circulate in the subarachnoid space and be absorbed normally via the arachnoid villi. The current literature is promising regarding the success of endoscopic third ventriculostomy in preventing permanent shunt placement in select individuals with noncommunicating hydrocephalus (Walker, Petronio, and Carey, 1994; Handler, Abbott, and Lee, 1994; Jones et al, 1994; McDermott, Ciricillo, and Edwards, 1995; Oka et al, 1994). Neuroendoscopy is also helpful in guiding shunt placement and creating communication between trapped ventricles or cysts and other CSF spaces (Walker, Petronio, and Carey, 1994).

Investigation continues in the use of drug therapy to prevent the need for permanent shunting (Gilmore, 1990; Hudgins et al, 1994). Acetazolamide (Diamox) and furosemide may be used to reduce the production of cerebral spinal fluid in individuals with slowly progressing hydrocephalus. Diamox is often used in combination with CSF drainage, either by serial lumbar punctures or tapping of a ventricular access device, to prevent progressive ventricular enlargement in preterm infants with intraventricular hemorrhage (Edwards and Derechin, 1988; Marlin and Gaskill, 1990; Rekate, 1994). These infants may eventually achieve compensation of posthemorrhagic hydrocephalus, and surgical treatment may therefore be delayed or avoided. Follow-up of preterm infants has shown that shunt complications, including infection and obstruction, are higher when shunts are placed in extremely premature neonates; therefore, prolonging permanent shunt placement may improve long-term outcome (Edwards and Derechin, 1988).

Occasionally, children with communicating hydrocephalus outgrow the need for a shunt (Rekate, 1991). Alternative pathways for absorption are believed to be established as a result of persistent increased intracranial pressure therefore compensating for the diminished absorption from the arachnoid villi in communicating hydrocephalus (Barkovich, 1995). This compensated or resolved hydrocephalus usually occurs during the first year of life with rapid growth of brain structures, though it may not be identified until later when lengthening of the shunt appears necessary as a result of growth. Compensated hydrocephalus is accompanied by stable ventricular size despite documented shunt obstruction. Shunt failure may be verified by the absence of flow after injection of a radioisotope into the shunt reservoir (shunt function study) or by radiologic confirmation of shunt disconnection (radiographic shunt series). In this situation, the shunt is left in place unless the risk of infection is high. The child is followed by periodic brain scans and neuropsychologic examinations. Annual neuropsychologic testing is recommended because intellectual deterioration has been associated with arrested hydrocephalus (Epstein, 1994).

Neuro-imaging of the brain is essential for the diagnosis and management of hydrocephalus. The three major imaging modalities include ultrasonography, computed tomography (CT) scan, and magnetic resonance imaging (MRI). Ultrasound is only possible in infants while the anterior fontanel remains open. CT scans are most commonly obtained if acute hydrocephalus or shunt malfunction is suspected. Although all techniques are reasonable for follow-up of ventricular size and shunt placement, MRI is superior in defining the etiology of hydrocephalus. MRI scans illustrate the central nervous system anatomy in multiple planes and allows for detailed imaging of the cerebrum and posterior fossa (Barkovich, 1995). One study compared findings on MRI with those identified previously by CT scans and noted that a new etiology for hydrocephalus was discovered in 11% of the subjects and additional information regarding the effects of hydrocephalus was obtained in 55% (Paakko et al, 1994). Advances in MRI technology can also be used to study CSF flow dynamics (Barkovich, 1994; Carey, Tullous, and Walker, 1995). This technique is useful in determining the success of third ventriculostomy in restoring CSF circulation.

In a small minority of children with hydrocephalus, ventricular size does not change with shunt malfunction (Epstein, 1994). These children may have apparent symptoms of increased intracranial pressure despite negative imaging. Further diagnostic evaluation must be performed before shunt malfunction is ruled out. Other diagnostic tools include radionuclide CSF shunt studies, shunt tap and culture for infection, and intracranial pressure monitoring either intermittently via the shunt reservoir or by placement of an intracranial pressure (ICP) monitor (Piatt, 1992). Keeping in mind the morbidity associated with a delay in the diagnosis of a shunt malfunction, the primary care provider must have a low threshold for ordering a brain scan or referring the child to the neurosurgeon when symptoms of increased ICP or shunt infection are apparent (Piatt, 1992).

RECENT AND ANTICIPATED ADVANCES IN DIAGNOSIS AND MANAGEMENT

Prevention should be a major goal in the treatment of hydrocephalus. It is difficult to prevent hydrocephalus directly because the cause is often variable and sometimes unknown. Advances in obstetric and neonatal intensive care, however, have decreased the incidence of hydrocephalus as a result of intraventricular hemorrhage and meningitis (Abdel-Rahman and Rosenberg, 1994; Edwards and Derechin, 1988; Rosseau, McCullough, and Joseph, 1992). In addition, nutritional guidelines recommending supplementation of folic acid in women of childbearing age may lower the incidence of hydrocephalus by decreasing the number of children born with myelomeningocele and other neural tube defects (Canadian Task Force on the Periodic Health Examination, 1994; Rieder, 1994).

Prenatal evaluation including high resolution ultrasound and measures of maternal alpha-fetoprotein (AFP) have increased the identification of fetal anomalies (Howell, 1994). Neural tube defects may be identified by elevated maternal AFP and fetal ultrasound. Ventriculomegaly may be diagnosed during routine prenatal ultrasound. The treatment options available to the family and the fetus with ventriculomegaly and spina bifida depend on the stage of pregnancy, the extent of brain and other anomalies, current laws and regulations regarding termination of pregnancy, and the family's individual beliefs (Clewell, 1990). Assessment for other congenital anomalies and follow-up ultrasounds to detect progressive ventricular enlargement are essential when counseling families (Clewell, 1990; Crombleholme, 1994). If severe brain dysfunction or other congenital anomalies are suspected, parents may decide to terminate the pregnancy; otherwise, the pregnancy is continued as close to term as possible and a shunt or ventricular access device is placed in the infant soon after birth (Hudgins and Edwards, 1990).

Prenatal treatment has been attempted with placement of a ventriculoamniotic shunt, however the risks are high for both the fetus and the mother (Crombleholme, 1994). Currently there is no evidence that the long-term outcome for these babies will improve significantly with in utero treatment; therefore, fetal surgery for hydrocephalus and spina bifida remains experimental and most studies are limited to exploration of surgical technique and outcome in animal studies (Hudgins and Edwards, 1990).

The standard treatment for hydrocephalus continues to be the placement of a CSF shunt. Shunt materials and systems continue to be modified to meet individual needs. Special antisiphon devices are available to treat symptoms of low pressure or "slit ventricle syndrome" and unified systems have decreased complications related to shunt disconnection (Rekate, 1994). Shunt placement can now be guided by the use of the endoscope allowing for real time visualization of the ventricular system and shunt placement (Manwaring, 1992). This is particularly helpful when treating individuals with complex hydrocephalus. Posthemorrhagic or postinfectious hydrocephalus may be complicated by the presence of septations or cystic areas within the ventricular system. Adequate CSF drainage may not be possible with one shunt, so these individuals may require multiple shunts with complex connecting systems, increasing the likelihood of shunt malfunction. Introducing the ventricular endoscope to fenestrate or making holes between these multiple compartments has been useful in reducing the number of ventricular catheters and simplifying the shunt system (Walker, Petronio, and Carey, 1994; Manwaring, 1992). As mentioned previously, endoscopic third ventriculostomy can obviate the need for shunt placement altogether in select individuals. As improvements are made in the handling and visual capabilities of the endoscope, indications for its use will probably increase (Walker, Petronio, and Carey, 1994).

ASSOCIATED PROBLEMS

Intellectual Problems

Intellectual function is difficult to predict early after diagnosis. The etiology of the hydrocephalus appears to be the most important determining factor, with uncomplicated hydrocephalus having a better cognitive prognosis than hydrocephalus associated with brain injury. Approximately 30% of the children with hydrocephalus in two recent long-term studies had mild-moderate mental retardation and 7% to 8% had severe retardation with some variability over time (Lumenta and Skotarczak, 1995; Villani et al, 1995). In children with IQs greater than 70, performance IQs, were lower than full-scale and verbal IQs, and there was evidence of speech impairment, visual motor integration deficits, memory deficits, and decreased performance in school (Blum and Pfaffinger, 1994; Lumenta and Skotarczak, 1995). These difficulties indicate a need for preschool and school counseling and testing to identify areas of learning disability.

Ocular Problems

As reported earlier, ocular abnormalities are often found at the time of diagnosis or during episodes of shunt malfunction. Increased intracranial pressure results in optic nerve pressure, limited upward gaze, extraocular muscle paresis, and papilledema (Gaston, 1991; Neville, 1993; Rudolph, 1987).

Even with a functioning shunt and controlled hydrocephalus, however, visual problems are common. Gaze and movement problems such as strabismus, astigmatism, nystagmus, and amblyopia are found in approximately 25% to 33% of the children (Gaston, 1991; Mankinen-Heikkinen and Mustonen, 1987). Refractive and accommodation errors are found in about the same percentage of children but not necessarily the same children. The optic disk is frequently found to be abnormally light or pale but papilledema is not found under normal conditions (Gaston, 1991; Mankinen-Heikkinen and Mustonen, 1987). Abnormalities in

---

ASSOCIATED PROBLEMS

- Intellectual problems
- Ocular problems
- Motor disabilities
- Seizures

---

vision are associated with lower intelligence scores and may help identify the child at higher risk for mental retardation and need for more careful follow-up and referral to infant stimulation programs (Donders, Canady, and Rourke, 1990; Riva et al, 1994). Correctable visual problems should be attended to as soon as possible so that poor vision does not interfere with learning potential.

Without prompt treatment for acute hydrocephalus or shunt malfunction, permanent visual damage is a definite risk. Before the era of successful CSF shunting, optic atrophy secondary to hydrocephalus was the leading cause of blindness from congenital malformations (Simpson and Hemmer, 1993).

Motor Disabilities

Unfortunately as many as 75% of the children with hydrocephalus will have some form of motor disability (Dennis et al, 1981; Fernell, Hagberg, and Hagberg, 1988a, 1988b). These disabilities vary from severe paraplegia to mild imbalance or weakness. The severity of the motor deficit is most often diagnosis related, with conditions such as porencephaly, Dandy-Walker malformation, and myelomeningocele having more serious motor defects than simple congenital hydrocephalus.

Hydrocephalus also affects fine motor control. Kinesthetic-proprioceptive abilities of the hands are often negatively affected, and this, coupled with the impaired bimanual manipulation and frequent visual deficits, makes it difficult for the child with hydrocephalus to perform well on time-limited, nonverbal intelligence tests (Blum and Pfaffinger, 1994; Riva et al, 1994).

Seizures

Because of increased intracranial pressure, seizures in infancy are common at the time of initial diagnosis. Fortunately, only 13% to 33% of the children with hydrocephalus continue to have seizures after the first year of life (Fernell, Hagberg, and Hagberg, 1988a, 1988b; Kokkonen et al, 1994; Villani et al, 1995). These seizures may be simple or complex, partial or generalized, and usually can be well managed with standard anticonvulsant therapy. Acquired hydrocephalus is more often associated with seizure activity because of the underlying reason for the development of hydrocephalus (e.g., brain tumor, CNS trauma, or infection). These seizures may be more focal in origin and more difficult to control. (For further discussion on seizure disorders, see Chapter 19).

PROGNOSIS

The outlook for children with hydrocephalus continues to improve with advances in shunt and surgical technology (Carey, Tullous, and Walker, 1994). Morbidity and mortality rates are variable determined by etiology of the hydrocephalus, number of shunt revisions, number and type of shunt infections, surgical complications, and environmental and social factors (Hirsch, 1994; Kokkonen et al, 1994; Lumenta and Skotarczak, 1995; Marlin and Gaskill, 1994; Vernet, Campiche, and de Tribolet, 1995). Five-year survival usually is greater than 80%, with the majority of deaths occurring as a result of severe congenital malformations or progressive brain tumors during the first year of treatment (Fernell, Hagberg, and Hagberg 1988a, 1988b; Hirsch, 1994; Kokkonen et al, 1994; Lumenta and Skotarczak, 1995; Marlin and Gaskill, 1994; Vernet, Campiche, and de Tribolet, 1995). Congenital hydrocephalus ranks eighth in congenital anomalies for years of potential life lost as measured by the National Center for Health Statistics (Centers for Disease Control, 1988). It is important for the primary care provider to remember that children with hydrocephalus remain at risk for increased morbidity and early mortality even after years of excellent progress and shunt function. Early detection and treatment of complications can greatly reduce morbidity and mortality.

Primary Care Management
HEALTH CARE MAINTENANCE

Growth and Development

Typically, measurements of a child seen in a primary care practice are done by minimally trained office or clinic personnel. In the case of the child suspected of having hydrocephalus or known to have hydrocephalus, the head circumference should be measured by the primary care provider. Until the cranial sutures are completely fused, which is often delayed in these children, growth of head size is a major diagnostic tool in evaluating the child's condition.

Once the diagnosis of hydrocephalus has been made and a shunt inserted, the head circumference may decrease 1 to 2 cm as the pressure is relieved. After this initial decrease the head should grow only in proportion to the child's body. Therefore, a newborn whose weight and height are in the 50th percentile for age and who has a head size of 40 cm when a shunt is placed shortly after birth may not resume head growth for 2 to 4 months (see Fig. 23-3). Resumption of growth before that time might indicate shunt malfunction. The significance of head size measurements in the child with a shunt cannot be overestimated, and daily measurements may be necessary during evaluation of the shunt-dependent infant for possible shunt malfunction. Weight gain must be assessed carefully as the increasing weight of the head in the infant with hydrocephalus may mask failure to thrive (Neville, 1993).

Endocrine dysfunction resulting in precocious puberty, short stature, delayed puberty, and amenorrhea have been reported in as many as 28% of children with hydrocephalus (Elias and Sadeghi-Nejad, 1994; Villani et al, 1995). Sexual development before the age of 8 years in girls and 10 years in boys is considered precocious and warrants further diagnostic study (Ott and Jackson, 1989; Pescovitz, 1990). Heights below the 5th percentile, if not compatible with family stature, indicate growth retardation. Treatment is available for both of these conditions, and children should be referred to an endocrinologist if these signs occur.

Standard early infant developmental assessment tools used in primary care practice, such as the Denver Developmental Screening Test, are of little help in assessing these infants. Tasks that require head

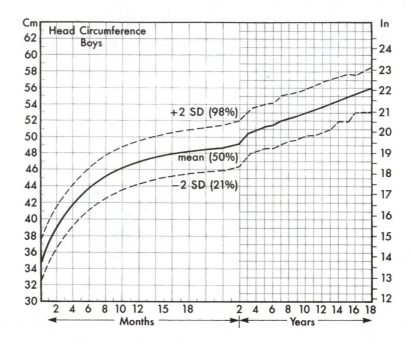

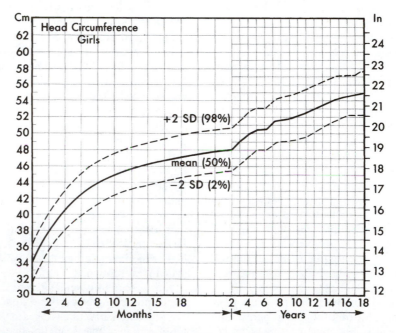

Fig. 23-3.   Head circumference charts from birth to age 18 years. (From Neilhaus G: Head circumference from birth to eighteen years, *Pediatrics* 41:106-114, 1968.)

control, such as elevating the head while in the prone position, rolling over, pulling to a sitting position without head lag, and even sitting unassisted, will be delayed in the infant with macrocephaly. It is important for the primary care provider to interpret developmental findings in light of other clinical observations to assist the parents in setting reasonable expectations for their infant.

Other motor delays can be expected during infancy and childhood given that approximately 75% of children with hydrocephalus have some form of motor disability. The primary care provider must carefully document motor skill acquisition, because a loss of skill may indicate shunt malfunction or progression of the primary etiology. This applies to the older school-aged child and the infant. Ataxia, slurred speech, lack of progression in school, incontinence, and so forth may indicate a deterioration in neurologic status and the need for further evaluation.

Children with hydrocephalus usually have verbal skills commiserate with their intellectual abilities and perform better on verbal tests than fine motor-visual perception tests. The primary care provider must assess speech carefully, however, because 25% to 35% of individuals with hydrocephalus develop a hyper verbal pattern of communication with good vocabulary and articulation but shallow intellect, poor social skills, and low academic attainment (Blum and Pfaffinger, 1994; Hendrick, 1993). This speech pattern is referred to as "cocktail party chatter" and may disguise a lower intelligence than is first apparent.

Often these children will benefit from infant stimulation programs or physical therapy, and the primary care provider must be familiar with the program offerings in the family's community to help them identify services that would be most beneficial for their child.

Diet

There are no special dietary requirements for children with hydrocephalus. Many parents become overly concerned about episodes of regurgitation or vomiting common in all infants, and clarification as to what is normal and what is pathologic vomiting should be made early after the diagnosis of hydrocephalus. The parents may be hesitant to burp the infant because of poor head control or concern over

dislodging the shunt. Alternate positions for burping can be demonstrated. If repeated regurgitation does occur, parents should be advised about using an infant seat for postfeeding positioning and introducing solids if age appropriate.

Safety

The primary care provider plays a major role in educating parents and children about safety. Families may be so overwhelmed with the task of parenting a child with a chronic condition that routine safety measures are overlooked.

The prolonged lack of head control in the child with hydrocephalus predisposes them to accidental head injury. In addition, car seat safety studies indicate infants should be positioned facing the rear in a semireclined position until the infant is able to sit upright fully supporting his or her head. Infants with hydrocephalus may not be able to attain head control or sit upright until late in their first year of life. This must be reviewed and parents encouraged to use the infant car seats properly to decrease the risk of head, neck, and abdominal injury (Bull, Stroup, and Gerhart, 1988). Transportation to and from day care or school must also be done with appropriate safety restraints to support the trunk and head in those children with severe disabilities (Paley et al, 1993).

As the child grows, activities should be limited as little as possible to encourage normal development and peer relationships. Helmets should be required for all activities which frequently result in falls, such as bike and skateboard riding.

The child's neurologic disabilities and visual perceptual integration may make competitive sports difficult and operation of motor vehicles hazardous. Each individual's ability must be assessed on a regular basis so the risks and benefits of activities can be determined. (Committee on Sports Medicine and Fitness, 1994).

Immunizations

Diphtheria, tetanus, and pertussis. Pertussis poses a special problem for infants with hydrocephalus. Infants and children with a history of seizures are at increased risk of seizures following receipt of pertussis (Committee on Infectious Diseases, 1994). As stated earlier, seizures at the time of diagnosis during the newborn period are often present in infants with hydrocephalus. It is difficult to determine which of these infants will continue to have recurrent seizures and which will not. Hence deferral of DTP immunization may be prudent until neurologic stability is ascertained. The infants neurologic status should be evaluated at each primary care visit to determine if the pertussis vaccine is still contraindicated. Children with a personal seizure history are at increased risk of seizures following pertussis immunization and must have their temperature monitored and controlled (Committee on Infectious Diseases, 1994). Because outbreaks of pertussis continue to occur in the United States, deferral of the vaccine must be weighed against the potential for disease and disease-related complications (Committee on Infectious Diseases, 1994).

Children in day care, attending special developmental programs, or receiving care in residential centers are exposed to other children who also may not be immunized and therefore are at increased risk of developing pertussis. In these difficult situations consultation with the child's neurosurgeon or neurologist may be advisable to help assess the child's seizure potential.

If the primary care provider, with parental consent, decides early in infancy that the pertussis immunization will be withheld, diphtheria and tetanus vaccines should be given on schedule. When an acellular pertussis vaccine becomes approved for infants, the incidence of neurologic side effects may be decreased. Hopefully infants with a history of seizures may then be immunized on schedule without increased risk.

Measles. Measles vaccine has also been implicated in postvaccination seizures, with a higher incidence occurring in infants and children with a personal history of seizures (Committee on Infectious Diseases, 1994). It is not believed these postvaccine seizures produce permanent neurologic damage, and the high ongoing risk of natural measles with its high morbidity rate justifies measles immunization in children with a personal history of convulsions (Committee on Infectious Diseases, 1994).

Haemophilus influenzae type b. The use of Hib vaccine is variable but generally much lower than the other recommended vaccinations (Gururaj and Rogers, 1987). Because of the increased risk of CNS infections in children with shunts, children with shunted hydrocephalus should definitely re-

ceive the conjugated vaccine starting at 2 months of age (Committee on Infectious Diseases, 1994). Children who have had a history of documented Hib disease before 2 years of age may not produce adequate antibodies to prevent a second infection and should therefore also be immunized. Chemoprophylaxis of household or day care contacts of children with Hib disease is required even with adequate immunization (Committee on Infectious Diseases, 1994).

Other immunizations. Vaccination for polio, hepatitis B, variccella, mumps, and rubella should be given as routinely scheduled. At this time there is no research on the efficacy of giving pneumococcal or influenza vaccines to these children (Committee on Infectious Diseases, 1994), but the primary care provider may elect to administer these additional vaccines to children with multiple shunt infections or severe motor disabilities.

Screening

Vision. Because of the high incidence of visual defects in children with hydrocephalus, the practitioner must pay particular attention to visual screening. The Hirschberg light reflex, cover test, tracking, and fundoscopic examinations should be performed at each office visit and the results carefully documented in the record. At approximately 6 months of age the child should be referred to a pediatric ophthalmologist for a thorough examination. Yearly examinations should be scheduled thereafter.

Frequently these children will need eye muscle surgery to correct esotropia or exotropia. The practitioner can be instrumental in completing preoperative examinations and preparing the family for surgery.

The primary care provider must remember that alterations in the fundoscopic examination, eye muscle control, or visual ability may be associated with shunt malfunction and must be evaluated carefully when shunt malfunction or infection is part of the differential diagnosis.

Hearing. In addition to routine office screening for hearing acuity, an auditory evoked response test should be ordered if the infant has had a history of CNS infection or antibiotic treatment with aminoglycocides. Subsequent shunt malfunctions or CNS infections require reassessment of hearing. Periodic evaluation by an audiologist is recommended.

Dental. Routine dental care is recommended. If the child is taking phenytoin (Dilantin) for seizure control, dental care may need to be more frequent because of hyperplasia of the gums. Poor dental hygiene and peridontal infections may produce bacteremia even in the absence of dental procedures (Dajani et al, 1990; Nunn, Gordon, and Carmichael, 1992). Antibiotic prophylaxis is recommended for all dental work likely to cause gingival bleeding including routine cleaning of teeth (Croll, Greiner, and Schut, 1979). The spontaneous shedding of primary teeth or simple adjustment of orthodontic appliances do not require prophylaxis (Dajani et al, 1990) to prevent bacterial endocarditis, (see Chapter 15).

Blood pressure. Blood pressure readings should be recorded on each clinic or office visit. Elevations in blood pressure occur in conjunction with elevations in intracranial pressure. Having an established baseline reading can help the practitioner assess the child for possible shunt malfunctions or progression of disease process.

Hematocrit. Routine screening is recommended.

Urinalysis. Routine screening is recommended.

Tuberculosis. Routine screening is recommended.

Condition-specific screening

HEAD CIRCUMFERENCE. Head circumference measurements should be taken at every clinic or office visit until the child's sutures are completely fused (see the discussion of growth and development).

COMMON ILLNESS MANAGEMENT

Differential Diagnosis

Unfortunately for the primary care provider, many of the symptoms of shunt malfunction or infection are the same symptoms commonly found with routine childhood illness. It is important to remember that these children will develop otitis media, gastrointestinal (GI) illnesses, and viral infections with fever just like their unaffected peers. The primary care provider must approach these children as children first. A calm manner, accompanied by a thor-ough history and examination, will be most reassuring to parents and most productive for the primary care provider.

Fever. Fevers associated with shunt malfunction or infection can be chronic or acute, mild or severe. The greater the time that has elapsed since the child's last shunt surgery, the less likely the fever is associated with shunt malfunction or infection. One recent study found the presence of fever was negatively associated with shunt malfunction in a cohort of children admitted to the hospital for evaluation (Watkins et al, 1994). Other symptoms, especially a change in sensorium or continued irritability or drowsiness after the fever has been controlled, are the most critical observations when trying to rule out shunt malfunction.

During the infant's first year when shunt infections are most common, parents should be encouraged to consult with the primary care provider whenever a temperature greater than 38.5° C occurs. The practitioner, with the consulting physician, can then evaluate the child early in the course of illness and note progression of symptoms.

If a focus of infection other than the shunt is identified, it should be treated appropriately. No

DIFFERENTIAL DIAGNOSIS

Fever—concern regarding shunt malfunction
Gastrointestinal symptoms—concern regarding:
    Peritoneal shunt placement and malfunction
    Abdominal infection may seed shunt
    Brain tumors may metastasize to abdomen via shunt
    Constipation may result in peritoneal shunt malfunction
Headaches—concern regarding increased intracranial pressure
Scalp infections—concern regarding infection spread to shunt reservoir
Alterations in behavior—concern regarding shunt malfunction

studies indicate that frequent antibacterial therapy for illnesses of questionable origin reduces the incidence of shunt malfunction. Children being treated for such bacterial infections as otitis media, pneumonia, or streptococcal sore throat should be seen in the office or clinic 24 to 48 hours after treatment is initiated to be carefully reassessed. Continued or worsening symptoms may indicate progression of the infection into bacteremia or a CNS infection caused by the increased susceptibility as a result of the shunt (Schutzman, Petryki, and Fleisher, 1991). Close follow-up is required.

If the child has a mild or moderate fever of unknown origin with other symptoms compatible with a common childhood illness and no obvious signs of shunt malfunction—such as erythema or edema along the tubing track, changes in sensorium, or meningeal signs—the primary care provider can assume a wait-and-see attitude. Arrangements for telephone follow-up or a return appointment in 24 hours should be made. The parents must be instructed on symptoms such as developing lethargy or recurrent vomiting that need to be reported immediately should they occur.

Children who have very high temperatures ($>40°$ C) and symptoms of moderate to severe illness must be assumed to have a shunt infection until proved otherwise. Consultation with the neurosurgeon or neurologist is advised. Blood cultures for both aerobic and anaerobic organisms should be drawn, though they often are not initially positive. A complete blood cell count is also indicated, but minimal leukocytosis does not rule out shunt infection. Cerebrospinal fluid can be obtained for culture via a lumbar puncture or through the shunt reservoir. A chest x-ray and urine culture are recommended to rule out pneumonia or urinary tract infection, but if the history and physical findings strongly suggest shunt involvement, those may be omitted. The neurosurgeon may prefer that all tests be done at the hospital because hospitalization is often required to complete the evaluation and treatment process.

Gastrointestinal symptoms. Nausea and vomiting are common clinical symptoms during childhood, often accompanying such diverse conditions as influenza, otitis media, and urinary tract infections. Diarrhea and abdominal pain are also frequent complaints in childhood. Children with hy-

drocephalus can be expected to have these common complaints as frequently as their unaffected counterparts.

When the child has mild GI symptoms, the practitioner must assess the presence or absence of other symptoms and history of exposure to GI illness. Mild to moderate fever is often present with both GI infections and shunt malfunction and therefore is not a good differentiating symptom. The presence or absence of swelling or inflammation along the catheter line or at the incision site is highly suggestive of shunt involvement. In addition, with a shunt malfunction the shunt reservoir may not pump and drain as expected and may be a key observation, though the sensitivity and predictive value of a shunt pumping test has recently come into question (Piatt, 1992). Probably most important to assess is a change in the child's sensorium and behavior, which indicates increased intracranial pressure. If the child appears normal to the parents or only a "little under the weather," the practitioner can again take a wait-and-see attitude as long as close follow-up can be maintained.

In children with shunts the primary care provider must recognize that abdominal symptoms may be the presenting symptom of peritoneal shunt malfunction. Abdominal pain, acute diarrhea, peritonitis, and tenderness associated with malfunctioning of the peritoneal tubing may mimic an acute condition of the abdomen (Klein, 1990). It may be impossible for the practitioner to differentiate the symptoms of an acute condition of the abdomen from peritoneal shunt malfunction, and consultation with and referral to the attending neurosurgeon are advised. In addition, children with peritoneal shunts are at risk for shunt infections originating in the abdominal cavity. Appendicitis and abdominal surgery must be managed in conjunction with the neurosurgeon (Pittman et al, 1992).

A recently published chart review reported constipation as the apparent cause of temporary peritoneal shunt malfunction (Bragg et al, 1994). Many children with hydrocephalus have other neurologic problems which may increase the incidence of constipation. Stool trapped in the colon may apply pressure on the peritoneal shunt resulting in a malfunction. Maintenance of regular stool patterns may prevent unnecessary hospitalization and possible shunt revision.

One unfortunate possible side effect of ventriculoperitoneal shunts is metastasis of brain tumor cells from the ventricular cavities into the abdominal cavity (Epstein, 1985). This must be considered when one is making a differential diagnosis in a child with more chronic or recurring abdominal complaints if the child has a history of a brain tumor. Appropriate referral is required to rule out this possibility after more common reasons for the complaint have been proved negative.

Headaches. Older children frequently complain of headaches. This too can occur in the child with a shunt and may have the same origin as in children without hydrocephalus. But if routine treatment with mild analgesics and rest does not relieve the symptom, if the headaches become frequent or chronic or associated with lethargy or irritability, evaluation by the neurologist and neurosurgeon is required (Rekate, 1991). Shunt malfunction can be partial or variable, depending on cerebral blood flow, CSF production, and the child's activity, and may result in periodic episodes of increased intracranial pressure (Schurr and Polkey, 1993).

Children with hydrocephalus occasionally experience headaches and vomiting in the early morning after sleeping all night. Usually these symptoms subside after the children have been up for a few hours; the symptoms may be caused by temporary partial blockage of the shunt from cellular debris, inactivity, and the horizontal sleeping position, which negates the beneficial effect of gravity for ventricular drainage. If these episodes are infrequent and self-limited, they do not require treatment other than acetaminophen for pain and possibly promethazine hydrochloride (Phenergen) or trimethobenzamide hydrochloride (Tigan) for nausea and vomiting. If the parents are reliable, prescriptions for these medications can be given in advance so that the parents will have them available when an episode occurs. Parents should be instructed to call the primary care provider if these symptoms continue for more than 6 hours or are associated with a decrease in the level of consciousness or loss of motor ability.

Scalp infections. A thin layer of skin covers the shunt reservoir on the scalp. If the skin around the shunt reservoir becomes infected, the integrity of the skin barrier may be broken and an infection of the shunt is possible. The primary care provider should manage scalp infections in conjunction with the neurosurgeon.

Alterations in behavior. All children experience mood swings and temporary behavior changes. In the child with hydrocephalus, a malfunctioning shunt may lead to the child "just not being right;" school performance may falter, normal interest in activities dwindle, and lethargy or irritability develop. If these changes persist beyond a few days, the child should be seen by the neurosurgeon for an evaluation.

Drug Interactions

No routine medications are prescribed for children with hydrocephalus. (See Chapter 19 for drug interactions with anticonvulsant therapy.)

DEVELOPMENTAL ISSUES

Sleep Patterns

Parents may be concerned about their infant or child sleeping in a position that might adversely affect the shunt. During the immediate postoperative period following shunt placement, the child should be positioned off the reservoir site to avoid skin breakdown. Except during this brief period, parents and caretakers need to be reassured their child can sleep in any position that is comfortable without fear of affecting the shunt. Infants and young children should be encouraged to assume a normal sleeping pattern at night.

Toileting

Children with neurologic deficits associated with hydrocephalus may have delayed ability to develop bowel and bladder control. Parents need to be counseled on the possibility of this difficulty and methods of toilet training reviewed. The neurologist and neurosurgeon following the child's development should be consulted concerning the neurologic capability of the child to attain satisfactory toilet training. If necessary, special bowel training and clean intermittent catheterization education should be provided and can usually be obtained through referral from the neurologist or neurosurgeon (see Chapter 27).

Discipline

Discipline for children with hydrocephalus should be managed as for normal children, recognizing the limitations of cognitive and motor development of the individual child. Some parents may have difficulty understanding the discrepancy between their child's verbal and performance skills and may have expectations that are too high for the child to attain. This may lead to inappropriate discipline. On the other hand, parents may be afraid to discipline their child and must be encouraged to set appropriate limits (Gardner, Tholcken, and Quay, 1991).

The practitioner must always be concerned with the increased possibility of child abuse in children with chronic conditions. Head injuries and abdominal injuries are common in child abuse and may result in further brain injury or shunt malfunction.

Child Care

The majority of mothers are currently working outside the home. Child care and preschool placement are major issues for all working parents but even more so when the child has a chronic condition. Fortunately the current shunt systems are self-maintained and do not require special care such as pumping periodically throughout the day. There are no special care needs for the child with hydrocephalus unless other disabilities such as cerebral palsy, seizures, or mental retardation are present.

If the child does have significant disabilities, child care arrangements will need to be evaluated for their ability to meet the child's needs. The passage of Public Law 101-476, the Individuals with Disabilities Education Act (1990) has extended services to children with disabilities from birth to school entry, so federally funded programs will now be accessible to children with disabilities (Fewell, 1993).

Children with hydrocephalus, however, are at greater risk for CNS infections than their peers because of the presence of the shunt. Parents must understand that children who attend day care or preschool will have more frequent exposure to childhood infections and will have more illnesses, usually respiratory or GI, than those who stay at home (Hurwitz et al, 1991; Takala et al, 1995; Thacker et al, 1992). Children less than 2 years of age have a higher shunt infection rate than older children (Odio, McCracken, and Nelson, 1984;

Yogev, 1985). For this reason it is advisable for children up to 2 years of age to receive child care at home or in a small home care program to minimize exposure to common pediatric pathogens. Limiting the child's exposure to upper respiratory and gastrointestinal infections will also reduce the frequency of illness and the question of shunt malfunction or infection requiring hospitalization or MRI/CT shunt evaluation.

Schooling

The primary care provider can be of great assistance in helping the family plan the child's individualized educational program (IEP) to assure appropriate interventions for the child. Although Public Law 94-142 requires the school district to assess the child's needs, financial constraints of the school district may limit neuropsychologic testing; therefore, any testing done before school may be very beneficial and should be forwarded to the school district on request. Parents may need assistance in obtaining medical records that would help in formulating the child's IEP.

Because of physical or intellectual limitations, some children with hydrocephalus will qualify for separate special education classes. Other children will be able to be mainstreamed into the regular classrooms and receive special services, such as adaptive physical education to help with motor control and balance, occupational therapy to assist with kinesthetic-proprioceptive deficits, speech therapy, or psychologic counseling to address emotional issues.

As the child reaches junior high school and high school some limitations should be made on competitive, high-impact sports. Tackle football, soccer, and ice hockey have a much higher risk of head and abdominal injury than track, swimming, or tennis. If the child has mild to moderate neuromotor deficits, an evaluation by a sports medicine professional may help identify sports activities the child will be able to perform with success. This is often beneficial to the child's self-esteem and encourages peer relationships, both of which may be problematic areas for the child with hydrocephalus.

Individuals with hydrocephalus but without significant motor and intellectual impairment may be caught in a Catch-22 of expectations. Their disabilities may not be recognized by teachers and peers who are unable to understand why the individual has difficulty in school or sports performance. The adolescent who is trying "not to be different" may not disclose his or her learning or motor deficit, but will not be able to compete successfully with nonaffected peers. The resulting incongruity between expectations and ability can lead to a sense of failure and lowered self-esteem.

The primary care provider should routinely ask the parents and child about school progress. If academic difficulties develop, the child should be referred for repeat neuropsychologic testing to rule out medical reasons for these problems. If the difficulty is assessed to be more emotional, which often happens during the adolescent years when the child struggles with his or her body image and identity, a referral for counseling should be made. It is advisable that the referral be made to a professional experienced in working with children with disabilities.

Sexuality

As previously mentioned, delayed or precocious puberty may occur in children with hydrocephalus. Their progression through puberty must be assessed and monitored (Ott and Jackson, 1989; Pescovitz, 1990). Counseling may be indicated to support the child or adolescent during this period. Research indicates children with precocious puberty may have lowered self-esteem, poor peer relationships, and have a higher incidence of sexual abuse than normally developing children (Jackson and Ott, 1990).

Sexuality and reproductive issues should be managed the same as with other children. Female adolescents receiving anticonvulsive therapy should be informed of the possible teratogenic effects of the medications they are taking (see Chapter 19). Adolescents with associated motor disabilities may have additional needs (see Chapters 19 and 27).

Transition into Adulthood

Beginning in the 1970s, improvements in shunt techniques and management of shunt complications have resulted in a dramatic increase in the survival of individuals with hydrocephalus. Researchers are following these young people as they make their transition into adulthood (Kokkonen et al, 1994; Simpson and Hemmer, 1993; Villani et al, 1995). These researchers have identified concerns

regarding how these young adults deal with vocational training, career placement, sexuality, and family roles.

Social outcome is highly influenced by associated disabilities, especially mental retardation and motor handicaps (Kokkonen et al, 1994). Many adults who were shunted during childhood have achieved full employment and successful personal relationships either because their disabilities were minor or because they were able to overcome them (Simpson and Hemmer, 1993). Results of studies assessing the employment rate of young adults with hydrocephalus associated with spina bifida have been less promising, with as many as 70% to 80% failing to maintain employment (Tew, Laurence, and Jenkins, 1990). Some of these subjects were described as lacking drive or initiative; however, both Tew and associates and Kokkonen and associates cite lack of an environment that fosters independence as a probable factor. Parents are often overcautious, overprotective, and fail to discipline appropriately. This inadvertently causes the child to be socially inappropriate and dependent (Gardner, Tholcken, and Quay, 1991).

A supportive climate that encourages independence, maturity, and responsibility is essential if young adults with hydrocephalus are to complete school, maintain employment, and function as adults. Professional guidance is often necessary to create this environment. The health professional should emphasize a positive prognosis for the young adult with hydrocephalus. Parents need to be prepared to face the normal problems of adolescence and to let their young children develop independence (Gardner, Tholcken, and Quay, 1991; Kokkonen et al, 1994; Simpson and Hemmer, 1993). The National Information Center For Handicapped Children and Youth (NICHY) can provide information and referrals for social skills programs that may be useful to parents, teachers, and others. At the college level, vocational training and special education resources can assist the young adult in preparing for job placement.

Young adults who are shunt dependent should be cautious about living alone. They could become acutely ill, confused, or even comatose during a shunt malfunction. It is recommended these young adults form a buddy system to assure their well-being and thereby minimize their risk of permanent brain injury from an unrecognized shunt malfunction (Rekate, 1991).

Issues regarding sexuality have been discussed previously. Hydrocephalus alone should not interfere with a woman's ability to conceive; however, recent reports suggest that shunt function can be affected by pregnancy (Wisoff et al, 1991). Wisoff and his associates reported the outcome of 16 pregnancies in women with hydrocephalus. Neurologic complications during pregnancy including seizures, headaches, nausea and vomiting, lethargy, ataxia, and gaze paresis occurred in 75% of the women with preexisting shunts. In most cases symptoms of increased intracranial pressure resolved postpartum, however four women required shunt revision during pregnancy or within 1 year of delivery. All infants were born without defects. The authors recommended that prenatal counseling and assessment include an evaluation of medications, especially anticonvulsants, genetic counseling, and review of family history for neural tube defects, and a complete assessment of shunt function (Wisoff et al, 1991). In addition, maternal supplementation with folic acid has been found to decrease the incidence of neural tube defects. Therefore, women in their child-bearing years should be encouraged to supplement their intake of folic acid before conception (Canadian Task Force, 1994; Rieder, 1994).

Securing health and life insurance may be difficult for young adults with hydrocephalus who are no longer covered by their parents' insurance benefits. Many insurance companies will deny coverage or charge exorbitant rates for individuals with preexisting conditions such as hydrocephalus. These young people should seek employment, if possible, with a large company that provides health coverage with few restrictions.

SPECIAL FAMILY CONCERNS AND RESOURCES

Parents of children with hydrocephalus constantly worry about continued shunt function. With every malfunction there is the need for surgery and the perceived threat of further brain damage. This constant worry and the daily responsibility and stress of caring for a child who may have multiple medical problems are very hard on families (Jackson,

1985). Financial strain from numerous medical visits or surgical procedures may deplete a family's financial reserve. Private insurance may not be obtainable unless offered through a large group employment policy. Concern about the child's ability to be self-supporting and independent in the future is also an issue for parents as the child grows into adolescence.

Parent-to-parent support groups can be very helpful offering parent support, publishing newsletters, and even hosting major medical conferences for both health professionals and parents. These organizations also enable a network for children with hydrocephalus, offering them the opportunity to make new friends, develop peer support, and exchange knowledge. The primary care provider should become familiar with the organizations in the community so that appropriate referrals can be made. It is better to make such a referral early after the child's diagnosis than to wait to see how the parents cope. All parents need support above and beyond what is reasonable for the physician or nurse to provide.

Organizations

National organizations
Hydrocephalus Association
  870 Market St #955
  San Francisco, CA 94102
  (415) 776-4713
HOPE (Hydrocephalus Opens People Eyes)
  104-47 120th St
  Richmond Hill, NY 11419
National Organization for Rare Disorders (NORD)
  PO Box 8923
  New Fairfield, CT 06812
  (203) 746-6518
National Information Center for Handicapped Children and Youth (NICHY)
  PO Box 1492
  Washington, DC 20013
Spina Bifida Association of America
  4590 MacArthur Blvd NW
  Suite 250
  Washington, DC 20007-4226
United Cerebral Palsy Association, Inc
  330 West 34th St
  New York, NY 10001
  (212) 947-5770

SUMMARY OF PRIMARY CARE NEEDS FOR THE CHILD WITH HYDROCEPHALUS

Health care maintenance

Growth and development

Height and weight are usually within normal range unless the child is severely handicapped.

If enlarged head size is diagnosed in infancy and a shunt is placed, head size should follow normal growth curve.

The head should be measured at each visit until the sutures are fused.

Both precocious puberty and short stature are reported.

Standard infant development tests may indicate delay because of poor head control.

Seventy-five percent of children will have some motor disability.

Need to assess verbal skills and compare to intellectual ability.

Diet

Normal diet indicated.

Concern and difficulty assessing infant vomiting as normal or as sign of increased ICP.

Safety

The risk of head injury is increased because of poor head control.

A rear-facing car seat should be recommended until the child is able to sit unsupported.

A helmet should be used for bike and skateboard riding.

Neurologic deficits may make competitive sports difficult and operation of motor vehicles hazardous.

Immunization

Pertussis vaccine may be deferred in infants with seizures.

Measles vaccine may cause seizures in children with seizure disorders but is recommended because of the prevalence of measles.

Haemophilus influenzae type b conjugated vaccine is strongly recommended.

Pneumococcal vaccine and influenza vaccine should be considered for children with multiple shunt infections.

Screening

Vision

Hirschberg's examination, cover test, ability to track, and fundoscopic examination should be done at each visit. The child should be examined by an ophthalmologist at 6 months of age and then yearly thereafter.

Alterations in eye examination may be associated with shunt malfunction.

Hearing

Routine office screening is recommended. Auditory evoked response test should be given to children with a history of CNS infection or who have been treated with aminoglycosides.

Dental

Routine dental care is recommended.

Children on phenytoin therapy require more frequent dental care.

Prophylactic antibiotics are recommended for dental procedures likely to cause bleeding.

Blood pressure

Blood pressure should be recorded at each visit.

Blood pressure increases with increased intracranial pressure.

Hematocrit

Routine screening is recommended.

Urinalysis

Routine screening is recommended.

Tuberculosis

Routine screening is recommended.

Condition-specific screening

HEAD CIRCUMFERENCE

Head circumference should be measured at each visit until the sutures are completely fused.

Common illness management

Differential diagnosis

Fever

Rule out shunt infection or CNS infection.

Gastrointestinal symptoms

Rule out increased intracranial pressure with nausea and vomiting.

Rule out peritonitis with abdominal pain or acute diarrhea.

Continued.

SUMMARY OF PRIMARY CARE NEEDS FOR THE CHILD WITH HYDROCEPHALUS—cont'd

Rule out shunt infection caused by abdominal infection.

Rule out constipation as cause of shunt malfunction.

Rule out metastatic abdominal tumor in children with primary brain tumors and ventriculoperitoneal shunts.

Headaches

Rule out shunt malfunction as the cause of acute or chronic headaches.

Scalp infections

Rule out possible infection spread to shunt reservoir.

Alterations in behavior

Rule out alterations in behavior as symptom of shunt malfunction.

Drug interactions

No routine medications are prescribed.

Developmental issues

Sleep patterns

Standard developmental counseling is advised.

Toileting

Delayed bowel and bladder training may occur because of neurologic deficit.

Constipation may cause peritoneal shunt malfunction.

Discipline

Expectations are normal, with recognition of the possible discrepancy between verbal and motor abilities. Physical punishment is a hazard because it may cause head or abdominal injury.

Child care

No special care needs are required except when the child has severe motor disability or seizures.

Home care or small day care programs are recommended during the child's first 2 years of life to reduce infections.

Schooling

Associated problems are often covered by Public Law 94-142.

Families should be assisted in IEP hearings.

Children may have possible adjustment problems during adolescence.

Children may need psychometric testing for poor school performance.

Low impact sports should be selected to prevent head trauma and abdominal injury.

Beware of the catch-22 of minor unseen disabilities.

Sexuality

Evaluate for delayed or precocious puberty.

Standard developmental counseling is advised unless associated problems warrant additional care.

Transition into adulthood

Research has identified difficulty with vocational training career, sexuality, and family roles associated with hydrocephalus and mental retardation and motor handicaps.

Need to foster independence from early age to prepare young adults for independence.

Shunt dependent individuals should develop a buddy system to assure shunt malfunction leading to acute illness, confusion, or coma does not go unrecognized.

Pregnancy may interfer with peritoneal shunt drainage. Securing independent health and life insurance may be difficult for individuals with hydrocephalus.

Special family concerns

ilies are concerned about continued shunt function and the possibility of brain damage caused by shunt failure or infection.

REFERENCES

Abdel-Rahman AM, Rosenberg AA: Prevention of intraventricular hemorrhage in the premature infant, *Clin Perinatol* 21(3):505-521, 1994.

Andretta G: Shunt infections in hydrocephalic children, *Int Pediatr* 2:242-244, 1987.

Barkovich AJ: Hydrocephalus. In Barkovich AJ, (editor): *Pediatric neuroimaging,* New York, 1995, Raven Press, pp 439-475.

Blum RW, Pfaffinger K: Myelodysplasia in childhood and adolescence, *Pediatr Rev* 15(12):480-484, 1994.

Bragg CL et al: Ventricloperitoneal shunt dysfunction and constipation: a chart review, *J Neurosci Nurs* 26(5):265-269, 1994.

Bull MJ, Stroup KB, and Gerhart S: Misuse of car safety seats, *Pediatrics* 81:98-101, 1988.

Canadian Task Force on the Periodic Health Examination: Periodic health examination, 1994 update: primary and secondary prevention of neural tube defect, *Can Med Assoc J* 151(2):159-166, 1994.

Carey CM, Tullous MW, and Walker ML: Hydrocephalus: etiology, pathologic effects, diagnosis, and natural history. In Check WR (editor): *Pediatric neurosurgery: surgery of the developing nervous system,* ed 3, Philadelphia, 1994, WB Saunders, pp 185-201.

Center for Disease Control: Premature mortality due to congenital anomalies–United States, *MMWR* 35:505-506, 1988.

Clewell WH: The fetus with ventriculomegaly: selection and treatment. In Harrison MR, Globus MS, and Filly RA, (editors): *The unborn patient: prenatal diagnosis and treatment,* Philadelphia, 1990, WB Saunders, pp 444-447.

Committee on Infectious Diseases: Report of the committee on infectious diseases, ed 23, Elk Grove Village, IL, 1994, The American Academy of Pediatrics.

Committee on Sports Medicine and Fitness: Medical conditions affecting sports participation, *Pediatrics* 94(5):757-760, 1994.

Croll TP, Greiner DG, and Schut L: Antibiotic prophylaxis for the hydrocephalic dental patient with a shunt, *Pediatr Dentistry* 1(2):81-85, 1979.

Crombleholme TM: Invasive fetal therapy: current status and future directions, *Semin Perinatol* 18(4):385-397, 1994.

Dajani AS et al: Prevention of bacterial endocarditis: recommendations by the American Heart Association, *JAMA* 264(22):2919-2922, 1990.

Dennis M et al: The intelligence of hydrocephalic children, *Arch Neurol* 38:607-615, 1981.

Donders J, Canady AI, and Rourke BP: Psychometric intelligence after infantile hydrocephalus, *Child's Nervous System* 6:148-154, 1990.

Edwards MSB, Derechin ME: Neurosurgical problems in the infant. In Ballard RA, (editor): *Pediatric care of the ICN graduate,* Philadelphia, 1988, WB Saunders, pp 196-205.

Elias ER, Sadeghi-Nejad A: Precocious puberty in girls with myelodysplasia, *Pediatrics,* 93(3):521-2, 1994.

Epstein FJ: How to get rid of the shunt: a comment, *Child's Nervous System* 10(5):342-343, 1994.

Fernell E, Hagberg B, and Hagberg G: Epidemiology of infantile hydrocephalus in Sweden. I. A clinical follow-up study in children born at term, *Neuropediatrics* 19:135-142, 1988a.

Fernell E, Hagberg B, and Hagberg G: Epidemiology of infantile hydrocephalus in Sweden. II. Current aspects of the outcome in preterm infants, *Neuropediatrics* 19:143-145, 1988b.

Fewell RR: Child care for children with special needs, *Pediatrics* 91(1):193-198, 1993.

Gardner R, Tholcken MF, and Quay NB: Psychosocial implications. In Leech RW, Brumback RA, (editors): *Hydrocephalus: current clinical concepts,* St Louis, 1991, Mosby, pp 181-196.

Gaston H: Ophthalmic complications of spina bifida and hydrocephalus, *Eye* 5:279-290, 1991.

Gilmore HE: Medical treatment of hydrocephalus. In Scott RM, (editor): *Hydrocephalus: concepts in neurosurgery,* Baltimore, 1990, Williams & Wilkins, pp 37-46.

Graham SM et al: Safety of percutaneous endoscopic gastrostomy in patients with ventriculoperitoneal shunt, *Neurosurgery* 32(6):932-934, 1993.

Gururaj VP, Rogers PF: *Haemophilus influenze* type b vaccine: use in the pediatric population, *Pediatrics* 80:731-735, 1987.

Handler MH, Abbott R, and Lee M: A near-fatal complication of endoscopic third ventriculostomy: case report, *Neurosurgery* 35(5):525-527, 1994.

Hendrick EB: Results of treatment in infants and children in hydrocephalus. In Schurr PH, Polkey CE (editors): *Hydrocephalus,* Oxford, 1993, Oxford University Press, pp 161-176.

Hirsch JF: Consensus: long-term outcome in hydrocephalus, *Child Nervous System* 10:64-69, 1994.

Howell LJ: The unborn surgical patient: a nursing frontier, *Nurs Clin North Am* 29(4):681-694, 1994.

Hudgins R, Edwards MS: The fetus with a CNS malformation: natural history and management. In Harrison MR, Globus MS, and Filly RA (editors): *The unborn patient: prenatal diagnosis and treatment,* Philadelphia, 1990, WB Saunders, pp 437-442.

Hudgins RJ et al: Treatment of intraventricular hemorrhage in the premature infant with urokinase: a preliminary report, *Pediatr Neurosurg* 20(3):190-197, 1994.

Hurwitz ES et al: Risk of respiratory illness associated with day care attendance: a nationwide study, *Pediatrics* 87(1):62-69, 1991.

Jackson PL: When the baby isn't perfect, *Am J Nurs* 85:396-399, 1985.

Jackson PL, Ott MJ: Perceived self-esteem among children diagnosed with precocious puberty, *J Pediatr Nurs* 5(3):190-203, 1990.

Jones RF et al: The current status of endoscopic third ventriculostomy in the management of noncommunicating hydrocephalus, *Minimally Invasive Neurosurg* 37(1):28-36, 1994.

Kast J et al: Time-related patterns of ventricular shunt failure, *Child's Nervous System* 10:524-528, 1994.

Klein DM: Shunt infections. In Scott RM, (editor): *Hydrocephalus: concepts in neurosurgery,* Baltimore, 1990, Williams & Wilkins, pp 87-98.

Kokkonen J et al: Long-term prognosis for children with shunted hydrocephalus, *Child's Nervous System* 10(6):384-387, 1994.

Lumenta CB, Skotarczak U: Long-term follow-up in 233 patients with congenital hydrocephalus, *Child's Nervous System,* 11:173-175, 1995.

Mankinen-Heikkinen A, Mustonen E: Ophthalmic changes in hydrocephalus: a follow-up examination of 50 patients treated with shunts, *Acta Ophthalmol* 65:81-86, 1987.

Manwaring KH: Endoscope-guided placement of the ventriculoperitoneal shunt. In Manwaring KH, Crone K, (editors): *Neuroendoscopy,* New York, 1992, Mariann Leibert, pp 29-40.

Marlin AE, Gaskill SJ: Cerebrospinal fluid shunts: complications and results. In Cheek WR (editor): *Pediatric neurosurgery: surgery of the developing nervous system,* ed 3, Philadelphia, 1994, WB Saunders, pp 221-233.

Marlin AE, Gaskill SJ: The etiology and management of

hydrocephalus in the preterm infant. In Scott RM (editor): *Hydrocephalus: concepts in neurosurgery,* Baltimore, 1990, Williams & Wilkins, pp 67-78.

McDermott MW, Ciricillo SF, and Edwards MSB: Neuroendoscopy, *Neurosurgery* 162(3):261-262, 1995.

Neville BGR: Clinical features of hydrocephalus in childhood and infancy. In Schurr PH, Polkey CE (editors): *Hydrocephalus,* Oxford, 1993, Oxford University Press, pp 100-118.

Nunn JH, Gordon PH, and Carmichael CL: Dental disease and current treatment needs in a group of physically handicapped children, *Comm Dental Health* 10:389-396, 1992.

Odio C, McCracken G, and Nelson J: CSF shunt infections in pediatrics, *Am J Dis Child* 138:1103-1106, 1984.

Oka K et al: Endoneurosurgical treatment for hydrocephalus caused by intraventricular tumors, *Child's Nervous System* 10:162-166, 1994.

Ott MJ, Jackson PL: Precocious puberty, *Nurs Pract* 14(11):21-30, 1989.

Paakko E et al: Information value of magnetic resonance imaging in shunted hydrocephalus, *Arch Dis Child* 70(6):530-534, 1994.

Paley K et al: Transportation of children with special seating needs, *South Med J* 86(12):1339-1341, 1993.

Pat Riarca P. and Lauer B: Ventriculoperitoneal shunt-associated infections due to Haemophilus influenza. *Pediatrics* 65:1007-1007, 1980.

Pescovitz OH: Precocious puberty, *Pediatr Rev* 11(8):229-237, 1990.

Piatt JH: How effective are ventriculopleural shunts, *Pediatr Neurosurg* 21(1):66-70, 1994.

Piatt JH: Physical examination of patients with cerebrospinal fluid shunts: is there useful information in pumping the shunt? *Pediatrics* 89(3):470-473, 1992.

Piatt JH, Carlson CV: A search for determinants of cerebrospinal fluid shunt survival: retrospective analysis of a 14-year institutional experience, *Pediatr Neurosurg* 19(5):233-241, 1993.

Pittman T et al: The risk of abdominal operations in children with ventriculoperitoneal shunts, *J Pediatr Surg* 27(8):1051-1053, 1992.

Punt J: Principles of CSF diversion and alternative treatment. In Schurr PH, Polkey CE (editors): *Hydrocephalus,* Oxford, 1993, Oxford University Press, pp 139-154.

Rekate H: Treatment of hydrocephalus. In Cheek WR (editor): *Pediatric neurosurgery: surgery of the developing nervous system,* ed 3, Philadelphia, 1994, WB Saunders, pp 202-220.

Rekate HL: Shunt revision: complications and their prevention, *Pediatr Neurosurg* 17:155-162, 1991–1992.

Rekate H, McCormick J, and Yamada K: An analysis of the need for shunting after brain tumor surgery. In Marlin AE (editor): *Concepts in pediatric neurosurgery* (11), Conn., 1991, S. Karger, pp 39-46.

Rennels MB and Wald ER: Treatment of Haemophilus influenzae type B meningitis in children with cerebrospinal fluid shunts, *J Pediatrics* 97:424-426, 1980.

Rieder MJ: Prevention of neural tube defects with periconceptional folic acid, *Clin Perinatol* 21(3):483-501, 1994.

Riva D et al: Intelligence outcome in children with shunted hydrocephalus of different etiology, *Child's Nervous System* 10(1):70-73, 1994.

Rosseau GL, McCullough DC, and Joseph AL: Current prognosis in fetal ventriculomegaly, *J Neurosurg* 77(4):551-555, 1992.

Rudolph A: *Pediatrics,* New York, 1987, Appleton-Century-Crofts.

Sainte-Rose C: Shunt obstruction: a preventable complication? *Pediatr Neurosurg* 19:156-164, 1993.

Schurr PH, Polkey CE: *Hydrocephalus,* Oxford, 1993, Oxford University Press.

Schutzman SA, Petryki S, and Fleisher GR: Bacteremia with otitis media, *Pediatrics* 87(1):48-53, 1991.

Scott RM: The treatment and prevention of shunt complications. In Scott RM (editor): *Hydrocephalus: concepts in neurosurgery,* Baltimore, 1990, Williams & Wilkins, pp 115-122.

Serlo W et al: Functions and complications of shunts in different etiologies of childhood hydrocephalus, *Child's Nervous System* 6:92-94, 1990.

Shapiro S et al: Origin of organisms infecting ventricular shunts, *Neurosurgery* 22(5):868-872, 1988.

Shiminski-Maher T, Disabato J: Current trends in the diagnosis and management of hydrocephalus in children, *J Pediatr Nurs* 9(2):74-82, 1994.

Simpson D, Hemmer R: Social aspects of hydrocephalus. In Schurr PH, Polkey CE (editors): *Hydrocephalus,* Oxford, 1993, Oxford University Press, pp 223-245.

Takala AK et al: Risk factors for primary invasive pneumococcal disease among children in Finland, *JAMA* 273(11):859-864, 1995.

Tew B, Laurence KM, and Jenkins V: Factors affecting employability among young adults with spina bifida and hydrocephalus, Zeitschrift fur Kinderchirurgie, *Surgery in Infancy and Childhood* 45:34-36, 1990.

Thacker SB et al: Infectious diseases and injuries in child day care, *JAMA* 268(13):1720-1726, 1992.

Vernet O, Campiche R, and de Tribolet N: Long-term results after ventriculo-atrial shunting in children, *Child's Nervous System* 11:176-179, 1995.

Villani R et al: Long-term outcome in aqueductal stenosis, *Child's Nervous System* 11:180-185, 1995.

Walker ML, Petronio J, and Carey CM: Ventriculoscopy. In Cheek WR (editor): *Pediatric neurosurgery: surgery of the developing nervous system,* ed 3, Philadelphia, 1994, WB Saunders, pp 572-581.

Watkins L et al: The diagnosis of blocked cerebrospinal fluid shunts: a prospective study of referral to a pediatric neurosurgical unit, *Child's Nervous System* 10:87-90, 1994.

Warnick RE, Edwards MSB: Pediatric brain tumors, *Curr Prob Pediatr* 21(4):129-166, 1991.

Wisoff JH et al: Management of hydrocephalic women during pregnancy. In Marlin AE (editor): *Concepts in Pediatric Neurosurgery* 3:60-68, Basel, Karger, 1991.

Yogev R: Cerebrospinal fluid shunt infections: a personal view, *Pediatr Infect Dis* 4:113-118, 1985.

Inflammatory Bowel Disease

24

Veronica Perrone Pollack

ETIOLOGY

The term inflammatory bowel disease (IBD) encompasses the diagnoses Crohn's disease and ulcerative colitis. These two diseases are distinct entities but are commonly discussed together because they share many of the same presenting signs and symptoms, as well as approaches to diagnosis and treatment.

Crohn's disease is a chronic inflammatory disease of the bowel that may occur at any point in the gastrointestinal (GI) tract, from mouth to anus. The inflammation is transmural; it may extend from the intestinal mucosal lining through the serosal layer. In this condition diseased segments of the bowel may border on segments of healthy tissue, which gave the condition its former name "regional enteritis." The disease most commonly affects the terminal ileum and proximal segments of the colon (50% to 60%); in about 20% of those individuals with Crohn's disease the terminal ileum alone is affected. Diffuse small bowel disease is seen in 20% of affected individuals, followed more rarely (approximately 10%) by colonic disease alone (Colenda and Grand, 1995). Oral, esophageal, and gastric manifestations of Crohn's disease are also seen (Kirschner, Schmidt-Sommerfeld, and Stephens, 1989). Perianal disease is not uncommon in Crohn's disease; affected children may have skin tags, fissures, hemorrhoids, and fistulas. Disease of the rectum, however, is unusual in Crohn's disease.

Ulcerative colitis is an inflammatory disease that affects the colonic and rectal mucosa. Pancolitis is reported in 50% to 60% of those individuals with this disorder. Disease limited to the descending colon occurs less often (22% to 35%), whereas rectal disease alone is seen still less frequently (15%) (Hyams, 1988; Kirschner, 1988a).

The etiology of IBD continues to be a fertile area for research. Increasing evidence suggests that these two forms of inflammatory bowel disease are partly and possibly wholly distinct in their initial pathogenic events, but it is also likely that they share important common pathophysiologic processes (Podolsky, 1991a). Environmental, genetic, and immunologic theories continue to be pursued as potential contributors to the development of both Crohn's disease and ulcerative colitis. Psychogenic causes of these illnesses have been disproved but stress may exacerbate a present illness. Current work directed toward a better understanding of the immunologic response of the gastrointestinal tract as well as ongoing research elucidating the genetic component of these conditions is potentially promising. The currently accepted framework for an explanatory model suggests that an environmental trigger (a virus or bacterium) may act as an antigen to induce a cellular reaction in the GI tract of the child. This response is thought to be one that is immunologically mediated and to which the individual may be genetically predisposed (Podolsky, 1991a).

INCIDENCE

The incidence of Crohn's disease has been increasing over the past 20 to 30 years, whereas that of ulcerative colitis appears to have remained stable. Although it is argued that the increase in cases of Crohn's disease may be explained by improved recognition, the figures seem to indicate that the increasing incidence is real (Kirschner, 1995). Incidence rates for Crohn's disease range from 1 to 7 cases per 100,000. Figures for ulcerative colitis range from 1 to 10 cases per 100,000 (Calkins and Mendeloff, 1995).

The risk for African Americans for IBD currently approximates that of white Americans. Asian populations are affected with approximately equal frequency as European and American populations. Additionally, contrary to previous reports, individuals of Jewish heritage are at no increased risk for IBD (Calkins and Mendeloff, 1995).

Approximately 25% of all new diagnoses of IBD are made during childhood (Berquist, 1991). Clinicians are becoming increasingly aware of the incidence of IBD in children less than 2 years of age (Gryboski, 1993, 1994).

CLINICAL MANIFESTATIONS AT TIME OF DIAGNOSIS

Crohn's disease and ulcerative colitis are similar in many presenting symptoms (see Table 24-1). These symptoms include abdominal pain, diarrhea, fever, blood in the stool, and weight loss. The symptoms noted are dependent on the location of the disease and its severity.

Classically the child who has ulcerative colitis complains of frequent, watery diarrhea that is grossly bloody. Often pus and mucus are noted as well. The diarrheal stools may be associated with abdominal cramping and, if rectal disease is present,

Table 24-1.   COMPARISON OF CROHN'S DISEASE AND ULCERATIVE COLITIS: PRESENTING SYMPTOMS

	Crohn's disease	Ulcerative colitis
Alteration in bowel pattern	Diarrhea is common; one may also see constipation, alternating with diarrhea	Diarrhea is a hallmark; an increase in frequency of bowel movements with urgency is often a component. Constipation may be seen if the disease is obstructive.
Blood in stool	Grossly bloody stools are occasionally seen, most often when colonic disease is present. Occult blood is not uncommon in Crohn's disease.	It is common to see grossly bloody diarrhea; one may also see pus or mucus
Abdominal pain	Abdominal pain is frequently present in association with meals; pain is often periumbilical	Abdominal cramping is often present in association with passage of stool. Pain is often noted in the lower part of the abdomen.
Fever	It is not uncommon to have intermittent, usually low-grade fever	Fever is sometimes seen
Onset of disease	Classically the signs of Crohn's disease are more subtle than those of ulcerative colitis, though in a smaller percentage onset may be abrupt	Onset may be insidious or abrupt
Weight loss	Weight loss is a common feature of Crohn's disease; it may have occurred for many months to years before diagnosis	It is not uncommon to see weight loss; typically it will be more abrupt than in Crohn's disease
Perianal disease	Perianal disease is common	Perianal disease is rarely seen

tenesmus (a cramping pain in the rectum accompanied by urgency, most commonly noted after the passage of a bowel movement). Fever, weight loss, and fatigue may also be seen in the child who has ulcerative colitis. Growth failure may be seen in 6% to 12% of children with ulcerative colitis before corticosteroid therapy (Kirschner, 1995). The onset of symptoms may be either abrupt or more insidious, occurring over weeks or months. The child may appear essentially well, or chronically or acutely ill.

As with ulcerative colitis, the symptoms of Crohn's disease may manifest in an array of fashions. The child may have an acute, severe attack or, more commonly, the symptoms of the disease are subtle and have been present for months or years before the diagnosis is made (Colenda and Grand, 1995). Symptoms of Crohn's disease affecting the small bowel are commonly obstructive in nature. A diffuse abdominal discomfort possibly associated with meals may be seen along with diarrhea or constipation, and blood may be noted in the stool. Usually the blood is occult, though the stool may be grossly bloody particularly in Crohn's disease of the colon. Fever, anorexia, and weight loss are more commonly seen in these children than in those with ulcerative colitis. Failure to grow or to develop sexually is a presenting symptom in approximately 40% of all children with Crohn's disease (Colenda and Grand, 1995) and may have been the original cue for the GI evaluation to commence.

Inflammatory bowel disease may manifest itself as symptoms other than those attributed to the GI tract alone (see Fig. 24-1). Children may have or may eventually develop extraintestinal symptoms of their disease. Extraintestinal manifestations of the disease not uncommonly seen at diagnosis include aphthous ulcers of the mouth, arthritic inflammation (especially of large joints), and dermatologic complications such as erythema nodosum and pyoderma gangrenosum. Clubbing is another extraintestinal manifestation seen most commonly in the child with Crohn's disease.

The diagnostic evaluation for IBD most often includes radiographic examination of the GI tract, endoscopy and biopsy, evaluation of growth parameters, and assessment of laboratory values. Common laboratory findings associated with IBD include an elevated erythrocyte sedimentation rate (ESR), low serum iron, low hematocrit value, and

low hemoglobin level. In Crohn's disease affecting the small bowel and in severe ulcerative colitis, hypoalbuminemia and a decreased total protein serum value may also be noted.

The severity of presenting symptoms may not be indicative of the disease course that is to follow for the child. Symptoms seen at diagnosis, such as the extraintestinal manifestations previously noted, may remain with the child, may reappear with exacerbations of the disease, or may never return. Also, new symptoms (GI or extraintestinal) may appear with exacerbations, which can be indicative of disease progression. An exacerbation of Crohn's disease or of ulcerative colitis may sometimes be preceded by an intercurrent illness, a dietary indiscretion, an emotional stress, or may occur for no apparent reason. Quite often children with IBD become adept at anticipating which activities may be most likely to trigger a flare of their disease; for example, an adolescent with IBD may find that during school examinations or around an important social event their symptoms worsen.

TREATMENT

The course of treatment for IBD is based on several modes of drug therapy (see Table 24-2), nutritional therapy, and nutritional supplementation. The specific treatment plan is dependent on the location and severity of the disease, the impact of disease on growth and development, and the degree of debilitation felt by the child. When standard, conservative medical treatment fails to adequately control symptoms, or when complications such as toxic megacolon, obstruction, or abscesses fail to respond to medical management, surgical intervention is indicated.

Drug Therapy

The mainstay of treatment for ulcerative colitis for years has been sulfasalazine (Azulfidine). Sulfasalazine is a compound that combines 5-aminosalicylic acid (5-ASA or mesalamine) with sulfapyridine. Sulfapyridine is useful primarily as a delivery agent which, when bound to 5-ASA, prevents its absorption in the proximal GI tract. Bacteria break apart this compound in the colon where 5-ASA exerts its local antiinflammatory effect. Unfortunately, up to 20% (Taffet and Das, 1983) of

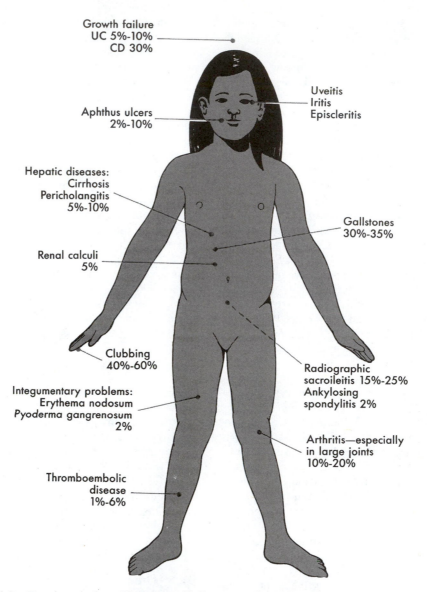

Growth failure
UC 5%-10%
CD 30%

Uveitis
Iritis
Episcleritis

Aphthus ulcers
2%-10%

Hepatic diseases:
Cirrhosis
Pericholangitis
5%-10%

Gallstones
30%-35%

Renal calculi
5%

Clubbing
40%-60%

Radiographic
sacroileitis 15%-25%
Ankylosing
spondylitis 2%

Integumentary problems:
Erythema nodosum
Pyoderma gangrenosum
2%

Arthritis—especially
in large joints
10%-20%

Thromboembolic
disease
1%-6%

Fig. 24-1.   Extraintestinal manifestations of inflammatory bowel disease.

individuals are unable to tolerate sulfasalazine because of significant side effects. The most common side effects of sulfasalazine are nausea, vomiting, and headache. Less common but more severe reactions are leukopenia, hemolytic anemia, and allergy. These side effects are attributed to sulfapyridine. Recently, several new 5-ASA agents have become available in the United States which are useful for treatment of children who have previously been unable to tolerate the sulfa component of the sulfasalazine. However, no notable therapeutic advantage has been found when comparing clinical efficacy of the newer 5-ASA formulations with that of sulfasalazine (Ogorek and Fisher, 1991).

Table 24-2.   **DRUGS USED FOR TREATMENT OF INFLAMMATORY BOWEL DISEASE**

Drug/dosage	Uses in IBD	Side effects in use with children with IBD	Special considerations
Sulfasalazine (Azulfidine) 50-75 mg/kg/ day	Treatment of ulcerative colitis Treatment of mild to moderate Crohn's disease, especially when there is colonic involvement	Common Headaches, GI upset, impaired folate absorption, male infertility Less common but significant Allergy (rash, bronchospasm) Leukopenia, worsening of disease	Fewer adverse reactions (allergy, headaches) may be noted if the dose is gradually increased to reach the planned therapeutic dosage Enteric coated tablets may alleviate GI upset It is available in suspension form Adverse reactions are generally noted within the first 3 months of therapy Monitor WBC count over first 3 months of treatment* It impairs folic acid absorption
Corticosteroids (prednisone) 1-2 mg/kg/ day	Useful in children who do not respond adequately to sulfasalazine Used in moderate to severe disease Available as foam (Cortifoam) and retention enema (Cortenema) for rectal disease	Common Growth retardation, cushingoid features, weight gain, striae, mood swings, acne, impaired calcium absorption, hypertension Less common but significant Cataracts	Alternate-day therapy at lowest possible dose is frequently used to minimize adverse effects The child should not discontinue corticosteroid use suddenly; this could result in not only hypocorticism but a flare-up of symptoms Ophthalmic examination should be done at each visit
Metronidazole (Flagyl) 15-20 mg/kg/day	Effective adjunct treatment of Crohn's disease May be useful in the management of perineal disease	Common GI upset, metallic taste, urticaria, darkening of the urine Less common but significant Paresthesia	Neurologic assessment should be done at each visit to monitor for any CNS effects† Paresthesia most commonly is reversible after discontinuation of medication or after reduction of dosage
6-Mercaptopurine (6-MP; Purinethol) 1.5 mg/kg/day Azathioprine (Imuran) 2.0 mg/kg/day	Used when sulfasalazine and corticosteroid therapy have failed Used when child is unable to be weaned from corticosteroids	Leukopenia Pancreatitis Possible risk of lymphoma in long-term use	If fever develops, drug should be discontinued It may take 3-6 months to achieve remission The WBC count should be monitored throughout therapy

*WBC, white blood cell.
†CNS, central nervous system.

Continued.

Table 24-2.   **DRUGS USED FOR TREATMENT OF INFLAMMATORY BOWEL DISEASE—cont'd**

Drug/dosage	Uses in IBD	Side effects in use with children with IBD	Special considerations
Oral 5-ASA agents 30-50 mg/kg/day	As with sulfasalazine	Common Diarrhea (especially olsalazine sodium), abdominal pain, nausea	Costly Fewer adverse reactions than sulfasalzine, useful for therapy in individuals unable to tolerate sulfasalazine Currently available preparations are unable to be divided or crushed to administer smaller doses for young children
Olsalazine sodium (Dipentum)	UC and Crohn's colitis,	Less frequent Headache, acne	
Mesalamine (Asacol, Pentasa)	UC and Crohn's colitis, Crohn's of small intestine	Rare but more serious Blood dyscrasias, nephritis, exacerbations of colitis	
Mesalamine (Rowasa)	Topical therapy for distal colitis, rectal disease	Pruritis, irritation	Costly Fewer adverse reactions than oral preparations

From Kirschner, BS 1995; Linn, FV, Peppercorn, MA, 1992; Geier, DL, Miner, PB, 1992.

Because sulfasalazine is less costly and equally efficacious, it remains the first line of therapy for mild to moderately active ulcerative colitis. Some clinicians, when initiating therapy, gradually increase the child's dosage to the therapeutic range (50 to 75 mg/kg/day) in an effort to alleviate or avoid the side effects of sulfasalazine. During the initiation of therapy, leukopenia and hemolytic anemia should be monitored every few weeks by a complete blood count (CBC). Should either of these occur the dosage should be decreased until the blood values return to normal. The dose may then be returned to the therapeutic range. Should this treatment be unsuccessful the drug may be discontinued and therapy with another 5-ASA preparation should be initiated.

Sulfasalazine inhibits folate absorption. Those children receiving sulfasalazine should be given supplemental folate (1 mg/day). Retention enemas and suppositories containing 5-ASA are also available. These topical preparations are useful for the child with disease limited to the rectum or descending colon. The systemic 5-ASA preparations have been better tolerated than sulfasalazine. Uncommon but reported side effects of both oral and topical preparations include: diarrhea, exacerbation of colitis, pneumonitis, pericarditis, pancarditis, and pancreatitis. Additionally, some individuals treated with topical mesalamine have complained of local irritation and burning (Ogorek and Fisher, 1991). As yet, pediatric dosages have not been established for the oral 5-ASA preparations. A suggested dosage schedule for 5-ASA is 30 to 50 mg/kg/day. One limitation in the use of oral mesalamine agents in younger children is that it is not possible to break apart or crush these preparations for delivery to young children requiring lower dosages.

In moderate to severe disease, as well as during exacerbations, corticosteroids given with sulfasalazine or an agent containing 5-ASA alone

TREATMENT

Drug therapy (see Table 24-2)

Nutritional therapy

Elemental diet—useful in reversing growth failure and attaining remission in children with Crohn's disease

Parenteral hyperalimentation—useful in reversing growth failure and attaining remission in Crohn's disease and ulcerative colitis. Generally reserved for those individuals with severe disease who cannot tolerate enteral feedings.

Surgical intervention

Indicated when disease activity or complications fail to respond to medical management

Crohn's disease: limited resection of diseased bowel segment

Ulcerative colitis: colectomy is the procedure of choice. For many individuals the option exists for reanastomosis and surgical construction of a "rectum" or pouch to retain contenance.

Stress management

have been found to be very effective in achieving remission. Children are first given a dosage ranging from 1 to 2 mg/kg/day, which is maintained until their symptoms diminish and they achieve their previous level of comfort and activity. The time period often allotted for this is 1 to 2 months (Kirschner, 1995). The dose is then gradually tapered to an alternate-day therapy while the child's symptoms and laboratory values, particularly the ESR and CBC, are monitored. This enables the child to continue to derive benefit from the drug while experiencing fewer side effects. The dose continues to be tapered until the child is able to function normally without its use. Side effects of prednisone include Cushingoid features, weight gain, hypertension, acne, striae, mood swings, calcium depletion, aseptic necrosis of the hip, and

cataracts. Another side effect of special significance to children with IBD is growth retardation. Although the impact of corticosteroids on growth in children is a concern, their contribution to growth failure in children with IBD remains controversial. Alternate-day corticosteroid use has been demonstrated to allow a normal growth rate to occur (Hyams and Carey, 1988). Alternative corticosteroid preparations such as retention enemas and foams for rectal instillation are also available. Rectal administration of the medication allows for local treatment of disease with fewer systemic side effects. Individuals with rectal disease, perianal disease, or disease of the descending colon may benefit from this therapy (Podolsky, 1991b).

Children with severe ulcerative colitis who are experiencing debilitating symptoms, pronounced abdominal pain or distension, severe electrolyte abnormalities, or anemia and hypoalbuminemia require aggressive medical intervention. They are hospitalized, placed on complete bowel rest, and receive intravenous (IV) hyperalimentation and corticosteroid therapy.

Management styles vary between practitioners with respect to the use of antispasmodic agents for the relief of chronic diarrhea in children with IBD (Kirschner, 1995). Drugs such as loperamide (Imodium) or diphenoxylate (Di-Atro) with atropine may be of use in controlling symptoms during daytime activities (Gitnick, 1989b; Hyams, 1988; Kirschner, 1995) but may be injudiciously used as a palliative measure. Bowel stasis, dilatation, and subsequently toxic megacolon may result (Barrett and Dharmsathaphorn, 1988; Reddy and Jeejeebhoy, 1988).

Crohn's disease is less responsive to sulfasalazine and the newer 5-ASA agents than ulcerative colitis. However, 5-ASA preparations such as Asacol, because they may be partially released in the intestine, play a role in treating Crohn's disease of the small intestine and are useful in maintaining clinical remission (Griffiths et al, 1993). They have also proven effective in therapy of Crohn's colitis and ileocolitis (Tremaine et al, 1994). Corticosteroids are more likely to be necessary as a first-line therapy in Crohn's disease.

Metronidazole has been found to be effective in the care of children with Crohn's disease. Of special interest is its effectiveness in the treatment of perianal disease. However, when the dosage is lowered or the drug is discontinued, it is common for the perianal disease to relapse. The effects of long-term use of metronidazole are not known. There is concern that it may potentially be carcinogenic or mutagenic, because this response has been identified in mice and rats (Brandt et al, 1982). There have been no cases in humans where either cancer or chromosomal aberrations have been proven to be attributable to metronidazole (Meyers and Sachar, 1995). The recommended pediatric dosage ranges from 10 to 15 mg/kg/day (Kirschner, 1995; Markowitz et al, 1991). Side effects of metronidazole include GI upset, urticaria, and a metallic taste. A more worrisome side effect of metronidazole is peripheral neuropathy. In one study up to 85% of those adolescents receiving metronidazole had abnormal nerve conduction studies (Duffy et al, 1985). Interestingly, far fewer than this percentage of individuals noted any loss of sensation. Several weeks to months after discontinuation of the drug almost all individuals will have reversal of the paresthesia (Duffy et al, 1985; Hyams, 1988).

6-mercaptopurine (6-MP) and azathioprine are immunosuppressive agents that are finding increased acceptance in the treatment of IBD in children. They are currently used as a second-line therapy in children for whom more conservative medical management has failed and for those individuals who have required long-term steroid use to control symptoms. The recommended dosage of 6-MP is 1.0 to 1.5 mg/kg/day (Kirschner, 1995) and for azathioprine 2 mg/kg/day (Markowitz et al, 1991). Response to these agents is not immediate, averaging 3 months (Geier and Miner, 1992). The most commonly cited complications of 6-MP and azathioprine are leukopenia and pancreatitis. A concern regarding the possible increased risk of lymphoma for individuals treated with these agents for IBD has been raised. In the results of one large study the risk for malignancy was found to be no greater than the background risk for individuals with IBD. The possibility of long-term teratogenic effects on the offspring of those who received 6-MP as children is another concern that causes hesitation when this therapy is prescribed for children. Other complications noted include allergy, hepatitis, and infectious complications (Present et al, 1989). For the first several months of therapy a CBC should be

checked every 2 weeks to assess for leukopenia. The WBC count should be checked monthly thereafter. The recommendation is to reduce the dosage or to terminate therapy if the WBC count falls below normal (Korelitz, 1992). Therapy may be reinstituted after the values return to normal. The primary care provider, family, and child must be aware that any fever during therapy with 6-MP or azathioprine is an indication for concern and needs to be evaluated. Discontinuing the drug may be necessary. Cyclosporine (Sandimmune) is an experimental therapy for IBD that has been finding increased acceptance in adults with refractory ulcerative colitis. It is hoped that cyclosporine will be another option as a second-line therapy for IBD that is refractory to more conservative treatment. Response to cyclosporine therapy has been inconsistent, and treated individuals have had a significant incidence of relapse while receiving therapy and reoccurrence when discontinuing the drug.

The role of cyclosporine in the therapy of Crohn's disease appears to be more limited. A major disadvantage to its use in Crohn's disease is the high rate of relapse after discontinuation along with the risks of toxicity (Meyers and Sachar, 1995). Side effects of cyclosporine include hypertension, tremor, hirsutism, seizures, and the potential for renal insufficiency. Lymphomas, which have been observed in children with transplants receiving cyclosporine, have not been reported in children with IBD treated with the drug.

Nutritional Therapy

The elemental diet, or formula providing total nutrition and supplying nitrogen in the form of simple amino acids, as therapy for IBD in children is a recent development. The elemental diet has been successful in attaining remission (Belli et al, 1988; Kleinman et al, 1989) and reversing growth failure in children with Crohn's disease (Belli et al, 1988). In some trials elemental diet has provided superior therapeutic results to the more traditional treatment with sulfasalazine and corticosteroids alone. In one study the intermittent use of elemental diet as the sole source of nutrition over a 1-year period resulted in decreased corticosteroid requirements and lower disease activity for the experimental group than during the year before therapy and lower than that of the controls (Belli et al, 1988). The children receiving elemental diets achieved significantly greater growth, and their height, weight, triceps skinfold, and midarm circumference were significantly increased relative to those not treated with elemental feedings. Pubertal change, as measured by Tanner scores, and bone age were not, however, significantly different from their peers in the control group. This finding indicates that there is potential for significant catch-up growth among those children who are treated in this fashion before puberty.

The superiority of this method of treatment must still be established. Studies comparing this mode of therapy with polymeric formulas, which are less costly and more palatable, are needed. Additionally, the long-term benefit of elemental diet as primary therapy for IBD has yet to be clearly established (Kirschner, 1995).

Nutritional therapy with parenteral hyperalimentation has also demonstrated improvement in disease activity and reversal of growth failure (Seidman et al, 1987). However, enteral feedings pose significant advantages over the parenteral route of nutrition because nasogastric feedings are less invasive, less costly, and pose fewer infectious risks than does the parenteral route.

Surgical Intervention

Indications for surgical intervention for the child with ulcerative colitis include intractable disease, refractory growth failure, toxic megacolon, hemorrhage, perforation, and cancer prophylaxis (Kirschner, 1995). Proctocolectomy is the procedure of choice for the child with ulcerative colitis requiring surgery. Historically, placement of a permanent ileostomy was necessary for individuals following total colectomy. During the past decade an alternative to this procedure, the ileoanal anastomosis (IAA), has been gaining wider acceptance by both clients and practitioners. This procedure provides continence without the need for a stoma. The IAA has been a welcome option for individuals facing total colectomy. Individuals undergoing this procedure have reported greater satisfaction in activities of daily living relative to the traditional ileostomy with collecting appliance (Pemberton et al, 1989). Some problems reported following IAA include soiling, most frequently during sleep, and numerous loose stools. More recently, variations on

this procedure have been developed in which a pouch is surgically constructed that acts as a reservoir. This procedure has offered the individual with ulcerative colitis improved continence and less frequent bowel movements. These newer procedures have resulted in even greater long-term satisfaction rates among children and adolescents (Telander et al, 1990).

The Kock pouch provides an abdominal reservoir that is emptied by the child using a catheter drainage appliance. The pouch opening is otherwise covered by a small dressing or bandage. This procedure is an alternative for the individual who, as a result of the disease or because of previous surgical resections, has anal sphincter control difficulties.

In one recent review 43% of children with Crohn's disease required surgery with 35% requiring reoperation (Gryboski, 1994). Most often resection of the diseased portion of the bowel is the approach chosen for the child with Crohn's disease who requires surgery. The likelihood of repeated surgical resections is high (Andrews, Lewis, and Allan, 1989). In addition, the likelihood of recurrence at the site of surgery makes the child with Crohn's disease ineligible for such procedures as the Kock pouch or the ileal anal anastomosis.

Stress Management

Because stress has been identified as a factor that may contribute to the exacerbation of IBD symptoms, some children find it helpful to master relaxation and stress management techniques for controlling or preventing flares of their disease and for managing daily stressors. The primary care provider may assist the family in finding programs that will promote the development of stress management and problem-solving skills.

RECENT AND ANTICIPATED ADVANCES IN DIAGNOSIS AND MANAGEMENT

Because of the significant overlap in clinical presentations and sometimes indeterminant histologic findings, distinguishing with certainty between these two conditions when disease is limited to the colon is sometimes difficult. Recently researchers have identified a genetic marker found in high levels in individuals with ulcerative colitis (Winter et al, 1994). The use of antineutrophil cytoplasmic antibodies (ANCA) has been restricted to research. This study may become a useful tool in the differentiation of Crohn's colitis and ulcerative colitis in children with indeterminant findings.

The most recent significant change in the clinical management of inflammatory bowel disease has been the introduction of newer mesalamine (5-ASA) preparations which do not contain the sulfa component found in sulfasalazine. This development benefits those individuals who previously would have benefited clinically from sulfasalazine but who were unable to tolerate the side effects most commonly attributed to its sulfa component. Another advantage of these agents over sulfasalazine is the finding that Asacol has been found to be useful in the treatment of Crohn's disease of the small intestine.

New corticosteroid preparations such as budesonide are currently undergoing clinical trials in the treatment of children with inflammatory bowel disease. It is hypothesized that because of their decreased suppression of hypothalamic-hypopituitary-adrenal axis, fewer of the more significant side effects seen in children—growth retardation and bone demineralization—would be experienced during long-term therapy (Gross et al, 1994).

Low-dose methotrexate administered weekly in both oral and intramuscular dosage forms has been explored in several studies (Baron, Truss, and Elson, 1993; Kozarek et al, 1991) as a treatment alternative for those individuals with steroid-dependent inflammatory bowel disease which is refractory to treatment with azathioprine or 6-mercaptopurine. Studies to date only have included adults and this mode of therapy remains within the realm of experimental trials. Continued study in larger groups with attention to side effects and potential benefit to children with IBD will hopefully provide exciting results.

ASSOCIATED PROBLEMS

Growth Failure

Growth failure and delayed onset of sexual maturation are common and significant problems for chil-

dren with IBD. At the time of diagnosis, 5% to 10% of children with ulcerative colitis and up to 30% of children with Crohn's disease have growth retardation (Kirschner, 1988a). A significant percentage of these children (approximately 50%) may have begun to demonstrate a decrease in height velocity an average of 12 months before the onset of any other symptoms attributable to Crohn's disease (Kanof, Lake, and Bayless, 1988).

Etiologic theories for growth failure have included malabsorption, excessive protein loss, and

---

ASSOCIATED PROBLEMS

Growth failure

Musculoskeletal problems

Osteoporosis
Peripheral arthritis
Ankylosing spondylitis
Sacroileitis

Dermatologic manifestations

Erythema nodosum
Pyoderma gangrenosum

Visual changes

Hepatobiliary complications

Primary sclerosing cholangitis
Pericholangitis
Cirrhosis
Gallstones

Renal changes

Renal calculi
Hydronephrosis

Fistulas and abscesses

Toxic megacolon

Lactese intolerance

Anemic

increased energy needs of children with IBD. The primary cause of growth failure in IBD is believed to be malnutrition. In one study the caloric intake of children with Crohn's disease was approximately 56% that of the recommended intake for height for age of the affected child (Kirschner et al, 1981). This caloric insufficiency may in part be the result of anorexia related to the association of pain with meals, to chronic illness, and to iatrogenic causes such as unnecessary dietary restrictions (Seidman et al, 1987).

Musculoskeletal Problems

Musculoskeletal problems associated with IBD include peripheral arthritis, ankylosing spondylitis, and sacroileitis. Peripheral arthritis is seen in approximately 20% of those individuals with IBD, usually in association with active intestinal disease (Kirschner, 1995). Inflammation and discomfort are noted in the large joints, especially those of the hip and the knee. Inflammation does not occur symmetrically. Unlike the other musculoskeletal manifestations of IBD, the arthritic symptoms often fluctuate with the activity of the bowel disease and respond to treatment of the disease. Other therapy for peripheral arthritis in IBD includes treatment with corticosteroids and nonsteroidal antiinflammatory agents. For selected individuals with active, refractory arthritis methotrexate may be useful (Kirschner, 1995). Ankylosing spondylitis may be seen in up to 11% of individuals with IBD and more commonly in those individuals with Crohn's disease (Retsky and Kraft, 1995). Sacroileitis may be noted on roentgenogram in 4% to 18% of those individuals with IBD, with far fewer than this percentage of individuals noting symptoms (Retsky and Kraft, 1995) such as low back pain. Although not an extraintestinal manifestation of IBD itself, osteoporosis is a significant risk for children with IBD because of their poor absorption of vitamin D and corticosteroid therapy (Retsky & Kraft, 1995).

Dermatologic Manifestations

Dermatologic manifestations occur in up to 5% to 15% of individuals with IBD (Retsky & Kraft, 1995). Erythema nodosum is a tender, reddened nodule that commonly appears on the anterior aspect of the lower leg, although it may be seen on the foot, the back of the leg, or on the arm. Erythema nodosum is seen more frequently with Crohn's disease (15%) than with ulcerative colitis (10%). Pyoderma gangrenosum is a more serious dermatologic condition that may be found in 1% to 12% of those individuals with ulcerative colitis. Pyoderma gangrenosum also is most frequently noted on the anterior aspect of the lower leg. It appears as one or many bullae bordered by an area of dark red or purple. Pyoderma gangrenosum may continue to penetrate into the tissues below and may result in osteomyelitis (Lewicki and Leeson, 1984). The child with this condition warrants immediate referral to a dermatologist.

Pyoderma gangrenosum is usually associated with severe bowel disease; however, the course of pyoderma gangrenosum is felt to be independent to that of the bowel disease (Retsky and Kraft, 1995). Despite any correlation between activity of the gastrointestinal and dermatologic conditions, most authorities recommend that treatment should include therapy directed at controlling the activity of the bowel disease.

Visual Changes

Ocular manifestations of IBD include iritis, episcleritis, uveitis, and conjunctivitis. It should also be noted that the child who is being treated with corticosteroids is at increased risk for cataracts and elevated intraocular pressure (Kirschner, 1995).

Hepatobiliary Complications

Other GI manifestations of IBD include hepatobiliary complications such as pericholangitis, cirrhosis, and primary sclerosing cholangitis. The physical examination should be closely monitored for hepatic enlargement or signs of portal hypertension. Gallstones are seen more frequently in Crohn's disease than in ulcerative colitis. They occur in from 13% to 34% of individuals with IBD, particularly in the client with extensive ileal disease or ileal resection. Their occurrence seems to be related to the malabsorption of bile salts with concomitant cholesterol precipitation and calculus formation (Retsky & Kraft, 1995).

Renal Changes

Renal calculi also may be seen in the individual with IBD. They have been noted in 8-19% of those individuals with IBD—the highest incidence occurring in people with Crohn's disease following small bowel resection or ileostomy. The child with severe ileal disease or resection of the ileum is at risk for the formation of calcium oxalate stones, which are the type seen more frequently in individuals with IBD (Retsky and Kraft, 1995). Hydronephrosis may also be seen in the child with IBD, particularly in those children who have had extensive scarring or inflammation of the small bowel or who have abscesses that may obstruct the ureter. Hydronephrosis associated with IBD is frequently asymptomatic; therefore, the primary care provider should be suspicious of this complication in a child with a history of fistulas or abscesses or who has a suspected abdominal mass.

Fistulas and Abscesses

Fistula and abscess formation are complications of Crohn's disease. Fistulas may form between the bowel and the surface of the skin or between the bowel and other organs or orifices. The clinician should question the child or parent about the passage of air or stool through the vagina or the urethra, because this may indicate a rectovaginal or rectourethral fistula.

Toxic Megacolon

Toxic megacolon is a life-threatening complication of IBD. It is most commonly associated with ulcerative colitis, but it may also occur early in the course of Crohn's disease. Toxic megacolon is an acute distension of the colon that may result in perforation, hemorrhage, and peritonitis. Signs of this complication are tachycardia, hypovolemia, fever, abdominal distension, decreased bowel sounds, and continuous, diffuse abdominal pain. The child taking corticosteroids, however, may have his or her fever suppressed. The child with suspected toxic megacolon should have all oral intake withheld and should be referred immediately to the gastroenterology team. Progression from severe disease to toxic megacolon and subsequent perforation may occur rapidly. The clinician should maintain a high index of suspicion for the likelihood of toxic megacolon in the child with worsening or severe disease. The evaluation includes radiologic assessment of the abdomen and clinical assessment. The role of the barium enema in precipitating a toxic megacolon remains controversial. It is recommended that flat plates of the abdomen are sufficient (Reddy, Jeejeebhoy 1988). Medical management includes bowel rest with nasogastric suction, parenteral hyperalimentation, and antibiotics given intravenously. If the toxic megacolon does not resolve within 24 to 72 hours, a colectomy is usually performed.

Lactose Intolerance

During periods of active disease some children with IBD may experience symptoms of lactose intolerance including bloating, abdominal cramping, and diarrhea related to the intake of dairy products. For this reason, some health care providers recommend that children eliminate lactose from their diet during their initial period of diagnosis and recovery to minimize confusion regarding the child's response to therapy. Kirschner, Defavaro, and Jensen (1981) found that when ethnicity was controlled, children with IBD had no greater incidence of lactose intolerance than a control sample. It was found that children who had African American or Jewish backgrounds had higher incidence of lactose intolerance. A breath hydrogen test may be performed to definitively diagnose lactose intolerance should such a clarification be desirable. Ultimately, a significant proportion of children with IBD will eventually be able to tolerate some amount of lactose in their diet.

Anemia

As a result of chronic malnutrition, malabsorption, the interference of sulfasalazine in the absorption of folates, and chronic blood loss, children with IBD are at increased risk for vitamin B_{12} deficiency and hypochromic microcytic or iron deficiency anemia. Daily supplementation with folic acid is recommended for them, as well as monitoring of CBC for all children with IBD. Also, iron supplementation is recommended for the symptomatic child.

PROGNOSIS

The overall life expectancy of individuals with IBD is essentially that of the general population (Harper et al, 1987); however, a significantly greater risk for intestinal malignancies exists among this group than among those who do not have IBD. It appears that in ulcerative colitis the risk of malignancy increases with the extent and duration of the disease. The risk of cancer begins to increase 10 to 15 years after the diagnosis of ulcerative colitis (Podolsky, 1991b). Those individuals diagnosed with ulcerative colitis at a younger age will remain at risk for cancer for a longer period of time, although age at diagnosis itself may not be a risk factor (Levin, 1995).

The issue of surveillance for cancer in individuals with long-standing ulcerative colitis is controversial. The efficacy of surveillance techniques is currently a matter of debate. Presently, those people who are considered high risk are recommended to undergo surveillance colonoscopy every 2 years (Podolsky, 1991b).

The prognosis is less clear for children with Crohn's disease. It is agreed that these individuals are also at greater risk for the development of an intestinal malignancy. The extent of that risk is not clear; the risk for colonic cancer may be similar to those with ulcerative colitis. The risk for small bowel malignancies is significantly greater than that of the general population (Feczko, 1987; Gitnick, 1989a). Because the incidence of these tumors in the general population is so low, however, this remains an uncommon complication of Crohn's disease (Podolsky, 1991b).

The information regarding the long-term impact of IBD on quality of life indicates that a significant percentage of adults with IBD report that their overall life satisfaction is low or affected negatively by their disease (Joachim and Milne, 1987). In Gryboski's recent reviews of children with IBD (1993, 1994), during the first 2 years after diagnosis of UC 75% of children or their parents felt that the child's quality of life was fair with 25% reporting a good quality of life. Interestingly, in individuals more than 24 months from diagnosis, these percentages were reversed with 75% of children's quality of life reported to be good. This is in contrast to those individuals diagnosed with Crohn's disease, 70% of whom reported their quality of life to be only fair, with 22% reporting a good quality of life, and 8% reporting a fair quality of life.

Primary Care Management
HEALTH CARE MAINTENANCE
Growth and Development

Children with IBD should have growth parameters measured and graphed on a National Center for Health Statistics chart at each primary care visit. For those children who have been recently diagnosed, it is helpful to go back through previous visits to calculate the child's growth curve in the years before the diagnosis was made. This will help the primary care provider assess for any deceleration in growth rate. Often school health or athletic offices may be of assistance in reconstructing the growth curve. Growth parameters of particular importance are both height and weight for age, Tanner stage, and arm anthropometry. Once growth retardation is identified as an actual or potential problem, a bone age should be obtained to identify the child's remaining growth potential. Continued careful measurement and graphing for growth parameters are essential. Catch-up growth is considered to be adequate if the child returns to his or her pre-illness growth percentiles.

Diet

No specific dietary restrictions have been documented to be helpful in controlling symptoms for the individual with IBD. Some individuals may feel most comfortable when they avoid certain foods; the child and family can be assisted in identifying such foods. The practitioner's fear is that the diet may become overly restricted by the anxious parent who feels able to attribute symptoms to multiple foods. This may result in a diet that is unappealing to the child and so restrictive as to provide too few calories to promote growth and development.

As a part of ongoing assessment of nutritional status, an evaluation of usual dietary intake is essential. If growth is unsatisfactory (i.e., less than 5 cm/year, height less than the 3rd percentile for age, or 2 standard deviations less than chronologic age), a referral should be made for a dietary consultation. The dietitian may assess the child's intake and nutritional status and counsel the child and family regarding ways in which caloric intake may be augmented. Commercially available calorically dense nutritional supplements may be a good adjunct to the child's diet in such circumstances.

If growth retardation associated with IBD is to be reversed, adequate nutritional supplementation is necessary. It is generally agreed that given adequate calories, a child or adolescent (before epiphyseal closure) may recover lost growth. As nutritional replenishment begins, a child or an adolescent with IBD may have greater caloric requirements than their unaffected peers. Recommendations for caloric intake range from 75 to 95 kcal/kg/day. Under routine circumstances it is not necessary for the child with IBD to receive more calories than a child without IBD (Kirschner, 1995).

During periods of active disease, many children, particularly those with Crohn's disease affecting the small bowel, may feel most comfortable on a low-roughage diet. Children with Crohn's disease of the small bowel are also more likely to experience some degree of lactose intolerance, which may persist even during periods of remission. During periods of inactive disease, these children may drink Lactaid milk or use lactase capsules and tablets which are readily available. For those children who feel especially deprived or set apart from their peers as a result of their dietary restrictions, such products may be of value. Experience has shown that these products are not helpful for all lactose-intolerant individuals, however. Children on milk-restricted diets and those taking corticosteroids should receive calcium supplementation because they are at risk for osteoporosis (Reid and Ibbertson, 1986).

Safety

The child with IBD requires no special restriction of activities. The child should be encouraged to participate in all sports he or she feels able to enjoy. Vigorous activities such as lacrosse or tackle football should pose no problem for the child in remission. The child with osteoporosis, however, should refrain from such sports. Because, as in many populations with special needs, there may be a tendency for anxious families to shelter their child from discomfort or tense situations, the primary care provider can play an integral role in advocating for a normal lifestyle for the child.

Alcohol consumption by the adolescent with IBD who is in remission is no more of a concern than is alcohol consumption by nonaffected peers. Alcohol ingestion may cause discomfort for some individuals with IBD. If this is the case, this individual should limit intake. Persons taking metronidazole should be informed that concomitant alcohol intake will induce a disulfiram (antiabuse) type of reaction.

Immunizations

No change from the normal immunization schedule is necessary unless the child receives maintenance therapy of corticosteroids or other immunosuppressive agents such as 6-MP or cyclosporine. These children should not receive live virus immunizations until they have been tapered from these drugs. If this is not feasible or exposure is of particular concern, a killed virus vaccine may be given, or condition-specific immunoglobulin. Children who receive maintenance therapy of immunosuppressive drugs should receive prophylaxis with varicella-zoster immune globulin for varicella exposure.

Screening

Vision. Ophthalmic examinations are necessary at each well-child visit because children with IBD are at risk for ocular manifestations of their disease. In the case of iritis, the examiner may note redness of the eye, eye pain, photophobia, or blurred vision. In uveitis, abnormal pupillary reaction may also be assessed. A reddened eye may be noted in episcleritis or conjunctivitis (Danzi, 1988). If the child is receiving prolonged corticosteroid therapy a yearly ophthalmology referral and assessment for cataracts is recommended. Any child with an abnormal ophthalmoscopic examination or who complains of the previously mentioned symptoms should be referred to an ophthalmologist and to the gastroenterology team.

Hearing. Routine screening is recommended.

Dental. Children who are being treated with cyclosporine are at risk for gingival hyperplasia. Proper dental hygiene and yearly dental visits should be reinforced at each well-child visit.

Blood pressure. Children who are taking cyclosporine or corticosteroids are at increased risk for hypertension. Their blood pressures should be measured every 6 months.

Hematocrit. Hemoglobin and hematocrit values should be measured yearly for children who are asymptomatic and who have no history of anemia. For any child with a history of anemia or who is experiencing increased symptoms of their disease, a CBC should be checked every 6 months or as needed.

Urinalysis. No change in the usual protocol for screening is necessary unless the history indicates renal involvement or the child is experiencing symptoms indicative of any of the previously mentioned conditions.

Tuberculosis. The child who is receiving immunosuppressive therapy may not respond to testing. Screening may be withheld until immunosuppressive drugs are discontinued. If exposure is suspected, a control may be placed along with the purified protein derivative of the tuberculosis to assess for anergy. Chest radiography may be necessary to screen for active disease.

Condition-specific screening

ERYTHROCYTE SEDIMENTATION RATE. An ESR should be measured yearly for the asymptomatic child. The ESR may be used for some children with IBD as an index of disease activity, in up to 90% of individuals with Crohn's disease and over 50% of those with ulcerative colitis (Colenda and Grand, 1995). The ESR should be normal in the child with inactive disease. A variation from baseline should be followed with close questioning regarding current disease activity, onset of new symptoms, or any recent dietary indiscretions.

FECAL OCCULT BLOOD TEST. For the child who is asymptomatic, stool should be monitored yearly for the presence of occult blood using a fecal-occult blood reagent (e.g., Hemocult). The results should, in most instances, be negative in the child with inactive disease. Some children with IBD will always carry a trace of blood in their stool. The child whose stool is routinely normal but has a positive occult blood result should be assessed more carefully for indications of increased disease activity.

CHEMISTRIES. The child taking cyclosporine, azathioprine, or 6-MP should have renal (blood urea nitrogen and creatinine levels) and liver function studies (fractionated bilirubin, aspartate aminotransferase, alanine aminotransferase, and alkaline phosphatase values) monitored at least every 6 months throughout his or her therapy. Liver function studies should be assessed every few years in the otherwise asymptomatic child with IBD. The child with Crohn's disease should also have albumin levels checked yearly.

LACTOSE INTOLERANCE. The diagnosis of lactose intolerance may be made empirically by eliminating lactose-containing products from the diet and monitoring for changes in symptoms such as cramping, distention, and diarrhea. The diagnosis may also be made by the breath hydrogen test. The clinician may also cursory screen for lactose intolerance in the office by testing stool for reducing substances or by testing the pH of the stool. An acidic pH (<6.5) would be indicative of lactose intolerance.

NEUROLOGIC EXAMINATION. Children who are being treated with metronidazole require close neurologic examination at each visit.

COMMON ILLNESS MANAGEMENT

Differential Diagnosis

The symptoms of IBD and its associated problems are varied. Symptoms of common childhood illnesses may be difficult to differentiate from exacerbations of the child's underlying disease process. Gastrointestinal symptoms are the ones that will most likely cause concern or alarm to the child, family, and primary care provider. An index of disease activity for some, but not all children, is the ESR. This may from time to time be of assistance in clarifying the child's symptoms.

Intercurrent illnesses, such as a viral or bacterial gastroenteritis or another illness that must be treated with antibiotic therapy, may contribute to the flare of the child's IBD. This may be a result of the alteration of the normal flora of the bowel, usually a predominance of *Clostridium difficile,* following antibiotic therapy.

Diarrhea. Children with IBD can and do have bouts of gastroenteritis similar to those of their peers and family members. The child's physical examination and history should include an evaluation of any IBD-like symptoms such as the presence of any blood, pus, or mucus in the stool; cramping or urgency associated with bowel movements; weight loss or anorexia; and the occurrence of any symptoms that might be extraintestinal manifestations of the disease. The child's abdomen should be closely examined for any change. Stool cultures should always be obtained because *Yersinia, Campylobacter, Shigella,* and *C. difficile* may mimic IBD. The child should be treated for any identified pathogen. Any child who has prolonged symptoms, significant hematochezia (with no identified pathogen), or weight loss should be referred to the gastroenterology team.

Abdominal pain. The child with abdominal pain should be examined for any changes that might indicate a progression of their disease, toxic megacolon, or an obstruction. The child should be questioned as to the similarity of the current pain to the pain previously experienced as a part of the IBD. Similarity to previous episodes, location of known disease, and a history of accompanying symptoms that would indicate disease rather than influenza or another acute condition of the abdomen should guide the practitioner. Pain that is acute in an ill-appearing child should be referred immediately to the gastroenterology team; less acute symptoms should be watched carefully, with referral if the symptoms fail to abate within 24 to 48 hours.

Vomiting. Vomiting in a child with Crohn's disease could indicate an obstruction. The history and physical examination should elicit information regarding distention, any associated pain and its relation to meals and nature of the emesis, and accompanying abdominal pain. As always, information should be gathered regarding the child's bowel pattern and the nature of the stools.

Skeletal complaints. Children who are receiving corticosteroid therapy are at increased risk for osteoporosis and aseptic necrosis of the hip. In addition, children with IBD have a greater likelihood of having peripheral arthritis, sacroileitis, and ankylosing spondylitis. The child with IBD who complains of back or hip pain requires radiologic examination to adequately assess the symptoms. When the child with IBD complains of joint pain, he or she should be questioned regarding the presence of erythema or swelling. If joint involvement is a concern, the child should also be assessed for any increased disease activity.

Drug Interactions

Sulfasalazine, the mainstay of traditional therapy for both ulcerative colitis and Crohn's disease, potentiates the action of both oral-form hypoglycemia agents, resulting in lower than anticipated blood glucose values, and phenytoin (Dilantin), resulting in higher than expected blood values of this drug and increased risk of drug toxicity. Sulfasalazine, metronidazole, and corticosteroids potentiate the action of warfarin (Coumadin). Increased prothrombin time has been reported in children taking warfarin and olsalazine (Dipentum) simultaneously (Physicians' Desk Reference, 1995). Finally, when administered along with digoxin (Lanoxin), sulfasalazine has been found to inhibit absorption, resulting in decreased blood levels of the drug. Metronidazole has a disulfiram (Antibuse) type of reaction when the individual ingests alcohol or alcohol-containing elixirs during drug therapy. Corticosteroids also diminish the efficacy of hypoglycemic agents taken orally, resulting in higher than desired blood glucose levels (Bradbury and Mehl, 1989).

DIFFERENTIAL DIAGNOSIS

Diarrhea

Rule out flare of disease: obtain cultures

Abdominal pain

Rule out flare of disease, toxic megacolon, and obstruction

Vomiting

Rule out flare of disease and assess for obstruction

Skeletal complaints

Rule out arthritic manifestations of the disease (sacroileitis, ankylosing spondylitis, peripheral arthritis) and osteoporosis

DEVELOPMENTAL ISSUES

Sleep Patterns

Children who are taking corticosteroids twice daily may feel agitated or euphoric at bedtime and may have some difficulty sleeping. Dosage times may be shifted somewhat to alleviate this problem. Once the dose is decreased, a single dose may be given in the morning. The child experiencing a flare of disease or whose disease is under poor control may be troubled by the need to use the bathroom many times during the night. This may make it difficult for the child to feel well rested and refreshed in the morning.

Toileting

Because the majority of children are diagnosed with IBD after the age at which toilet training is usually accomplished, families of children with IBD do not typically face this issue. For those children who are not trained, it is preferable to wait to begin toilet training until a time when the disease is quiescent and when the character of the bowel movement is as close to normal as possible.

Incontinence is an experience shared on occasion by many individuals with IBD; for those children who have frequent bowel movements accompanied by urgency, the fear of this occurrence is ever present. Children and families should be assisted in planning to prevent or to handle in a low-key fashion such an eventuality. In the context of an overview of the child's condition and its implications, the possibility of incontinence occurring should be shared with the school nurse and classroom teachers. They may then make plans to ensure that incidents will be handled with sensitivity and that the child may retain as much control and dignity as possible. The classroom teacher should be encouraged to move the child's seat nearer the door and to liberalize bathroom privileges so that he or she may leave the room unobtrusively. The primary care provider may suggest that an extra change of clothing be kept in the child's locker or in the nurse's office.

Discipline

Behavioral expectations for the child with IBD are similar to those of their nonaffected peers. One area of concern may be the issue of compliance for those children who are responsible or are assuming the responsibility for their treatment regimen. Those children in whom IBD remains in remission may not perceive the need for their medications because they may be essentially asymptomatic and feeling well. The concept of remission and disease being present but not discernable is a difficult one for the school-aged child or early adolescent to master. Because a large percentage of those children diagnosed with IBD are in their early to middle adolescence, rebellion and testing are normal development issues (Erikson, 1963). For adolescents with IBD, medications and treatment regimens become a fertile battleground for testing their independence. The primary care provider can help the family identify ownership of responsibility for the disease management.

Child Care

Parents of children with IBD should be encouraged to use the same guidelines for choosing child care arrangements for this child as they would their well siblings. Because the onset of IBD most commonly occurs in childhood, the increased risk of diarrheal illness secondary to diaper-changing areas and day care providers handling food does not often need to be addressed by these families. Should the child become infected, the illness should be promptly treated and the child monitored for signs of exacerbation of the disease. The overriding philosophy, however, is to not unduly isolate the child from normal activities of daily living.

Schooling

Children with Crohn's disease and ulcerative colitis are equally as able to achieve in the classroom as their nonaffected peers. As do many children with chronic conditions, children with IBD must juggle treatment schedules, and deal with stigma, pain, fatigue, and occasionally frequent or long school absences. Ultimately the child's struggle to overcome these hurdles may be reflected in his or her academic performance.

The nature of the disease processes and their treatment regimens often set children with IBD apart from their peers in significant ways. These include the Cushingoid faces of the child receiving corticosteroid therapy, the need for embarrassing treatments such as the instillation of rectal medications, and the use of nocturnal nasogastric feedings or restrictive diets. The isolation felt by the child experiencing these treatments may cause the child to limit participation in those activities that enrich the school experience. Alternatively, the child may choose not to comply with treatment regimens in an effort to fit in. This may set up a cycle of disease exacerbation and escalation of therapy which may affect the child's academic achievement and ultimately reinforce the child's sense of isolation. Sensitivity to these issues, creative problem solving, and anticipatory guidance by the primary care provider will support the child and family in achieving as normal a lifestyle as possible. An issue frequently faced by the individual with IBD is the common misunderstanding by lay people and some in the medical community that IBD is a psychologic disease. A primary role of the health care provider is that of educating school personnel and other significant adults in the child's life, such as club leaders, coaches, and day care providers.

Sexuality

Adolescence is a time when concerns regarding body image, interpersonal relationships with members of the opposite sex, and plans for one's future are paramount. It is not unusual then that adolescents or young adults with IBD would be concerned about the impact this diagnosis might have on their appeal as a sexual partner, their ability to perform sexually, and their fertility. The significant changes in appearance that the adolescent with IBD must withstand include, in many instances, the late onset of puberty, weight gain, and acne, all of which contribute to his or her feelings of self-consciousness and stigma. Individuals with Crohn's disease frequently have stomas or perianal involvement, which often is disfiguring. This, too, may affect the adolescent's feelings of sexual attractiveness or acceptability to another person. Positive feelings of self-worth and a sense of acceptance must be conveyed to the adolescent who has IBD. The option of joining a network of other adolescents who share common concerns should be offered whenever possible. Formal organizations or casual social gatherings may provide opportunities for teens and families to obtain support and acceptance.

Sulfasalazine has been demonstrated to cause infertility in men; a decrease in sperm count, dys-

motility, and malformation have been documented. These effects have been demonstrated to be reversible, however, when these men stop taking sulfasalazine for 3 months (Hanan and Kirsner, 1985; Korelitz, 1988). There have been no reports of infertility in men receiving the newer, oral 5-ASA preparations (Ogorek and Fisher, 1991). Neither ulcerative colitis nor Crohn's disease increases infertility in women with inactive disease. Some studies have indicated that women with Crohn's disease have higher rates of infertility than control populations. It is believed that the most common cause of infertility in women with Crohn's disease is the activity of the disease. Other factors include poor nutritional status, rectovaginal fistulas, fear of becoming pregnant, and advice from health care providers. Pelvic scarring is thought to be the cause of infertility in only a very small percentage of individuals (Burakoff, 1995).

The outcome of pregnancy in women with IBD approximates that of the general population, though some researchers have found a somewhat higher incidence of prematurity in infants born to mothers with IBD than in the general population (Burakoff, 1995).

Pregnancy does not increase the likelihood of a relapse of either ulcerative colitis or of Crohn's disease. In two thirds of all women with active IBD at conception, the disease will remain active or worsen during pregnancy.

Surgical resection for Crohn's disease or ulcerative colitis appears to affect neither fertility nor the outcome of pregnancy. Men who have undergone colectomy with ileostomy or one of the other continent ileostomy procedures have a low risk of impotence as a complication of the surgical procedure (Burakoff, 1995).

Transition into Adulthood

As with all adolescents with chronic conditions, the transition of responsibility for managing health care related issues is sometimes rocky. The primary care provider should begin facilitating these changes early in adolescence. Responsibility for specific tasks such as taking medicine can be assigned to the adolescent and gradually the adolescent's responsibility may be increased as both the teen and the family become comfortable. The practitioner can facilitate this transition through supportive counseling and appropriate referrals.

Individuals with IBD do not typically require a specialized environment or assistance with activities of daily living. The embarrassing nature of many of the required medical therapies and symptoms of active disease make private living facilities most desirable for many individuals with IBD. The practitioner may assist the individual in securing such accommodations.

There are no reports of specialized programs to transition adolescents with IBD to adult care. Many primary care providers have an informal policy of caring for their adolescent clients with IBD until they have weathered most of the anticipated developmental crises of late adolescence. It is best to wait to make this transition until a time when the individual's disease is quiescent.

SPECIAL FAMILY CONCERNS AND RESOURCES

Families of children with IBD, like families of children with other chronic conditions, may focus on the child's symptoms and treatment regimen. In the case of the family dealing with IBD, however, this often means disclosing such private and potentially embarrassing issues as toileting and personal hygiene. The invasion of privacy felt by the child may become a source of stress for the entire family. Common concerns shared by children with IBD include diet and their ability to fit in when sharing a meal or snacks with friends and family, personal appearance, and physical endurance. As the child enters adolescence, these issues are magnified as he or she seeks increased independence from the family and becomes increasingly self-conscious and concerned about body image and function. This may lead to poor communication and distrust between parent and child regarding disease activity and compliance with treatment regimens. If it is possible for the child to become relatively independent in disease management before this difficult time, the child and family may develop confidence and trust in one another and perhaps alleviate or avoid some of these conflicts. Another battle for control is often fought over the dietary habits of children with IBD who, because of individual sensitivity, disease activity, or parental misconception, use a restrictive diet. The primary care provider should anticipate such issues arising in the family

of a young adolescent with IBD and provide anticipatory guidance, ongoing counseling, and advocacy to achieve an individualized and manageable treatment regimen for the child.

IBD may affect children of many ethnic and religious backgrounds, at a wide range of ages and with varied clinical presentations and severity. When cultural or religious practices focus on food and special dietary practices, these children may feel conflicted if disease activity makes some foods difficult to tolerate. It should be emphasized that other than during times of disease activity it is not typically recommended that children limit their diet. Children should be encouraged to maintain a diet as unrestricted and palatable as possible to encourage adequate caloric intake to promote optimal growth and development. Sensitivity by members of the health care team regarding dietary issues as they relate to both everyday life and special celebrations or religious observance is important. Practitioners should work to develop a flexible plan of care which incorporates such individual cultural concerns such as religious feasts or times of fasting.

Organizations

Crohn's and Colitis Foundation of America, Inc
386 Park Ave S, 17th Floor
New York, NY 10016-8804
(800) 343-3637
(212) 685-3440

The Crohn's and Colitis Foundation of America (CCFA) is an organization with many chapters across the country that provides education and support for its members and for members of the community. Individuals with IBD and their families are encouraged to join and attend meetings and educational offerings. Many chapters have subcommittees that specifically deal with issues related to the needs of children with IBD and their families. The CCFA also publishes educational books, pamphlets, and newsletters written for the lay public. Professional memberships are also available. The CCFA holds seminars for health care providers and publishes newsletters, educational materials, and a scientific journal. The CCFA also produces audiovisual materials for use by professionals. Inquiries may be made regarding lists of publications and pamphlets, as well as chapter locations.

SUMMARY OF PRIMARY CARE NEEDS FOR THE CHILD WITH INFLAMMATORY BOWEL DISEASE

Health care maintenance

Growth and development

Growth failure is a common problem for children with IBD, more commonly seen in Crohn's disease than ulcerative colitis.

Growth parameters are important to measure and graph at each primary care visit.

Cognitive abilities are unimpaired by IBD.

Diet

No special diet is recommended; some children may be lactose intolerant particularly when disease is active. Some children during active disease may have less pain on a low roughage diet. Adequate caloric intake is essential for growth.

Safety

No special safety recommendations are necessary for the child with inactive disease. Children with osteoporosis should not participate in contact sports.

Immunizations

No change in the normal immunization protocol is indicated unless the child is taking maintenance doses of immunosuppressive agents; in this case no live vaccines should be administered but immune globulin may be used with exposures.

Screening

Vision

Ophthalmic examination is necessary at each visit. Some centers suggest yearly ophthalmologist visits for the child taking maintenance doses of corticosteroids.

Hearing

Routine screening is recommended.

Dental

Routine care is adequate, but children taking cyclosporine are at increased risk for gingival hyperplasia.

Blood pressure

Routine screening is recommended; if the child is taking cyclosporine or corticosteroids, blood pressure should be measured every 6 months.

Hematocrit

Hematocrit and hemoglobin values should be obtained yearly if the child is asymptomatic and has no history of anemia; otherwise a CBC should be obtained every 6 months or as necessary.

Urinalysis

Routine screening is recommended unless the child has a history of fistulas or abscesses.

Tuberculosis

Routine screening is recommended.

Condition-specific screening

ERYTHROCYTE SEDIMENTATION RATE

Check annually. Fecal occult blood test. Check stool yearly and with potential disease flare.

CHEMISTRIES

Liver function studies should be monitored every few years for the otherwise asymptomatic child with IBD. The child taking Dipentum, Asacol, or Pentasa should have renal functions studies monitored at least every 6 months. For children receiving cyclosporine, 6-MP, or azathioprine renal and liver function studies should be monitored every 6 months. For children taking 6-MP, amylase and lipase levels should be tested every 6 months.

LACTOSE INTOLERANCE

Check as indicated.

NEUROLOGIC EXAMINATION

Children receiving metronidazole should be assessed for paresthesia at each routine visit.

Common illness management

Differential diagnosis

Diarrhea

Rule out flare of disease: obtain cultures.

Abdominal pain.

Rule out flare of disease, toxic megacolon, and obstruction.

Vomiting

Rule out flare of disease and assess for obstruction.

Skeletal complaints

Rule out arthritic manifestations of the disease (sacroileitis, ankylosing spondylitis, peripheral arthritis) and osteoporosis.

Continued.

SUMMARY OF PRIMARY CARE NEEDS FOR THE CHILD WITH INFLAMMATORY BOWEL DISEASE—cont'd

Developmental issues

Sleep patterns

Generally children with IBD have no special needs; children receiving an evening dose of corticosteroids may have some difficulty sleeping. The child may also have some nighttime stooling, which interrupts sleep.

Toileting

Most children with IBD are diagnosed after toilet training has been accomplished. When toilet training is a concern it may be suggested that instituting toilet training be done at a time when the disease activity is quiescent. For older children with active disease, occasional incontinence may be an issue.

Discipline

Standard developmental counseling is advised.

Child care

Standard developmental counseling is advised.

Schooling

Children with IBD are equally as able to achieve in the classroom as their nonaffected peers. School personnel must be educated regarding special issues related to IBD; any misunderstandings regarding psychologic etiology of IBD should be alleviated.

Sexuality

Sulfasalazine may cause infertility in men while they are taking the drug. Pregnancy outcomes are similar to those of the general population. Self-esteem and body image issues are important to adolescents with IBD.

Transition into adulthood

Self-care responsibilities may be gradually taken on by the adolescent. Specialized environments and assistance with activities of daily living are not typically required by the young adult with IBD. The transition to a provider specializing in the care of adults is best done during periods of quiescent disease.

Special family concerns

Issues regarding compliance with the treatment regimen are commonly an area of concern for these families in light of the fact that the child has typically reached adolescence by the time of diagnosis and is experiencing the developmental problems associated with that stage of growth. Privacy issues regarding toileting are often difficult for children and families to deal with.

Cultural implications of care

Because IBD affects individuals of widely disparate backgrounds and varies in its clinical presentation and severity, it is especially important that the care of the child with IBD be individualized. The practitioner should be sensitive to the needs of those children and families whose cultural or religious practices focus on food if during periods of active disease dietary restrictions are indicated.

REFERENCES

Andrews HA, Lewis P, and Allan RN: Prognosis after surgery for colonic Crohn's disease, *Br J Surg* 76:1184-1190, 1989.

Baron TH, Truss CD, and Elson CO: Low-dose oral methotrexate in refractory inflammatory bowel disease, *Digestive Diseases and Sciences* 38:1851-1856, 1993.

Barrett KE, Dharmsathaphorn K: Pharmacological aspects of therapy in inflammatory bowel diseases: antidiarrheal agents, *J Clin Gastroenterol* 10:57-63, 1988.

Belli DC et al: Chronic intermittent elemental diet improves growth failure in children with Crohn's disease, *Gastroenterology* 94:603-610, 1988.

Berquist WE: Inflammatory bowel disease in childhood and adolescence. In Gitnick G (editor): *Inflammatory bowel disease: diagnosis and treatment,* New York, 1991, Igaku-Shoin Ltd, pp 227-238.

Bradbury K, Mehl B: Pharmacology focus: drug interactions, *Foundation Focus,* November 1989.

Brandt LJ et al: Metronidazole therapy for perineal Crohn's disease: a follow-up study, *Gastroenterology* 83:383-387, 1982.

Burakoff R: Fertility and pregnancy in inflammatory bowel disease. In Kirsner JB, Shorter RC (editors): *Inflammatory bowel disease,* Baltimore, 1995, Williams & Wilkins, pp 429-436.

Calkins BM, Mendeloff AI: The epidemiology of idiopathic inflammatory bowel disease. In Kirsner JB, Shorter RC (editors): *Inflammatory bowel disease,* Baltimore, 1995, Williams & Wilkins, pp 31-68.

Colenda K, Grand R: Clinical manifestations of pediatric inflammatory bowel disease. In Kirsner JB, Shorter RC, (editors): *Inflammatory bowel disease,* Baltimore, 1995, Williams & Wilkins, pp 380-389.

Danzi JT: Extraintestinal manifestations of idiopathic inflammatory bowel disease, *Arch Intern Med* 148:297-302, 1988.

Duffy LF et al: Peripheral neuropathy in Crohn's disease patients treated with metronidazole, *Gastroenterology* 88:681-684, 1985.

Erikson EH: *Childhood and society,* ed 2, New York, 1963, WW Norton.

Feczko PJ: Malignancy complicating inflammatory bowel disease, *Radiol Clin North Am* 25:157-174, 1987.

Geier DL, Miner PB: Treatment of inflammatory bowel disease, *Am J Med* 93:199-208, 1992.

Gitnick G: Inflammatory bowel diseases: Part 1. Classification and cancer risk, *Am Fam Phys* 39:216-220, 1989a.

Gitnick G: Inflammatory bowel diseases: Part 2. Extraintestinal involvement and management, *Am Fam Phys* 39:225-233, 1989b.

Griffiths A et al: Slow-release 5-aminosalicylic acid therapy in children with small intestinal Crohn's disease, *J Pediatr Gastroenterol Nutr* 17:186-192, 1993.

Gross V et al: Treatment of active Crohn's ileocolitis with eardragit coated budesonide, *Gastroenterol* 106:A694, 1994.

Gryboski JD: Crohn's disease in children 10 years old and younger: comparison with ulcerative colitis, *J Pediatr Gastroenterol Nutr* 18:174-182, 1994.

Gryboski JD: Ulcerative colitis in children 10 years old or younger, *J Pediatr Gastroenterol Nutr* 17:24-31, 1993.

Hanan IM, Kirsner JB: Inflammatory bowel disease in the pregnant woman, *Clin Perinatol* 12:669-682, 1985.

Harper RH et al: The long-term outcome in Crohn's disease, *Dis Colon Rectum* 30:174-179, 1987.

Hyams JS: Inflammatory bowel disease in children and adolescents. *Endosc Rev* 5:46-60, 1988.

Hyams JS, Carey DE: Corticosteroids and growth, *J Pediatr* 113:249-254, 1988.

Joachim G, Milne B: Inflammatory bowel disease: effects on lifestyle, *J Adv Nurs* 12:483-487, 1987.

Kanof ME, Lake AM, and Bayless TM: Decreased height velocity in children and adolescents before the diagnosis of Crohn's disease, *Gastroenterology* 95:1523-1527, 1988.

Kirschner BS: Inflammatory bowel disease in children. *Pediatr Clin North Am* 35:189-208, 1988a.

Kirschner BS: Medical management of inflammatory bowel disease in children. In Kirsner JB, Shorter RC (editors): *Inflammatory bowel disease,* Baltimore, 1995, Williams & Wilkins, pp 715-733.

Kirschner BS, Defavaro MV, and Jensen W: Lactose malabsorption in children and adolescents with inflammatory bowel disease, *Gastroenterology* 81:829-832, 1981.

Kirschner BS et al: Reversal of growth retardation in Crohn's disease with therapy emphasizing oral nutritional restitution, *Gastroenterology* 80:10-15, 1981.

Kirschner BS, Schmidt-Sommerfeld E, and Stephens JK: Gastroduodenal Crohn's disease in childhood, *J Pediatr Gastroenterol Nutr* 9:138-140, 1989.

Kleinman RE et al: Nutritional support for pediatric patients with inflammatory bowel disease, *J Pediatr Gastroenterol Nutr* 8:8-12, 1989.

Korelitz BI: Fertility and pregnancy in inflammatory bowel disease. In Kirsner JB, Shorter RC (editors): *Inflammatory bowel disease,* Philadelphia, 1988, Lea & Febiger, pp 319-326.

Korelitz BI: Use of steroids and 6-Mercaptopurine in inflammatory bowel disease. In Korelitz BI, Sohn N (editors): *Management of inflammatory bowel disease,* St Louis, 1992, Mosby, pp 262-271.

Kozarek RA et al: Methotrexate use in inflammatory bowel disease patients who have failed azathioprine or 6-mercaptopurine, *Gastroenterology* 100:A222, 1991.

Levin B: Gastrointestinal neoplasia in inflammatory bowel disease. In Kirsner JB, Shorter RC (editors): *Inflammatory bowel disease,* Baltimore, 1995, Williams & Wilkins, pp 461-473.

Lewicki LJ, Leeson MJ: The multisystem impact on physiologic processes of inflammatory bowel disease, *Nurs Clin North Am* 19:71-80, 1984.

Linn FV, Peppercorn MA: Drug therapy for inflammatory bowel disease: Part I, *Am J Surg* 164:85-89, 1992.

Markowitz J et al: Immunology of inflammatory bowel disease: summary of the proceedings of the subcommittee on immunosuppressive use in IBD, *J Pediatr GI Nutr* 12:411-423, 1991.

Meyers S, Sachar DB: Medical therapy of Crohn's disease. In Kirsner JB, Shorter RC (editors): *Inflammatory bowel disease,* Baltimore, 1995, Williams & Wilkins, pp 695-714.

Ogorek CP, Fisher RS: Current therapy for inflammatory bowel disease, *Compr Ther* 17:31-37, 1991.

Pemberton JH et al: Quality of life after Brooke ileostomy and ileal pouch-anal anastomosis, *Ann Surg* 209:620-626, 1989.

Physicians' Desk Reference, Montvale, 1995, Medical Economics Data Production Company.

Podolsky DK: Inflammatory bowel disease. Part 1, *New Engl J Med* 325:707-711, 1991a.

Podolsky DK: Inflammatory bowel disease. Part 2, *New Engl J Med* 325:1008-1016, 1991b.

Present DH et al: 6-Mercaptopurine in the management of inflammatory bowel disease: Short- and long-term toxicity, *Ann Intern Med* 111:641-649, 1989.

Reddy JB, Jeejeebhoy KN: Acute complications of Crohn's disease, *Crit Care Med* 16:557-561, 1988.

Reid IR, Ibbertson HK: Calcium supplements in the prevention of steroid-induced osteoporosis, *Am J Clin Nutr* 44:287-290, 1986.

Retsky JD, Kraft SC: The extraintestinal manifestations of inflammatory bowel disease. In Kirsner JB, Shorter RC (editors): *Inflammatory bowel disease,* Baltimore, 1995, Williams & Wilkins, pp 474-491.

Seidman EG et al: Nutritional therapy of Crohn's disease in childhood, *Dig Dis Sci* 32(suppl)82s-88s, December 1987.

Taffet SL, Das KM: Sulfasalazine: adverse effects and desensitization, *Digestive Diseases and Sciences* 28:833-842, 1983.

Telander RL et al: Long-term follow-up of the ileoanal anastomosis in children and young adults, *Surgery* 108:717-725, 1990.

Tremaine WJ et al: A randomized, double-blind, placebo-controlled trial of the oral mesalamine (5-ASA) preparation, Asacol, in the treatment of symptomatic Crohn's colitis and ileocolitis, *J Clin Gastroenterol* 19:278-282, 1994.

Winter H et al: Antineutrophil cytoplasmic antibodies in children with ulcerative colitis, *J Pediatr* 125:707-711, 1994.

Juvenile Rheumatoid Arthritis

25

Gail R. McIlvain-Simpson

ETIOLOGY

The diagnostic term juvenile rheumatoid arthritis (JRA) is the official term and the one most widely used in the United States (according to the American College of Rheumatology classification) to describe a form of chronic, idiopathic, inflammatory arthritis that differs in many respects from adult rheumatoid arthritis (RA) (Cassidy and Petty, 1995). Diagnostic criteria have been developed (Cassidy, Levinson, and Brewer, 1989) and are listed in the box on page 531.

Alternative nomenclature used by some researchers such as juvenile arthritis and juvenile chronic arthritis (preferred in Europe) continue to be controversial because of their lack of specificity (Singsen, 1993). JRA is the most widely used term and the only one studied in regards to criteria and classification (Singsen, 1990).

The etiology of JRA is unknown. Possible mechanisms include infection, autoimmunity, genetic predisposition, stress, and trauma. Although infections are known to cause multiple types of arthritis in children, isolation of specific infectious agents in JRA have not been achieved. The role of autoimmunity (immune response toward "self") in the pathogenesis of JRA is suggested by the very high prevalence of autoantibodies, such as antinuclear antibody (ANA) in JRA.

The mechanism by which genetics could lead to

arthritis is by defects in immunoregulation. Immunoregulatory imbalances are thought to be important in pathogenesis; however, it is still not clear which aberrations are primary and which are secondary (Lipnick and Tsokos, 1990). Recent studies of histocompatibility antigens have clearly indicated that specific genetic predispositions exist for JRA and its various subgroups (Lipnick and Tsokos, 1990). Human leukocyte antigen (HLA), the main histocompatibility complex (MHC) in humans is a chromosomal region containing genes that encode cell surface molecules to facilitate cell to cell recognition, critical for a regulated immune response. HLA studies have demonstrated that the clinical subgroups of JRA are distinct entities (Lang and Shore, 1990; Singsen, 1990). These subgroups can be differentiated on the basis of genetics and are clearly distinguishable from adult RA (Lotz and Vaughn, 1988; Albert, Woo, and Glass, 1990).

It is likely that certain genetic types code for surface receptors which can "handle" foreign or autoantigens in a way that promotes inflammation, which then leads to synovitis. The primary lesion in JRA and RA is synovitis which is the result of proliferation of synovial cells and bone marrow inflammatory cells. Synovial cells are extremely active immunologically and belong in two macrophage-fibroblast cell lines. These cells commonly get involved in diseases with an exacerbated immune response.

Additionally, trauma is thought to act as a localizing factor or to cause attention to an already in-

The editors and authors would like to acknowledge the work done by Patricia M. Reilly on this chapter in the first edition of the book.

530

CRITERIA FOR THE CLASSIFICATION OF JUVENILE RHEUMATOID ARTHRITIS

1. Age at onset <16 years
2. Arthritis (swelling or effusion, or presence of two or more of the following signs: limitation of range of motion, tenderness or pain on motion, and increased heat) in one or more joints
3. Duration of disease 6 weeks or longer
4. Onset type defined by type of disease in first 6 months:
   a. Polyarthritis: 5 or more inflamed joints
   b. Oligoarthritis: <5 inflamed joints
   c. Systemic: arthritis with characteristic fever
5. Exclusion of other forms of juvenile arthritis

From Cassidy JT and Petty PE: Textbook of pediatric rheumatology, ed. 3, Philadelphia, 1995, W.B. Saunders.

CLINICAL MANIFESTATIONS

Chronic joint inflammation (swelling, limited range of motion, heat)
Morning stiffness
Fatigue
Spiking fevers and rash (systemic onset only)
Anemia
Remissions and exacerbations

flamed joint. Psychosocial factors such as stress are common in families of children with JRA. It is not known, however, whether the stress factor comes before or after the diagnosis (Vandvik, Hoyeranl, and Fangertun, 1989).

INCIDENCE

Juvenile rheumatoid arthritis (JRA) is the most common rheumatic disease of childhood and also one of the most common chronic illnesses of childhood. Singsen (1990) reports that in six studies the mean incidence was 15.7/100,000 with a range of 9.2 to 25/100,000. There is an estimated 65,000 to 70,000 children in the United States affected with JRA (Singsen, 1990).

CLINICAL MANIFESTATIONS AT TIME OF DIAGNOSIS

JRA is a group of conditions characterized by the presence of chronic synovial inflammation (see Fig. 25-1). Signs of joint inflammation include swelling

with heat, redness, pain, or limited range of motion. The child may also have periarticular soft tissue edema, intraarticular effusion, or hypertrophy of the synovial membrane. Synovitis may develop insidiously and exist for months or years without causing joint destruction, or may damage cartilage, subchondral bone, or other joint structures in a relatively short period of time. Clinical features range from mild synovitis in one joint with no systemic symptoms to severe disease in many joints with fever, rash, lymphadenopathy, and organomegaly. Common clinical manifestations include morning stiffness, irritability, a limp, and fatigue. Although children do not often complain of pain, they can have it at rest or during passive or active range of motion. Extraarticular manifestations of JRA include growth retardation, iridocyclitis, and rheumatoid nodules (Malleson and Petty, 1990).

Manifestations at the time of onset and throughout the first 6 months allow classification into one of three major subtypes: systemic, polyarticular (>5 joints), and pauciarticular (<5 joints). These subtypes are based on the number of joints, variations in patterns and severity of joint disease, extraarticular manifestations, immunogenetic characteristics, age at onset, and sex of the child (Cassidy and Petty, 1995; Singsen, 1993; Jacobs, 1993) (see Table 25-1).

In disease of systemic onset, constitutional and systemic involvement may develop concurrently with arthritis or precede overt arthritis by many weeks or months. The most characteristic findings are high, daily, intermittent spiking fevers (>39°C)

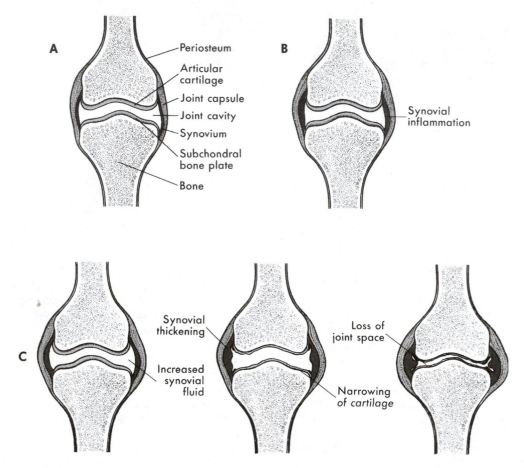

Fig. 25-1.   A, Normal diarthrodial joint. **B,** Early synovitis. **C,** Progressive destruction of an inflamed joint.

with a discrete, salmon-colored, evanescent, non-pruritic macular rash which commonly occurs on the trunk and proximal extremities (Jacobs, 1993; Cassidy and Petty, 1995). Laboratory findings typically show anemia of chronic disease, leukocytosis, and elevated acute phase reactants, such as the erythrocyte sedimentation rate (Cassidy and Petty, 1995). In polyarticular JRA, onset is generally gradual and most often associated with symmetric joint involvement. Children with a positive rheumatoid factor (RF) (15%) are the subgroup in JRA equivalent to those with classic adult RA. These children's arthritis is often severe with joint

destruction occurring rapidly in the first year (Lip-nick and Tsokos, 1990). RF negative arthritis exhibits less aggressive joint destruction.

Arthritis of pauciarticular onset develops predominantly in lower extremity joints, commonly in the knee. The ANA positive subgroup is at high risk for developing chronic uveitis, but mild articular involvement (Cassidy and Petty, 1995).

JRA is a disease characterized by exacerbations (flares) and remissions. Exacerbations may occur during episodes of acute illness or stress, with the frequency and duration of flares being unpredictable. Initially predicting when and how a child

Table 25-1.   CLINICAL MANIFESTATIONS OF JUVENILE ARTHRITIS

Mode of onset immunogenetics	Incidence		Sex (M:F)	Findings		Prognosis
	Frequency (% of all cases)	Age		Articular	Extraarticular	
Systemic (variable # of joints) ANA −(+ in 10%) RF − HLA −DR4 HLA −DR5 HLA −DR8	10	Any age (no peak)	M = F (1:1)	Multiple joint involvement; myalgia, arthralgia, or transient arthritis	High spiking fever, rash, hepatosplenomegaly, pericarditis pleuritis, abdominal pain, leukocytosis, anemia, thrombocytosis, mildly elevated LFTs, uveitis rare	Moderate to poor Severe disabling polyarthritis (20%-50%); good (40% remits); all disease mortality in this group (2%-4%)
Polyarticular (≥5 joints) Rheumatoid factor + ANA + (75%) RF + HLA-DR4 HLA-DR7	40	Late childhood (>8 years)	M < F (1:6)	Symmetrical involvement of large and small joints plus cervical spine. Early onset of erosive synovitis (unremitting).	Mild fever, mild to moderate hepatosplenomegaly and lymphadenopathy, other systemic symptoms generally mild, anemia, rheumatoid nodules, uveitis (5%)	Poor to moderately good. Severe persistent chronic polyarthritis resembling adult RA (50%).
Rheumatoid factor − ANA + (25%) RF − HLA-DpW3, HLA-DR8, HLA-DQW4		Any age (peak 2 years of age)	M < F (1:3)	Symmetrical involvement of large and small joints	Low grade fever, mild or absent systemic symptoms, anemia, uveitis rare	Severe polyarthritis (10%)
Pauciarticular (<5 joints) ANA +(65%-88%) RF − HLA-DR8, HLA-DR4 HLA-DRw6, HLA-DR5, HLA-PZW2	50	Early childhood (<5 years) (peak 1-2 years)	M < F (1:5)	Asymmetrical large joint involvement of knees, ankles, elbows. Hips and SI joint spared	Chronic uveitis, (20%) systemic symptoms usually not present	Excellent except for vision Polyarthritis (20%-30%). Loss of vision rare
Late onset ANA − RF − HLA − B27		Late childhood (>8 years) of age)	M > F (10:1)	Asymmetrical large joint involvement, hips and SI joint involvement common	Acute uveitis, occasional fever, anemia	Some may develop spondyloarthropathy

will flare is difficult; however, a pattern usually becomes clearer 1 year into the disease. Frequently flares of short duration do not require a change in the medication regimen. Flares of longer than 2-week duration may require adjustment of interventions.

Many children have complete remission of the disease without significant complications. Despite remission, others have residual problems such as contractures or visual impairment. Some children continue to have active disease into adulthood. Although criteria for remission vary among pediatric rheumatology centers, remission is commonly defined as no symptoms of active disease for at least 6 months on medications and for an additional 6 months after cessation of all medications.

TREATMENT

Maximizing a child's normal growth and development and minimizing deformity are the ultimate goals of early diagnosis and comprehensive therapy (Singsen, 1993). Management of JRA focuses on: relieving joint pain and inflammation, maintaining and increasing musculoskeletal function, promoting growth and development potential, supporting the psychological well-being of the child and family, and assisting the child to be as independent as possible in activities of daily living. Ideally, this is best achieved by a coordinated, multidisciplinary team including a pediatric rheumatologist, an advanced practice nurse, a primary care provider, an occupational and a physical therapist, and a social worker. Consultations with an orthopedist, an ophthalmologist, a psychologist, and a dietitian should be sought as indicated. The family should be the central component of this team.

Treatment should progress in a stepwise fashion beginning with the simplest, safest, and most conservative therapies to suppress inflammation and prevent deformity (Cassidy and Petty, 1995; Athreya and Cassidy, 1991). Recently the trend of pediatric rheumatology is for JRA to be treated earlier and more aggressively, thereby limiting the amount of disability the child may carry into adulthood (Levinson and Wallace, 1992).

The pharmacologic agents used in the treatment of JRA are identified in Table 25-2. Nonsteroidal antiinflammatory drugs (NSAIDs) are available in many forms and are replacing salicylate as the treatment of choice because NSAIDs have an easier dosing schedule (BID and TID versus QID) and have not been associated with Reye's syndrome. The predominant adverse reaction is gastrointestinal irritation so therefore the medication should be taken with meals.

The second group of medications has been referred to as both slow-acting antirheumatic drugs (SAARD) or disease-modifying antirheumatic drugs (DMARD). Medications within this group are gold (oral and injectable), hydroxychloroquine, sulfasalazine, d-penicillamine, and methotrexate, and are utilized when the disease is severe, persistent, or progressive despite the use of NSAIDs. The newest medication within this category is low-dose methotrexate which seems to be well tolerated and effective in treating JRA (Gabriel and Levinson, 1990; Giannini et al, 1992; Rose et al, 1990; Schaller, 1993).

Glucocorticoids (orally or intravenously as a pulse or bolus) are employed as a therapeutic bridge before disease control is obtained with other medications, to control serious systemic features and to act as an intraarticular injection in persistently inflamed joints (Schaller, 1993; Singsen and Rose, 1995; Wallace and Levinson, 1991). If required for longer than 6 months, glucocorticoids are tapered to an alternate-day schedule and discontinued as soon as possible.

TREATMENT

Nonsteroid antiinflammatory drugs (NSAID)/salicylates
Slow-acting antirheumatic drugs (SAARD) or disease-modifying drugs (DMARD)
Glucocorticoids
Immunosuppressive/cytotoxics
Physical therapy
Occupational therapy
Nutritional support
Surgery

Table 25-2.   MEDICATIONS COMMONLY USED IN TREATMENT OF JUVENILE RHEUMATOID ARTHRITIS*

Drug	Trade Name	Daily dose (mg/kg/day)	Side effects	Monitored parameters
Nonsteroidal antiinflammatory drugs				
Salicylates:				
Acetylsalicylate acid	Aspirin	60-100 mg/kg/d (qid) Maximum (4 gm/day pediatrics)	GI irritation and blood loss, mild hepatitis, hematuria, proteinuria, salicylism (tinnitus, hyperpnea, behavioral change), bleeding, anemia, oral ulcers, dental caries, allergic reaction, peptic ulcers	CBC, platelet count, UA, SGOT and SGPT levels 2 and 6 weeks after initiation of treatment and every 2-3 months thereafter SGOT and SGPT levels; for sustained elevations of enzyme levels or levels 5 times the normal, drug must be discontinued temporarily or dose reduced by 20% until levels are normal Occult blood in stools and PTT as required Salicylate levels (to guide correct dosage). Therapeutic range: 20-30 mg/dl 2 hours after dose.
Proprionic acid derivatives: Naproxen Ibuprofen	Naprosyn Advil, Motrin, Nuprin	15-20 mg/kg/d (bid) 20-45 mg/kg/d (bid/ tid)	Side effects common to all nonsalicylate NSAIDs: GI irritation and blood loss, proteinuria, hematuria, anemia, fluid retention, headache, dizziness, mild hepatitis, peptic ulcer, skin manifestations (pseudoporphyria with Naprosyn)	Initially: CBC, platelet count, UA, creatinine, BUN, SGOT, then q 1-3 months
Indoleacetic acid derivative: Tolmetin sodium	Tolectin	15-30 mg/kg/d (tid)	As above for Proprionic acid	As above for Proprionic acid
N-Phenylanthranilic acid derivative: Diclofenac sodium	Voltaren	2-3 mg/kg/d (bid/tid)	As above for Proprionic acid	As above for Proprionic acid

Continued.

Table 25-2.   MEDICATIONS COMMONLY USED IN TREATMENT OF JUVENILE RHEUMATOID ARTHRITIS*—cont'd

Drug	Trade Name	Daily dose (mg/kg/day)	Side effects	Monitored parameters
Nonsteroidal antiinflammatory drugs—cont'd				
Indoleacetic acid derivative:				
Indomethacin	Indocin	2-4 mg/kg/d (bid/tid) (qhs)	As Above	PT and PTT Follow-up laboratory not needed if asymptomatic
Slow-acting antirheumatic drugs				
Gold sodium thiomalate	Myochrysine	0.5-1.0 mg/kg/wk (after initial test dose) injectable maintenance dose for 20 weeks.	Nitritoid reaction, hematuria, proteinuria, stomatitis, exfoliative dermatitis, bone marrow suppression, photosensitivity, diarrhea	CBC, platelet count, UA, and liver function tests before initial dose, CBC, platelet count and UA before each injection or weekly with oral preparation. Initially then q 2-4 weeks thereafter.
Aurothioglucose	Solganal			
Auranofin	Ridaura	0.1-0.2 mg/kg/wk (oral preparation) (6-9 mg/d)		
D-Penicillamine	Cuprimine, Depen	3 mg/kg/d initially (qd-qid). Slowly increased to maximum 10 mg/kg/d (750 mg/day).	Proteinuria, thrombocytopenia, dermatitis, lupuslike syndrome, iron deficiency anemia, vitamin B_6 deficiency	CBC, platelet count, and UA before initial dose and weekly for 2 months, every other week for 6 months, then monthly. CPK every 6 months.
Sulfasalazine	Azulfidine	Initial therapy: 40-60 mg/kg/day in 3-6 doses Maintenance therapy: 30 mg/kg/day in divided doses	Anorexia, headache, nausea, vomiting, oligospermia, photosensitivity, blood dyscrasias, hypersensitivity reactions, hematuria crystalluria, folic acid deficiency, orange discoloration of urine and skin	CBC, UA monthly; liver function tests, BUN values, serum creatinine periodically
Hydroxychloroquine	Plaquenil	3-7 mg/kg/d (daily or bid)	Rashes, GI symptoms, headache, insomnia, decreased concentration,* blurred vision, corneal deposits, keratopathy, retinopathy	Retinal exam initially then every 6 months. CBC every 6 months.

Drug	Trade name	Dosage	Side effects	Laboratory monitoring
Methotrexate	Rheumatrex	5-15 mg/m² week, PO	Upper GI upset, diarrhea, abdominal pain. Mucosal ulcerations, hepatotoxicity, bone marrow suppression.	CBC, platelet count, SGOT & SGPT every week initially then monthly; creatinine initially and then every 3 months
Glucocorticoid drugs				
Systemic corticosteroid Prednisone		1-2 mg/kg/day for acute flare (lowest possible dose, preferred)	Acne, striae, Cushingism hirsutism, decreased growth velocity, osteopenia, increased likelihood of peptic ulceration, and infection. Hypertension mood and behavioral disturbances, cataracts.	CBC and other monitoring as needed for numerous side effects; ophthalmologic examinations yearly
Methylprednisolone		30 mg/kg/d (1 gm maximum every day × 3)		
Ophthalmic corticosteroids Dexamethasone Prenisolone		Doses vary according to degree of inflammation and magnitude of therapeutic response from 1 drop every 2 hr to 1 drop every other day	Cataracts, glaucoma, eye infections, Cushing's syndrome	Ophthalmologic examination every 2-3 weeks for several months and every 2-3 months thereafter
Immunosuppressive drugs				
Chlorambucil	Leukeran	0.1-0.2 mg/kg/day	Thrombocytopenia, leukopenia, mutagenics oncogenic potential sterility, bone marrow suppression, high rates of infection	CBC, monthly.
Azathioprine	Imuran	3-5 mg/kg/day		CBC, platelet count q 1-2 weeks, SGOT and SGPT
Cyclophosphamide	Cytoxan	Titrate dose up to 1-2 gm/M²		CBC, platelet count, UA, BUN, creatinine

*GI, gastrointestinal; CBC, complete blood cell count; UA, urinalysis; SGOT, glutamic oxaloacetic transaminase; SGPT, glutamic pyruvic transaminase; PTT, partial thromboplastin time; BUN, blood urea nitrogen; Cr, creatinine.
@Food and Drug Administration approval for use in children.

Immunosuppressive and cytotoxic agents are used for severe illness resistant to the aforementioned forms of therapy (Singsen and Rose, 1995). These medications include chlorambucil, cyclophosphamide, azathioprine, cyclosporine A, and y-interferon. They have significant short-term and long-term complications such as infertility, mutagenesis, and oncogenesis; therefore, their use is clinically limited (Gabriel and Levinson, 1990).

Physical and occupational therapy are critical to the successful management of the child with JRA. Therapists develop individualized exercise programs, teach the principles of joint protection and energy conservation, fabricate splints, recommend assistive devices, and suggest appropriate recreational activities (Melvin and Atwood, 1989; Scull, 1994). The child with arthritis, together with family members or other caregivers, is encouraged to carry out a recommended program of therapies at home. Although exercise programs carry potential risks for injury or overuse, preliminary evidence suggests that well-designed, individualized conditioning programs may benefit children with arthritis (Klepper and Giannini, 1994). These programs have the potential to increase muscular strength, endurance, and stamina for daily activities, without aggravating the joint disease (Klepper and Giannini, 1994). Periodic consultation with therapists is arranged as needed for early recognition of potential problems and to analyze the impact of any current limitation on present function (Scull, 1994). Depending on their level of involvement, children may need formal therapy 2 to 3 times per week.

Nutrition counseling is recommended for children who are systemically ill or on long-term steroids. For those children who are protein-energy malnourished, aggressive nutritional repletion including nocturnal nasogastric feeds has shown promise (Woo, White, and Ansell, 1990).

Orthopedic surgery plays a limited role within the management of the child with JRA (Cassidy and Petty, 1995). For a child with severe contracture of the knee or hip, soft tissue releases, posterior capsulotomy and tendon lengthening may be performed. Prophylactic synovectomies do not seem to alter long-term outcomes of the disease and are rarely performed (Jacobs, 1993; Woo,

White, and Ansell, 1990). As the child approaches adulthood and reaches bone maturity, reconstructive surgery plays a more vital role. Total joint replacements (hip and knee) have been of great benefit in young adults with marked disability (Cassidy and Petty, 1995; Hyman and Gregg, 1991). The materials and methods for fixation have greatly improved with the modern technology of joint replacement (Woo, White, and Ansell, 1990).

As a result of the chronicity, unpredictability, and sometimes relentless progression of the disease despite treatment, approximately 68% of parents having a child with JRA may be lured into utilizing an unconventional therapy, such as wearing copper bracelets, that gives them a sense of hope and purpose (Southwood et al, 1990; Panush, 1993). It is important to foster trust and create an accepting environment where frustrations with conventional treatment can be aired and unproven remedies openly discussed. The primary care provider should help families differentiate between harmless and potentially harmful interventions and assist them in evaluating the claimed efficacy of unconventional remedies (Manfred, Boutaugh, and Tehan, 1987).

RECENT AND ANTICIPATED ADVANCES IN DIAGNOSIS AND MANAGEMENT

The most recent model of pathogenetic mechanism for JRA involves trimolecular complexes comprised of a human leucocyte antigen (HLA) product, a T-cell receptor (TCR), and an antigen (Grom, Giannini, and Glaso, 1994). The interplay of certain genetically determined elements of the trimolecular complex is thought to trigger the inflammatory process. The researchers in genetics have concluded that the three clinically defined subsets are possibly three diseases all referred to by the same name—juvenile rheumatoid arthritis. Attempts to directly influence the interactions of the elements of the trimolecular complex, and tailoring management that takes into account the three subsets will provide the main guidance for future therapy.

ASSOCIATED PROBLEMS

Skeletal Abnormalities

In JRA, the growing skeleton is subjected to unique deformities. Chronic hyperemia in an inflamed joint is thought to stimulate accelerated maturation of the epiphyseal plates resulting in skeletal overgrowth of the extremity. This process is most characteristically seen in children with early onset pauciarticular disease who have unilateral knee involvement (Woo, White, and Ansell, 1990). Significant discrepancies in leg lengths can occur when overgrowth and subsequent elongation of the leg with arthritis occur simultaneously with delayed maturation of the opposite leg (Woo, White, and Ansell, 1990; Cassidy and Petty, 1995). In children over 9 years of age undergrowth of an extremity can result in premature closure of the growth plate (Woo, White, and Ansell, 1990). In addition, a severely ill child with JRA may have long periods of immobility yielding generalized osteoporosis.

Characteristic abnormalities of the cervical spine include apophyseal joint disease, associated with poor development of the vertebral body and impaired growth ultimately resulting in bony fusion (Espada et al, 1988; Cassidy and Petty, 1995). Children with a systemic onset and polyarticular course often have a C2-C3 subluxation as a result of the fusion of the vertebrae above and below them (Cassidy and Petty, 1995). Stiffness and pain of the cervical spine, with rapid loss of extension and rotation are common early findings in polyarticular JRA.

Children with JRA more commonly have scoliosis of the thoracolumbar spine than healthy children (Ross et al, 1987). Asymmetrical involvement of the knee joint with increased vascularity and increased epiphyseal growth can lead to a leg length discrepancy and a secondary scoliosis.

Hip pathology in the child with JRA is often masked by compensatory increased lumbar lordosis. Children with polyarticular disease experience limitation of full flexion, abduction, and rotation often as a result of iliopsoas and adductor spasm (Jacobs, 1993). In time, marked narrowing of the joint space occurs.

Children with arthritis of the knee joint can develop valgus of the knee with compensatory valgus deformity of the hindfoot and varus of the forefoot (Woo, White, and Ansell, 1990). Disturbances of

---

ASSOCIATED PROBLEMS

Skeletal abnormalities
  Joint deformities
  Cervical spine problems
  Scoliosis
  Hip, knee, and foot involvement
  Micrognathia
Uveitis
Anemia
Problems common with Systemic Onset
  Hepatosplenomegaly
  Lymphadenopathy
  Pericarditis
  Pleural effusion
  Renal problems
Nutritional problems

---

gait and balance can occur as a result of retarded growth and development of the feet with active persistent inflammatory disease (Woo, White, and Ansell, 1990). Children with long-standing disease may also experience overgrowth of the patella.

Micrognathia

Arthritis-induced abnormalities of the temporomandibular joint (TMJ) result in mandibular undergrowth, micrognathia, and malocclusion. The highest percentage of TMJ abnormalities (pain, tenderness, or crepitus) is found in the polyarticular subgroup. Combined orthodontic and reconstructive surgical procedures may improve function and esthetics in addition to decreasing pain in children with TMJ disease (Cassidy and Petty, 1995; Jacobs, 1993).

Uveitis

Uveitis (also known as iridocyclitis) is a chronic, nongranulomatous inflammation primarily affecting the anterior uveal tract (iris and ciliary body) (Cassidy and Petty, 1995; Petty, 1987). JRA-associated uveitis occurs in 2-20% of all children with JRA and is characterized by an insidious, asymptomatic, typically bilateral onset that infrequently precedes arthritis (Jacobs, 1993, Guidelines for opthalmic examinations in children with JRA, 1993). Its pattern of remissions and exacerbations does not parallel articular disease (O'Brien and Albert, 1989). Risk factors associated with developing uveitis include female gender, young age, antinuclear antibody (ANA) positivity, rheumatoid factor (RF) seronegativity, and pauciarticular onset. Slit-lamp examination is required for early detection. Early and aggressive treatment with topical steroids with or without a mydriatic drug and frequent ophthalmologic follow-up have been effective in preserving the vision of children without advanced disease. Uncontrolled uveitis results in glaucoma, cataracts, band keratopathy, posterior synechiae, and loss of vision (O'Brien and Albert, 1989).

Anemia

Microcytic, hypochromic anemia is a common feature of systemic and polyarticular JRA. The severity of anemia correlates with underlying inflammation and is an anemia of chronic disease. Microcytosis is associated with reduced levels of serum iron and serum iron-binding capacity and does not typically respond to iron supplementation (Harvey, Pippard, and Ansell, 1987). Children with poor nutrition or NSAID-induced gastrointestinal blood loss may also develop iron deficiency anemia (Mulberg et al, 1993; Henderson and Lovell, 1991).

Problems Associated with Systemic Onset or Course

Systemic onset of JRA can be accompanied by significant extraarticular manifestations. Hepatosplenomegaly and generalized lymphadenopathy occur in most children with active systemic disease. Pericarditis is a common cardiac finding among children with systemic onset or course. Clinical presentation varies from asymptomatic pericarditis with mild pericardial effusions to severe life-threatening cardiac involvement. Pleural effusions may present with an acute flare and can occur alone or concurrently with pericarditis. Renal manifestations unrelated to drug therapy are rare. Hematuria associated with glomerulonephritis and proteinuria may be present before drug therapy is initiated. In rare instances two other conditions can occur—amyloidosis and disseminated intravascular coagulation (Jacobs, 1993).

Nutrition

Of the children with juvenile rheumatoid arthritis, 10% to 50% can have protein energy malnutrition (Henderson and Lovell, 1991). Mechanical feeding problems can occur in 18% to 30% of affected children as a result of TMJ arthritis. This limits the opening of the mouth and causes pain. Hypoplasia of the mandible occurs in 20% to 30% of the children with JRA resulting in maldevelopment of the teeth and difficulty swallowing. Those with arthritis in the upper extremities may have difficulty in meal preparation or use of utensils (Henderson and Lovell, 1991).

PROGNOSIS

The prognosis for children with JRA is generally good with the majority (70% to 90%) of children going into spontaneous permanent remission or having satisfactory outcomes without serious disability (Cassidy and Petty, 1995; Malleson and Petty, 1990). The child at greatest risk for poor functional outcome develops polyarthritis of late age at onset, early involvement of small joints, rapid appearance of articular erosions, unremitting inflammatory activity or prominent systemic manifestations, rheumatoid nodules, and rheumatoid factor (RF) positivity (Cassidy and Petty, 1995; Schaller, 1993). Children with systemic disease are most prone to developing life-threatening complications. Children with pauciarticular disease fare best regarding joint disease, but worse with uveitis. In those children with chronic uveitis 25% have a good prognosis, 25% respond poorly to treatment, and 50% require prolonged treatment (Guidelines for Ophthalmologic Examinations in Children with Juvenile Rheumatoid Arthritis, 1993). Although visual outcomes are improving, functional blindness still occurs in 15% to 30% of these children (Cassidy and Petty, 1995).

Primary Care Management
HEALTH CARE MAINTENANCE

Growth and Development

The majority of children with mild JRA do not experience significant growth failure during the course of disease. Investigators have demonstrated periodic decreased growth velocity in children with JRA (Lovell and White, 1990). In children with systemic or polyarticular JRA, linear growth is retarded during periods of active disease. Catch-up growth usually occurs during remission or with suppression of disease activity by therapy. Height returns to normal within 2 to 3 years if premature epiphyseal fusion has not occurred. Children with JRA can have growth abnormalities which persist into adulthood. In one study 50% of those children having systemic onset had adult heights below the 5th percentile (Henderson and Lovell, 1991).

Corticosteroids do contribute to the growth problem by suppressing growth hormone production. Children with severe JRA who receive large daily doses of steroids (>5 mg/m^2 for 6 months or longer) exhibit the greatest degree of growth retardation (Jacobs, 1993). With cessation of steroids, height and weight return to near normal within 1 to 2 years. Importantly, the majority of adults with growth failure took no corticosteroids at any time for their JRA (Henderson and Lovell, 1991).

Combined results from several studies report that 60% of children with JRA improve their growth rate when given pituitary-derived or recombinant growth hormone (Henderson and Lovell, 1991). Adolescents on long-term corticosteroids may need to be evaluated by an endocrinologist for growth potential and use of growth hormone.

Gross motor delays or temporary regressions are not uncommon in the child with JRA. Fine motor skills are less likely to be delayed as long as the child is provided with toys and activities that encourage manipulation (Atwood, 1989a). Limited mobility and decreased opportunities to actively interact with the environment place a child at risk for cognitive and social delays. Language acquisition is generally unaffected unless a child has significant TMJ arthritis.

Children with severe JRA often fall behind in acquiring hygiene, toileting, dressing, and feeding skills. Regression in performance of these skills is common during acute illness and may be sustained during remissions as a result of lowered parental expectations and continued reinforcement of a child's dependent behaviors. Functional limitations in the child with arthritis can be assessed by two tools, the Childhood Health Assessment Questionnaire (CHAQ) and the Juvenile Arthritis Functional Assessment Scale (JAFAS) (Scull, 1994; Lovell, 1992). Demonstration by the child of personal care skills is preferred to child or parent report during evaluation of functional level. When parents habitually perform such duties for a child, neither parent nor child may have an accurate understanding of the child's abilities (Atwood, 1989a).

Standard infant and early childhood assessment tools, such as the Bayley Scales and Denver Developmental Screening Test II, may be of questionable value in evaluating delay in seriously affected children. An occupational and physical therapy team familiar with the impact of JRA on the child's overall development can be a valuable resource for the primary care provider.

Age appropriate physical activities for the child with JRA are important as with any child and should be based on the child's capabilities and energy level. Once guidelines regarding these activities have been put into place the child should be allowed to participate in activities to his or her tolerance.

Diet

Nutritional problems are common in JRA. Factors contributing to occurrence of these problems include: systemic disease (increase in inflammatory mediators), increased nutrient requirements as a result of fever, gastrointestinal side effects of medications, anorexia, depression, and limitations of TMJ or upper extremity joints. Excessive weight gain should be avoided to minimize stress on involved joints. Depression, poor food choices, increased appetite while on corticosteroids, and decreased physical activity from pain, stiffness, or deformity contribute to weight increase.

As many as 50% of children with JRA are at risk for protein and energy malnutrition (Henderson and Lovell, 1991). Decreased iron and calcium intake, as well as decreased calorie intake unrelated to disease activity, have been reported (Miller, Chacko, and Young, 1989). Evaluation by a dietitian will help to identify, treat, and monitor children at risk for dietary problems.

Corticosteroid therapy can cause increased appetite, fluid retention, weight gain, and osteoporosis secondary to calcium depletion. A low-sodium diet may be indicated. Calcium intake should be evaluated and supplementation considered if dietary sources are insufficient (Warady and Shields, 1987).

Up to 43% of individuals with JRA may use unconventional dietary remedies for arthritis (Southwood et al, 1990). Among the most popular are avoidance of nightshade vegetables, such as potatoes and eggplant, and acid foods such as tomatoes, diets with increased fish or fish oil, fasting, herbal remedies, and megavitamin therapy. Different researchers are reexamining the relationship between arthritis and diet (Panush, 1993). Given the current knowledge of JRA and diet, educating families about proper nutrition for a growing child with a chronic condition and evaluating potentially harmful dietary manipulations, especially those involving nutrient restrictions, are important responsibilities of the primary care provider.

Safety

Drug therapy is essential to the successful management of JRA. Education about medication safety is an important responsibility of the primary care provider. All medications must be kept in childproof containers out of reach of young children. This becomes especially important as older children assume responsibility for self-care. Children taking long-term immunosuppressant drugs are encouraged to wear Medic-Alert bracelets or necklaces.

Photosensitive skin reactions may occur with naproxen (Naprosyn), methotrexate (Rheumatrex), sulfasalazine (Azulfidine), and hydroxychloroquine (Plaquenil). Hypoallergenic sunblock lotion with a minimum sun protection factor (SPF) of 15 should be used on exposed skin.

Orthotic appliances are often recommended for joint protection. Important safety issues related to splint wearing include care of the splint to maintain integrity, proper skin care, signs and symptoms of an ill-fitting splint, and proper splint application. The splint should be checked at regular intervals to detect damage to the appliance and to ensure that the child has not outgrown it (Boutaugh and Tehan, 1987).

Superficial heat and cold modalities are frequently recommended to relieve pain and stiffness. Determining the type of applications used by the family and reviewing safety precautions specific to each type of application are important.

Adaptive equipment such as electric devices, lamp switch extenders, and elevated toilet seats are used by children with JRA to minimize joint stress and increase independence. Safety can often be maximized by such assistive devices. For example, bath safety can be improved by the use of safety strips, rubber mats, wall grab bars, tub chairs, and one-handed hose attachments (Scull, 1994). Adaptive equipment should be evaluated for the safety of all family members.

Immunizations

Children with JRA who are not taking immunosuppressive medications or experiencing systemic disease can receive routine immunizations. Children whose immunocompetence is altered by antimetabolites or large doses of corticosteroids should not receive live vaccines for at least 3 months after discontinuation of these drugs (Committee on Infectious Diseases, 1994). Live vaccinations may be administered to children with JRA whose only exposure to steroids are topically applied ophthalmic medication or intraarticular, bursal, or tendon injections (American Committee on Immunization Practices, 1994).

Children receiving long-term salicylate therapy may be at increased risk for developing Reye's syndrome in the presence of influenza and varicella infections (Forsyth et al, 1989; Rennebohm, et al, 1985). Yearly immunizations for types A and B influenza are recommended for children treated with aspirin and who are older than 6 months of age according to the dosage and schedule set out by the American Academy of Pediatrics Committee on Infectious Diseases (1994). These children should also receive the varicella immunizations. Aspirin should be stopped temporarily if a child develops chickenpox or influenza.

A widespread safety concern of many pediatric rheumatologists is that immunizations can lead to a flare of the underlying disease or immunologic disorder. Antecdotal experience in rheumatology views this as a potential problem; however, there is no scientific data to support this theory. These concerns should not discourage the primary care provider from immunizing children with JRA **after** consultation with the pediatric rheumatologist.

Screening

Vision. Thorough fundoscopic examination and acuity screening should be performed at each office visit. At the time of diagnosis every child must be examined for uveitis by an ophthalmologist. Frequent ophthalmologic examinations are recommended for children at risk for uveitis, glaucoma, and cataracts. Young children with pauciarticular and ANA positive arthritis are at greatest risk for development of ocular inflammation. The rheumatology section of the American Academy of Pediatrics has developed a opthalmologic screening schedule (See box on this page). More frequent follow-up is needed for children with active uveitis.

Corticosteroid-induced glaucoma or cataracts can occur at any time during treatment. Children started on topical corticosteroids should receive baseline intraocular pressure measurements on initiation of treatment with frequent reexamination during continued therapy (O'Brien and Albert, 1989; Wolf, Lichter, and Ragsdale, 1987).

Children taking hydroxychloroquine should have a baseline and bi-yearly ophthalmologic examination every 6 months, which includes a slit-lamp bimicroscopy, visual acuity, color vision, visual field determinations, and retinoscopy, because its toxicities affect the eye and can cause blindness (Cassidy and Petty, 1995).

Hearing. Routine screening is recommended; however, decreased acuity in children taking salicylates should be promptly investigated because tinnitus associated with salicylate toxicity may impair hearing.

Dental. Salicylates dissolved in the mouth cause erosion of the occlusal surfaces of the teeth and eruption of white, mildly inflamed, oral mucosal lesions (Christensen, 1984). Dental visits every 6 months, or more frequently if erosive signs develop, are recommended (Tanchyk, 1986). Prevention of lesions depends on the child avoiding overretention of salicylate preparations in the mouth and rinsing after ingestion of medication.

Increased incidence of dental caries can potentially occur in children with JRA, possibly because of poor oral hygiene secondary to TMJ or upper extremity limitations. Malocclusions and crowded mandibular teeth occur as a result of micrognathia (Jacobs, 1993). Children with JRA should be checked for bleeding gums and poor dental hygiene. Frequent dental visits, fluoride application, and sealants are recommended and orthodontic referrals made as needed.

OPHTHALMOLOGIC SCREENING SCHEDULE

High risk every 3-4 months

Pauciarticular—ANA+, onset <7 yr
Polyarticular—ANA+, onset <7 yr

Medium risk every 6 months

Pauciarticular—ANA+, onset ≥7 yr
Pauciarticular—ANA−, any age onset
Polyarticular—ANA+, onset ≥7 yr
Polyarticular—ANA−, any age onset

Low risk yearly

Systemic—any age onset

Prophylactic antibiotic coverage for dental work or other surgeries is indicated for children with total joint replacements (any prosthesis) or those taking corticosteroids (see Chapter 15 for prophylactic schedule).

Dental work for children taking sulfasalazine (Azulfidine) who develop thrombocytopenia or leukopenia should be postponed until blood counts have returned to normal (U.S. Pharmacopeia, 1995). Consultation with the pediatric rheumatology team and the dentist in these situations is necessary.

Blood pressure. Routine screening is recommended. Mild hypertension may occur in children taking NSAIDs and SAARDs. Steroid-induced hypertension can occur although it is less frequent with current treatment regimens (Singsen and Rose, 1995).

Hematocrit. Hematologic testing is done frequently by the pediatric rheumatology team so therefore routine screening is not required.

Urinalysis. Urinalysis is recommended at the start of treatment and at intervals of 6 to 12 months. Periodic and mild proteinuria and hematuria occur in many children with JRA. Urinalysis screening tests with protein >1+, RBCs >5, and casts should be called to the pediatric rheumatologist immediately.

Tuberculosis. Routine screening is recommended.

Condition-specific screening

Erythrocyte sedimentation rate, complete blood count with differential, platelet count, urinalysis, and liver function tests are routinely reviewed by the staff of the pediatric rheumatology center to monitor disease activity, response to therapy, drug toxicity, and anemia. Routine salicylate levels are not indicated unless underdosing or overdosing is suspected.

COMMON ILLNESS MANAGEMENT

Differential Diagnosis

Fever. Children with JRA may have fevers as a response to an infectious process or as a result of their chronic condition. The classic JRA fever is characterized by daily or twice daily temperature elevation to 39°C or higher, usually in the afternoon or evening, with a rapid return to baseline without intervention. Remittent and low grade fever are less frequently seen patterns. Children often appear very ill during febrile periods and well when afebrile (Cassidy, 1995). Fever occurs typically at disease onset and may recur with arthritis flares. Moderate or mild temperature elevations occur with polyarticular and pauciarticular disease. A careful history and complete physical examination will usually determine the source of the fever.

Dermatologic symptoms. The classic systemic JRA fever is usually accompanied by a rash consisting of 2 to 6 mm evanescent, salmon pink, generally circumscribed macular lesions. The rash may become confluent with larger lesions developing pale centers and pale periphery. It is most commonly seen on the trunk, extremities, and over pressure areas; however, face, palms, and soles may also be involved. The rash is most prominent during fever spikes and may be visible only after rubbing or scratching the skin. A hot bath or stress may also induce the rash (Cassidy and Petty, 1995; Jacobs, 1993).

Otologic symptoms. TMJ arthritis may cause referred pain to the ear and this should be considered when evaluating children for otitis media.

Respiratory symptoms. Aspirin intolerance, characterized by acute bronchospasm, severe rhinitis, or generalized urticaria/angioedema occurring within 3 hours after ingestion of aspirin or other NSAID, has been reported. Any child with recurrent rhinitis or asthma must be considered at risk for bronchoconstriction when exposed to aspirin or other NSAIDs (Morassut, Yang, and Karsh, 1989). Tachypnea occurs with aspirin toxicity. A serum salicylate level should be drawn immediately when a child on aspirin therapy presents with an increased respiratory rate. Salicylates should be withheld pending laboratory results.

Cricoarytenoid arthritis (laryngeal arthritis) can cause stridor, dyspnea, and cyanosis in systemic JRA (Jacobs, 1993). Side effects of methotrexate such as cough, wheezing, and chronic x-ray changes should be monitored for in those children receiving the medication.

Gastrointestinal symptoms. Gastrointestinal tract disease is rarely described in children with JRA. However, gastrointestinal symptoms may be difficult to evaluate because NSAIDs cause some degree of nausea, dyspepsia, abdominal pain, and diarrhea. A number of adverse reactions are being noted in children (Lindsley, 1993). In children experiencing major gastrointestinal problems, inflammatory bowel disease should be ruled out (Cassidy and Petty, 1995). See Chapter 24. A careful history and physical examination, as well as consultation with the pediatric rheumatologist as needed, will assist the primary care provider in the evaluation of differential diagnoses.

Drug-induced or stress-induced gastrointestinal bleeding must also be considered in children receiving NSAIDs or steroids (Barrier and Hirschowitz, 1989). Peptic ulcers may present as chronic anemia secondary to occult blood loss or as acute gastrointestinal hemorrhage. The classic symptom of epigastric pain that improves with eating and worsens with an empty stomach is more common in the adolescent but may be absent in the young child (Steinhorn and Berman, 1987).

Renal symptoms. Children taking aspirin may experience increased urinary urgency and frequency; however, this problem is generally temporary. Urinary tract infection must be ruled out first. Microcytic hematuria and low grade proteinuria are renal side effects of many JRA medications. Urine cultures are typically the most reliable diagnostic test for infection.

Drug Interactions

Many potential interactions exist between medications commonly used to treat JRA and over-the-counter and prescription drugs used to manage other common pediatric conditions. The box that follows identifies the major interactions of which the primary care provider must be aware in providing care to these children. As a result of the complexity of possible drug interactions, it is advised that the primary care provider work in conjunction with the rheumatology team when recommending any medications.

The primary care provider should not discontinue the child's condition-specific medications without consulting the pediatric rheumatologist. Conditions warranting possible temporary cessa-

tion of medications include: (1) exposure to chicken pox or influenzalike illness, (2) significant bleeding of the nose or gums or gastrointestinal tract, (3) dehydration as a result of illness (may result in possible salicylate toxicity), and (4) rapid, deep breathing, until salicylate toxicity is ruled out (Mahy, 1987).

DEVELOPMENTAL ISSUES

Sleep Patterns

Active disease causes increased wakefulness at night. A child fatigues more readily during flares and requires longer periods of rest during the day. The severity and duration of morning stiffness increases. Recommendations to alleviate morning symptoms include the use of flannel sheets, thermal underwear, joint comforters, warmed clothing, and a sleeping bag. An electric blanket with a timer

---

POTENTIAL DRUG INTERACTIONS IN CHILDREN TREATED FOR JUVENILE RHEUMATOID ARTHRITIS

Aspirin plus salicylate-containing medications can cause salicylate toxicity

Antacids may alter the absorption rate of NSAIDs, glucocorticoids, or penicillamine resulting in subtherapeutic serum levels

Antacids can alter renal excretion of aspirin, leading to higher serum levels of salicylate with antacid withdrawal or subtherapeutic levels with antacid addition

Corticosteroids decrease plasma concentration of salicylates

Methotrexate concentrations are increased by salicylates and NSAIDs, salicylates may displace methotrexate from binding sites and decrease renal clearance, leading to toxic methotrexate plasma concentration

Sulfonamides may displace or be displaced by other highly protein-bound drugs, such as NSAIDs, salicylates, and methotrexate. Monitor children for increased effects of highly bound drugs when sulfonamides are added.

Folic acid with methotrexate may interfere with antifolate effects of methotrexate

Sulfonamides plus methotrexate may yield increased hepatotoxicity

Concurrent use of NSAIDs and salicylates, glucocorticoids, or NSAIDs may increase risk of gastrointestinal side effects (i.e., ulceration and hemorrhage)

Estrogen-based oral contraceptives may alter the metabolism or protein binding leading to decreased clearance, increased elimination, half-life and increased therapeutic or toxic effects of glucocortosteroids

NSAIDs plus acetaminophen increase the risk of adverse renal defects

Concomitant use of NSAIDs and alcohol may increase the risk of gastrointestinal side effects including ulceration and hemorrhage

Data from Drug information for health care professions, 15th edition, United States Pharmacopeia of Drugs (USPD), 1995.

set to warm the blanket 1 hour before a child is scheduled to awaken can also reduce morning stiffness. Warm waterbeds may be helpful. Finally, administering medications with food 30 to 60 minutes before rising and exercising in a warm bath before starting daily activities can increase range of motion (Boutaugh and Tehan, 1987).

Toileting

The acquisition of self-care skills may be delayed in the child with JRA. Toilet training should be postponed during periods of active disease because the child may lack the motivation and physical capability to perform tasks necessary for successful toileting.

Limitations in upper and lower extremities create difficulty in transferring on and off the toilet, managing toilet paper, and dressing and undressing for toileting. Safety bars and elevated toilet seats are reliable assistive devices for children with lower extremity involvement. For children with upper extremity limitations, effective aids for wiping after toileting are difficult to locate. Occupational therapists will be helpful in devising solutions to this problem. A bidet can be attached to a toilet, thereby circumventing the need for paper. Adaptive clothing and dressing aids can facilitate toileting (Atwood, 1989b).

Consideration should be given to toilet hygiene in facilities outside the home where assistive devices will not be available. In addition, bedpans and urinals may be required at night if pain and stiffness limit mobility.

Discipline

Parents of children with JRA may experience difficulty with discipline. Overly protective parents impose unnecessary limitations on activities or enforce excessive safety precautions. Feelings of guilt, sorrow for a child in pain, or fear that stress will trigger a flare-up cause some parents to adopt an overly permissive discipline style. In addition, overindulgence during periods of active disease alternating with normalization of discipline practices during remissions fosters inconsistent limit setting (Erlandson et al, 1987).

Parent education about every child's need for clear, reasonable, and consistent limits should include a review of alternatives to physical punishment. Guidance regarding age-specific developmental tasks and the effect of JRA on the acqui-

sition and performance of self-care, language, motor, and social skills offers parents a framework for making decisions about discipline (Atwood, 1989a).

Child Care

Parents of children receiving medications may have difficulty locating child care providers who are willing to administer medications. For caregivers who accept this responsibility, parents should prepare a list that includes the name, dose, time, and method of administration, and side effects of each drug. The name and telephone number of the person to contact for questions or problems should be provided.

It is important for caregivers to understand that exacerbations and remissions characterize the JRA disease pattern and that a child's functional capacity, energy level, and developmental progress may fluctuate. Education about JRA and about a child's actual or anticipated limitations is likely to decrease anxiety among day care staff and promote appropriate interactions between caregivers and a child affected by JRA.

Schooling

Children with JRA face many potential difficulties in school. Inattention and distractibility have been most highly related to school performance (Stoff, Bacon, and White, 1989). The primary care provider should periodically question children and parents about school-related problems with fatigue, distractibility, limited mobility, absences, and medications, and work with the family, school staff, and pediatric rheumatology team to identify and remedy problems before and when they occur.

Discrepancies may exist between what teachers, parents, and students perceive to be obstacles. Parents and teachers more often identify limitations in activities of daily living and physical health as primary difficulties. Affected children focus on self-concept and peer relations and prefer to solve peer issues by themselves (Taylor, Passo, and Champion, 1987).

Many students will require only minor adjustments in school programs. Surgery or disease flares may necessitate temporary home tutoring and should be planned for in a child's individualized education plan (IEP). Public Law 101-476 requires that special services such as occupational therapy, physical therapy, adaptive physical education, and transportation between home and school be available to students with JRA attending federally funded schools.

A student with JRA can participate in modified school athletic programs. It is important to individualize appropriate amounts and forms of exercise depending on the number, type, and severity of joints involved.

Sexuality

Sexual maturation may be delayed in adolescents with JRA, particularly in those with systemic disease. Menarche has been shown to occur later in girls with JRA (mean age 13.2 years) than in unaffected controls (mean age 12.5 years), although no clear etiology for this difference was identified (Fraser et al, 1988). Development of secondary sexual characteristics may be delayed in both boys and girls.

Contraceptive advice should include discussion of interactions among arthritis medications and various oral contraceptives, as well as the effects, if any, of arthritis medications on fertility and fetal development. If mechanical methods of birth control are difficult to use for adolescents with hand or hip involvement, a review of alternative birth control methods and consultation with the occupational therapist on the pediatric rheumatology team are indicated. Specific issues regarding sexuality and arthritis are addressed in the pamphlet *Living and Loving: Information about Sex* which is published and distributed by the Arthritis Foundation.

In a retrospective study of 76 pregnancies in 51 women with JRA two major conclusions were reached: (1) pregnancy had no adverse effects on the signs and symptoms of JRA, and (2) maternal and fetal outcome of pregnancy were good (Ostensen, 1991).

Transition into Adulthood

As outlined by Rettig and Athreya (1991), transition programs are an important service in the management of older adolescents with rheumatic disease. These programs must be knowledgeable about adolescent development and committed to providing necessary services. These programs must be staffed by adult practitioners with an interest in providing care to individuals with pediatric onset chronic conditions. Given the limited number of pediatric rheumatology programs associated with adult tertiary centers, current health care reimbursement issues, and adult practitioners knowledgeable and willing to accept older adolescents as clients, it can be very difficult to provide a viable transition solution.

Another issue for young people with arthritis involves the change from secondary school to higher education or work environment. Two agencies that work together to help adolescents make a successful transition from student to independent adult are (1) the Department of Education and (2) Vocational Rehabilitation (VR). Students and their parents need to check with their school counselor and local VR regarding transition programs. The Arthritis Foundation provides a pamphlet that outlines many of these services. Adolescents attending college can often access the Office of Americans with Disabilities to obtain services such as special scheduling and priority housing. HEATH, a national clearinghouse on postsecondary education for individuals with handicaps provides excellent resources; their address is as follows: HEATH, One DuPont Circle, Suite 800, Washington, DC 20036-1193. An additional resource is the National Center for Youth with Disabilities (NCYD) University of Minnesota, Box 721, UMHC Harvard Street at East River Road, Minneapolis, MN 55455.

SPECIAL FAMILY CONCERNS AND RESOURCES

Miller (1993) reviewed recent studies on the psychosocial factors related to rheumatic diseases in childhood. The general consensus was that most children with a rheumatic disease survive the stress of the disease with good psychosocial adjustment, utilizing denial as a needed coping mechanism. Demographic factors and stresses related to poor maternal function and depression were viewed as major risk factors (Miller, 1993). The mother's sense of mastery was seen as a beneficial factor (Miller, 1993). Psychosocial interventions targeting high risk families and encouraging families to be self-advocates will provide for good utilization of resources.

Community Resources

American Juvenile Arthritis Organization (AJAO)
Arthritis Foundation
1314 Spring Street NW
Atlanta, GA 30309
(404) 872-7100

AJAO is a national membership association of the Arthritis Foundation which serves the special needs of young people with arthritis or rheumatic diseases and their families. Videotapes, quarterly newsletters, educational materials for children, parents, and health professionals, as well as information about summer camps, pen pal clubs, and family support groups are available through the national office of AJAO or through local chapters of the Arthritis Foundation.

SUMMARY OF PRIMARY CARE NEEDS FOR THE CHILD WITH JUVENILE RHEUMATOID ARTHRITIS

Health care maintenance

Growth and development

Linear growth may be retarded during active systemic disease.

Catch-up growth occurs with suppression of disease activity or during remission.

Corticosteroids may suppress growth.

Poor weight gain may be as a result of systemic disease.

Excessive weight gain may occur as a result of inactivity, depression, poor nutrition.

Gross motor delays and temporary regressions are not uncommon.

Fine motor skills are less likely to be affected.

Language acquisition is affected only with severe TMJ arthritis.

Standard infant development screening tests may be of questionable value in evaluating severely affected children.

Age appropriate physical activities are important and should be based on the child's capabilities and energy level. Participation should be allowed up to tolerance.

Diet

Increased risk of protein-caloric malnutrition.

Improper nutrition, depression, corticosteroid usage, and decreased physical exercise may contribute to problems of underweight or overweight.

Addition of daily vitamin and iron supplementation is recommended.

Evaluate "arthritis diets" for nutritional adequacy and educate family about proper nutrition for a growing child with a chronic disease.

Safety

Use childproof containers for medications.

Medic-Alert bracelet or necklace for child taking immunosuppressive agents.

Review safety issues related to splintwearing, heat and cold applications, and adaptive equipment.

Immunizations

Routine immunizations for children who are not taking immunosuppressive drugs.

In the absence of neurologic symptoms, a child with classic, intermittent JRA fever can be immunized during febrile episodes.

No live viruses should be given to children receiving antimetabolites or large doses of corticosteroids.

Yearly immunizations for types A and B influenza are recommended for children older than 6 months who are being treated with aspirin.

Screening

 Vision:

Fundoscopic examination and acuity screening each visit.

Continued.

SUMMARY OF PRIMARY CARE NEEDS FOR THE CHILD WITH JUVENILE RHEUMATOID ARTHRITIS—cont'd

Ophthalmologic examination for uveitis. Children on topical or systemic steroids require close ophthalmologic follow-up.

Hearing:

Routine office screening.

Dental:

For children taking salicylates, dental visits every 6 months or more frequently if erosive signs develop. Frequent dental visits for children with micrognathia. Prophylactic antibiotics for dental work in children with total joint replacements or those on steroids.

Blood pressure:

Routine screening.

Hematocrit:

Frequent screening done by rheumatology team to rule out anemia.

Urinalysis:

Frequent screening may be done by rheumatology team as a result of toxicity profile of some medications used to treat JRA.

Tuberculosis:

Routine screening is recommended.

Condition-specific screening:

CBC, differential, ESR, platelet count, and liver function tests are routinely drawn and reviewed by pediatric rheumatology staff.

Common illness management

Differential diagnosis

Fever:

Differentiate classic, intermittent JRA fever from fevers of infectious origin.

Dermatologic symptoms:

Rule out rheumatoid rash in systemic JRA; rule out drug-related photosensitivity reactions.

Otologic symptoms:

Differentiate TMJ arthritis with referred ear pain from otitis media.

Respiratory symptoms:

Rule out salicylate-induced tachypnea or bronchospasm; differentiate cold from influenza symptoms and treat all type A influenza with amantadine; colds and flu may cause arthritis

flares necessitating increased dosage of antiinflammatory medications.

Gastrointestinal symptoms:

Rule out nonspecific pain of JRA-related mesenteric adenopathy, drug-induced peptic ulcer, drug-related gastrointestinal symptoms.

Renal symptoms:

Increased urinary urgency or frequency in a child on aspirin therapy may be temporary drug side effects, but UTI must be ruled out first.

Developmental issues

Sleep patterns

Recommendations to alleviate morning stiffness should be discussed with the family.

Toileting

Postpone training during periods of active disease.

Utilize assistive devices to compensate for upper and lower extremity limitations.

Anticipate situations in public facilities where assistive devices are not available.

Bedpans and urinals may be necessary if pain and stiffness limit mobility at night.

Discipline

Identify overprotection, overindulgence, and inconsistent limit setting.

Give guidance regarding the effect of JRA on age-specific developmental tasks to offer parents a framework for decision making about discipline.

Child care

Caregiver must be capable of giving medications, using assistive devices, applying splints.

Parents should prepare caregiver with information about child's medications.

Educate caregivers about effect of JRA on child's functional capacity, energy level, and developmental progress.

Home-based, single provider day care setting rather than group child care is recommended for child on steroids or immunosuppressants.

Continued.

SUMMARY OF PRIMARY CARE NEEDS FOR THE CHILD WITH JUVENILE RHEUMATOID ARTHRITIS—cont'd

Most infants and young children with JRA are eligible for Public Law 99-457 educational programs.

Schooling

Public Law 101-476 entitles most students with JRA to occupational therapy, physical therapy, adaptive physical education, and transportation between school, home, and facilities where services are provided.

Most students with JRA can participate in modified school athletic programs.

Sexuality

Pubarche may be delayed in children with JRA. Refer to physical and occupational therapists with

pediatric rheumatology team for difficulties with sexual postures or with problems related to use of mechanical birth control devices.

Transition into adulthood

Advise adolescent of transitional programs and vocational rehabilitation.

Special family concerns

Divergent views regarding perceptions and impact of JRA may exist.

REFERENCES

Albert E, Woo P, and Glass DN: Immunogenetic aspects. In Woo P, White PH, and Ansell BM (editors): *Paediatric rheumatology update,* Oxford, 1990, Oxford University Press, pp 6-20.

American Academy of Pediatrics. In Peter G (editor): *Red book: report of the committee on infectious diseases,* ed 23, Elk Grove Village, IL, 1994, American Academy of Pediatrics.

American Commitee on Immunization Practices (1989). General recommendations on immunizations. *Morbidity and Mortality Weekly Report, 38,* 205-227.

Athreya BH, Cassidy JT: Current status of the medical treatment with juvenile rheumatoid arthritis, *Rheumatic Dis Clin North Am* 17:871-889, 1991.

Atwood M: Treatment consideration. In JL Melvin, (editor): *Rheumatic disease in the adult and child: occupational therapy and rehabilitation,* Philadelphia, 1989a, FA Davis, pp 215-234.

Atwood M: Treatment consideration. In Melvin JL (editor): *Rheumatic disease in the adult and child: occupational therapy and rehabilitation,* Philadelphia, 1989b, FA Davis, pp 215-234.

Barrier, C.H., Hirschowitz, B.I. (1989). Controversies in the detection and management of nonsteroidal anti-inflammatory drug induced side effects of upper gastrointestinal tract. *Arthritis and Rheumatism, 32,* 926-932.

Boutaugh ML, Tehan N: Saving joints and energy. In Arthritis Foundation (editor): *Understanding juvenile rheumatoid arthritis: a health professional's guide to teaching children and parents,* Atlanta, 1987, The Arthritis Foundation, pp 7-1 to 7-D.

Cassidy JT: Juvenile rheumatoid arthritis. In Kelley WN et al (editors): *Textbook of rheumatology,* ed 3, Philadelphia, 1989, WB Saunders, pp 1289-1311.

Cassidy JT, Levinson JE, and Brewer EG: The development of classification criteria for children with juvenile rheumatoid arthritis, *Bulletin on the Rheumatic Disease,* The Arthritis Foundation 38:1-7, 1989.

Cassidy JT, Petty RE: *Textbook of pediatric rheumatology,* ed 3, Philadelphia, 1995, WB Saunders.

Christensen, J.R. (1984). A soft tissue lesion related to salacylate treatment of juvenile rheumatoid arthritis: Clinical report, *Pediatric Dentistry, 6,* 159-161.

Erlandson D et al: *Psychosocial issues and JRA.* In Arthritis Foundation (editor): *Understanding juvenile rheumatoid arthritis: a health professional's guide to teaching children and parents,* Atlanta, 1987, Arthritis Foundation, pp 13-1 to 13-E.

Espada G et al: Radiologic review: the cervical spine in juvenile rheumatoid arthritis, *Semin Arthritis Rheum* 17:185-195, 1988.

Forsyth BW et al: New epidemiologic evidence confirming that bias does not explain the aspirin/Reye's syndrome association, *JAMA* 261:2517-2524, 1989.

Fraser PA et al: The timing of menarche in juvenile rheumatoid arthritis, *J Adolesc Health Care* 9:483-487, 1988.

Furst DE: Toxicity of antirheumatic medications in children with juvenile arthritis, *J Rheum* 19(suppl 33):11-15, 1992.

Gabriel CA, Levinson JE: Advanced drug therapy in juvenile rheumatoid arthritis, *Arthritis Rheum* 33:587-589, 1990.

Giannini EH et al: Methotrexate in resistant juvenile rheumatoid arthritis—results of the USA-USSR double-blind, placebo-controlled trial, *New Engl J Med* 326:1043-1049, 1992.

Giannini EH, Cassidy JT, and Brewer EJ: Comparative efficiency and safety of advanced drug therapy in children with juvenile rheumatoid arthritis, *Semin Arthritis Rheum* 23:34-46, 1993.

Grom AA, Giannini EH, and Glaso DN: Juvenile rheumatoid arthritis and the trimolecular complex (HLA, T-cell receptor, and antigen), *Arthritis Rheum* 37:601-607, 1994.

Guidelines for ophthalmologic examinations in children with juvenile rheumatoid arthritis, *Pediatrics* 92:295-296, 1993.

Harvey AR, Pippard MJ, and Ansell BM: Microcytic anemia in juvenile chronic arthritis, *Scand J Rheumatol* 16:53-59, 1987.

Henderson CJ, Lovell DJ: Nutritional aspects of juvenile rheumatoid arthritis, *Rheum Dis Clin North Am* 17:403-413, 1991.

Hyman BS, Gregg JR: Arthroplasty of hip and knee in juvenile rheumatoid arthritis, *Rheum Dis Clin North Am* 17:971-983, 1991.

Jacobs JC: *Pediatric rheumatology for the practitioner,* New York, 1993, Springer-Verlag.

Klepper SE, Giannini MJ: Physical conditioning in children with arthritis. *Arthritis Care Res* 7:226-236, 1994.

Lang BA, Shore A: Pathogenesis of juvenile arthritis more recent immunologic studies. In Woo P, White PH, and Ansell BM (editors): *Paediatric rheumatology update,* Oxford, 1990, Oxford University Press, pp 21-37.

Levinson JE, Wallace CA: Dismantling the pyramid, *J Rheumatol* 19(suppl 33):6-10, 1992.

Lindsley CB: Uses of nonsteroidal antiinflammatory drugs in pediatrics, *AJDC* 147:229-236, 1993.

Lipnick RN, Tsokos GC: Immune abnormalities in the pathogenesis of juvenile arthritis, *Clin Experimental Rheumatol* 8:177-186, 1990.

Lotz M, Vaughn JH: Rheumatoid arthritis. In Samter M (editor): *Immunological diseases,* ed 4, Boston, 1988, Little, Brown, pp 1365-1416.

Lovell DJ: New functional outcome measurements in juvenile rheumatoid arthritis: a progress report, *J Rheumatol* 19(suppl 33):28-31, 1992.

Lovell DJ, White PH: Growth and nutrition in juvenile rheumatoid arthritis. In Woo P, White PH, and Ansell BM (editors): *Paediatric rheumatology update,* Oxford, 1990, Oxford University Press, pp 47-56.

Mahy, M. (1987). Medications. In Arthritis Foundation, ed: Understanding juvenile rheumatoid arthritis: A health professional's guide to teaching children and parents, Atlanta, The Arthritis Foundation, 4-1 - 4H16.

Malleson PN, Petty RE: Remodeling the pyramid—a pediatric perspective, *J Rheumatol* 17:867-868, 1990.

Manfred SM, Boutaugh ML, and Tehan N: Unproven remedies. In Arthritis Foundation (editor): *Understanding juvenile rheumatoid arthritis: a health professional's guide to teaching children and parents.* Atlanta, 1987, The Arthritis Foundation, pp 9-1 to 9-A.

Melvin JL, Atwood M: Juvenile rheumatoid arthritis. In Melvin JL (editor): *Rheumatic disease in the adult and child: occupational therapy and rehabilitation,* Philadelphia, 1989, FA Davis, pp 135-187.

Miller JJ: Psychosocial factors related to rheumatic diseases in childhood, *J Rheumatol* 20A(suppl 38):1-11, 1993.

Miller, M.L., Chacko, J.A., and Young, E.A. (1989). Dietary deficiencies in children with juvenile rheumatoid arthritis. *Arthritis Care Research, 2,* 22-24.

Morassut, P., Yang, W., and Karsh, J. (1989). Aspirin intolerance. *Semin Arthritis Rheum, 19,* 22-30.

Mulberg AE et al: Clinical and laboratory observations—identification of nonsteroidal antiinflammatory drug-induced gastroduodenal injury in children with juvenile rheumatoid arthritis, *J Pediatr* 122:647-649, 1993.

O'Brien JM, Albert DM: Therapeutic approaches for ophthalmic problems in juvenile rheumatoid arthritis, *Rheum Dis Clin North Am* 15:413-337, 1989.

Ostensen M: Pregnancy in parents with a history of juvenile rheumatoid arthritis, *Arthritis Rheum* 34:881-887, 1991.

Panush RS: Reflections on unproven remedies, *Rheum Dis Clin North Am* 1a:201-206, 1993.

Petty RE: Current knowledge of the etiology and pathogenesis of chronic uveitis accompanying juvenile rheumatoid arthritis, *Rheum Dis Clin North Am* 13:19-36, 1987.

Rennebohm RM et al: Reye syndrome in children receiving salicyclate therapy for connective tissue disease, *J Pediatr* 107:877-880, 1985.

Rettig P, Athreya BH: Adolescents with chronic disease, *Arthritis Care Res* 4:174-180, 1991.

Rose CD et al: Safety and efficacy of methotrexate therapy for juvenile rheumatoid arthritis, *J Pediatr* 117:653-659, 1990.

Ross AC et al: Scoliosis in juvenile chronic arthritis, *J Bone Joint Surg* 69B:175, 1987.

Schaller JG: Therapy for childhood rheumatic diseases, *Arthritis Rheum* 36:65-70, 1993.

Scull SA: Juvenile rheumatoid arthritis. In Campebell SK (editor): *Physical therapy for children,* Philadelphia, 1994, WB Saunders, pp 207-225.

Singsen BH, Rose CD: Juvenile rheumatoid arthritis and the pediatric spondyloarthropathies. In Weissan MH, Weinblatt ME (editors): *Treatment of the rheumatic diseases.* Companion to the Textbook of Rheumatology, Philadelphia, 1995, WB Saunders, pp 217-240.

Singsen BH: Rheumatic disease of childhood, *Rheum Dis Clin North Am* 16:581-590, 1990.

Singsen BH: Juvenile rheumatoid arthritis. In Schumacher HR, Klippel JH, and Koopman WS (editors): *Primer on the rheumatic diseases,* ed 10, Atlanta, 1993, Arthritis Foundation.

Southwood TR et al: Unconventional remedies used for patients with juvenile arthritis, *Pediatrics* 85:150-153, 1990.

Steinhorn D, Berman WF: Gastrointestinal hemorrhage. In Hoekelman RA (editor): *Primary pediatric care,* St Louis, 1987, Mosby, pp 974-978.

Stoff E, Bacon MC, and White PH: The effects of fatigue, distractibility and absenteeism on school achievement in children with rheumatic disease, *Arthritis Care Res* 2:49-53, 1989.

Tanchyk AP: Prevention of tooth erosion from salicylate therapy in juvenile rheumatoid arthritis, *Gen Dent* 34:479-480, 1986.

Taylor I, Passo MH, and Champion VL: School problems and teacher responsibilities in juvenile rheumatoid arthritis, *J Sch Health* 57:186-190, 1987.

United States Pharmacopeia of Drug Information: *Drug Information for the Health Care Professional,* Rockville, MD: ed. 15, 1995.

Vandvik IH, Hoyeranl HM, and Fangertun H: Chronic family difficulties and stressful life events in recent onset of juvenile arthritis, *J Rheum* 16:108, 1989.

Wallace CA, Levinson JE: Juvenile rheumatoid arthritis: outcome and treatment for the 1990s, *Rheum Dis Clin North Am* 17:891-905, 1991.

Warady B, Shields C: Nutrition management. In Arthritis Foundation (editor): *Understanding juvenile rheumatoid arthritis: a health professional's guide to teaching children and parents.* Atlanta, 1987, The Arthritis Foundation, pp 8-1 to 8-P.

Wolf, M.D., Lichter, P.R., and Ragsdale, C.G. (1987). Prognostic factors in the uveitis of juvenile rheumatoid arthritis. *Ophthalmology, 94,* 1242-1248.

Woo P, White PH, and Ansell BM (editors): *Paediatric rheumatology update,* Oxford, 1990, Oxford University Press.

Learning Disabilities and/or Attention Deficit Hyperactivity Disorder

26

Janice Selekman
and Marybeth Snyder

ETIOLOGY

Great confusion exists in the literature regarding the causes, symptoms, and interventions for attention deficit hyperactivity disorder (ADHD) and learning disabilities (LD), because no literature differentiated between LD and ADHD until recently, especially for etiology. Many of the manifestations and treatments, however, are significantly different. Although the conditions are distinct, they do overlap (see Fig. 26-1).

The current diagnoses of LD and ADHD were preceded by many other labels, which combined the two conditions, including: brain damaged, minimal brain dysfunction, hyperactive child syndrome, and attention deficit disorder (Barkley, 1990).

The term "learning disability" was introduced in 1963 and revised to refer to a heterogeneous group of disorders manifested by significant difficulties in the acquisition and use of listening, speaking, reading, writing, reasoning, or mathematical abilities, or of social skills (The Interagency Committee on Learning Disabilities [ICLD], 1987).

The definition of ADHD continues to change but is currently defined by the *Diagnostic and Statistical Manual of Mental Disorders IV* (DSM) as a "persistent pattern of inattention and/or hyperactivity-impulsivity that is more frequent and severe than is typically observed in individuals at a comparable level of development" (American Psychiatric Association [APA], 1994, p 78).

These disorders are intrinsic to the individual and presumed to be the result of central nervous system dysfunction. Even though ADHD or a learning disability may occur concomitantly with other handicapping conditions (e.g., sensory impairment, mental retardation, social and emotional disturbance), or untoward socioenvironmental influences (e.g., cultural differences, insufficient or inappropriate instruction, psychogenic factors, an impoverished environment), LDs and ADHDs are not the direct result of those conditions or influences (ICLD, 1987; Castellanos and Rapoport, 1992; Hammill, 1993).

The cause and the exact mechanisms involved remain unknown. There is a genetic predisposition for both LD and ADHD in a significant number of cases (Castellanos and Rapoport, 1992; Duane, 1993; Faraone et al, 1993; Rourke and Del Dotto, 1994). Although central nervous system dysfunction is often cited as the general cause for both conditions, no substantial findings exist at this time related to specific defects. However, there has been a recent increase in activity exploring neurobiologic and neuroanatomic causes for LD and ADHD (Hynd et al, 1990; Galaburda, 1991; Hechtman, 1994).

The neurobiologic hypothesis pertains primarily to children with ADHD. The hypothesis

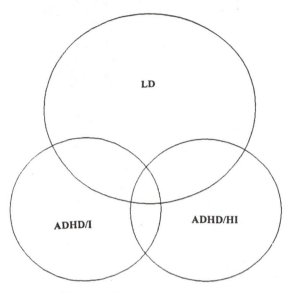

LD - Learning Disability

ADHD/I - Attention Deficit
             Hyperactivity Disorder-Inattention

ADHD/HI - Attention Deficit
               Hyperactivity Disorder-
               Hyperactivity/Impulsivity

Fig. 26-1.   Relationship of diagnostic classifications.

focuses on neurotransmitters, especially cate-cholamines. Because most of the medications that have proven efficacy with ADHD increase dopamine release and inhibit reuptake of neuro-transmitters, the suggestion is strong that deficits in this system are one of the primary causes of ADHD (Castellanos and Rapoport, 1992; Dulcan, 1990).

The neuroanatomic hypothesis attempts to identify structural anomalies of, or damage to, the brains of children with LD and ADHD. Beginning research is now concentrating on frontal lobe anatomy, cerebral glucose metabolism, and orbital-limbic pathways (Barkley, et al 1990; Hechtman, 1994; Riccio, Gonzalez, and Hynd, 1994; Zametkin et al, 1990). Thus far, autopsy findings, CT scans, and MRIs have been futile in identifying these pro-posed structural defects.

There is no empirical support for chemicals and allergies as causes for LD or ADHD (Silver, 1992b),

excluding the permanent damage done by chemicals such as lead. Diets high in sucrose or aspartame have also been ruled out as causes of hyperactivity and be-havioral problems (Wolraich et al, 1994). Brain dam-age with resulting LDs or ADHD is known to occur as a result of infections or trauma.

Other suggested causes include: (1) offspring of mothers with high antinuclear antibody titers, and (2) effects of smoking, drinking, and medica-tion use (prescribed or illicit) during pregnancy on the developing child (Barkley, et al 1990; Castel-lanos and Rapoport, 1992; Duane, 1993).

Specific groups appear to be at increased risk for developing learning disabilities, including: (1) very-low-birth-weight infants, some of whom later develop difficulty with spatial relations and vi-sual motor integration (Bauchner, Brown, and Pe-skin, 1988), and (2) persons with late effects of cancer treatment from cranial irradiation and in-trathecal chemotherapy, although signs are not evi-denced until years after the treatment (Foley, Focht-man, and Mooney, 1993). Learning disabilities may, in fact, be multifactorial rather than the result of a single etiologic determinant.

INCIDENCE

Between 5% and 10% of school-aged children have been identified as having a learning disability; however, it is suggested the number may be twice as high (Silver, 1993b) because many children have not yet been identified and the criteria for the diag-nosis differs between states and over time. Half of all children enrolled in federally supported special education programs receive services for learning disabilities (Shapiro and Gallico, 1993). In addi-tion, "between 35% and 50% of children seen in mental health clinics have learning or language dis-abilities" (Silver, 1993b, p. xiii).

ADHD has been diagnosed in 3% to 5% of chil-dren, but some authorities believe the incidence could be as high as 20% (Barkley, et al. 1990). Ap-proximately 20% to 25% of children with LD also have ADHD (Silver, 1993a). Of the children with ADHD, 19% to 26% have at least one type of LD (Barkley, et al. 1990). Therefore, approximately 4 to 10 million children in the United States have LD and/or ADHD.

More boys than girls have been diagnosed with these conditions. Although the ratios differ by the setting, with an increased ratio of males to females in clinic-referred samples, the general ratio of male to female with LD and ADHD is 3:1 (Barkley, et al., 1990).

CLINICAL MANIFESTATIONS AT TIME OF DIAGNOSIS

Learning Disability

There are two frameworks that have been used to identify learning disabilities. The first is the DSM-IV (APA, 1994) which refers to learning disabilities as learning disorders (formerly called academic skills disorders) and identifies them as "disorders . . . characterized by academic functioning that is substantially below that expected given the person's chronological age, measured intelligence, and age-appropriate education" (p 38). These disorders are subdivided into reading disorder, mathematics disorder, disorder of written expression, and a learning disorder not otherwise specified. Unfortunately this format only views learning as academic related and does not incorporate its impact on the child's life.

Diagnosis is multidimensional and includes standardized testing and academic achievement that are significantly below that expected given the person's chronologic age, measured intelligence, and age-appropriate education (APA, 1994; Silver and Hagin, 1993). There is usually a significant gap of 1.5 to 2.0+ standard deviations between the child's achievement on individually administered standardized tests of reading, math, and written expression, and intelligence (APA, 1994; Silver and Hagin, 1993). Handicapping conditions that may result in learning disabilities must be ruled out, for example, vision and hearing deficits, mental retardation, psychosocial problems, and environmental conditions.

Reading disorders include deficits in reading accuracy, speed, or comprehension. Mathematics disorders evaluate the child's ability in mathematical calculations and reasoning. Disorders of written expression involve evaluation of writing skills. No differentiating features exist for the category identified as "learning disorder not otherwise specified."

Although the previously mentioned learning disorders are based on academic tasks and test results, the basic problem for children with an LD is processing information, especially if it involves more than one process (Silver, 1993a). A second, and more conceptual approach, is to view alteration in the areas of sensory-receptive/input, integrative/memory, motor/output, and diffuse abilities (Selekman, 1988; Silver, 1993a).

Alterations in sensory-receptive/input. Alterations in sensory-receptive intake involve deficiencies in using and processing information received via the senses, including visual perceptual, auditory perceptual, and sensation-related deficits.

Visual perceptual deficits involve difficulty in decoding or comprehending (or both) written language because of reversals of letters or words (dyslexia), difficulty in visual memory and perception of symbols such as musical notes, or misperception of distance and depth. These children may have difficulty copying and identifying letters or shapes, differentiating right from left, and drawing a clock. The dyslexic child's eyes may not be able to move evenly across a printed line, but instead jump from line to line, causing the child to lose his or her place. This child may also have difficulty with figure-ground visual perception, that is, difficulty differentiating an object from its background (Selekman, 1988; Silver, 1993a).

The child with an auditory perceptual deficit has difficulty with phonetics, recitation from memory (e.g., the alphabet), understanding and following directions (especially multistep instructions), and interpreting tone of voice. Because of this, the child may be erroneously judged to be emotionally disturbed, retarded, or a "problem child" who does not do as he or she is told. This deficit will also present as an inability to differentiate similar-sounding words, such as pit and pet (Selekman, 1988).

Children who have difficulty in perceiving tactile or body sensations may be unable to read their own body cues. Sensations such as the need to toilet or the onset of menses may be missed or misread, leading to difficulty in toilet training, resolving enuresis or encopresis, and establishing self-care behaviors. They may dislike or misperceive how they are being touched or be supersensitive to the tags on shirts or certain types of materials.

CLINICAL MANIFESTATIONS

Learning disability

Reduced academic achievement

(1.5-2.0 standard
  deviations below that
  projected for age,
  intelligence, and education)
  in reading, math, written
  expression

Alterations in sensory-receptive processing

Visual perceptual deficits
Decoding language
Visual memory
Perception of symbols,
  depth, distance
Auditory perceptual deficits
Phonetics
Directions
Tone of voice
Discrimination of sounds
Tactile perceptual deficits
Kinesthetic

Alteration in integrative processing

Multitask coordination
Memory problems

Alteration in motor-expressive performance

Clumsy, uncoordinated
Speech disorders
Fine motor skill delays

Diffuse alterations

Heterogenous manifestations

Attention deficit hyperactivity disorder

Predominately inattentive
Predominantly hyperactive-
  impulsive
Combined
*See box on p. 558 for DSM-IV
  criteria)*

Kinesthetic misperception can result in difficulty understanding the body language and facial expressions of others as well as awareness of their own body movements (Silver, 1993a).

Alterations in integrative processing. The child with an alteration in integrative processing can receive stimuli adequately, but has difficulty in retrieving and using this information accurately. This manifests itself in several ways, including: difficulty sequencing data or parts of a story; difficulty understanding the concepts of time and space, parts and whole, and cause and effect; disorganization of thought and planning; a slowness in the speed with which he or she can process problem solving; and difficulty in analysis and abstract thinking. The child may become lost easily and have difficulty reading maps. Children with this condition are limited in the amount of general knowledge they can process from their environment (e.g., knowing the number or sequence of the days in a week, holidays and relating seasons of the year to the calendar or following directions). They have difficulty with short-term memory (e.g., memorizing spelling words or multiplication tables) (Selekman, 1988; Silver, 1993a).

Older school-age children with integrative difficulties frequently find it difficult to process multiple intake stimuli at the same time. To listen to a lecture, observe visual aids, and take notes simultaneously may prove to be confusing, because they may be easily distracted and have difficulty identifying the important points. In addition, these children may find it difficult to understand humor, clichés, and puns because they interpret language literally. Their limited understanding of concepts may result in their perception being worse than the reality of the problem (Selekman, 1988).

Alterations in motor-expressive performance. Alterations in the motor-expressive aspects of developmental tasks is a third classification of LDs. This ranges from (1) difficulty in performing gross or fine (or both) motor tasks, resulting in the labels of "clumsy," "noncoordinated," or "accident-prone"; to (2) speech disorders, including dysphasia, stuttering, poor articulation; to (3) difficulties in skills such as handwriting, spelling, arithmetic, drawing, and sports activities. These children may try to avoid hobbies and extracurricular activities that require physical activity (Silver, 1993a).

Diffuse alterations. The final category is diffuse alterations, which is a combination of the other three categories. This heterogeneous form is more commonly seen in girls. Frequently this diagnosis is delayed because the signs of dyslexia and hyperactivity are more common in boys and learning disabilities are rarely considered as a differential diagnosis for girls. These children may appear to be daydreaming or may appear to drift off in the middle of an activity. They are highly distractible by activity or noise. Overlap occurs in this category with the signs and symptoms of ADHD-inattention.

ADDITIONAL FINDINGS. One controversial set of findings is that of "soft neurologic signs." These in-

dividual minor abnormalities are identified during neurologic assessment and history taking. They consist of motor findings (clumsiness, posturing, repetitive finger tapping), mirror movements, poor directionality (especially left-right orientation), and poor gross motor skills. The incidence of soft signs in children who appear otherwise normal is so high that they have very limited use in diagnosing LDs (Gerber, 1993). If a child has soft signs and is happy and doing well, it is recommended that no further intervention be made other than routine follow-up. If a diagnosis of LD has already been made, the presence or absence of soft signs has not been noted to alter the prognosis (Shapiro and Gallico, 1993).

ADHD

The past emphasis on hyperactivity has now been replaced by giving equal importance to impulsivity and inattention. These manifestations occur in all facets of the child's life and frequently worsen in situations requiring sustained attention. The subtypes of ADHD are the predominantly inattentive type, the predominantly hyperactive-impulsive type, and the combined type (APA, 1994).

In order to be labeled ADHD, predominantly inattentive, at least six of the nine symptoms must have persisted for at least 6 months (see box on diagnostic criteria, p. 558). For ADHD, predominantly hyperactive-impulsive, at least six of the nine characteristics in that category need to have persisted for at least 6 months. A diagnosis of the combined type requires at least six symptoms from each of the sets of categories. Most children have the combined type (APA, 1994).

Although symptoms may be identified in early childhood, the symptoms may be missed until after the child enters a structured school environment. The DSM-IV (APA, 1994) also begins to address symptoms that may assist in diagnosing an adolescent or adult with ADHD.

No one test or tool is able to diagnose a child as having an LD or ADHD. Multiple data sources are used over a period of time to make the diagnosis. These include a family history, perinatal history, developmental history with current developmental assessment, assessment of past and current temperament of the child, health history, assessment of academic performance, comprehensive

DIAGNOSTIC CRITERIA FOR ATTENTION DEFICIT HYPERACTIVITY DISORDER

A. Either (1) or (2):

(1) Six (or more) of the following symptoms of inattention have persisted for at least 6 months to a degree that is maladaptive and inconsistent with developmental level:

Inattention

a. Often fails to give close attention to details or makes careless mistakes in schoolwork, work, or other activities

b. Often has difficulty sustaining attention in tasks or play activities

c. Often does not seem to listen when spoken to directly

d. Often does not follow through on instructions and fails to finish schoolwork, chores, or duties in the workplace (not due to oppositional behavior or failure to understand instructions)

e. Often has difficulty organizing tasks and activities

f. Often avoids, dislikes, or is reluctant to engage in tasks that require sustained mental effort (such as schoolwork or homework)

g. Often loses things necessary for tasks or activities (e.g., toys, school assignments, pencils, books, or tools)

h. Is often easily distracted by extraneous stimuli

i. Is often forgetful in daily activities

(2) Six (or more) of the following symptoms of hyperactivity-impulsivity have persisted for at least 6 months to a degree that is maladaptive and inconsistent with developmental level

Hyperactivity

a. Often fidgets with hands or feet or squirms in seat

b. Often leaves seat in classroom or in other situations in which remaining seated is expected

c. Often runs about or climbs excessively in situations in which it is inappropriate (in adolescents or adults, may be limited to subjective feelings of restlessness)

d. Often has difficulty playing or engaging in leisure activities quietly

e. Is often "on the go" or often acts as if driven by a motor"

f. Often talks excessively

Impulsivity

g. Often blurts out answers before questions have been completed

h. Often has difficulty awaiting turn

i. Often interrupts or intrudes on others (e.g., butts into conversations or games)

B. Some hyperactive-impulsive or inattentive symptoms that caused impairment were present before age 7 years

C. Some impairment from the symptoms is present in two or more settings (e.g., at school [or work] and at home)

D. There must be clear evidence of clinically significant impairment in social, academic, or occupational functioning

E. The symptoms do not occur exclusively during the course of a pervasive developmental disorder, schizophrenia, or other psychotic disorder and are not better accounted for by another mental disorder (e.g., mood disorder, anxiety disorder, dissociative disorder, or a personality disorder)

Data from American Psychiatric Association: Diagnostic and statistical manual of mental disorders, ed. 4, p.83-85, Washington, D.C., 1994, APA.

age-appropriate psychological and intelligence testing, and a comprehensive physical assessment with an emphasis on neurologic and motor abilities. It is helpful for the primary care provider to arrange time to observe the child's performance and behavior in school compared with performance and behavior at home or during unstructured activities. Although all of these data are needed to make the diagnosis of an LD or ADHD, it is important to reevaluate the child on these same parameters every 2 to 3 years to identify changes and new areas for needed intervention.

The primary care provider is responsible for initiating the diagnostic process for the child who has been identified as being at risk. The history and the physical and developmental assessments are within the abilities and responsibilities of the primary care provider. Psychological testing may have to be referred to specially trained individuals. Regardless of the amount of input the primary care provider makes toward the diagnostic process, he or she must assume the role of the child's advocate to initiate and collaborate in the diagnostic process. The diagnostic period is a difficult one for the parents, and guidance and support for them are especially helpful.

TREATMENT

Cognitive, behavioral, and psychosocial strategies are used in treating LD and ADHD. Pharmacologic intervention may also be very helpful in treating children with ADHD. Just as no one test can identify a child with an LD or ADHD, no one approach works for all children. Working with the child and family does, however, require an interdisciplinary team approach. This team may include some or all of the following individuals: (1) the nurse and physician (one of whom is the primary care provider), (2) the psychologist, (3) occupational and physical therapists, (4) specialists in vision, hearing, and speech and language, (5) educators, and (6) the child and his or her parents (Silver, 1992b).

Different strategies may be needed at different ages. It is important for both parents and the team to identify the child's strengths and how the child learns best, and to use that modality as the initial approach throughout the routine health care teach-

TREATMENT

LD

Multiple modalities are needed to counter the area of deficit
Pharmacologic treatment not generally used for LD, unless associated psychiatric problems coexist

ADHD

Pharmacologic intervention is used for ADHD
Treatment determined by type of ADHD and the severity of symptoms
(See Tables 26-1 and 26-2 for pharmacologic management of ADHD)

Both

Multidisciplinary approach is most effective
Interventions for both child and family members helpful
Cognitive, behavioral and psychosocial strategies are used for both

ing and treatment implementation. The primary care provider can then recommend these generalized approaches for both the home and the school environment to meet the specific needs of each child.

For the child with a visual perceptual deficit, presenting material verbally in addition to using hands-on experiences is important. This is an appropriate intervention for the clinician who is trying to provide information for or to promote compliance in this child. The child with an auditory perceptual deficit will need health education materials presented in writing and pictorially, as well as tactily. For this child, a short list of directions should be provided with either pictures of a procedure or demonstration on a model (Selekman, 1988).

The child with integrative deficits may need multisensory approaches. Directions can be written down and explained with the child watching; charts can be used if the child can read them. Feedback should constantly be elicited from the child to check his or her understanding. Calendars and lists can be used to help the child organize specific tasks or daily health-related activities. These children need shorter learning periods and more time for repetition before mastering a task.

Interventions for the child with motor deficits are similar to those for the child with cerebral palsy. Steps of a particular skill need to be broken down to component parts and verbally described. These children will need extra time to perform or verbalize. The meaning of their comments must be validated because they may have a limited expressive vocabulary.

Pharmacologic management is effective for approximately 70% to 75% of children with ADHD (Greenhill, 1992; Simeon and Wiggins, 1993). Medications utilized for ADHD currently include psychostimulants, alpha$_2$ noradrenergic agonists, and tricyclic antidepressants. The drugs of choice for treatment of ADHD are the psychostimulants: methylphenidate (Ritalin), dextroamphetamine (Dexedrine), pemoline (Cylert), and methamphetamine (Desoxyn) (see Table 26-1). Some psychostimulants come in both short-acting and long-acting preparations, whereas others are only available in the long-acting form. The effectiveness of stimulant use is measured by behavioral changes, such as decreased motor activity and increased attention span and concentration. Behavioral changes can be identified 30 to 90 minutes after ingestion. The mechanism of action for these drugs is presumed to be at the CNS transmitter level by increasing the availability of dopamine and norepinephrine at the neural synapse (Weiss and Hechtman, 1993; McEvoy, 1995). Psychostimulants can increase attention span and short-term memory, reduce distractibility, reduce motor activity, and improve cognitive performance (Greenhill, 1992; Weiss and Hechtman, 1993). These medications do not alter learning disabilities, if present, but do allow the child with ADHD to be more cognitively available for learning.

Children vary widely in both their response to dose and across domains of behavior and learning (Greenhill, 1992). Actual dosage for each child should be individually titrated for optimal effects using side effects and therapeutic responses as

guides (McEvoy, 1995). Emotional lability and a dazed, glassey-eyed appearance indicate a dose that is too high (Silver, 1992b). Refer to Table 26-1 for pharmacologic treatment guidelines for specific stimulants.

Methylphenidate (Ritalin) has been the predominantly prescribed psychostimulant for ADHD, although use of the other stimulants is increasing. Ritalin should be given with or after meals to prevent appetite suppression. A long-acting form of Ritalin is available, Ritalin-SR; however, its onset and variability in response and duration have been questioned by some (Dulcan, 1990). The Ritalin-SR 20 tablet must be swallowed, not chewed, or erratic absorption may occur. The slower rate of absorption of Ritalin-SR may reduce plasma peak concentrations and absorption phase slopes, which seem to provide less beneficial effects in children with ADHD (Greenhill, 1992). The most beneficial effects of psychostimulants do not seem to correlate with plasma peak drug levels, but rather during the period of most rapid absorption (Dulcan, 1990); therefore blood levels have little relationship to clinical effect.

Dextroamphetamine doses are generally half those of Ritalin (Dulcan, 1990). D-amphetamine is available as an elixir of 5 mg/5 cc, as well as in time-release capsules in 5 mg, 10 mg, and 15 mg strengths. The reports of increased duration of action of time-release capsules are only anecdotal and not supported by controlled studies (Dulcan, 1990; McEvoy, 1995).

Pemoline is another long-acting stimulant which is usually given only in the morning. It has varying rates of metabolism and absorption and behavioral changes may not be seen for 2 weeks unless the dosage is calculated and initiated at 1 to 2 mg/Kg (Sallee, Stiller, and Perel, 1992).

Methamphetamine (Desoxyn) is a newer long-acting stimulant, with a duration of action of 8 to 12 hours, which has 5 mg, 10 mg, and 15 mg formulations. Sources identify Desoxyn gradumets as effective for once-daily dosing, a plus for students who do not want to take medicine at school (Adderall and Other Drugs for ADHD, 1994; Wender, 1993). There are very few studies of its use in children, and Desoxyn does not appear to be the therapy of choice because of the public stigma related to its potential for substance abuse. Wender (1993) contends that

Table 26-1.   **PSYCHOSTIMULANTS USED FOR ADHD**

Drug	Dosage (individualized)	Maximum	Onset	Duration	Dosing schedule
Methylphenidate (MPH) Generic MPH tablets Ritalin tablets	Start with 5 mg bid (2.5 mg for preschoolers; 10 mg for child >30 Kg) with breakfast and lunch; increase by 5 mg/week; a third dose may be required with dinner Usual: 0.6-1.0 mg/Kg/day	Rarely need >60 mg/day	30-60 min	3-6 hr	2-3 x/day
Ritalin-SR 20 mg	Still may need bid dosing		Variable: up to 3 hr	4-6 hr (variable)	1-2 x/day
Dextroamphetamine Generic Dexedrine tablets Dexedrine elixir 5 mg/5 ml Dexedrine spansules (sustained release)	Start with 2.5 mg (5 mg for child >30 Kg) with breakfast and lunch; increase by same increments/week; third dose may be needed with dinner Usual: 0.15-0.5 mg/Kg/dose	Rarely need >40 mg/day	30-60 min	3-6 hr 4-6 hr (variable)	2-3 x/day 1-2 x/day
Pemoline Cylert	Start at 18.75 mg (37.5 mg for large child); increase dose/week to 0.5-3.0 mg/Kg/day	112.5 mg	Gradual	8-9 hr	Daily in AM
Methamphetamine Desoxyn tablets	Start with 2.5-5.0 mg each AM; raise by 5 mg increments/week		Gradual	3-6 hr	Once or twice daily
Desoxyn gradumets (time release)	Usual dose: 20-25 mg/day		Gradual	8-12 hr	Daily in AM

Dulcan, 1990; Greenhill, 1992; Koda-Kimble et al, 1992); Silver, 1992b; Simeon and Wiggins, 1993; McEvoy, 1995.

any of the stimulants carry abuse potential, and he has found Desoxyn preferable to other stimulants because of the long duration of action.

Stimulant use in preschool children appears more variable, with more adverse reactions and less research available on its safety and efficacy. Psychostimulant use in this age group should be reserved for severe cases or for when parent training and behavioral programs have been ineffective (Simeon and Wiggins, 1993).

Tricyclic antidepressants (TCAs) are considered second-line drugs for treating children with ADHD, although with slightly less effective results (Green, 1992; McEvoy, 1995). See Table 26-2. For children who failed to respond to psychostimulants or in whom adverse effects occurred, the TCAs may offer longer duration of action, less behavioral rebound and insomnia, and no risk of abuse (Simeon and Wiggins, 1993). In treating ADHD, desipramine (Norpramin), imipramine (Tofranil), amitriptyline (Elavil), nortriptyline (Pamelar), and clomipramine (Anafranil) are all effective; desipramine and imipramine have been studied to a greater degree. TCA use in children has recently come under scrutiny after reports· arose of sudden death as a result of cardiac arrest in four children being treated with desipramine (Riddle, Geller, and Ryan, 1993). Although a specific mechanism has not been identified, conduction slowing with arrhythmia potentiation is suspected. ECG monitoring after establishing a baseline is recommended for children treated with TCAs (Scahill and Lynch,

1994). A baseline ECG, followed by monitoring at dose intervals of 1 mg/kg, 3 mg/kg, and 5 mg/kg, and every 3 months is recommended (Weiss and Hechtman, 1993).

The dosages for TCA use in ADHD are lower than those for depression and the onset of response may be more rapid (see Table 26-2). TCA use is effective in reducing hyperactivity, improving mood, and enhancing sleep, but does not seem to positively affect concentration (Green, 1992). Recommendations for starting doses are presented in Table 26-2. Begin at a low, subtherapeutic dose and

Table 26-2.   SECOND-LINE MEDICATIONS FOR TREATING ADHD

Drug	Dosage*	Maximum	Side effects
Imipramine (Tofranil)	Start 10-25 mg/day (1.5-5.0 mg/Kg/day)	2.5 mg/Kg/day (children)	Common: cardiac conduction slowing, mild tachycardia, anticholinergic effects
Desipramine (Norpramin)	Start 10-15 mg/day (2.5-5.0 mg/Kg/day)	150 mg	Uncommon but serious: Heart block or arrhythmias, induction of psychosis, confusion, seizures, hypertension
Amitriptyline (Elavil)	Start 10-25 mg/day (Average: 20-150 mg/day)	300 mg/day (adolescents)	
Nortriptyline (Pamelor)	10-25 mg/day	75 mg	
Clomipramine (Anafranil)	Start 25 mg/day (Average: 85 mg/day)	200 mg or 3.0 mg/Kg/day, whichever is less	Occasional: rash, tics, photosensitization, gynecomastia
Clonidine (Catapres)	8-12 yrs: 0.25-0.3 mg/day Adolescents: 0.3-0.4 mg/day Give tid with meals and at HS	Rarely >0.5 mg/day	Common: sedation, hypotension (usually not clinically significant), headache and dizziness, stomach ache, nausea, and vomiting
Transdermal patches	5-7 day application		Uncommon but serious: rebound hypertension depression, Occasional: enhances appetite, Raynaud's phenomena

*Schedule of dosing—consider dividing dose into 2 to 3 doses to minimize adverse effects; otherwise may use daily dosing; initiating at bedtime can reduce sedative effects. Onset of effect is 4 days.
(Ryan, 1990; Koda-Kimble et al, 1992; Scahill and Lynch, 1994; Green, 1992; McEvoy, 1995)

titrate up until the maximum dose, total serum drug, or metabolite levels, or untoward effects are observed. The recommendation that TCAs be administered in two or three doses to minimize untoward effects seems prudent. Drugs should be tapered over a 10 day period when discontinuing to prevent withdrawal effects (nausea, vomiting, fatigue, abdominal pain).

Another second-line drug used for ADHD (but not attention deficit without hyperactivity) is clonidine (Catapress), an alpha-adrenergic antagonist. Clonidine primarily increases frustration tolerance and task orientation and decreases impulsivity, whereas stimulants decrease distractibility and improve focusing of attention (Green, 1992). Transdermal patch availability is a plus for some children. Beneficial effects occur with single clonidine use and combined use with stimulants. Combined pharmacotherapy for ADHD may be useful for the 30% to 40% of children who do not respond to a single agent (Wilens et al, 1995).

Despite the fact that ADHD is a chronic condition, controversy exists over what hours to cover with medication. Some children are maintained on medication for attention only during school hours, not after school or on weekends; however, many benefits are gleaned when the interactions with family, siblings, and peers are covered. Not all learning takes place in the classroom and many children benefit from continual medication. The use of medication during weekends, holidays, and vacations can assist the child to handle situations that will tend to be less structured, and therefore usually more difficult for the child with ADHD.

The effectiveness of stimulant medication should be evaluated periodically and may involve prescribing "drug holidays" during which time no medications are taken. Although the beginning and end of the school year have been proposed as evaluation times, school activities then are either new or less predictable and also more difficult for the child with ADHD to manage. Therefore, evaluations by parents, teachers, and the primary care providers are essential to determine whether the medication is still needed and should occur at a "neutral" time of the school year. Summer drug holidays give children a break from dependency on drugs that affect their behavior and may allow for catch-up growth in those children for whom ap-

petite suppression is a significant adverse effect (Murphy and Hagerman, 1992). Some researchers, however, question the efficacy of removing children from their medications (Weiss and Hechtman, 1993). They believe that because learning does not stop outside the classroom, children who need pharmacologic support need it continuously. Children who continue taking medication during vacations may have fewer accidents and improved social-emotional growth (Weiss and Hechtman, 1993). Occasionally drug holidays occur accidentally when there has been a failure to take the prescribed medications; these provide excellent opportunities for evaluating the child.

Although pharmacotherapy can significantly improve the behavior of the child with ADHD, education of the child, parents, and teachers is a key component of treatment (Shealy, 1994). Academic and social adjustments are most difficult for these children because of deficient behavioral and cognitive skills. Behavioral interventions are helpful adjuncts to pharmacotherapy, and combined use can offer synergistic and cost-effective benefits (Pelham and Sams, 1992). Children with ADHD or LDs need assistance in learning the steps involved in problem solving, self-control, and decision making, as well as how to use past learning to process new environmental information. These children should be encouraged to be actively involved in the learning process, rather than passively receiving new data. Health care professionals, educators, and parents must help these children set appropriate goals and then guide them in organizing and prioritizing strategies to obtain them.

Multimodal, multidisciplinary approaches have traditionally been proposed as most effective in meeting the needs of children with ADHD and LDs (Weiss and Hechtman, 1993; Ostrander and Silver, 1993). Few controlled studies evaluate the efficacy of multimodal "packaged" therapy; however, one study has found that the combination of cognitive behavior modification and medication was no more effective than medication alone (Abikoff, 1991). The support of professionals for child-parent training is important in helping the family and child cope effectively with a chronic, difficult situation. Many interdisciplinary team members work with the child and family at the same time, and it is important for the primary care provider to ensure that a case manager is coordinating interventions and serving as educator and advocate. Initially, this case manager will be the primary care provider, ensuring comprehensive care and coordinating efforts. The long-term strategy, however, should be to transfer the case manager role first to parents, and then to the child who should ultimately assume a self-advocacy role.

Controversial Therapies

Numerous therapies have been recommended to correct LDs and hyperactive behavior. A number of these therapies have received support from small groups of parents and special interest groups, but none has been empirically supported by controlled clinical studies. In addition, none is supported by the American Academy of Pediatrics as treatment. The different controversial approaches include cognitive-behavioristic approaches, neurophysiologic retraining, megavitamins, diet modification, and allergen avoidance.

Cognitive-behavior modification approaches teach these children cognitive techniques that can be used to control their own behavior. The goal is to promote self-controlled behavior through problem-solving strategies. Although improvement has been identified on cognitive laboratory tasks, these have not translated into changes in home and school performance (Barkley, et al 1990; Pelham and Sams, 1992).

Neurophysiologic retraining is based on the premise that "by simulating specific sensory inputs or by exercising specific motor patterns one can retrain, recircuit, or in some way improve the functioning of a part of the central nervous system" (Silver, 1993c, p 340). This approach includes patterning, optometric visual training, cerebellar-vestibular dysfunction, and applied kinesiology.

Patterning, or sensory integration, is based on the concept that individuals follow a set sequence in the development of skills. Failure to pass through these stages in sequential fashion results in poor neurologic organization. This type of therapy, primarily performed by occupational therapists, is aimed at stimulating the appropriate motor pathway with a frequency and intensity greater than what is normally experienced. No empirical data exists to support efficacy of patterning approaches as a treatment for LDs or children with cerebral palsy (Silver, 1993c).

Optometric visual training is based on a similar premise. Proponents state that vision follows developmental steps and that learning is primarily a visual task. Treatment consists of using ocular skills to improve the child's ability to read. Although no eye defects have been identified as the cause of visual perceptual deficits and claims of success with this treatment are without empirical support, some optometrists have convinced school districts to relinquish control of the LD programs to their specialty. The danger for children is that only one form of LD (visual perceptual deficit) is assessed and addressed.

The cerebellar-vestibular approach treats dyslexia with antimotion sickness medication. Applied kinesiology proports bony manipulation as a resolution to certain LDs. Neither of these approaches have any research-based support (Silver, 1993c).

Perhaps the best known treatment for hyperactivity is the Feingold diet, also known as the Kaiser-Permanente diet. Approximately 1% of children placed on this dietary management respond positively (Castellanos and Rapoport, 1992). The diet is not well received by children and is difficult to follow at school cafeterias or eateries catering to school-age children. The diet consists of the following restrictions: (1) omit foods containing natural salicylates (almonds, apples, cherries, cucumbers, grapes [raisins], oranges, peaches, tea, tomatoes), (2) omit foods and medications containing artificial colors and flavors (most types of bacon, margarine, ice cream, chocolate syrup, luncheon meats, soft drinks, catsup, bakery goods, chips), and (3) omit toothpaste, tooth powder, and compounds containing aspirin and food additives such as BHA and BHT. The generalized effectiveness of this diet cannot be supported in crossover testing measures and is no longer being recommended (Silver, 1992b).

The use of megavitamins or trace element replacements has not been empirically supported and the American Academy of Pediatrics has warned that large amounts of fat-soluble vitamins and vitamin B_6 may result in damage to the nervous system (Silver, 1993c). Other unsupported diet modifications include the elimination of sorbitol (an artificial sweetener), caffeine, and refined sugars. In repeated studies, parents' observations of the hyperactive reactions of these substances on their children's behavior cannot be supported.

The final controversial therapy proposes that children previously described as "hyperactive" are actually "allergic" to foods, chemicals, and other environmental allergens. This may be true for a small number of children, but a complete allergy workup should be able to rule this out or provide needed allergy control.

RECENT AND ANTICIPATED ADVANCES IN DIAGNOSIS AND MANAGEMENT

Further research to delineate the various etiologic factors of LD and ADHD will perhaps permit attention to focus on the areas of prevention and certainly early detection. With increased technologic ability to study the genetic, neurobiologic, and neuroanatomic basis for LD and ADHD, potential new avenues of treatment should emerge. Recognition of the life-span impact of LD and ADHD, coupled with federal support for individuals with disabilities, should broaden treatment options and opportunities for children who are diagnosed as hyperactive and learning impaired who have "grown up."

ASSOCIATED PROBLEMS

Psychologic Sequelae

Children who are misdiagnosed or not diagnosed in grade school may experience many years of academic failure. The psychologic sequelae of multiple failures can result in altered self-esteem and altered social interactions with peers. Chronic school failure can result in anxiety and depression, leading to school absenteeism or resignation. Hechtman (1992) described adolescents with hyperactivity as having significant academic, social, and emotional problems. Moffit (1990) described significant differences in delinquents and nondelinquent children with and without ADD; significantly more motor skill deficits, more family adversity, lower verbal intelligence, and poorer reading skills were reported in the delinquent group with ADD. Klein and Mannuzza (1991) reviewed longitudinal studies of boys with ADD diagnosed in childhood, reporting that 70% have ADD into adolescence and 50% had conduct disorders. Rates of arrests and in-

carcerations were significantly higher for subjects with ADHD than control groups. All of these factors can result in children who fail to reach their potential and become undereducated and underemployed (Hechtman, 1992).

A number of children with LDs or ADHDs have difficulty with peer relationships, especially those who have significant psychomotor dysfunction, whose use of language is restricted, who are in special education classes, or who are singled out and labeled as "different" in a regular classroom (Silver, 1992b). However, a similar number of children who are learning disabled are quite popular. Some of the social behavior problems may be the result of the child's impulsivity and difficulty in reading nonverbal social cues, resulting in misjudgement of acceptance or rejection (Shapiro and Gallico, 1993).

One of the problems in identifying children as LD or ADHD is the impact of labeling. The label allows the child to receive services to compensate for deficits and adjust to the consequences, but it also may result in a self-fulfilling prophesy. Educators must be careful not to use the label to separate or identify children in a mainstreamed classroom.

Psychosomatic Complaints

Children who are frustrated and stressed by their inability to perform in an academic or motor task

---

ASSOCIATED PROBLEMS

- Psychologic sequelae: low self-esteem, inadequate social skills, anxiety, depression, conduct disorders
  Academic difficulties
  Motor skill deficits
  Family conflict
  Failure to reach potential
  Labeling
- Psychosomatic complaints
- Medication side effects
- Increased risk of accidents

may develop psychosomatic symptoms when those skills are the focus in school. As with any psychosomatic disorder, all other physical causes must be ruled out. The primary care provider must assess the pattern of development of the symptoms (time of day, subject being taught in class, activity being required). Treatment involves addressing the specific needs and referring to members of the interdisciplinary team to develop a plan for intervention.

Pharmacologic Sequelae

Stimulant medication is generally well tolerated. Many side effects are dose related. In general, the stimulants produce several frequent, but short-lived adverse effects. These include: anorexia, weight loss or less than expected weight gain, headache, stomachache, tachycardia at rest, irritability or crying, abdominal pain, mild hypertension, and insomnia (Barkley, et al 1990; Greenhill, 1992; McEvoy, 1995). These symptoms generally disappear when the drug is stopped. A common side effect is behavioral rebound, manifested by exaggerated ADHD symptoms when medication is wearing off. Uncommon, but more serious adverse effects, include tic symptoms, depression, height growth impairment (more common with long-term use of dextroamphetamine), and psychotic-like symptoms (Dulcan, 1990; McEvoy, 1995). Pemoline can impair liver functioning and cause neuropsychiatric adventitious movements. Theoretical adverse effects of stimulants that have not been substantiated include a lowering of seizure threshold and increased recreational use of medications (Greenhill, 1992; McEvoy, 1995). As with any medication use, the benefits gained must be weighed against the side effects. Fewer than 4% of children need to have stimulants stopped because of adverse effects (Greenhill, 1992).

Clinically, to prevent or minimize side effects of stimulants, the following recommendations were advised by Dulcan (1990): (1) rule out a child and family history of tic disorders and adventitious movements, (2) use long-acting stimulants other than pemoline, or use antidepressants, if daily dosing is desired, (3) use the lowest effective dose and drug holidays to allow catch-up in height if taking dextroamphetamine, (4) perform liver function tests when Pemoline is initiated and every 3 to 6

months throughout the course of treatment (toxic symptoms are usually reversed when the drug is withdrawn), and (5) take medication with or following meals to alleviate appetite suppression.

Side effects of the tricyclic antidepressants that commonly occur are cardiac conduction slowing, mild tachycardia, and anticholinergic effects. The potentially serious adverse effects, although uncommon, include heart block and arrhythmias, tachycardia, confusion, lowering of the seizure threshold (primarily in children with some concomitant neurologic disorder), and hypertension (Ryan, 1990; Weiss and Hechtman, 1993; McEvoy, 1995). Obtaining a baseline ECG and periodic monitoring are essential for safe use (Green, 1992). Selection of alternative medications, if possible, would be preferable in children with higher risk of seizure activity. If withdrawal effects are observed in children on daily dosing of antidepressants (more likely as a result of the higher metabolism of medication), then divided dosing throughout the day is advised (Ryan, 1990). The potential risk for death from accidental or deliberate overdose is high with the tricyclic antidepressants; therefore these medications should be prescribed in limited quantities, secured, and kept under careful supervision.

Common adverse effects of Clonidine include: sedation, hypotension, headache and dizziness, stomachache, and nausea and vomiting. These effects are usually transient, or not clinically significant when therapeutic doses are used and dose increases are made slowly. Rebound hypertension is a serious adverse effect which can develop after high dose or chronic therapy; sudden discontinuation of Clonidine should be avoided by tapering the drug slowly (about 0.5 mg/day). Clonidine use should be avoided in children and adolescents with mood disorder histories, because its use can induce depression (Hunt, Capper, and O'Connell, 1990). Dermatitis can preclude the transdermal patch use in some children.

PROGNOSIS

A significant number of children diagnosed as learning disabled continue to be affected into adulthood. About half of today's high school graduates with LDs will fail to make a successful transition to employment (Faas, 1992). Many of these individuals have difficulty choosing occupations or professions that match their strengths and succeeding in professions, and are more likely to be underemployed and undereducated, even though their intelligence is at least average or above average. Others have learned to compensate for their areas of weakness and to build on their strengths.

Approximately 70% of children with ADHD are still manifesting symptoms as adolescents (Barkley, et al 1990; Hechtman, 1992). Recently, the diagnosis of ADHD has been applied to adults as well, dispelling even further the concept that children outgrow ADHD (Silver, 1992b). Studies of long-term outcome in ADHD demonstrate considerable variation in results. Some adults with ADHD resemble normal controls, whereas others demonstrate considerable problems with concentration and socioemotional and impulsive behaviors. Still others retain a hyperactivity component with significant psychiatric and antisocial behaviors (Hechtman, 1992). Positive or negative outcomes appear to be mediated by such factors as socioeconomic status, mental health of family members, intelligence, comorbidity of aggression and conduct disorder, and persistence of symptoms (Hechtman, 1992).

It should be noted, however, that many children with LDs and ADHD grow up to become very successful adults and have learned to compensate for their disability. A number of them have become members of the health care team by entering such fields as dentistry, psychology, medicine, and nursing. Because section 504 of the Rehabilitation Act (1973) indicates that "if otherwise qualified" these individuals must be provided entrance to jobs and continuing education, their potential is limitless.

Primary Care Management
HEALTH CARE MAINTENANCE

Growth and Development

Careful attention to measuring weight and physical growth parameters must be done routinely, approximately every 6 months, if the child is taking stimulant medication for hyperactivity. The effect of stimulant medication on growth is somewhat controversial but may result in growth suppression in some children (Vincent, Varley, and Leger, 1990).

Learning disabilities and ADHDs have not routinely been diagnosed until the child begins school. With the initiation of Public Law 99-457, the Education of the Handicapped Amendments of 1986, however, assessment of children at risk for developing LDs or ADHD must be completed in the first 3 years of life if signs and symptoms are evident. This will place more responsibility on health care providers to develop and use tools that can measure cognitive abilities and hyperactivity at an earlier age.

Because children learn to compensate for their disability, and in some cases the nature of their disability changes as they grow and develop, it is important to reevaluate the child's cognitive, motor, and psychosocial level of development every few years. Parents may request this as part of the child's individualized education plan (IEP). This provides a baseline for changing the IEP and accessing other members of the interdisciplinary team.

Diet

There are no dietary restrictions. Children on stimulant medication may have a decreased appetite, and their increased activity level may warrant an increased caloric intake. Therefore, foods high in protein and calories should be encouraged to enhance the quality of their nutritional status.

Safety

There are a number of safety issues for children and adolescents with LDs and ADHD. Because of an increase in impulsive behavior and an alteration in judgment in some children, they are at higher risk for acting without thinking and engaging in unsafe activities. Children with learning disabilities may have increased frequency of getting lost because of problems in processing information about their environment. Those children who have difficulty understanding directions may be unable to safely complete tasks or to take appropriate action in an emergency.

The primary care provider may need to help families and older children develop plans to structure their environment and their activities. Breaking down activities into component parts and using checklists may help children be more aware of their behavior. Parents should be advised that normal activities may take more time and they should keep the child's schedule simple to prevent it from becoming overloaded.

A significant number of adolescents with ADHD and LD have decreased judgment of space and distance. This deficit, plus decreased ability to pay attention to such things as conditions of the road and driving speed, results in an increase in motor vehicle accidents in this population (Barkley et al, 1993). Driving is an activity that requires multiple tasks and decision making simultaneously. Adolescents who have difficulty in these areas are advised to delay driving for a few years.

Although no data support abuse of stimulant medications, medication safety should always be a consideration in teaching. Using containers that mark the pills for each day of the week may be helpful for children who are self-administering their medications. Standard precautions for keeping medications safely secured should be followed.

Immunizations

No changes in the routine schedule of immunizations are needed.

Screening

Vision. Comprehensive vision testing should be performed, especially if a child is suspected of having a visual perceptual deficit. The child who has a problem with letter reversals may have difficulty when being tested on the Snellen E chart where the direction of the letter *E* has to be determined. It is also helpful to perform a short reading test (if age appropriate) to assess reading comprehension and whether a line can be read across without skipping words or losing place.

Hearing. Comprehensive audiometric testing should be performed at diagnosis, especially if a child is suspected of having an auditory perceptual deficit.

Speech and language. Speech and language assessments should be initiated for children demonstrating receptive or expressive language disorders (Johnson, 1993).

Dental. Routine screening is recommended.

Blood pressure. Routine screening is recommended except for children receiving stimulants, tricyclics, or Clonidine. These children may experience changes in blood pressure and should be monitored every 6 months unless dosage changes; they may also have an increased pulse rate.

DIFFERENTIAL DIAGNOSIS

Effects of stimulant therapy

Anorexia or weight loss
Insomnia
Short stature

Developmental/behavioral deviations

Adjustment disorders
Cognitive delay
Visual and auditory problems
Global delays

Increased injuries

Comorbidity

Conduct disorder
Major depression
Anxiety disorders

Hematocrit. Routine screening is recommended.

Urinalysis. Routine screening is recommended.

Tuberculosis. Routine screening is recommended

Condition-specific screening

LIVER FUNCTION. Children taking Pemolin will need liver function tests every few months.

CARDIAC FUNCTION. Children taking antidepressants will need baseline ECGs, repeated with dose increments and semiannually (Green, 1992).

COMMON ILLNESS MANAGEMENT

Differential Diagnosis

Effects of stimulant therapy. It is important to differentiate between the clinical manifestations of LD and ADHD from other problems of childhood, such as the irritability and inability to attend to a task, that are common when a child is ill. Side effects of stimulant medications may mask the symptoms of physical and psychologic illness such as anorexia, weight loss, and insomnia. Prepubertal children who have been taking stimulant medications for a number of years and who experience growth retardation should be evaluated for other causes of short stature in addition to considering the side effects of the stimulants.

Developmental/behavioral deviations. Numerous developmental deviations, including adjustment disorders, cognitive delay, visual and auditory problems, and global delays, may be mistaken for ADHD. Children must be evaluated carefully to rule out these conditions before a diagnosis is made.

Psychologic conditions such as chronic anxiety, fear of failure, and those that develop from being in a dysfunctional family (divorce, illness and death in the family, teen pregnancy, poverty, and malnutrition) may result in difficulty attending to academic tasks but should not be confused with a worsening of the disability.

Increased injuries. Children with ADHD or LDs who are frequently seen for mild trauma care and are thought to have possibly experienced abuse need to be reassessed from the perspective of their LD or ADHD. Children with difficulty following safety directions or those who lack hand-eye coordination may be more prone to environmental injury.

Comorbidity. Comorbidity is common in children with ADHD. These associated diagnoses include conduct disorder, major depression, and anxiety disorders. These conditions, having occurred, have clouded the literature regarding symptomatology, etiology, and treatment outcomes. ADHD and conduct disorder occur together in 30% to 50% of the cases (Biederman, Newcorn, and Sprich, 1991; Biederman, Faraone, and Lapey, 1992). There is a 25% overlap of ADHD with anxiety disorders (Biederman, Faraone, and Lepay, 1992).

Drug Interactions

Medications used to treat ADHD have a number of interactive effects when given with other drugs (see Table 26-3). Psychostimulants, when administered simultaneously with sympathomimetic medications used for cold and allergy symptoms (ephedrine and pseudoephedrine) or other stimu-

lants, can result in a dangerously heightened stimulant effect (Greenhill, 1992). In addition, monoamine oxidase inhibitors (MAOI) retard the metabolism of psychostimulants, which can lead to toxic effects, and the coadministration of these two types of medications leading to a potentially lethal hypertensive crisis (Greenhill, 1992). Amphetamines can impair the hypotensive effects of guanethidine (Ismelin), possibly resulting in arrhythmias. Clearance of amphetamines is enhanced by urinary acidifiers resulting in lower levels of the amphetamine; alkalinizers result in impaired renal tubular clearance.

Each of the psychostimulants has specific precautions that need to be addressed. Methylphenidate (1) elevates the levels of oral anticoagulants (e.g., dicumarol), (2) increases serum phenytoin, phenobarbital, and phenylbutazone levels, resulting in an increase in the pharmacologic and toxic effects of phenytoin, and (3) increases the serum concentration of tricyclic antidepressants (McEvoy, 1995). Dextroamphetamine interacts with furazolidone (Furoxone), causing the body to respond more sensitively to the stimulant drug, thus resulting in amphetamine toxicity. It also impedes the action of beta blockers. Phenothiazides and dextroamphetamine together result in decreased action of both (Tatro, 1990). Pemoline causes a decrease in the seizure threshold in children currently taking antiepileptic medications. Methamphetamine may decrease insulin requirements in children with diabetes mellitus (Sallee, Stiller, and Perel, 1992; McEvoy, 1995).

Tricyclic antidepressants can cause increased effects with stimulants, central nervous system depressants (MAOI, sympathomimetics, alcohol, or other substance abuse medications), anticholinergics, thyroid preparations, seizure-potentiating medications, and phenytoin. Tricyclic antidepressants can decrease the effects of guanethidine and clonidine. The effects of the tricyclics are increased by phenothiazines, cimetidine, and oral contraceptives (McEvoy, 1995). The effects of the tricyclics are decreased by lithium, barbiturates, chloral hydrate, and smoking (Ryan, 1990). Combined use of tricyclics and marijuana may cause significant sinus tachycardia.

Clonidine increases the effects of CNS depressants and anticholinergic preparations, although

Table 26-3.   **DRUG INTERACTIONS RELEVANT IN TREATING ADHD**

Drug A	Combined with drug B	Interaction
Stimulants	Sympathomimetics, other stimulants	(↑↑) Significantly increased stimulant effect
	MAO inhibitors	(↑↑) Toxic stimulant effect Hypertensive crisis; may be lethal
Amphetamines	Urinary acidifiers	↓ Amphetamine effect
	Urinary alkalinizer	↑ Amphetamine effect
	Guanethidine	↓ Guanethidine effect (arrhythmias)
Methylphenidate	Oral anticoagulants	↑ Anticoagulant level
	Phenytoin	↑ Phenytoin levels
	Phenylbutazone	↑ Phenylbutazone levels
	TCA	↑ TCA levels
Dextroamphetamine	Furazolidone	↑ Amphetamine effect
	Beta blockers	↓ Beta blocker action
	Phenothiazine	↓ Action of both drugs
Pemoline	Antiepileptic medications	↓ Seizure threshold
Methamphetamine	Insulin	↓ Requirements of insulin
TCA	Stimulants	↑ Effects of stimulants
	CNS depressants (MAOI, alcohol sympathomimetics)	↑ CNS depressant effect
	Anticholinergics	↑ Effect of anticholinergics
	Thyroid preparations	↑ Thyroid activity
	Seizure potentiating medications	↑ Seizure potentiation
	Phenytoin	↑ Phenytoin levels
	Guanethidine	↓ Effect of guanethidine
	Clonidine	↓ Effect of clonidine
	Phenothiazines	↑ TCA effect
	Oral contraceptives	↑ TCA effect
	Lithium	↓ TCA effect
	Barbiturates	↓ TCA effect
	Chloral hydrate smoking	↓ TCA effect
	Smoking	↑ TCA effect
	Marijuana	Sinus tachycardia
Clonidine	CNS depressants	↑ Drug B
	Anticholinergic preparations	↑ Drug B
	Beta-adrenergic blockers	↓ Drug B effect
	Fenfluramine	↑ Clonidine effect
	Thiazide diuretics	↑ Clonidine effect
	Antihypertensive agents	↑ Clonidine effect
	CNS depressants	↑ Sedative effect of Clonidine
	TCAs	↓ Hypotensive effect of Clonidine
	Sympathomimetic drugs	↓ Hypotensive effect of Clonidine
	NSAIDS	↓ Hypotensive effect of Clonidine

usually less in children than adults. It decreases the effects of β-adrenergic blockers, which heightens the rebound hypertension that can occur when it is discontinued. The effect of clonidine is enhanced with fenfluramine, thiazide diuretics, and other antihypertensive agents. The sedative effect of Clonidine is increased with concurrent use of other CNS depressants. The hypotensive effects of Clonidine are impaired with tricyclic antidepressants, sympathomimetic drugs, and nonsteroidal antiinflammatory agents (Hunt, Capper, and O'Connell, 1990; McEvoy, 1995).

DEVELOPMENTAL ISSUES

Sleep Patterns

Learning disabilities have no affect on sleep unless emotional problems are present. In the child with ADHD, medication timing or inability to settle down may affect falling asleep. Assessment of drug administration schedule should be completed. Insomnia is a common side effect of stimulant medication and frequently resolves as a tolerance to the medication develops. If this does not resolve, decreasing the dosage or scheduling administration earlier in the day may help. Medication rebound may necessitate adding a small bedtime dose of stimulant (Dulcan, 1990).

Toileting

No impact on toileting exists unless the child experiences sensory or tactile deficits. In this case, the child needs to be walked through the sensations involved in toileting. Routine toilet breaks should be a part of the daily schedule. Elementary schools should also be sensitive to this need and incorporate toileting into the day's activities.

Discipline

All children act out and misbehave at various intervals in the developmental process. As with other children, discipline should fit the seriousness of the misbehavior. However, children with an LD or ADHD do not learn well from past experiences and may not be able to understand cause and effect or verbal sequences of directions (Pfiffner and Barkley, 1990). Even after these children have done something wrong, they may not relate their activity to the punishment and will need frequent clarifica-

tion from adults. Frequent feedback related to progress is important (Shelton and Barkley, 1992).

Behavior modification techniques may help the child develop self-control. If time-out is used, the child needs to be told when the period of restriction has ended. He or she needs to be reminded of the reasons for the punishment and consistently helped to differentiate between "the act being wrong or bad" and "the child being bad." Identification and reward for good behavior is effective. For the hyperactive child, parents need assistance in determining to what degree the child's normal behavior requires discipline. Parenting classes may be helpful in making this differentiation.

Discipline should be part of the daily routine for these children and it must be consistent. Limit setting is an important component of their day. Structuring the daily routine of the home environment will help these children establish acceptable patterns of behavior. Parents should be reminded to teach the recommended behavioral approaches to the child's significant others, such as grandparents and babysitters.

Child Care

If day care is a component of child care, a program that has a small class size, a structured and safe environment, constant adult supervision, and an opportunity to engage in gross motor play outdoors should be selected. Children with hyperactivity will need to develop a medication regimen that best fits their needs. Predictability of schedule is reassuring to the child with ADHD or an LD, since he or she does not handle surprises or changes very well.

Schooling

A major issue is that of school readiness. The appropriateness of the child for a kindergarten class at age 5 years needs to be evaluated. A number of children with LDs spend 2 years in kindergarten or first grade, thus giving them time to develop the psychosocial and cognitive skills needed to be successful. It is important to assess for prerequisite deficits in knowledge or skills and to plan remediation for them. The primary care provider may play a key role in emotionally supporting parents through the difficult decision of holding their child back. Focusing on the long-term gains will help diminish the parents' initial disappointment and grieving.

Making the child feel special and giving attention to his or her accomplishments will be beneficial to the child.

Children with LDs and ADHD may be mainstreamed into regular classrooms, use the resource room, attend special education classes, be tutored, or a combination thereof. The goal is to mainstream these children into normal classrooms, but special education classrooms and resource rooms are also very acceptable therapies. In resource rooms (supplementary help) and special education (self-contained) classrooms, teachers can limit the number of students in the classroom, decrease the amount of distraction, and provide specific interventions based on the child's needs.

According to Public Law 101-476, every child with a learning disability or ADHD should have an individualized education plan (IEP) developed specifically for them. It should include the type of classroom, and the type and length of services the child will use. The educational objectives and the plan for intervention will be identified in the IEP. The primary care provider should be a key member on the education team and have input into the IEP recommendations.

Parents should participate in the IEP development and be encouraged to meet with each member of the interdisciplinary team who will interface with their child. These meetings should occur throughout the year to update the parents and enhance communication between the parents and teachers. The primary care provider functions as health care coordinator, educator, and consultant for the IEP team.

A significant part of the educational plan is to help children learn to compensate for their particular disability. Children need to understand which learning modalities work best for them and then to have material presented (or available) to them in that modality. For children with visual perceptual deficits, tape recording class lectures may be more helpful than manual note taking.

The child with altered coordination and difficulty in motor skills may shy away from participation in age-appropriate activities. Being involved in noncompetitive sports, being given a different role in a group activity so as to continue being a member of the group, and finding alternative motor activities such as using a computer rather than being required to use script, will enhance the child's self-concept and make him or her less fearful of participation.

Classroom teachers who are unfamiliar with the special needs of these children will require specific information as to their role in education, assessment, and control measures (if necessary). The Conners Teacher Rating Scale (Conners, 1987) provides important information in the periodic assessment of hyperactive children. It assesses behavior in the classroom, group participation, and attitude toward authority. This assessment will prove to be essential to the primary care provider in determining whether stimulant medication should be continued or should be changed.

Children with LDs and ADHD may be highly distractible. Educational strategies and environmental modifications that have proved beneficial for these children in a regular classroom are listed in the box on page 573.

The child with an LD or ADHD and his or her family will need to readjust to the child's condition at every new developmental stage. The psychologic impact of LDs or ADHD results in specific psychosocial needs. Building a child's self-esteem and self-confidence, as well as an accurate self-perception, become even more important when the child is experiencing chronic academic difficulty.

The child who continues to have academic difficulty resulting in failure will need counseling support and assistance in dealing with the related stress. By high school, the inattention of ADHD may be manifested as chronic academic underachievement and motivation problems (Werry, 1992). Children with LDs and ADHD need to understand that even though they failed a course (or examination), they are not a failure. It is not appropriate to tell a child to "try harder." The child's decreased performance is often not a lack of effort or anyone's fault. These children need to be reassured that they are not stupid and that requests for repetition of directions and clarification of content are not a nuisance.

It is important to assist the child in developing strategies for coping. These should build on the child's strengths and compensate for his or her weaknesses. In addition, encouraging social interaction with peers is another goal of the primary care provider. Adolescents find it very difficult to adjust

EDUCATIONAL AND ENVIRONMENTAL STRATEGIES FOR THE CHILD WITH LD/ADHD

Muted wall colors

Decreased clutter

Seat child in front of room, away from doors, windows, and distractions

Seat child near on-task peer

Structured environment preferred over open, unstructured environment

Use of calendar; assignment books; structured schedule; untimed testing; testing orally; testing in separate quiet room

Use technology assistive devices—tape recorders, word processors

Verbal and written instructions

Positive reinforcement for effort and achievement

Adequate feedback; divide large projects down into parts

Complex, important subjects early in the day for children on medication

Second set of books at home for those with memory problems

to a chronic condition. This is a time of conformity rather than having to meet special needs. Young people need the opportunity to express their feelings about having a disability, but also being different, especially if they are taking stimulant medication.

Medication administration during school hours has presented some problems for children. Legal guidelines for school personnel administering drugs and for keeping medications in the school vary with each state. These guidelines should be shared with parents so that they can plan accordingly. In addition, some children forget to come for their lunchtime dose because they often (1) have to leave their friends to go to the infirmary or office, (2) are involved in group activities, or (3) may feel guilty or self-conscious about having to take pills, especially if "Just say No to drugs" information is being promoted.

The primary care provider must have communication with members of the IEP team, the family,

and the child at least twice each year to assess and modify the plan of care. These interactions can be much more frequent (every 2 to 4 weeks) as the need arises.

Sexuality

Sex education for children and adolescents is an important role for the primary care provider. Using the learning techniques previously identified, sex education must be individualized to the child's specific learning abilities.

Transition into Adulthood

The transition of older adolescents into adulthood is a critical point for families of children with ADHDs and LDs (Dane, 1993). The underlying condition and its associated risks do not go away. Therefore the adolescent who is working on the developmental tasks of separation from parents and family, establishing a sense of identity, and formulating personal and occupational goals will often require professional help. Youths with LDs and ADHD often have unresolved issues from earlier developmental phases, less developed problem-solving skills, and may have limited awareness of the ramifications of their disability (Dane, 1993). Having someone who believed in them (counselor, parent, teacher, or therapist) was identified as having helped these young adults the most in their process of growing up (Greenfield, Gottlieb, and Weiss, 1992).

Interventions that will assist in the transition include: (1) fostering an awareness and acceptance in young adults of their ADHD or LD and their individual strengths and weaknesses, (2) developing strategies to adapt to their disability, (3) developing self-advocacy skills, (4) fostering the development of external support systems (mentors, support groups, counselors), (5) vocational counseling, (6) selecting a college with a program providing academic or "life skills" support for students with LDs or ADHD, and (7) encouragement and support in attempting new challenges (Brinckerhoff, 1993; Greenfield, Gottlieb, and Weiss, 1992; Spekman, Herman, and Vogel, 1993; Weller et al, 1994).

It is encouraging to note that many young adults with LDs and ADHDs describe satisfaction in aspects of social life with family, friends, and peers (Spekman, Goldberg, and Herman, 1992), and report successful completion of college and career goals (Vogel, Hruby, and Abelman, 1993).

ADHD and LDs are not just academic disabilities; the ramifications pervade every area of the child's life and keep the child from functioning at an optimal level. By accepting the diagnosis, children can begin to take control of their lives. Children with ADHD and LD can develop accommodation strategies to compensate for their learning difference. These children can learn; they just learn differently. In essence, they have a living disability. With appropriate intervention, their goal of growing into adulthood using their full potential can be accomplished.

SPECIAL FAMILY CONCERNS AND RESOURCES

Before a diagnosis of LD or ADHD is made, parents are often confused, concerned, and even anxious as to why their child is having difficulties. Once a diagnosis is made, parents will grieve for the wished-for "perfect" child and may respond to the diagnosis with embarrassment, frustration, guilt, self-blame, anger, or even relief that the problem has been identified and is not imagined.

Before parents can begin to accept their child and work toward resolution of the treatment objectives, they need to be educated about this disability. In this endeavor, the family can be empowered to assume control of the plan developed for their child and for guiding their child's development. Routine anticipatory guidance is also provided. It should be kept in mind that often a child with an LD or ADHD has a parent with the same condition. Therefore, teaching about child care and other developmental issues should use the same approaches as discussed earlier, depending on the parent's specific needs.

Environmental control in the home is similar to that discussed for the classroom. Decreasing clutter, developing routines, scheduling ample time for activities, and providing clear directions in the format that best meets the child's needs may prove beneficial. These parents typically give more commands, directions, and supervision to their child than for a "normal" child. They are concerned about the child's future potential for schooling and vocational choices, as well as the child's ability to assume an independent lifestyle. This results in increased parental stress, depression, and marital discord. Parents, as well as their children, need coping strategies and consistent support.

There can be a significant impact on the siblings of a child with LDs or ADHD. Siblings may resent the amount of time and attention paid to the child with special needs and the embarrassment that their sibling often causes them. Younger siblings will need to be sensitive to the feelings of the child with special needs as the younger sibling matches and often surpasses the academic level of the child with an LD or ADHD.

The only cultural implication related to LDs and ADHDs is the culture of poverty. Children who attend schools where educational standards are not high or where issues such as malnutrition or neglect interfere with learning must be carefully assessed to accurately differentiate these causes from a true LD or ADHD. Although there may not be a difference in the incidence of LDs or ADHD across cultures, culture may play a role in how families and the affected child handle the diagnosis and interventions (Barkley, 1990).

Books on learning disabilities and ADHD: for parents

Fowler M: *Maybe you know my kid: A parent's guide to identifying, understanding and helping your child with ADHD,* New York, 1990, Birch Lane Press.

Silver L: *The misunderstood child: A guide for parents of children with learning disabilities,* Blue Ridge Summit, PA, 1992, TAB Books.

Silver L: *Dr. Larry Silver's advice to parents on attention-deficit hyperactivity disorder,* Washington, DC, 1993, American Psychiatric Press.

Books on learning disabilities and ADHD: for children

Gehret J: *Eagle eyes,* Fairport, NY, 1991, Verbal Images Press.

Gordon M: *Jumpin' Johnny: Get back to work,* DeWitt, NY, 1991, GSI Publications.

Mosa D: *Shelly, the hyperactive turtle,* Bethesda, MD, 1989, Woodbine House.

Quinn P, Stern J: *Putting on the brakes,* New York, 1991, Magination Press.

Organizations

Children and Adults with Attention Deficit Disorders (CHADD)

499 Northwest 70th Ave
Suite 101
Plantation, FL 33317
305-587-3700
National Center for Learning Disabilities
381 Park Ave S
Suite 1420
New York, NY 10016
212-545-7510
Learning Disabilities Association
4156 Library Rd
Pittsburgh, PA 15234
412-341-8077
Council for Exceptional Children
1920 Association Dr
Reston, VA 22091-1589
703-620-3660

Council for Learning Disabilities
PO Box 40303
Overland Park, KS 66204
913/492-8755

Vocational rehabilitation services for individuals with learning disabilities

Although Public Law 101-476 provides educational services for the individual under the age of 21, the recognition by the American Psychiatric Association that many of these children continue to exhibit symptoms of their chronic condition into adulthood has led to their being eligible for state and federal vocational rehabilitation services. Primary care providers should remember that many vocational counselors have had no experience in counseling young people with these conditions. Consequently, the primary care provider may need to instruct the counselor.

SUMMARY OF PRIMARY CARE NEEDS FOR THE CHILD WITH LEARNING DISABILITIES OR ATTENTION DEFICIT HYPERACTIVITY DISORDER

Health care maintenance

Growth and development

Manifestations of an LD or ADHD vary with development.
Medications for hyperactivity cause appetite suppression—assess height and weight.
Toddlers and preschoolers are eligible for diagnostic and intervention services under PL 101-476.

Diet

Children may be poor eaters because of distraction and decreased appetite if they are taking stimulant medication. A nutritious diet with adequate protein and calories for growth is important.

Safety

There is a risk of injury because of impulsive behaviors. Drivers with LD and ADHD may have automobile accidents because of spatial perception difficulties.

Medication should be safely kept out of reach of young children.

Immunizations

Routine schedule is recommended.

Screening

Vision
Comprehensive visual testing is done to identify acuity problems and rule out other causes of a visual perceptual deficit.
Children may have difficulty using standard *E* chart.
Hearing
Comprehensive audiometric testing is done to identify hearing loss and rule out other causes of an auditory perceptual deficit.
Children may have difficulty with audiometric testing because of directionality problems.
Speech and language
Specialized testing is done if a problem in this area is observed, there is a high incidence of speech

Continued.

SUMMARY OF PRIMARY CARE NEEDS FOR THE CHILD WITH LEARNING DISABILITIES OR ATTENTION DEFICIT HYPERACTIVITY DISORDER—cont'd

and language problems in children with ADHD.

Dental

Routine screening is recommended.

Blood pressure

Routine screening is recommended. If the child is taking stimulant medication, screening must be done more frequently because of possible hypertension. Clonidine may cause slight hypotension and an increase in the pulse rate.

Hematocrit

Routine screening is recommended.

Urinalysis

Routine screening is recommended.

Tuberculosis

Routine screening is recommended.

Condition-specific screening

Liver function tests are necessary for children taking Pemoline.

ECG monitoring is necessary for children on tricyclic antidepressants.

Common illness management

Differential diagnosis

Irritability

Rule out illness or medication effect.

Anorexia, weight loss, and insomnia

Rule out illness or need for a change in dosage or dosing schedule for medications.

Drug interactions

Stimulant medications inhibit liver metabolism of other drugs.

Methylphenidate affects anticoagulants, quanethidine, phenytoin, phenobarbital, MAO inhibitors, and tricyclic antidepressants.

Dextroamphetamine affects furazolidone, quanethidine, beta blockers, phenobarbital, phenytoin, and phenothiazides. These medications should not be given with MAO inhibitors.

Clonidine affects CNS depressant agents, anticholinergic agents, beta blockers, fenfluramine, antihypertensive agents, thiazide diuretics, tricyclic antidepressants, sympathomimetic agents (allergy preparations), and nonsteroidal antiinflammatory analgesics.

Tricyclic antidepressants affect any CNS stimulant or depressant drug (including MAO inhibitors, sympathomimetic drugs, and alcohol), anticholinergics. thyroid medication, seizure-potentiating medications, phenytoin, clonidine, and guanethidine.

Phenothiazines, methylphenidate, oral contraceptives, lithium, barbiturates, chloral hydrate, and smoking affect the tricyclics.

Do not give tricyclics with MAO inhibitors.

Developmental issues

Sleep patterns

Children with ADHD on stimulant medication may have insomnia if given late in the day or in large doses.

Toileting

No impact unless child has sensory tactile deficits.

Discipline

Children may have difficulty responding to directions. They may not understand discipline. Consistency is important.

Child care

Administration of medication may be necessary in the day care setting. Children perform better in a small, structured safe environment with constant adult supervision.

Schooling

Education strategies to decrease distraction in a regular classroom plus creative teaching modalities appropriate to the specific learning needs of the child should be implemented. Building a child's self-esteem and confidence is essential. Children should be helped to learn to compensate for their disability. Development of the individualized education plan (IEP) is a team effort.

Continued.

SUMMARY OF PRIMARY CARE NEEDS FOR THE CHILD WITH LEARNING DISABILITIES OR ATTENTION DEFICIT HYPERACTIVITY DISORDER—cont'd

Sexuality

Learning techniques individualized for the particular adolescent must be used when teaching sexuality and birth control material.

Transition into adulthood

Professional help may be necessary to facilitate the transition to more autonomous living and work situations.

Career development counseling may be helpful in identifying a vocation appropriate for young adults to accept personal strengths and weaknesses in learning style.

Special family concerns and resources

The child and the family need to readjust to this disability at every new developmental stage. Family counseling can provide information and emotional support. A learning disability is a living disability.

Other factors such as poverty, poor nutrition, and inadequate schooling must be assessed for their responsbility or relationship to learning difficulties.

REFERENCES

Abikoff H: Interaction of methylphenidate and multimodal therapy in the treatment of attention deficit hyperactivity disorder. In Osman B, Greenhill L (editors): *Ritalin: theory and patient management,* New York, 1991, Mary Ann Liebert, pp 147-154.

Adderall and other drugs for attention deficit hyperactivity disorder, *The Medical Letter* 36(936):109-110, 1994.

American Psychiatric Association: *Diagnostic and statistical manual of mental disorders,* ed 4, Washington, DC, 1994, Author.

Barkley R: *Attention deficit hyperactivity disorder: a handbook for diagnosis and treatment,* New York, 1990, The Guilford Press.

Barkley R et al: Driving related risks and outcomes of attention deficit hyperactivity disorder in adolescents and young adults: a 3- to 5-year follow-up survey, *Pediatrics* 92(2):212-218, 1993.

Bauchner H, Brown E, and Peskin J: Premature graduates of the newborn intensive care unit: a guide to follow up, *Pediatr Clin North Am* 35(6):1207-1226, 1988.

Biederman J, Faraone S, and Lapey K: Comorbidity of diagnosis in attention deficit hyperactivity disorder, *Child Adolesc Psychiatr Clin North Am* 1(2):335-360, 1992.

Biederman J, Newcorn J, and Sprich S: Comorbidity of attention deficit hyperactivity disorder with conduct, depressive, anxiety, and other disorders, *Am J Psychiatr* 148(5):564-577, 1991.

Brinckerhoff L: Self-advocacy: a critical skill for college students with learning disabilities, *Fam Community Health* 16(3):23-33, 1993.

Castellanos FX, Rapoport J: Etiology of attention deficit hyperactivity disorder, *Child Adolesc Psychiatr Clin North Am* 1(2):373-384, 1992.

Conners CK: How is a teacher rating scale used in the diagnosis of attention deficit disorder? *J Child Contemp Society* 19 (1-2):33-40, 1987.

Dane E: Family fantasies and adolescent aspirations: a social work perspective on a critical transition, *Fam Community Health* 16(3):34-45, 1993.

Duane D: The medical and neurological diagnostic process, *Child Adolesc Psychiatr Clin North Am* 2(2):283-293, 1993.

Dulcan M: Using psychostimulants to treat behavioral disorders of children and adolescents, *J Child Adolesc Psychopharmacol* 1(1):7-20, 1990.

Faas L: WAIS-R subtest regroupings as predictors of employment success and failure among adults with learning disabilities, *J Rehabil* (4):47-50, 1992.

Faraone SV et al: Evidence for the independent familial transmission of attention deficit hyperactivity disorder and learning disabilities: results from a family genetic study, *Am J Psychiatr* 150(6):891-895, 1993.

Foley GV, Fochtman D, and Mooney KH: *Nursing care of the child with cancer,* Philadelphia, 1993, WB Saunders.

Galaburda AM: Anatomy of dyslexia: argument against phrenology. In Duane DD, Gray DB (editors): *The reading brain: the biological basis of dyslexia,* Parkton, MD, 1991, York Press.

Gerber A: *Language-related learning disabilities: their nature and treatment,* Baltimore, 1993, Paul H Brookes.

Green W: Nonstimulant drugs in the treatment of attention deficit hyperactivity disorder, *Child Adolesc Psychiatr Clin North Am* 1(2):449-465, 1992.

Greenfield B, Gottlieb S, and Weiss G: Psychosocial interventions: individual psychotherapy with the child, and family and parent counseling, *Child Adolesc Psychiatr Clin North Am* 1(2):481-504, 1992.

Greenhill L: Pharmacotherapy: stimulants, *Child Adolesc Psychiatr Clin North Am* 1(2):411-447, 1992.

Hammill D: A timely definition of learning disabilities, *Fam Community Health* 16(3):1-8, 1993.

Hechtman L: Genetic and neurobiological aspects of attention deficit hyperactive disorder: a review, *J Psychiatr Neuroscience* 19(3):193-201, 1994.

Hechtman L: Long-term outcome in attention deficit hyperactivity disorder, *Child Adolesc Psychiatr Clin North Am* 1(2):553-566, 1992.

Hunt R, Capper L, and O'Connell P: Clonidine in child and adolescent psychiatry, *J Child Adolesc Psychopharmacol* 1(1):87-102, 1990.

Hynd GW et al: Brain morphology in developmental dyslexia and attention deficit disorder hyperactivity, *Arch Neurol* 47:919-926, 1990.

Interagency Committee on Learning Disabilities: *Learning disabilities: a report to the US congress,* Washington, DC, 1987, US Department of Health and Human Services.

Johnson D: Language disorders, *Child Adolesc Psychiatr Clin North Am* 2(2):233-248, 1993.

Klein RG, Mannuzza S: Long-term outcome of hyperactive children: a review, *J Am Acad Child Adolesc Psychiatr* 30:383-387, 1991.

Koda-Kimble MA et al: *Handbook of applied therapeutics,* ed 2, Vancouver, WA, 1992, Applied Therapeutics Inc.

McEvoy GK, (editor): *American hospital formulary service drug information,* Bethesda, MD, 1995, American Society of Health-System Pharmacists Inc.

Moffit TE: Juvenile delinquency and attention deficit disorder: boy's developmental trajectories from age 3 to age 15, *Child Dev* 61:893-910, 1990.

Murphy M, Hagerman R (1992). Attention deficit hyperactivity disorder in children: Diagnosis, treatment, and followup. *Journal of Pediatric Health Care* 6(1)2-11.

Ostrander R, Silver L: Psychological interventions and therapies for children and adolescents with learning disabilities, *Child Adolesc Psychiatr Clin North Am* 2(2):323-337, 1993.

Pelham WE, Sams SE: Behavior modification, *Child Adolesc Psychiatr Clin North Am* 1(2):505-518, 1992.

Pfiffner L, Barkley R: Educational placement and classroom management. In Barkley R (editor): *Attention deficit hyperactivity disorder: a handbook for diagnosis and treatment,* New York, 1990, The Guilford Press, pp 498-539.

Riccio C, Gonzalez J, and Hynd G: Attention deficit hyperactivity disorder (ADHD) and learning disorders, *Learn Disabil Q* 17:311-322, Fall 1994.

Riddle M, Geller B, and Ryan N: Another sudden death in a child treated with desipramine, *J Am Acad Child Adolesc Psychiatr* 32:792-797, 1993.

Rourke BP, Del Dotto JE: *Learning disabilities: a neuropsychological perspective,* Thousand Oaks, CA, 1994, Sage.

Ryan ND: Heterocyclic antidepressants in children and adolescents, *J Child Adolesc Psychopharmacol* 1(1):21-31, 1990.

Sallee FR, Stiller RL, and Perel JM: Pharmacodynamics of pemoline in attention deficit disorder with hyperactivity, *J Am Acad Child Adolesc Psychiatr* 31(2):244-251, 1992.

Scahill L, Lynch K: Tricyclic antidepressants: cardiac effects and clinical implications, *J Child Adolesc Psychiatr Nurs* 7(1):37-39, 1994.

Selekman J: The learning disabled child: another frontier for nursing, *Holistic Nurs Pract* 2(2):1-10, 1988.

Shapiro B, Gallico R: Learning disabilities, *Pediatr Clin North Am* 40(3):491-505, 1993.

Shealy A: Attention deficit hyperactivity disorder: etiology, diagnosis, and management, *J Child Adolesc Psychiatr Nurs* 7(2):24-36, 1994.

Shelton T, Barkley R: The role of parent training groups in the treatment of attention deficit hyperactivity disorder, *Child Adolesc Psychiatr Clin North Am* 1(2):519-537, 1992.

Silver AA, Hagin RA: The educational diagnostic process, *Child and Adolesc Psychiatr Clin North Am* 2(2):265-281, 1993.

Silver L: Diagnosis of attention deficit hyperactivity disorder in adult life, *Child Adolesc Psychiatr Clin North Am* 1(2):325-334, 1992a.

Silver L: *The misunderstood child,* Blue Ridge Summit, PA, 1992b, TAB Books.

Silver L: Introduction and overview to the clinical concepts of learning disabilities, *Child Adolesc Psychiatr Clin North Am* 2(2):181-192, 1993a.

Silver L: Preface, *Child Adolesc Psychiatr Clin North Am* 2(2):xiii-xiv, 1993b.

Silver L: The controversial therapies for treating learning disabilities, *Child Adolesc Psychiatr Clin North Am* 2(2):339-350, 1993c.

Simeon JG, Wiggins DM: Pharmacotherapy of attention deficit hyperactivity disorder, *Can J Psychiatr* 38(6):443-448, 1993.

Spekman N, Goldberg R, and Herman K: Learning disabled children grow up: a search for factors related to success in the young adult years, *Learning Disabilities Research and Practice* 7:161-170, 1992.

Spekman N, Herman K, and Vogel S: Risk and resilience in individuals with learning disabilities: a challenge to the field, *Learning Disabilities Research and Practice* 8(1):59-65, 1993.

Tatro D (editor). (1990). *Drug interaction facts.* St. Louis: Lippincott.

Vincent J, Varlay C, and Leger P: Effects of pethylphidate on early adolescent growth, *Am J Psychiatr* 147:501-502, 1990.

Vogel SA, Hruby PJ, and Adelman PB: Educational and psychological factors in successful and unsuccessful college students with learning disabilities, *Learning Disabilities Research and Practice* 8(1):35-43, 1993.

Weiss G, Hechtman L: *Hyperactive children grown up: ADHD in children, adolescents, and adults,* New York, 1993, The Guilford Press.

Weller C et al: Adaptive behavior of adults and young adults with learning disabilities, *Learn Dis Q* 17(Fall):282-295, 1994.

Wender P: Editorial: methamphetamine in child psychiatry, *J Child Adolesc Psychopharmacol* 3(1):iv-vi, 1993.

Werry J: History, terminology, and manifestations at different ages, *Child Adolesc Psychiatr Clin North Am* 1(2):297-310, 1992.

Wilens TE et al: Combined pharmacotherapy: an emerging trend in pediatric psychopharmacology, *J Am Acad Child Adolesc Psychiatr* 34(1):110-112, 1995.

Wolraich M et al: Effects of diets high in sucrose or aspartame on the behavior and cognitive performance of children, *New Engl J Med* 330(5):301-307, 1994.

Zametkin AJ et al: Cerebral glucose metabolism in adults with hyperactivity of childhood onset, *New Engl J Med* 323(20):1361-1366, 1990.

Myelodysplasia

27

Judith A. Farley
and Mary Jo Dunleavy

ETIOLOGY

The classification of neural tube defects pertains to the malformation of the central nervous system during embryonic development. The embryologic development of the central nervous system begins early in the third week of gestation. During this time, the neural plate invaginates and folds together forming the neural tube. The process of neurulation produces the functional nervous system or the future brain and spinal cord. If the neural tube fails to close, the process of neurulation is interrupted, which results in the imperfect formation of the brain and spinal cord at a focal point (Warkany and Lemire, 1986).

Myelodysplasia is one form of a neural tube defect, which refers to the defective formation and subsequent development and function of the spinal cord. This defect can occur at any level of the spinal cord; the extent of nerve tissue and spinal cord involvement varies. The malformation results in altered body function at and below the level of the defect (see Table 27-1 on p. 582).

The etiology of neural tube defects is unknown. Many potential causes or factors have been considered, but none has been confirmed as an isolated cause. At this time there is insufficient data in the literature to link a specific drug exposure with the development of neural tube defects (Moore, 1987; McLone and Naidich, 1986; Humphreys, 1991).

INCIDENCE

The incidence of neural tube defects is approximately 0.7 to 1.0 for every 1000 live births in the United States each year. A higher incidence of neural tube defects exists in affected families, as well as an overall increased risk of birth defects with poor prenatal care and maternal nutritional deficiencies. The strong association of fetal demise with neural tube defects reduces the actual prevalence of neural tube defects at birth (Wallander, Feldman, and Varni, 1989; Shaw et al, 1994).

CLINICAL MANIFESTATIONS AT TIME OF DIAGNOSIS

Clinical presentation at the time of diagnosis will vary depending on the extent of involvement of the spinal cord and surrounding structures of nerve, bone, muscle, and skin. Myelodysplasia is classified based on the pathophysiology of the lesion or defect (see Fig. 27-1).

Spina bifida occulta is the failed fusion of the vertebral arches that surround and protect the spinal cord. This may involve a small portion of one vertebra or the complete absence of bone. Absence of the vertebral arches is commonly associated with cutaneous abnormalities such as tufts of hair, hemangiomas, and dermoid cysts located on the surface at the area of the defect. Usually no

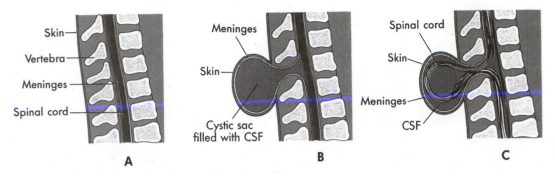

Fig. 27-1.   Diagram showing section through **A,** normal spine; **B,** meningocele; **C,** myelomeningocele.

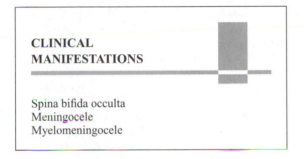

CLINICAL
MANIFESTATIONS

Spina bifida occulta
Meningocele
Myelomeningocele

neurologic deficits present at the time of birth; however, a child with such a defect may develop bowel, bladder, and musculoskeletal difficulties later in life (American Association of Neuroscience Nurses [AANN], 1990).

Another example of myelodysplasia is the meningocele in which the neural tube fails to close resulting in a cystic dilatation of meninges through the vertebral defect and around the malformed tube. This defect does not involve the spinal cord and the condition of hydrocephalus can be associated with this diagnosis (AANN, 1990). At birth the infant presents with a protruding sac on the back at the level of the defect evident at birth. The sac may be covered by a thin layer of muscle and skin and usually appears as raw, fluid-filled tissue. The child may or may not have abnormal neurologic findings at birth. Manipulation of the sac, surgical closure, and infection may lead to neurologic changes. Functional implications are dependent on the level and severity of the defect (see Table 27-1).

Myelomeningocele is the failure of the neural tube to close resulting in a cystic dilatation of meninges and protuberance of the spinal cord through the vertebral defect (AANN, 1990). Hydrocephalus is present in virtually all children afflicted with this condition (AANN, 1990). Approximately 85% will require an internal shunt system to control the hydrocephalus (McLone and Naidich, 1986; Dias and McClone, 1993). (See Chapter 23). The actual involvement of the spinal cord has greater implications for overall function throughout growth and development (see Table 27-1).

TREATMENT

Initial treatment for meningocele and myelomeningocele is early surgical closure of the defect (Humphreys, 1991; Thomas, 1993). Specific tissue malformation and involvement and the presence of hydrocephalus can only be determined through further diagnostic tests such as ultrasonography, CT (computerized tomography) scan, and MRI (magnetic resonance imaging). Careful assessment of the infant during the surgical closure often aids in determining the depth and extent of involvement. This information is important for habilitative planning and potential outcome.

The multisystem involvement of this diagnosis requires a comprehensive multidisciplinary team approach to treatment. This team may include nurses, neurosurgeons, urologists, orthopedists, pediatricians, physical therapists, occupational therapists, and social workers.

Table 27-1.
FUNCTIONAL ALTERATIONS IN MYELODYSPLASIA RELATED TO LEVEL OF LESION

Level of lesion	Functional implications
Thoracic	Flaccid paralysis of lower extremities
	Variable weakness in abdominal trunk musculature
	High thoracic level may have respiratory compromise
	Absence of bowel and bladder control
High Lumbar	Voluntary hip flexion and adduction
	Flaccid paralysis of knees, ankles, feet
	May walk with extensive braces and crutches
	Absence of bowel and bladder control
Midlumbar	Strong hip flexion and adduction
	Fair knee extension
	Flaccid paralysis of ankles and feet
	Absence of bowel and bladder control
Low Lumbar	Strong hip flexion, extension and adduction, knee extension
	Weak ankle and toe mobility
	May have limited bowel and bladder function
Sacral	"Normal" function of lower extremities
	"Normal" bowel and bladder function

RECENT AND ANTICIPATED ADVANCES IN DIAGNOSIS AND MANAGEMENT

Because the pathophysiology of myelodysplasia is determined early in gestation, prenatal diagnosis is possible. The presence of a neural tube defect may result in an elevation in the maternal serum alpha-fetoprotein (AFP) levels. It is important to note that

TREATMENT

Assess level of involvement:
Ultrasonography
CT scan
MRI scan
Surgical closure of deformity

a closed neural tube defect may not alter the AFP levels. When maternal serum AFP levels are elevated, further testing is indicated (Humphreys, 1991). The amniotic fluid can be obtained for evaluation through amniocentesis. Additionally, high-resolution ultrasonography is a noninvasive study to evaluate pregnancies at risk or suspect for neural tube defects (Hogge et al, 1989).

The purpose of antenatal diagnosis is two-fold. First it offers the parents the option to terminate the pregnancy. If the parents choose to continue the pregnancy, prenatal diagnosis provides the family and health care team the opportunity to prepare both physically and emotionally for the birth of the child. Delivery by cesarean section may limit trauma to the open myelomeningocele (Luthy et al, 1991). Genetic counseling should be offered at this time as well.

Recent studies indicate that ingestion of multivitamins with folic acid before conception or early in the pregnancy may offer protection against the occurrence of neural tube defects (Milunsky et al, 1989). Repeated studies demonstrate a 60% to 86% reduction of risks for neural tube defects with the periconceptional ingestion of vitamins containing the U.S. recommended daily allowance of 0.4 mg to 0.8 mg folic acid (Mulinare, 1993; Werler, Shapiro, and Mitchell, 1993).

The Centers for Disease Control has determined that women who have had a pregnancy resulting in a neural tube defect are at increased risk for recurrence. These women should be counseled and advised that folic acid supplements may substantially reduce this risk. The recommended dose for women

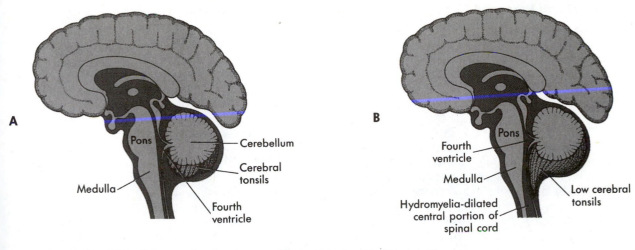

Fig. 27-2.   Diagram showing **A,** normal brain; **B,** brain with Chiari malformation.

in this category, unless contraindicated, is 4 mg per day of folic acid periconceptionally (Centers for Disease Control [CDC], 1991).

ASSOCIATED PROBLEMS

Arnold Chiari II Malformation

One associated problem of myelodysplasia is the Chiari II malformation. This deformity involves the downward displacement of the cerebellum, brain stem, and fourth ventricle (see Fig. 27-2). The exact pathogenesis of the malformation is not known (Madsen and Scott, 1993). The area of the brain involved is the posterior fossa region which is primarily responsible for vital functions including respirations and protective reflexes directed by the twelve cranial nerves. The downward displacement of this area results in compression and elongation of nerves and tissue which restricts neuronal performance to varying degrees (Madsen and Scott, 1993).

Skin Integrity

The newborn is at great risk for developing infection secondary to the altered skin integrity over the malformed spine. This is a possible complication until the lesion has completely healed. The risk of skin breakdown continues throughout the child's

ASSOCIATED PROBLEMS

Arnold Chiari II malformation
Maintaining skin integrity
Hydrocephalus
Seizures
Visual and perceptual problems
Cognitive deficit
Altered motor and sensory function
Musculoskeletal deformities
Urinary dysfunction
Latex allergic reactions

life span as a result of altered sensory function below the level of the lesion.

Hydrocephalus and Seizures

Hydrocephalus occurs in approximately 85% of cases (Dias and McClone, 1993). Seizures occur in approximately 30% of those children with myelodysplasia (Reigel, 1993). See Chapters 23 and 27 for additional information.

Visual and Perceptual Problems

Visual and perceptual problems including ocular palsies, astigmatism, and visual perceptual deficits are common (Lollar, 1993b). Pressure on cranial nerves that control eye movements—CN III (oculomotor), CN IV (trochlear), CN VI (abducens)—may result in a mild disconjugate gaze or esotropia.

Cognitive Deficit

Children born with myelodysplasia have mean intellectual quotients (IQ) in the average range (Lollar, 1993b). Children who are shunted as a result of the associated diagnosis of hydrocephalus have been reported to have IQs in the range of low-average or below (Lollar, 1993b). Hydrocephalus, especially complicated by frequent shunt revisions, malfunctions, or infections, may limit intellectual function (Lollar, 1993b). (Refer to Chapter 23.) These children often exhibit strength in verbal skills; however, limited cognitive skills such as memory, speed of response, acquired knowledge, integrated functioning, and coordination are common and must be considered in the intellectual assessment of these children (Lollar, 1993b).

Altered Motor and Sensory Function

Invariably motor and sensory functions below the level of the lesions are altered. This dysfunction may include paralysis, weakness, spasticity of lower extremities, and sensory loss. Altered motor and sensory function may also impair peristalsis leading to constipation, impaction and incontinence of feces. These associated problems may worsen as the child grows and the cord ascends within the vertebral canal, pulling primary scar tissue and tethering the spinal cord. As a result, tethering of spinal cord is present in virtually all cases (Humphreys, 1991).

Musculoskeletal Deformities

Musculoskeletal deformities related to myelomeningocele may include club feet, dislocated hips, and improper musculoskeletal alignment from altered embryonic development. Spinal deformities such as scoliosis, kyphosis, and gibbus are also common. Muscle group imbalance occurs with growth and development and may cause further deformities over time (Mazur and Menelaus, 1991; Ryan, Ploski, and Emans, 1992).

Urinary Dysfunction

Depending on the level of defect, neurogenic bladder may occur. Other potential complications of the urinary system include dyssynergy, hydronephrosis, incomplete emptying of the bladder, urinary reflux, urinary tract infections, and incontinence. Presentation of any of these findings may indicate deterioration of urinary function and could lead to renal damage (Bauer, 1989; Kreder et al, 1992).

Latex Allergic Reactions

Approximately 18% to 40% of individuals with myelodysplasia have a sensitivity to latex (CDC, 1991; Leger and Meeropol, 1992). These individuals are at risk for anaphylaxis during operations and procedures where latex is used (Slater, 1989; Slater 1994; Young et al, 1992; Brown, 1994; Leger and Meeropol, 1992). Therefore, it is absolutely essential that the primary care provider inform and educate the parents and individual of this potential sensitivity, observe for signs, and document the allergy. Examples of products that may contain latex are surgical gloves, balloons, catheters, and bandages (an updated list of such products and alternatives for use is available from the Spina Bifida Association of America). It is recommended that individuals with latex sensitivity carry an epi-pen, a letter documenting the allergy, nonlatex gloves, and wear a Medic-Alert bracelet indicating the allergy.

PROGNOSIS

Myelodysplasia is a chronic condition. The prognosis is dependent on the success of prophylactic and acute treatment for potential and actual complications that affect each body system. These children are at risk for sudden death as a result of a shunt malfunction or problems related to the Chiari II malformation (Madsen and Scott, 1993). Improved ventricular shunt systems have helped to minimize infections that may potentially lead to central nervous system damage. Also, the advent of new urologic interventions such as early urodynamic assessment and intermittent catheterization greatly reduce the risk of renal damage (Bauer, 1994). Further treatments and interventions will be necessary throughout the child's life span. Procedures are individualized to the child's needs and are rendered when indicated by the clinical presentation, assessment, and evaluation.

Primary Care Management
HEALTH CARE MAINTENANCE

Growth and Development

The deformity, degree of motor impairment, cognitive function, and personal motivation all influence the growth and development of each child (Mazur and Menelaus, 1991; Tappit-Emas, 1989; Ryan, Ploski, and Emans, 1992). As with all children, monitoring growth and development by obtaining routine heights and weights and plotting them on a standardized growth chart is crucial. Obesity is a common problem seen in children with myelodysplasia as a result of decreased levels of activity. Because obesity may lead to problems with skin breakdown, brace fittings, and the ability to ambulate, education for parents and children is essential (Ryan, Ploski, and Emans, 1992). Obesity may also interfere with development of a positive self-image.

Obtaining heights may be difficult, depending on the child's ability to stand. If needed, the primary care provider should measure the full body length with the child supine or by using arm span. Because of shortening of the spine or muscle atrophy, these children often fall below the 10th percentile in height.

Head circumference should be monitored closely by the primary care provider during the infancy and early childhood period. If a progressive enlargement in size is noted, referral to the neurosurgeon should be made (refer to Chapter 23).

Motor development may or may not be affected and is directly related to the level of the lesion (see Table 27-1). The degree of weakness, paralysis, and decreased sensation will vary. Early orthopaedic and physical therapy assessment and intervention are extremely important to prevent contractures, minimize deformities, and monitor muscle strength and flexibility. This assessment aids in planning for the child's future mobility and independence (Ryan, Ploski, and Emans, 1992).

The rate at which cognitive and intellectual skills are acquired depends greatly on the child's interaction with the environment and the severity of the defect. The orthopedist and physical therapist can assist the child by ensuring that the physical developmental sequence proceeds normally (Bunch, 1986). For instance, if the child is not able to stand by age 10 to 18 months, using a standing frame or a parapodium allows the child to accomplish various developmental tasks and stand with his or her hands free for play (Ryan, Ploski, and Emans, 1992; Bunch, 1986).

As the child grows and develops, other adaptive equipment (i.e., braces, wheelchairs) is used to increase mobility and independence. Each child's treatment program will vary because of differences in motivation and variability of social resources. Age-related goals are most important (Ryan, Ploski, and Emans, 1992).

Surgical intervention is often recommended and sometimes required to achieve proper muscle balance and body alignment for problems common to this population such as dislocated hips, scoliosis, kyphosis, and club feet which would limit the child's potential.

Precocious puberty has been noted in a number of children with myelodysplasia and hydrocephalus. The cause is not known, but may be related to early pituitary gonadotropin secretion activated by the hydrocephalic brain (Elias and Sadeghi-Nejad, 1994).

Diet

Infancy is an excellent time to guide and educate the parents regarding nutritional needs. It is important to teach parents early about the dangers of overfeeding especially in the child who is less mobile and therefore has less caloric needs. Avoiding obesity is a primary goal in the nutritional management of these children as well as avoiding the pattern of using food as a reward.

The child's diet should include plenty of fluids to lessen the chance of constipation and the incidence of urinary tract infections. Dietary management is important in controlling the consistency of stools and in avoiding constipation. A diet high in fiber and low in constipating foods is usually recommended. Early nutritional assessment and guidance are an essential part of the care of the child with myelodysplasia.

Poor feeding and prolonged feeding time are common presenting symptoms of the Chiari II malformation in affected children (Madsen and Scott, 1993). In children with severe symptomatology, a gastrostomy tube may be required to avoid malnutrition and aspiration.

Safety

Issues regarding safety that are particular to the infant and child with myelodysplasia are numerous. Because the neurologic system is the primary system involved, parents must be educated to the changes that may occur and threaten their child's safety. The potential for limited cognitive ability and altered judgment exists in these children. An awareness of limitations is essential in order to assist the child with issues such as independence, decision making, self-care, and sexuality. Instructions regarding proper use of equipment for mobility such as wheelchairs, braces, and crutches should be appropriate to the child's developmental and cognitive abilities.

The congenital defect affects nerve function at and below the level of the defect on the spine. This alters mobility and sensation of bone, muscle, and skin tissue below the level of the defect. This decreased sensation puts the child at greater risk for injuries such as burns, fractures, and skin breakdown. With proper body positioning, frequent position changes, and assurance that adaptive equipment fits properly and is used correctly, this risk can be minimized. Tepid water should be used for bathing to prevent burns. The condition of the child's skin should be monitored at least twice a day for redness and irritation. As soon as the child is competent to assume this responsibility, she or he should be taught how to perform a thorough skin check.

In children with seizures, parents should be instructed on how to intervene safely and appropriately during a seizure (refer to Chapter 19).

Immunizations

The recommended schedule for routine immunizations is suggested, although it may be altered as a result of frequent hospitalizations (Raddish et al, 1993). The primary care provider should attempt to keep the child up to date with the routine immunizations. Alterations in the immunization schedule for children with hydrocephalus and seizures are addressed in Chapters 19 and 23.

Screening

Vision. Routine screening is recommended. Because of the high incidence of visual and perceptual deficits, ocular palsies and astigmatism in children with myelodysplasia, the practitioner should consider these during routine screening. Referral to an ophthalmologist is indicated for any positive visual findings.

Hearing. Routine screening is recommended. The authors of this chapter have observed that children with myelodysplasia who are shunted for hydrocephalus are hypersensitive to loud noises. Awareness of this finding may alleviate parental concern. Use of aminoglycocides may cause hearing deficits (refer to Chapter 23).

Dental. Routine dental screening and care are recommended. Dentists should be notified of the risk of latex allergy. Children with shunted hydrocephalus should receive prophylactic antibiotics before any dental care that may result in bleeding. (See Chapter 15.)

Hematocrit. Routine screening is recommended.

Tuberculosis. Routine screening is recommended.

Blood pressure. Routine screening is recommended. Children with known renal problems such as urinary reflux or a history of hypertension should have more frequent assessment. Persistent elevated readings should be communicated to the child's urologist.

Urinalysis. Baseline urinalysis and urine cultures are obtained in the newborn period. After this time, routine cultures should be obtained every 4 to 6 months. If a urinary tract infection is suspected, a urine culture and sensitivity should be obtained by catherization (bag specimens have been noted to have a higher chance of contamination). A positive urine culture should be reported to the child's urologist.

Condition-specific screening (See box.)

COMPLETE BLOOD COUNT. If an individual is on long-term antibiotic therapy for prevention of urinary tract infections (i.e., sulfonamides), he or she should have complete blood counts checked approximately every 6 months to monitor changes (Kirulata, Gillingham, and Squires, 1986).

SERUM CREATININE. This should be checked routinely in the newborn period as a baseline study for renal function and should be repeated yearly.

SCOLIOSIS. Screening for scoliosis in children with myelodysplasia should begin during the first year of life and continue throughout adolescence. Spine x-rays should be obtained yearly or as indicated.

**CONDITION-SPECIFIC
SCREENING**

Complete blood count
Serum creatinine
Scoliosis
Latex allergy

DIFFERENTIAL DIAGNOSIS

Chiari II malformation
Tethering of the spinal cord
Hydrocephalus
Urinary tract infections
Fevers
Gastrointestinal symptoms

LATEX ALLERGY. Careful history should be elicited regarding signs and symptoms of latex allergy. There are two types of reactions that may occur. Type IV is a less serious reaction and may include symptoms such as watery eyes, eczematous skin eruptions, or dermatitis. Type I reaction is an immediate hypersensitivity to exposure and may include symptoms such as rhinitis, conjunctivitis, wheezing, bronchospasm, facial swelling, tachycardia, laryngeal edema, and hypotension. Individuals with Type I reaction to latex are at extreme risk for developing anaphylaxis. Those who experience Type IV are at lower risk for developing anaphylaxis, but constant sensitization may predispose them to anaphylaxis. Avoidance of latex products is extremely important in preventing allergic reactions. Refer to an allergist if latex allergy suspected.

COMMON ILLNESS MANAGEMENT

Differential Diagnosis

Chiari II. Chiari II is a serious, potentially life-threatening malformation that invariably occurs with myelodysplasia. The Chiari II malformation may be a clinically silent phenomenon, or cause catastrophic events such as cardiac or respiratory arrest. The malformation compresses and essentially stretches the posterior region of the cerebellum and brain stem downward through the foramen of magnum into the cervical space. Seldom do these children show immediate signs at birth but become symptomatic during the first days to weeks of life. In other children manifestations of the condition may not become obvious until 4 to 5 years of age or older (Madsen and Scott, 1993).

The brain stem houses the 12 cranial nerves (CN) (see Table 27-2). Pressure on this region results in altered function of these vital nerves or actual palsies. Dysfunction of the lower cranial nerves is common. The infant may present with apnea, respiratory difficulties, stridor, and the classic barking cough of croup. The primary care provider must be cautious not to dismiss these findings as a simple upper respiratory infection, but must consider the possibility that these symptoms result from pressure on CN IX (glossopharyngeal), CN X (vagus), and CN XII (hypoglossal). A depressed or absent gag may be present leading to possible aspiration pneumonia. Feeding difficulties and symptoms of failure to thrive may also be present.

Pressure on the cranial nerves that control eye movements—CN III (oculomotor), CN IV (trochlear), CN VI (abducens)—may result in a mild disconjugate gaze or esotropia.

Subtle complaints and changes in hand function or strength, increased upper extremity spasticity, neck pain, or behavior changes such as irritability, necessitate immediate consultation with the neurosurgeon. Treatment is focused on the symptomatic relief of the presenting problems (i.e., gastrostomy tube and tracheostomy may be placed for absent gag and cough). Surgical decompression of the cervical region is controversial, and to date has not been proven a reliable solution (Madsen and Scott, 1993).

Tethering of the spinal cord. Tethering of the spinal cord will develop with growth. Symptoms related to this problem may include scoliosis, altered gait pattern, changes in muscle strength and

Table 27-2.
IMPLICATIONS OF CRANIAL NERVE DYSFUNCTION IN MYELODYSPLASIA

Cranial nerve	Functional implications
I olfactory	Sense of smell
II optic	Visual acuity, visual fields
III oculomotor	Raises eyelids
	Constricts pupils
	Moves eyes up, down, and in
IV trochlear	Moves eyes down
V trigeminal	Sensory innervation to face, tongue
	Opens and closes jaw
VI abducens	Moves eyes laterally (out)
VII facial	Closes eyelids
	Motor and sensory for facial muscles
	Secretion of lacrimal and salivary glands
VIII acoustic	Hearing; equilibrium
IX glossopharyngeal	Gag, swallow
	Taste
X vagus	Muscles of larynx, pharynx, soft palate
	Parasympathetic innervation
XI spinal accessory	Shoulder shrug
XII hypoglossal	Moves tongue

tone at or below the lesion, disturbance in urinary and bowel patterns, and back pain. The primary care provider should be alert to these findings and refer to the neurosurgeon for further evaluation which may include urodynamic studies and MRI. Surgical release may be indicated based on evaluation and symptoms.

Hydrocephalus. The majority of individuals will have an internal shunt system to treat hydrocephalus. The differential diagnosis of shunt malfunction and infection must be considered in the presence of lethargy, fever, gastrointestinal distress, and headache (refer to Chapter 23).

Urinary tract infections. Urinary tract infections (UTIs) are common among children with myelodysplasia. Fever associated with UTIs may be mild or severe. Other symptoms may include ab-

dominal pain, vomiting, cloudy, malodorous urine, and increased wetting. Frequency and burning may be masked because of decreased sensation. The presence of these symptoms should alert the primary care provider to obtain a urine specimen by catheterization for culture. A positive culture should be reported to the child's urologist, especially in cases with urinary reflux. Treatment of positive cultures may vary depending on the individual's urologist but is usually initiated only in the presence of symptoms or urinary reflux (Bauer, 1994). Recommendations for treatment may include a short course of appropriate antibiotics and instillation of an antibiotic solution into the bladder via catheterization. Those children with urinary reflux need continuous antibiotic coverage and frequent urine cultures. Repeat cultures should be obtained once during the course of treatment and again approximately 1 week after treatment.

Fevers. Fever of unknown origin may be the result of an undetected fracture of an insensate extremity. Osteoporosis associated with paralysis, decreased weight bearing and inactivity, especially after immobilization in a cast, may contribute to the occurrence of fractures (Ryan, Ploski, and Emans, 1992). An undetected burn of insensate areas may also result in fever. Careful examination of the area for swelling, redness, or abrasions should be undertaken by the practitioner. Obtaining a complete history from the individual and the parents may assist in determining if there has been recent trauma. Other causes include, but are not limited to, shunt infection and malfunction, urinary tract infection, skin breakdown and cellulitis. Particular consideration must be given to the presence of a fever since it may lower the seizure threshold in these children.

Gastrointestinal symptoms. Nausea, vomiting, and diarrhea are all common symptoms in the pediatric population. In the child with myelodysplasia, however, a heightened concern and consideration to the cause should be assessed. Nausea and vomiting may be symptomatic of shunt malfunction. Urinary tract infections may be the cause of gastrointestinal distress. A child with a neurogenic bowel may become impacted with stool leading to gastrointestinal distress. The presence of diarrhea may be misleading as liquid stool passes around the impacted stool. A KUB may help differentiate diarrhea versus impaction (Leibold, 1991).

In the child with a high lesion, the practitioner should consider the possibility of appendicitis as a cause of nausea or vomiting. The classic symptom of pain may be altered as a result of the decreased sensation.

Drug Interactions

Many of these children are on routine medication therapy. Potential interactions among these and other medications need to be carefully considered when additional pharmotherapeutics are prescribed. Commonly used drug categories are:

1. Antibiotics for treatment of UTIs or prophylaxis. These include amoxicillin (Amoxil), trimethoprim and sulfamethoxazole (Bactrim), sulfisoxazole (Gantrisin), and nitrofurantoin (Furadantin). If a child requires other antibiotic therapy for common childhood illness such as ear infections, the antibiotic for the UTI is discontinued during the needed course of treatment.

2. Anticholinergics to assist in urinary continence and reduce high bladder pressure. These include oxybutynin chloride (Ditropan) and propantheline bromide (Pro-Banthine). Oxybutynin chloride can cause heat prostration in the presence of high environmental temperatures. Anticholinergics may delay absorption of other medications given concomitantly in these children (Physician's Desk Reference [PDR], 1990).

3. Sympathomimetics to increase urethral resistance. These include ephedrine (Gluco-Fedrin), pseudoephedrine hydrochloride (Sudafed), and phenylpropanolamine. The practitioner should determine if the child is taking any of these drugs before treating cold symptoms.

4. Stool softeners, stimulants, and bulk formers to aid in evacuation of stool. Many products are used for this purpose, and most are over-the-counter drugs. None of these should be administered in the presence of abdominal pain, nausea, vomiting, or diarrhea.

5. Anticonvulsants to control seizure activity. These include phenobarbital, phenytoid sodium (Dilantin), and carbamazepine (Tegretol). Concomitant administration of carbamazepine with erythromycin may result in toxicity (PDR, 1990) (see Chapter 19).

DEVELOPMENTAL ISSUES

Sleep Patterns

Individuals with Chiari II malformation may experience sleep apnea, increased stridor, and snoring with sleep. These children are at increased risk for sudden respiratory arrest. It is, therefore, recommended that children with such symptoms wear a cardiac/apnea monitor during sleep. Parents must also be capable to perform cardiopulmonary resuscitation in the event of an arrest.

Alteration in the child's normal sleep pattern (longer naps, increased frequency of naps), may indicate increased intracranial pressure from a shunt malfunction (refer to Chapter 23 on hydrocephalus).

In addition, sleep may be interrupted if a child needs to be repositioned during the night to prevent pressure sores and skin breakdown from developing.

Toileting

Mastery of bowel and bladder continence is crucial to optimal functioning and is of major importance for social acceptance (King, Currie, and Wright, 1994; Leibold, 1991; Sloan, 1993; Younoszai, 1992). The child's physical abilities and psychologic readiness for toileting should be assessed. Children who are unable to sit independent of adaptive devices or who are unable to master self-dressing skills will need special consideration when toileting is introduced. A physical or occupational therapist should be consulted regarding the use of bars, adaptive seats, etc. Special clothing or underwear may be helpful to make access to the perineum easier.

Clearly, it is desirable for the child to master self-care methods of toileting before entering school. Urinary and fecal incontinence may partly explain the poor social adjustment experienced by many children with myelodysplasia (Leibold, 1991). Bowel management should be monitored from birth to avoid constipation and impaction. At age 2 to 3 years the concept of toileting should be introduced to the child. The goal of bowel management is to maintain soft-formed stools and to develop a regular schedule of evacuation on the toilet every 1 to 2 days to avoid impaction or soiling in between bowel movements. This can be accomplished by sitting on the toilet at regular times, taking advantage of the gastrocolic reflex by toileting after meals, and increasing abdominal pressure by methods such as having the child blow bubbles, tickling the child to make him or her laugh, or by placing the child's legs on a stool to increase pressure by hip flexion.

Stool consistency is crucial to developing a good bowel program. Bulking agents such as psyllium taken with increased fluids are a key factor in avoiding constipation and eventual impaction (Leibold, 1991). The child should assume responsibility for timed evacuation and good perineal care as physical and cognitive development allows. Some children will not be able to assume toileting responsibilities and will require continued assistance by parents or caretakers.

The use of medicinal aids may also be necessary to control the consistency or to aid in evacuation. A number of agents are available including stimulants, softeners, and lubricants. Biofeedback, behavior modification techniques, and the use of an enema continent catheter have also been used with some success in this population for treatment of fecal incontinence (Younoszai, 1992; Blair et al, 1992; Liptak and Revell, 1992).

It is important to remember that each program of management will vary from child to child. A sympathetic manner in working with the child will help to avoid feelings of guilt and blame for unavoidable accidents. Accidents can be avoided with careful attention to diet and timed defecation (Leibold, 1991). Despite a successful continence program, some individuals may need to wear a diaper during sleep.

Clean intermittent catheterization is the most commonly used method to help achieve urinary continence. If catheterization has not been started for other reasons, it may be started in the child who is 2 to 3 years of age in an attempt to get the child out of diapers when most other children have achieved this milestone (Bauer, 1989; Rudy and Woodside, 1991; Vereecken, 1992). If the child has been catheterized from birth, the concept of using the toilet for the procedure should be introduced at this time. Ideally, the procedure is taught to the parents and other individuals involved in the child's direct care. Often, instituting this procedure causes a resurfacing of emotions in parents related to the child's disabilities. Fear of injuring the child, diffi-

culties with genital touching, and frustration with the mechanics of the procedure are common. Psychologic and emotional concerns are usual and must be addressed before the parent can be expected to understand and comply with the recommendations (Brown, 1990).

Self-catheterization is a realistic goal for most children with myelodysplasia. An individualized approach including the child's readiness will be of great benefit in achieving this goal (Smith, 1990; Brown, 1990). Often, providing the young child with an anatomically correct doll and catheter will help the child master the skill. The goal is to have this task accomplished by early school age. In children with limited cognitive abilities and poor manual dexterity, continued assistance may be necessary. Noncompliance with self-catheterization may become an issue in adolescence when catheterization is used as a focus in the fight for independence.

If continence is not attained by catheterization alone, medications such as anticholinergics and sympathomimetics may be used in conjunction with the procedure. Continence may also successfully be achieved through use of bladder stimulation and surgical interventions such as artificial urinary sphincter, bladder neck reconstruction, bladder augmentation, and creation of continent stomas (Selzman, Elder, and Mapstone, 1993; Bauer, 1994; Aprikian et al, 1992; Leonard, Gearhart, and Jeffs, 1990).

Discipline

A child with such a complex chronic condition is at increased risk for experiencing psychosocial adjustment problems (Wallander, Feldman, and Varni, 1989). This may affect the parents and family members' response to discipline. The need for discipline, direction, and encouragement of independence should be addressed early in the child's life (Lollar, 1993b). Referral for parent counseling may be necessary to assist with the particular needs and challenges that may arise (Kazak and Clark, 1986).

Child Care

The primary care provider should be familiar with resources available for referral since early intervention programs for infants will vary from state to state. The preschooler is eligible for placement in public programs that meet his or her physical and educational needs. It is important that the day care or educational setting be notified in advance about a prospective student to allow for education of day care staff and facilitate a smooth transition (Palfrey, Haynie, and Porter, 1989) (refer to Chapter 5).

The child with myelodysplasia and a ventriculoperitoneal shunt may exhibit signs of shunt malfunction while in the care of someone other than a parent. That individual should be aware of the signs and alert the parent or guardian. Additional concerns related to the issue of hydrocephalus can be found in Chapter 23.

Knowledge of the child's specific bladder and bowel program should be communicated. Any procedures necessary to carry out the particular program must be taught to the care provider. This is not usually necessary in the birth to 3 year programs unless the child is also in day care. If so, a trained person should perform the procedure. Care providers should be informed of all medications the child requires and of latex sensitivity.

Many children with myelodysplasia will have adaptive equipment to aid in mobilization, maintain appropriate body alignment, prevent further deformity, and increase independence. The primary care provider should be aware of proper application and fit of the equipment. It is also important to communicate the child's actual motor and sensory capacity to prevent injury.

A list of emergency telephone numbers must accompany the child. If possible, the primary care provider should be available to answer questions and concerns from child care staff.

Schooling

Learning disabilities are common in children with myelodysplasia. Problems may occur in perceptual motor performance, comprehension, attention, activity, memory, organization, sequencing, and reasoning. These areas need to be assessed early in the educational process so particular needs may be met and adaptations made to minimize educational problems and frustrations by the child, family, and educators. Neuropsychologic testing is recommended to support this process (Lollar, 1993a; Burke and Meeropol, 1994). School performance is

further compromised by frequent absences as a result of illnesses or medical treatment.

Federal laws protect the rights of children with disabilities to have access to an appropriate education (refer to Chapter 5). Individualized education plans (IEPs) must be formulated to take care of each child's specific needs including educational and physical requirements. The primary care provider, the child, and the family must actively collaborate with the school in this planning process. Each child's particular needs must be addressed in the IEP including the need for catheterization, timed toileting, administration of medication(s), physical, occupational and speech therapy, and individual counseling. On occasion, these particular needs may require assistance from an aide.

Adaptive equipment may be necessary and is dependent on the child's degree of disability. School personnel should be aware of what adaptive equipment the child has, how it functions, and what to monitor with regard to fit, skin irritation, and so on (Ryan, Ploski, and Emans, 1992). Elevators are also helpful in assisting the child to get to classes in a timely manner and to minimize fatigue.

As children age, they may choose to use a wheelchair for mobilization in the school building. This should be viewed as an increase rather than a decrease in independence. Ideally, the school should be free of structural barriers to enable the child to move freely and to participate in all activities. Special provisions must be made for safe departure from the building in the event of an emergency, as well as transportation to and from home (i.e., wheelchair van or bus). Those with known latex allergy will need to have adaptations made in all aspects of the school setting to avoid exposure. Common sources of latex in the school environment include art supplies, pencil erasers, and gym mats or floors. Clinical personnel or allergists are possible resources to assist in this process.

Children with chronic conditions and physical disabilities are at risk for experiencing adjustment problems (Lollar, 1993a). Children with myelodysplasia often have low self-concepts, low levels of general happiness, and high levels of anxiety (Kazak and Clark, 1986). Awareness of these potential problems will be helpful to those working with children with myelodysplasia. Emotional independence is the foundation that supports the successful development of physical independence. Appropriate referrals for further psychologic intervention and support may be advised. The primary care provider should encourage the child to be involved in extracurricular activities such as clubs, scouting, and sporting activities to enhance peer relationships, self-esteem, and independence (Loller, 1993b).

Academic planning and career counseling must take into consideration the individual's physical as well as cognitive abilities. Education and vocational training should prepare the individual to be successful in employment, independent living, and in social relationships (Edwards, et al, 1994).

Sexuality

The issue of sexuality is a major area of concern for parents and children with myelodysplasia. Education, information, and an opportunity to address concerns regarding sexuality and reproductive function should be discussed early in the child's life (Sloan, 1993). Urodynamic studies in the newborn period may help to determine prognosis regarding sexual function (Bauer, 1989). Maximizing urinary and fecal continence, fostering self-esteem, and promoting self-care are all beneficial to the child in developing a sexual identity (Sloan, 1993).

The usual sources of sexual information available to adolescents may be difficult to access by individuals with myelodysplasia as a result of limited mobility and poor peer relationships (Bunch, 1986; Sloan, 1993). The practitioner should provide anticipatory guidance during routine health maintenance visits and assess for signs of early sexual development associated with precocious puberty (Elias and Sadeghi-Nejad, 1994). If the primary care provider does not feel skilled in gynecologic care, the child should be referred to a sensitive specialist with experience examining individuals with disabilities.

Women with myelodysplasia are capable of normal fertility. Birth control methods must be evaluated carefully on an individual basis. The risk of blood clots and pelvic inflammatory disease make oral contraceptives and intrauterine devices more hazardous (Sloan, 1993). The high incidence of latex allergies in this population prohibits the use of latex condoms and diaphragms. Nonlatex condoms are available but do not protect from AIDS or other sexually transmitted diseases. Because of increased risk of urinary tract infection with intercourse, those women not on routine antibiotics should take prophylactic antibiotics before and after intercourse.

Although individuals with myelodysplasia have normal sex drives, unless sensation exists in the bulbourethral, bulbocavernosus, and perineal muscles of both sexes, orgasm is not likely (Sloan, 1993). Women may benefit from use of additional lubricating gels when attempting intercourse as vaginal lubrication in response to sexual arousal does not occur with lower spinal cord injury.

Severe spinal deformities or complex urologic problems may increase the risk for complications during pregnancy. These women are also at risk for having a child with a neural tube defect. Genetic counseling should be available to these individuals and encouraged by their primary care provider (Sloan, 1993). The American College of Obstetrics and Gynecology has guidelines on pregnancy and delivery for women with myelodysplasia.

In men with myelodysplasia, the level of spinal lesion will predict their capacity for erection and ejaculation. Because this functional ability will vary among individuals, the reproductive potential is much less predictable than in women (Elder and Feetham, 1987). Past erections and ejaculations are an important part of the sexual history in the male client. Penile implants or collection of sperm by electric stimulation may be indicated for this population (Sloan, 1993). Technologic advances may offer more possibilities in the future.

Transition into Adulthood

Transition planning is a process mandated by law (Section 204 of the Carl D. Perkins Act) that must begin by age 14 years (Rowley-Kelly, 1993). Amendments under the Individual with Disabilities Education Act (PL 101-476) require that goals and objectives related to employment and postsecondary education, independent living, and community participation be included in IEPs no later than age 16 years (Burke and Meeropol, 1994).

Of utmost importance for parents and school personnel is beginning as early as possible to work together in fostering necessary skills and traits in the adolescent for successful transition from high school to college or to the workplace (Rowley-Kelly, 1993; Edwards et al, 1994).

The survival rate of individuals with myelodysplasia has greatly increased with medical advances; thus a new population of adults with myelodysplasia has emerged (Rauen and Aubert, 1992). These young adults often find themselves at a loss for accessing appropriate health care (Schidlow and Fiel, 1990). Depression, chemical addiction, obesity, contractures, decreased ambulation, pressure ulcers, osteoporosis, joint pain, and hydronephrosis are some of the common secondary disabilities seen in this population (Rauen and Aubert, 1992; Kaufman et al, 1994). As in the pediatric multidisciplinary care model, coordinated care remains of utmost importance in the adult population. In a recent symposium on preventing secondary conditions associated with spina bifida, the recommendation to health care professionals was to "provide a single point entry to a system that coordinates the needed care" (Marge, 1994). Primary health care should be directed by providers interested and committed to working with this high-risk population. This necessary transition of care has been met with reluctance by many adult health care providers for a number of reasons including lack of familiarity of the complex needs of individuals with myelodysplasia. The providers may perceive this population as having negative economic impact on their practice.

Coordinated multidisciplinary care, education of health care providers and clients, costs, and promotion of client-directed care are issues that need to be addressed. A few adult programs have been developed in various parts of the country. Further information can be obtained from the Spina Bifida Association of America.

SPECIAL FAMILY CONCERNS AND RESOURCES

Families of children born with myelodysplasia suffer chronic grief for the "loss of the normal" child at birth. This grief is expressed repeatedly as the child fails to achieve developmental milestones (Burke, 1989).

The risk for sudden death as a result of a shunt malfunction or of complications related to the Chiari II malformation is a chronic and intense stress on the family system. This stress, in addition to the other complex needs of these children, often results in families becoming overprotective (Lollar, 1993b). Families may be hesitant or fearful of allowing others to care for their child because of the child's special needs. Parents should be encouraged to meet their own individual needs and, as a couple, to participate in activities outside the home independent of the child and to seek respite care if other caretakers are not available (Pavin et al, 1994; Samuelson, Foltz, and Foxall, 1992).

The multisystem involvement of this condition requires frequent hospitalizations, surgeries, outpatient services, and multidisciplinary care. These factors, in addition to such items as special equipment or medications that may be needed by these children, place a tremendous financial burden on parents. Many children with myelodysplasia are eligible for social security benefits. Social service involvement with these families is crucial in providing guidance and support.

The health care system recognizes empathy to the multitude of needs for children with myelodysplasia and their families and offers physical, emotional, spiritual, and social care. Nevertheless, no individual understands or feels the problems these children and families face during their day-to-day lives as well as another child or family with the same disorder. For this reason, support groups and opportunities available to provide this network of support within the community are not only necessary but have proven to be a major factor in coping and adaptation for these families (Wallander and Varni, 1989). The following are a few of the support systems available to families. Each region has its own community-based network or local chapter. It is important that the primary care provider be aware of available local resources.

Spina Bifida Association of America
    4590 MacArthur Blvd NW, Suite 250
    Washington DC 20007-4226
    202-944-3285 or 1-800-621-3141
Northeast Myelodysplasia Association
    c/o New England Regional Genetics Group
    Joseph Robinson, coordinator
    P.O. Box 670
    Mt. Desert, ME 04660
    207-288-2705
Arnold-Chiari Family Network
    c/o Kevin and Maureen Walsh
    67 Spring St
    Weymouth, MA 02188

SUMMARY OF SPECIAL PRIMARY CARE NEEDS FOR THE CHILD WITH MYELODYSPLASIA

Health care maintenance

Growth and development

Obesity is common in these children.

Head size may be enlarged if diagnosed with hydrocephalus; measure head each visit.

Motor delays are common.

Both precocious puberty and short stature are reported.

Diet

Need to evaluate regurgitation, vomiting, and difficulties with gag reflex for increased intracranial pressure and Chiari II malformation.

Monitor caloric intake to minimize potential for obesity.

Diet should include increased fluids to lessen chance of constipation and urinary tract infections.

Safety

Recommend education on emergency care with seizures.

Increased risk of injuries as a result of decreased sensation and mobility

Recommend proper body positioning, frequent position changes, and proper fit of adaptive equipment.

Immunizations

Pertussis vaccine may be deferred in infants with seizures.

Measles vaccine may cause seizures in children with seizure disorder but recommended because of prevalence of disease.

Screening

Vision

Routine screening is recommended.

These children have a high incidence of visual deficits such as ocular palsies, astigmatism, and visual perceptual deficits.

Hearing

Routine screening is recommended. They may have hypersensitivity to loud noises if shunted.

If exposed to aminoglycocides, hearing should be evaluated by an audiologist.

Dental

Routine care is recommended. Latex allergy should be considered before dental work. If the child is shunted for hydrocephalus, he or she will need antibiotic prophylaxis before dental work that may result in bleeding.

Hematocrit

Routine screening is recommended.

Tuberculosis

Routine screening is recommended.

Blood pressure

Routine monitoring. Children with renal problems may develop hypertension and should have more frequent monitoring.

Urinalysis

Baseline urinalysis and cultures should be obtained in the newborn period.

Bladder catheterization recommended for obtaining urine for cultures

Condition-specific screening

BLOOD TESTS

CBCs should be obtained frequently on children treated with sulfonamides. Serum creatinine should be done on newborns and then yearly to monitor renal function.

SCOLIOSIS

Screening for scoliosis should be done yearly from birth through adolescence.

LATEX ALLERGIES

Monitor for signs and symptoms.

Common illness management

Differential diagnosis

If the child presents with:

- Respiratory difficulties, stridor, croupy cough: rule out Chiari II malformation.
- Scoliosis, altered gait pattern, changes in muscle strength and tone, disturbance in urinary and bowel patterns and back pain: rule out tethered cord.
- Headaches: rule out shunt malfunction.
- Fevers: rule out shunt or CNS infection; urinary tract infection; fracture or injury of insensate area.

Continued.

SUMMARY OF SPECIAL PRIMARY CARE NEEDS FOR THE CHILD WITH MYELODYSPLASIA—cont'd

- Gastrointestinal symptoms: rule out increased intracranial pressure with nausea and vomiting; urinary tract infection; fecal impaction.

Drug interactions

No routine drug therapy therefore any intereactions are specific to the individual and any medications they must be taking.

Developmental issues

Sleep patterns

Apnea, increased stridor, and snoring may occur in the child with symptomatic Chiari II malformation.
Lethargy may indicate increased intracranial pressure.

Toileting

Delayed bowel and bladder training may occur as a result of neurologic deficit.
Encourage independence when developmentally and physically appropriate.
Bowel regimens will vary.
Intermittent catheterization is common, compliance may be an issue during adolescence.

Discipline

These children are at an increased risk of psychosocial adjustment problems.
They have a need for discipline and encouragement toward independence.

Child care

Special medical needs may be necessary with severe physical involvement.

Early intervention programs are ideal for infants and toddlers.

Schooling

Federal laws protect children with disabilities.
Assist families in IEP hearings.
Children may have possible adjustment problems.
Neuropsychologic testing is recommended.
Special provisions may be necessary for adaptive equipment, transportation, and accessibility.
Special physical needs must be tended to during school hours.

Sexuality

Precocious puberty may occur.
Sexual functioning may be altered.
Genetic counseling may be necessary.
In choosing birth control, must consider risks of latex allergy and blood clots associated with OCS.

Transition into adulthood

Issue dependent on severity of associated problems: primary health care, independent living, vocational training, socialization.

Special family concerns

Parents suffer chronic grief for loss of "normal" child.
Stress related to frequent hospitalizations, surgeries, and need for multidisciplinary care.
Caring for these children can be a financial burden on families.

REFERENCES

American Association of Neuroscience Nurses: *Core curriculum for neuroscience nursing* ed 3, Park Ridge, IL, 1990, AANN.

Aprikian A et al: Experience with the AS-800 artificial urinary sphincter in myelodysplastic children, *Can J Surg* 35(4):396-400, 1992.

Bauer SB: Urologic management of the myelodysplastic child. In Webster G, Galloway N (editors): *Problems in urology,* Philadelphia, 1989, JB Lippincott, pp 86-101.

Bauer SB: Urologic care of the child with spina bifida, *Spina Bifida Spotlight,* Washington, DC, 1994, Spina Bifida Association of America, pp 1-4.

Blair GK et al: The bowel management tube: an effective

means for controlling fecal incontinence, *J Pediatr Surg* 27(10):1269-1272, 1992.

Brown JP: Latex allergy requires attention in orthopaedic nursing, *Orthop Nurs* 13(1):7-11, 1994.

Brown JP: A practical approach to teaching self-catheterization to children with myelomeningocele, *J Enterostomal Ther* 17(2):54-56, 1990.

Bunch W: Myelomeningocele. In Lovell WW, Winter RB (editors): *Pediatric orthopaedics, vol I,* ed 2, Philadelphia, 1986, JB Lippincott, pp 402-403.

Burke M, Meeropol E: The student with myelodysplasia. In Schwab N (editor): *Guidelines for the management of students with genetic disorders: a manual for school nurses* ed 2, Mt Desert, ME, 1994, New England Regional Genetics Group, pp 101-166.

Burke ML: Chronic sorrow in mothers of school-age children with a myelomeningocele disability, *Doctoral dissertation,* 50:233-234B, Boston University, 1989, Dissertation Abstracts International.

Centers for Disease Control: *Morbidity and Mortality Weekly Review* 40(30):513-516, 1991.

Dias MS, McClone DG: Hydrocephalus in the child with dysraphism, *Neurosurg Clin North Am* 4(4):715-726, 1993.

Edwards G et al: Recommendations for vocational and educational professionals. In Lollar DJ (editor): *Preventing secondary conditions associated with spina bifida or cerebral palsy; proceedings and recommendations of a symposium,* Washington, DC, 1994, Spina Bifida Association of America, pp 108-112.

Elias ER, Sadeghi-Nejad A: Precocious puberty in girls with myelodysplasia, *Pediatrics* 93(3):521-522, 1994.

Hogge WA et al: The role of ultrasonography and amniocentesis in the evaluation of pregnancies at risk for neural tube defects, *Am J Obstet Gynecol* 161:520-523, 1989.

Humphreys RP: Current trends in spinal dysraphism, *Paraplegia* 29(2):79-83, 1991.

Kaufman B et al: Disbanding a multidisciplinary clinic: effects on the health care of myelomeningocele patients, *Pediatr Neurosurg* 21:36-44, 1994.

Kazak AE, Clark MW: Stress in families of children with myelomeningocele, *Dev Med Child Neurol* 28:220-228, 1986.

King JC, Currie DM, and Wright E: Bowel training in spina bifida: importance of education, patient compliance, age, and reflexes, *Arch Phys Ther Rehabil* 75(3):243-247, 1994.

Kirulata HG, Gillingham D, and Squires D: Long-term cotrimoxazole prophylaxis in spina bifida: effects on folic acid. Presented at the annual meeting of the Urology Section of the American Academy of Pediatrics, Washington, DC, Oct 1986.

Kreder K: Anomalies associated with myelodysplasia, *Pediatr Urol* 39(3):248-250, 1992.

Leger RR, Meeropol E: Children at risk: latex allergy and spina bifida, *J Pediatr Nurs* 7(6):371-376, 1992.

Leibold S: A systematic approach to bowel continence for children with spina bifida, *Eur J Pediatr Surg* 1(supp)1:23-24, 1991.

Leonard MP, Gearhart JP, and Jeffs RD: Continent urinary reservoirs in pediatric urological practice, *J Urol* 144(2):330-333, 1990.

Liptak GS, Revell G: Management of bowel dysfunction in children with spinal cord disease or injury by means of the enema continence catheter, *J Pediatr Surg* 120(2):190-194, 1992.

Lollar DJ: Educational issues among children with spina bifida, *Spina bifida spotlight,* Washington, DC, 1993a, Spina Bifida Association of America, pp 1-4.

Lollar DJ: Learning among children with spina bifida, *Spina Bifida Spotlight,* Washington, DC, 1993b, Spina Bifida Association of America, pp 1-6.

Luthy DA et al: Cesarean section before the onset of labor and subsequent motor function in infants with myelomeningocele diagnosed internally, *New Engl J Med* 324(10):662-666, 1991.

Madsen JR, Scott RM: Chiari malformation, syringomyelia, and intramedullary spinal cord tumors, *Curr Opin Neurol Neurosurg* 6:559-563, 1993.

Marge M: Toward a state of well-being: promoting healthy behaviors to prevent secondary conditions. In Lollar DJ (editor): *Preventing secondary conditions associated with spina bifida or cerebral palsy: proceedings and recommendations of a symposium,* Washington, DC, 1994, Spina Bifida Association of America, pp 87-94.

Mazur JM, Menelaus MB: Neurological status of spina bifida patients and the orthopedic surgeon, *Clin Orthop Related Res* (264):54-64, 1991.

McLone DG, Naidich TP: Myelomeningocele. In Hoffman HJ, Epstein F (editors): *Disorders of the developing nervous system: diagnosis and treatment,* New York, 1986, Praeger.

Milunsky A et al: Multivitamin/folic acid supplementation in early pregnancy reduces the prevalence of neural tube defects, *JAMA* 24:2847-2852, 1989.

Moore K: *The developing human,* Philadelphia, 1987, Lippincott.

Mulinare J: Epidemiologic association of multivitamin supplementation and occurrence of neural tube defects, *Ann New York Academy of Sciences* 678:130-136, 1993.

Palfrey JS, Haynie M, and Porter SM: *Children assisted by medical technology in educational settings: guidelines for care,* Boston, 1989, Children's Hospital, pp 13-14.

Pavin M et al: Recommendations for parents and families. In Lollar DJ (editor): *Preventing secondary conditions associated with spina bifida.or cerebral palsy: proceedings and recommendations of a symposium,* Washington, DC, 1994, Spina Bifida Association of America, pp 101-107.

Physcian's Desk Reference, ed. 44 Gradell, NJ: 1994 Barnhart.

Raddish M: The immunization status of children with spina bifida, *Am J Dis Child* 147:849-853, 1993.

Raucn K, Aubert E: A brighter future for adults who have myelomeningocele—one form of spina bifida, *Orthop Nurs* 11(3):16-26, 1992.

Reigel DH: Infancy through the school years. In Rowley-Kelly F, Reigel DH (editors): *Teaching the student with spina bifida,* Baltimore, 1993, Brookes, pp 3-30.

Rowley-Kelly F: Transition planning to adulthood. In Rowley-Kelly F, Reigel DH (editors): *Teaching the student with spina bifida,* Baltimore, 1993, Brookes, pp 305-323.

Rudy DC, Woodside JR: The incontinent myelodysplastic patient (review), *Urol Clin North Am* 18(2):295-308, 1991.

Ryan KD, Ploski C, and Emans JB: Myelodysplasia—the musculoskeletal problem: habilitation from infancy to adulthood, *Phys Ther* 71(12):935-946, 1992.

Samuelson JJ, Foltz J, and Foxall MJ: Stress and coping in families of children with myelomeningocele, *Arch Psychiatr Nurs* 1(5):287-295, 1992.

Schidlow DV, Fiel SB: Life beyond pediatrics, *Med Clin North Am* 75(5):1113-1120, 1990.

Selzman AA, Elder JS, and Mapstone TB: Urologic consequences of myelodysplasia and other congenital abnormalities of the spinal cord (review), *Urol Clin North Am* 20(3):485-504, 1993.

Shaw GM et al: Epidemiologic characteristics of phenotypically distinct neural tube defects among 0.7 million California births, 1983–1987, *Teratology* 49:143-149, 1994.

Slater JE: Rubber anaphylaxis, *New Engl J Med* 320:1126-1129, 1989.

Slater JE: Latex allergy, *J Allergy Clin Immunol* 94(2 pt1):139-149; quiz 150, Aug 1994.

Sloan SL: Sexuality issues in spina bifida, *Spina bifida spotlight,* Washington, DC, 1993, Spina Bifida Association of America, pp 1-3.

Smith KA: Bowel and bladder management of the child with myelomeningocele in the school setting, *J Pediatr Health Care* 4(4):175-180, 1990.

Tappit-Emas E: Spina bifida. In Tecklin J (editor): *Pediatric Physical Therapy,* Philadelphia, 1989, JB Lippincott, pp 106-140.

Thomas CV: Closure of large spina bifida defects: a simple technique based on anatomical details, *Ann Plastic Surg* 31(6):522-527, 1993.

Vereecken RL: Bladder pressure and kidney function in children with myelomeningocele: review article, *Paraplegia* 30(3):153-159, 1992.

Wallander JL, Varni JW: Social support and adjustment in chronically ill and handicapped children, *Am J Comm Psychol* 17:185-201, 1989.

Wallander JL, Feldman WS, and Varni JW: Physical status and psychosocial adjustment in children with spina bifida, *J Pediatr Psychol* 14:89-102, 1989.

Warkany J, Lemire RJ: Pathogenesis of neural tube defects. In Hoffman HJ, Epstein F (editors): *Disorders of the developing nervous system: diagnosis and treatment,* Boston, 1986, Blackwell.

Werler MM, Shapiro S, and Mitchell AA: Peroconceptual folic acid exposures and risk of occurrent neural tube defects, *JAMA* 269(10):1257-1261, 1993.

Young MA et al: Latex allergy: a guideline for perioperative nurses, *AORN J* 56(3):488-493, 1992.

Younoszai MK: Stooling problems in patients with myelomeningocele (review), *South Med J* 85(7):718-724, 1992.

Organ Transplants

28

Eileen McNamara, Nancy Pike, Candace Gettys, and Beverly Corbo-Richert*

ETIOLOGY

Organ transplantation is a complex surgical procedure performed in children with life-threatening conditions as a result of failure of a particular organ. The three most prevalent organ transplant procedures for children are renal, liver, and heart replacement. A summary of the diseases and conditions that lead to end-stage organ failure in children is listed in Table 28-1.

During the past three decades, host and graft survival rates have improved as a result of the introduction of new immunosuppressive agents. Graft rejection continues to be a major obstacle to successful organ transplantation. Immunosuppressive protocols used at transplant centers include multiple drugs: cyclosporine (Sandimmune), prednisone (Deltasone), and azathioprine (Imuran) or tacrolimus (Prograf), with or without prednisone. Complications and side effects of immunosuppressive agents continue to present a medical challenge, encouraging researchers to continue their efforts to discover better immunosuppressive drugs.

In 1994, tacrolimus was approved by the FDA for use as an immunosuppressant agent in transplantation. Tacrolimus has been shown to be as effective as cyclosporine in both adult and pediatric liver transplant recipients (McDiarmid et al, 1995). Additionally, there are significantly fewer episodes of acute rejection that are corticosteroid-resistant or refractory to treatment in patients receiving tacrolimus. However, there has been a higher incidence of nephrotoxicity and neurotoxicity that has required discontinuation of the drug (US Multicenter FK506 Liver Study Group, 1994).

Renal Transplants

The first successful pediatric renal transplantations were performed in the early 1960s. The most common diagnosis requiring transplantation was chronic glomerulonephritis (Starzl et al, 1966). The procedure became more prevalent in the late 1960s and early 1970s. Today renal transplantation is the treatment of choice for end-stage renal disease. From 1987 to 1992, 3438 renal transplants were performed in 3176 individuals below 21 years of age (North American Pediatric Renal Transplant Cooperative Study, 1994).

Liver Transplants

After many years of animal research, experimentation with human liver orthotopic (replacement of an organ in its normal position) transplantation began in the early 1960s with both adults and children. In 1963, the first pediatric liver transplantation was

*The editors and authors would like to acknowledge the work done by Karen E. Zamberlan on this chapter in the first edition of the book.

Table 28-1.   COMPARATIVE INDICATIONS FOR TRANSPLANTATION IN CHILDREN BY ORGAN*

Renal	Liver	Heart	Dual transplants
Congenital disease	**Cholestatic disease**	**Cardiomyopathy**	**Heart and liver**
Renal hypoplasia	Biliary atresia	Dilated	Familial hypercholester-
Renal dysplasia	Familial cholestasis	Hypertrophic	olemia with isch-
Prune belly syndrome	Alagille's syndrome	Restrictive	emic cardiomyopa-
Congenital nephrotic	Byler's syndrome	**Congenital heart**	thy
syndrome	**Parenchymal disease**	defects (se-	Intrahepatic biliary
Wilms' tumor	Budd-Chiari syndrome	lect lesions)	atresia and dilated
Obstructive uropathy	Congenital hepatic fibrosis		cardiomyopathy
Acquired disease	Cystic fibrosis		**Liver and kidney**
Glomerulonephritis	Neonatal hepatitis		Cystinosis
lupus nephritis	Acute fulminant hepatic		Oxalosis
membranous glomeru-	failure		**Heart and lung**
lonephritis	Hepatitis B		Primary pulmonary hy-
focal segmental	Hepatitis C		pertension
glomerular sclerosis	**Metabolic disorders**		Congenital heart defects
IgA nephropathy/	α_1-antitrypsin deficiency		with elevated pul-
Henoch-Schönlein purpura	Wilson's disease		monary vascular re-
Hemolytic uremic syndrome	Glycogen storage disease,		sistance
Chronic pyelonephritis	type IV		
Renal infarct	Tyrosinemia		
Sickle cell nephropathy	**Hepatomas**		
Hereditary disease			
Alport's syndrome			
Juvenile nephrophthisis			
Polycystic kidney disease			
Metabolic disorders			
Cystinosis			
Oxalosis			

*These are a few of the more common conditions leading to end-stage organ failure; the list is not all inclusive.

performed on a 3-year-old child with extrahepatic biliary atresia; however, the child died as a result of hemorrhage on the operative day (Starzl et al, 1982). In 1967, the first child who experienced extended survival after a liver transplantation was a 1½-year-old girl with hepatocellular carcinoma who lived for 13 months (Starzl et al, 1982). In the 1960s the 1-year survival rate for children was 34% (Starzl et al, 1979). In the 1990s the 1-year survival rate for the pediatric recipient of a liver has increased to 87% (Esquivel et al, 1991). Research efforts to improve procurement and surgical techniques and the preservation of donor organs are in part responsible for the

improved survival currently being experienced by the recipients, as well as the introduction of new immunosuppressants such as tacrolimus. Because the demand for donor organs far exceeds the number of donated organs, the available donor pool has been expanded by the use of living-related donor livers, reduced size livers, and by splitting livers so that one adult liver may be used for two recipients.

Heart Transplants

Heart transplantation in humans also began in the 1960s. A significant breakthrough was the development of successful orthotopic surgical techniques involving the removal of the recipient's ventricles, leaving the posterior atrial walls and the ridge of the interatrial septum intact (Lower and Shumway, 1960). The first pediatric heart transplantation was performed on an 18-day-old infant with Ebstein's anomaly who died 6 hours later from complications (Kantrowitz et al, 1968).

In 1985, neonatal transplantation was introduced as a treatment option for infants with hypoplastic left heart syndrome which is lethal within the first few months of life (Bailey et al, 1986). The 1-year survival rate of people receiving heart transplants has improved from 72% during 1981 to 1985 to 80% during 1988 to 1993 (Hosenpud et al, 1994).

Dual-Organ Transplants

Dual-organ transplantations involve the replacement of a combination of organs such as heart-liver, heart-lung, or liver-kidney. The first heart-lung transplantation was attempted on a 2-month-old girl with atrioventricular canal defect whose condition was terminal. Although the child survived the surgery, she died 14 hours later of pulmonary insufficiency (Cooley et al, 1969). The first successful pediatric heart-liver transplantation was performed in 1983 on a 6-year-old girl with ischemic cardiomyopathy secondary to familial hypercholesterolemia. This girl subsequently underwent a retransplantation of the liver in 1990 for rejection; however, 9 months later she succumbed to rejection of the heart.

The most common indications for heart-lung transplantation is congenital heart disease (46%) either surgically corrected or uncorrected which is associated with end-stage pulmonary vascular disease and primary pulmonary hypertension (19%) (Hosenpud et al, 1994; Conte et al, 1995; Spray, 1993). The 1-year survival rate for people receiving heart-lung transplants has increased slightly from 56% during 1981 to 1987 to 60% during 1988 to 1993, along with a decreasing number of recipients as a result of the advancements in single/double lung transplants and congenital heart surgery (Hosenpud et al, 1994).

INCIDENCE

Today in the United States, approximately 11 children per 1 million population under age 19 years begin end-stage renal disease (ESRD) treatment. Over 50% of the children presenting with ESRD are between the ages of 11 and 15 years (Ettenger, Grimm, and Firzli, 1992). The most common congenital diagnoses are hypoplastic/dysplastic kidneys and obstructive uropathy. Focal segmental glomerulosclerosis is the third most common primary diagnosis and continues to be the most common lesion among acquired renal diseases (NAPRTCS, 1994).

Approximately 500 children per year await a liver transplant in the United States (United Network for Organ Sharing [UNOS], 1995). The incidence varies according to the specific liver disease. Biliary atresia is the most common indication for liver transplant, with 400 to 600 cases identified each year (Whitington and Balisteri, 1991).

The incidence of cardiomyopathy in children less than 15 years of age is approximately 39 per 1 million population in the United States annually (Gillum, 1986).

Congenital heart disease occurs in approximately 8 out of every 1000 live births each year (American Heart Association, 1994). Most children with congenital heart disease can be helped surgically with an estimated 10% being incorrectable, thus requiring heart or heart-lung transplantation.

According to the United Network for Organ Sharing (UNOS), the number of children 16 years of age or less on the waiting list as of January 1995 was (1) 473 children awaiting renal transplants, (2) 524 children awaiting liver transplants, (3) 158 children awaiting heart transplants, (4) 38 awaiting heart-lung transplants, and (5) 115 awaiting lung transplants (UNOS, 1995).

The largest percentage of deaths among the pediatric population awaiting a liver transplant is found in infants less than 1 year of age. Nearly 18% of those children died while waiting for a suitable donor organ (UNOS, 1994). To alleviate the problem of mortality associated with the lengthy wait for a cadaveric donor from an infant less than 15 kg, transplantation using reduced size livers, split livers, and segments from living-related donors have become alternative methods of liver transplantation in the 1990s. Survival of the children receiving reduced size grafts and the hepatic functions of those grafts are not statistically different from those recipients who receive full size graft (Esquivel et al, 1991).

CLINICAL MANIFESTATIONS AT TIME OF DIAGNOSIS

The presenting symptoms of children experiencing end-stage organ failure vary according to the affected organ and to the specific disease. The severity of the symptoms is contingent on the particular disease, the age of the child at the time of diagnosis, medical management, and the individual response of the child to treatment. Table 28-2 presents the comparative clinical manifestations of end-stage organ disease in children.

Renal Disease

Children who have undergone transplantation for any of the indications listed in the renal column of Table 28-1 may have experienced many of the clinical manifestations of chronic renal failure.

As ESRD progresses, children are faced with two treatment options, dialysis or transplantation. Transplantation is considered the treatment of choice in ESRD. For children to proceed from ESRD directly to transplant without maintenance on dialysis is referred to as preemptive transplantation.

There are no medical or psychosocial benefits to a child's being dialyzed before renal transplant (Cohn, 1994). Dialysis is only a temporary measure in children who will proceed to transplant. With dialysis there are also many potential complications, such as growth delay, anorexia, chemistry imbalances, and hypertension. Manifestations of chronic renal failure are discussed in Chapter 32. Not all children are candidates for preemptive transplant but, when possible, it should be pursued. In 1994, almost 30% of the children receiving renal transplants received preemptive transplants (NAPRTCS, 1994).

Liver Disease

Children with liver disease may have serious clinical manifestations. The condition can be acute or chronic, and depending on the specific disease etiology, the symptoms will vary. The more common manifestations of a failing liver in children with congenital biliary atresia are jaundice, hepatomegaly, splenomegaly, ascites, recurrent spontaneous bacterial peritonitis, cutaneous xanthomas with pruritus, and a history of variceal bleeding (see Fig. 28-1). Other chronic congenital or hereditary liver diseases in children can result in delayed growth, malnutrition, rickets or fractures, coagulopathies, and encephalopathy.

Table 28-2.   COMPARATIVE CLINICAL MANIFESTATIONS OF END-STAGE RENAL, LIVER, AND HEART DISEASE IN CHILDREN*

Renal	Liver	Heart
Electrolyte abnormalities	Jaundice	Respiratory distress
Sodium retention	Ascites	Tachypnea
Hyperkalemia	Hepatomegaly	Congestive heart failure
Hypokalemia	Splenomegaly	Cardiomegaly
Metabolic acidosis	Portal hypertension	ST- and T-wave abnormalities
Hyperglycemia	Hypercholesterolemia	Cardiac murmurs
Hyperlipidemia	Hyperammonemia	Growth retardation
Anemia	Hypoalbuminemia	Arrhythmias
Congestive heart failure or pericarditis	Hypoglycemia	
Peripheral neuropathy	Prolonged prothrombin time	
Renal osteodystrophy	Hormone imbalance	
Growth retardation	Encephalopathy	

*These are a few of the more common manifestations; they are not all inclusive.

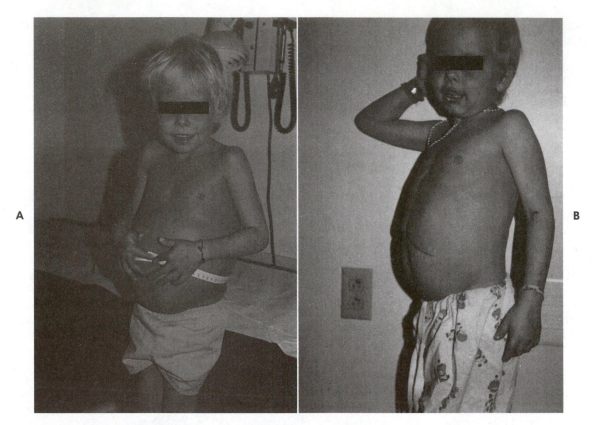

Fig. 28-1.   **A,** Boy, four and a half years old, with biliary cirrhosis of unknown etiology at clinic evaluation for liver transplant. **B,** Same boy, follow-up clinic visit, 3 months after liver transplant.

Acute end-stage liver disease caused by fulminant failure or acute hepatitis may be insidious in onset, with rapid progression of the clinical course in children over a few days to a few months. It is characterized by rapidly increased jaundice, shrinkage of the liver, fetor hepaticus, coagulopathy, renal failure, hepatic encephalopathy, and eventual coma or death (Iwatsuki et al, 1989). Chronic liver disease may progress more slowly, with symptoms appearing gradually over a period of several months. Transplantation is clearly indicated if the child has demonstrated any life-threatening complications such as bleeding, recurrent encephalopathy, coagulopathy, malnutrition, deep jaundice, profound growth and development retardation, or metabolic bone disease. Liver transplantation may also be indicated for children who

have primary unresectable tumors of the liver without metastases.

Heart Disease

The clinical manifestations and long-term outcome in children with cardiomyopathies have been described in recent studies (Ciszewski et al, 1994; Burch et al, 1994). Younger age at onset for dilated cardiomyopathy has been associated with better outcomes, with children less than 2 years having a better prognosis (Ciszewski et al, 1994; Burch et al, 1994). The clinical manifestations of dilated cardiomyopathy include symptoms of congestive heart failure as a result of decreasing myocardial contractility. Other common clinical signs include an enlarged heart by chest radiography, nonspecific ST-T wave changes and sinus tachycardia on electrocardiography, and a gallop rhythm is often heard on auscultation. Some nonspecific symptoms may include fever, vomiting, weight loss, or failure to thrive (Baker, 1994).

The clinical manifestations of hypertrophic cardiomyopathy differ somewhat from the dilated cardiomyopathies. The clinical manifestations include symptoms of congestive heart failure, systolic ejection murmur, dyspnea on exertion, dizziness or syncope, left ventricular hypertrophy or left bundle branch block on electrocardiography, and cardiomegaly or left ventricular hypertrophy on chest radiography. The majority of children discovered to have hypertrophic cardiomyopathy outside of infancy do not have prominent cardiac symptoms and are at considerable risk for sudden death.

TREATMENT

Renal Disease Management

In chronic renal failure the use of continuous ambulatory peritoneal dialysis or hemodialysis should be considered if the glomerular filtration rate approaches 5 ml/min per 1.73 m^2 (Fine, 1990). The indications for initiating dialysis in an infant, child, or adolescent with chronic renal failure vary and are contingent on the clinical status of the child (see Chapter 32). Dialysis is an expedient therapy to maintain life until successful transplantation can be accomplished.

Liver Disease Management

Children with chronic liver disease may be managed at home with attention to the liver's synthetic function, supplemental nutrition support from total parental nutrition, lipids or enteral feedings, and medical management of the complications of liver disease (i.e., coagulopathy, ascites, rickets, encephalopathy, and malabsorption of fat-soluble vitamins). If the child's condition worsens, stabilization may be achieved by hospitalization, followed by urgent transplantation of an available organ.

Portal hypertension, which often develops with biliary atresia, may require repeated endoscopy with sclerotherapy or banding, or the use of vasopressors to control bleeding from esophageal and gastric varices or hypersplenism. If there is a sudden decrease in the hematocrit level, the child should be hospitalized and an endoscopy performed to rule out gastrointestinal (GI) bleeding. Esophageal endosclerosis is accomplished by the injection of a sclerosant, usually 5% sodium morrhuate, into the distal esophageal varices.

Recurrent use of sclerotherapy to control esophageal hemorrhage can lead to formation of strictures, ulcers, and perforations. Several liver transplant centers are presently looking at the feasibility of the use of the transjugular intrahepatic portosystemic shunt (TIPSS) procedure to provide long-term treatment for the child with recurrent variceal bleeds.

If endoscopy is not possible, the careful introduction of a Sengstaken-Blakemore tube to decompress varices may be used. Vasopressin (Pitressin) administered intravenously may aid in prevention of hemorrhage by reducing the portal and mesenteric blood flow. The Kasai operation for biliary atresia establishes biliary drainage and may offer an option before liver transplantation.

Cholangitis caused by biliary stasis and bacterial contamination is a frequent complication for children with biliary atresia. Any fever (temperature >38°C), elevation of white blood cell count, increase in serum bilirubin concentration, and positive blood cultures may indicate its presence. Wanek and colleagues (1989) suggested the use of third-generation cephalosporins and aminoglycosides intravenously because of the difficulty in identifying the causative organism of cholangitis.

Heart Disease Management

Children with cardiomyopathy may be managed medically on oral medications if symptoms of heart failure are controlled. Medical management of dilated cardiomyopathy consists of maximizing cardiac output and controlling symptoms of heart failure with digoxin, diuretics, and afterload reduction. Angiotensin-converting enzyme inhibitors (i.e., captopril or enalapril) for afterload reduction have proven to be beneficial in optimizing cardiac function and decreasing the workload of the heart. Antiarrhythmics may be needed in some children. Anticoagulation therapy may also be needed to prevent thrombus formation in a dilated and poorly contracting heart. Heart transplantation is the alternative when medical management fails.

In contrast, medical management for hypertrophic cardiomyopathy consists of maintaining a normal preload and afterload while reducing ventricular contractility. This is usually accomplished with calcium channel blockers as well as beta blockers to decrease the septal muscle from obstructing the left ventricular outflow tract. Antiarrhythmics may also be needed for ventricular arrhythmias but has not shown to prevent sudden death. Surgical intervention can be attempted to remove muscle bundles in the left ventricular outflow tract in an attempt to relieve obstruction. Surgical intervention is not recommended until medical management has failed because of the possibility of recurrent obstruction. Heart transplantation is the alternative when medical and surgical management have failed.

Evaluation for Transplantation

Evaluation for organ transplantation involves a multidisciplinary approach. Many institutions involve members from nursing, neurology, psychiatry, physical therapy, dentistry, and social services in the evaluation process, as well as the specialty medical services. Frequently, the evaluation is completed on an outpatient basis. In children who have more advanced disease, hospitalization may be indicated for the evaluation and continued until a donor can be found.

The primary care provider has an important role in the evaluation process. Continuity of care encompassing psychosocial aspects and family preparation for the evaluation can be facilitated by the referring primary care provider. The provider is in an optimal position to assess the child and family's previous illness and hospital experiences, life stressors, coping abilities, and level of knowledge and to communicate such information to the transplant center staff. This knowledge equips the hospital staff to best explain the transplant process to the child on an appropriate developmental level and to the family in the context of their life experiences. The provider might encourage both parents or parent and significant other to attend the evaluation session so that two adults may hear the information together. If it is not possible for at least two adults to attend, one parent may tape record the sessions for the absent partner, thus including them and also allowing for further reflection on the information. Regardless, parents are encouraged to bring note pads and pencils to take notes and record their own thoughts and questions.

For the child being evaluated for an organ transplant, there are few contraindications to his or her acceptance as a candidate. General exclusion criteria should include evidence of systemic infections, diseases that will recur after transplant, multisystem organ failure, and an expectation of poor quality of life outcome (Whitington and Balisteri, 1991). Pulmonary vascular resistance (PVR) is evaluated on all heart transplant candidates by cardiac catheterization. If the PVR is greater than 8 wood units and is unresponsive to oxygen or nitroprusside, this is a contraindication for isolated heart transplantation. The child would then be evaluated for a heart-lung transplant (Sarris et al., 1994; Baum et al., 1991). Each child is evaluated on an individual basis, and the child's suitability for the particular organ is weighed against the presence of other ongoing problems.

Multiple diagnostic tests, cultures (blood, urine, and secretions), blood work evaluation, and radiologic examinations may assist in the evaluation of the child for transplant candidacy.

All children who are transplant candidates should be screened for prior exposure to cytomegalovirus (CMV) and Epstein-Barr virus. Screening for tuberculosis and varicella has also been advocated. Epstein-Barr screening is performed because it has been associated with the development of lymphoma after transplantation (Cox et al, 1995). In certain circumstances attempts may be made to match donors and recipients according to CMV status. Without such matching these organisms could seriously infect recipients who have not been previously exposed. Hepatitis and HIV screens are completed before the transplantation.

Donor matching for heart and liver transplantation is primarily by ABO blood type and body size. In renal transplant ABO blood type and human leukocyte antigen (HLA) matching with donor is necessary for transplantation. Pretransplant screening of child candidates includes HLA tissue typing, cytotoxic antibody cross-match compatibility, and ABO blood typing, in addition to percent panel reactive antibody (PRA). Percent panel reactive antibody is determined by having the recipient's serum react with normal human lymphocytes and reveal whether a recipient has developed antibody to histocompatible antigens.

A PRA of 0% indicates the child has not been exposed to a sensitizing event and developed antibodies. Sensitizing events would include previous transplants, graft rejection, blood transfusions, and pregnancy. All of these events can lead to the formation of histocompatible antibodies, thus increasing the PRA. The higher the PRA, the more difficult it becomes to find a crossmatch negative kidney (Terasaki, Park, and Danovitch, 1992).

RECENT AND ANTICIPATED ADVANCES IN DIAGNOSIS AND MANAGEMENT

The past decade has brought many changes in transplantation. Children with organ transplants enjoy an improved quality of life as a result of better immunosuppressant drugs, surgical techniques, and medical management. Rejection continues to be a challenge in the field of transplantation. Ongoing research is focused on finding better drugs to combat rejection and achieve physiologic tolerance.

CellCept (mycophenolate mofetil) has recently been approved by the FDA as an immunosuppressant. CellCept blocks the de novo pathway of purine biosynthesis, on which lymphocytes are dependent (Kaufman, Jones, and Matas, 1992). CellCept is an isolate of the mold penicillin glaum (Roche product monograph, 1995).

Cyclosporine and corticosteroids are used with CellCept as immunosuppressant therapy. Trials in the United States showed a lower rejection in individuals with kidney transplants on CellCept, cyclosporine, and corticosteroids versus azathioprine, cyclosporine, (Roche product monograph, 1995). A second study showed CellCept was effective at reversing acute rejection. The principal side effects associated with CellCept include diarrhea, leukopenia, sepsis, and vomiting (Roche product monograph, 1995).

Rapamycin is a macrolide antibiotic from the bacterium streptomyces hygroscopius (Kaufman, Jones, and Matas, 1992). Studies have shown rapamycin works by inhibiting human T-cell proliferation. Rapamycin has been shown to have synergistic effects with cyclosporine and low-dose tacrolimus, allowing for lower drug dosing (Kaufman, Jones, and Matas, 1992). Lower drug dosages decrease potential toxic side effects of these agents. The toxicity of rapamycin affects the gastrointestinal tract and the central nervous system (Kaufman, Jones, and Matas, 1992).

15-Deoxyspergualin (15-DS) is a bacillus lactosporus, an antitumor antibiotic with immunosuppressant properties (Kaufman, Jones, and Matas, 1992). 15-DS has been used successfully in experimental models to prolong graft survival, yet its mechanism of action is not fully understood (Ferraresso and Kahan, 1994). Several randomized trials have found 15-DS to be effective in treating acute rejection of renal allografts. Side effects associated with 15-DS include leukopenia, thrombocytopenia, nausea, vomiting, anorexia, and headache (Ferraresso and Kahan, 1994).

Small Bowel Transplantation

Significant progress has been made in the area of small bowel transplantation in children with short gut syndrome in recent years. A few centers in the United States are now offering this procedure to children who have no other alternative therapy. Although the use of total parenteral nutrition has improved the outcome for children with short gut syndrome, associated long-term complications include TPN-related liver failure, venous access problems, infection, and thrombosis. Clinical trials have produced encouraging results (Reyes et al, 1993). In clinical trials at Children's Hospital of Pittsburgh, 41 children have received isolated small bowel, liver/small bowel, or multivisceral transplants from July 1990 through July 1995. Overall survival during this 5-year period is 56% with nearly all patients at home and free of TPN (Kosmach, 1995).

Along with drug research, other advances on the horizon in transplantation are induction of chimerism by simultaneous bone marrow transplantation as well as xenografting.

Chimerism

Following transplantation, donor cells migrate throughout the recipient's body with an exchange of a type of leukocytes from the grafted organ into recipient tissues and a replacement of the same type of leukocytes from the recipient into the donor tissue. This coexistence of donor and recipient cells, called chimerism, is believed to be necessary for the body to accept the transplanted organ and is dependent on effective immunosuppression (Starzl et al, 1993). The theory is that if chimerism can be maintained, chronic rejection may be avoided and less immunosuppression will be required long term (Starzl et al, 1993). Additionally, findings indicate that chimerism can be augmented in the recipient by the infusion of donor bone marrow during transplantation (Rao et al, 1994).

Chimerism is achieved when the recipient takes on cellular characteristics of the donor. Immunohistochemistry has established that cells can carry the HLA type and sex of the donor rather than the recipient (Kocoshis et al, 1993). Chimerism has been well accepted in the population of liver transplantation. Long-term graft acceptance without immunosuppression has been described in a small group of recipients with liver transplants (Kocoshis et al, 1993). This group showed prominent systemic chimerism.

As chimerism is better understood it may lead to more sophisticated early immunosuppression and less intense long-term immunosuppression (Kocoshis et al, 1993). A new possibility to create chimerism may be simultaneous bone marrow transplantation, with solid organ transplantation. Preliminary experience suggests engraftment of the solid organ is more likely when simultaneous bone marrow transplantation is performed (Kocoshis et al, 1993).

Tolerance

Achieving a chimeric state is thought to lead to the development of tolerance. Although it is presumed that children who have received a transplanted organ will require immunosuppression for the remainder of their lives, some individuals have been able to achieve tolerance of the transplanted organ after successful weaning of maintenance immunosuppression. Ramos and colleagues (1995) have followed 59 long-surviving liver transplant recipients, ages 12 to 68 years. Sixteen individuals (27%) were completely weaned from immunosuppression and 28 patients (48%) were at various stages of weaning without any complications. Weaning has failed in 15 patients (24%), but without graft losses. This study suggests that a significant percentage of appropriately selected transplant recipients can achieve tolerance, but advises appropriate selection of long-term survivors with close monitoring and follow-up.

Xenotransplantation

Bone marrow transplantation may also show to be effective in xenotransplantation. Xenotransplantation is cross-species transplantation. During the past 10 years xenotransplantation has occurred in humans with baboon organs. Kidney transplants, heart transplants, and liver transplants have been performed on humans with baboon organs. Although the surgeries were sometimes successful, all of the individuals receiving the baboon organs died from complications. The baboon is believed to be resistant to hepatitis B. Two individuals with hepatitis B have received baboon liver transplants. They died shortly after transplant, but there was no evidence of recurrent hepatitis or rejection in the xenograph. Baboon organs have been used in xenotransplant even though theoretically the chimpanzee is believed to be a better immunologic match with humans. Chimpanzees were used initially in xenotransplantation because of their almost identical chromosome match with humans. They are now an endangered species so they cannot be considered in xenotransplantation.

ASSOCIATED PROBLEMS AFTER TRANSPLANTATION

Immunosuppression

The routine primary immunosuppressive regimen for children with renal, liver, and heart transplants may vary from institution to institution. The box on page 608 lists the drugs used at a major transplant center. The major maintenance immunosuppressive agents used alone or in combination therapy to prevent rejection are cyclosporine, tacrolimus, azathioprine, and prednisone.

Cyclosporine has been the primary immunosuppressant drug used since 1981 to prevent rejection of transplanted organs. Generally the children take maintenance doses of cyclosporine orally every 12 hours. Cyclosporine is absorbed in the intestinal tract therefore predicting absorption of this drug is difficult. The level of drug metabolites in the blood should be based on 12-hour trough levels.

Tacrolimus (formerly FK-506), a recent addition to transplant immunonology, is a macrolide produced from a strain of soil fungus, Streptomyces tsukubaensis. This is a potent immunosuppressant recently approved by the FDA for use in the liver transplant population. The drug is taken at 12-hour intervals and because it is absorbed primarily in the stomach, the drug manufacturer recommend that the drug be administered 1 hour before eating or 2 hours after eating.

Careful monitoring of side effects of cyclosporine or tacrolimus is required to maintain adequate immunosuppression, as well as to prevent toxicities. These two immunosuppressants are not used in combination because of their synergistic and nephrotoxic effects (Prograf product monograph, 1994). Children may require therapy of cyclosporine and prednisone; triple-drug therapy consisting of cyclosporine, azathioprine, and prednisone; or tacrolimus either alone or in combination with corticosteroids to maintain their functioning graft. Long-term maintenance may consist of cyclosporine alone in some children. Recently, children who have experienced chronic rejection taking cyclosporine and prednisone have had their immunosuppression therapy changed to tacrolimus and have had positive early results. Long-term outcomes have yet to be determined. Recent results of newborns after heart transplantation suggest that they tolerate an immunosuppressive regimen without corticosteroids (Boucek et al, 1990). These newborns were treated with cyclosporine and azathioprine for the first year and then treated with only cyclosporine. Corticosteroids were used only in the immediate postoperative period unless a diagnosis of graft rejection was made.

Some of the more common side effects of cyclosporine are hypertension, renal dysfunction, gum hyperplasia, hirsutism, diarrhea, seizures, and tremors (Sandimmune product monograph, 1993). Side effects experienced after taking tacrolimus orally include headache, insomnia, tremors, sensation of racing, hair loss or increased hair growth, nausea, vomiting, diarrhea, and anorexia.

Other complications of immunosuppressive therapy include hypertension, lymphoproliferative disease, coronary vascular disease, and corticosteroid-induced diabetes. The complication of corticosteroid-induced diabetes is uncommon and usually transient. At least 50% of recipients will experience one or more of these complications (Sandimmune product monograph, 1993). The exception has been with infants from one center treated with cyclosporine after heart transplantations with no evidence of hypertension (Boucek et al, 1990). High-dose corticosteroids are also implicated as a cause of hypertension by promoting sodium and water retention (Baluarte, Braas, and Kaiser, 1994; Starnes et al, 1992).

Posttransplant hypertension is associated with cyclosporine therapy and high-dose corticosteroids. Calcium channel blockers have been shown to effectively control hypertension from cyclosporine therapy (Baluarte, Braas, and Kaiser, 1994). β-adrenergic blockers, with their vasodilatory actions, have also been proven to be effective in controlling hypertension.

Nephrotoxicity secondary to cyclosporine therapy includes transient or chronic increases in blood urea nitrogen and creatinine levels. This is one of the major side effects of cyclosporine (Ettenger,

---

ASSOCIATED PROBLEMS

Immune Suppression	Side effects of medications
	Potential for infection
	Nephrotoxicity of cyclosporine
	Lymphoproliferative disease
Seizures	
Lymphoproliferative disease	
Rejection	Acute—first 6 months posttransplant
	Reversible
	Chronic—slower process lasting months to years; leading cause of late graft loss
Infection	Bacterial
	Viral
	Fungal
	Protozoan
	Symptoms of infection masked by immunosuppressive therapy

MAINTENANCE ROUTINE IMMUNOSUPPRESSIVE REGIMENS FOR CHILDREN WITH ORGAN TRANSPLANTS*

Renal transplants

Azathioprine 2 mg/kg/day for 1 month
     1-1.5 mg/kg/day thereafter
Cyclosporine 14-20 mg/kg/day—divided into 2 doses
     Trough levels first month 300-350 ng/ml
     Months 2-3 300 ng/ml
     Months 4-6 250 ng/ml
     Over 6 months 200-250 ng/ml
Tacrolimus 0.15 mg/kg per day, divided in bid dosing

Prednisone	Dose for wt .20 kg	Dose for wt .20 kg
Days 3-7	2 mg/kg	1.5 mg/kg
Days 7-14	1.5 mg/kg	1 mg/kg
Days 15-21	1 mg/kg	0.75 mg/kg
Days 22-30	0.75 mg/kg	0.6 mg/kg
Months 2-3	0.5 mg/kg	0.4 mg/kg
Months 4-6	0.4 mg/kg	0.3 mg/kg
Months 7 on	0.3 mg/kg	0.2 mg/kg
M.D. option if doing well	0.2 mg/kg	0.2 mg/kg

Liver transplants

Azathioprine 1-3 mg/kg/day
Cyclosporine 17.5 mg/kg/day or twice daily
Prednisone 2.5-10 mg/day or every other day
Tacrolimus 0.15 mg/kg twice daily†

Heart transplants

Azathioprine 2 mg/kg/day
Cyclosporine 10-20 mg/kg/day (3 divided doses)
Prednisone 0.6 mg/kg/day (2 or 3 divided doses)
OKT3 0.1 mg/kg/day IV for 14 days

*All medications taken orally. Dosages vary widely depending on the individual's blood levels. For cyclosporine, TDx levels of less than 400 ng/ml of whole blood is desirable.

†Because of the synergistic effect of cyclosporine and tacrolimus, children receive only one of the two drugs. Tacrolimus blood levels are measured by a whole blood assay, Abbott IMX. Therapeutic levels 5-10 ng/ml.

Data from Lucile Salter Packard Children's Hospital at Stanford Immunosuppressive regimen for children with renal transplants.

Grimm, and Firzli, 1992). The incidence and severity of chronic cyclosporine nephrotoxicity following renal transplantation has declined as maintenance doses of cyclosporine have been reduced (Baluarte, Braas, and Kaiser, 1994).

Serum creatinine level usually returns to baseline about 1 month after transplantation and then increases slowly to reach a plateau at about 1 year. More sophisticated measures of renal function may need to be done to determine long-term impairment from cyclosporine.

Seizures

There have been reports of seizures in children with transplants with no history of previous epilepsy. The incidence of seizures remains low (Sandimmune product monograph, 1993), but the cause remains controversial; the seizures may result from a drug interaction of high dose methylprednisone and cyclosporine, or hypertension may play a role in posttransplant seizures. Effective therapy consists of antiseizure medications. Importantly, many antiseizure medications decrease the blood level of cyclosporine (Sandimmune product monograph, 1993). See Chapter 19 for more information on seizure management.

Lymphoproliferative Disease

Lymphoproliferative disease has occurred in children who are immunosuppressed who test positively for Epstein-Barr virus infection. It has been seen in children taking azathioprine and prednisone, as well as cyclosporine. The frequency of occurrence in pediatric transplant recipients has been estimated at 4% (Ho et al, 1988); however, the cumulative incidences may be as high as 20% in children taking cyclosporine who had transplantations 7 years earlier (Malatack, 1990). The usual manifestations in children have been enlarged tonsils, enlarged cervical lymph nodes, and GI bleeding. The diagnosis is confirmed by biopsy of the lymph nodes or the mass.

The usual treatment is to reduce or discontinue immunosuppressive therapy. Providers at several transplant centers also recommend to begin treatment with ganciclovir for a period of 4 to 6 weeks and on discontinuing the ganciclovir, acyclovir should be instituted for a long-term period (Cox, 1993).

Rejection

Rejection can be divided into two categories: acute and chronic. Acute rejection is the most frequent form of rejection seen after transplantation (Friedman, 1994). Acute rejection is most commonly seen in the first 6 months following transplantation and is reversible. In renal transplantation acute rejection affects 50% of living-related donor transplants and 65% of cadaver transplants (Friedman, 1994). Chronic rejection is a much slower process that occurs over months to years. Chronic rejection is the most common cause of late graft loss. Symptoms of organ specific rejection can be seen in Table 28-3.

Meticulous monitoring of laboratory blood values for elevations in serum transaminases, bilirubin, alkaline phosphatase, and creatinine, as well as the child's physical status, can detect any problems with functioning of the liver or renal graft. Signs and symptoms of rejection include fever, swollen graft, abdominal pain, and irritability. Rejection of a transplanted kidney is usually determined by decreased blood flow on renal flow scan, whereas rejection of the liver is usually confirmed by biopsy. Fluid retention, ascites, and oliguria may be other accompanying signs of rejection.

Rejection in the liver transplant recipient may appear at any time after the fifth postoperative day. The clinical manifestations can include fever, elevated white blood cell count, lethargy and fatigue, irritability, and elevated liver enzymes. When a rejection episode is suspected, always check the trend of the liver enzymes because many of the symptoms associated with rejection are similar to symptoms seen with an infectious process or a bile ductal problem (e.g., obstruction). Therefore, a percutaneous liver biopsy may be necessary to make the definitive diagnosis of rejection. Approximately 20% of children require retransplantation of the kidney or liver with the majority necessary because of graft rejection (Fung et al, 1990). Changing the child from cyclosporine to tacrolimus may be of benefit in controlling persistent rejection episodes.

The clinical signs of rejection of a cardiac transplant include: symptoms of heart failure, enlarged heart, perihilar edema, pleural effusions on chest radiography, increase in heart rate above the normal resting rate, cardiac arrhythmias, gallop rhythm heard on auscultation and diminishing QRS voltage on electrocardiography. Other nonspecific findings have been fever, irritability, and poor feeding (Bailey et al, 1988). Most rejection is detected on routine endomyocardial biopsy or suspected on clinical assessment (including echocardiography) and confirmed by biopsy (Sarris et al, 1994). Biopsies are performed weekly for the first month, every other week for the second month, and then every 1 to 3 months, varying by institution. Infants are biopsied less frequently because of risk factors as well as limitations in venous access (Starnes et al, 1992). Infants are monitored more closely by clinical assessment and routine echocardiograms.

Persistent rejection episodes in infants and children are treated initially with methylprednisolone

Table 28-3.   CLINICAL SIGNS OF ORGAN REJECTION

Liver	Kidney	Heart
Fever	**Rejection in kidney**	**Heart rejection**
Elevated WBCs (Eosinophils)	Fever	Clinical signs:
Pain and swelling over graft site	↑ BUN	Heart failure
Lethargy/fatigue	↑ Creatinine	Enlarged heart
Elevated liver enzymes (alkaline phosphatase/GGT)	Pain/tenderness over abdomen	Atrial arrhythmias
Changes in stool color (becomes white, clay colored)	Swollen graft	S3 and/or S4 on auscultation
Scleral jaundice	Irritability	Diminished QRS voltage
Dark urine	Weight gain	Fever, nonspecific

intravenously for two courses and then with antirejection drugs in children older than 1 month (Sarris et al, 1994; Merrill et al, 1991; Bailey et al, 1988, Fullerton et al, 1995).

Approximately 3% of children having heart transplants and 10% of children having heart-lung transplants will need to be retransplanted (Hosenpud et al, 1994).

Infection

Infection is a major cause of graft failure and death in children who have undergone transplantation. Bacterial, fungal, viral, and protozoan infections leading to renal, heart, and liver dysfunction are well documented (Baum et al, 1991; Sarris et al, 1994; Starnes et al, 1992). Bacterial infections have occurred early after transplantation and tend to be associated with the site of organ transplantation (Reitz, 1992; Sarris, et al, 1994). Viral infections have been caused primarily by CMV, with a significant incidence of graft loss and death (Reitz, 1992). The use of ganciclovir (Cytovene) for acute symptomatic CMV infections has improved the outcome in these children (Reitz, 1992). Other important causes of viral infections include adenovirus and Epstein-Barr virus. Fungal infections, primarily *Candida* species, have also significantly contributed to morbidity and mortality.

Prophylaxis against protozoan infections such as Pneumocystis carnii (PCP) is accomplished through the use of Septra or Dapsone. In those children with allergies to sulfa, the use of Pentamidine intravenously or via inhalation may be indicated. See Chapter 22 for further discussion.

The difficulty in diagnosis is complicated by the use of immunosuppressive therapy, which may mask infections. Any child who has a fever and other generalized signs suggestive of infection should undergo physical and laboratory examination to determine any obvious source. Cultures for bacteria, fungi, and viruses obtained from blood, oral secretions, and urine should be performed when possible.

In general, medications are prescribed to all children for approximately 3 months to 1 year after transplantation to prevent viral, fungal, and protozoan infections. Since this protocol has been instituted, the incidence of serious infection from these organisms has decreased.

PROGNOSIS

Survival Statistics

Although the overall prognosis varies depending on the particular organ that is transplanted, the survival outcomes have improved dramatically for children needing renal, liver, or heart transplants.

Improvements in pediatric renal transplantation and dialysis procedures are contributing factors to the excellent physical survival of children with end-stage renal disease. One major center reports 1-year recipient survival rates to be 100%, with 1-year graft survival rates at 98% (Aluzri et al, 1994). Another major center reports 3-year graft survival rates in living-related and cadaver renal transplants to be 86% and 75%, respectively (Laine et al, 1994).

Currently, survival rates for children receiving liver transplants are 87% at 1 year and 85% at 3 years (Esquivel et al, 1991). New immunosuppressants and innovative surgery techniques have contributed to the improvement of the survival of children after liver transplantation.

The prognosis for children with cardiomyopathy is variable depending on the age of onset and etiology of the myopathy; the 1-year survival rate is 46% to 86% and the 5-year rate is 50% (Fowles, 1990; Abelmann and Lorell, 1989). Thus many of these children are candidates for heart transplants. The International Heart Registry reported more than 1800 children up to age 18 years received heart transplants and more than 200 children up to age 18 years received heart-lung transplants during 1983 to 1993. The 2-year actuarial survival for all individuals receiving (orthotopic) heart transplants is 76%, whereas the 2-year survival for infants less than 1 year of age is 63%, children 1 to 5 years of age is 70%, and children 6 to 18 years of age is 76% (Hosenpud et al, 1994).

One center, which specializes in cardiac transplantation in infancy, reported that 21 of 25 infants (84%) who had transplantations in the past 3 years are alive (Boucek et al, 1990). The most common diagnosis in this group was hypoplastic left heart syndrome.

Primary Care Management
HEALTH CARE MAINTENANCE

Growth and Development

The inhibitory effect of corticosteroids on growth in children is well established (Harmon and Jabs, 1992). Cyclosporine in combination with low-dose steroids has improved the growth in children posttransplant. Corticosteroids are rarely discontinued in children with transplants on cyclosporine (Harmon and Jabs, 1992). The majority of children with transplants on cyclosporine who have corticosteroids discontinued, undergo some form of rejection

and must resume corticosteroids (Harmon and Jabs, 1992). However, children with transplants on tacrolimus have been successfully weaned off corticosteroids.

Physical growth after liver transplantation has been shown to be enhanced in those children who are able to have their steroids discontinued in the posttransplant period. One study (Falkenstein et al, 1992) measured the growth and development of a group of children pretransplant and found that a number of them were below the 5th percentile for height and weight before receiving a liver transplant. The same group of children was studied posttransplant after their steroid therapy had been stopped. Over half of the group (66%) experienced an acceleration in their growth rate and were measured in the 25th percentile for height. Presently a number of liver transplant centers are using very-low-dose steroid therapy or are discontinuing steroids altogether in the early posttransplant period to help the pediatric recipient achieve a normal growth pattern.

Impaired growth from renal insufficiency in children improves little with dialysis (Ettenger, Grimm, and Firzli, 1992). A successful transplant can allow for better growth. Growth after transplant is affected by age at transplant, severity of pretransplant growth suppression, bone age, graft function and immunosuppressant medications (Rees, 1994).

Renal transplantation is the treatment of choice for children with chronic renal failure, principally because it can normalize physiologic status and provide these children with the potential for normal growth (Harman and Jabs, 1992).

In children receiving heart transplants, linear growth, neurologic outcome, and development are normal in the majority of infants who undergo transplantation before 6 months of age (Baum et al, 1993; Trento et al, 1989).

All children with organ transplants should have their height and weight documented at each clinic visit. Growth measures should be plotted on growth charts to monitor the rate and consistency of the child's growth and should be compared with normal percentile curves. Linear growth, anthropometrics of skin fold thickness, and nutritional measurements are important.

Research on cognitive functioning and development of children after transplantation are new areas of investigation. Cognitive functioning appears to be minimally affected after a child receives a liver transplant. There were no significant differences in IQs of 29 children tested before and after liver transplantation; about 20% of the children improved to the normal range, and 10% decreased from superior to normal (Zitelli et al, 1988). However, one study (Zamberlan, 1992) revealed deficits in school-aged children who tended to forget and were slow to finish school work.

After heart transplantation, infants were achieving normal developmental milestones more than 1 year after surgery (Bailey et al, 1988). In comparison with other groups of children who are chronically ill, liver transplant recipients show deficits in areas such as visual-spatial skills and abstract-reasoning skills (Stewart et al, 1991a). Variables such as the type of liver disease (e.g., biliary atresia), early age onset of the disease, severity of the disease, and the postoperative medications (immunosuppressants) can affect the child's cognitive development posttransplant (Stewart et al, 1992 and Stewart et al, 1991b).

The majority of children after heart or heart-lung transplant return to school, participate in sports, in age-appropriate activities, and are in the New York Heart Association Functional Class I (Conte et al, 1995; Sarris et al, 1994). One study of 65 children revealed delays in cognitive and emotional development after transplantation (Wray et al, 1994). Wray and colleagues attribute the delays to missed school, frequent hospitalizations, peer reactions, and fear of organ rejection and death.

Several quality-of-life studies of children who have had liver transplantations have been conducted (Kosmach, 1990; Zamberlan, 1992; Zitelli et al, 1988). As many as 5 years later, Zitelli and coworkers (1988) documented objective lifestyle changes in 65 children who had improved from pretransplant status. Zamberlan assessed 20 school-aged children 3 to 6 years after liver transplantation. Although the children perceived their quality of life to be good to excellent, they related negative changes and feelings about physical appearance, expressed feelings of insecurity, loneliness, and difficulties in peer relations, and had higher anxiety levels than the norm group. In a related descriptive study, seven adolescents who had survived liver transplantation for 1 to 4 years re-

ported a satisfactory quality of life but desired to make changes, perceived limitations, and were concerned about physical appearance and rejection (Kosmach, 1990). Overall, many of the issues expressed by transplant recipients are similar to those of children with chronic conditions and relate to developmental tasks.

Diet

Many children experience excessive weight gain after transplantation. Prednisone increases the appetite and causes the body to make fat and lose muscle. Also, children may overeat because most dietary restrictions are now lifted. Before discharge from the hospital, parents and children meet with a dietitian to discuss a well-balanced meal plan that includes the basic food groups. Children who take maintenance doses of cyclosporine and are hypertensive may require a low-sodium diet.

Children with heart transplants should be on a low-salt, low-fat diet because of the increased incidence of atherosclerosis. Children under 2 years of age should not be on a low-fat diet because dietary fat is needed for normal tissue and neurologic development.

Safety

Even though children are immunosuppressed after transplantation, routine hand washing and general cleanliness are all that are required. Most parents and children are sensitized to good hand-washing techniques during hospitalization, and such techniques should be continued in the home. Families who own cats as pets should avoid having the transplant recipient change the cat's litter box because of the possibility of being infected with the *Toxoplasma* organism found in the animal's feces.

Children taking prednisone may have more photosensitive skin. Use of sunscreen with sun protection factor of at least 15 is recommended.

Children with previous problems of rickets pretransplant may be at risk for bone fractures. This problem can be exacerbated by the use of prednisone, because steroids are well known to contribute to the development of osteoporosis.

When children or families are planning to travel, certain precautions should be taken. The transplant team should be notified before departure. They can inform the family of the transplant center nearest to their destination. Transplant recipients should always take all medications with them on trips and carry them onto airplanes rather than checking medications with luggage. Also, children should wear their Medic-Alert bracelets and carry an identification card that identifies them as a transplant recipient and has the name and telephone number of the transplant physician.

Exercise. In the child with a heart or heart-lung transplant it is important to understand that the incisions in the heart sever the sympathetic and parasympathetic nerves which ordinarily regulate heart rate. This lack of neural connections is known as denervation. Without the direct control of the central nervous system, the transplanted heart will beat faster in a resting state (e.g., 90 to 110 bpm). This faster than normal rate is associated with normal cardiac function and the capability of sustaining vigorous physical activity. The transplanted heart depends on circulating adrenalin and related hormones produced by the adrenal gland to change the heart rate instead of a direct impulse from the brain. In response to exercise, it may take up to 10 minutes to see an increase in heart rate and about 1 hour after stopping exercise to see a decrease in rate. Another effect of denervation is that chest pain or angina pectoris cannot be perceived should the new heart develop coronary artery disease. Thus coronary arteriograms are part of the pediatric transplant annual studies before reaching adulthood.

For the child with a heart/heart-lung transplant, activity restrictions are needed for the first 6 to 8 weeks after surgery to allow the sternum to heal. Recipients should avoid lifting, pushing or pulling heavy objects, bike riding, climbing, sit-ups, push-ups, roller skating, and contact sports during this time period. After 8 weeks, all activities can be resumed as well as gym class at school. Children will be instructed by a physical therapist before leaving the hospital on an exercise program. This consists of a 5-minute warm-up and cool-down period before and after peak physical activity. If the child shows signs of increased shortness of breath or fatigue, then the cool-down period should begin. It is important for gym teachers to be informed of the above information before returning to gym class after transplantation. Exercise should also be decreased during periods of rejection.

Exercise in the child with a liver or kidney transplant is encouraged, but there are some limitations. Recipients should avoid lifting heavy objects for at least 6 months. Push-ups or sit-ups, as well as activities that stretch or put pressure on the abdomen and incision, are to be avoided after liver or renal transplantation. Contact sports are not recommended. Children are encouraged to resume previous activities; however, it is recommended that they progress slowly.

Immunizations

Whenever possible, all recommended immunizations should be given before transplant surgery when the immune system will be better able to respond (Gershon, 1993).

Inactivated vaccines are not a risk to children who are immunocompromised although the efficacy of these vaccines is reduced.

Children who have had diphtheria, pertussis, and tetanus (DPT), IPV, or Hib immunization schedules disrupted because of chronic conditions can resume a schedule of treatment after the transplantation. Usually the child should be able to resume the immunization schedule within 3 months following the transplantation once minimal immunosuppressant therapy has been achieved.

Hepatitis B is an infrequent but important cause of decreased graft survival, morbidity, and mortality after transplantation. Children waiting for transplants should be vaccinated. All children on dialysis should be vaccinated as well. Pretransplantation vaccination may be achieved by administration of the inactivated Hib vaccine Heptavax-B, Recombivax, or Energix-B.

Live virus vaccines are contraindicated in children who are immunosuppressed because of the risk of contracting the disease. Enhanced inactivated polio is recommended for the child with a transplant and all household contacts who need to be immunized (Committee on Infectious Diseases, 1994). Unfortunately, no inactivated form of vaccination for measles, mumps, rubella and varicella exists. Each transplant center will determine the immunization policy for the children in their practice and the primary care provider should contact the transplant center to determine the desired immunizations for the affected child as well as household contacts. It is usually recommended that household contacts receive the MMR and Varivax to decrease the exposure potential for the child with a transplant (Committee on Infectious Diseases, 1994).

During epidemics of vaccine-preventable diseases or known exposure to someone with active disease, disease-specific immunoglobulin may be offered to a child or immunosuppressive therapy to bolster the child's antibodies against the specific disease (Committee on Infectious Diseases, 1994). Children who are exposed to chicken pox must receive human varicella-zoster immune globulin (VZIG) within 72 hours following contact exposure if they do not have a positive history of varicella. If children are hospitalized at the time of exposure, they are placed in isolation from day 10 to day 28 after exposure to chicken pox and treatment with VZIG. Children who develop lesions despite VZIG should also receive acyclovir intravenously within 24 hours of eruption of the skin rash and continued for 7 to 10 days (Committee on Infectious Diseases, 1994).

Screening

Vision. Children should have their eyes examined with an ophthalmoscope at clinic visits, as well as yearly ophthalmology checkups to monitor for changes such as cataracts, glaucoma, or pseudotumor cerebri, all potential side effects to immunosuppressant drugs.

Hearing. Children should have yearly audiograms because they receive many ototoxic drugs to treat infections during the postoperative period. The cumulative effects of the drug therapies should be monitored monthly during the immediate postoperative period and then yearly to evaluate any hearing loss.

Dental. Routine dental visits (twice yearly) are recommended for children after transplantation. It is usual practice for prophylactic antibiotics to be administered before dental care to prevent infection (see box on p. 306, in Chapter 15). In addition, children taking cyclosporine may develop gum hyperplasia requiring gingivectomy. Bonding of the teeth has been successful in restoring a natural finish to permanent teeth stained in utero for children with biliary atresia.

Blood pressure. Home blood pressure readings should be taken and recorded twice daily by par-

ents. The primary care provider should carefully evaluate home results and current blood pressure reading at the clinic visit. Children with hypertension may take nifedipine hydralazine or clonidine for blood pressure control.

Hematocrit. Hematocrit is done with monthly laboratory work at the request of the transplant center so additional screening is not necessary.

Urinalysis and urine culture. Urinalysis and urine cultures are performed frequently as part of the posttransplant management of children with renal, and to a less extent, heart and liver transplants. Many children who have undergone renal transplantation have underlying urologic problems that would predispose them to urinary tract infections and pyelonephritis. The immunosuppressant medications can mask early symptoms of urinary tract infections; therefore, frequent urinalysis and cultures help to identify infections before symptoms occur.

Tuberculosis. Before transplantation all children should receive the purified protein derivative (PPD) 5 U/0.1 ml test dose intradermally with anergy control to evaluate exposure. A positive skin test reaction is followed by chest radiograph before treatment. Children who are chronically ill are at greatest risk for tuberculosis pneumonia. Children with a history of tuberculosis who are PPD positive or who demonstrate other symptoms should take isonizid (INH) maintenance therapy for life.

Condition-specific screening

BLOOD WORK. Blood work is drawn at every clinic visit. Most of the following tests are performed: complete blood cell count with differential and platelets, serum potassium, glucose levels, enzymes levels (aspartate aminotransferase [AST], alanine aminotransferase [ALT], phosphate, lactic dehydrogenase [LDH], creatine phosphokinase [CPK], and gamma-glutamyl transpeptidase), uric acid concentration, ammonia level, BUN level, and serum creatinine. Patterns and trends are evaluated for each child. Children on immunosuppressive therapy may develop anemia requiring iron supplements.

Drug levels of cyclosporine or tacrolimus are obtained each time the child has blood work done. The tubes with blood samples are packaged and mailed to the transplant center for consistent monitoring of the child's response to the immunosuppressant drug. Adjustments in immunosuppressant management are made by the transplant center staff.

GRAFT EVALUATION. Children return to the transplant center usually on a yearly basis for follow-up care by the transplant team. A complete history and physical examination are performed. Organ-specific tests such as abdominal ultrasound of the liver, echocardiography, renal flow scan, computerized tomography scan of the abdomen, or biopsy (renal, liver, or endomyocardial) are performed if needed. With any invasive procedure (e.g., cardiac catheterization) the child may require overnight admission to monitor for any complications following the procedure.

COMMON ILLNESS MANAGEMENT

Differential Diagnosis

Fever. Within 3 months of transplantation, these children are at increased risk for bacterial infections related to surgery or viral illness, which can be manifested by a fever. Once the source of the fever is determined, appropriate treatment is instituted. The occurrence of fever may be upsetting to the child and family who fear potential loss of the organ as a result of rejection because fever accompanies rejection. Support, comfort, and explanations of other possible causes should be discussed with the child and family.

Abdominal symptoms. The primary care provider should be aware that children who have renal or liver transplants have not usually had incidental appendectomies along with the transplant surgery. Thus appendicitis cannot be automatically ruled out when symptoms of such occur. Also, children who receive liver transplants have their native gallbladder removed and a cholecystectomy is performed on the donor organ. However, it is possible for children to develop stones that can obstruct the common bile duct, resulting in abdominal pain, jaundice, or fever. Children with abdominal pain should also be screened for complications caused by rejection, ulcers, possible small bowel obstruction, or infection from spontaneous bacterial peritonitis.

Viral illnesses that cause vomiting and diarrhea may result in poor absorption of the immunosup-

---

DIFFERENTIAL DIAGNOSIS

Fever—Common childhood conditions vs rejection

Abdominal symptoms—Common childhood conditions vs obstruction in common bile duct, ulcers, small bowel obstruction, peritonitis, or rejection. Vomiting and diarrhea may result in poor absorption of medications

Metabolic abnormalities—Hyperkalemia, hyperglycemia, and low CO_2 levels may be related to immunosuppressant medications

---

pressant medications, leading to nontherapeutic blood levels. Hydration of the child should be maintained through fluids given orally or intravenously, and intravenous drug therapy considered if the child is unable to orally take and retain their immunosuppressant medication(s).

Metabolic abnormalities. Children usually do not experience metabolic abnormalities when a transplanted graft is functioning properly. Imbalances such as hyperkalemia, hyperglycemia, and low CO_2 levels may be related to high levels of immunosuppressant medications.

Drug Interactions

Cyclosporine absorption can be affected by phenytoin, phenobarbital, ketoconazole (Nizoral), fluconazole (Flucon), diltiazem (Cardiazem), and erythromycin (Erythrocin). Children who have required anticonvulsant drug therapy for seizure control may need higher doses of cyclosporine. Tacrolimus absorption may be affected by some of these same drugs (Prograf product monograph, 1994). In general, over-the-counter medications are to be avoided without the approval of a transplant team professional because the medications may interact with the immunosuppressant therapy. Acetaminophen (Tylenol) rather than aspirin is recommended for fever or headache.

Ibuprofen is excreted by the kidneys and increases creatinine levels in children with renal transplants so therefore should be avoided. Decongestants should also be avoided if the child is on antihypertensive medication. Pseudoephedrine, a common ingredient in decongestants, increases blood pressure.

DEVELOPMENTAL ISSUES

Sleep Patterns

Some children have experienced long hospitalizations before and after the transplantation and may have developed erratic sleep patterns and fears. In addition, nightmares and hallucinations may be precipitated by certain drugs such as tacrolimus, corticosteroids, the stresses of hospitalization, or separation from parents. Corticosteroids have been implicated in impaired sleep, including the decreased need for sleep (Watts et al, 1984). Parents may need to reinstitute familiar home routines and rituals and provide continued emotional support and reassurance until normal patterns return. Professional counseling sessions may be necessary to assist the child to assimilate his or her experiences.

Toileting

The initiation of urine flow in the child with a kidney transplant is often a time of great excitement for the family. The establishment of urinary continence will require support and time for the child to learn to identify the body cues needed for continence. Episodes of incontinence and enuresis are to be expected.

Regression in toileting may be expected in the toddler and preschool age child during and after hospitalization for illness or surgery. Care providers must be understanding of this temporary regression and support the child in regaining toileting skills.

Discipline

For many children who were chronically ill for long periods during the pretransplant phase, certain family role patterns are established. Once the transplant restores children to "health," it is sometimes difficult for families to make the transition from parenting a sick child to parenting a well child. Many parents tend to continue patterns of overprotectiveness. They may have difficulty allowing the child more freedom and insist on setting tight limits that may no longer be warranted.

Noncompliance with immunosuppressive medications resulting in graft loss can occur in adolescents and preadolescents as well as in young adults. Efforts should be made to identify and provide counseling for the child, adolescent, and family who may be at high risk for noncompliance.

Child Care

In general, children who receive transplants are not restricted from day care. However, during the first 2 months after the transplant, children are taking the highest doses of immunosuppressants and are the most susceptible to infections. Accordingly, children should be kept away from people with measles, mumps, varicella, shingles, herpes stomatitis, or influenza. Crowded areas such as airports, movie theaters, or public transportation terminals should be avoided when possible.

Children receiving maintenance doses of immunosuppressants should have adequate immunity to fight the common cold. Thus exposure to other children is of minimal risk. However, parents should be kept informed by the child care provider of any outbreaks of common childhood illnesses, particularly measles or varicella, because contraction of these illnesses places the child at serious risk. When outbreaks occur, home care is advised during the incubation period.

Schooling

It is important for children of school age to return to school as soon as possible. Because of lengthy hospitalization, children often need to repeat a grade in school, attend summer classes, or both. Learning disabilities acquired pretransplant or posttransplant will further complicate the goal of school reentry. Once in the school setting, children are confronted by peers who tease them about their appearance (Kosmach, 1990; Zamberlan, 1989) at an age when peer acceptance and uniformity are critical to self-esteem.

Although most children are receiving maintenance corticosteroid doses by the time of school reentry, corticosteroid-induced mood changes are possible, particularly if the child is being treated with corticosteroid boluses for organ rejection. A school-based practitioner is in an optimal position to meet with these children to assess their current treatment needs and to provide emotional support and reassurance. The nurse's knowledge of the transplant process and the routine medications children are taking may help to develop the child's confidence in the nurse. In addition, such children may benefit from individualized or family counseling to assist them in understanding and coping with the stresses they face. Restrictions on activity are discussed under Safety in this chapter.

Sexuality

As older school-aged children and adolescents recover after transplantation, their bodies undergo often dramatic changes because of the surgery and medications that may result in lifelong alterations in body image. Transplant surgery usually results in extensive incisional scars.

Sternotomy incisions in heart/heart-lung transplant recipients are difficult to conceal. Asymmetry of the breasts is sometimes seen with the sternotomy incision in females. One breast may rest higher than the other or one breast may be slightly smaller in size.

In addition, physical appearance is altered by medication side effects, including hirsutism, obesity, Cushingoid faces, and discoloration of teeth. Thus it is not surprising that some adolescents who have organ transplants infrequently engage in dating and display a cautious attitude toward sexuality (Kosmach, 1990). Such adolescents may be at risk for psychosocial and emotional difficulties (Kosmach, 1990) and may benefit from professional counseling. Remedies such as electrolysis and cosmetic surgery, though costly, may be helpful to improve self-esteem.

As more pediatric transplant recipients survive to reach childbearing age, concerns about contraception and childbearing become more prominent. For contraceptive management, barrier methods of birth control are recommended because oral contraceptives may precipitate thrombus formation. The effects of long-term use of immunosuppressive agents by transplant recipients on the unborn child are not well known. Women have had successful pregnancies after renal transplantation and reports suggest that women who have undergone liver transplantation and immunosuppressive therapy are able to safely have children, although with an increased risk of premature and cesarean births. The majority of the offspring have had normal physical and mental development thus far (Scantlebury et al, 1990).

Sexually active teenagers with heart transplants worry about the strain of sexual activity and childbearing on the new heart. Sexual activity can resume 6 to 8 weeks after surgery. Childbearing in the heart transplant recipient has been discouraged in the past (Wagoner et al, 1994). A recent study of 194 heart transplant centers found 32 known pregnancies in heart and heart-lung transplant recipients. The results showed 29 children born in good health with prematurity (41%) and low birth weight (17%) as the most common complications (Wagoner et al, 1994).

Transition into Adulthood

Transition from adolescence into adulthood is often difficult and challenging for healthy individuals. The adolescent with a transplant struggles with the same issues of independency and separation in an attempt to define his or her identity and plan for the future. Parental conflicts over autonomy verses dependency are often seen in families of children with chronic illness as they approach adulthood. Parental coping and peer validation play an important part in this transition. Concerns of sexuality, pregnancy, fear of organ rejection, infection, and death continue to be important for this population. The psychologic incorporation of the donor organ into the self image may be a difficult task for the recipient. Issues of body image as a result of long-term immunosuppression drugs are important to the adolescent transplant pursuing career goals or a potential life partner. A negative body image can often lead to noncompliance with medications in an attempt to alter drug-induced changes. Employability and insurability are of concern because of a preexisting condition and any physical limitations. Financial issues become more realistic to the young adult when childhood health care coverage is discontinued. The social workers involved with the transplant programs can help the adolescent transition into adulthood by providing vocational guidance, self-acceptance, and individual/family counseling through this difficult period.

SPECIAL FAMILY CONCERNS AND RESOURCES

Parents are often concerned about the effect of the transplant process on the entire family and wonder how to reestablish a normal home life after transplantation. Fears of organ rejection and the possibility of an unsuccessful search for another donor organ, leading to the child's death, are paramount (Weichler, 1990). Also, the psychologic incorporation of the donor organ into the self-image may be a difficult task for the recipient. Another concern for families is the financial impact of the transplant process. Hospitalization, surgery, immunosuppressive and other medications, housing near the transplant center, and day-to-day living expenses amass to a major financial burden for many families. Financial support can come from third-party health insurance payers, community fund raising, state funding, or self-pay through the family's own resources. Families are in need of information and emotional support from the transplant team and primary care providers to cope with their fears, future milestones, and financial aspects of organ transplantation.

Some families, as a result of cultural or religious beliefs, may refuse to accept organ transplantation as a medical option or donate organs for living-related transplants or cadavar transplants. In some cultures keeping the physical body intact is important because it houses the "spirit" of the person. Health care providers must be sensitive to these cultural beliefs.

Organizations

American Liver Foundation
1425 Pompton Ave
Cedar Grove, NJ 07009
(800) 223-0179

National Heart Assist and Transplant Fund
PO Box 258
Bryn Mawr, PA 19010
(610) 527-5056

American Kidney Fund
6110 Executive Blvd, No 1010
Rockville, MD 20852
(301) 881-3052(212) 867-4486

National Disease Research Interchange
1880 JFK Blvd
6th Floor
Philadelphia, PA 19103
(215) 557-7361

National Kidney Foundation
30 East 33rd St.
New York, NY 10016
(212) 889-2210

Renal Physicians' Association
1101 Vermont Ave, NW, No 500
Washington, DC 20005-3547
(202) 835-0436

United Network for Organ Sharing
3001 Hungary Spring Rd
PO Box 28010
Richmond, VA 23228
(804) 330-8500

Transplant Recipients' International Organization
244 N Bellefield Ave
Pittsburgh, PA 15213
(412) 734-5698

SUMMARY OF PRIMARY CARE NEEDS FOR THE CHILD WITH AN ORGAN TRANSPLANT

Health care maintenance

Growth and development

Height and weight should be measured each visit.

Linear growth may be affected by long-term corticosteroid use.

Catch-up growth may be attained after transplantation.

Improved physical development after transplantation has a positive effect on psychosocial development.

Cognitive functioning should be monitored.

Diet

Prednisone may cause overeating, leading to weight gain; dietary planning is needed for well-balanced meals and possibly sodium-restricted diets.

Children with heart transplants should reduce cholesterol and saturated fats.

Safety

Precautions with animal feces, especially cat litter boxes, is recommended to prevent transmission of disease to children who are immuno-suppressed.

Prednisone predisposes to sunburn.

No contact sports.

Medic-Alert bracelets are recommended.

Exercise restrictions are necessary for the first 6 to 8 weeks to allow for healing. Activity should decrease when fatigue occurs.

Immunizations

Immunodeficient children should receive DPT and IPV immunizations.

The MMR vaccine is safe for children after transplantations.

Haemophilus influenzae type b vaccine is recommended for children starting at 2 months.

Varicella-zoster immune globulin must be administered within 72 hours of exposure to varicella for seronegative children.

Varicella vaccine is contraindicated in children with transplants.

Pretransplant immunization against hepatitis B is recommended.

Screening

　Vision

Yearly examinations should be given for changes in eyesight, blurry vision, cataracts, glaucoma or pseudotumor cerebri from immunosuppressants.

　Hearing

Audiograms should be done yearly to evaluate hearing loss from ototoxic drugs.

　Dental

Dental screening should be done at minimum every 6 months, with prophylactic antibiotics used. Cyclosporine and extended release nifedipine may cause gingival hyperplasia.

　Blood pressure

Blood pressure should be checked at each visit; the effectiveness of antihypertensive medication should be evaluated.

　Hematocrit

Routine screening is deferred because of posttransplant blood tests.

　Urinalysis

UAs done as part of posttransplant assessment.

Additional routine screening is not necessary unless symptomatic.

　Tuberculosis

Routine screening is recommended.

　Condition-specific screening

BLOOD WORK

At each follow-up transplant clinic visit multiple blood tests are done and assessed for patterns and trends. Serum drug levels are also tested.

GRAFT EVALUATION

Diagnostic testing is done yearly to evaluate graft function.

Common illness management

Differential diagnosis

　Fever

Normal childhood illnesses should be ruled out; fever may indicate organ rejection or infection.

Continued.

SUMMARY OF PRIMARY CARE NEEDS FOR THE CHILD WITH AN ORGAN TRANSPLANT—cont'd

Abdominal symptoms

Abdominal pain should be investigated to rule out appendicitis or intestinal obstruction, ulcers, and peritonitis; vomiting and diarrhea may lower therapeutic blood levels of immunosuppressant drugs.

Metabolic abnormalities

Hyperkalemia can result from drug therapy; hyperglycemia may result from immunosuppressant medications.

Drug interactions

Cyclosporine and tacrolimus absorption is altered by phenytoin, phenobarbital, ketoconazole, erythromycin, fluconazole, and diltiazem.

Higher doses of cyclosporine may be needed to achieve therapeutic range when it is administered with anticonvulsants.

Use acetaminophen instead of aspirin or ibuprofen.

Avoid decongestants if hypertensive.

Developmental issues

Sleep patterns

Hospitalization or drugs may alter sleep patterns.

Toileting

Urinary continence may require support in children with kidney transplants.

Discipline

Parental overprotectiveness is likely; parents may need help to promote independence in their children.

Noncompliance with medications may occur with adolescents.

Child care

The children may attend day care; precautions should be taken to limit exposure to communicable diseases.

Schooling

Normal schooling should be resumed after transplantation.

Alterations in body image may negatively affect peer interactions.

Sexuality

The transplant experience may affect body image and self-esteem.

Barrier methods of birth control are recommended.

Childbearing after transplantation has produced normal children.

Transition into adulthood

Difficulty attaining independence.

Body image and intimacy may be negatively affected.

Concerns over employment and health insurance develop.

Special family concerns

Special family concerns include fear of rejection, search for a new organ, organ donor issues, and finances.

REFERENCES

Abelmann W, Lorell B: The challenges of cardiomyopathy, *J Am Coll Cardiol* 13:1219-1239, 1989.

Aluzri A et al: Aggressive early cyclosporine therapy is desirable in pediatric renal transplantation, *Trans Proc* 26:88-90, 1994.

American Heart Association: If your child has a congenital heart defect, 1-49, 1994.

Bailey L et al: Method of heart transplantation for treatment of hypoplastic left heart syndrome, *J Thorac Cardiovas Surg* 92:1-5, 1986.

Bailey L et al: Orthotopic transplantation during early infancy as therapy for incurable congenital heart disease, *Ann Surg* 208:279-286, 1988.

Baker A: Acquired heart disease in infants and children, *Crit Care Nurs Clin of North Am* 6:175-185, 1994.

Baluarte H, Braas C, and Kaiser B: Postoperative management of pediatric transplant patient. In Tejani A, Fine R (editors): *Pediatric renal transplantation,* New York, 1994, Wiley-Liss, pp 23-27.

Baum D et al: Pediatric heart transplantation at Stanford: results of a 15-year experience, *Pediatrics* 88:203-214, 1991.

Baum M et al: Growth and neurodevelopmental outcome of infants undergoing heart transplantation, *Journal of Heart and Lung Transplantation* 12(6 Pt 2):S211-217, 1993.

Boucek M et al: Cardiac transplantation in infancy: donors and recipients. *J Pediatr* 116:171-176, 1990.

Broelsch CE et al: Evolution and future perspectives for reduced sized hepatic transplants, *Surgery, Gynecology and Obstetrics* 171, Oct 1991.

Buckingham S: Personal communication, April 30, 1995.

Burch M et al: Dilated cardiomyopathy in children: determinants of outcome, *Br Heart J* 72:246-250, 1994.

California Pacific Medical Center Department of Transplant: *Quarterly progress report,* July 1993.

Cellcept (mycophenolate mofetil) Roche Laboratories. product monograph, Nutley, NJ, May 1995.

Ciszewski A et al: Dilated cardiomyopathy in children: clinical course and prognosis, *Pediatr Cardiol* 15:121-126, 1994.

Cohn R: Preemptive transplantation. In Tejani A, Fine R (editors): *Pediatric renal transplantation,* New York, 1994, Wiley-Liss, pp 23-37.

Committee on Infectious Diseases: *Report of the committee on infectious diseases,* ed 23, Elk Grove Village, IL, 1994, The American Academy of Pediatrics.

Conte J et al: Pediatric heart-lung transplantation: intermediate term results, Publication pending 1-20, 1995. Journal of Heart Lung Transplantation-submitted.

Cooley D et al: Organ transplantation for advanced cardiopulmonary disease, *Ann Thorac Surg* 8:30-46, 1969.

Cox K: Personal communication, Mar 1993.

Cox K et al: An increased incidence of Epstein-Barr virus infection and lymphoproliferative disorder in young children on FK-506 after liver transplantation, *Transplantation* 59:524-529, 1995.

Esquivel CO et al: Impact of liver reduction in pediatric liver transplantation, Arch Surg 1286, Oct 1991.

Ettenger R, Grimm P, and Firzli E: Kidney transplant in children. In Danovitch G (editor): *Handbook of kidney transplantation,* Boston, 1992, Little, Brown, pp 305-337.

Falkenstein K et al: Impact of steroid withdrawal on growth in the pediatric liver transplant, *Journal of Transplant Coordination* 2:1-3, 1992.

Ferraresso M, Kahan B: Immunosuppressive strategies for the pediatric population. In Tejani A, Fine R (editors): *Pediatric renal transplantation,* New York, 1994, Wiley-Liss, pp 23-37.

Fine R: Recent advances in the management of the infant, child,

and adolescent with chronic renal failure, *Pediatr Rev* 11:277-283, 1990.

Fowles R: Natural history and prognosis of overt dilated cardiomyopathy. In Baroldi G, Camerini F, and Goodwin J, (editors): *Advances in cardiomyopathies,* Berlin, 1990, Springer-Verlag, pp 337-346.

Friedman A: Diagnosis of acute rejection. In Tejani A, Fine R (editors): *Pediatric renal transplantation,* New York, 1994, Wiley-Liss, pp 269-276.

Fullerton D et al: Heart transplantation in children and young adults: early and intermediate-term results, *Ann Thorac Surg* 59:804-812, 1995.

Fung J et al: Conversion from cyclosporine to FK-506 in liver allograft recipients with cyclosporine-related complications, *Transplant Proc* 22(suppl 1):6-12, 1990.

Gershon A: Immunizations for pediatric transplant patients, *Kidney International* 44(Supp 43):S87-90, 1993.

Gillum R: Idiopathic cardiomyopathy in the United States, 1970–1982, *Am Heart J* 111:752-755, 1986.

Harmon W, Jabs K: Factors affecting growth after renal transplantation, *J Am Soc Nephrol* 2:S295-S303, 1992.

Ho M et al: The frequency of Epstein-Barr virus infection and associated lymphoproliferative syndrome after transplantation and its manifestations in children, *Transplantation* 45:719-727, 1988.

Hosenpud J et al: The registry of the international society for heart and lung transplantation: eleventh official report— 1994, *J Heart-Lung Transplantation* 13:561-570, 1994.

Iwatsuki S et al: Liver transplantation for fulminant hepatic failure, *Transplant Proc* 21:2431-2434, 1989.

Kantrowitz A et al: Transplantation of the heart in an infant and an adult, *Am J Cardiol* 22:782-790, 1968.

Kaufman D, Jones J, and Matas: New immunosuppressive agents: FK-506, rapamycin, RS-61443, 15-deoxyspergualin, *J Transplant Coordination* 2:20-27, 1992.

Kocoshis S et al: Pediatric liver transplantation history, recent innovations and outlook for the future, *Clin Pediatr* 7:386-391, 1993.

Kosmach B: *Adolescents' responses to quality of life issues following liver transplantation,* master's thesis, Pittsburgh, 1990, University of Pittsburgh.

Kosmach D: Personal communication, Children's Hospital of Pittsburgh, Department of Transplant Surgery, August 17, 1995.

Laine J et al: Renal transplantation in children with emphasis on the young patient, *Pediatr Nephrol* 8:313-319, 1994.

Lower RR, Shumway NE: Studies on orthotopic transplantation of the canine heart, *Surg Forum* 11:18-19, 1960.

Malatack J: Personal communication, June 29, 1990.

McDiarmid S et al: FK-506 (tacrolimus) compared with cyclosporine for primary immunosuppression after pediatric liver transplantation. Results from the US Multicenter Trial, *Transplantation* 59:530, 1995.

Merrill W et al: Heart transplantation in children, *Ann Surg* 5:393-398, 1991.

North American Pediatric Renal Transplant Cooperative Study Annual Report, 1994, pp 1-10.

Prograf (tacrolimus) product monograph, Deerfield, IL, Oct 1994, Fujisawa.

Ramos H et al: Weaning of immunosuppression in long-term liver transplant recipients, *Transplantation* 59(2):212-217, 1995.

Rao A et al: Augmentation of chimerism in whole organ recipients by simultaneous infusion of donor bone marrow cells. Transplantation Proceedings, XVth World Congress of the Transplantation Society, Kyoto, Japan, 1994.

Rees L: Growth posttransplantation in children: steroid and growth inhibition. In Tejani A, Fine R (editors): *Pediatric renal transplantation,* New York, 1994, Wiley-Liss, pp 423-436.

Reitz B: Heart and heart-lung transplantation. In Braunwald E (editor): *Heart disease: a textbook of cardiovascular medicine,* Philadelphia, 1992, WB Saunders, p 527.

Reyes J et al: Postoperative care of small bowel transplant recipients, *Care of the Crit Ill* 9(5):193-198, 1993.

Sandimmune (cyclosporine) product monograph, East Hanover, NJ, 1993, Sandoz Pharmaceutical

Sarris G et al: Pediatric cardiac transplantation: The Stanford experience, *Circulation* 90(5)(supp 2):51-55, 1994.

Scantlebury V, Gordon R, Tzakis A, et al: Childbearing after liver transplantation. *Transplantation* 49:317-321, 1990

Sollinger H (editor): *Recent developments in transplant medicine: new immunosuppressant drugs,* 1994, Physician's and Scientist's Publishing Co.

Spray T: Projections for pediatric heart-lung and lung transplantation, *J Heart-Lung Transplant* 12:S337-S343, 1993.

Starnes V et al: Heart, heart-lung, and lung transplantation in the first year of life, *Ann Thorac Surg* 53:306-310, 1992.

Starzl T et al: Evolution of liver transplantation, *Hepatology* 2:614-636, 1982.

Starzl T et al: Fifteen years of clinical liver transplantation, *Gastroenterology* 77:375-388, 1979.

Starzl T et al: The role of cell migration and chimerism in organ transplant acceptance and tolerance induction, *Transplantation Science* 3(1):47-50, 1993.

Starzl T et al: The role of organ transplantation in pediatrics, *Pediatr Clin North Am* 13:381-420, 1966.

Stewart S et al: Cognitive patterns in school-age children with end-stage liver disease, *Dev Behav Pediatr* 13:331-338, 1992.

Stewart S et al: Neurophysiologic function in young children who have undergone liver transplantation, *J Pediatr Psychol* 16:569-583, 1991a.

Stewart S et al: Neuropsychologic outcome of pediatric liver transplantation, *Pediatrics* 87:367-376, 1991b.

Terasaki P, Park M, and Danovitch G: Histocompatability testing, crossmatching, allocation of cadaver kidney transplants. In Danovitch G (editor): *Handbook of kidney transplantation,* Boston, 1992, Little, Brown, pp 43-65.

Trento A et al: Lessons learned in pediatric heart transplantation, *Ann Thorac Surg* 48:617-623, 1989.

United Network for Organ Sharing (UNOS) Update: 1994 Annual Report of the US Scientific Registry of Transplant Recipients and the Organ Procurement and Transplantation Network, 11(3), 1995.

US Multicenter FK-506 Liver Study Group: A comparison of tacrolimus (FK-506) and cyclosporine for immunosuppression in liver transplantation, *New Engl J Med,* 331(17):1110-1115, 1994.

Wagoner L et al: Immunosuppressive therapy, management, and outcome of heart transplant recipients during pregnancy, *J Heart-Lung Transplant* 13:993-1000, 1994.

Wanek EA et al: Biliary atresia, *Pediatr Rev* 11:57-62, 1989.

Watts D, Freeman A, McGiffin D et al: Psychiatric aspects of cardiac transplantation. *Heart Transplant* 3:243-247. 1984.

Weichler N: Information needs of mothers of children who have liver transplants. *J Pediatr Nurs* 5:88-96, 1990.

Whitington P, Balisteri W: Liver transplantation in pediatrics: indications, contraindications, and pretransplant management. *J Pediatr* 118(2), 1991.

Wray J et al: Cognitive function and behavioral status in pediatric heart and heart-lung transplant recipients: the harefield experience, *BMJ* 309:837-841, 1994.

Zamberlan K: Quality of life in school age children following liver transplantation, *Matern Child Nurs J,* fall/winter 1992.

Zitelli B et al: Changes in lifestyle after liver transplantation, *Pediatrics* 82:173-180, 1988.

Phenylketonuria

29

Kathleen Schmidt Yule

ETIOLOGY

Phenylketonuria (PKU) is an autosomal recessive inherited metabolic disorder that causes plasma phenylalanine (phe) levels to rise to more than $1000 \mu M$ (16.5 mg/dL).[1] Phenylketonuria is caused by a mutation of the phenylalanine hydroxylase (PAH) gene and exposure to elevated blood phe. Clinically less harmful than PKU, mild hyperphenylalaninemia (HPA) is a related disorder in which phe levels are greater than $120 \mu M$ but less than $1000 \mu M$. Phenylketonuria is clinically distinguished from non-PKU HPA by a lower tolerance for dietary phe (<500 mg/day). Mild HPA can have the same effects as PKU in some cases (Scriver et al, 1995).

The metabolic pathway for phe is in the liver: PAH, an enzyme, converts phe by hydroxylation to tyrosine (tyr) in the hepatocyte for use in the biosynthesis of (1) protein, (2) melanin, (3) thyroxine, and (4) the catecholamines in the brain and adrenal medulla. Loss of PAH activity causes an accumulation of normal phe metabolites, phenylpyruvic acid, and derivatives (phenylketones), which the kidney has a finite capacity to excrete when plasma phe reaches $1000 \mu M$. There are no abnormal metabolites in PKU, only normal metabolites in abnormal amounts. A high level of phe inhibits the entry of large neutral amino acids into the brain; essential

cellular processes of myelination and protein synthesis in the brain are disrupted causing a deficient neurotransmitter supply to the brain and the neuropathology of PKU (Kaufman, 1989; Hommes, 1991; Scriver et al, 1995).

In a growing child the recommended dietary allowance (RDA) for phe is used by the body in two major ways: (1) up to 60% is used for new tissue protein synthesis, decreasing with age, and (2) 40% is hydroxylated to form tyr. Homeostasis of phe in the body reflects the interaction among (1) a dietary intake of phe; (2) turnover of the body's tissue protein; and (3) outflow by means of hydroxylation (to form tyr), transamination (to form pheynlypyruvic acid and derivatives), and conversion to other minor metabolites under the control of multiple independent genes and the PAH gene (Scriver et al, 1995; Treacy et al, 1994).

The phe hydroxylation system is a complex biochemical reaction that requires the presence of tetrahydrobiopterin (BH_4), oxygen, and phe. Three enzymes responsible for the synthesis and regeneration of BH_4 are also necessary for the hydroxylation of phe (see Fig. 29-1). A deficiency of any one of these enzymes causes a deficiency of BH_4 and HPA. Characterized by progressive neurologic deterioration, BH_4-deficient disorders are phenotypically and genotypically distinct from PKU, require different modes of therapy, and have a different prognosis (Blau et al, 1993; Blau et al, 1995).

Because both PKU and the BH_4-deficient disorders present with neonatal HPA, screening for

---

[1]To convert phe from μM (same as μmol/L) to mg/dL, multiply [x phe μM] by .0165. To convert phe from mg/dl to μM, multiply mg/dl by 60.53.

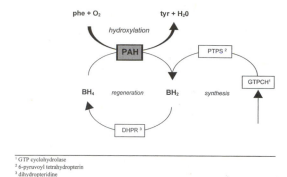

Fig. 29-1.   The phenylalanine hydroxylation system.

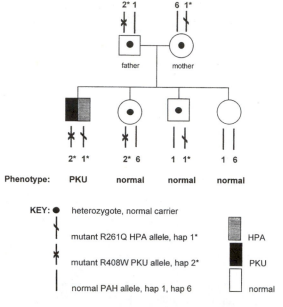

Fig. 29-2.   Hypothetical family pedigree showing segregation of mutant PKU and mutant HPA alleles with haplotype.

BH$_4$ deficiency should be done in all newborns with HPA. Older children with microcephaly, mental retardation, convulsions (grand mal or myoclonic), disturbances of tone and posture, abnormal movements, drowsiness, diurnal fluctuation of alertness, irritability, hypersalivation, swallowing difficulties, or recurrent hyperthermia without infection should also be tested for HPA and the BH$_4$-deficient disorders (Blau et al, 1993).

Phenylketonuria is the result of over 100 different mutations in the PAH gene on chromosome 12. Because all cases of true PKU and 95% of all cases of mild HPA are the result of a mutation at the PAH locus, this locus is the PKU locus in humans. A mutation changes the DNA code for PAH protein, creating an unstable enzyme with varying degrees of activity, less than 1% of normal activity for PKU and 2% to 5% for mild HPA (Scriver et al, 1995). This high degree of genetic diversity at the PAH locus partially accounts for the clinical spectrum of HPA observed in PKU and mild HPA.

All individuals inherit two PAH alleles at the PAH locus—one from each parent. PAH alleles that encode for the abnormal production of little or no functional PAH enzyme are mutant PKU alleles. If both alleles inherited carry identical mutations for PKU, the individual is homozygous for PKU at the locus; if each allele carries a different mutation, the individual is compound heterozygous for PKU at the locus. Mutation analysis of DNA has revealed that approximately 75% of PKU cases are compound heterozygotes for PKU alleles; each parent contributed a different PKU mutation. Alternatively, because PKU alleles and mild HPA alleles are allelic, an individual can inherit them together and be compound heterozygous for both PKU and mild HPA (Fig. 29-2). Clinically this explains why individuals with PKU, mild HPA, and even affected siblings have different degrees of HPA (Svensson et al, 1992; Scriver et al, 1995).

Of the individuals with PKU, 10% to 15% have no identifiable mutation by present methods of DNA analysis (Scriver et al, 1995). All individuals have identifiable normal variations in the DNA surrounding the PAH locus on chromosome 12 called *restriction fragment length polymorphisms* (RFLPs). Because eight specific RFLPs segregate with the PKU mutation on the PAH gene, when they do they act as markers for PKU and are called *PKU haplotypes* (haps); out of 384 possible PKU haps, hap analysis to date has identified 70 and assigned a hap number to each (Scriver et al, 1995).

Because PKU and mild HPA follow the Mendelian autosomal recessive pattern of inheritance, PKU hap analysis can trace the segregation pattern of the PKU alleles in a family at 25% risk for PKU with each offspring (see Fig. 29-2) without direct mutation analysis. The sensitivity of DNA testing for PKU is lower than testing for plasma HPA; polymorphic markers in gametic association with a PKU mutation are used together for the fetal diagnosis of PKU; currently, prenatal diagnosis can be 90% to 95% informative. Direct DNA mutation analysis for PKU is indicated for sperm and ovum donors, with or without phenotypic expression of HPA (Scriver et al, 1995; Jones, 1994).

Direct DNA analysis in a newborn with PKU is a valuable tool for identifying the specific mutation and further defining the severity of PKU so that therapy can be optimized and long-term prognosis anticipated and enhanced (Scriver et al, 1995). Mutation analysis of 12 haps characterized 56.5% of the PKU alleles in 112 children with PKU in the Midwest; both PKU alleles were identified in 35% of the children, 9.4% were homozygous for the R408W mutation, the rest were compound heterozygotes for this specific mutation with another PKU mutation (Kaul et al, 1994).

INCIDENCE

PKU is prevalent in many populations. The incidence of PKU ranges from 5 to 385 cases per 1 million live births (see Table 29-1). The worldwide incidence of PKU in Caucasian populations is 1:10,000. Based on this incidence, 1 out of 50 Caucasians carries the PKU gene and the PKU gene frequency in Caucasians is 1%, the same as in the Chinese. Carriers, or gene frequency in populations, remain constant from generation to generation despite availability of carrier testing and prenatal diagnosis. The incidence of PKU in the black population in the United States is 1:50,000 (Hofman et al, 1991).

Both PKU and mild HPA are currently screened for using nonselective newborn screening (NBS) in all 50 states and in more than 30 countries. There will continue to be individuals of all ages who may or may not know whether they were previously screened, diagnosed, and treated for PKU or even that they have mild HPA. It is estimated that at least 10% of individuals with untreated PKU may have near normal intelligence quotients (IQ's).

Women with PKU are a clinically significant group because their offspring are at risk for maternal PKU (MPKU) syndrome. Over 50% of all

Table 29-1.

INCIDENCES OF HYPERPHENYLALANINEMIA VARIANTS BY PHENOTYPE, REGION, AND ETHNIC GROUP

Variant	Geographic region or ethnic group	Incidence (per 10^6 births)
PKU	Turkey	385
	Yemenite Jews	190
	Scotland	190
	Eire	190
	Czechoslovakia	150
	Poland	130
	Hungary	90
	France	75
	Scandinavia	
	Denmark	85
	Norway	70
	Sweden	25
	Finland	5
	England (London region)	70
	Italy	60
	China	60
	Canada	45
	Japan	7
	Ashkenazi Jews	5
Non-PKU HPA	All regions except Finland	15-75
BH_4-deficient HPA	Panethnic and panregional	1-2

Adapted from Scriver CR et al: The hyperphenylalaninemias. In Scriver CR, (editors): *The Metabolic and Molecular Bases of Inherited Disease,* ed 7, New York, 1995, McGraw-Hill, vol I, pp 1037.

births in North America and Europe are to women unscreened for PKU. Women with mild HPA can produce offspring with severe MPKU embryopathy. Mothers of newborns with transient HPA, as well as mothers who have delivered infants with any of the features of MPKU syndrome, should be tested for PKU (Hanley, 1994).

Case findings for PKU, mild HPA, and MPKU syndrome should be paramount in the primary care provider's mind when (1) a presumptive positive

PKU NBS test result is reported, even if the newborn is found negative on recall testing (mild HPA); (2) the newborn is premature, (3) a child has unexplained microcephaly, intrauterine or postnatal growth delay, dysmorphic facial features, congenital anomalies, particularly a congenital heart defect or harsh systolic murmur (MPKU syndrome); (4) an infant has unexplained developmental delay or a child has any degree of mental retardation; (5) the family immigrated to the United States; and (6) the maternal history includes a spontaneous abortion (SAB), stillbirth, rash, seizures, poor coordination of unknown etiology, any degree of mental retardation, or when the mother was born before 1967 (Acosta and Wright, 1992).

Newborn screening (NBS) programs are the greatest referral of HPA cases. The primary care provider's role in NBS is critical (Buist and Tuerck, 1992). The lack of universal NBS standards, tests or legislation, and different technologies available for the testing of phe make uniform recommendations for providers difficult. Knowledge about specific regional NBS program practices (Council of Regional Networks for Genetic Services [CORN], 1994; Kling, 1993) and consultation with the regional NBS coordinator are mandatory for the follow-up protocol of presumptive positive HPA NBS test results. Different conditions, treatments, and other biologic variables at the time of testing can alter the phe level; the provider must be alert to the causes of false-negative and false-positive results in the newborn (Schmidt, 1989). Discharging newborns early from the hospital after birth can affect NBS testing for HPA. The follow-up varies depending on the methodology employed by the regional NBS program Jew, 1995; (Jew et al, 1994; Lorey and Cunningham, 1994; Arnopp et al, 1995).

CLINICAL MANIFESTATIONS AT TIME OF DIAGNOSIS

The NBS test alone does not establish the diagnosis of PKU: a positive PKU test result does not constitute the diagnosis of PKU; nor does a negative PKU test result dismiss the possibility of PKU. Further investigation for PKU is warranted in a child with manifestations of untreated PKU. Berg (1984) states:

CLINICAL MANIFESTATIONS

Normal appearance at birth
Fair pigmentation
Irritability
Neonatal vomiting
Infantile spasms
Generalized epilepsy
Microcephaly
Atopic dermatitis
Mousey odor of urine and sweat
Increased deep tendon reflexes
Plantar responses variable
Tailor's sitting position
Fine rapid irregular tremor
Parkinson's-like movements
Bony changes in growth plate
Decreased height in males
Increased weight in females
Delayed motor skills
Delayed intellectual skills
Delayed speech and language skills
Decreased IQ
Hyperphenylalaninemia

Affected infants usually appear normal at birth, but within several months become irritable and may have recurring vomiting. Though milestones may be reached at a normal time, they are usually delayed in both motor and intellectual skills. Acquisition of speech and language is delayed. Seizures occur in at least 25% of untreated PKU patients and in early life are typically infantile spasms. As the patients become older, the convulsions assume other forms of generalized epilepsies. Microcephaly is common and increased muscle tone with hyperreflexia is generally present. Patients often assume an unusual seated position, "schneidersitz" (tailor's position) and many children have a fine, rapid and irregular tremor at rest as well as with outstretched arms. The plantar responses are variable. Electroencephalograms are usually abnormal and hypsarrhythmia is commonly found, sometimes when no clinical convulsive activity has been noted.

If untreated, the toxic effects of phe in a child with PKU cause a drop in developmental quotient to 50 points by 1 year of age and to 30 points by 3 years of age (Koch and Wenz, 1987). Since the advent of NBS and earlier diagnosis and treatment, it has been demonstrated that an average of 10 intelligence quotient (IQ) points are lost if phe homeostasis is not achieved during the first month of life and an additional 10 points is lost if it is not achieved by the second month (Fishler et al, 1987; Smith, Beasley, and Ades, 1990).

Boys with untreated PKU have measurements for height that are consistently 2 SDs less than the mean when compared with boys without PKU. In contrast, mean height and weight measurements for girls with untreated PKU are consistently 2 SDs more than the mean when compared with girls without PKU (Fisch, Gravem, and Feinberg, 1966). Characteristic mesodermal changes in the growth plate of long bones of intrauterine origin are characteristic in neonates and children with PKU, both untreated and early treated (Fisch et al, 1991a).

Of the children with untreated PKU, 20% to 40% have eczema, an atopic dermatitis with predilection for flexural creases on the arms and legs, indistinguishable from that in children who do not have PKU (Irons and Levy, 1986). A lingering musty odor sometimes described as mousey, barn-like, or old urine is commonly present and is secondary to the urinary excretion of phenylacetic acid, which accumulates over the first month of life. Typically the child with PKU has a fairer complexion than the composite coloring of other family members, which is related to inhibitions of tyr metabolism and reduced melanin production. In ethnic backgrounds where black hair is expected, this feature will be expressed as hair that is brown or even reddish. Caucasians will typically have blonde hair and blue eyes. Because these manifestations are not pronounced at birth, their expression may not be evident until irreversible brain damage has already occurred.

The results of complete blood cell count, routine urinalysis, and liver, renal, and endocrine function tests are normal in children with untreated PKU (Koch and Wenz, 1987). The concurrence of PKU with other genetic disorders is relatively uncommon, though can occur, such as with Down syndrome (author's experience), and less com-

---

TREATMENT

Phe-restricted diet
Supplement tyr if low
Provide nutrients to support normal growth and
    development

---

mon with Goldenhar syndrome (Tokatli et al, 1994) is possible.

TREATMENT

Treatment for PKU is simple in theory but difficult in practice. It involves restricting phe in the diet to maintain a nontoxic level of plasma phe between 2 and 6 mg/dl while allowing optimum growth and brain development by supplementing the diet with adequate sources of energy, protein, and other nutrients. Tyrosine is supplemented when plasma tyr levels are less than 0.33 mg/dl. Optimal management is a phe-restricted diet initiated within the first 2 weeks of life and continued throughout childhood, adolescence, and adulthood, especially before conception and throughout pregnancy for the benefit of the offspring.

Clinical tolerance of phe distinguishes PKU from mild HPA. The phe requirement for infants and young children with PKU is between 250 and 500 mg/day and not more than 1.5 times greater than this level in the older child. Children with PKU have a narrower tolerance between the lower and upper limits of required phe than individuals with greater PAH activity. An individual with HPA requiring dietary restriction of phe to maintain a plasma phe level of less than 10 mg/dl needs treatment regardless of the distinction made between PKU and mild HPA. Tolerance of phe is observed over time and can change within weeks, months, or even years. Rarely, PKU and mild HPA can be transient, and a child's tolerance for phe can increase to normal levels because of either a regulatory defect affecting PAH activity or a transient disorder of biopterin metabolism. Careful and continuous monitoring of individuals whose phe intake is restricted is necessary to avoid phe deficiency when tolerance changes because of these rare cases or because of changes related to growth rate.

Dietary restriction of phe is accomplished by the use of commercially available elemental medical foods (EMFs). These products are modified protein hydrolysates in which phe is removed or are mixtures of free amino acids that do not contain phe. EMFs provide the essential amino acids in suitable proportions for the given age of the individual (see Table 29-2). Because natural protein contains 2.4% to 9% of phe by weight, adequate protein cannot be obtained from natural foods without ingesting excess phe. Therefore, phe-restricted diets are usually designed so that EMF products provide the majority of the essential nutrients with the exception of the caloric requirement, which is derived from no-protein or low-protein, high-calorie natural sources. Nutrient intakes must be sufficient to meet the anabolic requirements of the individual and maintain essential conversion reactions (Acosta and Yannicelli, 1993).

Phenylalanine-restricted diets are prescribed by the medical genetics PKU treatment center team who continually monitor the child's phe tolerance. Individuals' phe requirements depend on PAH activity, age, growth rate, adequacy of energy and protein intakes, and state of health (see Table 29-3).

The greatest benefits of continuing the diet are in those areas of cognitive functioning measured by IQ tests and by the reading and spelling subtests of the Wide Range Achievement Test (WRAT). There is a strong relationship between the IQ of the child and the age at which dietary control is lost (blood phe level consistently more than 15 mg/dl) (see Table 29-4). The best predictor of IQ in a child with PKU and of the deficit in IQ between the child and unaffected siblings or parents is the age when dietary control is lost. The IQ deficit is greatest when phe control is lost before 6 years of age. If phe control continues past 8 years of age to at least 12 years of age, IQ remains at the national average; there is virtually no change in IQ between 6 and 12 years of age (Fishler et al, 1987; Azen et al, 1991; Koch et al, 1993).

Children with late-diagnosed PKU should also be placed on the phe-restricted diet no matter how

Table 29-2.

MEDICAL FOODS USED IN THE TREATMENT OF PKU ACCORDING TO DEVELOPMENTAL STAGE

Developmental stage	Medical food
Infant/Toddler:	Phenex-1*
	PKU 1†
	Lofenalac†
	XP Analog‡
Child:	Phenex-2*
	(Red Punch and Grapefruit Flavonex optional)
	PKU 2†
	Phenyl-Free†
	XP Maxamaid‡
	(Unflavored and Orange flavor)
	Periflex‡
	(Unflavored and Orange-pineapple flavor)
	Maxamaid XP Bar‡
	(Apricot flavor)
	Phenyl Ade** (Vanilla, Orange Creme and Strawberry
	Phenyl Ade Amino Acid Bar** (Chocolate and Chocolate Crispy)
Adult:	Phenex-2*
	PKU 3†
	Phenyl-Free†
	XP Maxamum‡
	(Unflavored and Orange flavor)
	Maxamaid XP Bar‡
	(Apricot flavor)
	Phenyl Ade** (Vanilla, Orange Creme and Strawberry
	Phenyl Ade Amino Acid Bar** (Chocolate and Chocolate Crispy)
Maternal PKU:	Phenex-2*
	PKU 3†
	Phenyl-Free†
	XP Maxamum‡
	(Unflavored and Orange flavor)
	Maxamaid XP Bar‡
	(Apricot flavor)
	Phenyl Ade** (Vanilla, Orange Creme and Strawberry
	Phenyl Ade Amino Acid Bar** (Chocolate and Chocolate Crispy)

*Ross Laboratories   ‡Scientific Hospital Supplies, Inc.
†Mead Johnson   **Foodtek Manufacturing, Inc.

Table 29-3. **RECOMMENDED DAILY NUTRIENT INTAKES (RANGES) FOR INFANTS, CHILDREN, AND ADULTS WITH PKU**

Age	Nutrient				
	PHE[1] (mg/kg)	TYR[1] (mg/kg)	Protein (g/kg)	Energy (kcal/kg)	Fluid (ml/kg)
Infants					
0 to <3 mo	25-70	300-350	3.50-3.00	120 (145-95)	160-135
3 to <6 mo	20-45	300-350	3.50-3.00	120 (145-95)	160-130
6 to <9 mo	15-35	250-300	3.00-2.50	110 (135-80)	145-125
9 to <12 mo	10-35	250-300	3.00-2.50	105 (135-80)	135-125
	(mg/day)	(g/day)	(g/day)	(kcal/day)	(ml/day)
Girls and boys					
1 to <4 yr	200-400	1.72-3.00	30	1300 (900-1800)	900-1800
4 to <7 yr	210-450	2.25-3.50	35	1700 (1300-2300)	1300-2300
7 to <11 yr	220-500	2.55-4.00	40	2400 (1650-3300)	1650-3300
Women					
11 to <15 yr	250-750	3.45-5.00	50	2200 (1500-3000)	1500-3000
15 to <19 yr	230-700	3.45-5.00	50	2100 (1200-3000)	1200-3000
≥19 yr	220-700	3.75-5.00	50	2100 (1400-2500)	2100-2500
Men					
11 to <15 yr	225-900	3.38-5.50	55	2700 (2000-3700)	2000-3700
15 to <19 yr	295-1100	4.42-6.50	65	2800 (2100-3900)	2100-3900
≥19 yr	290-1200	4.35-6.50	65	2900 (2000-3300)	2000-3300

From Acosta PB and Yannicelli S: *The Ross metabolic formula system nutrition support protocols,* Columbus, Ohio, 1993, Abbott Laboratories, USA.
[1]Modify prescription based on frequently obtained blood and/or plasma values and growth in infants and children and frequently obtained plasma values and weight maintenance in adults.

late they are identified as having PKU. Improvement in behavior and cognitive functioning has been seen in severely retarded individuals who had untreated PKU (Clarke et al, 1987; Koch and Wenz, 1987; Pietz et al, 1993; Potocnik and Widhalm, 1994).

RECENT AND ANTICIPATED ADVANCES IN DIAGNOSIS AND MANAGEMENT

The correlation of the clinical phenotype of individuals with PKU with their genotype continues in populations worldwide with hopes of improving the clinical outcome of PKU (Guldberg et al, 1994; Lichter-Konecki et al, 1994; Scriver et al, 1993). Other modes of therapy for PKU continue to be investigated. Based on research of the depletion of dopamine in the prefrontal cortex, supplementation of the large neutral amino acids could offset the effects on the brain of persisting phe levels of 2 to 6 mg/dl (Diamond, 1993; Diamond et al, 1994). Pioneers in hepatic gene therapy are aiming to restore enough PAH enzyme activity to make phe restriction unnecessary; the PAH gene has successfully been delivered to the hepatocyte of the PKU mouse model (Cristiano, Smith, and Woo, 1993; Kay and Woo, 1994). Phenylalanine tolerance was restored to a 10-year-old boy with PKU who

Table 29-4.   MEAN 12 YEAR WISC-R, WRAT, AND PARENT WAIS
IQ SCORES* FOR PKU COLLABORATIVE STUDY
CHILDREN** GROUPED BY AGE AT LOSS
OF DIETARY CONTROL

Loss of dietary control, age in years:	<6	6 to 10	>10	ANOVA P
WISC-R[1] IQ scores	n = 23	n = 47	n = 25	
Verbal	85 ± 15	95 ± 14	101 ± 11	.0004
Performance	92 ± 15	95 ± 14	101 ± 11	.0499
Full scale	87 ± 14	96 ± 14	101 ± 11	.0028
WRAT[2] standard scores	n = 22	n = 46	n = 20	
Reading	92 ± 13	97 ± 11	105 ± 12	.0029
Spelling	87 ± 17	92 ± 13	98 ± 17	.0452
Arithmetic	80 ± 11	82 ± 11	84 ± 10	.6033
Parent WAIS IQ[3] scores	n = 23	n = 43	n = 25	
Full scale	104 ± 10	109 ± 9	108 ± 14	.1905

Adapted from Azen CG, Koch R, Friedman EG et al: *Am J Dis Child,* 145:35-39, 1991.
*Values are means ± SDs.
**The PKU Collaborative Study supported by grant 4-RO1-HD-09543 and contract N01-HD-4-3807 from NICHHD, NIH.
[1]Weschler Intelligence Scale for Children-Revised
[2]Wide Range Achievement Test
[3]Weschler Adult Intelligence Scale

received a liver transplant for concurrent active cirrhosis (Vajro et al, 1993). Liver transplantation may potentially benefit the BH_4-deficient disorders, but because early lifelong dietary restriction of phe improves the prognosis of PKU, it is not warranted.

ASSOCIATED PROBLEMS

Neurologic Changes

Parents and children must be appraised of the lifelong vulnerability of the nervous system to HPA. In a recent study (Thompson et al, 1993), abnormal findings in cerebral white matter are common on cranial magnetic resonance imaging (MRI) of children treated early or late for PKU; abnormalities in the periventricular and subcortical white matter have been demonstrated in children with PKU aged 7 years and older. Clinically there was no evidence of neurologic deterioration of the 25 early treated children with PKU studied by MRI, although 40% showed brisk lower limb reflexes.

ASSOCIATED PROBLEMS

Neurologic

Abnormal cerebral white matter
Demyelinization
Brisk lower limb reflexes

Cognitive deficits

Mathmatical deficits
Visual perception deficits
Linquistic deficits

Gamma globulinaemia

Allergic sensitizations

Pyloric stenosis

Peptic ulcers

The extent of MRI and single-photon emission computed tomography (SPECT) changes of the brain do not correlate with the start, duration, or quality of dietary treatment, as much as the degree of HPA at the time of the studies and the number of years since the phe-restricted diet was stopped (Thompson et al, 1993; Leuzzi et al, 1993; O'Tuama and Treves, 1993). Immature myelin, demyelinization, and edema respond within a few weeks or months of reinstituting phe restriction. In young children still receiving a well-controlled, phe-restricted diet, the clinical risk appears to be predominately of impairment of intellectual function, whereas in older individuals with PKU on relaxed or normal diets, the risk is progressive damage to the white matter. The risk of myelin damage increases the longer the individual is exposed to unrestricted amounts of phe. Demyelinization is the extreme manifestation of more generalized myelin changes and could explain irreversible neurologic deterioration.

Cognitive Deficits

Deficits in cognitive function relative to mathematical conceptualizations is a troubling finding in children with PKU who have maintained good phe control since birth. When tested at 12 years of age, children with well-controlled PKU scored 17 points lower on the Wide Range Achievement Test (WRAT) for arithmetic than previous baseline levels. This does not indicate gross deficits in the intellectual status of treated children with PKU but is evidence of subtle deficits that become more pronounced over time (Table 29-4).

Children with PKU who have maintained good phe control often have difficulty with visual perception and linquistic development (Brunner, Berch, and Berry, 1987). Neither the age at which treatment was initiated nor the phe level during the early years of life correlate with a discrepancy in skills of children with PKU compared with their siblings at 5 years of age on tests of visual perception and at 7 years of age on tests of psycholinguistic abilities (Fishler et al, 1987). In a study of 16 young adults with PKU, ages 13 to 20 years old, whose phe level ranged between 300 to 500 μM, their mutation genotype correlated with MRI findings of frontal white matter changes and with deficits in visuospatial learning and memory and visuomotor functioning suggesting that there are

limitations to the effect of dietary treatment in HPA (Lou et al, 1992, 1994). In another study (Craft et al, 1992), boys treated early for PKU (mean age 9.76 ± 2.97 years) exhibited right visual field impairment in disengaging attention, indicative of left hemisphere dysfunction, and overall slowed reaction times. The lifelong outcome for children with well-treated PKU is yet to be observed because the history of treated PKU is relatively short (O'Flynn, 1992).

Gammaglobulinaemia

Environmental factors and genetic factors affect IgE synthesis in children with PKU. PKU appears to be a metabolic disorder with particular immunologic features such as low IgG levels and high IgE levels but, when treated with diet therapy, the high rate of allergic pathology, specifically asthma, does not occur. Elevated IgE levels in children with PKU must be considered a gammaglobulinaemic disorder, similar to some inherited primary immunodeficiencies in which asthma is exceptional, despite high IgE levels, (e.g., common variable immune deficiency, Job syndrome, and Wiskott-Aldrich syndrome). Allergic sensitizations are more frequent in children with PKU (Riva et al, 1994).

Pyloric Stenosis

Pyloric stenosis has been observed more frequently in males with PKU than in the general male newborn population (male/female ratio is 5:1). Children of either sex identified with pyloric stenosis should be retested for PKU (Koch and Wenz, 1987).

Peptic Ulcer

Peptic ulcer, with the uncommon complication of bleeding or perforation, has been documented in both sexes of individuals (11 to 25 years of age) with PKU. The relationship of peptic ulcer to PKU is not clear. Elevated blood phe concentrations secondary to PAH deficiency may lead to increased gastric secretion, which in some individuals results in peptic ulceration; vomiting, which was formerly a common presenting symptom in untreated children with PKU, could possibly be explained by this same mechanism (Scriver, et al, 1995). Peptic ulcer could be related to the dietary treatment; L-amino acid supplements can stimulate gastric acid secretion (Greeves, Carson, and Dodge, 1988).

PROGNOSIS

The phenotypic expression of PKU represents the degree of homeostasis achieved given the variables (1) at the PKU locus, (2) the collective genotype at other loci that can neutralize the PKU allele at the PKU locus, and (3) in the environment. "The most relevant environmental variable for PKU is food intake which can be influenced by culture, income, and family structure. If the family environment does not support compliance to a special diet, the outcome of a normally predictable course can drastically change" (Valle and Mitchell, 1994, pp 4-5). Imperfections in the dietary treatment of PKU as it is currently known (Sanjurjo et al, 1994), and delays in treatment are all factors evidenced by neuropsychologic and cognitive functions that are slightly less than average in treated individuals with PKU.

Primary Care Management
HEALTH CARE MAINTENANCE

Growth and Development

Growth and development are normal for children with PKU on a controlled, phe-restricted diet. Head circumference, weight, and length are measured at scheduled monthly intervals for the first year, then every 3 months until after the prepubertal growth spurt, and then every 6 months throughout adolescence to monitor adequacy of diet. There is a tendency toward obesity in children with PKU (McBurnie et al, 1991), which is related to the high caloric density of natural food sources necessary to meet the child's RDA for calories, the free sugar in the EMF product, and the free foods high in carbohydrates.

Children with PKU are at risk for having low self-esteem. The fact that they require a special diet and the fact that they are different from others are obvious causes. The possible consequences of being taken off the diet and the effect that high blood phe levels has on their behavior contribute to this risk (Pietz et al, 1993; Potocnik and Widhalm, 1994). Children with PKU older than age 4 years are at risk for having immature social interaction and interpersonal skills (Kazak, Reber, and Snitzer, 1988). Continuing the phe-restricted diet, becoming involved in PKU peer support groups, promoting self-control of the diet at an early age, and de-

emphasizing that children with PKU are "different" are easier said than done. Art therapy with younger children and role playing for older children are only some of the creative ways to elicit the child's attitudes about having PKU. As children approach school age, parents need to be encouraged to enhance their child's social development by allowing them to spend increasing amounts of time outside the immediate family.

Affective disorders and acting out behaviors are not the norm for well-managed children with PKU; the psychologist on the medical genetics PKU treatment team is a resource for dealing with these issues and knowing when professional intervention is required.

Diet

Dietary support at all developmental stages of the individual with PKU is an important component of therapy. Monitoring of phe concentrations with weight and diet changes will need to occur throughout the individual's life. It is important to initiate self-management of the phe-restricted diet early in childhood (Gleason et al, 1992; Trahms, 1992). Some reasons for failure to achieve long-term adherence to the phe-restricted diet include poor family coping skills, increasing independence of children, limited food choices, and unpalatable EMF products.

In the infant, protein is initially prescribed in an amount greater than the RDA. When the EMF is the primary source of protein, the requirement for protein increases because of rapid absorption, early and high peak of plasma amino acids, and rapid catabolism of amino acids. Mature human breast milk (>15 days' lactation) is an ideal source of whole protein for the infant with PKU (Greve et al, 1994). Breast milk, compared with cow's milk, contains an amino acid composition that supports adequate growth at a lower protein intake (0.9 to 1.0 versus 3.3 g/dl) and enhances bioavailability of minerals and trace elements (especially zinc) because of the greater percentage of protein (70% versus 20%) from the predominant whey fraction. Breast milk has a lower phe content per ounce compared with other formulas.*

---

*Breast milk = 12.3 mg of phe/oz; Enfamil = 17 mg of phe/oz; Similac[20] = 22 mg of phe/oz; SMA = 24 mg of phe/oz; Isomil and Prosobee = 29 mg of phe/oz; and cow's milk = 104 mg of phe/oz.

Infants with PKU should be given a variety of foods at the appropriate ages so that these foods become part of their diet later in life. It is recommended to ingest ⅓ of the total amount of EMF with the main meals to optimize utilization of total protein intake by the body (Herrmann et al, 1994). A system of food exchanges where phe content is used as the basis for providing specific amounts of foods by food group is employed. Foods of similar phe content are grouped together and are exchanged, one for another, within the list to give variety to the diet (Acosta and Yannicelli, 1993).

Elemental medical food products are sensitive to heat and a prolonged shelf life. These products should not be heated beyond 54.5°C because of the Maillard reaction; amino acids, peptides, and proteins condense with sugars, forming bonds for which no digestive enzymes are available. The reaction is characterized by initially a light brown color, followed by buff yellow and then dark brown; caramel-like and roasted aromas develop. Any amino acid preparation should be inspected for these changes and the expiration date checked before use. The shelf life for EMF products is generally 2 years. The vitamin C content diminishes initially, followed by the vitamin A and D content, which can decrease to as much as 30% below labeled values after the expiration date. In addition, the fats in EMF products become rancid after the expiration date. Products containing L-amino acids taste best when they are served cold (frozen to a slush) to disguise the sulfurous bitter taste. There is no contraindication for freezing EMF products or warming them to less than 54.5°C. Terminal sterilization of an infant's EMF formula is contraindicated (Acosta and Yannicelli, 1993).

Activities other than those that revolve around food can be promoted with peers. It is quality peer relationships that are important, not that an individual has to eat the same things to be accepted. Food is a social instrument for a child of any age, and every effort should be made to use the available tips from an experienced nutritionist to approximate the visual, textural, and taste appeal of the unrestricted diet.

Safety

Children with PKU are not at an increased risk of acute safety hazards. Chronic ingestion of excess dietary phe is more deleterious to the health of the child than the accidental intake of a product containing aspartame. A Medic-Alert bracelet or necklace that indicates "special PKU diet" is added assurance that a child with PKU will receive proper care in case of an emergency.

Because chronic ingestion of EMF products can lead to nutritional deficiencies, they are contraindicated for any individual not diagnosed as needing a phe-restricted diet.

Pigmented lesions—melanin spots that are light brown to black—occur in individuals with PKU. The oculocutaneous pigmentary dilution observed even in children with PKU who adhere to a phe-restricted diet is a systemic mechanism related to the disturbed phe/tyr ratio in the circulation. The pigmentary activity of the epidermal melanocytes is unimpaired in individuals with PKU and is normal at the skin level peripherally. Erythema response and ability to tan after exposure to artificial or natural light for individuals with PKU have been demonstrated to be no different than for individuals without PKU who are blonde (Bolognia and Pawelek, 1988; Hassel and Brunsting, 1959). Limiting exposure to the sun and using sunblocks are recommended for the child with PKU as they are for any child.

Immunizations

The immunization schedule for children with PKU is the same as it is for any child. The child with PKU must be closely observed for a reaction to the immunization. A febrile reaction can lead to a catabolic state, increasing plasma phe levels. Any illness should be supported with adequate hydration and calories.

Screening

Vision. Routine screening is recommended.

Hearing. Routine screening is recommended.

Dental. The diet for PKU contains sufficient carbohydrate to present more than the usual potential for dental decay. The phe-restricted diet relies on frequent intake of carbohydrates to meet the daily requirement for calories. Explanations to parents about the role that frequency of carbohydrate consumption has and the effects of extremes, such as nursing bottle caries or uncontrolled access to candy, helps focus their efforts. Practical goals include weaning the child with PKU to a glass as soon as possible, starting with sips at 6 months of age; retentive foods should be followed by fibrous ones to effect food removal; liquid forms of carbohydrate should be used when possible to promote oral clearance; free foods such as fruits should be offered in place of more retentive forms of refined sugars; and dental hygiene and screening should be initiated at the eruption of the first tooth with close follow-up thereafter (Casamassimo et al, 1984).

Blood pressure. Routine screening is recommended.

Hematocrit. Iron status is monitored by plasma ferritin levels at 6, 9, and 12 months of age and then every 6 months thereafter. Hemoglobin and hematocrit values are evaluated at 6 and 12 months of age and annually thereafter. The child with anemia will have a falsely low phe level, and the newborn with polycythemia can have a falsely high phe level.

Breast-fed infants with PKU have exaggerated physiologic anemia of infancy, requiring iron supplementation when the hematocrit value approaches 30% (McCabe et al, 1989).

Urinalysis. Routine screening is recommended.

Tuberculosis. Routine screening is recommended.

Condition-specific screening

URINE SCREENING FOR PHENYLKETONURIA. The analysis of pterins in urine is done in all newborns with HPA to differentiate PKU and mild HPA from the BH$_4$-deficient disorders. This selective screening test is best collected by the primary care provider taking caution not to expose the clean catch urine to light and delivering by next-day courier at room temperature to the metabolic genetics laboratory designated by the medical genetics PKU treatment center.

The qualitative urine test for PKU (ferric chloride reaction or Phenistix) measures phenylpyruvic acid, which is not excreted in the urine until blood phe levels reach 1000 μM. Care must be taken in the interpretation of a ferric chloride reaction because of false-positive and false-negative test results caused by instability of urine specimens and interfering metabolites (Nystaform-HC ointment or iodochlorhydroxyquin, salicylates, phenothiazines derivatives, isoniazid, and L-dopa metabolites).

BLOOD PHE MONITORING. The blood test for phe (newborn, child, and adult), whether for screening or diet monitoring, is a capillary blood sample obtained from a free-flowing puncture wound using a semiautomated lancet (Burns, 1989) 2 to 4 hours postprandially. Only a blood specimen is reliable in detecting quantitative or semiquantitative levels of phe; phe content can be measured by different laboratory techniques. A fluorometric assay of blood spotted directly onto filter paper is most sensitive to mild HPA yielding a phe level higher than a spot from a capillary tube, dorsal vein, or from a serum sample (Jew et al, 1994; Lorey and Cunningham, 1994).

Immediately after birth (0 to 2 hours) the mean phe value in newborns without PKU is 2.75 mg/dl, quickly rises to a peak of 3.06 mg/dl at 7 to 9 hours of age, and slowly tapers off to 2.73 mg/dl at 24 hours; after 24 hours of age the mean phe value is 2.66 mg/dl by fluorometric assay (Arnopp et al, 1995). For infants the upper limit of normal phe is <120 μM, for children 62 ± 18 μM, for teenagers 60 ± 13 μM and for adults 58 ± 15 μM (Scriver et al, 1993).

Plasma phe and tyr levels are evaluated twice weekly by quantitative methods in the newborn with PKU until concentrations are stabilized and approximate dietary phe and tyr requirements are known. Thereafter, blood phe is evaluated twice weekly with dietary changes or weekly without dietary changes in both the infant and child. The plasma phe and tyr levels are evaluated by the medical genetics PKU treatment center team.

NUTRITIONAL INDICES SCREENING. Nutrient intake is recorded for 3 days before each blood phe

CONDITION-SPECIFIC SCREENING

Urine pterin screening
Blood phe monitoring
Nutritional indices screening
Auscultation for dysrhythmias
DNA analysis

test on forms provided and evaluated for phe, tyr, protein, and energy intake by the nutritionist on the PKU treatment team. Protein status is evaluated by plasma albumin of prealbumin levels (or both) every 3 months in the infant and every 6 months in the child and adolescent. Individuals on semisynthetic diets are at high risk for deficiencies in the trace elements. Insufficient intake of iron, zinc, and selenium and the interaction of iron with copper and zinc at the intestinal level can cause deficiencies. Safe ranges of fluoride, selenium, and molybdenum are also monitored by the medical genetics PKU treatment team. Overall balance of nutrients is critical in the child with PKU.

AUSCULTATION. Regular auscultation of heart sounds of children with PKU on a phe-restricted diet is advisable for detection of a dysrhythmia. Selenium deficiency related to a low protein diet and altered bioavailability can cause ventricular tachycardia that is corrected by selenium supplementation (Greeves et al, 1990).

DNA ANALYSIS. Nucleic acid analysis can be done from blood spotted onto filter paper as described above. Caution should be taken in prepping the skin with alcohol, not betadine, and blood should not be collected in heparinized (lithium) tubing and transferred to the filter paper. The filter paper should be properly identified and mailed to the DNA lab specified by the medical genetics PKU treatment center team.

PHENYLALANINE TOLERANCE TESTING. The practice of phe challenges is no longer warranted with the advent of DNA mutation analysis.

COMMON ILLNESS MANAGEMENT

Differential Diagnosis

Management during illness and surgery. If a child with PKU has a negative nitrogen balance for any reason, the blood phe content can be elevated because body tissue protein catabolism occurs, releasing phe. The paradox of phe-restricted diets is in the transient elevations of plasma phe when phe is overrestricted; protein synthesis is blocked by nutrient deficiency (negative nitrogen balance), resulting in impaired flow of phe to anabolic nitrogen pools. An elevated temperature is just one of many reasons for a negative nitrogen balance. An accurate history of the child's illness and dietary intake before the illness may help distinguish the cause of a catabolic reaction.

During common childhood illnesses the blood phe level is not tested until the child is well as long as the illness is less than 3 weeks' duration. During the illness supportive measures should be undertaken to limit protein catabolism. In the infant or adolescent energy intake should be enhanced by allowing (1) as much fruit juice as tolerated; (2) liquid-flavored gelatin; (3) polycose glucose polymers (liquid or powder) added to the fruit juices; and (4) caffeine-free, nondiet soft drinks. With close consultation with the medical genetics PKU treatment team, the child with PKU is returned to the EMF and preillness diet plan as rapidly as tolerated; usually the EMF product is initiated at one half original strength, then full strength as tolerated (Acosta and Yannicelli, 1993).

Minor uncomplicated surgery (e.g., tonsillectomy, hernia repair, cytoscopy) with the child under general anesthesia does not cause major alteration in the blood phe level. The highest blood phe levels ($\leq$17 mg/dl) occur approximately on the second postoperative day and decline on the fourth postoperative day ($\leq$10 mg/dl). Because the elevation in phe level is transient, no special dietary measures are needed (Fiedler et al, 1982).

Skin lesions. Localized or generalized eczema and peeling of the soles of the feet and the palms of the hands occur after a long-term catabolic state.

DIFFERENTIAL DIAGNOSIS

Management during illness/surgery negative nitrogen balance due to fever or illness may result in catabolic reaction requiring diet change. Minor surgery does not require special diet.
Skin lesions
   Eczema
   Scleroderma

Skin lesions related to an amino acid imbalance and disturbed phe/tyr ratio need to be distinguished from other rashes by accurate history of the lesion and diet. Establishing phe homeostasis will resolve eczema and peeling that are not responsive to topical medications.

Children with skin lesions suggestive of scleroderma, severe localized induration of the skin, subcutaneous tissue, and muscle should be tested for PKU. Scleroderma, a rare, often familial, connective tissue disorder and untreated PKU both have a common secondary biochemical deficiency of tryptophan. Tryptophan is an immediate precursor of serotonin and the catecholamines in the tyrosine metabolic pathway. An increased concentration of phe decreases that availability of tyr and tryptophan. The scleroderma-like changes observed in PKU present earlier (first year of life), have a different distribution and histologic pattern in the child in contrast to true scleroderma, but become indistinguishable with age (Irons and Levy, 1986; Nova, Kaufman, and Halperin, 1992).

Drug Interactions

Aspartame. Aspartame (APM) is contraindicated in individuals with PKU and care must be taken to read content labels of food, beverages, vitamins, and medicines for its presence. Marketed under the brand name NutraSweet, the high-intensity artificial sweetener is no longer solely distributed by NutraSweet Company; the familiar NutraSweet swirl logo alerting individuals with PKU to APM in the product may not be displayed on the packaging. The FDA requires the statement "PHENYLKETONURICS: CONTAINS PHENYLALANINE" on the label of all products containing the white, odorless, crystalline powder consisting of two amino acids: L-phenylalanine and L-aspartic acid.

For children with PKU, ingesting 34 mg of APM per kg of body weight will elevate the plasma phe level to approximately 850 μM; a quart of APM-sweetened Kool Aid contains 280 mg of phe, approximately half the child's daily allowance of phe (Scriver et al, 1995). For individuals with mild HPA who tolerate 50 to 100 mg of phe/kg, APM is not recommended; the acceptable daily intake of APM for individuals without PKU or mild HPA is 40 mg/kg. Individuals who carry the PKU gene and

ingest APM have safe levels of phe that persist longer in their bodies than in individuals who are not carriers (Curtius, Endres, and Blau, 1994). The use of APM by women with PKU during pregnancy is not recommended because of a 1:2 concentration gradient for phe between the maternal and fetal blood (Scriver et al, 1995).

Check the *Physicians' Desk Reference* (PDR) and *Drug Facts and Comparisons* before prescribing medications to a child with PKU for the ingredient phenylalanine or L-aspartyl-L-phenylalanine methyl ester (APM). Caution parents about APM in over-the-counter medications and vitamins. The exact amount of phe in medications needs to be calculated as part of the child's daily phe intake (Schuett, 1995).

Any drug that affects the neurotransmitters in the central nervous system should be thoroughly investigated before prescribing in the child or young adult with PKU. For example Daraprim tablet, pyrimethamine, is listed in the PDR as causing HPA and contraindicated in individuals with PKU. Great care must be taken when individuals with PKU are on any medication, especially when blood phe levels change and when medication is withdrawn (Dolan, Koch, and Bekins, 1995).

Monoamine oxidase inhibitors. Individuals with PKU who receive monoamine oxidase (MAO) inhibitors will have elevated levels of phenylethylamine, a phenylketone, in the urine and tissues without a detectable level in the cerebrospinal fluid and without signs of clinical deterioration. Use of MAO inhibitors for the treatment of a psychiatric disorder in an individual with PKU is controversial because of conflicting reports of the neurotoxicity of phenylethylamine (Kaufman, 1989).

Oral contraceptives. Fluctuations can occur in plasma amino acids during the menstrual cycle. Plasma phe and tyr levels should be monitored when women with PKU are using oral contraceptives.

DEVELOPMENTAL ISSUES

Sleep Patterns

There are diurnal variations of phe and tyr levels in children who have and do not have PKU. The difference in children with PKU is an elevation of the tyr level in the evening, like children without PKU, but a decrease in the phe level at night, unlike nonaffected children. The implications of this variation in the phe/tyr ratio are in their relationship to tryptophan, the precursor of serotonin. In the presence of low phe levels, the tryptophan level is elevated. Elevation of tryptophan markedly reduces the total time in rapid eye movement (REM) sleep to 3% (normal REM time in children is 29.5% ± 4.8%). During lower levels of tryptophan, REM sleep is increased to 8% to 11%. Approximately 10% of children with PKU had paroxymal abnormalities, particularly during the night in a study of EEG patterns (Campistol, 1994). Children with PKU are more susceptible to sleep disturbances, which can be expressed as insomnia or hyperactivity at night. Children who have elevated levels of phe can often have disturbed sleep patterns with nightmares. Any alteration in the ratios of phe, tyr, and tryptophan can cause sleep disturbances; a phe-restricted diet balanced throughout the 24-hour time period optimizes sleep patterns in the child with PKU (Guttler, Olesen, and Wamberg, 1969; Herrero et al, 1983; Wyatt et al, 1971; Hayaishi, 1994).

Toileting

Infants with PKU who are prone to eczema may experience more problems with diaper dermatitis. Careful, explicit instructions on standard management techniques should be given and follow-up appointments made for evaluation of treatment success. Toileting habits become an issue when phe control is lost. When the blood phe level is elevated for any reason, phenylketones are present in the urine and sweat, causing the characteristic musty odor of PKU. Attention to and training of the child in his or her hygiene needs at all ages will avoid unnecessary embarrassment.

Discipline

Consistent discipline for children with PKU is as, if not more, important as it is for any child. Food is a very major social component in any child's life and how it is managed from the very beginning by parents can determine the success of the only current therapy for PKU, dietary restriction of phe. A major pitfall in disciplining children with PKU is to use food as a reward system and to use the need for blood tests as punishment. Strategies helping children to adhere to special diets are available.

Child Care

More than one individual in the child's home environment should be knowledgable about the phe-restricted diet and the preparation of EMF products. Materials about PKU written specifically for baby-sitters, grandparents, and teachers, as well as creative ideas on how to deal with these issues, can be found in National PKU News.

Schooling

Children with treated PKU experience difficulties in school more frequently than nonaffected children; 33% of children with PKU are 1 or more years below grade level compared with 14% of children in the general white population. For grades 1 through 4, 38% of girls with PKU are 1 or more years below compared with 29% of boys with PKU (Fishler et al., 1987).

Children with PKU need comprehensive integrated psychodiagnostic and neuropsychologic assessments. Developmental testing is performed ideally at the medical genetics PKU treatment center at scheduled intervals starting at 6 months of age and every 6 months until 2 years of age, then annually thereafter. It is important for optimal performance that the child's blood phe level be in maintenance range on the day of testing.

Anticipatory guidance in the development of visual-spatial skills may be required. Computer games and software programs that train and stimulate the development of visual-spatial skills and hand-to-eye coordination are ideal. Attention to proper lighting is important so that contrasts are clear; black on a white background is perceived better than grey or a monotone by children with PKU (Diamond, unpublished work). Special education in math and language acquisition may also be necessary. Teacher involvement at all stages of the child's schooling is important.

Sexuality

Sexual development and curiosity are no different for the child with PKU than for any other child. Genetic counseling specifically for the child with PKU is individualized to the child's understanding of PKU and assessment of readiness. The medical genetics PKU treatment team works closely with families on this issue, and often PKU peer support groups and videos specific to the developmental stage of the child or adolescent with PKU are beneficial.

For the female adolescent with PKU, the onset of menses can cause fluctuations in the plasma amino acid pattern, specifically the tyr level. Monitoring the quantitative plasma amino acid levels is important to ensure that excesses or deficiencies can be alleviated by dietary intervention. Discussions of contraception and the implications of being a woman with PKU should be individualized and approached with sensitivity. Again, PKU peer support groups and written materials and videos designed specifically for female adolescents with PKU are available.

Transition to Adulthood

Individuals with PKU can successfully adjust to society (Koch, Yusin, and Fishler, 1985). Worldwide, few adults with PKU are on a phe-restricted diet. It has only been since the 1990s that a *lifelong* diet (Levy, Waisbren, and Shiloh, 1994; Potocnik and Widhalm, 1994) has been advocated through the developmental stages of adulthood. The first successful pregnancy outcomes from MPKU surveillance were being realized in 1990, as the children enrolled in the PKU Collaborative Study reached 12 years of age demonstrating that the best performance profiles were by children with PKU who adhered to phe restriction the longest and maintained phe levels (<6 mg/dl) more closely approximating phe homeostasis. These results show the protective benefits of long-term dietary therapy. To realize optimal psychologic and behavior benefits, adults with PKU should not completely stop the diet, but can liberalize phe intake (Pietz et al, 1993). There is roughly a 30% reduction of serum phe levels with advancing age (Pitt and Danks, 1994).

Although some of the effects of PKU are directly related to phe levels, others seem to be unaffected by institution or reinstitution of phe restriction. A study (Ris et al, 1994) of the late effects of PKU demonstrated that although IQs were normal in adults (>18 years) who benefited from early treatment in childhood, their IQs and performance on measures of attention and complex visuoconstructional ability were lower than their unaffected siblings. Both the age at which blood phe levels rose >1200 μM and the age the EMF was discontinued correlated with intellectual and, to a lesser

extent, neuropsychologic variables. This study validates previous observations by others that concurrent elevation of blood phe levels are strongly correlated with lowered, reversible neuropsychologic measures indicative of selective impairment of executive functions: set maintenance, planning, impulse control, organized search, and flexibility of thought and action.

The hazards of losses experienced off dietary control are observed from both the chronic and acute effects of PKU. The natural history of untreated PKU in individuals ages 28 to 72 years (Pitt and Danks, 1994) suggests that PKU does not generally cause a progressive loss of abilities in adult life beyond the irreversible effects sustained in childhood. General health problems, other than those previously associated with untreated PKU in childhood, are not remarkable in the adult with PKU; their causes of death are the same as for individuals without PKU and not related to PKU. A vigilant study (Dolan, Koch and Bekins, 1995) of untreated older adults with PKU started very slowly on a personalized lowering of dietary phe observed a reduction of behavioral manifestations that previously interfered with abilities, and an enhancement of social skills.

Young adults with PKU, especially women, are at risk for depression, anxiety, and agoraphobia that lessen with reinstitution of phe restriction (Waisbren and Levy, 1991). Emotional effects can persist despite reductions in phe levels. Women with PKU who are treated early in childhood and later go off the diet tend to seek professional help or be on medications for emotional problems that begin in the teens. The biochemical difficulties in PKU, rather than the fact of having a chronic medical problem are related to personality psychopathology (Waisbren and Zaff, 1994). Although all individuals treated early for PKU function normally within a social context, those individuals who continue or reinstitute phe homeostasis, especially women, benefit in measurable and immeasurable ways. Participation in a Maternal PKU Camp or program is a supportive activity for women with PKU.

Maternal PKU. The first generation of identified and treated infants with PKU are now between the ages of 15 and 25 years old. The incidence of undiagnosed MPKU is about 1 in 30,000. Sexual activity among adolescents and young women with

HPA is no different than it is for their peers without PKU; 42% of all never-married 15- to 19-year-old girls have experienced sexual intercourse, two thirds either inconsistently or never use a form of contraception (Platt et al, 1992). The success of dietary therapy in arresting the neurologic deficits caused by HPA has inadvertently produced an increasing number of non-HPA mentally retarded offspring with MPKU syndrome; the possibility exists that in one generation the incidence of PKU-related mental retardation could return to the level it was before NBS and treatment were available.

A minimal teratogenic effect of HPA occurs when maternal blood phe levels are maintained between 2 and 6 mg/dl. Women with PKU who do not maintain blood phe control before and throughout an entire pregnancy may have infants without PKU, but with other birth defects. The fetus is at great risk for the teratologic effects of phe exposure because of a positive transplacental gradient of phe approximately 1.13 to 2.19 times higher than the maternal blood phe level. The results of high maternal blood phe levels (>10 mg/dl) in the fetus, especially in the first trimester, are mental retardation, microcephaly, intrauterine and postnatal growth delay, left outflow tract cardiac defects, and a constellation of facial dysmorphic features (MPKU syndrome) (see Fig. 29-3). Compared to women who do not have PKU, 24% of the offspring born to mothers with PKU had abnormal head circumferences (HCs), and had decreased weight and length, 11% respectively (Platt et al, 1992). Deceleration of head growth after birth is evident in the first year of life, even if not microcephalic at birth, in offspring of women with PKU who maintained phe levels <600 μM. Women with mild HPA who maintained blood phe levels <360 μM without phe restriction throughout pregnancy had offspring with HCs in the 43rd percentile (Matalon et al, 1994). Dose-related effects of phe on pregnancy are evident.

Of women with PKU whose phe levels were >20 mg/dl throughout pregnancy, 90% had offspring who were microcephalic and whose weight, length, and HC were all below the 3rd percentile; 97% of their offspring had at least one dysmorphic feature (Platt et al, 1992). All offspring of women with PKU had at least one dysmorphic feature regardless of how well phe restriction was controlled;

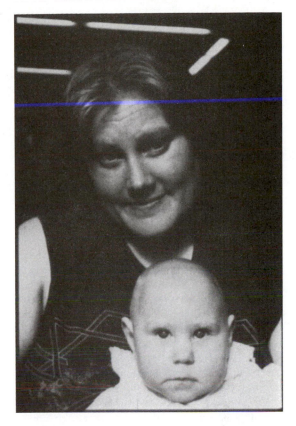

Fig. 29-3.   Mother with 8-month-old daughter with MPKU syndrome.

facial appearance included epicanthal folds, prominent ears, long philtrum, upturned nose, micrognathia, and wide, depressed nasal bridge. None of the mothers with PKU who maintained their phe level <10 mg/dl had children with cardiac defects found in the offspring of the mothers with higher phe levels. Defects included ventricular septal defect, hypoplastic left ventricle, coarctation of the aorta, and tetrology of Fallot. The risk of cardiac defects in children born to mothers with PKU whose phe levels are not in control by 10 weeks' gestation is 7.2% compared to 0.5% to 1.0% risk for the general population (Koch et al, 1993).

Pregnancy in the women with PKU is a medical challenge. The goals of diet are similar to pregnant teenagers without PKU with respect to normal and appropriate weight gain based on height, prepregnancy weight, and gestational age, with indices of nutritional status in the normal range. Concentration of blood phe and tyr is between 2 and 4 and 1.65 mg/dl, respectively. The phe requirements vary in the same woman throughout pregnancy depending on age, weight gain, trimester of pregnancy, adequacy of energy and protein intakes, and state of maternal health. At 20 weeks' gestation the phe requirements increase dramatically. Magnesium, copper, and cholesterol levels are significantly lower in MPKU (Acosta and Yannicelli, 1993), and special EMF products (see Table 29-2) have been developed to meet these needs.

Paternal PKU. Historically, few males with PKU have been followed to age 18; therefore, primary care providers must educate them on the importance of remaining on diet for the benefits of lessening depression, agitation, and aggressiveness, and improving attention span and concentration (Waisbren and Levy, 1991). Fertility does not appear to be affected in men with PKU. However, an inverse correlation between plasma phe level and semen volume and between plasma phe level and sperm count has been observed, indicating another benefit of achieving phe homeostasis (Fisch, et al, 1991b). Investigation of paternal PKU is ongoing as part of the nationwide MPKU Collaborative Study.

SPECIAL FAMILY CONCERNS AND RESOURCES

PKU is prevalent in all populations. Because PKU is a universal disorder, the cultural and ethnic implications will be just as diverse. Cultural and ethnic preferences will need to be considered when planning the diet, when providing genetic counseling, and when discussing family planning options. Maternal PKU is one example of how two different cultures perceive PKU. In a study comparing attitudes of women with PKU in the United States with those in Israel, Israeli women perceived PKU more negatively and had less knowledge about MPKU than women in the United States. Yet because Israeli women shun premarital sex and utilize oral contraception more frequently, the number of MPKU pregnancies treated before conception in Israel is proportionately greater than those treated in the United States (Shiloh et al, 1993).

Mutation analysis has provided insights into the population genetics of PKU. A founder effect, genetic drift and heterozygote advantage in the origins and distribution of mutant PAH alleles in the human population have all been proposed (Eisensmith et al, 1995; Scriver et al, 1995). Significant correlations exist between some RFLP haps and HPA phenotypes within specific populations (Scriver et al, 1993; Scriver et al, 1995). Haps 1 through 6 together account for over 80% of all mutant chromosomes in many European populations; however, it is not an exclusive relationship. Haps 1 and 4 are common among chromosomes in both normal individuals and those with PKU, as is the case with hap 4 which is exclusively found in the Asian population. Most individuals with PKU in northern European populations who have any combination of mutant PAH alleles of hap 2 or 3 exhibit a severe form of PKU, whereas if they have mutant PAH alleles on hap 1 or 4 they display a wide range of HPA phenotypes (Scriver et al, 1995). Genotype-phenotype correlations are less well characterized in the United States and cannot be inferred until further research is completed.

Currently the degree of HPA in PKU cannot be predicted from hap and DNA mutation analysis. Parents must live with the knowledge that their child's intellectual development depends on how well the diet is managed. Outcome is directly related to the effectiveness of dietary control, and genetic potential inherited from the parents. Families with children who have PKU perceive themselves to be less adaptable and cohesive than other families. Mothers of children with PKU particularly feel separated rather than connected within the family structure and feel rigid rather than structured. More rigid family systems may be an adaptive response to children whose daily routine is less flexible than most children. Helping the family discover ways in which to provide a flexible, yet structured organization of the child's management of PKU would be supportive, allowing them to let go of their perceived need for rigidity. On other measures of family stress, parents of children with PKU did not report significantly greater degrees of parental psychologic distress, marital dissatisfaction, or parenting stress than other parents, although the tendency for stress in these areas was present (Fehrenbach and Peterson, 1989; Kazak, Reber, and Snitzer, 1988).

Reproductive patterns in families after birth of a child with PKU are affected by the birth order of that child, the age of the parents at the time of the birth of the child with PKU, and the expressed intentions of the parents whether to have additional children (Burns et al, 1984). Having a child with PKU does not appear to limit parental reproductive plans. Since the advent of prenatal diagnosis for PKU, another factor that contributes to the reproductive decision-making process includes the parents' perception of the progress of the child with PKU. For families with at least one child with PKU who decided not to have more children, family size was the primary limiting factor (35%), followed by concern about PKU (25%), and finances (20%) (Jew, Williams, and Koch, 1988).

The financial burden of PKU is variable for parents of a child with PKU or a young adult with PKU living on his or her own. An estimated annual cost for a 1- to 2-year-old child with PKU is roughly $2000 (EMF costs $1800/yr and natural foods $200/yr) compared to the lowest cost estimate by the USDA for the 1- to 2-year-old child without PKU of $818. Nineteen states have some legislation for the provision of EMF and medical foods; others are in the process of passing legislation. Five states require insurance companies to pay for the EMF (Massachusetts, Minnesota, Montana, New York, and Washington). At least 43 states have some kind of program that provides EMF either through Medicaid, WIC, or some other program (Velazquez, 1994). A number of insurance companies and health maintenance organizations (HMOs) will partially or fully cover expenses of EMF, special low-protein medical foods, and blood phe monitoring, but usually after a great deal of parental anguish and negotiating with the given insuring group in the first weeks after the diagnosis of the infant, at a time that is already emotionally traumatic for families (Awiszus and Unger, 1990; Black, 1993).

Information about nonselective NBS is optimally given to all expectant parents prenatally (Holtzman et al, 1983). Information should be given to the newborn's parents at least before discharge from the birth facility, assuming the newborn is less than 1 week of age. If information about the significance of NBS for the child's health and the NBS testing process is not sufficient, parents experience a greater degree of anxiety and de-

pression about their child's health than about the fact that their child needs to be tested again for a presumptive positive NBS test result (Sorenson et al, 1984). If the child is ultimately diagnosed with PKU, the parents experience guilt over their genetic contribution as a carrier to their child with PKU. The stigma of being a carrier is powerful, but the knowledge that the entire human population carries at least one recessive gene for a disorder such as PKU, excluding only 0.01% of all couples that do not, may dispel the myth of this stigma for future generations (Burn, 1994). A primary care provider who is astute about PKU can greatly alleviate parents' anxieties of being a carrier.

Informational Materials

Audiovisual materials

Ahn S, Velazquez K, Ojeda N, Cunningham GC producers: *PKU and you: Young women share their thoughts,* Berkeley, CA, ©1988, Maternal PKU Project, Genetic Disease Branch, California Department of Health Services. *The purpose of this program is to convey the issues that concern young women with PKU. This video, filmed at California's Maternal PKU Camp, shows young women with PKU, 13 years and older, sharing their experiences of growing up with PKU, giving each other support to stay on or return to the diet, and discussing the importance of returning to diet before and throughout pregnancy.* Running time is 20 minutes VHS videotape. To order call the GeneHELP Resource Center (510)540-2972.

Helmore JD, producer: *A message to PKU parents,* Berkeley, CA, ©1989, Genetic Disease Branch, California Department of Health Services. *The purpose of this program is to help parents of children newly diagnosed with PKU understand the condition and to show that children with PKU can grow to healthy adulthood, leading normal lives.* Produced in cooperation with Kathleen Jew, RN, MPH and Julian C. Williams, MD, Children's Hospital of Los Angeles. Running time is 21 minutes and 23 seconds VHS videotape. To order call the GeneHELP Resource Center (510)540-2972.

Dunn SP, James J, and Eckert-Smith K: *Maternal PKU: A new crisis on the horizon,* ©March 1995. *This video explains the history of PKU from its discovery through the creation of the special medical diet, and how the newborn screening process essentially eliminated the mental retardation caused by PKU. This historical perspective leads naturally into the introduction of MPKU and complications for the fetus. The latter half of the program explains how a multidisciplinary medical team participates in the treatment of successful MPKU pregnancies and how the evidence provided by the 10-year collaborative study of MPKU has led to its successful treatment. The audience is health care providers and policymakers, although informative for the general public.* Directed by Sean P. Dunn, contributors are NICHD, with a supplemental grant from Scientific Hospital Supplies. Running time is 28 minutes, 30 seconds. The cost is $24.95 for a VHS videotape; $34.95 for the video and the companion MPKU booklet. Distributed by Boathouse Row Entertainment, Inc, (formerly Octus Entertainment) 11901 Santa Monica Blvd, Suite 494, Los Angeles, CA 90025. To order call (310) 289-5628.

Satter E, producer: *Child of mine: feeding with love and good sense,* Bull Publishing Co, PO Box 208, Palo Alto, CA, ©1989. *A series of four videotapes of real parents, child care providers, and children shows what works and what does not work in helping children to eat well, stay out of struggles with eating, understand feeding from the child's perspective, and know when and when not to hold the line.* Video is based on the producer's book by the same title. Running time is 15 minutes for individual tape (*The Infant; The Older Baby; The Toddler;* and *The Preschooler*); 60 minutes for set of four on one VHS videotape. The cost of an individual tape is $54.95; the set of four on one tape costs $164.95; the book costs $14.95. To order call 1-800-676-2855.

Written materials for adults

Acosta PB and Yannicelli S: *A Guide for the Family of the Child With Phenylketonuria.* Ross Products Division, Abbott Laboratories, Columbus, Ohio, 1994. *This comprehensive guide introduces parents to PKU and its management.* Provided free by local representative for Ross. *Metabolic Formula Systems, 625 Cleveland Ave., Columbus, OH 43215. (800)551-5838.*

Dolan BE, Koch R, and Bekins C: *Guidelines for adults with untreated PKU: late treatment and dietary intervention,* 1995. *This guide outlines the process for converting and transitioning untreated adult individuals with classical PKU to diet.* To obtain a copy of the guidelines contact Barbara Dolan, RN, MSN, Redwood Coast Regional Center, 1116 Airport Park Blvd, Ukiah, CA 95482-3832, or call (707) 462-3832.

GeneHELP Resource Center, Berkeley, CA. *The center maintains a database of public education materials produced nationwide and support groups for PKU, maternal PKU, and other genetic disorders across the USA.* For information or to order available materials, write the Gene-HELP Resource Center, Genetic Disease Branch, State of California Department of Health Services, 2151 Berkeley Way, Annex 4, Berkeley, CA 94704, or call (510)540-2972.

Henderson RA, Castiglioni L, Koch R, et al: *Education of students with phenylketonuria (PKU): information for teachers, administrators and other school personnel,* Washington, DC, US DHHS, Public Health Service, NIH Pub. No. 92-3318, 1991. *This book acquaints teachers, school nurses, administrators, and other school personnel with current knowledge about PKU, and identifies the psychoeducational implications of the condition. Lists additional resource materials for PKU.* To order write the National Center for Education in Maternal and Child Health, 8201 Greensboro Dr, Suite 600, McLean, VA 22102, or call (703) 821-8955 x254.

Mead Johnson: *Living with PKU,* 1994. *This booklet includes a discussion of what PKU is, the genetics and management of PKU, interviews with families, and helpful hints from experienced parents.* Provided free by local representative for Mead Johnson Nutritional Group, Medical Affairs, Evansville, IN 47721, Technical Pediatric Product Information (812) 429-5599.

New York State Department of Health: Neonatal Screening Blood Specimen Collection and Handling Procedure and Simple Spot Check, 1994. These posters are provided free by Schleicher and Schuell, Inc, 10 Optical Ave, PO Box 2012, Keene, NH 03431-2012, 1-800-245-4024.

NutraSweet® in Foods and Beverages: *Information About PKU and Diet,* and *A Guide to Phenylketonuria for Parents and Health Care Profession-*

als. Both brochures are provided free by The Nutrasweet® Center, Box 830, Deerfield, IL 60015-0830, Consumer Affairs Department, (800) 321-7254.

PHE Forum: *The California maternal PKU program newsletter,* Berkeley, 1989–present. *This newsletter is published twice a year and contains articles and dietary tips relevant to the young adult with PKU and information about the California Maternal PKU Camp activities.* To order write the Maternal PKU Program Coordinator, Genetic Disease Branch, State of California Department of Health Services, 2151 Berkeley Way, Annex 4, Berkeley, CA 94704, or call (510) 540-2727.

Satter E: *How to get your kid to eat . . . but not too much,* Bull Publishing Co, PO Box 208, Palo Alto, CA 94302-0208, ©1991. *The topics covered include: Quit when the job is done, Pressure doesn't work, What is normal eating, Nutritional tactics for preventing food fights, Is your toddler jerking you around at the table? The popular preschooler, The industrious schoolager, The individualistic teenager, The child who grows poorly, Helping all you can to keep your child from being fat, and Eating disorders.* The cost is $14.95. To order call (800) 676-2855.

Schuett V: *Low protein cookery for PKU,* 1993. *This cookbook contains over 450 recipes, plus helpful hints for managing the PKU diet.* The cost of the cookbook is $19.86 (postage included). To order write Marketing Department, University of Wisconsin Press, 114 North Murray Street, Madison, WI 53715, or call (608) 265-2792.

Schuett V: *Low protein food list for PKU,* 1995. *This book lists the phenylalanine content of over 3000 natural and brand name specific foods. This is a flexible, well-designed system for calculating phenylalanine, protein, and calories for both weight of food and household measures; easy for children to use.* The cost is $35 US, $37 US for Canada, and $40 US for foreign address. To order write or send check, drawn on a US bank, payable to Dietary Specialties, Inc, PO Box 227, Rochester, NY 14601, or call (800) 544-0099.

Scientific Hospital Supplies, Inc and Schuett V: *International PKU Cookbook,* 1993. *This cookbook contains over 100 simple-to-follow recipes from around the world, with complete phenylalanine content listed. Advice on eating out and holiday meals is given.* The cost is $23. To order write SHS, PO Box 117, Gaithersburg, MD 20884, or call (800) 365-7354 or FAX (301) 963-7026.

Taylor JF and Latta S: *Why can't I eat that!: Helping kids obey medical diets,* Saratoga, CA, R&E Publishers, 1993. *For parents and members of the helping professions, this book details the psychology of getting children to observe any prescribed diet, and is designed to supplement the dietary measures outlined by the physician and dietitian. The book lists over 50 organizations concerned with children's disorders involving dietary considerations and has over 700 indexed entries.* To order write ADD Plus, 1095-25th St SE #107, Salem, OR 97301, or call (800) 847-1233, or FAX (503) 364-7454. The cost is $11.95 (add 10% shipping & handling).

Written materials for children

Taylor M and Schuett VE: *You and PKU,* 1993. *This is a 50-page spiral-bound notebook, with appealing illustrations, for children ages 3 to 8 years. Presented in storybook fashion, the notebook contains information about the PKU diet, blood drawing, and clinic visits. Included are suggestions for parents about teaching their child about PKU.* The cost is $5.00. To order write University of Wisconsin Press, 114 N Murray St, Madison, WI 53715, or call (608) 262-8782.

Wessler KW: *A Journey into the world of PKU,* Johns Hopkins University, 1991. *A fantasy story, appropriate for the school-age child, that describes PKU and responsibility toward self-care.* The cost is $12.00 including postage; check payable to JHU, Center for Medical Genetics. Mail order to Kenneth W. Wessel, EdD, JHU Center for Medical Genetics, CMSC 1004, 600 N Wolfe St, Baltimore, MD 21205.

Wyatt D: *All about PKU. Developed by a registered nurse, this 18-page cartoon coloring book is designed to help children ages 4 to 9 years old understand their diet and PKU.* The cost is $1.50 each, or $10.00 for 10 or more. To order write Children's Hospital Research Foundation, Division of Inborn Errors of Metabolism, Elland and Bethesda Avenues, Cincinnati, OH 45229.

Community Resources

Children's PKU Network. *This is a national nonprofit organization dedicated to working together for the benefit of all people involved in the treatment of PKU and other metabolic disorders. As a support service organization, activities include an express "care package" of information to new parents of a child with PKU, a crisis intervention service to children or adults in need, and the sale of dietary gram scales. The Network administers an educational scholarship program and the Regional Coordinator Network Council for PKU parents' groups nationwide.* Children's PKU Network, 8388 Vickers St, Suite 113, San Diego, CA 92111, Phone (619) 569-9881, FAX (619) 450-5034.

Maternal PKU Camps/Programs. *Three separate Maternal PKU Camps run annual summer educational programs for young women with PKU. The goals of Maternal PKU Camp are to foster social support among young women with PKU, positive attitudes toward treatment and self-management of the phe-restricted diet and knowledge about maternal PKU.* For information about the California Maternal PKU Camp contact the Maternal PKU Program Coordinator, Genetic Disease Branch, State of California Department of Health Services, 2151 Berkeley Way, Annex 4, Berkeley, CA 94704, (510) 540-2727; for the Northeast Regional Maternal PKU Camp, contact the PKU CORPS Coordinator, Children's Hospital, The PKU CORPS, 300 Longwood Ave, Boston, MA 02115, (617) 355-7346; and the Illinois Maternal PKU Program, Hazel Vespa, LCSW, Social Work #130, Children's Memorial Medical Center, Division of Social Services, 2300 Children's Plaza, Chicago, IL 60614, (312) 880-4486.

National PKU News©. *This national nonprofit organization publishes a newsletter 3 times a year to promote exchange of information about PKU. Regular columns include: Research Review, Special Features, Food and Nutrition Notes, The Learning Place, Connections, Just for Kids, and Hang in There . . . the teens and young adults column. Edited by Virginia Schuett.* The cost is $14 US, $20 Canadian currency, and $24 (US currency or bank draft) for foreign subscription. Make check payable to National PKU News, 6869 Woodlawn Ave NE #116, Seattle, WA 98115, FAX (206) 525-5023.

New England Connection for PKU and Allied Metabolic Disorders. *This is a nonprofit organization formed and directed by those affected by PKU and other inborn errors of metabolism and by parents and professionals involved with the treatment of these disorders. Organized to provide support and necessary services and educate those affected, to influence research, and to increase public awareness of these disorders.* Contact Trish Mullaley, President, 16 Angelina Lane, Mansfield, MA 02048, (508) 261-9671.

The PKU CORPS (Community Outreach Resource Program). *Model programs have been designed to provide community and family-centered support to meet the need for continued follow-up of individuals with PKU as they reach adolescence and young adulthood.* The Phe Buddy Program of the PKU CORPS, *are peer counselors with PKU (>16 years old) who provide support to children with PKU (6 to 15 years old).* The Resource Mothers Program, *matches mothers of younger children with PKU to young women with PKU who are planning a pregnancy or who are already pregnant.* The organization's regional activities are published four times a year in The PKU CORPS Bulletin, Children's Hospital, The PKU CORPS, 300 Longwood Ave, Boston, MA 02115, Phone (617) 355-7346.

PRODIGY, Online Bulletin Board PKU Parent Support. *Access by computer with modem: select Jump, Medical support bb, select topic Rare diseases, select subject Metabolic disorders. "Chat" by computer with other parents of children with PKU for support maintaining phe levels, recipe sharing, meeting information or about whatever is on your mind.* Initiated by superhighway pilots Virginia Crimarco and Barbara Rowe, phone and/or FAX (716) 838-3452.

Medical Food Products

Dietary Specialties
PO Box 227
Rochester, NY 14601
Customer Service:
800/544-0099

Mead Johnson Nutritional
   Group
Medical Affairs
2400 W Lloyd Expressway
Evansville, IN 47721
Customer Service:
   800/457-3550

Ener-G Foods, Inc
6901 Fox Ave, South
PO Box 24723
Seattle, WA 98124
Customer Service:
  206/767-6660

Foodtek Manufacturing, Inc.
Custom Medical Foods
273 Franklin Ave
Randolf, NJ 07869
Customer Service: 800-605-0410

Med Diet
3050 Ranchview Lane
Plymouth, MN 55447
Customer Service:
  800/MED-DIET

Ross Laboratories
Ross Products Division
625 Cleveland Ave
Columbus, OH 43215
Metabolic Formula Systems
Customer Service: 800/551-5838

Scientific Hospital Supplies, Inc
PO Box 117
Gaithersburg, MD 20884
Customer Service: 800/365-7354

SUMMARY OF PRIMARY CARE NEEDS FOR THE CHILD WITH PHENYLKETONURIA

Health care maintenance

Growth and development

Growth and development are normal on a phe-restricted diet.
Caloric intake of high CHO-free foods controlled to avoid obesity.
Adequate protein intake to promote greater dietary phe tolerance.
Children with PKU may have underdeveloped social skills.

Diet

Phe-restricted diet is for life.
Blood phe monitoring with weight and diet changes for life.
Self-management of phe-restricted diet should be initiated early in childhood.
For optimum availability of nutrients, EMF products should be prepared as prescribed and taken with meals.
Sensitivity to the social and cultural importance of food at each developmental stage is needed.

Safety

Medic-Alert bracelet or necklace specifying phe-restricted diet advisable.
Only individuals with a diagnosis of PKU should ingest EMF products as prescribed.
Children and teens need sun protection.

Immunizations

Routine immunizations are recommended.
Any catabolic reaction should be supported with hydration and calories.

Screening

Vision
Routine screening is recommended.
Hearing
Routine screening is recommended.
Dental
Screening should be initiated at eruption of the first tooth and closely followed thereafter.
Frequent CHO intake decreases the risk of caries.
Blood pressure
Routine screening is recommended.
Hematocrit
Hematocrit and hemoglobin values are assessed at 6 and 12 months of age and then annually.
Plasma ferritin levels are checked at 6, 9, and 12 months of age and every 6 months thereafter.
Breast-fed infants have exaggerated physiologic anemia of infancy and require iron supplements.
Urinalysis
Routine screening is recommended.
Tuberculosis
Routine screening is recommended.
Condition-specific screening
All children with persistent HPA require a urine pterin screening test.

Continued.

SUMMARY OF PRIMARY CARE NEEDS FOR THE CHILD WITH PHENYLKETONURIA—cont'd

Blood phe should be monitored with weight and dietary changes for phe tolerance.

Nutritional indices that should be monitored include tyr, vitamins, prealbumin, albumin, essential fatty acids, selenium, and other trace elements and metals.

Regular auscultation of heart sounds is advisable to identify selenium deficiency.

DNA mutation analysis of blood on filter paper.

Common illness management

Differential diagnosis

Differentiate elevated blood phe caused by illness or by intake of too little or too much dietary phe by an accurate history.

Prevent catabolic state related to common childhood illness with adequate hydration and caloric intake.

Minor surgery results in only a transient level of blood phe.

Differentiate skin lesions from allergic sensitivities, eczema, and scleroderma related to imbalance of blood phe, tyr, or tryptophan.

Limit sun exposure and use sun blocks as for any child.

Drug interactions

Aspartame ingestion is contraindicated.

Care should be taken to read food labels and medication ingredients for aspartame.

Monoamine oxidase inhibitors are contraindicated.

Daraprim (pyrimethamine) is contraindicated.

Caution should be taken in prescribing drugs that alter neurotransmitters.

Plasma tyr levels of women taking oral contraceptives should be monitored.

Developmental issues

Sleep patterns

Disturbed sleep patterns or nightmares may occur during loss of phe homeostasis.

Toileting

Infants may be more prone to diaper dermatitis.

Daily hygiene is important, especially for musty odor related to loss of phe homeostasis during illnesses and changes in diet and activity levels.

Discipline

Avoid use of food as a reward system and blood tests as punishment.

Expectations are normal based on age and developmental level.

Child care

Providers should be aware of the need for special diet and hydration and calories during illness and trauma.

Schooling

Visual spatial skills should be promoted.

Good lighting and contrasts of dark on light backgrounds (not greys) promote visualization of detailed subject matter (i.e., letters and numbers).

Annual developmental testing is recommended.

Math and language skills may require tutoring.

School personnel may be made aware of a child's special dietary needs at the parents' discretion.

Sexuality

Young women with PKU should be educated about the risks of MPKU.

Fertility is unaffected in men with PKU, although phe homeostasis is recommended.

Genetic counseling should be provided at the time appropriate for each individual with PKU.

Gamete donors should be tested for PKU by DNA analysis.

Transition into adulthood

Recommend that all individuals remain on phe-restricted diet for life.

Phe homeostasis throughout the lifetime improves the neuropsychiatric executive functions.

Participation in PKU support groups and professional counseling as needed are

Continued.

SUMMARY OF PRIMARY CARE NEEDS FOR THE CHILD WITH PHENYLKETONURIA—cont'd

recommended for adults with PKU and their families.

Psychotropic medication should be a last resort in an individual with PKU, after phe homeostasis is achieved.

Special family concerns

Special family concerns include delays in diagnosis after NBS positive result for PKU, the vigilant supervision of the child's 'diet for life,' the parental guilt at having passed a *hidden gene* on to their child, genetic counseling of immediate and extended family members, family planning and prenatal diagnosis options, inability to predict severity of HPA, financial support of the lifelong need for EMF products and medical care. Cultural and ethnic sensitivity in planning phe-restricted diet and all aspects of medical care to foster a positive attitude toward PKU in the child that will last a lifetime.

REFERENCES

Acosta PB, Wright L: Nurses' role in preventing birth defects in offspring of women with phenylketonuria, [published erratum appears in *JOGNN,* 21:352, 1992], *JOGNN,* 21:270-276, 1992.

Acosta PB, Yannicelli S: Protocol 1-Phenylketonuria. In Cameron AM (editor): *Ross metabolic formula system nutrition support protocols,* Columbus, OH, 1993, Division of Abbott Laboratories, pp 1-135.

Arnopp JJ et al: Results of screening for phenylketonuria using a lower cutoff value in early collected specimens, *Screening* 3:193-199, 1995.

Awiszus D, Unger I: Coping with PKU: results of narrative interviews with parents, *Eur J Peds* 149(suppl 1):S45-S51, 1990.

Azen CG et al: Intellectual development in 12-year-old children treated for phenylketonuria, *Am J Dis Child* 145:35-39, 1991.

Berg BO: *Child neurology,* Greenbrae, CA, 1984, Jones Medical Publications.

Black PR: Seeking legal advice for PKU-related insurance disputes, *National PKU News* 4(3):4-5, Winter 1993.

Blau N et al: A missense mutation in a patient with guanosine triphosphate cyclohydrolase I deficiency missed in the newborn screening program, *J Peds* 126:401-405, 1995.

Blau N et al: Tetrahydrobiopterin deficiency: from phenotype to genotype, *Pteridines* 4:1-10, 1993.

Bolognia JL, Pawelek JM: Biology of hypopigmentation, *J Am Acad Dermatol* 19:217-254, 1988.

Brunner RL, Berch DB, and Berry H: Phenylketonuria and complex spatial visualization: an analysis of information processing, *Dev Med Child Neurol* 29:460-468, 1987.

Buist NR, Tuerck JM: The practitioner's role in newborn screening, *Pediatr Clin North Am* 39:199-211, 1992.

Burn J: Relevance of the human genome project to inherited metabolic disease, *J Inher Metab Dis* 17:421-427, 1994.

Burns ER: Development and evaluation of a new instrument for safe heelstick sampling of neonates, *Lab Med* 20:481-483, 1989.

Burns JK et al: Impact of PKU on the reproductive patterns in collaborative study families, *Am J Med Genet* 19:515-524, 1984.

Campistol J: Neuropsychological problems in hyperphenylalaninemic patients. In *Proceedings of An International Symposium on the Occasion of the 60th Anniversary of Føllig's Discovery of Phenylketonuria,* Elsinore, Denmark, 1994.

Casamassimo PS et al: *Dental health in children with phenylketonuria and other inborn errors of amino acid metabolism managed by diet,* Publication No HRS-D-MC 84-1, Rockville, MD, 1984, US Department of Health and Human Services.

Clarke JTR et al: Neuropsychological studies on adolescents with phenylketonuria returned to phenylalanine restricted diets, *Am J Ment Retard* 92:255-262, 1987.

Council of Regional Networks for Genetic Services (CORN), Newborn Screening Committee: *National Newborn Screening Report-1991,* CORN, New York, 1994.

Craft S et al: Lateralized deficits in visual attention in males with developmental dopamine depletion, *Neuropsychologia* 30:341-351, 1992.

Cristiano RH, Smith LC, and Woo SL: Hepatic gene therapy: adenovirus enhancement of receptor-mediated gene delivery and expression in primary hepatocytes. In Proceedings of the *National Academy of Sciences of the United States of America* 90:2122-2126, 1993.

Curtius HC, Endres W, and Blau N: Effect of high-protein meal plus aspartame ingestion on plasma phenylalanine concentrations in obligate heterozygotes for phenylketonuria, *Metabolism* 43:413-416, 1994.

Diamond A: Prefontal cortex cognitive deficits in early-treated

PKU: results of a longitudinal study in children and of an animal model, *Soc for Neuroscience Abstracts* 18:1063, 1993.

Diamond A et al: An animal model of early-treated PKU, *J Neuroscience* 14:3072-3082, 1994.

Dolan BE, Koch R, and Bekins C: Dramatic behavioral and medical benefits of two adults with untreated PKU: dietary intervention and guidelines for late treatment. In *Proceedings of American Association on Mental Retardation Conference,* San Francisco, CA, 1995.

Eisensmith RC et al: Recurrence of the R408W mutation in the phenylalanine hydroxylase locus in Europeans, *Am J Hum Genet* 56:278-286, 1995.

Fehrenbach AM, Peterson L: Parental problem solving skills, stress, and dietary compliance in PKU, *J Consult Clin Psychol* 57:237-241, 1989.

Fiedler AE et al: Phenylalanine levels in PKU following minor surgery, *Am J Med Genet* 11:411-414, 1982.

Fisch RO, Gravem HJ, and Feinberg SB: Growth and bone characteristics of phenylketonurics: Comparative analysis of treated and untreated phenylketonuric children, *Am J Dis Child* 112:3-10, 1966.

Fisch RO et al: Bony changes of PKU neonates unrelated to phenylalanine levels, *J Inher Metab Dis* 14:890-895, 1991a.

Fisch RO et al: Children of fathers with phenylketonuria: an international survey, *J Pediatr* 118:739-741, 1991b.

Fishler K et al: Psychoeducational findings among children treated for phenylketonuria, *Am J Ment Defic* 92:65-73, 1987.

Gleason LA et al: A treatment program for adolescents with phenylketonuria, *Clinical Peds* 31:331-335, 1992.

Greeves LG, Carson DJ, and Dodge JA: Peptic ulceration and phenylketonuria: a possible link? *Gut* 29:691-692, 1988.

Greeves LG et al: Potentially life-threatening cardiac dysrhythmia in a child with selenium deficiency and phenylketonuria, *Acta Paediatr Scand* 79:1259-1262, 1990.

Greve LC et al: Breast feeding in the management of the newborn with phenylketonuria: a practical approach to dietary therapy, *J Am Diet Assoc* 94:305-309, 1994.

Guldberg P et al: Mutation analysis in families with discordant phenotypes of phenylalanine hydroxyase deficiency. Inheritance and expression of the hyperphenylalaninemias, *J Inher Metab Dis* 17:645-651, 1994.

Guttler F, Olesen ES, and Wamberg E: Diurnal variations of serum phenylalanine in phenylketonuric children on low phenylalanine diet, *Am J Clin Nutr* 22:1568-1570, 1969.

Hanley WB: Prenatal testing for maternal phenylketonuria (MPKU), *Int Pediatr* 9(suppl 2):33-39, 1994.

Hassel CW, Brunsting LA: Phenylpyruvic oligphrenia: an elevation of the light-sensitive and pigmentary characteristics of seventeen patients, *AMA Arch Dermatol* 79:458-465, 1959.

Hayaishi O: Tryptophan, oxygen, and sleep, *Annu Rev Biochem* 63:1-24, 1994.

Herrero E et al: Inhibition by L-phenylalanine of tryptophan transport by synaptosomal plasma membrane vesicles: impli-cations in the pathogenesis of phenylketonuria, *J Inher Metab Dis* 6:32-35, 1983.

Herrmann ME et al: Dependence of the utilization of a phenylalanine-free amino acid mixture on different amounts of single dose ingested: a case report, *Eur J Peds* 153:501-503, 1994.

Hofman KJ et al: Phenylketonuria in US blacks: molecular analysis of the phenylalanine hydroxylase gene, *Am J Hum Genet* 48:791-798, 1991.

Holtzman NA et al: Effect of informed parental consent on mothers' knowledge of newborn screening, *Pediatrics* 72:807-812, 1983.

Hommes FA: On the mechanism of permanent brain dysfunction in hyperphenylalaninemia, *Biochem Med Metab Bio* 46:277-287, 1991.

Irons M, Levy HL: Metabolic syndromes with dermatologic manifestations, *Clin Rev Allergy* 4:101-124, 1986.

Jew K, Williams JC, and Koch R: Reproductive decision making in PKU families. In *Proceedings of the 6th National Neonatal Screening Symposium,* Portland, OR, 1988.

Jew K et al: Validity of screening early collected newborn specimens for phenylketonuria using a fluorometric method, *Screening* 3:1-9, 1994.

Jones SL: Assisted reproductive technologies: genetic and nursing implications, *JOGNN* 23:492-497, 1994.

Kaufman S: An evaluation of the possible neurotoxicity of metabolites of phenylanine, *J Pediatr* 114:895-900, 1989.

Kaul R et al: Frequency of 12 mutations in 114 children with phenylketonuria in the midwest region of the USA, *J Inher Metab Dis* 17:356-358, 1994.

Kay MA, Woo SL: Gene therapy for metabolic disorders, *Trends in Genet* 10:253-257, 1994.

Kazak AE, Reber M, and Snitzer L: Childhood chronic disease and family functioning: a study of phenylketonuria, *Pediatrics* 81:224-283, 1988.

Kling S: *Newborn screening—an overview of newborn screening programs in the United States and Canada 1993,* Illinois Department of Public Health, Springfield, IL, 1993.

Koch R et al: The North America collaborative study of maternal PKU, *AJDC* 147:1224-1230, 1993.

Koch R, Wenz E: Phenylketonuria, *Ann Rev Nutr* 7:117-135, 1987.

Koch R, Yusin M, and Fishler K: Successful adjustment to society by adults with phenylketonuria, *J Inher Metab Dis* 8:209-211, 1985.

Leuzzi V et al: Neuroradiological (MRI) abnormalities in phenylketonuric subjects: clinical and biochemical correlations, *Neuropediatrics* 24:302-306, 1993.

Levy HL, Waisbren SE, and Shiloh S: PKU in adolescents: rationale and psychological factors in diet continuation. In *Proceedings of An International Symposium on the Occasion of the 60th Anniversary of Føllig's Discovery of Phenylketonuria,* Elsinore, Denmark, 1994.

Lichter-Konecki U et al: Relation between phenylalanine hydroxylase genotypes and phenotypic parameters of diagnosis and treatment of hyperphenylalaninaemic disorders, *J Inher Metab Dis* 17:362-365, 1994.

Lorey FW, Cunningham GC: Effect of specimen collection methods on newborn screening for PKU, *Screening* 3:57-65, 1994.

Lou HC et al: An occipito-temporal syndrome in adolescents with optimally controlled hyperphenylalaninemia, *J Inherit Metab Dis* 15:687-695, 1992.

Lou HC et al: Brain magnetic resonance imaging in children with optimally controlled hyperphenylalaninemia. In *Proceedings of An International Symposium on the Occasion of the 60th Anniversary of Føllig's Discovery of Phenylketonuria,* Elsinore, Denmark, 1994.

Matalon R et al: Maternal collaborative study: pregnancy outcome and postnatal head growth, *J Inher Metab Dis* 17:353-355, 1994.

McBurnie MA et al: Physical growth of children treated for phenylketonuria, *Annals Human Bio* 18:357-368, 1991.

McCabe L et al: The management of breast feeding among infants with phenylketonuria, *J Inherited Metab Dis* 23:467-474, 1989.

National Committee for Clinical Laboratory Standards: Blood collection on filter paper for neonatal screening programs, ed 2, *NCCLS Document LA4-A2,* 1992.

Nova MP, Kaufman M, and Halperin A: Sclerodermalike indurations in a child with phenylketonuria: a clinicopathologic correlation and review of the literature, *J Am Acad Derm* 26:329-333, 1992.

O'Flynn ME: Newborn screening for phenylketonuria: 30 years of progress, *Current Problems in Peds* 22(4):159-165, 1992.

O'Tuama LA, Treves ST: Brain single-photon emission computed tomography for behavior disorders in children, *Seminars in Nuc Med* 23:255-264, 1993.

Pietz J et al: EEGs in phenylketonuria: I. follow-up to adulthood, II. short-term diet-related changes in EEGs and cognitive function, *Dev Med Child Neuro* 35:54-64, 1993.

Pitt DB, Danks DM: The natural history of untreated phenylketonuria over 20 years, *J Paediatr Child Health* 27:189-190, 1994.

Platt LD et al: Maternal phenylketonuria collaborative study, obstetrical aspects and outcome: the first 6 years, *Am J Ob Gyn* 166:1150-1162, 1992.

Potocnik U, Widhalm K: Long-term follow-up of children with classical phenylketonuria after diet discontinuation: a review, *J Am College Nutr* 13:232-236, 1994.

Ris MD et al: Early treated phenylketonuria: adult neuropsychologic outcome, *J Peds* 124:88-392, 1994.

Riva E et al: PKU-related dysgammaglobulinaemia: the effect of diet therapy on IgE and allergic sensitization, *J Inher Metab Dis* 17:710-717, 1994.

Sanjurjo L et al: Polyunsaturated fatty acid status in patients with phenylketonuria, *J Inher Metab Dis* 17:704-709, 1994.

Schmidt K: Primer to the inborn errors of metabolism for perinatal and neonatal nurses, *J Perinat Neonatal Nurs* 2:60-71, 1989.

Schuett V: *National survey of treatment programs for PKU and other selected inherited metabolic diseases,* Washington, DC, US DHHS Pub; No. HRS-MCH-89-5, 1990.

Scriver CR et al: Associations between populations, phenylketonuria mutations, and RFLP haplotypes at the phenylalanine hydroxylas locus: an overview, *Dev Brain Dysfunct* 6:11-25, 1993.

Scriver CR et al: The hyperphenylalaninemias. In Scriver CR et al (editors): *The metabolic and molecular bases of inherited disease,* New York, 1995, McGraw-Hill, vol I, pp 1015-1075.

Shiloh S et al: Cross-cultural perspectives on coping with the risks of maternal phenylketonuria, *Psych Health* 8:435-446, 1993.

Smith I, Beasley MG, and Ades AE: Intelligence and quality of dietary treatment in phenylketonuria, *Arch Dis Child* 65:472-478, 1990.

Sorenson JR et al: Parental response to repeat testing of infants with 'false positive' results in a newborn screening program, *Pediatrics* 73:183-187, 1984.

Svensson E et al: Two missense mutations causing mild hyperphenylalaninemia associated with DNA heplotype 12, Human Mutation 1:129-137, 1992.

Thompson AJ et al: Brain MRI changes in phenylketonuria, *Brain* 116:811-821, 1993.

Tokatli A et al: Classical phenylketonuria associated with Goldenhar's syndrome: a case report, *Turk J Peds* 36:153-156, 1994.

Trahms CM: Self-management skills: the key to successful PKU treatment, part I. First steps: teaching your young child the basics, *National PKU News* 3(3):4-5, Winter 1992.

Trahms CM: Self-management skills: the key to successful PKU treatment, part II. Moving ahead and walking strong: promoting self-management for the school-aged child, *National PKU News* 4(1):4-5, Spring/Summer 1992.

Trahms CM: Self-management skills: the key to successful PKU treatment, part III. Standing on your own two feet: the adolescent years and beyond, *National PKU News* 4(2):4-5, Fall 1992.

Treacy E et al: Phenylalanine metabolism in vivo in mild phenylketonuria, the effect of multiple loci, abstract 106, *Am J Hum Genet* 55 (suppl):A22, 1994.

Vajro P et al: Correction of phenylketonuria after liver transplantation in a child with cirrhosis, *NEJM* 329:363, 1993.

Valle D, Mitchell G: Introduction to genetic disorders: sources of variability. In *Dietary Management of Persons With Metabolic Disorders,* Evansville, IN, 1994, Mead Johnson and Company, pp 4-5.

Velazquez K: Legislative Update. In *Proceedings of The 16th PKU Parents Conference,* Walnut Creek, CA, 1994.

Waisbren SE, Levy HL: Agoraphobia in phenylketonuria, *J Inher Metab Dis* 14:755-764, 1991.

Waisbren SE, Zaff J: Personality disorder in young women with treated phenylketonuria, *J Inher Metab Dis* 17:584-592, 1994.

Wyatt RJ et al: Effects of 5-hydroxytryptophan on the sleep of normal human subjects, *Electroencephalogr Clin Neurophysiol* 30:505-509, 1971.

Prematurity

30

Diane J. Goldman, Steven L. Goldman,
and Toshiko Hirata

ETIOLOGY

The population of premature, low-birth-weight
(LBW) infants represents a heterogeneous group.
At one end of the spectrum are infants who spend
their first weeks of life critically ill and, if they survive, require lifelong chronic care. At the other end,
are those infants who have little or no problems
during the perinatal period and require no special
long-term care.

The terminology used to describe premature or
LBW infants is not uniformly applied, which can
result in confusing overlap. Premature, or preterm,
generally refers to infants born before 38 weeks'
gestation; however, the World Health Organization
uses birth at less than 37 weeks as the definition of
prematurity. Low birth weight refers to infants
whose birth weight is less than 2500 g, very low
birth weight (VLBW) refers to infants less than
1500 g, and extremely low birth weight (ELBW)
refers to infants less than 1000 g. Historically the
term "low birth weight" has been used almost syn-
onymously with the term "premature." This usage
can be misleading. For example, some term infants
have birth weights less than 2500 g (these infants
are small for gestational age, or SGA), and some
premature infants have birth weights greater than
2500 g (these infants are large for gestational age,
or LGA). Appropriate for gestational age infants
(AGA) have a birth weight within the normal range
for their gestational age. Many of the references

cited in this chapter vary in the terminology used.
The term "premature" will be used preferentially in
this chapter. Where the use of this term is not consistent with a reference, however, other terms will
need to be used as well.

The causes of prematurity are varied, and many
are interrelated. In simplest terms, infants are born
prematurely for one of two reasons: either the delivery was iatrogenically caused (pharmacologic
induction or cesarean section) or the delivery could
not be stopped (spontaneous preterm delivery).
Some of the known causes or risk factors are listed
in the accompanying box on page 651. In many
cases, a specific cause or risk factor cannot be identified (Creasy, 1994).

INCIDENCE

Because birth certificate gestational data are unreliable, birth weight is used to estimate the incidence
of prematurity. In 1992, the incidence of LBW infants in the United States was 8.4%; VLBW infants
comprised 1.3% of births. A racial disparity in birth
weight continues: the incidence of black LBW infants is approximately 2.5 times that of white LBW
infants (Wegman, 1994).

CLINICAL MANIFESTATIONS

The condition of prematurity is definitively diagnosed at the time of birth. The degree of prematu-

CAUSES OF PRETERM BIRTH

Iatrogenic preterm delivery

Maternal indications

Severe preeclampsia
Infection placing mother or infant at risk
Bleeding (previa, abruption)
Cardiovascular instability
Uncontrolled diabetes

Fetal indications

Death of an identical twin
Poor growth
Unstable biophysical profile
Hydrops

Spontaneous preterm delivery

Maternal risk factors

Prior premature birth
Pariety = 0 or >4
Incompetent cervix
Abnormal placentation
Infection
Drug use (alcohol, cocaine, tobacco, etc.)
Preterm rupture of membranes
Short interval since last live born
Previous cesarean section

Fetal risk factors

Multiple gestation
Fetal anomalies

rity is most accurately assessed using reliable maternal history. Occasionally when the date of the last menstrual period is uncertain, the gestational age can be confirmed using the measurements obtained at an early ultrasound examination. In the absence of reliable dates or if there are conflicting data, the objective assessment of physical and neurologic findings in the neonate can estimate the gestational age to within ±2 weeks (Ballard et al, 1991; Constantine et al, 1987; Dubowitz, Dubowitz, and Goldberg, 1970).

Instruments that have been developed for the clinical assessment of gestational age take advantage of the profound physical and neurologic changes that occur in the fetus during the last trimester. For example, an infant of 24 weeks' gestation is extremely hypotonic, with fragile, thin, gelatinous skin. The skin breaks down and the subcutaneous tissue bleeds with minimal trauma. Because the chest wall is so flexible at this gestational age, respiratory effort results in substernal retractions. As the fetus matures, there is a global increase in resting tone, a flexed posture develops, the skin thickens, and bone and cartilage become firmer.

CLINICAL MANIFESTATIONS

- Low, very low, or extremely low birth weight
- Premature neurologic development
- Premature physiologic and metabolic development

TREATMENT

The most desirable treatment for prematurity is prevention, but if the preterm birth is inevitable, treatment should begin in utero. Corticosteroids given to the mother before delivery will accelerate fetal lung maturation and decrease the risk of respiratory distress syndrome (RDS) and significantly reduce the incidence of intraventricular hemorrhage. If time permits, the mother and fetus should be transferred to a center with expertise in the

TREATMENT

Prevention of prematurity
- Prevention of premature births
- Corticosteroids given to mother to increase fetal lung maturation
- Birth at a center for high-risk pregnancies

Management of complications of prematurity
- Metabolic
- Infections
- Respiratory
- Neurologic
- Hematologic
- Cardiovascular
- Gastrointestinal

management of high-risk deliveries and in caring for high-risk infants.

After the infant is born, treatment is tailored to existing or anticipated problems. Often, prophylactic treatment modalities are used in infants at highest risk. For example, exogenous surfactant can be given at birth to prevent or lessen the severity of RDS (Corbet et al, 1991), indomethacin (Indocin) may be given before signs of patent ductus arteriosus are clinically apparent, and respiratory stimulants such as caffeine or theophylline may be given before apnea occurs.

RECENT AND ANTICIPATED ADVANCES IN DIAGNOSIS AND MANAGEMENT

Prematurity itself does not cause long-range problems for the affected infant; rather, the complications associated with prematurity cause, in some cases, irreparable damage.

The most important advance in this area would be to decrease the incidence of premature births. Society has the means (e.g., providing universal access to prenatal care), but not the resolve to

commit the resources at present. Advances in managing the complications associated with premature birth will lessen the incidence of poor outcomes. Such advances will come in the form of improving on techniques now in use. For example, liquid ventilation may decrease the lung damage seen with conventional ventilation. Ways to stabilize capillaries may further decrease the risk of periventricular-intraventricular hemorrhage (PIVH).

ASSOCIATED PROBLEMS

As outlined in Table 30-1, the potential clinical problems associated with prematurity are many. Any, all, or none of these clinical problems can develop, and many of these represent risk factors for the development of other problems. For example, an infant with severe RDS is more apt to develop a periventricular-intraventricular hemorrhage (PIVH) than an infant without respiratory disease; an infant with prolonged feeding intolerance or necrotizing enterocolitis (NEC) is more likely to develop rickets. Recognizing that these problems are possible allows the clinician to anticipate the long-term implications.

Periventricular-Intraventricular Hemorrhage

Periventricular-intraventricular hemorrhage (PIVH) often begins with bleeding into the subependymal germinal matrix. The bleeding can extend into the ventricular system or into the nearby brain parenchyma. PIVH has been classified into four grades according to Papile, Munsick-Bruno, and Schaefer (1983): grade I, subependymal hemorrhage; grade II, intraventricular hemorrhage; grade III, intraventricular hemorrhage with ventricular dilation; and grade IV, intraventricular hemorrhage with parenchymal hemorrhage.

The germinal matrix is a metabolically active, highly vascularized area that persists until term and is predisposed to hemorrhage for several reasons. Because there is poor autoregulation of blood flow to this area in premature infants, the delicate capillaries of the germinal matrix are vulnerable to damage from acute changes in systemic arterial or venous pressure. Perinatal asphyxia, metabolic problems, or respiratory problems can also damage the

Table 30-1.   ASSOCIATED PROBLEMS

	Metabolic	Infection	Respiratory	Neurologic	Hematologic	Cardiovascular	GI*
Early onset (≤2 wk)	Decreased calcium level Decrease or increase in glucose level Poor temperature regulation	Perinatally acquired (e.g., group B *Streptococcus*)	RDS TTN† Meconium aspiration Apnea	PIVH‡	Anemia (usually iatrogenic)	Patent ductus	Nonspecific feeding intolerance Necrotizing enterocolitis
Late onset (>2 wk)	Rickets	Hospital acquired (e.g., *Staphylococcus*, gram-negative rods)	BPD§ Apnea	Posthemorrhagic hydrocephalus Periventricular leukomalacia	Exaggerated anemia of prematurity		Postparenteral nutritional cholestasis

*GI, gastrointestinal.
†TTN, transient tachypnea of the newborn.
‡PIVH, periventricular-intraventricular hemorrhage.
§BPD, bronchopulmonary dysplasia.

capillary bed and further predispose toward hemorrhage.

The reported incidence of PIVH varies considerably depending in part on the population studied and method of diagnosis. It is clear that the risk of PIVH increases with decreasing gestational age and with a host of risk factors, most of which are a reflection of how ill the infant is. Periventricular or intraventricular hemorrhage of any grade occurs in approximately 40% of infants with birth weight less than 1500 g (Volpe, 1995).

Treatment is supportive, and risk factors thought to contribute to further hemorrhage are minimized. Serial ultrasound examinations are necessary to document the resolution of the hemorrhage and to detect the development of hydrocephalus. If hydrocephalus develops, treatment must be instituted to minimize brain damage (see Chapter 23).

Mortality from PIVH is related to severity. Whereas there is no mortality associated with minimal hemorrhage, as many as 50% of infants with the most extensive hemorrhage do not survive (Volpe, 1995). In most reports of those who do survive, infants with the higher grades of PIVH have the worst outcome. In the series of VLBW infants by Papile, Munsick-Bruno, and Schaefer (1983), the incidence of major disability at 1 to 2 years of age was approximately 8% for infants with no, grade I, or grade II PIVH. However, 25% of those with grade III PIVH and 60% of those with grade IV PIVH had major disabilities. In many reports, infants with posthemorrhagic hydrocephalus tend to have the worst outcome (Krishnamoorthy et al, 1990). Papile, Munsick-Bruno, and Lowe (1988) have reported improvement over time in this group of infants, suggesting that the outcome for infants with larger hemorrhages is not as dismal as once thought.

Retinopathy of Prematurity

Retinopathy of prematurity (ROP), also known as retrolental fibroplasia, affects the retina of the premature infant. Vascularization of the retina may not be complete until after approximately 42 to 44 weeks' postconceptual age. For reasons that are not clear, in some premature infants, abnormal vascularization of the retina develops. In most cases the retinopathy resolves without sequelae;

however, in a few infants a proliferative neovascularization can develop, accompanied by fibrosis and retinal detachment. This leads to total or partial blindness.

The following stages of ROP have been described: stage 1, demarcation line between vascularized and avascular retina; stage 2, ridge (raised demarcation line); stage 3, ridge with extraretinal fibrovascular proliferation; stage 4, partial retinal detachment; stage 5, total retinal detachment (International Committee for the Classification of the Late Stages of Retinopathy of Prematurity, 1987).

With increasing survival of infants with birth weight less than 1000 g, there are increasing numbers of infants with ROP. Risk factors for the development of ROP have been identified (Purohit et al, 1985), but clear cause and effect relationships remain to be confirmed. The most important risk factors appear to be prematurity and length of time in supplemental oxygen. The risk of ROP increases with decreasing gestational age, but the precise risk varies considerably from center to center. Infants with birth weight greater than 1500 g have an approximate 0.6% to 3% risk, whereas in some series those infants with birth weight less than 1000 g have as high as a 50% risk. A small proportion of affected infants progress to the most severe stages (Phelps, 1995). Other factors that may increase risk are sepsis, apnea, and blood transfusion with adult blood. Most infants with stage 1 or 2 ROP experience regression and have no significant visual sequelae. Infants with ROP stages 3 and higher are likely to have vision problems ranging from myopia to retinal detachment and blindness.

Historically treatment results had been uniformly poor. Vitamin E remains a controversial treatment. The role of cryotherapy (localized hypothermia) has been evaluated in a nationwide randomized trial. Enrollment was halted in 1988 after preliminary results demonstrated definite benefit, underscoring the importance of making a timely diagnosis (Multicenter Trial of Cryotherapy for Retinopathy of Prematurity, 1988). More recently, laser photocoagulation has been found to be at least as effective as cryotherapy and potentially better at preventing progression to retinal detachment. It appears to have less adverse side effects as well, including less pain, swelling, and less likelihood of damage to the eye (Landers, 1990; McNamara et al, 1993).

Anemia

No single, specific definition for anemia exists in this population. The hemoglobin level or hematocrit value must be assessed in light of the infant's age. For example, a hematocrit value of less than 40% at birth would be considered anemia. It is normal, however, for the hematocrit value to decrease to less than 40% over the weeks after birth. Anemia of prematurity is an exaggeration of the normal newborn's "physiologic" anemia.

Infants with anemia documented soon after birth should be evaluated for hemolysis, chronic blood loss in utero, or acute perinatal blood loss. Common causes of anemia that develop after the immediate perinatal period in the premature infant are iatrogenic blood loss and anemia of prematurity. The blood volume of an infant is only 80 to 100 ml/kg. Even with microtechniques, laboratory tests in a sick infant can easily deplete this blood volume. Anemia of prematurity results from a failure of the erythropoietin feedback system. When the tissues sense inadequate oxygen delivery, the kidney should manufacture erythropoietin. In the newborn and especially the premature newborn, the set point is temporarily too low, probably reflecting the normal hypoxemia of the environment in utero. Early iatrogenic anemia in very small, very sick premature infants is virtually universal. Most such infants will require at least one blood transfusion.

The decision to treat a premature infant for anemia is not based on absolute hematocrit values. Tachycardia, tachypnea, poor weight gain, and acidosis are nonspecific symptoms of anemia. Presence of any of these symptoms in the face of a low hematocrit value may indicate the need for a transfusion of packed red blood cells (Sacher, Luban, and Strauss, 1989). Treatment is not without risk. Transfusion reactions are rare but can occur in neonates. Despite screening, infectious complications include cytomegalovirus, hepatitis, and human immunodeficiency virus (HIV). The risk of HIV virus exposure decreased significantly after 1985 when screening became common (see Chapter 22).

Genetic engineering has made human erythropoietin readily available. Clinical trials are ongoing to determine if erythropoietin is a safe, effective treatment for anemia in premature infants. Anemia of prematurity is a self-resolving condition; the infant should be provided with oral supplemental iron if breast feeding or if insufficient iron is being supplied in the formula (see section on diet in this chapter). Many premature infants are discharged from the hospital with hematocrit values much lower than those of term infants. This distinction makes follow-up and screening more important in the premature infant.

Nutrition

Nutrition remains a major problem for the smallest premature infants. Generally infants with birth weight greater than 1250 g without significant medical problems tolerate enteral feedings easily. For those with acute problems and for smaller infants, however, enteral feedings are often delayed for days or weeks.

Parenteral nutrition consisting of dextrose, emulsified fat, and amino acids can provide infants with adequate calories for growth. Early complications of parenteral nutrition include hyperglycemia, protein intolerance reflected by hyperammonemia or acidosis, and difficulties related to prolonged intravenous access such as infiltrates and infection. Occasionally these complications prevent the infant from receiving adequate nutrition for long periods. Late complications of parenteral nutrition include cholestatic jaundice, often with elevated liver enzymes, which affects 30% to 40% of infants who weigh less than 1500 g who receive parenteral nutrition for more than 2 weeks (Bell et al, 1986). The jaundice may be prolonged, lasting several weeks or more, but eventually resolves.

Enteral feeding practices have changed over the past decade. Because premature infants have special nutritional needs (increased need for protein, calcium, phosphate, and sodium), formulas have undergone many changes to meet as many of these needs as possible while maintaining an acceptably high caloric density and an acceptably low osmolality and solute load. Preterm mother's milk supplemented with human milk fortifiers has been shown to be highly suited to the infant's nutritional needs. Despite the availability of parenteral nutrition, fortified breast milk, and premature formulas, most small premature infants do not receive adequate calcium and phosphorous intake. Hence the incidence of rickets in VLBW infants may be as high as 32% (Callenbach et al, 1981; Committee on Nutrition, 1985, 1993).

The process of weaning parenteral nutrition and slowly introducing breast milk or formula can be frustrating. Feedings are often "not tolerated," a catchall phrase that includes vomiting, abdominal distention, and large gastric residuals. Because these nonspecific symptoms may be early signs of NEC, feeding is often temporarily discontinued. This on again–off again phase of enteral feeding results in a period of poor nutrition.

Necrotizing enterocolitis is a condition most common in premature infants and is characterized by ischemic damage to the submucosal layer of the bowel. This condition accounts for approximately 2% of deaths in premature infants. It probably has many etiologies. The long list of risk factors include asphyxia, hypertonic feedings, umbilical vessel catheterization, exchange transfusion, and polycythemia. In severe cases of NEC, intestinal perforation—an absolute indication for surgery—can occur. Whether or not perforation occurs, stricture and obstruction, along with symptoms of abdominal distention and vomiting, occur weeks later in approximately 15% of affected infants. Lifelong problems may develop in those infants with postoperative short bowel syndrome (Vanderhoof et al, 1994).

Respiratory Problems

Lung damage. Respiratory distress occurs in approximately 10% of all neonates. Of those, 60% to 70% of the infants have transient respiratory problems. Approximately 10% each will have RDS, aspiration of meconium, blood, or amniotic fluid, or congenital pneumonia (Martin, Fanaroff, and Klaus, 1993; Kopelman, Mathew, 1995).

A wide range of treatment modalities is available, and treatments are tailored to the infants' needs. Most infants require little supportive therapy, such as supplemental oxygen given through a hood. Others require positive pressure as continuous positive airway pressure or mechanical ventilation through an endotracheal tube. Treatment with positive pressure and supplemental oxygen, though lifesaving, may damage the lungs and airways. This

damage must be viewed as a continuum. The extreme example of this is bronchopulmonary dysplasia (BPD) (see Chapter 10). Premature infants who require mechanical ventilation but do not develop BPD have evidence of lung and airway damage (Coates et al, 1977). This damage may be subclinical, demonstrated only with pulmonary function testing, or may be reflected in increased airway reactivity or increased pulmonary infections in the first years of life.

Apnea. Of LBW infants, 25% to 30% have apnea, mostly attributable to respiratory center immaturity (apnea of prematurity). The incidence increases with decreasing gestational age. In most cases, apnea resolves by the time the infant reaches 40 weeks' maturational age. For many VLBW infants, persistence or recurrence of apnea at this stage would suggest gastroesophageal reflux. Diagnosis and treatment of reflux result in resolution of the apnea.

There is no evidence that apnea of prematurity increases the risk for sudden infant death syndrome (SIDS). Graduates of intensive care nurseries (ICNs), however, are statistically at much higher risk for SIDS, a risk that appears to be magnified by other factors such as BPD, maternal drug abuse (especially cocaine), and VLBW. Unfortunately there is no way to predict which infant will go on to develop SIDS. Nevertheless, many centers perform pneumograms on LBW infants as a diagnostic tool to decide which infants should be sent home with a cardiorespiratory monitor.

The premature infant who continues to have apnea, when in all other respects he or she is ready for discharge, presents a management problem. There appears to be no consensus on treatment. Some care providers keep the infant in the hospital indefinitely, whereas others send the infant home with a cardiorespiratory monitor with or without theophylline or caffeine therapy. Parents of infants at higher risk for apnea or SIDS should be taught infant cardiopulmonary resuscitation (CPR) before the infant is discharged from the hospital.

Gastrointestinal Problems

The incidence of inguinal hernias is higher in LBW newborns than in term neonates. Inguinal hernias occur more frequently in those infants born at less than 32 weeks' gestation or who weigh less than

1250 g; for SGA male infants born at less than 32 weeks' gestation, the risk is even higher. Preterm infants requiring inguinal hernia repair may have increased risk of incarceration, recurrent apnea, anesthesia morbidity, and postoperative complications (Peevy, Speed, and Hoff, 1986). Surgical repair should be accomplished as soon as possible by a qualified pediatric surgeon (DeLorimier, 1988).

Genitourinary Problems

Low birth weight and premature male infants have a higher rate of undescended testes than full-term newborns. Nearly 100% of infants weighing approximately 900 g exhibit bilateral undescended testes. In most of these tiny infants, the testes descend during the first year of life. Medical and surgical intervention is indicated soon after 1 year of age for those children with undescended testes because there is evidence of decreased spermatogonia if the testes remain in the abdomen (Hawtrey, 1990).

PROGNOSIS

Probably in no other area is the question of survival and quality of life so important. The "morality of drastic intervention" (Avery, 1994) can be discussed at length without a uniform consensus being reached. Because centers (and individuals) differ in what is considered to be appropriate therapy, the published reports of outcome in terms of morbidity and mortality are not easily compared. However, some generalities can be made. Infant mortality continues to decrease. In 1992, the infant mortality rate in the United States was 8.5/100 live births. Prematurity and LBW, and their associated problems are responsible for many of these deaths. According to the Centers for Disease Control (CDC), "Disorders relating to short gestation and unspecified low birth weight" account for 11.7% of deaths; respiratory distress syndrome for 6%; and maternal complications of pregnancy (which often leads to prematurity) for 4.2% (Centers for Disease Control (CDC), 1994; Wegman, 1994).

Overall, survival is related directly to gestational age or birth weight, and there has been improved survival over the past 15 years. The reason for the improved survival in the smaller infants is, in part, the result of scientific and technologic improvements in many areas such as ventilatory and nutritional support. In addition, however, the application of available technology to infants previously thought to be nonviable has been an important reason for improved survival rates.

With increasing survival there are increasing numbers of infants with significant morbidity. Poor outcome is related to the associated complications of prematurity. Because the smallest infants are those with the most complications, the worst outcome is in the smallest infants.

One measure of the increased morbidity is the higher use of medical resources by LBW infants during the first year of life. Low birth weight infants are twice as likely and VLBW infants 4.5 times as likely to be hospitalized during the first year of life compared with normal birth weight infants (McCormick, 1985; McCormick, Shapiro, and Starfield, 1980). At 5 years of age, VLBW children have an increased number of hospital admissions and days in the hospital as compared with normal birth weight children. Respiratory tract problems and ear, nose, and throat surgery are the most common reasons for readmission (Kitchen et al, 1990).

Primary Care Management
HEALTH CARE MAINTENANCE

Growth and Development

The growth pattern of the majority of preterm AGA infants when plotted by corrected age rather than chronologic age follows the same pattern as full-term infants (Brandt, 1978). Corrected age is the postnatal age less the number of weeks the infant was premature. Moderately premature infants without serious medical illness show maximal catch-up growth earlier than extremely premature infants or those with serious medical problems. "Healthy" premature infants exhibit catch-up growth within the first year, whereas small or sicker infants may not reach their growth potential until 3 or more years of age (Hack and Fanaroff, 1988; Hirata et al, 1983).

Several studies have shown that LBW and VLBW infants demonstrated lower growth patterns during the first 12 months and remain smaller as a group than normal children at 3 years of age, even when corrected age is used (Casey et al, 1990). A study by Ross, Lipper, and Auld (1990), however, showed that a group of VLBW premature children who had been smaller than full-term peers at the first and third years of life had caught up to the normal population by 8 years of age. Even ELBW infants reach their genetic potential in stature by adolescence (Hirata and Bosque, 1994).

Premature SGA infants tend to have poor neonatal growth, with the period of rapid catch-up growth occurring between 40 weeks' corrected age and 8 months of age (Hack et al, 1984). However, approximately one half of these infants have subnormal weights at 8 months of age with no further catch-up growth during the second or third year. Approximately one fourth of SGA premature infants born with subnormal head circumference at birth continue to have small head circumferences at 33 months of age. The SGA infants with normal head circumference at birth tend to have normal weights at 33 months (Hack et al, 1984).

Head circumference of the LBW infant must be followed closely. Catch-up growth, usually occurring in the first 6 weeks after birth and continuing until 6 to 8 months, will result in disproportionately high head circumference percentiles, especially in the first 3 months after term. The primary care provider must be aware of those infants with intracranial hemorrhage during the neonatal course to differentiate catch-up growth from developing hydrocephalus. Cranial ultrasound or computerized tomography of the head is indicated when the signs of hydrocephalus are present (see Chapter 23) (Bernbaum et al, 1989).

Early postnatal head growth is an indicator of positive neurodevelopmental outcome. Lack of catch-up growth or initial catch-up growth followed by slow head growth are ominous signs (Hack and Fanaroff, 1988).

The parameters of growth must be followed closely to determine that the infant is thriving. Corrected age should be used until 2 to 3 years of age when measurements are plotted on standard growth charts. The length for weight graph on the National Center for Health Statistics growth chart is helpful in determining proportional growth in those infants with weights and lengths below the 5th percentile. Infants who fail to grow within their established growth curves should be investigated for failure to thrive.

Infants with birth weights of less than 1500 g are at greatest risk for high morbidity. Outcomes have improved over time in these infants. In ELBW infants, there has been dramatic increase in survival but no increase in the incidence of disabilities, and if adjustments are made for severity of illness, there is significant improvement in the disability rate as well (Perlman et al, 1995; Robertson et al, 1992).

Bauchner, Brown, and Peskin (1988) in summarizing the developmental literature, report that for infants with birth weights less than 1000 g approximately 50% will demonstrate normal-range cognitive (developmental quotient ≥85) and motor development at 2 years of age. For infants with birth weights between 1000 and 1500 g, 75% can be expected to be within the normal range at 2 years of age. For infants weighing more than 1500 g, approximately 90% will be developmentally normal.

Perinatal risk factors for poor developmental outcome include LBW, outborn, low gestational age, use of mechanical ventilation, asphyxia, intraventricular hemorrhage, and infection (Bauchner, Brown, and Peskin, 1988). Research suggests that premature infants are also more vulnerable to environmental deprivation, resulting in abnormal developmental outcomes (Escalona, 1982) and disabilities are more severe than those found in their more advantaged peers (Leonard et al, 1990).

The types of developmental disabilities associated with being VLBW include mental retardation, low-average intelligence, static motor disorders (with the spectrum ranging from incapacitating cerebral palsy to motor clumsiness and incoordination), seizure disorders, behavior disorders, learning disabilities, speech delay, and peripheral or central visual and auditory impairments. Many children have multiple problems, with the most pervasive and global disabilities becoming evident early (Desmond et al, 1980). Early intervention may be able to maximize the developmental potential of the high-risk infant (Als et al, 1994).

Neuromuscular abnormalities. Low birth weight infants often show signs of neuromuscular abnormalities that resolve during the second year of life and therefore do not carry the same prognostic importance as in the full-term infant. The most common neurologic abnormalities include increased extensor tone of the lower extremities, shoulder retractions caused by hypertonicity of the shoulder girdle and trapezius muscles, mild or transient asymmetry in tone, mild to moderate hypotonicity, and hypertonicity of the upper or lower extremities or trunk (Bernbaum et al, 1989; Dubowitz, 1988). It is essential that the primary care provider perform thorough neurologic assessments during the first 2 years of life to determine the presence and progress of abnormalities.

A child with extreme tone abnormalities and delays must be identified so that intervention can be initiated, but one must be cautious about labeling a child as having cerebral palsy before 18 months' corrected age (see Chapter 12). Experts differ about recommendations for physical therapy during the first 2 years of life. Bernbaum and colleagues (1989) suggest that formal physical therapy is necessary when an abnormality is sufficient enough to adversely affect the infant's functional status or delay the achievement of key developmental milestones.

An essential component of primary care of the premature infant is developmental assessment and anticipatory guidance concerning developmental expectations. Although it is often difficult to do formal testing in an office setting, the Denver Developmental Screening Test II can help the clinician effectively screen and formulate a clinical impression of the infant's developmental capabilities. When premature infants are tested, corrected age is commonly used until 2 to 3 years of age. Allen and Alexander (1990) suggest that using chronologic age in assessing gross motor abilities will lead to overdiagnosis of motor delay in ELBW preterm infants. But others advise that chronologic age be used for more accurate referral and follow-up decisions and that corrected age be used to allay undue parental anxiety (Elliman et al, 1985). Corrected age should be used when more specific and comprehensive developmental tests are used.

Further evaluation is necessary when a delay is evident or the parents are extremely worried about mental development. Referrals can be made to high-risk follow-up clinics, child development centers, regional developmental services, Easter Seal centers, or developmental pediatricians with training in assessment of premature infants.

Data suggest that combining early child development and family support services with pediatric follow-up shows substantive promise of decreasing the number of LBW premature infants at risk for later developmental disabilities (Infant Health and Development Program, 1990; Resnick et al, 1987). Public Law 99-457 offers states the option to provide services to handicapped, developmentally delayed, or at-risk children from birth to 3 years of age. The primary care provider must be familiar with local early intervention programs and criteria and processes for admission, so that appropriate referrals can be initiated.

Diet

Breast and bottle feeding. The use of an electric pump every 3 hours on each breast helps mothers to maintain an adequate milk supply while their infants are hospitalized. Premature infants are now often given the opportunity to suckle as early as age 32 weeks' gestation, with positive effects for both mother and infant (Meier and Anderson, 1987). It is essential for the primary care provider to determine the mother's breast-feeding desires. Anxiety, fatigue, and emotional stress may inhibit lactation, and mothers need support, guidance, and breast-feeding education while in the hospital, as well as after discharge, to ensure adequate nutritional intake and a healthy feeding environment for the infant-mother dyad (see Fig. 30-1). Many communities and hospitals have lactation counselors who are able to work with mothers to establish a successful breast-feeding regimen.

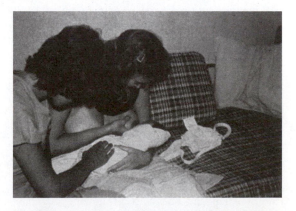

Fig. 30-1.   Nurse assisting mother with breast feeding her preterm infant.

Feeding the premature infant can be difficult because the mouth is small, oral musculature is weak, and the sucking mechanism is disorganized. Certain premature infants may benefit from any or all of the following interventions: frequent, small-volume feedings; soft bottle nipples; support of head, neck, and hips in slight flexion; minimal talking during eye contact, and a quiet, slightly darkened room (Gorski, 1988).

Abnormal feeding behaviors such as tonic bite reflex, tongue thrust, hyperactive gag reflex, or oral hypersensitivity can also be seen. Hypersensitivity secondary to intubation, repeated suctioning, or use of nasogastric or orogastric tubes can make the infant resistant to any type of oral stimulation, including nipples, spoons, and cups (Bernbaum et al, 1989). It is important for the primary care provider to continually assess the infant's feeding capabilities and parental concerns about feeding. Referral to a therapist (speech, physical, or occupational) familiar with feeding disorders is warranted when a significant or prolonged problem is identified.

Gastroesophageal reflux is a common problem in preterm infants with characteristics and therapy similar to those described for full-term infants. Treatment is dependent on the clinical findings and degree of severity (Bernbaum et al, 1989).

The AAP dietary guidelines for full-term infants are usually appropriate for healthy preterm infants after discharge if the corrected age is used (Bernbaum et al, 1989; Committee on Nutrition, 1993). By the time of discharge, mature breast milk is usually nutritionally adequate for the preterm infant. The use of regular commercial formula (20 kcal/30 ml) is also appropriate for the healthy premature infant, and recommended amounts can be based on corrected age. Increasing the caloric density of formula for infants who fail to exhibit catch-up growth can be achieved by adding medium-chain triglycerides, glucose polymers or milk enhancers, or less water to the concentrate or powder. Increasing the caloric density should be considered only after consultation with a neonatologist or pediatric dietitian (Bernbaum et al, 1989; Peterson and Frank, 1987).

Solid foods can be introduced to the premature infant when any one of the following criteria is met: (1) the infant consistently consumes more than 32 oz of formula per day for 1 week, (2) the in-fant weighs 6 to 7 kg, or (3) the infant's corrected age is 6 months. The AAP does not recommend feeding solids before 4 months' chronologic age (Bernbaum et al, 1989).

A multivitamin supplement is often used until the infant is consuming more than 300 kcal/day or when the body weight exceeds 2.5 kg. Infants with poor growth because of recurrent or chronic illness or poor caloric intake should continue to receive a multivitamin supplement until they are consuming a well-balanced diet (Bernbaum et al, 1989).

The AAP Committee on Nutrition recommends that LBW infants receive supplemental iron (2 mg/kg/day to a maximum of 15 mg/day) starting at 2 months' chronologic age (Committee on Nutrition, 1985, 1993). Infants' vitamin E status must be considered because use of iron in vitamin E-deficient infants can result in a hemolytic anemia (Committee on Nutrition, 1985, 1993). Sufficient iron can be supplied by iron-fortified formulas (12 mg/L), multivitamin preparations containing iron, or ferrous sulfate drops. Most authors agree that iron supplementation should continue for 6 to 12 months until the child is eating iron-rich solid foods on a regular basis (Bernbaum et al, 1989; Hagedorn and Gardner, 1991; Koerper, 1988).

If iron deficiency is suspected by history or documented by laboratory testing, the LBW infant may require increased supplementation (3 to 4 mg/kg/day). Higher doses may be poorly tolerated and do not result in a more rapid response (Dallman, 1988).

Safety

Anticipatory guidance about safety must be adjusted to the child's developmental level rather than to chronologic age. Because many parents continue to consider their children weak or vulnerable, they must be encouraged not to restrict activities but to allow exploration and social interaction within a safe setting.

Recommendations (Committee on Injury and Poison Prevention and Committee on Fetus and Newborn, 1991) for the safe transportation of premature infants include the following: (1) Place the infant in the car seat in a location that allows for observation by an adult during travel. All infants weighing less than 17 to 20 lb must ride facing the rear. (2) Use blanket rolls inside the car seat to improve head and trunk control. Blanket rolls can be placed on both sides of the infant's trunk for lateral support and between the crotch strap and the infant to reduce slouching. (3) If the infant's head drops forward, tilt the seat back and/or wedge a cloth roll under the safety seat base so that the baby reclines at a 45-degree angle. (4) Avoid using convertible car seats with a shield, abdominal pad, or arm rest if the infant's face or neck could directly contact these objects during impact. Position the car seat's retainer clip on the infant's chest (see Fig. 30-2).

Specific recommendations regarding travel for infants at possible risk of respiratory problems include (1) counseling families to minimize travel for infants at risk for respiratory compromise, (2) having an appropriate hospital staff person conduct a period of observation of the infant in a car seat before discharge to monitor for possible apnea, bradycardia, or oxygen desaturation on infants of less than 37 weeks' gestation, (3) having infants with prescribed home cardiac and apnea monitors use this monitoring equipment during travel with portable, self-contained power for twice the expected transport duration, (4) restraining all portable medical equipment with adjacent seat belts, wedged on the floor, or under the seats, and (5) using alternative child restraint devices for infants who must ride prone, supine, or in a less upright position (Committee on Injury and Poison Prevention and Committee on Fetus and Newborn, 1991).

Immunizations

Studies have demonstrated that preterm infants immunized with diphtheria, pertussis, and tetanus (DPT) at routine intervals (2, 4, and 6 months after birth) are capable of producing a protective serologic response with fewer side effects than are full-term infants (Bernbaum et al, 1985). Therefore, the AAP recommends that full doses of DPT be administered to premature infants at the same chronologic ages as recommended for full-term infants (Committee on Infectious Diseases, 1994). The same contraindications for pertussis vaccine in the term infant apply to the premature infant.

Polio vaccine should be administered orally to premature infants at the same chronologic ages as recommended for full-term infants. If the infant remains hospitalized, this vaccine should be withheld until discharge to prevent cross-infection or,

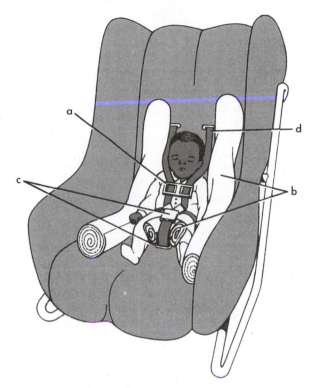

Fig. 30-2.   Positioning of premature infant in car seat: *a,* retainer clip positioned on child's chest; *b,* blanket rolls on both sides of trunk, and between crotch strap and infant; *c,* distance of 5½ inches or less from crotch strap to seat back; *d,* distance of 10 inches or less from lower harness strap to seat bottom.

alternatively, inactivated polio vaccine (IPV) can be given (Committee on Infectious Diseases, 1994). Measles, mumps, rubella, varicella, and *Haemophilus influenzae* type b (Hib) vaccine should be administered at the chronologic ages recommended by the AAP.

Hepatitis B vaccine.   The AAP recommends that all infants receive hepatitis B (HB) vaccination. Infants born to mothers with positive HB surface antigen should be given HB immunoglobulin (HBIG) at birth and HB vaccine within 7 days after birth and at 1 and 6 months. These same recommendations apply to preterm infants, although data on the effectiveness of HB vaccine are not available for infants with birth weights of less than 2000 g. The administration of the HB vaccine may be delayed if necessary (not HBIG) but should be given within 1 month if possible. If administration of the vaccine is delayed for as long as 3 months, a second dose of HBIG (0.5 ml) should be given (Committee on Infectious Diseases, 1994).

Varicella-zoster immune globulin. Because of the poor transfer of antibodies across the placenta early in pregnancy, the AAP recommends that all infants born before 28 weeks' gestation (or who weigh <1000 g) who still require hospitalization for treatment of prematurity and related conditions and are exposed to varicella should receive varicella-zoster immune globulin (125 U). The recommendation also applies to premature infants born after 28 weeks' gestation whose mothers have a negative history of past infection (Committee on Infectious Diseases, 1994).

Screening

Vision. Ophthalmologic problems, including ROP, myopia, and strabismus, occur with increased frequency among premature infants (Bull et al, 1986). According to AAP recommendations, all oxygen-exposed infants with birth weights less than 1800 g (or <35 weeks' gestation) and all infants weighing less than 1300 g at birth (or born at <30 weeks' gestation) regardless of oxygen exposure should have an ophthalmologic examination before discharge or at 5 to 7 weeks after birth to assess for ROP (AAP, 1992). Because of the significant risk of early and late sequelae, infants who have ROP and, by virtue of their immature retinae, those who are still at risk for ROP should receive close ophthalmologic follow-up after discharge (Bernbaum et al, 1989; Gardner and Hagedorn, 1990).

The eye examination of the LBW infant by the primary care provider should include assessment of the vision, the fundus (red reflex), and the alignment of the eyes. Visual assessment includes the infant's ability to fixate and follow objects. This response should be present by 6 weeks' corrected age (Day, 1988). Continued yearly assessment of visual acuity in this population is important to identify more subtle refractive errors that may affect scholastic achievement. Anisometropia (unequal refraction) may lead to amblyopia.

Hearing. The incidence of sensorineural hearing loss in preterm infants is usually reported to be 1% to 3%. Factors associated with prematurity

such as hypoxia, hyperbilirubinemia, environmental noise levels, concomitant antibiotic and diuretic therapy, and congenital infections place LBW infants at particular risk for hearing problems (Bernbaum et al, 1989).

All VLBW infants or infants with any other risk factors should be screened for hearing loss preferably under the supervision of an audiologist. Optimally screening should be performed before discharge from the newborn nursery but no later than 3 months of age. Initial screening should include auditory brainstem response (ABR) (American Speech-Language-Hearing Association, 1989). If the results of an initial screening are equivocal, the infant should be referred for general medical, otologic, and audiologic follow-up which should include a repeat ABR and a behavioral auditory testing when the child is 4 to 6 months corrected age. Ongoing testing is necessary when there are conditions which increase the probability of progressive hearing loss, such as family history of delayed onset of hearing loss, degenerative disease, meningitis, or intrauterine infections (Joint Committee on Infant Hearing, 1991).

Health care providers should be alerted to those children who have delays in speech development, poor attentiveness, and absent or abnormal responses to sound. These findings may indicate hearing loss and require more thorough investigation.

Dental. Prolonged orotracheal intubation affects the palate and possibly the dentition; very high arched palates and deep palatal grooves have been observed. In mild cases these deformities usually resolve within the first year of life. Abnormally shaped teeth with notching have been observed in some infants. Dental eruption is usually mildly delayed in premature infants (even allowing for corrected age), with greater delays seen in chronically ill infants (Piecuch, 1988). Staining of deciduous teeth as a result of neonatal illness such as hyperbilirubinemia and cholestatsis may be evident. Consultation with a pediatric dentist may be required (Rosenthal et al, 1986; Herbert and Delcambre, 1987). Specific guidelines for fluoride use in premature infants do not exist; however, routine fluoride supplementation is not recommended for the first 6 months of life (American Academy of Pediatrics, 1995).

Blood pressure. Premature infants may be at risk for developing hypertension. Several studies attribute the hypertension to complications of umbilical arterial catheters. Hypertension screening should be done at 1, 2, 6, 12, and 24 months of age and then routinely in childhood (Cohen and Taeusch, 1987). Infants with a blood pressure greater than the 95th percentile for age on three separate visits should be considered hypertensive and evaluation of etiology should be initiated (Sheftel, Hustead, and Friedman, 1983).

Hematocrit. The hematocrit values of the preterm infant should be checked monthly until the infant is 6 months of age and then every 2 months throughout the first year of life (Koerper, 1988). As in the immediate neonatal period, there is no one hematocrit value that indicates anemia during the months following birth. Between 2 and 3 months of age, the hematocrit value can fall as low as 21% and still be considered nonpathologic. The drop in hematocrit value is an exaggerated physiologic anemia and is rarely related to iron deficiency (Committee on Nutrition, 1985). As in term infants, if the drop in hematocrit value is more extreme or fails to increase over time, other causes for anemia must be considered and treated as needed.

Urinalysis. Routine screening is recommended.

Tuberculosis. Routine screening is recommended.

Condition-specific screening

HERNIA AND TESTICULAR SCREENING. At each primary care visit the infant's caretaker must be asked about the presence of inguinal swelling that increases in size with coughing or crying. The inguinal area and canal must be palpated for any swelling or masses. Because of the increased incidence of undescended testicles in premature male infants, a thorough testicular examination is warranted.

COMMON ILLNESS MANAGEMENT

Differential Diagnosis

Infection. Respiratory viruses such as respiratory syncytial virus (RSV), parainfluenza viruses, and influenza viruses are a major cause of morbid-

DIFFERENTIAL DIAGNOSIS

Infections
- Increased susceptibility to viral respiratory illnesses
- Increased incidence of wheezing and bronchiolitis
- Infections associated with birth—HSV, group B *streptococcus, Chlamydia, Staphlococcus aureus,* and *E. coli* require appropriate antibiotics

ity for the ICN graduate. Although the clinical symptoms of RSV infection in the term infant may be the expected ones of pneumonia or bronchiolitis, the symptoms in the premature infant may be nonspecific, with apnea being a prominent finding (Arvin, 1988).

Viral respiratory disease is particularly dangerous for infants with residual lung disease, and those infants must be monitored closely by the primary care provider for signs of respiratory distress (see Chapter 10). The risk of acquiring lower respiratory tract disease secondary to infection is related to the age at acquisition of the primary infection, with reduced morbidity in the second and third years of life. Since older siblings and adults usually bring viral pathogens into the home, direct contact with the infant by symptomatic individuals should be minimized when symptoms are present, especially during the first year of life (Arvin, 1988).

Herpes simplex virus (HSV) and late-onset group B streptococcal infection are two examples of pathogens that infants are exposed to in the perinatal period that cause rapidly progressive illness in an infant who was considered to be doing well. The incubation period for infants with perinatal exposure to HSV is variable, ranging from 2 days to 6 weeks. Because the attack rate for HSV is increased with prematurity, the diagnosis of HSV should be considered in the high-risk premature infant who has any symptoms compatible with HSV, including lethargy, poor feeding, herpetic lesions, and transient low-grade fever. Because the effects of HSV type 1 can be as devastating to the high-risk infant as HSV type 2, it is necessary to advise parents to avoid exposing the infant to individuals with fever blisters or cold sores (Arvin, 1988).

Organisms such as *Chlamydia,* group B *Streptococcus, Staphylococcus aureus,* or *Escherichia coli* can colonize in an infant during birth or hospitalization and become invasive, causing serious infection after discharge. In addition, premature infants may be at special risk from organisms such as *Streptococcus pneumoniae* (pneumococcus) and Hemophilus influenza type b (Hib). The major sites of infection are the central nervous system, bones, joints, and respiratory system.

Healthy premature infants who have unexplained fever should be assessed according to their corrected ages. The work-up is the same as that of term infants. Antibiotic selection must take into account possible neonatal sources of infection. Parents need to be instructed about signs and symptoms of infection, which include lethargy, poor feeding, irritability, fever, respiratory distress, and bowel changes. Because some of these symptoms may be characteristics of the well premature infant's baseline behavior, awareness of changes in this baseline may help to identify illness.

Drug Interactions

There are no specific drug interactions.

DEVELOPMENTAL ISSUES

Sleep Patterns

The sleep patterns of the premature infant differ from those of the full-term infant. Premature infants can wake up as frequently as every 2 hours until 4 months' corrected age and may not be able to sustain an 8-hour sleep period at night until 8 months' corrected age. This immature sleep organization may be the result of neurologic immaturity, nutritional demands, and metabolic differences (Gorski, 1988).

Whereas full-term infants may be able to sleep through any distraction, many premature infants appear to be hypersensitive to sights and sounds (Gorski, 1988). Conversely, many premature children become habituated to the noise and lights of the ICN and have difficulty adjusting to the quiet

and dark of the home environment. The use of a night light or radio is often recommended for these infants to ease their transition to the home.

An infant's ability to sleep through the night is also determined by many factors, such as age, nutritional status, temperament, and previous sleep patterning. Premature infants should not be expected to sleep through the night earlier than 2 to 4 months of corrected age. Parents must be supported during this period and provided with realistic guidelines for sleep patterning of the premature infant (Ferber, 1985).

Toileting

Signs of toileting readiness are more likely to appear at the appropriate corrected rather than chronologic age. Abnormal neurologic findings such as increased muscle tone may have a negative effect on the toilet training process, and training may be more effectively done when muscle tone has decreased.

Discipline

The stress of having an infant in the ICN leaves many parents prone to what Green and Solnit (1964) have called "the vulnerable child syndrome." These attitudes about the child may result in overindulgence and overpermissiveness. Families often have difficulties setting limits, which can interfere with normal development; the child may exhibit dependent, demanding, or uncontrolled behavior (Bernbaum et al, 1989).

Premature infants are often more difficult to care for than full-term infants. Their sleep-wake cycle is disturbed by their long hospital stays. Many become agitated or nonresponsive to what is considered average stimulation. These infants are often difficult to soothe, have trouble eating, have delayed milestones, and require more care and patience from their parents.

It has been suggested that families try to normalize the caretaking and daily activities of their premature infant. This normalization process is seen as critical to the development of a healthy relationship between parents and child. Families should also be encouraged to set disciplinary limits and schedules that enable them to be in control (Bernbaum and Hoffman-Williamson, 1986).

Child Care

Many studies have demonstrated the increased incidence of infectious diseases such as diarrhea and respiratory illnesses in infants and children attending day care centers compared with children cared for in the home. Because LBW infants have greater and more prolonged immune deficiencies, the transmission of infectious diseases within day care centers may affect the morbidity of the LBW infant attending these facilities. Based on these considerations, home child care would be preferable to other day care situations. Unfortunately many of the women who have LBW infants are least likely to be able to afford child care in the home. For those families unable to afford a one-to-one situation, a small home care program would be more desirable than a large day care center. Parents must also consider their role in educating the day care provider about the special needs of the LBW infant (e.g., nutrition, stimulation, sleep habits).

Schooling

Many studies have documented an increased frequency of educational problems in children who have received ICN care. Some investigators have found premature infants more likely to have lower school achievement and greater need for special class placements. Often these problems manifest as subtle visual-motor, perceptual, language, reading difficulties or hyperactive behavior (McCormick, Gortmaker, and Sobol, 1990; Vohr and Coll, 1985). School readiness is often delayed (particularly in boys) in the VLBW infant, and early school problems may be avoided by starting these children in school a year behind their full-term peers.

The prevalence of learning problems in preterm infants of normal intelligence emphasizes the need for early identification and implementation of individual intervention programs (Hunt, Cooper, and Tooley, 1988; Klein et al, 1985; Sell et al, 1985). Ideally these children should be longitudinally followed in high-risk clinics into the school years. If these services are not available, the primary care provider should assess the neurodevelopmental progress of the child, including the presence of soft signs that may be an indication of poor academic performance (Blondis, Snow, and Accardo, 1990). School performance and progress should be discussed with parents and school personnel; referral

for educational testing should be initiated if a problem is suspected.

Sexuality

Women who were born SGA have been found to be at increased risk for giving birth to both growth retarded and preterm infants (Klebanoff, Meirik, and Berendes, 1989). Appropriate counseling and early prenatal referral to parents and adolescents are necessary with regard to these findings.

Transition into Adulthood

Transition into adolescence and adulthood may be more difficult for the VLBW premature child, depending on earlier developmental and behavioral problems. Fortunately, most VLBW and ELBW children experience a more rapid catch-up growth during adolescence, and reach stature closer to their genetic potential. However, VLBW children appear to have lower social competence and higher behavior problems in their school years compared to their peers (Ross, Lipper, and Auld, 1990).

Any preexisting developmental or behavioral problems may become more exaggerated during the turbulence of adolescence. Feelings of not measuring up to their peers may surface if growth has been poor, and health problems have interfered with their quest for independence. Parental overprotection may add to feelings of low self-esteem. During adolescence, children are more sensitive about personal appearance, and any cosmetic deformities and scars from their hospital experience (IV, chest tube, surgery scars) may cause extreme anguish. Efforts toward cosmetic repair of more pronounced problems should be made.

If concerns during adolescence are addressed with good parental communication, support, and encouragement, the transition into adulthood should be less problematic and more comparable to that of their full-term peers. In some cases, professional psychologic intervention may need to be provided.

SPECIAL FAMILY CONCERNS AND RESOURCES

Families with premature infants have multiple issues to address (Able-Boone, Stevens, 1994). Parents must deal with the grief of delivering a preterm infant while going through the attachment process. The transition from hospital to home is a period of extreme anxiety; parents are faced with caring for their infant without the support of hospital staff. Parents have financial issues, as well as concerns involving the health and developmental outcome of the infant. It is often difficult for parents to appreciate the progress of their premature infant while friends, relatives, and strangers continually make comparisons to full-term infants. Education and support from primary care providers will enable parents to create an environment that will encourage infants to attain their full potential.

The American family is always changing and the family of the premature infant is an exaggerated reflection of that change. Increasing numbers of children are being cared for in one-parent, minority, low-income, and immigrant families. Premature children are disproportionately represented in these statistics. In the 1990 census, minority children represented 31% of the U.S. children and were projected to be 48% by the year 2025. The most rapidly increasing minorities are Latinos and Asians, bringing language barriers to the obstacles (The Future of Children, 1994). The main obstacles to adequate care for these children are associated with poverty and poor access to medical and social services. Premature children in these cultural categories need special attention to developmental care because they are quite vulnerable to environmental risk and poor outcome. These children would benefit from enrollment in programs directed toward development and behavior enhancement.

Resources are available for families with premature infants. Many hospitals have parent support groups that work with the family during hospitalization and after discharge. Many ICNs have a follow-up clinic that employs an interdisciplinary team for ongoing evaluation of infants identified as high risk for physical and developmental problems.

Informational Materials

Harrison H: *The premature baby book,* 1983, New York, St Martin's Press.

Jason J, Van der Meer A: *Parenting your premature baby,* 1989, New York, H Holt.

Lieberman A, Sheagren T: *The premie parents' handbook,* 1984, New York, EP Dutton.

Organizations

Local parent-to-parent groups

SUMMARY OF PRIMARY CARE NEEDS FOR THE PREMATURE OR LOW BIRTH WEIGHT INFANT

Health care maintenance

Growth and development

Use corrected age to plot height, weight, and head circumference.

Preterm infants who are AGA follow similar growth patterns as full-term infants.

Infants who are SGA tend to be smaller children.

Catch-up growth occurs within the first year to after 3 years of age; may be prolonged in ELBW infants.

Monitor head circumference for abnormal growth.

Premature infants are at high risk for neurologic and cognitive abnormalities.

The incidence of abnormal development increases with decreasing birth weight.

Transient neuromuscular abnormalities can be present in the first year.

Diet

Breast feeding or iron-fortified formula is recommended.

Use of multivitamins should be encouraged for infants who weigh less than 2.5 kg or infants who have chronic illness or poor growth. Beginning at 2 months of age, infants should receive 2 mg of iron/kg/day.

Feeding problems such as oral hypersensitivity and gastroesophageal reflux are common.

Safety

Anticipatory guidance is based on developmental age.

Recommendations for car seat use include using blanket rolls for support, observing while driving, and avoiding models with lap pads or shields.

Immunizations

All immunizations should be administered at chronologic ages recommended by the AAP.

Infants may be given OPV after discharge.

Screening

Vision

Assessment of fixation, following alignment and fundoscopic examination are recommended.

Ophthalmologic follow-up is necessary for infants with ROP or positive visual finding.

Hearing

Screening is necessary for infants with identified risk factors within 3 months of age.

Dental

Prolonged intubation affects palate and dentition. Tooth eruptions may be delayed.

Routine fluoride supplementation is recommended.

Blood pressure

Hypertension screening should be done at 1, 2, 6, 12, and 24 months of age and then routinely in childhood.

Hematocrit

Hematocrit values should be checked monthly until 6 months, then every 2 months through 1 year of age.

Urinalysis

Routine screening is recommended.

Tuberculosis

Routine screening is recommended.

Condition-specific screening

HERNIA AND TESTICULAR SCREENING

Infants should be screened for inguinal hernia and undescended testicles.

Common illness management

Differential diagnosis

These infants have an increased risk of infection.

Herpes simplex virus, *Chlamydia,* group B *streptococcus, Staphylococcus aureus,* and *Escherichia coli* must all be considered possible pathogens.

Drug interactions

No routine medications are given.

Continued.

SUMMARY OF PRIMARY CARE NEEDS FOR THE PREMATURE OR LOW BIRTH WEIGHT INFANT—cont'd

Developmental issues

Sleep patterns

Children may have disorganized sleep patterns.

Toileting

Toileting readiness is based on developmental age. Increased muscle tone may impede toilet training.

Discipline

Children should be assessed for vulnerable child syndrome.

Child care

Home care or small day care programs are recommended.

Schooling

These children have an increased incidence of educational problems. School readiness should be ascertained before the child enters kindergarten.

Psychometric testing is indicated for poor school performance.

Sexuality

Standard developmental counseling is advised. There is an increased incidence of SGA and prematurity in offspring of women who were SGA at birth.

Transition into adulthood

Preexisting developmental or behavior problems may become more exaggerated. Concerns of parental overprotection, adolescent low self-esteem, correction of cosmetic deformities, and parental communications should be addressed.

Special family concerns

Special family concerns include grief, attachment issues as a result of prolonged hospitalization, financial considerations, and concerns about developmental outcomes.

REFERENCES

Able-Boone H, Stevens E: After the intensive care nursery experience: families' perceptions of their well-being, *Child Health Care* 23:99-114, 1994.

Allen M, Alexander G: Gross motor milestones in preterm infants: correction for degree of prematurity, *Pediatrics* 116:955-959, 1990.

Als H et al: Individualized developmental care for the very low birth weight preterm infant, *JAMA* 272:853-858, 1994.

American Academy of Pediatrics and American College of Obstetrics and Gynecology: *Guidelines for perinatal care,* ed 3, Elk Grove, IL, 1992, American Academy of Pediatrics and American College of Obstetrics and Gynecology.

American Academy of Pediatrics, Committee on Nutrition. Fluoride supplementation for children: interim policy recommendations, *Pediatrics* 95:777, 1995.

American Speech-Language-Hearing Association: Guidelines for audiologic screening of newborn infants who are at-risk for hearing impairment, *ASHA* 31:89-92, 1989.

Arias F, Tomich P: Etiology and outcome of low birth weight and preterm infants, *Obstet Gynecol* 60:277-281, 1982.

Arvin A: Infectious disease issues in the care of the ICN gradu-

ate. In Ballard R (editor): *Pediatric care of the ICN graduate,* Philadelphia, 1988, WB Saunders, pp 216-225.

Avery GB: The morality of drastic intervention. In Avery GB, Fletcher MA, and MacDonald MG (editors): *Neonatology: pathophysiology and management of the newborn,* Philadelphia, 1994, JB Lippincott, pp 8-11.

Ballard JL et al: New ballard score, expanded to include extremely premature infants, *J Pediatr* 119:417-23, 1991.

Bauchner H, Brown E, and Peskin J: Premature graduates of the newborn intensive care unit: a guide to followup, *Pediatr Clin North Am* 35:1207-1226, 1988.

Bell RL et al: Total parenteral nutrition-related cholestates in infants, *J Parenter Enteral Nutr* 10:356-359, 1986.

Bernbaum JC et al: Preterm infant care after hospital discharge, *Pediatr Rev* 10:195-206, 1989.

Bernbaum JC et al: Response of preterm infants to diphtheria-tetanus-pertussis immunizations, *J Pediatr* 107:184-188, 1985.

Bernbaum J, Hoffman-Williamson M: Following the NICU graduate, *Contemp Pediatr* 3:22-37, 1986.

Blondis T, Snow J, and Accardo P: Integration of soft signs in academically normal and academically at-risk children, *Pediatrics* 85(suppl):421-425, 1990.

Brandt I: Growth dynamics of low birth weight infants with emphasis on the perinatal period. In Falkner F, Tanner JM (editors): *Human growth,* vol 2, *Postnatal growth,* New York, 1978, Plenum Press, pp 557-617.

Bull MJ et al: Follow-up of infants after intensive care, *Perinatol Neonatol* 23-28, 1986.

Callenbach JC et al: Etiologic factors in rickets of very low birth weight infants, *J Pediatr* 98:800-805, 1981.

Casey PH et al: Growth patterns of low birth weight preterm infants: a longitudinal analysis of a large, varied sample, *J Pediatr* 117:298-307, 1990.

Centers for Disease Control: Infant mortality-united states–1992, *MMWR* 43:905-909, 1994.

Coates AL et al: Long-term pulmonary sequelae of premature birth with and without idiopathic respiratory distress syndrome, *J Pediatr* 90:611-616, 1977.

Cohen M, Taeusch HW: Primary care for the neonatal intensive care unit graduate. In Taeusch HW, Yogman MW (editors): *Follow-up management of the high-risk infant,* Boston, 1987, Little, Brown, p 70.

Committee on Infectious Disease: Report of the Committee on Infectious Disease, ed 23, Elk Grove Village, IL, 1994, The American Academy of Pediatrics.

Committee on Injury and Poison Prevention and Committee on Fetus and newborn: Safe transportation of premature infants. Pediatrics 87:120-122, 1991.

Committee on Nutrition: Nutritional needs of low birth weight infants, *Pediatrics* 75:976-986, 1985.

Committee on Nutrition: *Pediatric nutrition handbook,* ed 3, Elk Grove Village, IL, 1993, The American Academy of Pediatrics.

Constantine NA et al: Use of physical and neurologic observations in assessment of gestational age in low birth weight infants, *J Pediatr* 110:921-928, 1987.

Corbet A et al: Decreased mortality rate among small premature infants treated at birth with a single dose of synthetic surfactant: a multicenter controlled trial, *J Pediatr* 118:277-84, 1991.

Creasy RK: Preterm labor and delivery. In Creasy RK, Resnik R (editors): *Maternal-fetal medicine, principles and practice,* Philadelphia, 1994, WB Saunders, pp 494-520.

Dallman PR: Nutritional anemia of infancy: iron, folic acid, and vitamin B12. In Tsang RC, Nichols BL (editors): *Nutrition during infancy,* Philadelphia, 1988, Hanley & Belfus, pp 216-235.

Day S: The eyes of the ICN graduate. In Ballard R (editor): *Pediatric care of the ICN graduate,* Philadelphia, 1988, WB Saunders, pp 121-126.

DeLorimier AA: Care of ICN graduates after neonatal surgery. In Ballard R (editor): *Pediatric care of the ICN graduate,* Philadelphia, 1988, WB Saunders, pp 187-195.

Desmond M et al: The very low birth infant after discharge from intensive care: anticipatory health care and developmental course, *Curr Probl Pediatr* 10:1-59, 1980.

Dubowitz LMS: Neurologic assessment. In Ballard R (editor): *Pediatric care of the ICN graduate,* Philadelphia, 1988, WB Saunders, p 84.

Dubowitz LMS, Dubowitz V, and Goldberg C: Clinical assessment of gestational age in the newborn, *J Pediatr* 77:1-10, 1970.

Elliman A et al: Denver developmental screening test and preterm infants, *Arch Dis Child* 60:20-24, 1985.

Escalona S: Babies at double hazard: early development of infants at biologic and social risk, *Pediatrics* 70:670-676, 1982.

Ferber R: *Solving your child's sleep problems,* New York, 1985, Simon & Schuster.

The Future of Children: Critical health issues for children and youth, vol 4, The Center for the Future of Children, The David and Lucille Packard Foundation, 1994.

Gardner SL, Hagedorn MI: Physiologic sequelae of prematurity: the nurse practitioner's role, part II. Retinopathy of prematurity, *J Pediat Health Care* 4:72-76, 1990.

Gorski PA: Fostering family development after preterm hospitalization. In Ballard R (editor): *Pediatric care of the ICN graduate,* Philadelphia, 1988, WB Saunders, pp 27-32.

Green M, Solnit A: Reactions to the threatened loss of a child: a vulnerable child syndrome, *Pediatrics* 34:58-66, 1964.

Hack M, Fanaroff A: Growth patterns in the ICN graduate. In Ballard R (editor): *Pediatric care of the ICN graduate,* Philadelphia, WB Saunders, pp 33-39, 1988.

Hack M et al: Catch-up growth in very low birth weight infants, *Am J Dis Child* 138:370-375, 1984.

Hagedorn MI, Gardner SL: Physiologic sequelae of prematurity: the nurse practitioner's role, part IV. Anemia, *J Pediat Health Care* 5:3-10, 1991.

Hawtrey C: Undescended testis and orchiopexy: Recent observations, *Pediatr Rev* 11:305-308, 1990.

Herbert FL, Delcambre TJ: Unusual case of green teeth resulting from neonatal hyperbilirubinemia, *ASDC J Dent Child* 54(1):54-6, 1987.

Hirata T, Bosque E: When they grow up: the long-term growth of extremely low birth weight infants from birth to adolescence, *Clin Res* 42:1, p 69A, 1994.

Hirata T et al: Survival and outcome of infants 501 to 750 gm: a 6-year experience, *J Pediatr* 102:741-748, 1983.

Hunt JV, Cooper BAB, and Tooley WH: Very low birth weight infants at 8 and 11 years of age: role of neonatal illness and family status, *Pediatrics* 82:596-603, 1988.

Infant Health and Development Program: Enhancing the outcomes of low birth weight, premature infants, a multisite, randomized trial, *JAMA* 263:3035-3042, 1990.

International Committee for the Classification of the Late Stages of Retinopathy of Prematurity: An international classification of retinopathy of prematurity II. The classification of retinal detachment, *Arch Ophthalmol* 105:906-912, 1987.

Joint Committee on Infant Hearing (1991): 1990 position statement, *ASHA* 33(suppl 5):3-6, 1991.

Kitchen WH et al: Health and hospital readmissions of very low birth weight and normal birth weight children, *Am J Dis Child* 144:213-218, 1990.

Klebanoff M, Meirik O, and Berendes H: Second generation consequences of small-for-dates birth, *Pediatrics* 84:343-347, 1989.

Klein N et al: Preschool performance of children with normal intelligence who were very low birth weight infants, *Pediatrics* 75:531-537, 1985.

Kliegman RM, Fanaroff AA: Necrotizing enterocolitis, *N Engl J Med* 310:1093-1102, 1984.

Koerper M: Anemia in the ICN graduate. In Ballard R (editor): *Pediatric care of the ICN graduate,* Philadelphia, 1988, WB Saunders, pp 46-47.

Kopelman AE, Mathew OP: Common respiratory disorders of the newborn, *Pediatr Rev* 16:209-217, 1995.

Krishnamoorthy KS et al: Periventricular-intraventricular hemorrhage sonographic localization, phenobarbital, and motor abnormalities in low birth weight infants, *Pediatrics* 85:1027-1033, 1990.

Landers III MB et al: Argon laser photocoagulation for advanced retinopathy of prematurity, *Am J Ophthalmol* 110(4):429-431, 1990.

Leonard CH et al: Effect of medical and social risk factors on outcome of prematurity and very low birth weight, *J Pediatr* 116:620-626, 1990.

Martin RJ, Fanaroff A, and Klaus M: Respiratory problems. In Klaus M, Fanaroff A (editors): *Care of the high-risk neonate,* Philadelphia, 1993, WB Saunders, pp 228-259.

McCormick MC, Gortmaker SL, and Sobol AM: Very low birth weight children: behavior problems and school difficulty in a national sample, *J Pediatr* 117:687-93, 1990.

McCormick MC: The contribution of low birth weight to infant mortality and childhood morbidity, *N Engl J Med* 312:82-90, 1985.

McCormick MC, Shapiro S, and Starfield B: Rehospitalization in the first year of life for high-risk survivors, *Pediatrics* 66:991-999, 1980.

McNamara JA et al: Diode laser photocoagulation for retinopathy of prematurity, *Arch Ophthalmol* 110(12):1714-1716, 1993.

Meier P, Anderson GC: Responses of small preterm infants to bottle and breast feeding, *Matern Child Nurs J* 12:97-105, 1987.

Multicenter Trial of Cryotherapy for Retinopathy of Prematurity: Preliminary results: cryotherapy for retinopathy of prematurity cooperative groups, *Arch Ophthalmol* 106:471-479, 1988.

Papile LA, Munsick-Bruno G, and Lowe J: Grade III and IV periventricular, intraventricular hemorrhage (PIVH): longitudinal neurodevelopment outcome, *Pediatr Res* 23:4 (part 2):453A, 1988.

Papile LA, Munsick-Bruno G, and Schaefer A: Relationship of

cerebral intraventricular hemorrhage and early childhood neurologic handicaps, *J Pediatr* 103:273-277, 1983.

Peevy KJ, Speed FA, and Hoff CJ: Epidemiology of inguinal hernia in preterm neonates, *Pediatrics* 77:246-247, 1986.

Perlman M et al: Secular changes in the outcomes to 18 to 24 months of age of extremely low birth weight infants, with adjustment for changes in risk factors and severity of illness, *J Pediatr* 126(1):75-87, 1995.

Peterson K, Frank D: Feeding and growth of premature and small-for-gestational age infants. In Taeusch HW, Yogman MW (editors): *Follow-up management of the high-risk infant,* Boston, 1987, Little, Brown, pp 187-204.

Phelps DL: Retinopathy of prematurity, *Pediatr Rev* 16:50-56, 1995.

Piecuch R: Cosmetics, skin, scars, and residual traces of the ICN. In Ballard R (editor): *Pediatric care of the ICN graduate,* Philadelphia, 1988, WB Saunders, pp 50-56.

Purohit DM et al: Risk factors for retrolental fibroplasia: experience with 3025 premature infants, *Pediatrics* 76:339-344, 1985.

Resnick MB et al: Developmental intervention for low birth weight infants: improved early developmental outcome, *Pediatrics* 80:68-74, 1987.

Robertson CMT et al: Population-based study of the incidence, complexity, and severity of neurologic disability among survivors weighing 500 through 1250 g at birth: a comparison of two birth cohorts, *Pediatrics* 90(5):750-754, 1992.

Rosenthal P et al: Management of children with hyperbilirubinemia and green teeth, *J Pediatr* 108(1):103-5, 1986.

Ross G, Lipper EG, and Auld PAM: Growth achievement of very low birth weight premature children at school age, *J Pediatr* 117:307-309, 1990.

Ross G, Lipper EG, and Auld PAM: Social competence and behavior problems in premature children at school age, *Pediatrics* 86:391-397, 1990.

Sacher RA, Luban NLC, and Strauss RG: Current practice and guidelines for the transfusion of cellular blood components in the newborn, *Transfusion Med Rev* 3(1):39-54, 1989.

Sell E et al: Early identification of learning problems in neonatal intensive care graduates, *Am J Dis Child* 139:460-463, 1985.

Sheftel D, Hustead V, and Friedman A: Hypertension screening in the follow-up of premature infants, *Pediatrics* 71:763-766, 1983.

Vanderhoof JA, Zach TL, and Adrian TE: Gastrointestinal disease. In Avery GB, Fletcher MA, and MacDonald MG (editors): *Neonatology: pathophysiology and management of the newborn,* Philadelphia, 1994, JB Lippincott, pp 614-616.

Vohr BR, Coll CTG: Neurodevelopmental and school performance of very low birth weight infants: a 7-year longitudinal study, *Pediatrics* 76:345-350, 1985.

Volpe JJ: *Neurology of the newborn,* ed 3, Philadelphia, 1995, WB Saunders.

Wegman ME: Annual summary of vital statistics—1993, *Pediatrics* 94:792-803, 1994.

31

Prenatal Cocaine Exposure

Elizabeth A. Kuehne
and Marianne Warguska Reilly

ETIOLOGY

The problem of substance abuse during pregnancy is a long-standing one within our society (Chasnoff, 1989b). However, it was not until 1973, when the term fetal alcohol syndrome was first used to describe a distinctive pattern of malformations in infants born to alcoholic mothers (Jones et al, 1973), that these problems began to receive attention from health care professionals and the general public.

Since this time the effects of alcohol, opiates, marijuana, and other noncocaine substances on the developing fetus have been studied and described extensively. A summary of these effects is shown in the box on p. 672. Over the past 10 years the patterns of use of these drugs have changed very little (Chasnoff, 1988), while cocaine has emerged as a widely used recreational drug.

An estimated 22 million Americans have tried cocaine once, and 6 million are believed to use it on a regular basis (National Institute on Drug Abuse, 1990). With cocaine's rise in popularity among the general public has come a rise in use by women of childbearing age (Azuma and Chasnoff, 1993). Cocaine is now the illicit substance most frequently used by pregnant women and is commonly used in combination with tobacco, alcohol, and marijuana (Chasnoff, 1991).

Cocaine can be administered in a variety of ways: intranasal snorting, intravenous (IV) injec-

tion, and smoking (Wootton and Miller, 1994). Currently the most popular form of cocaine is "crack." Crack consists of alkaloid crystals of cocaine that are smoked in a water pipe. Crack became available in the mid-1980s, and its popularity shows no signs of diminishing.

Crack differs from cocaine hydrochloride (the preparation used intranasally) in three ways. First, because it is smoked and not sniffed, the "high" is reached within 10 seconds and lasts approximately 5 to 15 minutes. Second, crack is absorbed more effectively from the highly vascular surface of the lung, creating a more intense and powerful high. Third, crack is relatively inexpensive, costing a few dollars per "rock" (Gold, 1987; Howard, 1989a; Hutchings, 1993). These factors and eliminating the need for IV injection are believed to contribute to crack's popularity among both young people and women of childbearing age.

Because of crack's dramatic effects on users, a few patterns of use have emerged. Many women use crack to abort an unwanted pregnancy, or they use it in the belief that it will ease their deliveries. Some women use crack to induce labor thinking that early delivery will prevent further fetal exposure to cocaine. In addition, many women addicted to crack turn to prostitution for themselves or their children to support their habit (Lowe, 1989). This situation has many grave social and public health implications, which include sexually transmitted

EFFECTS OF DRUG USE ON FETAL DEVELOPMENT

Cocaine

Cocaine causes placental and uterine vasoconstriction, resulting in fetal hypoxia. Associated problems include prematurity, low birth weight, hypertonicity, irritability, tremors, central nervous system (CNS) abnormalities, neurodevelopmental problems, and congenital anomalies.

Heroin

Newborns undergo a true withdrawal syndrome that includes irritability, tremors, hypertonicity, and fever. Infants have increased risk of sudden infant death syndrome (SIDS) and are vulnerable to many neonatal infections, including human immunodeficiency virus (HIV).

Alcohol

Infants undergoing withdrawal from alcohol may have tremors, irritability, hypertonicity, muscle twitching, and restlessness. The term fetal alcohol syndrome is used to describe a similar pattern of malformations noted in the offspring of alcohol-abusing women. Features of this syndrome include intrauterine growth retardation, slow postnatal growth, microcephaly, mental retardation, and craniofacial abnormalities.

Marijuana

Infants may have tremors, altered visual responses, low birth weight, growth retardation, and neurobehavioral abnormalities. Severity of symptoms is probably related to the quantity of drug used by the mother.

Barbiturates

Severe and prolonged withdrawal syndrome may occur. Symptoms include hyperactivity, restlessness, excessive crying, and hyperreflexia. Sudden withdrawal by the mother or infant can result in seizures.

Tobacco

Smoking in pregnancy is associated with spontaneous abortion, low birth weight, prematurity, and increased perinatal mortality

---

diseases (STDs), congenital infections, unwanted pregnancy, and the abandonment and physical and sexual abuse of children.

INCIDENCE

Each year in the United States, it is estimated that between 350,000 and 739,200 infants are exposed to one or more illicit substances (Chasnoff, 1991). Prevalence reports from around the country have documented cocaine use in 8% of women giving birth at a Chicago hospital (Neerhof et al, 1989), 12% of infants delivered at a Bronx hospital (Wingert et al, 1994), 17% of women in a prenatal care program in Boston (Frank et al, 1988), and in 31% of newborns in a Detroit hospital (Ostrea et al, 1992). A Rhode Island survey detected illicit drug use in 7.5% of women sampled, with cocaine found in 2.6% of that group (Hollinshead et al, 1990).

The study conducted in Rhode Island (Hollinshead et al, 1990) showed that cocaine was detected more often in women who were nonwhite, were classified as living in poverty, used public health insurance, and delivered in a regional perinatal center. In contrast, Chasnoff (1989c) reported the overall prevalence of illicit drug use by pregnant women in Pinellas County, Florida, to be 14.8%, with a rate of 16.3% among women using public clinics and a rate of 13.1% for women in the private health care sector. Moreover, he found similar percentages of positive toxicologic results among black women and white women (14.1% versus 15.4%).

It is prudent to address illicit drug use with all pregnant women. Drug use is often denied by users. Accordingly, the clinician can expect an underestimation of drug use when relying entirely on maternal self-report (Ostrea et al, 1992). Other maternal factors that may assist the clinician in identifying children who have been exposed to cocaine in utero are history of drug use, previous birth of a drug-exposed infant, STD, signs of intoxication, lack of prenatal care, physical indications of drug use, and suspicious or erratic behavior.

Because of the unreliability of maternal self-report, many hospitals in communities with known drug abuse problems routinely screen all high-risk mothers and their newborns for prenatal drug exposure.

Screening for cocaine and its metabolites can be performed using a variety of methods. Thin layer chromatography is the least sensitive method and has the possibility of producing false-negative results. Techniques such as the enzyme immunoassay (EIA) or the radioimmunoassay (RIA) are widely used and can detect benzoylecgonine (a cocaine metabolite) for 24 to 48 hours after use. Gas chromatography/mass spectroscopy provide the most specific and unchallengable information; they are also the most expensive (Hawks and Chiang, 1986; Udell, 1989).

Because urine toxicologic screening of newborns is feasible only during the immediate postpartum period, primary care providers will find its usefulness limited. It is important to remember that a negative urine toxicologic result is in no way conclusive evidence of lack of prenatal exposure, because of the rapid metabolism and excretion of cocaine.

Neonatal meconium and hair sample tests are believed to be reliable indicators of maternal drug use (Ostrea, 1992; Ostrea et al, 1992; Wingert et al, 1994). These tests have the advantage of reflecting drug use during the entire pregnancy instead of only the few days before delivery. More widespread use of these tests will assist the primary care provider in identifying children prenatally exposed to drugs.

For those clinicians working in the newborn nursery, toxicologic screening must be performed within institutional policy and protocol.

CLINICAL MANIFESTATIONS AT TIME OF DIAGNOSIS

Pharmacology and Physiologic Effects of Cocaine

Cocaine is benzoylmethylecgonine, a local anesthetic and CNS stimulant prepared from the extract of the leaves of the coca plant (Erythroxylon coca) (Ritchie and Greene, 1980). Cocaine readily crosses from maternal to fetal circulation, and because of metabolic differences, it may remain in the fetal system long after it has been excreted by the mother. It is absorbed from all sites of application and is metabolized by liver and plasma cholinesterases into two major metabolites that are excreted in the urine: benzoylecgonine and ecgoine methyl ester (Hawks and Chiang, 1986; Kennedy and Haddox, 1986; Ritchie and Greene, 1980).

Another metabolite, norcocaine, has been identified in humans and is believed to be biologically active. Norcocaine is water soluble with a high level of CNS penetration. Because of these characteristics, norcocaine does not easily reenter the maternal circulation, and theoretically the fetus may continue to be exposed to this metabolite by ingestion of the amniotic fluid (Chasnoff and Lewis, 1988; Wootton and Miller, 1994).

Cocaine is a CNS stimulant that can cause feelings of well-being, euphoria, restlessness, and excitement. Overdosage can lead to convulsions, CNS depression, and respiratory failure (Kennedy and Haddox, 1986; Ritchie and Greene, 1980).

Cocaine inhibits the reuptake of neurotransmitters at the adrenergic nerve terminals, producing increased levels of norepinephrine and dopamine. These elevated levels of catecholamines result in increased blood pressure, tachycardia, and vasoconstriction. Cocaine also causes elevations in body temperature. Large doses are directly toxic to the myocardium and may result in cardiac failure (Kennedy and Haddox, 1986; Ritchie and Greene, 1980).

Prenatal Effects of Cocaine

Because cocaine readily crosses the placenta, its physiologic effects, such as CNS stimulation, vasoconstriction, tachycardia, and blood pressure elevations, are believed to occur in both the mother and the fetus. In animal studies the fetal complications of cocaine use have included cardiovascular changes and changes in fetal oxygenation resulting from reduced uterine blood flow and impaired oxygen transfer (Woods, Plessinger, and Clark, 1987).

Prenatal manifestations of maternal cocaine use are fetal death, spontaneous abortion, preterm labor, precipitous labor, fetal distress, meconium staining, in utero cerebrovascular accidents and possibly abruptio placenta (Bingol et al, 1987; Chasnoff, Burns, and Burns, 1987; Chasnoff et al, 1986; Chasnoff, MacGregor, and Chisum, 1988; Hadeed and Siegel, 1989; Hutchings, 1993; MacGregor et al, 1987; Ryan, Ehrlich, and Finnegan, 1987).

Manifestations at Birth

Abundant literature describes the manifestations of intrauterine cocaine exposure exhibited at birth, including (1) prematurity, intrauterine growth retardation, microcephaly, and low birth weight*; (2) CNS abnormalities such as tremors, seizures, electroencephalographic (EEG) abnormalities, hyper-

tonicity, and cerebral infarct (Chasnoff et al, 1986; Chasnoff, MacGregor, and Chisum, 1988; Doberczak et al, 1988); (3) poor feeding (Udell, 1989); (4) necrotizing enterocolitis (NEC) (Porat and Brodsky, 1991; Czyrko et al, 1991).

The adverse effects manifested in cocaine-exposed infants probably are not indicative of a true withdrawal syndrome as seen with infants exposed to narcotics. Some believe that these signs of cocaine exposure represent either CNS hyperexcitability as a result of the direct effects of cocaine or indications of CNS damage.

TREATMENT

Infants who have been exposed to cocaine in utero can be identified based on maternal history, urine or meconium toxicologic screening, and clinical presentation.

Although pharmacologic therapy, including the use of phenobarbital, paragoric, and diazepam, has been advocated for narcotic withdrawal (Besunder and Blumer, 1990), infants who have been prenatally exposed to cocaine do not require such therapy. Pacification techniques such as swaddling and decreasing environmental stimuli are used to treat the symptoms of irritability and tremors often seen when cocaine is used in combination with other drugs.

Details of discharge planning for infants with prenatal exposure to cocaine will depend on who their caretakers will be after discharge. Planning for discharge is generally done in conjunction with hospital social service staff and in some cases child protective workers. Once the caretaker has been

---

CLINICAL MANIFESTATIONS

CNS stimulation
  tremors
  seizures
  hypertonicity
Vasoconstriction
Tachycardia
Blood pressure elevation
Prematurity
Intrauterine growth retardation
Microcephaly
Poor feeding/soothing

TREATMENT

Narcotic withdrawal therapy if indicated
Pacification techniques
Assessment of safety and competence of
  caretaker

---

*Bingol et al (1987), Cherukuri et al (1988), Chouteau, Namerow, and Leppert (1988), Fulroth, Phillips, and Durand (1989), Hadeed and Siegel (1989), Jacobson et al (1994) Kaye et al (1989), Kliegman et al (1994) and Zuckerman et al (1989).

identified, he or she must be provided with routine discharge information, as well as information regarding behavioral patterns to expect and pacification techniques. A referral to or consultation with a primary care provider who is familiar with drug addiction and its associated problems is ideal. These infants should be seen often, perhaps monthly, by the same provider.

RECENT AND ANTICIPATED ADVANCES IN DIAGNOSIS AND MANAGEMENT

Over the past decade, the issues surrounding prenatal exposure to cocaine have received attention both in the medical literature and in the mass media. Initial media reports described a "lost" generation of children who were "permanently damaged," and who would never function well in society. The term "crack baby" was coined and urban schools braced themselves for classrooms full of disturbed children (Coles, 1993; Zuckerman and Frank, 1992).

Health care providers, particularly those involved in providing obstetric, neonatal, and foster care services, saw increasing numbers of children who were prenatally exposed to cocaine. In the absence of solid research findings, these practitioners had to develop creative ways of providing health care services to these children and their families.

Since the mid-1980s much has been learned about prenatal cocaine exposure, including: (1) most of these children go on to do well and to function within normal limits for their appropriate age; (2) most women who use cocaine do so in combination with other drugs such as alcohol, tobacco, and marijuana, hence it is difficult to separate the effects of cocaine on the developing fetus from the effects on the mother (Robins and Mills, 1993). Richardson and Day (1994) collected data on 267 women who used cocaine or crack in the first trimester and 227 infants born to enrollees. They reported that women who use cocaine prenatally are also likely to use alcohol, marijuana, or tobacco. They concluded that the effects of prenatal drug exposure reported to date were the result of polydrug use and a disadvantaged lifestyle; and (3) there probably is a "dose related effect" on the fe-

tus, that is, women who use cocaine often and in large doses may have a worse perinatal outcome than the casual user (Hutchings, 1993; Jacobson et al, 1994).

Areas of ongoing research in prenatal cocaine exposure include: (1) animal studies in which the effects of confounding variables such as lifestyle, diet, and polydrug use can be controlled; (2) larger and better designed research studies to determine cocaine's effect on the human fetus; (3) long-term studies of neurodevelopmental and behavioral outcomes; and (4) use of meconium and hair samples to detect prenatal drug use (Robins and Mills, 1993).

In summary, the verdict is not yet in on children exposed to cocaine in utero. Although health and developmental problems are seen in some of these children, it has proven very difficult to separate cocaine's effects from those related to a drug-using lifestyle. At this juncture, it seems cocaine alone may not be responsible for all of the problems reported in exposed children; unfortunately, conclusive data and studies of long-term outcome are not available. It is helpful to view maternal cocaine use as a "marker" for other health and developmental risk factors, including inadequate prenatal care, poor nutrition, polydrug use, poverty, violence, foster care placement, inadequate parenting, and a chaotic home environment.

ASSOCIATED PROBLEMS

Prematurity

Infants exposed to cocaine in utero have an increased risk of preterm birth and consequently require appropriate neonatal intervention and long-term follow-up (see Chapter 30).

Congenital Infections and Infectious Diseases

The general use of illicit drugs has become increasingly associated with infectious diseases, STDs, and AIDS (Glaser, 1994; Wootton and Miller, 1994). Accordingly, the offspring of women using drugs can be expected to have increased rates of congenitally acquired infections. In particular, congenital syphilis has reached epidemic proportions in many areas (Glaser, 1994).

Many crack users will exchange sex for drugs; this frequent sexual activity with multiple partners is believed to be responsible for the recent explosion in the number of syphilis cases. This pattern of behavior also places the mother and the infant at increased risk for HIV infection. Many users of crack also inject cocaine or may use heroin to bring themselves down from periods of prolonged cocaine use, thus increasing their risk of HIV infection from contaminated needles.

In addition to syphilis and HIV infection, the primary care provider must consider infectious diseases such as hepatitis B, tuberculosis, and TORCH (toxoplasmosis, rubella, cytomegalovirus, herpes) infections, as well as other STDs such as gonorrhea and chlamydia, when assessing the health status of an infant or child of a cocaine-abusing mother.

ASSOCIATED PROBLEMS

Prematurity
Exposure to congenital infections
Growth retardation
Microcephaly
Congenital anomalies
Sudden Infant Death Syndrome
Neurologic/development problems
Feeding difficulties
Continued exposure to drugs
Parenting adequacy

Growth Retardation

Intrauterine growth retardation in cocaine-exposed infants has been well documented and is believed to be related to chronic uterine and placental hypoxia secondary to cocaine-induced vasoconstriction. Poor maternal nutrition is probably also a factor, especially in light of the anorectic effects of cocaine.

Microcephaly

A potentially worrisome finding of prenatal cocaine exposure is that of microcephaly. Currently the causes for this manifestation remain speculative. The clinician must recognize that children with microcephaly may be at risk for poor long-term developmental outcome (Griffith, Azuma, and Chasnoff, 1994).

Congenital Anomalies

Cocaine may be a teratogen. The most common congenital malformations associated with maternal cocaine use are those involving the genitourinary (GU) tract. Other malformations include: renal vascular abnormalities, congenital heart disease, skull defects, limb reduction defects, and intestinal atresia (Bingol et al, 1987; Chavez, Mulinare, and Cordero, 1989; Hoyme et al, 1990; Lipschultz, Frassica, and Orav, 1991; Ho, Afshani, and Stapleton, 1994). It is thought that vascular compromise or fetal hypoxia resulting from cocaine-induced vasoconstriction may be responsible for the appar-

ently increased rate of congenital malformations in these infants (Bingol et al, 1987; Hoyme et al, 1990).

Sudden Infant Death Syndrome

At this juncture it is not clear whether infants exposed to cocaine prenatally are at an increased risk for SIDS. Chasnoff and colleagues (1989) described a retrospective review of 66 cocaine-exposed infants. They discovered 10 deaths which were attributed to SIDS, for an overall incidence of 15%. This incidence is significantly greater than that among the general population and greater than the risk previously described for narcotic-exposed infants. A subsequent prospective study by the same authors revealed no deaths from SIDS (Chasnoff et al, 1989). Bauchner and associates (1988) studied 175 infants exposed to cocaine in utero and also found no deaths as a result of SIDS.

Recently, Kandall and associates (1993) reviewed SIDS cases among 1.2 million infants born in New York City between 1979 and 1989. After controlling for high-risk variables such as ethnicity, maternal age, parity, maternal smoking, and low birth weight, the authors found that opiate use was associated with a 2.3 to 3.7-fold increase in SIDS. They also demonstrated a significant, yet more modest, increase in the rate of SIDS after intrauterine exposure to cocaine. In addition, they noted that cocaine-associated SIDS seems to be increasing.

This may be related to the introduction of "crack" in the mid-1980s.

Although no causative relationship between drugs and SIDS has been established, the clinician should be aware that infants of substance abusing mothers do seem to be at an increased risk for SIDS and may have other risk factors such as prematurity and exposure to cigarette smoke.

Neurologic and Developmental Effects

The effects of intrauterine cocaine/polydrug exposure on the developing CNS that have been reported include seizures, perinatal cerebral infarction, and EEG abnormalities. Neurodevelopmental abnormalities described include irritability, tremulousness, and hypertonicity. In addition, these infants demonstrate depressed interactive abilities and poor state control when compared with drug-free infants of the same ages (Chasnoff et al, 1985; Schneider, Griffith, and Chasnoff, 1989). Four common behavioral patterns have been described in cocaine-exposed infants: (1) a deep sleep state, (2) an agitated sleep state, (3) vacillating extremes of state during handling, and (4) a panicked awake state (Schneider, Griffith, and Chasnoff, 1989). These unusual patterns of behavior, combined with inconsolability and irritability, may interfere with appropriate caregiver-infant interactions, potentially hindering the process of bonding and attachment.

Motor behavior in these infants is characterized by an increase in extensor tone, which interferes with children's ability to explore the environment and their own bodies. When supine, these children will often lie in an extended posture, and when held upright, they will stiffen and extend their ankles, knees, and hips, resulting in a weight-bearing position on their toes. These children have difficulty bringing their arms to midline and are poorly coordinated. Children with truncal hypertonicity often have difficulty with balance and may not be able to sit. These motor findings are mild or transient in some children and persistent in others, making general predictions of long-term outcome difficult.

There seems to be a consensus in the literature that intrauterine exposure to drugs alone does not seriously affect neurologic or cognitive develop-ment. Complicating factors such as lack of prenatal care, poor maternal nutrition, prematurity, poverty, poor parenting skills, and placement in foster care can adversely affect neurodevelopmental outcome (Neuspiel and Hamel, 1991; Chasnoff, 1993).

Griffith, Azuma, and Chasnoff (1994) reported a 3-year outcome study comparing three groups of children: group I—exposed to cocaine and poly-drugs, group II—exposed to polydrugs with no cocaine, and group III—controls with no prenatal drug exposure. Using the Stanford Binet Intelligence Scale, ed 4, they found no differences on global measures of intellectual development among the two drug-exposed groups and the controls.

The literature suggests that follow-up studies of children exposed to cocaine throughout pregnancy and cared for in middle-class adoptive homes would eliminate postnatal environmental risks and provide better outcome data.

Further studies are needed to examine school-age children with a history of cocaine exposure to evaluate intellectual function when more complex cognitive skills are necessary for learning. Other problems such as learning disabilities or attention deficit disorders may be uncovered.

Feeding Difficulties

Feeding difficulties and gastrointestinal (GI) symptoms such as poor suck-swallow response, vomiting, diarrhea, and constipation have been reported among infants exposed to cocaine in utero (Newald, 1986; Udell, 1989). From our experience at the Children's Aid Society Foster Care Medical Clinic, we have noted another feeding characteristic of these children—a voracious appetite. Caretakers will report that an infant will take a full feeding every 2 hours around the clock. The infants are unable to be consoled by anything other than food; they seem genuinely hungry.

Postnatal Exposure to Cocaine/Other Drugs

Children of cocaine-using parents can potentially be exposed to cocaine after birth as well as before. Cocaine and its metabolites are detectable in breast milk, and infants can be exposed to large doses of cocaine by breast feeding. Irritability, tremulousness, and other signs of CNS stimulation are seen in infants who ingest cocaine via breast milk (Chasnoff, Douglas, and Squires, 1987).

In addition, children who have been passively exposed to the smoke of crack have manifested such neurologic symptoms as seizures, drowsiness, and unsteady gait (Bateman and Heagarty, 1989). The possibilities for later cocaine exposure via breast feeding, passive inhalation, and accidental ingestion should be considered by the caretaker when caring for the children of drug-using parents. Because of the known frequency of polydrug use (Richardson and Day, 1994), signs and symptoms of exposure to other drugs, including secondhand smoke, must be evaluated by the primary care provider.

Parenting Issues

Parents dealing with their own addiction may have multiple medical and social problems that interfere with their ability to care for their children. They themselves may have been children of substance-abusing parents (Howard, 1989b). These parents, often single, may have had few positive parenting experiences in their own lives. If interventions such as preventive social service supports prove to be inadequate, the courts may move to terminate parental rights so that a permanency plan can be made for the young child. Many of these infants are at risk for biologic vulnerability from intrauterine drug exposure exacerbated by inadequate parenting (Chasnoff, 1993).

PROGNOSIS

Conclusive information regarding the prognosis for children with prenatal exposure to cocaine is unavailable at this time. However, two correlates of prenatal drug exposure—HIV infection and preterm birth—have significant effect on morbidity and mortality and must be considered when determining the prognosis for such a child.

New York City birth certificate data show that the infant mortality rate for cocaine-exposed infants is about 3 times that for other infants (Robbins and Mills, 1993), but as stated above, it is currently impossible to determine the direct effect of cocaine exposure from those related to a family drug-using lifestyle.

Primary Care Management
HEALTH CARE MAINTENANCE

Growth and Development

It is imperative that the primary care provider closely monitor the physical growth of these infants and young children. Monthly evaluations are prudent during infancy. Accurate measurements for weight, length, and head circumference require using the same scale and measuring tools at each visit. It is especially important that head size be measured accurately because of the high incidence of microcephaly. Data should be plotted on a standard National Center for Health Statistics growth chart. Data on infants with a history of prematurity should be plotted using the corrected age.

Recent data indicate that by the age of 2 years, cocaine-exposed infants "catch up" in height and weight when compared to nondrug-exposed children from a similar background. However, those children prenatally exposed to cocaine display smaller head circumferences than nonexposed children (Chasnoff, 1993; Griffith, Azuma, and Chasnoff, 1994).

Developmental assessment of an infant exposed to cocaine poses a challenge to the primary care provider. Routine office screening tools such as the Denver Developmental Screening Test II may or may not be helpful. Validity will depend on the stability of the infant's state control during testing. In addition, these infants may exhibit problems with motor development that can effect results.

It is useful to assess the infant's development at monthly intervals during the first 6 months of life and every 2 months during the second 6 months of life. Frequent assessments by the same provider offers valuable information about the child's developmental progress. Early referrals for a more detailed assessment by a developmental psychologist may prove useful if problems are suspected or before school entry.

For some infants, simultaneous visual and voice stimuli may prove to be too stressful and may interfere with parent-infant interaction. Without appropriate guidance, bonding and attachment may be seriously jeopardized. Parents should be advised to make full use of the infant's quiet and alert states. They also need to know that the attainment of developmental milestones can be unpredictable and is generally slower in these fragile infants.

When the cocaine-exposed infant is evaluated, a complete physical assessment is essential. Abnormal neurologic findings are common in these young children. The examiner should observe for irritability, tremors, extended postures, limb stiffness, hyperreflexia, clonus, persistence of primitive reflexes, subtle signs of infantile spasms, jerky eye movements, the inability to track visually, and the inability to respond to sound.

A neurologic consultation is necessary if seizures or other withdrawal symptoms such as persistent hypertonicity, irritability, or disturbance in the sleep-wake state are noted in the newborn period. Moreover, early assessment and intervention by a neurodevelopmentally trained physical therapist can provide the parent with helpful advice about handling and positioning "stiff" infants.

Diet

As mentioned earlier, breast feeding is not recommended for women using cocaine because the metabolites remain in the breast milk 12 to 60 hours after the last use (Hurt, 1989).

Because cocaine-exposed infants often have low birth weights, careful monitoring of caloric intake and feeding behavior is required. In addition, caretakers may tend to overfeed the irritable infant. These infants tend to have poor coordination of sucking and swallowing reflexes, tongue thrusting, and tongue tremors, as well as general oral hypersensitivity (Lewis, Bennett, and Schmeder, 1989; Schneider, Griffith, and Chasnoff, 1989).

Parents need continued support in introducing solid foods because the tongue thrust and oral hypersensitivity may persist beyond 6 months. Forced feeding is not appropriate and should be avoided. The primary care provider should encourage the parents to give food and fluids that are tolerated well.

Proper positioning and handling are essential for satisfactory feeding. A gentle, calm approach with a soothing voice while maintaining the infant in a relaxed, flexed posture will assist with feeding. If vomiting or spitting up occurs after feeding, frequent feedings of small amounts may be better tolerated. A side-lying swaddled position after feeding is recommended.

Safety

Because the chronic use of mind-altering drugs by the parent can interfere with memory, attention, and perception, safety of the child is a major concern for the provider (Howard et al, 1989). Home visits by health or social service professionals will help provide assessment of the home situation and limited parental supervision for these vulnerable children.

Often the primary interest of parents who are addicted, especially those using crack, is the drug, not their children. When they are high, they may be completely unaware of their child's presence. In addition, the children may be living in unstable, dangerous environments with parents who are unable to function as protectors. Because of this, it is important to keep the child visible in the community. Social service case workers can recommend infant stimulation programs, day care programs, and after-school and weekend recreational programs that are appropriate for these children and that will allow community workers to assess the child's health and emotional status on a regular basis.

Substance-abusing parents should also be warned about the danger of passive inhalation or accidental ingestion of the drugs by their children.

Immunizations

No reports have yet been published with regard to immunizing children who have been exposed to cocaine prenatally. Until such recommendations are available, the primary care provider must assess each child's health status, social situation, and immunization needs on an individual basis. In general the recommendations published by the American Academy of Pediatrics (AAP) should be followed.

Oral polio virus vaccine. Children born with prenatal drug exposure are at an increased risk for congenital HIV infection, and the AAP guidelines should be followed with regard to the administration of the live oral polio vaccine. In a child whose HIV status is seronegative or unknown but who is living with an immunocompromised caretaker, the inactivated polio virus (IPV) is recommended (Committee on Infectious Diseases, 1994). If there is any question as to the immune status of the parent, the IPV is the prudent choice.

Measles. For children living in areas where measles epidemics are likely to occur, such as large urban areas or areas with high concentrations of unimmunized children, it is prudent to give the measles, mumps, and rubella vaccine at 12 months of age and again before entry to school. Immunogenicity among children immunized at the earlier age has been shown to be adequate (Committee on Infectious Diseases, 1994). During measles epidemics, infants at risk in the community may be immunized at 6 months with repeat immunization at 12 months (Committee on Infectious Diseases, 1994).

Pertussis. Children who have been exposed to cocaine in utero often show CNS manifestations of this exposure, and a small number of these children may have seizures. Infants and children with a history of seizures have an increased risk of seizures after receipt of pertussis-containing vaccines (Committee on Infectious Diseases, 1994). Because seizure activity in cocaine-exposed infants is limited generally to the early neonatal period, it is recommended that the pertussis component of the diphtheria, pertussis, tetanus vaccine be given to all of these infants except those who have persistent, uncontrolled seizures. Consultation with the child's neurologist is recommended for those cocaine-exposed children whose neurologic status is not yet clearly understood.

Hepatitis B. Hepatitis B infection is a problem common among cocaine-using parents (Chasnoff, 1988). Generally, mothers are tested during the prenatal or immediate postpartum period. Infants of hepatitis B surface antigen (HBSAg)-negative mothers should receive three doses of hepatitis B vaccine according to AAP/CDC guidelines. Those infants of HBSAg-positive mothers should receive immunoprophylaxis with 0.5 ml hepatitis B immune globulin (HBIG) within 12 hours of birth, and 0.5 ml of either Recombivax HB or Engerix-B at a separate site. These infants should receive the second dose of vaccine at 1 month of age and the third at 6 months "At last..." (*Contemporary Pediatrics,* 1995).

Unfortunately a child's health care maintenance may not be a high priority for a drug-using parent. Every effort should be made to encourage the parent to keep the child's immunizations up to date and to keep the immunization record intact and in a safe place. The clinician may choose to administer several immunizations when the child is seen for health care because there may be no guarantee of compliance with follow-up visits. The AAP guidelines should be followed in doing this.

Screening

Vision. Routine screening is recommended.

Hearing. Routine screening is recommended unless there is a speech delay, in which case a complete audiologic evaluation is warranted.

Dental. Routine screening is recommended.

Blood pressure. Four extremity blood pressures at birth and yearly screening are recommended as a result of the possibility of renal vascular abnormalities.

Hematocrit. Routine screening is recommended.

Urinalysis. Routine screening is recommended.

Tuberculosis. There is a higher incidence of tuberculosis among the drug-using population, especially if the users are HIV infected. Yearly screening with purified protein derivative (PPD), 0.1 ml intradermally, is recommended beginning at age 12 months.

Condition-specific screening

TOXICOLOGY SCREENS. If a mother is a suspected substance abuser or has not received prenatal care, the newborn's urine/meconium is screened for drugs using one of the laboratory methods previously described.

CONGENITAL. Because substance abusers are also at high risk for contracting infectious diseases, obtaining TORCH titers to rule out congenital infections such as cytomegalovirus and a maternal syphilis serologic test may be prudent.

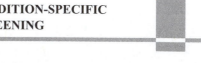

CONDITION-SPECIFIC SCREENING

Toxicology screens
Congenital infections
Cardiac abnormalities
Neurologic abnormalities
Genitourinary abnormalities

GENITOURINARY ABNORMALITIES. The urologist may recommend a renal ultrasonogram or a voiding cystourethrogram to evaluate the urologic system.

CARDIAC ABNORMALITIES. The cardiologist may recommend an electrocardiogram (ECG) and echocardiogram (ECHO) to evaluate for heart disease.

NEUROLOGIC ABNORMALITIES. The neurologist may recommend any of the following studies: brainstem auditory evoked response (BAER), magnetic resonance imaging (MRI), EEG, and skull x-ray studies to evaluate the nervous system.

COMMON ILLNESS MANAGEMENT

Differential Diagnosis

Infections. During the first 3 months of life it is often difficult to diagnose illness because of the subtle signs and symptoms the newborn exhibits when ill. A change in behavior is often a key factor in the assessment of the child. This complicates diagnosing illness in infants exposed to cocaine in utero because of the great variability in their sleep-wake state control. The primary care provider should carefully assess the irritable or deeply sleeping infant for signs of concomitant illness.

Parents should be taught how to take temperatures. They should be encouraged to call the pediatric office or clinic with any concerns. Frequent telephone contact will help the parent manage the child at home. If the parent is a poor historian or seems overly concerned on the telephone, the child should be seen in the office or the clinic.

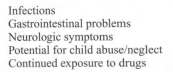

DIFFERENTIAL DIAGNOSIS

Infections
Gastrointestinal problems
Neurologic symptoms
Potential for child abuse/neglect
Continued exposure to drugs

The practitioner needs to be aware of the increased risk of HIV infection in this population. Accordingly, frequent infections may warrant an immunologic consultation.

Gastrointestinal symptoms. Gastrointestinal symptoms such as poor feeding, vomiting, diarrhea, or constipation are common in the first 6 to 9 months of life (Lewis, Bennett, and Schmeder, 1989). Parents should be advised to report any GI symptoms to their primary care provider. Once serious illness is ruled out, routine advice for handling these problems is helpful. The diarrhea described by most parents consists of loose stools with a water ring; dietary changes usually help to control the consistency of the stool. Small frequent feedings are usually well tolerated.

Neurologic symptoms. As mentioned earlier, seizures may occur in the neonatal period. Parents need to be advised about injury prevention when the child is having a seizure and the importance of having the child evaluated by the provider immediately (see Chapter 19). As children enter preschool or school, an evaluation for learning disabilities should be undertaken if there is any indication of difficulty processing information or attending to tasks. These children are considered "at risk" and are therefore eligible for evaluative services under Public Laws 99-457 and 101-476.

Child abuse. These potentially difficult children are at increased risk for child abuse. The provider should be alert to this possibility and thoroughly examine the skin for marks or bruises. Parents who did not have appropriate parenting role models may have difficulty knowing how to care for themselves and may have no understanding of how to care for an irritable infant.

Parental drug use. The provider should also keep in mind that a parent who is high on drugs may not follow directions appropriately. Therefore, any potentially serious condition warrants an office visit, and children who are ill may need to be hospitalized or placed in temporary foster care to ensure appropriate medical management.

Drug Interactions

If a child is taking anticonvulsants for seizure activity, the same precautions outlined in Chapter 19 should be followed.

DEVELOPMENTAL ISSUES

Sleep Patterns

Because of these infants' variable sleep-wake control state patterns, establishing regular sleeping patterns is difficult. Techniques that assist parents with sleep problems include swaddling, slow rhythmic rocking, offering a pacifier, and holding the infant in a relaxed, flexed position. In addition, keeping the lights low and reducing noise in the environment are helpful. Fortunately, few sleep problems are reported after the first year. Since drug-exposed infants may have an increased risk of SIDS, they should be placed on their backs or sides for sleep.

Toileting

Persistent motor delays, hyperactivity, and behavioral problems may cause difficulty with toilet training. Parents need a great deal of patience and support for their efforts with the child. Early counseling with the parents may help to avoid potential difficulties.

Children with persistent enuresis may require urologic evaluation because of the increased incidence of urinary tract anomalies found in cocaine-exposed children.

Discipline

Behavior in these infants and young children may be characterized by irritability, excessive crying, and hyperactivity. The primary care provider can suggest techniques for pacifying these children such as swaddling, offering pacifiers, and decreasing environmental distractions. Older children, especially slow learners, require patient limit setting, and discipline must be developmentally appropriate. To date, few resources exist with expertise in managing children with difficult behaviors. The primary care provider will need to assess mental health and developmental services in their home communities for appropriate referrals.

Child Care

Working parents often place children in day care and preschool nursery programs. At this point, there is no evidence that children with a history of drug exposure need placement in special or therapeutic settings.

Schooling

Children who experience drug exposure during the neonatal period may be at risk for learning problems. It is wise to make early referrals to Head Start or licensed preschool programs. Enrollment in these programs gives the child the added benefit of supervision by child care professionals on a daily basis. Problems such as abuse, neglect, or poor academic performance can be addressed in a timely fashion.

Public Law (PL) 99-457 provides for public education and related services for handicapped preschoolers ages 3 to 5 years old. Public Law 101-476 provides these services for school-age children through age 21.

Substance abusing parents may not be able to assist their children with homework assignments and are sometimes lax about making sure their children attend school on a regular basis. Referrals to after school and tutorial programs will encourage these children to recognize their strengths, increase their self-esteem, develop appropriate peer relationships, and provide on-going supervision during the school years.

The long-term educational needs of these children have not been determined. Any child performing below grade level should be evaluated for learning disabilities, and a specialized educational program should be developed to meet their needs.

Sexuality

Besides giving routine advice to adolescents, the primary care provider must be aware of the potential for desperate drug users to prostitute their children for drugs. In addition, there is the added risk of sexual abuse in these highly dysfunctional families. The provider should be alert to any physical or psychologic indications of sexual abuse and, if suspected, report the situation to the appropriate authorities.

Transition into Adulthood

Adolescents in foster care should be encouraged to utilize "independent living" programs which focus on smoothing the transition between foster care and life on their own. When providing anticipatory guidance for these teens, the primary care provider should discuss reducing their health risk, taking responsibility for their own health, and accessing health care. These young adults should also be encouraged to apply for Medicaid or private health insurance before discharge from foster care and to locate an appropriate primary care provider. Discharge with a medical summary and a current immunization record will promote continuity of care.

Children treated for congenital syphilis will continue to have a positive serum treponemal test (fluorescent treponemal antibody absorption [FTA-ABS] or microhemagglutination assay for T. pallidium [MHA-TP]). It is believed that this will persist into adulthood. Adolescents should be made aware of this fact and have documentation of treatment on their permanent medical record or immunization card.

SPECIAL FAMILY CONCERNS AND RESOURCES

The family court system may deem parents to be unfit. In some states, a neonatal drug screen test result that is positive for illicit drugs triggers a report to the Child Welfare Administration as evidence of neglect. Neuspiel and colleagues (1993) found that only 38% of cocaine-exposed infants in one New York City hospital were discharged to their mothers, 28% went to other family members, and 36% entered agency foster care. This situation forces relatives, often elderly grandparents, to assume full responsibility for these drug-addicted infants and their siblings while the parents seek treatment in the limited number of available programs. Few drug treatment programs will accept pregnant addicts.

Before being placed in either a kinship or temporary foster home, these infants may stay in the hospital for 2 to 4 weeks in the boarder nursery. In other cases children are moved quickly to preadoptive homes. There is now a growing movement among health and social service professionals to have family assessments made early to improve the potential for family recovery.

Foster and kinship foster parents need respite. The social service agency responsible for the child should be contacted. In addition, foster parents need ongoing positive reinforcement. Practitioners must empower them with the strength and resources to cope with these needy children. Professionals also need to examine their own feelings of

attachment to the children of substance-abusing parents. It may be difficult to maintain empathy and concern for these parents without becoming judgmental. As Weston and associates (1989) have noted, "Stereotypes can blind us to the unique characteristics that both infants and mothers bring to their relationship, despite the impact of drugs."

Substance-abusing parents who continue to use illicit drugs must be warned about the possibility of losing custody of their children if they fail to adequately care for them or if they endanger them in any way.

The low income, and women of color, may be more likely to be tested for illicit substances during their pregnancies; however, drug use crosses all ethnic and socioeconomic boundaries. All women should be treated respectfully, and judgments about drug use and fitness as a parent should not be based solely on their ethnicity or economic status.

Despite careful counseling by health care professionals, adoptive parents will often have expectations about the infant or child that they accept into their home. Since long-term outcomes are unknown in the cocaine-exposed population, adoptive parents must be advised accordingly. Many of these infants who have had a difficult first few months look "normal" to adoptive parents who so eagerly want a child. It is important to follow the child's progress with the adoptive parents while remaining objective and realistic about the outcome.

Across the nation communities are responding to the devastating problems associated with drug addiction. NAPARE provides information on the dangers of substance abuse during pregnancy and on treatment options. In addition, many government and private agencies have substance abuse hotlines.

Organizations

National Association for Perinatal Addiction Research and Education (NAPARE)
200 N Michigan Ave
Suite 300
Chicago, IL 60601
(312) 541-1272

This national organization is a resource center for individuals and groups concerned with perinatal addiction.

The Family Center
Thomas Jefferson University Hospital
1201 Chestnut St
11th Floor
Philadelphia, PA 19107
(215) 955-8577

This center provides pregnant addicts and their children with medical, psychiatric, and social services, as well as a variety of clinical assessments.
National Institute on Drug Abuse (NIDA)

Cocaine Helpline
(800) COCAINE

SUMMARY OF PRIMARY CARE NEEDS FOR THE CHILD WITH PRENATAL COCAINE EXPOSURE

Health care maintenance

Growth and development

Growth parameters, particularly weight and head circumference, should be monitored monthly for the first 6 months and every 2 months for the next 6 months.
Attainment of developmental milestones is unpredictable and generally slower than normal.
Motor problems are common.

Diet

Breast feeding is not recommended for cocaine-using women because cocaine metabolites are present in breast milk.
Caloric intake and feeding behavior should be monitored.
To enhance feeding, parents should be taught proper positioning and handling techniques.

Safety

Home visits are recommended if parents are suspected substance abusers.
Social service involvement and referrals to after school and recreational programs are recommended to keep the child visible in the community.
Parents should be warned about the dangers of passive inhalation of crack fumes and the potential for accidental ingestion of drugs by the children.

Immunizations

Routine immunizations are recommended.
If the child tests HIV seropositive, the guidelines in Chapter 22 should be followed.
Infants with limited history of seizures in the neonatal period can receive the pertussis vaccine. Infants with persistent seizures require consultation with a pediatric neurologist.
Hepatitis B immune globulin is given if the mother is infected.
Drug-using parents may not be compliant with well-child care visits; the clinician may choose to give several immunizations at one visit.

Screening

Vision
Routine screening is recommended.
Hearing
Routine office screening is recommended unless there is a speech delay, in which case a complete audiologic evaluation is warranted.
Dental
Routine screening is recommended.
Blood pressure
Yearly four extremity screening in the neonatal period is recommended.
Hematocrit
Routine screening is recommended.
Urinalysis
Routine screening is recommended. The high incidence of urologic abnormalities in these

Continued.

SUMMARY OF PRIMARY CARE NEEDS FOR THE CHILD WITH PRENATAL COCAINE EXPOSURE—cont'd

children may require referral to a urologist for testing.

Tuberculosis

Yearly screening with PPD beginning at 12 months is recommended.

Condition-specific screening

TOXICOLOGY

Urine toxicologic screening should be done if the mother is a suspected substance abuser or did not receive prenatal care.

INFECTIONS

Syphilis serologic testing and TORCH titers should be considered.

GENITOURINARY SCREENING

May be done in infancy because of a high rate of anomalies.

CARDIAC SCREENING

Both ECG and ECHO may be obtained if a heart murmur is detected.

NEUROLOGIC SCREENING

If neurologic problems are suspected, BAER, MRI, EEG, and skull films may be obtained.

Common illness management

Differential diagnosis

Infections

The irritable or deeply sleeping infant should be carefully assessed.

Parents should be taught to take temperatures.

An office visit should be scheduled if any questions exist about the child's condition.

These children are at high risk for contracting congenital infections, including HIV.

Gastrointestinal problems

Gastrointestinal symptoms such as vomiting, diarrhea, and constipation may persist for the first 6 to 9 months. Other illnesses need to be ruled out.

Neurologic problems

The child should be evaluated immediately if a seizure occurs.

Child abuse

Behavior should be observed and the skin checked closely for signs of abuse.

Parental drug use

If the parents are abusing drugs, the child may need to be hospitalized or placed in temporary foster care during periods of illness to ensure medical management.

Drug interactions

No routine medications are prescribed. If the child is taking seizure medication, see Chapter 19.

Developmental issues

Sleep patterns

Trouble with regulation of the sleep-wake state may occur in the first year of life.

Pacification techniques, low lighting, and a relatively quiet environment are helpful.

Infant should be placed on back or side to sleep.

Toileting

Persistent motor delays, hyperactivity, and behavior problems may interfere with toilet training.

Children with persistent enuresis may need genitourinary work-up.

Discipline

Parents should be encouraged to be consistent, firm, and patient in their disciplinary efforts.

Child care

Routine placement is advised.

Early identification and referrals to programs such as Head Start are helpful.

Schooling

These children may be at high risk for learning problems.

Sexuality

These children are at high risk for sexual abuse.

Continued.

SUMMARY OF PRIMARY CARE NEEDS FOR THE CHILD
WITH PRENATAL COCAINE EXPOSURE—cont'd

Transition into adulthood

Teens in foster care should be enrolled in independent living programs.

Discuss access to health care, risk reduction, and health insurance.

Document treatment for congenital syphilis on immunization card.

Special family concerns

Foster and kinship foster parents need respite.

Adoptive parents require ongoing counseling because long-term outcomes are generally unknown.

Health care providers must try to remain empathic and nonjudgmental.

REFERENCES

At last: A unified schedule for childhood immunizations, *Contemp Pediatr* 12:19-20, 1995.

Azuma SD, Chasnoff IJ: Outcome of children prenatally exposed to cocaine and other drugs: a path analysis of 3-year data, *Pediatrics* 92:396-402, 1993.

Bateman DA, Heagarty MC: Passive freebase cocaine ('crack') inhalation by infants and toddlers, *Am J Dis Child* 143:25-27, 1989.

Bauchner H et al: Risk of sudden infant death syndrome among infants with in utero exposure to cocaine, *J Pediatr* 113:831-834, 1988.

Besunder JB, Blumer JL: Neonatal drug withdrawal syndromes. In Koren G (editor): *Maternal-fetal toxicology: a clinician's guide,* New York, 1990, Marcel Dekker, pp 161-190.

Bingol N et al: Teratogenicity of cocaine in humans, *J Pediatr* 110:93-96, 1987.

Centers for Disease Control: Syphilis and congenital syphilis—United States, 1985–1988, *MMWR* 37:486-489, 1988.

Chasnoff IJ: Drug use in pregnancy: parameters of risk, *Pediatr Clin North Am* 35:1403-1412, 1988.

Chasnoff IJ: Drug use and women: establishing a standard of care, *Ann NY Acad Sci* 562:208-210, 1989a.

Chasnoff IJ: Drug use in pregnancy, *NY State J Med* 89:255, 1989b.

Chasnoff IJ: The incidence of cocaine use. In *Special currents: cocaine babies,* Columbus, OH, 1989c, Ross Laboratories.

Chasnoff IJ: Drugs, alcohol, pregnancy, and the neonate: pay now or pay later, *JAMA* 266:1567-1568, 1991.

Chasnoff IJ: Missing pieces of the puzzle, *Neurotoxicol Teratol* 15:287-288, 1993.

Chasnoff IJ, Burns KA, and Burns WD: Cocaine use in pregnancy: perinatal morbidity and mortality, *Neurotoxicol Teratol* 9:291-293, 1987.

Chasnoff IJ, Douglas EL, and Squires L: Cocaine intoxication in a breast-fed infant, *Pediatrics* 80:836-838, 1987.

Chasnoff IJ et al: Cocaine use in pregnancy, *N Engl J Med* 313:666-669, 1985.

Chasnoff IJ et al: Perinatal cerebral infarction and maternal cocaine use, *J Pediatr* 108:456-459, 1986.

Chasnoff IJ et al: Prenatal cocaine exposure is associated with respiratory pattern abnormalities, *Am J Dis Child* 143:583-587, 1989.

Chasnoff IJ, Lewis DE: Cocaine metabolism during pregnancy, *Pediatr Res* 23:257a, 1988 (abstract).

Chasnoff IJ, MacGregor S, and Chisum G: Cocaine use during pregnancy: adverse perinatal outcome, *Nat Inst Drug Abuse Res Monogr Ser* 81:265, 1988.

Chavez GF, Mulinare J, and Cordero JF: Maternal cocaine use during early pregnancy as a risk factor for congenital urogenital anomalies, *JAMA* 262:795-798, 1989.

Cherukuri R et al: A cohort study of alkaloidal cocaine ("crack") in pregnancy, *Obstet Gynecol* 72:147-151, 1988.

Chouteau M, Namerow PB, and Leppert P: The effect of cocaine abuse on birthweight and gestational age, *Obstet Gynecol* 72:351-354, 1988.

Committee on Infectious Diseases: *Report of the committee on infectious diseases,* Evanston, IL, 1994, The American Academy of Pediatrics.

Coles CD: Saying "goodbye" to the "crack baby," *Neurotoxicol Teratol* 15:290-292, 1993.

Czyrko C et al: Maternal cocaine abuse and necrotizing enterocolitis: outcome and survival, *J Pediatr Surg* 26:414-421, 1991.

Doberczak TM et al: Neonatal neurologic and electroencephalographic effects of intrauterine cocaine exposure, *J Pediatr* 113:354-358, 1988.

Frank DA et al: Cocaine use during pregnancy: prevalence and correlates, *Pediatrics* 82:888-895, 1988.

Fulroth R, Phillips B, and Durand DJ: Perinatal outcome of infants exposed to cocaine and/or heroin in utero, *Am J Dis Child* 143:905-910, 1989.

Glaser J: Detecting congenital syphilis, *Contemp Pediatr* 11:57-66, 1994.

Gold M: Crack abuse: its implications and outcomes, *Resident and Staff Physician* 33:45-52, 1987.

Griffith DR, Azuma SD, and Chasnoff IJ: Three-year outcome of children exposed prenatally to drugs, *J Am Acad Child Adolesc Psychiatr* 33:20-27, 1994.

Hadeed AJ, Siegel SR: Maternal cocaine use during pregnancy: effect on the newborn infant, *Pediatrics* 84:205-210, 1989.

Hawks R, Chiang CN: Examples of specific drug assays, *Nat Inst Drug Abuse Res Monogr Ser* 73:84-114, 1986.

Ho J, Afshani E, and Stapleton FB: Renal vascular abnormalities associated with prenatal cocaine exposure, *Clin Pediatr* 32:155-156, 1994.

Hollinshead WH et al: Statewide prevalence of illicit drug use by pregnant women—Rhode Island. *MMWR* 39:225-227, 1990.

Howard J: Cocaine and its effects on the newborn, *Dev Med Child Neurol* 31:255-257, 1989a.

Howard J: Long term development of infants exposed prenatally to drugs, In *Special currents: cocaine babies,* Columbus, OH, 1989b, Ross Laboratories, pp 1-2.

Howard J et al: The development of young children of substance abusing parents: insights from 7 years of intervention and research, *Zero to three: bulletin of national center for clinical infant programs* 9:8-12, 1989.

Hoyme HE et al: Prenatal cocaine exposure and fetal vascular disruption, *Pediatrics* 85:743-747, 1990.

Hurt H: Medical controversies in evaluation and management of cocaine exposed infants, In *Special currents: cocaine babies,* Columbus, OH, 1989, Ross Laboratories, pp 3-4.

Hutchings DE: The puzzle of cocaine's effects following maternal use during pregnancy: are there reconcilable differences? *Neurotoxicol Teratol* 15:281-286, 1993.

Jacobson JL et al: The effects of alcohol use, smoking, and illicit drug use on fetal growth in black infants, *J Pediatr* 124:757-764, 1994.

Jones KL et al: Pattern of malformation in offspring of chronic alcoholic mothers, *Lancet* 1:1267-1271, 1973.

Kandall SR et al: Relationship of maternal substance abuse to subsequent sudden infant death syndrome in offspring, *J Pediatr* 123:120-126, 1993.

Kaye K et al: Birth outcomes for infants of drug abusing mothers, *NY State J Med* 89:256-261, 1989.

Kennedy RL, Haddox JD: Local anesthetics. In Craig CR, Stitzel RE (editors): *Modern pharmacology,* ed 2, Boston, 1986, Little, Brown, pp 480-490.

Kleigman RM et al: Relation of maternal cocaine use to the risk of prematurity and low birth weight, *J Pediatr* 124:751-756, 1994.

Lewis KD, Bennett B, and Schmeder NH: Care of infants menaced by cocaine use, *MCN* 14:324-329, 1989.

Lipschultz SE, Frassica JJ, Orav EJ: Cardiovascular abnormalities in infants prenatally exposed to cocaine, *J Pediatr* 118:44-51, 1991.

Lowe C, (editor): Maternal drug abuse—New York City, *City Health Information* 8:1-4, 1989.

MacGregor SN et al: Cocaine use during pregnancy: adverse perinatal outcome, *Am J Obstet Gynecol* 157:686-690, 1987.

National Institute on Drug Abuse: 1990 National Household Survey on Drug Abuse, US Dept of Health and Human Services (unpublished).

Neerhof MG et al: Cocaine abuse during pregnancy: peripartum prevalence and perinatal outcome, *Am J Obstet Gynecol* 161:633-638, 1989.

Neuspiel DR, Hamel SC: Cocaine and infant behavior, *Dev Behav Pediatr* 12:55-64, 1991.

Neuspiel DR et al: Custody of cocaine-exposed newborns: determinants of discharge decisions, *Am J Public Health* 83:1726-1729, 1993.

Newald J: Cocaine infants: a new arrival at hospital's step? *Hospitals* 60:96, 1986.

Ostrea EM et al: Drug screening of newborns by meconium analysis: a large prospective epidemiologic study, *Pediatrics* 89:107-113, 1992.

Ostrea EM: Detection of prenatal drug exposure in the pregnant woman and her newborn infant, *Nat Inst Drug Abuse Res Monogr Ser* 117:61-79, 1992.

Porat R, Brodsky N: Cocaine: a risk factor for necrotizing enterocolitis, *J Perinatol* 11:30-32, 1991.

Richardson GA, Day NL: Detrimental effects of prenatal cocaine exposure: illusion or reality: *J Am Acad Child Adolesc Psychiatr* 33:28-34, 1994.

Ritchie JM, Greene NM: Local anesthetics. In Gilman AG, Goodman LS, Gilman A (editors): *The pharmacological basis of therapeutics,* New York, 1980, MacMillan, pp 300-308.

Robins LN, Mills JL, (editors): Effects of in utero exposure to street drugs, *Am J Public Health Suppl* 83:17, 1993.

Ryan L, Ehrlich S, and Finnegan LP: Cocaine abuse in pregnancy: effects on the fetus and newborn, *Nat Inst Drug Abuse Res Monogr Ser* 76:280, 1987.

Schneider JW, Griffith DR, and Chasnoff IJ: Infants exposed to cocaine in utero: implications for developmental assessment and intervention, *Infants Young Child* 2:25-36, 1989.

Udell B: Crack cocaine. In *Special currents: cocaine babies,* Columbus, OH, 1989, Ross Laboratories, pp 5-8.

Weston DR et al: Drug exposed babies: research and clinical issues, *Zero to three: bulletin of the national center for clinical infant programs* 9:1-7, 1989.

Wingert WE et al: A comparison of meconium, maternal urine, and neonatal urine for detection of maternal drug use during pregnancy, *J Forensic Sci* 39:150-158, 1994.

Woods JR, Plessinger MA, and Clark KE: Effect of cocaine on uterine blood flow and fetal oxygenation, *JAMA* 257:957-961, 1987.

Wootton J, Miller SI: Cocaine: a review, *Pediatr Rev* 15:89-92, 1994.

Zuckerman B, Frank DA: "Crack kids": not broken, *Pediatrics* 89:337-339, 1992. Zuckerman B et al: Effects of maternal marijuana and cocaine use on fetal growth, *N Engl J Med* 320:762-768, 1989.

Renal Failure, Chronic

32

Judy H. Taylor*

ETIOLOGY

More than 8 million Americans have renal disease, and children represent approximately 10% of this population, which is a small but significant percentage of the total group. Early recognition and management are essential to minimize the potentially devastating consequences of renal failure.

Progression of Chronic Renal Failure (CRF)

CRF is a broadly used term that is measured by glomerular filtration rate (GFR) and may be described in four stages: (1) early renal failure with a GFR of 50% to 75% normal, characterized by decreased renal reserve but with fairly normal excretory and regulatory functions; (2) chronic renal insufficiency (CRI), with a GFR of 25% to 50% normal, and associated impairment of excretory and regulatory functions; (3) chronic renal failure (CRF), with a GFR of 10% to 25% normal, and increasing clinical manifestations of renal failure; and (4) end-stage renal disease (ESRD), with a GFR of 10% and renal replacement therapy (RRT) with dialysis or transplantation necessary to sustain life (Foreman, Tsuru, and Chan, 1990; Kher, 1992).

Etiologies of CRF are varied and can be broadly categorized as congenital or hereditary, or by patho-

physiology including: obstructive uropathy, glomerulopathies, collagen vascular, metabolic or cystic diseases, and malignancies. Refer to Table 32-1 for elaboration of etiology in children related to age, sex, race, and incidence. Glomerulonephritis accounts for the largest single group (36.4%) of children with ESRD, followed by congenital and other hereditary/cystic diseases (23.6%). Race-related patterns are demonstrated with hypertension being more common among children who are of African American descent, as in adults, and congenital/other hereditary and cystic diseases more common in children of Caucasian and Native American descent (U.S. Renal Data System [USRDS], 1994).

Children with congenital disorders, or whose renal disease begins in infancy are at greatest risk of significant growth failure and progression to ESRD. Children with congenital renal anomalies will frequently have abnormalities of other organ systems as well, according to the period of embryonic development and gestational stage in which the problem occurred. Genetic counseling is recommended for future family planning.

It is important to establish the exact etiology of CRF in a child whenever possible, because (1) disorders may require different treatments and have varying prognoses; (2) genetic counseling and early diagnosis and treatment of similarly affected siblings should be initiated if a hereditary or metabolic disease is involved; and (3) the timing of renal transplantation may be altered in those diseases with a high incidence of recurrence in renal allografts.

*The editors and author would like to acknowledge the work done by Elizabeth San Luis on this chapter in the first edition of the book.

689

Table 32-1.   INCIDENCE OF TREATED ESRD BY DETAILED PRIMARY DISEASE, AGE, RACE, SEX AND ONE-YEAR TRANSPLANT AND DEATH STATUS FOR PEDIATRIC PATIENTS AGE < 20, 1988-1991

Primary disease	Total incident count 1988–91*	% of Total**	Median age	% Male	% of race				%***	
					White	Black	Asian	Native Amer.	Transplant in 1st year	Died in 1st year
All ESRD, (reference)	3475	100	15	57.6	100	100	100	100	43.3	4.2
Diabetes	39	1.2	18	51.2	1.3	1.1	0.0	2.5	33.3	2.5
Hypertension	156	5.1	17	57.0	3.4	11.0	1.2	5.1	31.4	7.0
Glomerulonephritis	1097	36.3	16	55.4	33.1	44.8	41.7	41.0	42.7	3.5
Cystic kidney diseases	138	4.5	11	54.3	5.8	0.7	2.5	7.6	54.3	7.2
Interstitial nephritis	127	4.2	16	55.9	4.8	2.1	5.0	2.5	48.0	0.7
Obstructive nephropathy	208	6.8	13	75.4	7.9	3.8	6.3	5.1	48.5	3.8
Collagen vascular diseases	287	9.5	16	28.5	8.5	11.2	18.9	5.1	20.2	3.8
Malignancies	12	0.3	4	66.6	0.4	0.2	0.0	0.0	16.6	16.6
Metabolic diseases	41	1.3	10	46.3	1.6	0.7	0.0	0.0	82.9	2.4
Congenital/other Hereditary diseases	578	19.1	11	72.8	21.8	12.2	11.3	17.9	55.1	4.3
Sickle cell disease	8	0.2	16	50.0	0.1	0.7	0.0	0.0	25.0	0.0
AIDS-Related	1	<0.1	13	100.0	0.0	0.1	0.0	0.0	0.0	100.0
Other ESRD	35	1.1	8	42.8	1.3	0.4	0.0	2.5	22.8	11.4
Cause labeled as "unknown"	294	9.7	16	58.8	9.2	10.5	12.6	10.2	42.8	3.0
Missing information	454		14	57.7					41.4	5.2

Patients in Puerto Rico and U.S. Territories are included. Medicare patients only. Rows sum to "All ESRD (reference)" row for total incident count, percent of total and percent of race categories.

*Divide total by 4 to determine the average annual count of children new to ESRD between 1988 and 1991.

**Patients with missing information (13% of total) are excluded from this column.

***In these two columns, "1st year" refers to 1st year of ESRD therapy.

Modified from U.S. Renal Data System, USRDS 1994 Annual Data Report, The National Institutes of Health, National Institute of Diabetes and Digestive and Kidney Diseases, Bethesda, MD, July 1994.

Early surgical intervention may slow the progression of renal disease. Reimplantation of ureters may prevent further vesicoureteral refluxing and renal scarring from pyelonephritis. Early ablation of posterior urethral valves may delay renal failure and positively affect growth and later sexual development in males (Lyon, Marshall, and Baskin, 1992; Reinberg, de Castano, and Gonzales, 1992). Unfortunately, it is not always possible to determine etiology, especially when a child presents already in CRF. A renal biopsy may be indicated for diagnosis, prognosis, and treatment recommendations.

INCIDENCE

In the most comprehensive collection of data available, the United States Renal Data Service (USRDS, 1994) identified 822 newly diagnosed cases of children, age birth to 19 years, beginning renal replacement therapy for ESRD during 1991. This incidence rate, 1/100,000 U.S. children, has remained fairly constant over the past 10 years, in contrast to the increased incidence seen in adults with ESRD. The adjusted rate of incidence per million population was 11 for 0 to 19 years, 96 for 20 to 44 years, 392 for 45 to 64 years, and continues to increase with age. Males have a higher incidence of CRF than females in all age groups, but especially in the under 5 years age group. By race, incidence rates in children per million population were 10 for Caucasian, 17 for African Americans, 9 for Asian/Pacific Islanders, and 14 for Native Americans. In the 15 to 19 year group, CRF occurs twice as often in African Americans than in Caucasians; in adult groups, this rate increases to 3 times more in African Americans and 4 times more in Native Americans than Caucasians. The disparity is largely attributed to the increased incidence in hypertension and diabetes mellitus associated CRF in adolescents and adults. Pediatric prevalence counts for 1989 through 1991 show a 4% overall increase, compared to the previous period, which reflects improved survival in children with CRF.

CLINICAL MANIFESTATIONS AT TIME OF DIAGNOSIS

Presenting symptoms at the time of diagnosis vary depending on the primary renal disease and the amount of renal function present. The child with CRF may exhibit few or many common signs and symptoms of renal failure.

Fluid, Electrolyte, Acid-Base Abnormalities

As renal function decreases, solute, fluid, and toxin accumulate in the blood (uremia). Impairment of bicarbonate reabsorption and ammonia excretion causes metabolic acidosis, manifested as tachycardia, hyperpnea, hyperkalemia, lethargy, and growth impairment.

Hyperkalemia occurs as a result of catabolism, acidosis, and reduced renal excretion, and if

---

CLINICAL MANIFESTATIONS

Anemia, pallor
Anorexia, vomiting, weight loss
Metabolic acidosis
Electrolyte imbalance
Renal osteodystrophy, rickets, myopathy
Dry, scaly, itchy skin, poor hair texture
Fluid imbalance, usually overload, edema
Headache, confusion, poor concentration

Fatigue
Growth retardation
Delayed sexual development
Gross/fine motor delay
Secondary hyperparathyroidism
Peripheral neuropathy
Congestive heart failure
Pericarditis

untreated, may be fatal, causing lethal ventricular fibrillation and cardiac standstill (Lancaster, 1991). Hypokalemia, although less common, can result from potassium-wasting diuretic therapy or dietary restriction in a child with polyuria or tubular disorders (Fine, 1990a).

The kidney's ability to conserve sodium and to concentrate urine decreases as renal failure progresses. Sodium and water retention, edema, hypertension, pericarditis, and pericardial effusion can occur secondary to impaired sodium excretion. Congenital renal abnormalities such as hypoplasia and dysplasia, however, can produce a "salt-wasting" state requiring sodium chloride supplementation (Rodriquez-Soriano et al, 1986). In children with salt-losing nephropathy, serum sodium levels may remain within normal limits because of volume contraction. Dietary sodium restrictions may lead to further deterioration in GFR as a result of decreased renal perfusion.

Metabolic Abnormalities

Decreased GFR and tubular defects result in retention of phosphate wastes and impaired vitamin D synthesis. Hyperphosphatemia causes calcium resorption from bone and increased stimulation by the parathyroid gland to secrete more parathormone (PTH) to enhance phosphate excretion. This circular mechanism ultimately results in secondary hyperparathyroidism. As more calcium is removed from bone, it is deposited in soft tissues, joints, and arteries, which causes (1) pain and decreased mobility, (2) dry, itchy, and scaly skin, (3) decreased vascular contractility, and (4) cardiac dysfunction. Disturbance in the calcium/phosphorus/bone metabolism relationship causes renal osteodystrophy, delayed bone growth, renal rickets and other bone deformity, hyperparathyroidism, and metastatic calcifications (Lancaster, 1991). Hypertriglyceridemia and hypercholesterolemia can occur as CRF worsens.

Decreased Hormone Secretion

Decreased erythropoietin production and a shorter life span of red blood cells result in anemia, manifesting as pallor, fatigue, dizziness, tachycardia, bruising, dyspnea on exertion or at rest, and exercise intolerance. Decreased renin secretion, coupled with sodium and fluid imbalance, may alter

blood pressure control. Hypertension is more common than hypotension in CRF.

Progression of Uremia

Initially, the child with CRF may have a loss of normal energy and increased fatigue on exertion. Such fatigue often develops gradually and goes unnoticed. The child may prefer sedentary activities rather than active play. Physical examination may reveal a slightly listless, pale child whose hemoglobin is low. Blood pressure may be high or normal. Secondary amenorrhea is common in adolescent girls. Urine output may decrease or remain normal in volume but with decreased solute clearance.

As renal failure worsens, manifestations become more pronounced. The child will become more fatigued, disinterested in play, with poor appetite, and less capable of accomplishing schoolwork as attention span diminishes and memory becomes erratic from toxin accumulation.

Uremic toxicity is characterized by anorexia, nausea, vomiting, malaise, somnolence, and headache (Papadopoulou, 1990). If untreated, the child's symptoms can progress to malnutrition and wasting, gastrointestinal bleeding, convulsions, and coma. Pericarditis, congestive heart failure, and arrhythmias may develop.

TREATMENT

Treatment goals include restoring and maintaining the child's health and developmental level of function to the highest degree possible. As psychosocial stressors and coping mechanisms affect physical health, the child and family should be included in planning care and treatment to elicit best compliance (Richie, Mapes, and Dailey, 1991). Treatment is based on the severity of clinical manifestations of CRF. Approaches include conservative management and, eventually, renal replacement therapy.

Conservative Management Therapy

Fluid, electrolyte, and blood pressure control. Early recognition and management of biochemical imbalances may prevent adverse consequences. Fluid overload and hypertension may be controlled by limiting total fluid intake to total output volume plus insensible losses, restricting salt intake, and us-

TREATMENT

Conservative management

Fluid, electrolyte, and blood pressure control
Anemia management
Hypertension control
Metabolic control and calcium homeostasis

Renal replacement therapy

Peritoneal dialysis
Hemodialysis
Transplantation

ing diuretic and antihypertensive medications. Loop diuretics help control the volume-dependent hypertension seen in CRF; angiotensin-converting enzyme inhibitors reduce glomerular capillary pressure which may slow the progression of CRF (Hockenberry, 1991). Although β-adrenergic blockers, α-adrenergic antagonists, peripheral vasodilators, calcium channel blockers, and ACE inhibitors are groups of drugs available for CRF-associated hypertension, some drugs are not acceptable for use in young children. Hypertension control must be managed primarily, or in consultation with, a pediatric nephrologist. Less common conditions are hypovolemia and hypotension, which may be seen in some salt-wasting disorders or overly aggressive fluid restriction (Fine, 1990a).

Hyperkalemia can be controlled through dietary restriction of high-potassium foods, use of bicarbonate for intracellular mobilization and acidosis prevention, and use of polystyrene sulfonate (Kayexalate) 1 Gm/Kg once or twice daily to remove potassium from the body (Fine, 1990a). Hypokalemia may occur less commonly with particular renal tubular disorders, prolonged vomiting, or overly aggressive hyperkalemia control. Potassium-restoring medications and dietary supplementation will correct the problem. Metabolic acidosis may be controlled by use of alkalinizing medications such as sodium bicarbonate, Bicitra, or Polycitra.

Anemia control. Anemia treatment is aimed at increasing red blood cell (RBC) production and decreasing RBC loss. Oral iron supplementation is prescribed if the serum ferritin is <20 ng/L or serum iron level is <50 G/dl (or both). Blood transfusions carry associated risks of iron overload, as defined by serum ferritin >300 ng/ml (Eschbach and Adamson, 1985), hepatitis-acquired immunodeficiency syndrome, and sensitization to histocompatibility antigens (Campos and Garin, 1992). If transfusions are required, filtered, washed, leukocyte-poor RBC mass, instead of whole blood, is usually preferred.

Until recently, children with ESRD required frequent to periodic blood transfusions to maintain acceptable hematocrit levels. Administration of synthetic human recombinant erythropoietin, epoetin alfa, produced by recombinant DNA technology, is now the gold standard for treatment of anemia associated with CRF. Multicenter studies report variations in frequency (1 to 3 times weekly) and dosage (50 to 150 U/Kg according to desired hematocrit) (Aufricht et al, 1993; Campos and Garin, 1992; Morris et al, 1993). The dose must be carefully titrated to prevent a rapid rise in hematocrit and possible hypertensive crisis (Morris et al, 1993). Rare seizures and iron/ferritin deficiency from increased erythropoiesis have also been reported (Kirlin, 1993). Oral iron may continue to be needed for optimal benefit. Reticulocyte count and RBC indices should be monitored. Common positive effects reported include an increase in sense of well-being, energy and endurance levels, exercise tolerance, and appetite, as well as improvement in concentration ability, school performance, and active play (Painter and Carlson, 1994). Significant improvement in cognitive function, IQ testing, and fewer symptoms of anxiety and depression were also reported (Corea, 1993; Schira, 1994). The present trend is toward earlier use of epoetin alfa in children with renal insufficiency before ESRD develops (Scharer et al, 1993).

Metabolic control and calcium homeostasis. Control of calcium and phosphate balance is necessary to prevent renal osteodystrophy and secondary hyperparathyroidism. Dietary phosphate restrictions are imposed, which significantly limit the child's dairy product intake. Medications include calcium-based phosphate binders to remove excess phosphate from the blood, calcium supplementation, vitamin D replacement therapy with calcitriol (Rocaltrol) or dihydrotachysterol (DHT) to allow better utilization of available calcium (Bruiner, 1994).

Renal Replacement Therapy

As GFR drops to 5% to 10% normal, conservative management is no longer adequate and treatment with either dialysis or transplantation is required (Ritz, 1991). As ESRD approaches, discussing the future and presenting options for dialysis and transplantation to the child (if of suitable age) and parents are important. Educating about the different modalities of therapy (hemodialysis, peritoneal dialysis, and transplant), touring the pediatric dialysis center, and networking child and parent with one or more well-adjusted families on dialysis or posttransplant are helpful ways to prepare children and families. Indications for timing of renal replacement therapy (RRT) are individualized, with consideration given to the following factors: (1) age of child, (2) GFR < 10% or creatinine clearance <10 ml/min/1.73 M^2, (3) primary renal disease and impact of comorbid conditions, (4) deviation from expected growth curve, (5) failure to thrive, (6) developmental delay, (7) inability to function at school, and (8) inadequate control of blood pressure, electrolyte, and metabolic parameters despite aggressive medical management (Fine, Salusky, and Ettenger, 1987). Absolute indicators include congestive heart failure, uncontrollable hypertension, pericarditis, uremic encephalopathy, and peripheral neuropathy (Fine, 1990a).

Peritoneal dialysis. Peritoneal dialysis (PD) incorporates the peritoneum as a filtering membrane to remove wastes and excess fluid from the vascular system. Silastic peritoneal catheters, curled or straight with one or two dacron cuffs, are surgically implanted in children (Prowant and Gallagher, 1991; Ash and Daugirdas, 1994). Through the catheter, a sterile solution of electrolytes and glucose is instilled into the peritoneal space. Waste particles are removed from the blood across the peritoneal membrane by diffusion, and excess water is removed with the ultrafiltration gradient by osmosis (Prowant and Gallagher, 1991).

Ideally, PD is performed at home. Continuous ambulatory peritoneal dialysis (CAPD) delivers 4 to 6 dialysate bag exchanges daily into the peritoneum, with dwell times of 3 to 4 hours during the day and a long dwell overnight. With CAPD, no machine is required, and the greatest freedom with dialysis is allowed. Taking time during the day to perform 4 to 6 exchanges, however, is time consuming and inconvenient at work and school.

Continuous cycling peritoneal dialysis (CCPD) utilizes a similar concept, but by using an automated cycler, all exchanges can be performed at night while the child and parents sleep, leaving the daytime with a long dwell and free of exchanges.

With both CAPD and CCPD, meticulous care is crucial to prevent contamination and infections at the catheter exit site and within the peritoneum. Peritonitis is the most common problem associated with PD, with a rate of one episode per 7.1 patient-months reported by a large multicenter study of 534 children on PD (Alexander et al, 1993). Most peritonitis is caused by gram positive organisms, usually *Staphylococcus epidermidis* or *Staphylococcus aureus*. Intraperitoneal antibiotics are instilled to treat the infection, which usually resolves without catheter replacement. Repeated peritonitis, however, will result in loss of membrane permeability by scarring, often requiring a change to hemodialysis. Other problems associated with PD include fluid overload or dehydration, membrane failure unrelated to infection, hernia development, bleeding or leaking, catheter exit site or tunnel infection, catheter obstruction by fibrin or omentum, and catheter perforation.

Peritoneal dialysis has several advantages over hemodialysis. It is a simple and safe procedure that can be carried out at home without the psychologic trauma associated with repeated fistula needle punctures. Near steady-state biochemical and fluid control is maintained, thereby avoiding the nausea, vomiting, and disequilibrium associated with hemodialysis. In addition, fewer restrictions are needed with regard to diet, fluid intake, or physical activity (Alexander, 1989). Perhaps the most attractive features of CAPD and CCPD are that they interfere less with normal daily activities and offer more control to child and family. A child on peritoneal dialysis can attend school every day with little or no interruption. Family vacations are easier to arrange. Home monitoring support services are important in promoting successful peritoneal dialysis at home (Berkoben and Schwab, 1995; Ponferrada et al, 1993).

Hemodialysis. Hemodialysis (HD) utilizes an artificial semipermeable membrane to allow filtration of wastes and excess fluid directly from the vascular system. Hemodialysis treatments are performed 3 to 4 times per week for 3 to 5 hours in a pediatric dialysis center.

Vascular access is the most difficult part of hemodialysis, and may be considered the "lifeline" of the child. An internal or external vascular access is necessary to deliver blood to the extracorporeal dialysis circuit for solute and fluid removal. (see Fig. 32-1.) Internal accesses include the arteriovenous (AV) fistula or synthetic graft, created surgically and, after a maturation time to develop, accessed through special fistula needle cannulation (Lumsden et al, 1994). External access devices include silastic shunts (rarely used today) and central venous catheters, temporary or permanent. A permanent type of catheter will be of soft, silastic tubing with a dacron cuff, tunneled under the skin, and will likely reside in the top of the right atrium of the heart. An internal fistula or graft is preferred for larger children ($>$12 to 15 Kg) because it affords greater freedom for the individual, with less risk of infection, but does require a maturation time and cannot be used immediately. (see Fig. 32-2.) Infants and small children have smaller blood vessels, limiting them to catheter access. The external catheter or shunt creates a higher risk for infection, sepsis, and clotting, and poses greater restrictions in physical activity of the individual (Berkoben and Schwab, 1995; Ruble, Long, and Connor, 1994; Hartigan, 1991).

For infants and small children, peritoneal dialysis is technically easier to perform than hemodialysis. In many cases, however, PD may be medically contraindicated. Even very small infants can be successfully hemodialyzed, using central venous, umbilical, or femoral catheters as access and special equipment and supplies adaptable to neonatal volume requirements (Knight et al, 1993). Infants and small children are hemodynamically more fragile and therefore respond more quickly to sodium and fluid depletion or excess associated with dialysis procedures. Careful and continuous monitoring is absolutely critical (Taylor, 1994a). Pediatric hemodialysis should be performed in a pediatric dialysis center by a multidisciplinary team of qualified pediatric nephrology personnel. Because of distance, adolescents may be dialyzed in adult centers, but risk the lack of comprehensive assessment and therapies provided by a pediatric center. In these cases, the pediatric primary care provider's role becomes more important in ensuring continuity of care for the child with ESRD. On an individual basis, very stable children might be considered for home hemodialysis with a dialysis nurse or very well-trained parents.

Hemodialysis offers advantages of more rapid correction of fluid, electrolyte, and metabolic abnormalities than does PD. Risks associated with hemodialysis include dialysis disequilibrium, hypotension, accidental blood loss from clotting or dialyzer membrane leak, air embolism, and pyrogenic or hemolytic reactions related to dialysate problems. Hemodialysis procedures can be threatening to both child and family; therefore, it is wise to take time to give basic explanations and elicit cooperation as much as possible (Frauman and Gilman, 1990; Neff, 1987).

Renal transplantation. Renal transplants are usually preferred for children with ESRD and, with careful planning, may be primary therapy bypassing the need for dialysis. Children may receive a kidney transplant from live-related or cadaveric donors, either of which are histocompatibly matched. Adult kidneys may be transplanted into small children using intraabdominal placement (Haggerty and Sigardson-Poor, 1990). Apart from surgical techniques, careful medical management is the key to maintaining a successful kidney transplant. See Chapter 28. With a successful renal transplant, children have a better chance at achieving desired growth and development, attending school regularly, and leading a more normal life.

RECENT AND ANTICIPATED ADVANCES IN DIAGNOSIS AND MANAGEMENT

Early detection of potential renal problems by the primary care provider and referral to pediatric nephrology can often prevent irreversible renal damage. Earlier and closer monitoring of vesicoureteral reflux, including periodic urine cultures, voiding cystourethrograms to monitor degree of

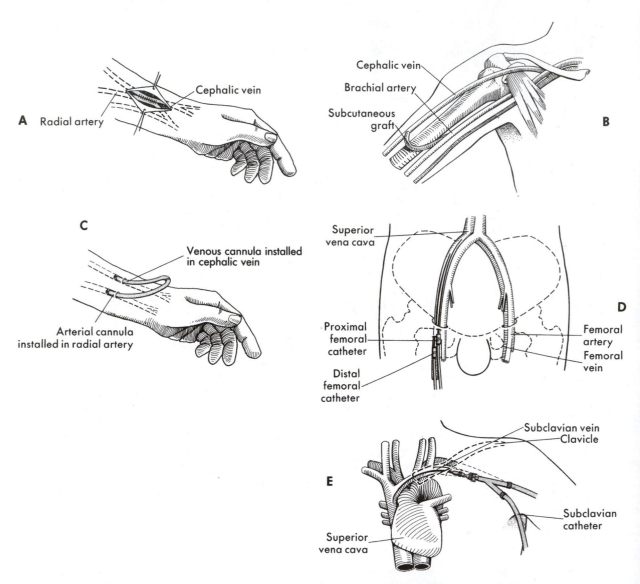

Fig. 32-1. Frequently used methods for gaining vascular access for hemodialysis include **A,** arteriovenous fistula, **B,** arteriovenous graft, **C,** external arteriovenous shunt, **D,** femoral vein catheterization, and **E,** subclavian vein catheterization. *(From Phipps WJ, Sands J, Lehman MK, and Cassmeyer VL: Medical-surgical nursing: concepts and clinical practice, ed 5, St Louis, 1995, Mosby.)*

reflux, and renal scans to detect scarring can prevent permanent damage. Antibiotic prophylaxis to prevent recurrent urinary tract infections, monitoring for improvement of reflux, and surgical ureteral reimplantation if indicated, may result in preventing renal deterioration and failure (Barakat, 1990). Corrective action based on prenatal sonography detection of posterior urethral valves, and in utero stenting to decrease fetal hydronephrosis may delay or prevent renal failure, frequently associated with

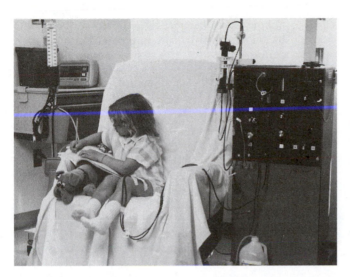

Fig. 32-2.   Child undergoing hemodialysis. *(From Whaley LF, Wong DL: Nursing care of infants and children,* ed 4, St Louis, 1991, Mosby.)*

posterior urethral valves (Bernhardt, 1993; Reinberg de Castano, and Gonzales, 1992)

The past decade has witnessed significant development of technical advances in the treatment of infants and children with chronic renal failure. More children are receiving therapy for ESRD, surviving longer, and living a higher quality of life. This longevity and improved quality can be credited to some of the following developments: use of epoetin alfa and growth hormone in children with CRF, with mode of administration broadened to include subcutaneous, intravenous, and intraperitoneal; greater adherence to kinetic modeling calculations and biochemical parameters, as well as subjective responses, for individual tailoring of dialysis adequacy and improved efficiency; early and aggressive correction of electrolyte and metabolic imbalances; and prevention of associated consequences of ESRD. Peritoneal dialysis innovations include various disconnect alterations by competitive suppliers and design of smaller suitcase-size portable PD cyclers which propose to decrease risk of infection, promote easier PD exchanges, and improve quality of life. Hemodialysis equipment is more technologically advanced with greater computerization capability.

Large multicenter studies of various aspects of pediatric nephrology care are providing more data for analysis of current treatment, problems, and recommendations (Alexander et al, 1993; Fine

et al, 1994). Increased use of computers for database management, calculations, and projected versus actual response to new therapies show potential in improving state of the art therapy assessment and planning by serving as on-line consultation and communication (Summar and Hakim, 1990).

ASSOCIATED PROBLEMS

Electrolyte Abnormalities

Electrolyte disturbances are probably the most common abnormalities found in renal failure. Hyperkalemia is a frequent problem in CRF management, even after dialysis initiation. Children with ESRD are frequently nonadherent to a low-potassium diet. Aggressive infant nutrition for improved developmental potential may provide higher dietary potassium than desired. Hyperkalemia should be avoided, if possible, through dietary restriction of foods high in potassium, providing additional dialysis time or treatments, and oral administration of sodium bicarbonate or Kayexalate (Fine, 1990a). Hypokalemia is less likely to be a problem in children with CRF; however, it can occur from use of potassium-wasting diuretics or excessive removal of potassium during either hemodialysis or peritoneal dialysis. Potassium supplementation through diet or medication may be needed. Overall, better electrolyte control can be established by CAPD or CCPD because of the

---

ASSOCIATED PROBLEMS

Electrolyte abnormalities
Anemia
Hypertension
Cardiovascular disorders
Neurologic problems
    Aluminum toxicity
    Uremic neuropathy
    Encephalopathy
Calcium/Phosphate disorders and renal
    osteodystrophy
Growth retardation
Intercurrent illness

---

continuous steady state of dialysis clearance, rather than the intermittent clearance of hemodialysis.

Anemia

The anemia of CRF (hematocrit <30) is generally normocytic, normochromic, with a low reticulocyte index. The primary cause of anemia in CRF is decreased red blood cell (RBC) production as a result of decreased production and release of erythropoietin (Josblena, 1990). Other contributing factors include shorter RBC life span because of uremic toxins, blood loss as a result of platelet adhesiveness in uremia, retention of uremic toxins and inhibitors, microcytic anemia caused by aluminum toxicity and folate deficiency (Korbet, 1989; Szromba, 1992), and blood loss associated with hemodialysis treatments and lab testing (Paganini, 1989). Infection, malnutrition, and nephrectomy may further aggravate the decreased erythropoietin production (Papadopoulou, 1990).

Epoetin alfa can be administered subcutaneously for children with CRF, intravenously after each hemodialysis treatment, and intraperitoneally with CAPD or CCPD. Problems associated with use of epoetin alfa include hypertension and occasional clotting of vascular access and dialyzer from increased RBC mass, rare seizures, and iron/ferritin deficiency from increased erythropoiesis (Kirlin, 1993). Management of side effects are problem-specific, including antihypertensive medications, increased heparinization to prevent clotting with careful monitoring of clotting times to prevent bleeding, and use of oral or intravenous iron supplementation to promote efficacy of epoetin alfa.

Hypertension

The medical management of hypertension associated with CRF depends on the underlying etiology if known, the degree of renal impairment, the relative contributions of extracellular fluid (ECF) volume overload, renin-angiotensin system, and the severity of the hypertension (Bazilinski and Dunea, 1994). Management of hypertension in children on dialysis includes dietary salt and fluid restriction, and dialytic ultrafiltration of excess extracellular fluid volume. Persistent or uncontrolled hypertension can accelerate the decline in renal function, in addition to risking the possibility of hypertensive encephalopathy, seizures, stroke, and death (Bazilinski and Dunea, 1994). Effective long-term control of hypertension is necessary to prevent cardiac complications common with dialysis and transplantation.

Cardiovascular Disorders

Abnormal cardiac function associated with CRF can be attributed to hypertension, anemia, and uremia. Congestive heart failure can occur as a result of fluid overload, severe hypertension, or uremic myocardiopathy (Fine, 1990a). The presence of anemia and arteriovenous shunting (vascular access) can increase the cardiac workload and contribute to congestive heart failure (Papadopoulou, 1990). Heart murmurs are common in children with CRF as a result of anemia, hypertension, and volume overload. Electrocardiographic abnormalities include left ventricular hypertrophy, elevated T waves, and widened QRS complexes (Morris et al, 1994).

Uremic pericarditis is a late manifestation of CRF, with such presenting signs and symptoms as fever, precordial pain, friction rub, sudden drop of hemoglobin level, cardiomegaly, cardiac arrhythmias, and cardiac failure (Papadopoulou, 1990).

Neurologic Disorders

Progressive encephalopathy, developmental delay, microcephaly, and EEG and CT scan abnormalities have been reported in 80% of children with CRF in infancy (Elzouki et al, 1994). Aluminum toxicity, hyperparathyroidism, undernutrition, and psychosocial problems may be contributing factors in the developmental delays. Fennell and associates (1990) found a deterioration in the verbal performance of children 6 to 11 years related to the length of time in renal failure, but it was not found in an older age group. Renal insufficiency may have deleterious effects on verbal development during this time of language skill acquisition.

Aluminum toxicity. A syndrome of progressive neurologic deterioration in children with CRF has been linked to aluminum toxicity (Coburn and Alfrey, 1995; Rotundo, Nevins, and Lipton, 1982; Salusky et al, 1991). It is indistinguishable from the dialysis dementia seen in adults and is characterized by speech disorders, seizures, and dementia. Aluminum toxicity can result in mental retardation or death. Use of calcium-based phosphate binders instead of aluminum-containing agents not only is safer but has been reported to be more effective as a phosphate-binding agent and will hopefully reduce the incidence of mental retardation and other neurologic dysfunction in the future (Salusky et al, 1991). Aluminum-based antacids as phosphate binders *are not* recommended for children under age 10 years (Salusky et al, 1991). Other agents implicated in possibly attributing to aluminum toxicity include total parenteral nutrition (TPN), repeated albumin use, and infant formulas (Salusky et al, 1990). Deferoxamine (Desferal) administration intravenously as a chelating agent is being used without adverse effects in infants and children whose aluminum levels are high despite use of calcium-based phosphate binders (Salusky, 1990).

Uremic neuropathy. Uremic neuropathy often affects the lower extremities and involves both motor and sensory function (Papadopoulou, 1990). Signs of neuropathy caused by uremia include muscle weakness; postural hypertension; loss of deep tendon reflexes (especially patellar and Achilles); "restless legs" syndrome, including peculiar creeping, crawling, prickly sensations, and pruritus; and loss in the sensation of pain, light touch, vibration, and pressure. Uremic neuropathy may be improved with more efficient or adequate dialysis.

Encephalopathy. Encephalopathy may be seen in advanced renal failure. Early symptoms include headache, fatigue, and listlessness. The child may have memory loss, decreased attention span, drowsiness, and impaired speech with further deterioration in renal function. Metabolic and biochemical abnormalities associated with CRF may be particularly detrimental to the still-developing central nervous system of the child (Uysal et al, 1990). Rapid reduction of urea from blood through highly efficient hemodialysis may cause cerebral edema. Symptoms are headache, disorientation, muscle cramps, nausea, and vomiting. If left untreated, seizures, coma, and death may occur (Leichter and Kher, 1992). With a high BUN, initial dialysis treatments should be gentle, slow, and not overly efficient for urea clearance.

Calcium/Phosphorus Disorders and Renal Osteodystrophy

Despite the encouraging outlook for children with ESRD brought about by improved dialysis techniques and control of anemia without blood transfusions, growth retardation and renal osteodystrophy remain significant problems (Chesney, 1992).

Loss of renal function has a profound effect on calcium and phosphorus homeostasis, and thus on bone integrity (Bruiner, 1994). Bones contain 99% of total body calcium. Dietary phosphorus restriction in renal children is difficult because it curtails intake of dairy products and meat. Phosphorus restriction and use of calcium-based phosphorus binders help to keep the serum concentration of phosphorus within the normal range to prevent renal osteodystrophy and secondary hyperparathyroidism (Bruiner, 1994).

Renal osteodystrophy is common, occurring in approximately 60% to 80% of children with uremia (Papadopoulou, 1990). This is a significant complication in growing children because of their open epiphyses and rapid bone mineralization and remodeling. The two most common types of bone disease are osteitis fibrosa and osteomalacia (Fine, 1990a). Osteitis fibrosa is secondary to hyperparathyroidism, hyperphosphatemia, and high serum alkaline phosphatase activity. Osteomalacia is caused by vitamin D deficiency, resulting from the kidney's inability to convert 25-hydroxyvitamin A to 1α, 25-dihydroxyvitamin D_3. Renal bone disease can also manifest as myopathy, which can be mistakenly interpreted as malaise (Papadopoulou, 1990).

These children will usually not complain of bone pain but often restrict their physical activity to protect a painful extremity. They may develop subtle gait abnormalities. Clinical manifestations of renal osteodystrophy include valgus deformities, fractures, rickets, myopathy, growth retardation, bone pain, and, in severe bone disease, epiphyseal slipping of the femoral head and metaphyseal fractures (Kher, 1992, Mehls and Ritz, 1989). Renal osteodystrophy may be improved by aggressive therapy with calcium and vitamin D therapy, and adequate metabolic control by diet, medication, and adequate dialysis (Fine and Tejani, 1992).

Growth Retardation

Growth retardation is a significant consequence of CRF and occasionally the symptom that leads to the diagnosis of renal disease (Fine et al, 1994). The majority of children with ESRD are >2 SDs below the mean height for age (Barratt et al, 1986; Stablein, 1992). Age of onset of CRF appears to be an important variable affecting growth. The lowest growth rates and greatest loss of growth potential are evident in infants whose CRF occurred at, or shortly after, birth (Rizzoni et al, 1986). Other factors associated with poor growth in CRF include protein and calorie malnutrition, anorexia, electrolyte imbalance, uremic toxicity, and renal osteodystrophy (Claris-Appiani et al, 1989; Fine et al, 1994). Dietary manipulations to avoid exacerbation of uremic symptoms such as protein restrictions, can further compromise growth (Fine et al, 1994). Data support that growth retardation continues to be an unresolved consequence of CRF despite optimal clinical management (Chan et al, 1994; Fine et al, 1994).

Researchers conducting a double-blind study of 125 children with chronic renal failure using recombinant growth hormone (rhGH) in two thirds of the children and a placebo in one third, concluded that growth rate and height were accelerated in the children with CRF receiving rhGH without significant side effects or decrease in creatinine clearance noted (Fine et al, 1994). Many studies concur that using recombinant human growth hormone has significant potential for improving the stature of children with CRF and growth retardation without advancing bone disease (Daughaday and Harvey, 1994; Fine et al, 1994; Koch et al, 1989; Scharer, 1990; Tonshoff et al, 1990; Van, 1991).

Intercurrent Illness

Development of intercurrent illnesses in children with CRF must be assessed thoroughly and managed appropriately to prevent further complications and promote optimal health. Infection is a frequent and common complication, especially infection of the vascular access and peritoneum (Lindholm and Bergstrom, 1989). Heart failure, pericarditis, pulmonary edema, and gastrointestinal disease may occur with uremia. Some common childhood viral diseases may be particularly hazardous to children on immunosuppressive therapy for conditions such as lupus and nephrotic syndrome, or to children having received a transplant (Cherry and Flegin, 1989).

PROGNOSIS

Infants and younger children are more likely to be on peritoneal dialysis (PD) than hemodialysis (HD). After 2 years of ESRD treatment, this trend reverses with 11% of children on PD and 19% on HD. Younger children are more likely to receive a transplant and to spend less time on dialysis than older children and adults. Of these children, 53% have a functioning transplant graft after 2 years of ESRD therapy (USRDS, 1994).

In the U.S., children with ESRD, 0 to 19 years, the 2-year overall survival rate in 1992 was 79.7%. Of the pediatric deaths reported in the 1994 USRDS report, nearly 7% of the deaths occurred within 2 years of ESRD onset. Not unexpectedly, the lowest 2-year survival is experienced in the 0 to 4 year age group. Survival of children with ESRD between the ages of 5 and 9 years is 93% at 2 years and 82% at 10 years. Survival of children between 10 and 14 years is 96% at 2 years and 78% at 10 years. According to USRDS data reported in 1994, overall death rates in children on all forms of renal replacement therapy were considerably lower than all adult age groups. Cardiac problems led the list in cause of death among children (17.5%), followed by sepsis (15.3%). The highest survival rates in children are reported in children with transplants with 97.7% for live-related and 94.6% for cadaver recipients (USRDS, 1994).

If transplant rejection occurs, children must return to either peritoneal dialysis or hemodialysis while waiting for another transplant. Unfortunately, many children develop reactive antibodies to a large potential donor pool. Consequently, the wait for a second or third transplant may be long.

Primary Care Management
HEALTH CARE MAINTENANCE

Growth and Development

Incorporation of development and behavioral assessments into primary health care evaluation can result in significant advances in early identification and intervention of developmental or behavioral problems (Finney and Weist, 1992). Children with renal disease may not have any clinical signs other than retarded growth. Many children exhibit growth retardation at the time of referral to the pediatric nephrologist. Despite advances in dialytic therapy for children with ESRD, inadequate growth is still a problem. Poor growth in children undergoing dialysis has been related to poor appetite (characteristic of CRF) resulting in inadequate caloric intake, poor vitamin D uptake from the gastrointestinal tract, metabolic acidosis, and malaise. The effect of epoetin alfa on appetite stimulation and energy level has resulted in weight gain and more energy but without significant increases in height velocity (Fine, 1990b). With aggressive nutritional supplementation, infants have achieved better but still suboptimal growth (Abitbol et al, 1990).

Accurate growth measurements should be taken at the initial visit and at least every 3 to 6 months thereafter, and plotted on National Center for Health Statistics growth charts. The weight/height index provides a measure of muscle and adipose tissue relative to height. A low weight/height index may be an indication of malnutrition. Caution should be paid to true values that may be obscured by an increase in ECF volume. Skinfold thickness at the biceps and subscapular sites should be obtained at least every 6 months and with any major change in the mode of treatment (Barratt and Chantler, 1987; Papadopoulou, 1990). It should also be noted that the child's height may be altered because of renal osteodystrophy and the development of rickets.

Neurologic status should be carefully ascertained. Head circumference should be obtained on all children less than 3 years of age and must be accurately recorded at 3- to 6-month intervals.

The significance of increasing head circumference as a measure of continued brain growth cannot be overstressed in children under 3 years. Developmental assessment should be done with the onset of CRF and repeated at 2- to 9-months intervals, depending on the child's age and disease severity. The Denver Developmental Screening Test II can be used as a screening tool, but the infant with CRF should be referred to a developmental pediatrician or child psychologist for thorough evaluation. The impact of the disease process on the child's psychologic status, school attendance, intellectual performance, and social development should be assessed every 6 to 9 months. Pubertal staging using the Tanner Scale (Tanner, 1962) should be determined every 6 to 12 months for the school-aged child until adult staging is reached.

Diet

Protein restriction may delay progression of CRF (Locatelli et al, 1991; Raymond et al, 1990). Although protein restriction is a common practice with adults with CRF, it is not acceptable in children. In addition to growth and developmental delay in children, poor nutrition is associated with increased morbidity and mortality (Moore, 1991). Nutritional problems are manifest long before ESRD is reached and continue after initiation of renal replacement therapy. Children on peritoneal dialysis experience a feeling of fullness soon after eating small amounts because of abdominal distention from the volume of peritoneal fluid, which may be more apparent with CAPD and daytime dwells. In addition, obligatory protein losses occur through the peritoneum, as the pore size is easily permeable to albumin transfer (Blake, 1994; Moore, 1991).

Parents of infants and small children soon become frustrated over the unsuccessful efforts to get children to eat the recommended calories and protein. Children with renal failure are often poor feeders, which increases stress in the family. Supplemental tube feedings by orogastric, nasogastric, or gastrostomy tube/button may be instituted early in renal insufficiency as an important and useful therapy to ensure better nutritional intake with less stress to the family (Balfe et al, 1990; Brewer, 1990; O'Regan and Cearel, 1990). Nonpalatable additives of MCT oil and polycose can be easily instilled by tube along with medications as needed to supplement the child's oral feedings. The formula calculation for supplemental feedings should be frequently reevaluated and adjusted for growth and changes in renal function and treatment (Cunningham, 1990). The current recommendation is to aggressively treat infants with caloric and protein intake above the RDA to help improve physical and cognitive growth. The primary care provider should obtain the dietary management plan from the nephrology team to reinforce family education.

Safety

Although children with CRF should be encouraged in the pursuit of normal childhood activities, some considerations and limitations must be kept in mind. Delay in cognitive and gross motor development may result in the child being academically and physically slower than classmates, as well as being smaller in size. Attempting to keep up with larger and faster children in active play may result in injury to the child with CRF. The child with CRF may become the brunt of jokes and unkind comments. In response to the challenge, the child may attempt to perform activities which he or she is not capable, possibly incurring injury in the process.

Some children require special occupational and physical therapy programs to enhance physical ability and improve skills and stamina. Bike helmets and knee guards may help prevent easy bruising. Children should be encouraged to wear a Medic-Alert bracelet or necklace to alert other health care providers of the CRF status, medication needs, and other possible complications.

Children on immunosuppressive therapy are more at risk for infections—bacterial and viral—and heal more slowly. Those with indwelling central venous catheters should not be allowed to swim, to prevent serious infection developing through the catheter. Children with a hemodialysis internal vascular access (AV fistula or graft) must be cautioned against wearing restrictive clothing or accessories that can lead to venostasis and clotting, engaging in activities that may cause bleeding soon after dialysis while they are still heparinized, and disallowing blood pressure measurement or venipuncture in the affected arm. Swimming with PD catheters is controversial, and may require special procedures for catheter/exit site care.

Renal osteodystrophy may predispose children to fractures or cause bone pain on exertion. Physical activity, however, should be encouraged to promote physical and mental health. Group aerobic exercise programs, camping, group games at picnics, and other outings are excellent ways to promote controlled exercise, encourage independence, and help raise self-esteem.

Health care workers should follow universal precautions according to CDC guidelines when handling blood and body fluids of children on dialysis, even though the status of hepatitis and HIV positivity is usually known on children with ESRD.

Immunizations

Routine immunizations should be given to children with CRF except for a few specific disease conditions and therapies. Immunosuppressive therapy, used in treating some renal conditions, including glomerulonephritis, nephrotic syndrome, and lupus nephritis, is generally an indication for withholding live virus immunizations (Committee on Infectious Diseases, 1994; Weiss, 1988). Immunizations should be withheld until the child is in remission and off immunosuppressive therapy for 6 months; exceptions are determined by weighing risks/ benefits on an individual basis for children who are steroid resistant or have frequent relapses. Inactivated polio vaccine (IPV) is preferred for children who are immunosuppressed (Committee on Infectious Diseases, 1994). Unfortunately, no killed measles vaccine presently exists, and the MMR is not for individuals who are immunosuppressed. Disease specific immunoglobulin may be given after known exposure. As with other live virus vaccines, Varivax is not recommended in individuals who are immunosuppressed (Center for Disease Control, 1994). Children with CRF or immunosuppressive therapy should continue to receive VZIG upon exposure because widespread immunity in the general public will not be realized for several years.

Pneumococcal and influenza vaccines are recommended for children with CRF and active nephrotic syndrome because of the children's increased susceptibility to infections (Committee on Infectious Diseases, 1994; Travis, Brouhard, and Kalia, 1984).

Even though epoetin alfa use has decreased the need for blood transfusions in children with ESRD, hepatitis B is still a risk. Hepatitis surface antigen and antibody status should be ascertained before starting dialysis (Shusterman and Singer, 1987). If a child is hepatitis A or B antigen negative, the hepatitis vaccine series should be started as soon as possible to complete the series before transplant. Because these children's antibody response to the hepatitis B vaccine may be diminished with CRF, they may require repeated doses until seroconversion is achieved (Committee on Infectious Diseases, 1994; Drachman et al, 1987). Serum antibody concentrations should be measured every 6 months because protection from the vaccine may be less complete, which may also be true for response to other immunizations such as the HIB vaccine (Fivush et al, 1993).

Screening

Vision. In addition to routine vision screening, a yearly eye examination by a pediatric ophthalmologist is recommended. Eyes should be examined for scleral calcification caused by hypercalcemia or uncontrolled hyperphosphatemia. The fundus should be examined for arterial narrowing, hemorrhages, exudates, and papilledema secondary to hypertension. Cataract assessment should be included for any child having been treated with steroid therapy.

Hearing. Children with CRF should be referred to an audiologist for annual assessment. High-frequency sensorineural deafness is characteristic of Alport's syndrome (Barratt and Chantler, 1987). Hearing loss can also result from use of ototoxic drugs such as furosemide and gentamicin.

Dental. Routine dental care at 6-month intervals is recommended for children with CRF. Dental procedures may cause breaks in the skin and mucous membrane with bleeding, and release of microorganisms into the blood stream, causing infective endocarditis or colonization of the vascular access (Durack and Phil, 1995). The pediatric nephrologist should be consulted before dental procedures on children who are immunosuppressed or on those with a vascular access. The American Heart Association's standard prophylaxis protocol for dental, oral, and upper respiratory tract procedures now advises amoxicillin using the schedule outlined in Table 32-2.

Children with congenital renal disease will frequently have enamel defects. Poor nutritional intake may lead to poor mineralization of teeth. In an effort to improve nutrition, the small child with CRF may be allowed to use a bottle for a longer time, resulting in deformities of the primary teeth. Use of oral iron for anemia may cause staining of teeth; liquid preparations should be placed in the mouth past the teeth.

Drug-induced gingival hyperplasia may occur in children with CRF receiving drugs such as phenytoin (Dilantin) for seizures, calcium channel blockers such as nifedipine (Procardia) or verapamil (Calan) for hypertension, and cyclosporine (Sandimmune) for immunosuppression used in transplant, lupus, and nephrotic syndrome treatment. Prevention may be helped by good dental and oral hygiene with mechanical stimulation by daily brushing and flossing, gingival massage, plaque

Table 32-2.   AMERICAN HEART ASSOCIATION STANDARD PROPHYLAXIS PROTOCOL

Child's weight	Amoxicillin initial dose: 1 hr before procedure	Amoxicillin follow-up dose: 6 hr after initial dose
<15 Kg	750 mg	375 mg (one half initial dose)
15-30 Kg	1500 mg	750 mg (one half initial dose)
>30 Kg	3000 mg—full adult dose	1500 mg (one half initial dose)
	OR calculate at 50 mg/Kg	one half initial dose

For amoxicillin-penicillin allergies, erythromycin or clindamycin may be used (Adapted from: Committee on Infectious Diseases, 1994).

control, and use of folate rinses. Gingivectomy treatment by surgical excision or laser may be needed periodically (Rossman, Ingles, and Brown, 1994).

Blood pressure. Blood pressure measurements should be taken at each primary care visit, and at periodic intervals, depending on the clinical condition. Many children with CRF develop some degree of hypertension during the course of their illness, with about 79% requiring antihypertensive therapy (Scharer and Ulmer, 1987). Use of epoetin alfa, resulting in increased RBC mass, may contribute to high blood pressure. Because some antihypertensive medications are less suitable for children and interact adversely with other CRF medications or further impair renal function, initiation and follow-up of antihypertensive therapy should be done in consultation with the pediatric nephrologist.

The "white coat phenomenon" (of blood pressure being higher in clinics) is eliminated by use of automated monitoring devices (Khoury et al, 1992). Small, computerized, automated blood pressure monitors are available to be worn 24 to 48 hours. They can give better insight to the true overall blood pressure at daily rest and activity and facilitate more ideal medical management (American College of Physicians, 1993).

Hematocrit. Routine screening may be deferred if a recent complete (CBC) blood count is included with the other renal function tests. Anemia is a chronic problem and is usually followed by the nephrology team.

Urinalysis. Routine screening is not necessary because of the frequent urine analysis done by the renal team. Some children with CRF have little to no urine output; therefore, urinalysis is not indicated.

Tuberculosis. Yearly screening is recommended by PPD testing.

Condition-specific screening

BLOOD WORK. The nephrology team will regularly monitor the CBC, serum ferritin, iron, transferrin, folate, and reticulocyte count to assess anemia management. Serum electrolytes, urea nitrogen (BUN), creatinine, calcium, phosphorus, alkaline phosphatase, protein, albumin, cholesterol, and liver function tests help monitor renal function and treatment efficacy. Metabolic acidosis must be identified and treated promptly to prevent bone demineralization and growth retardation. Parathy-

roid hormone levels (PTH) should be monitored every 3 to 6 months and correlated with radiologic findings for prevention/management of renal osteodystrophy. Fasting blood levels are best for monitoring cholesterol and triglycerides, but this is difficult in the small child or infant. Viral titers for VZV, CMV, HSV, EBV, hepatitis profile (HAV, HCV, HBV, antibody to HBV), rubella, rubeola, and HIV should be monitored initially as a baseline, before transplant, and then periodically, as determined by the pediatric nephrologist.

CARDIAC SCREENING. A chest radiograph and baseline electrocardiogram and echocardiogram should be performed initially and every 6 to 12 months to assess the cardiovascular status of children with CRF.

RADIOLOGIC SCREENING. Radiologic bone studies can show evidence of secondary hyperparathyroidism, rickets or osteomalacia, osteosclerosis, and delayed bone age as distinct patterns in children with renal osteodystrophy (Kher, 1992). Examination of hands and knees should be obtained initially and at 6-month intervals to assess for evidence, improvement, or worsening of renal osteodystrophy, and to compare bone age with chronologic age to determine growth potential. Bone density studies and bone biopsy are less commonly used methods to assess bone mineralization in children.

COMMON ILLNESS MANAGEMENT

Differential Diagnosis

Infections. Because of a compromised immune system, children with CRF may be at greater risk for routine infections which may linger or result in secondary complications. The pediatric primary care provider should manage routine pediatric problems and evaluate for influenza, urinary tract or gastrointestinal infections, and fever. The primary care provider should consult the pediatric nephrologist regarding the child's hydration status and residual renal function, as well as antibiotic selection and dose related to the child's renal disease and residual function. Temporary alterations in the child's dialysis program may be needed during periods of illness.

If other common benign causes of fever have been ruled out, fever related to a dialysis access infection or peritonitis should be managed directly by the pediatric nephrologist.

Gastrointestinal symptoms. Nausea and vomiting are common symptoms in childhood. Worsening renal function must be ruled out in children with mild renal failure, especially in the absence of associated fever.

Headaches and facial palsy. Uncontrolled hypertension should be ruled out in children with CRF complaining of frequent headaches or facial palsy.

Drug Interactions

The most important factors to consider in pharmacokinetics is the extent to which the drug is excreted by the kidney, the degree of renal impairment, and drug interactions with various other medications needed in the ESRD treatment regimen.

Drug dose regimens are altered with GFRs less than 30 to 40 ml/min (Trompeter, 1987). The initial loading dose of drugs excreted by the kidneys, however, is the same as it is for children without renal failure. Maintenance doses must be adjusted by either lengthening the interval between doses or by reducing individual doses. Cardiac glycosides or aminoglycoside antibiotics are examples of drugs that are almost entirely dependent on renal excretion for elimination, thus requiring dosage adjustment even in mild renal failure. CRF may predispose to bleeding and easy bruising, therefore, acet-aminophen is preferred over aspirin for pain and fever control.

Antibiotics that are excreted by both renal and hepatic metabolism may require no dose adjustment until renal function is severely decreased. Anticonvulsants may require dosage adjustments. The child with anemia and CRF receiving a calcium-based phosphate binder (not aluminum), given with food or within 30 minutes after eating, should wait 1 hour before taking oral iron as the two medications are antagonistic to each other, compromising the desired effect. All pediatric medication calculations should be based on weight rather than age of the child with CRF. Medications that are removed by dialysis (vitamins, some antihypertensive medications, and antibiotics) should generally be given after dialysis. The pediatric nephrologist should be consulted for appropriate medication selection and dosage adjustment.

DEVELOPMENTAL ISSUES

Sleep Patterns

Infants and young children, even those using CAPD or CCPD, should be encouraged to assume a normal sleeping pattern at night. Most children are able to sleep undisturbed using nocturnal CCPD treatment. An increased need for sleep and lethargy or depression may be indications of worsening renal failure and should be reported to the nephrology team.

Toileting

Children with CRF may be oliguric, anuric, or have normal urine output, as determined largely by the etiology of the renal disorder. Some congenital abnormalities require bladder augmentation or creation of a type of urinary diversion with an appliance worn over the stoma. Families and children need instruction in care of the stoma (Garvin, 1994).

Even after corrective urologic surgery, some children may be unable to achieve urinary continence. Often toilet training for urinary continence is deferred until after transplant if the capability for urinary continence is present. Proper wiping in females is an important focus of teaching to prevent urinary tract infections. Bowel training should be initiated when the toddler is developmentally ready.

Discipline

Parental anxiety, guilt, and despondency over their child's chronic condition may lead to ambivalent feelings toward child rearing or the treatment program, resulting in child behavior problems or nonadherence with the treatment regimen (Grupe et al, 1986). Parents need honest answers to their questions about their child. They need encouragement and support in setting and holding limits and behavioral expectations for their child. Frequently, children with CRF may not be well disciplined because they are "sick" and therefore allowed to get by with behaviors not tolerated in siblings. Parental overprotection of the child with CRF may further reinforce lack of discipline.

Children on hemodialysis can have difficulty accepting the painful procedure of venipuncture required for each treatment. For pain associated with procedures, management techniques such as play therapy, guided imagery, hypnosis, and progressive muscle relaxation can be taught to the child and his or her parents. Topical anesthetics such as EMLA cream used 1 hour before fistula cannulation to lessen the pain is a common practice in many pediatric dialysis centers. The child should be encouraged to participate in his or her care, through performance of achievable tasks and decision making. Cooperation can be gained by allowing even a 3-year-old to help select the venipuncture site, remove the tourniquet, rotate the blood tubes, and help place the tape. Singing and other diversions also elicit cooperation. Many children on hemodialysis self-cannulate their needles or set up their own dialysis machines for treatment. They can become competitive with one another in the dialysis center with independent tasks and self-control. Children on CCPD or CAPD can learn to do their own exchanges and exit site care. Children may be taught to self-administer subcutaneously their own epoetin alfa or growth hormone (Salmon and Broyan, 1991).

Child Care

Children with CRF are not restricted from day care. Children receiving corticosteroid therapy are more susceptible to infections and heal more slowly from infection or injury (Cherry and Geigin, 1989). Home care or small group child care will decrease the risk of infection. When child care is used, the caregiver must be taught about the child's dietary restriction, medications, and any special treatment regimen. Very specific instructions should be given in writing, with a phone contact if there are questions. Children on CAPD and their parents are encouraged by the nephrology team to arrange the dialysis schedule around the child care hours whenever possible. If the child has a vascular or peritoneal dialysis access, those entrusted as caregivers must be given instructions regarding potential emergencies and action to be taken.

Schooling

Every effort must be made to encourage the school-aged child to attend school full time. The CAPD exchanges should be scheduled around school activities with least interference whenever possible, or CCPD might be preferable for the school-aged child. Changes in schedules to accommodate after-school activities can be discussed with the pediatric nephrology team. Pediatric hemodialysis centers

should include a school teacher, provided by the district school board, or tutor to assist children with missed schoolwork. A dual school-home bound educational program may be established with both teachers communicating for continuity of the child's learning. Teachers need to know the child's strengths, weaknesses, abilities, and limitations in the classroom as well as in physical education, on the playground, and to and from school. Children with renal disease may need a note to be allowed extra bathroom trips because of a small bladder capacity or infection, or to drink more or less fluids, or to receive assistance with ureterostomy or central venous catheter care. The pediatric nephrology team may need to provide educational materials on specific CRF management and in-service presentations to school personnel regarding a particular child's physical or emotional needs.

Poor school performance must be evaluated for contributing factors and an IEP developed to support the child's learning needs. Cognitive deficits have been correlated with more advanced CRF and with congenital etiologies.

Adolescence can be a time of turbulence associated with transition, maturational crises, and adjustment (Wong, 1995). Table 32-3 highlights some of the differences, problems, and interventions related to cognitive, physical, and psychosocial development in adolescents with ESRD.

Sexuality

Delayed sexual development is common among children with CRF as a result of insufficient production of gonadal steroids and elevated gonadotropin levels (Fine, 1990b). More than half of female adolescents with ESRD have delayed development of secondary sex characteristics and menarche. There are large individual variations in the time course of menstrual bleeding and the occurrence of amenorrhea and irregular bleeding among adolescent females with CRF (Scharer et al, 1990). Although menstrual abnormalities (amenorrhea, oligomenorrhea, and menorrhagia) and infertility have been described, successful pregnancies in women who were on dialysis have been reported (Scharer et al, 1990). Adolescent males with ESRD may show delayed development of genitalia or pubic hair. Testicular size may also be reduced. These adolescents need to be counseled about birth control, sexually transmitted diseases, and acquired immune deficiency syndrome, as do their healthy counterparts.

The primary care provider must explore with the adolescent issues related to delayed development, such as poor body image because of short stature, surgical scars from dialysis accesses, peritoneal catheters, malformed extremities caused by large vascular fistulas, and delayed pubertal development.

Transition into Adulthood

Children with chronic renal failure will become adults with chronic renal failure. Independence and career development are difficult to attain unless a successful renal transplant has occurred. The individual with short stature, from years of poor nutrition, may require assistive devices to drive an automobile. Hypertension, diabetes, and impaired vision may result in other long-term health problems. These individuals will need to be encouraged not to smoke, to eat a healthy diet, and to avoid alcohol and drug abuse.

SPECIAL FAMILY CONCERNS AND RESOURCES

The impact of CRF in a child is felt by the child's entire family. Parents must deal with (1) feelings of shock and disbelief, (2) anger, (3) loss, (4) possible guilt at causing renal failure, (5) depression, (6) fatigue and burnout associated with constant care and appointments, (7) inadequacy at not being able to heal or fix the problem, (8) frustration with medical establishment for no cure, (9) overprotection versus being too lenient, (10) marital stress, and (11) financial worries. Siblings also feel the impact of the child's CRF, feeling overprotective or resentful, angry, and responsible for the ill child. Frequent trips to the dialysis center or clinic, daily or nightly PD treatments, and additional physical care that is needed tend to interfere with family schedules, siblings' school and extracurricular activities, and family outings.

Family coping and adaptation is improved through maintaining open communication, actively participating in care planning and decision making, and by the presence of supportive extended family, friends, church members, or renal-focused support or advocacy groups (Travis, 1976). Providing networking sessions is often helpful, grouping new

children and families with a client who has adjusted well to the dialysis or transplant routine and is willing to share information (Frauman and Gilman, 1990). Families should be encouraged to continue normal activities such as family outings, camps for children, and vacations with priorly arranged transient dialysis scheduling at a pediatric dialysis center if necessary.

The family's belief system must be taken into account. Religious practices may prohibit use of blood transfusions, even in life-threatening situations, or challenge that faith healing alone is all that is needed. With children of the Jehovah Witness faith, it may be advisable to start early use of epoetin alfa administration before renal failure reaches end stage, to use microtainers for lab tests whenever possible, and to advise use of cell-saver reinfusion during surgery.

Some renal diseases are linked to race and ethnicity. Overall statistics show increased morbidity and mortality in African Americans with ESRD and transplants, especially in the early posttransplant period (Lopes et al, 1993; Ojo et al, 1994). Some children who are African American or Hispanic wait longer on dialysis for an acceptable transplant match, firstly, because of ABO compatibility and major histocompatibility complex matching difficulties. The possibility of a better match is secured with a member of the same race, for both live-related and cadaveric transplantation. Secondly, there are fewer African-American and Hispanic donor organs available (Kasiske et al, 1991).

An understanding of the family's background, religious and cultural beliefs and practices, dietary beliefs associated with health care, and identification of the primary leader of the family (e.g., a great-grandmother) is valuable to the primary care provider when effective interventions require altering the individual's or family's health care practices (Richie, Mapes, and Dailey, 1991).

Families will need support as they make decisions about their child's care that will have long-range implications. Even the smallest, very ill infant can now be treated with life-sustaining dialysis, but at a high cost. Extracorporeal membrane oxygenation (ECMO) with integrated hemofiltration is more widely performed today with positive results. Equipment, supplies, and professional

Table 32-3.   COGNITIVE, PHYSICAL AND PSYCHOSOCIAL DEVELOPMENT OF ADOLESCENTS WITH ESRD

Expected difference from normal development	Manifestations or potential problems	Prevention and interventions
COGNITIVE ASPECTS: Should move from concrete to abstract thinking at 12 to 15 years of age. May have excessive school absences for medical reasons, slower or accelerated learning, which must be individualized Academic achievement less affected with later CRF onset. RF affects new skills acquisition and attention and speed of processing data.	Advanced education requires greater ability to abstract, reflected in competency or scholastic testing and academic scores. Concrete thinkers lack ability to apply general principles from one event to another. Academic delay may result in school disinterest anddropout. Hearing/vision problemsmay be CRF related. More difficultyin learning new skills. Attention and responses aided by good biochemistry, control, worsened by nonadherence.	Concrete thinkers need care plans that realize immediate goals; abstract thinkers can work with long-range goals. Incorporate results from academic/neuropsychomotor skills testing to guide improvement. Encourage school attendance and participation in extracurricular activities Encourage adherence to care plan Encourage opportunities for responsible decision making, problem solving, and development of own beliefs and values Prepare for transition into adulthood
PHYSICAL ASPECTS: Linear growth retardation is affected by treatment modality and steroids. Decreased effect/production of growth and sex hormones. Delayed puberty onset (refer to Tanner staging, 1962).	Short stature—1 to 3 SDs below norm. Does not follow HT/WT curve pattern of puberty. Compares size to peers. Girls: delay in breast enlargement, pubic hair, menarche onset (hallmark of womanhood)	Early diagnosis and RRT. Adolescent/family education about normal growth/development and expected alterations. Encourage diet and medications, adherence, physical activities and exercise, and physical independence.

Girls—10.5 to 14 years, with menarche onset about 13 years. Boys—12 to 16.5 years. Delay in development of secondary sexual characteristics and sexually active behavior.

Nutritional needs vary with sex/age: protein—0.8 to 1.0 gm/Kg gm needed; calories—38 to 60cal/Kg needed; Phosphates restricted

Anemia present

Boys: delay in testes/scrotal growth, pubic hair, penile size and ability to erect and ejaculate, muscle mass increase, voice change to deeper pitch

May be under/overweight. May rebel at ESRD treatment regimen through dietary indiscretions, especially in peer groups.

May be nonadherent with medications, especially those causing visible side effects

May develop renal osteodystrophy with rickets or fractures; hypocalcification by bone x-rays. Fatigue or SOB from anemia.

Consider use of growth hormone; teach self-administration. Encourage self-participation in care plan. Provide sexuality education at individual level of understanding.

Encourage optimal nutrition to promote best growth potential. Encourage dietary adherence, work with dietitian to include as many favorite foods as possible. Consider meal pattern of school lunches, fast food stops with peers. Focus on positive, not negative nutrition. Encourage taking phosphate binders. Consider early use (preRRT) of epoetin alfa; teach self-administration; monitor.

PSYCHOSOCIAL ASPECTS:

Interruption or inability in mastery of adolescent developmental tasks; dependency vs. independency conflict; identity quest; body image dissatisfaction; peer group identity desired; future planning.

Self-esteem influenced by actual and perceived image and peer response. Risk of lower self-esteem greater with negative body image, poor peer and family relationships, strong family dependence.

Delayed psychosexual development

Coping behaviors used: denial, regression, projection, displacement, anger, acting out, increased risk taking, disruptive, resentment, argumentative, challenging authority Vacillates between child-compliant and rebel-noncompliant. May sublimate poor academic performance with physical prowess. Fears peer rejection, loneliness, depression, withdrawal; despite strong need for friends and social support.

May avoid sexual relationships and activity, or experiment to prove sexual worth

Promote achievement of developmental tasks, foster independence and autonomy. Allow controlled choices. Encourage activities that enhance positive self-esteem and self-worth.

Encourage healthy group activities in community, school, church, camps, support groups. Evaluate self-concept through assessment tools (Piers-Harris, Vineland, State-Trait Anxiety instruments).

Encourage ventilation of feelings of sexuality, and provide education for understanding

Assist in preparation for transition into adulthood

Characteristics of ESRD Adolescent Development by Domain, Adapted from Taylor, 1994b.

expertise are more costly for the infant with ESRD. Many of these infants have other congenital anomalies; morbidity and mortality are high in this early period. Children with mental retardation are being dialyzed and transplanted. Quality of life issues, rights of parents versus rights of minor children are being discussed with no black-and-white answers (Currier, 1994). Some infants will not become productive members of society; others have demonstrated adequate growth and development with early and aggressive renal replacement therapy and are attending regular school full time and living fairly normal lives. Children with severe developmental or mental delays require considerable comprehensive and long-term care. Repeated noncompliance to prescribed therapy with some adolescents may result in loss of the transplanted kidney. All of these issues will have a significant impact on the family.

In addition, families must deal with members of medical and legislative committees who argue that many children should not receive all ESRD services because of cost containment. Reduction in services through capitation of financial resources may decidedly affect children with ESRD, a special population of ESRD consumers.

Resources

The cost of ESRD treatment is very expensive, ranging from $20,000 to $35,000 per year. On July 1, 1973, the Social Security Act was amended to provide Medicare benefits for persons <65 years of age who were certified to have chronic kidney failure and require dialysis or transplantation (HR-1, Public Law 92-603, Section 2001). The family should be referred to the nephrology social worker for assistance in accessing available services.

Individual states may have a specialized medical care and rehabilitation program (such as Children's Medical Services or crippled children's programs provided by Title V SSA state funding) for children <21 years of age diagnosed as having a severe, chronic, or disabling disorder.

Additional financial assistance information is available through the National Kidney Foundation affiliates, the American Kidney Fund, and the American Association of Kidney Patients.

Summer camp programs, such as the Moncrief Mountain Ranch Camp in Colorado, provide fun activities for children undergoing dialysis or who have been transplanted and respite for families. Pediatric nephrology centers will also have information on local camps, other recreational programs, and patient/family support groups.

American Association of Kidney Patients (AAKP)
100 S Ashley Dr, Suite 250
Tampa, FL 33602
813/223-7099
Newsletter and quarterly journal, *Renalife*. Contact local chapter for educational assistance, summer camps, support groups, and financial information.

National Kidney Foundation (NKF)
30 E 33rd St
11th Floor
New York, NY 10016
1-800-622-9010
Contact local chapter for educational assistance, summer camps, support groups, and financial information.

American Kidney Fund (AKF)
6110 Executive Blvd, Suite 1010
Rockville, MD 20852
1-800-638-8299
Free educational materials are available.

HCFA ESRD Networks
Divided into geographic regions, Networks are assigned to coordinate and review dialysis and transplant facilities to ensure the best possible care. Call AAKP or NKF for location in your state.

Renal Physicians' Association (RPA)
2011 Pennsylvania Ave
Suite 800 NW
Washington, DC 20006
202/835-2746

American Nephrology Nurses Association (ANNA)
National Office
East Holly Ave, Box 56
Pitman, NJ 08071-0056
609/256-2320

SUMMARY OF PRIMARY CARE NEEDS FOR THE CHILD WITH CHRONIC RENAL FAILURE

Health care maintenance

Growth and development

Despite advances in medical management, dialysis and transplant, growth retardation is a major problem in children with CRF (majority >2 SDs below mean height for age).

Achievement of developmental milestones (all ages) is delayed; sexual maturation is delayed.

Monitor anthropometric measurements, developmental assessment, and Tanner staging.

Aggressive nutrition, adequate dialysis efficiency, and growth hormone injections may improve growth.

Diet

Protein and caloric requirements in children with CRF are greater than the normal RDA to enhance growth and development and offset losses (protein in PD).

Consider supplemental oral, NG, or G-tube feedings to improve nutrition.

Safety

Children with CRF should be encouraged to live as normal and as active lives as possible, incorporating modification and assistive devices as necessary.

Immunizations

Routine immunizations are recommended; however, the child on immunosuppressive therapy may not receive live vaccines.

Influenza, pneumococcal, and hepatitis vaccines are recommended.

Screening

Vision

Routine annual examinations by a pediatric ophthalmologist to assess for calcification, arterial hemorrhages, and cataracts (if child is on steroid therapy), as well as vision testing are recommended.

Hearing

Routine annual examinations are recommended; monitor hearing when using ototoxic drugs.

Dental

Routine dental care at 6-month intervals; child with vascular access or immunosuppressed is at risk for endocarditis and needs prophylactic antibiotic coverage for dental procedures.

Monitor for gingival hyperplasia, enamel defects, poor mineralization.

Blood pressure

Blood pressure should be taken at all medical visits; frequency of measurement depends on BP value. Use correctly sized cuff.

Antihypertensive therapy should be managed by the pediatric nephrologist.

Hematocrit

Anemia is a problem; monitor CBC.

Urinalysis

Routine screening is done by pediatric nephrology team if indicated.

Tuberculosis

Tine test or PPD is needed annually.

Condition-specific screening

Blood work—CBC, RBC indices and folate studies, electrolytes, BUN, creatinine, calcium, phosphorus, alkaline phosphatase, albumin, and ferritin are monitored monthly.

PTH and viral titers are monitored periodically.

Cardiac screening—chest x-ray, ECG, and echocardiogram every 6 months.

Radiologic screening—monitor chest x-ray, bone x-ray for skeletal growth, and renal osteodystrophy.

Common illness management

Differential diagnosis

Routine pediatric care should be provided by a pediatrician in collaboration with the pediatric nephrologist.

Fever should always be assessed for cause; a fever related to a vascular access or PD catheter infection should be managed by the pediatric nephrologist.

Continued.

SUMMARY OF PRIMARY CARE NEEDS FOR THE CHILD WITH CHRONIC RENAL FAILURE—cont'd

Drug Interactions

For all medications, know the route of excretion, degree of renal impairment, and interaction with other medications in CRF management.

Calculate dosage by weight, not age, of the child.

Renal-excreted drugs may require dosage adjustment.

Use calcium-based phosphate binders rather than aluminum preparations.

Use acetaminophen rather than aspirin for pain or fever.

Developmental Issues

Sleep patterns

Increased fatigue and need for sleep may indicate worsening renal failure.

Toileting

The child with CRF may have normal urine output, oliguria, or anuria. Urinary diversion may be present; not all children can achieve urinary continence.

Begin bowel training when child is developmentally ready.

Discipline

Parents' own emotions may interfere with discipline of the child, resulting in parents being overprotective or too lenient without discipline. Parents need honest answers and encouragement. Nonadherence with plan of care is a source of conflict.

Child with CRF should learn self-care and take responsibility for independence as much as possible.

Child care

The child care provider must be instructed on diet, medications, special treatment regimen, and emergency measures.

Schooling

Encourage school attendance when possible, or provide alternative means (home bound, tutor, teacher in dialysis).

Instruct teacher about child's care plan and needs.

Poor school performance must be evaluated for physical versus psychologic causative factors.

Adolescence, sexuality, and transition into adulthood

Adolescent characteristics differ between early, middle, and late adolescence; assess areas of growth, cognition, identity, sexuality, emotionality, family and peer relationships across the age span.

Encourage ventilation of emotions; physical activity for emotional health, independence, and support groups.

Promote responsibility toward transition into adulthood.

Special family concerns

CRF affects the entire family; work to strengthen total family unit.

Provide networking with other families of children with CRF.

Ethnic, cultural, and racial factors impact on adjustment to CRF and care.

Ethical issues

Closely related to economics and highly controversial.

Health care team practices patient advocacy.

Cost containment has impact on care.

REFERENCES

Abitbol CL et al: Linear growth and anthropometric and nutritional measurements in children with mild to moderate renal insufficiency: a report of the Growth Failure in Children with Renal Diseases Study, *J Pediatr* 116(2):S46-54, 1990.

Alexander SR: Peritoneal dialysis in children. In Nolph KD (editor): *Peritoneal dialysis,* ed 3, The Netherlands, 1989, Dordrecht, pp 343-364.

Alexander SR et al: Maintenance dialysis in North American children and adolescents: a preliminary report. North American Pediatric Renal Transplant Cooperative Study (NAPRTCS), *Kidney Int* 43:S104-109, 1993.

American College of Physicians: Automated ambulatory blood pressure and self-measured blood pressure monitoring devices: their role in the diagnosis and management of hypertension, *Annals of Intern Med* 118(11):889-892, 1993.

Ash SR, Daugirdas JT: Peritoneal access devices. In Daugirdas JT, Ing RS (editors): *Handbook of dialysis,* ed 2, Boston, 1994, Little, Brown.

Aufricht C et al: Subcutaneous recombinant human erythropoietin in children with renal anemia on continuous ambulatory peritoneal dialysis, *Acta Paediatrica* 82(11):959-962, 1993.

Balfe JW et al: Tube feeding in children on chronic peritoneal dialysis, *Advances Peritoneal Dialysis* 6:257-261, 1990.

Barakat AY: The role of early diagnosis and intervention in the prevention of kidney disease. In Barakat AY (editor): *Renal disease in children—clinical evaluation and diagnosis,* New York, 1994, Springer-Verlag.

Barratt TM, Chantler C: Clinical evaluation. In Holliday MA, Barratt TM, and Vernier RL (editors): *Pediatric nephrology,* ed 2, Baltimore, 1987, Williams & Wilkins, pp 275-281.

Barratt TM et al: Assessment of growth, *Am J Kidney Dis* 7:340-346, 1986.

Bazilinski N, Dunea G: Hypertension. In Daugirdas JT, Ing RS (editors): *Handbook of dialysis,* ed 2, Boston, 1988, Little, Brown.

Berkoben M, Schwab SN: Maintenance of permanent hemodialysis vascular access patency, *ANNA Jrnl* 22(1):17-24, 1995.

Bernhart J: Renal/genitourinary disorders. In Beachy P, Deacon J (editors): *Core curriculum for neonatal intensive care nursing,* Philadelphia, 1993, WB Saunders.

Blake PG: Malnutrition in peritoneal dialysis—part II, *Contemp Dialysis Nephr* 15(11):20-21, 1994.

Brewer ED: Growth of small children managed with chronic peritoneal dialysis and nasogastric tube feedings: 203-month experience in 14 patients, *Advances Peritoneal Dialysis* 6:269-272, 1990.

Bruiner GM: Calcium/phosphorus imbalances, aluminum toxicity, and renal osteodystrophy, *ANNA Jrnl* 21(4):171-177, 1994.

Campos A, Garin EH: Therapy of renal anemia in children and adolescents with recombinant human erythropoietin (rHuEPO), *Clin Pediatr* 31(2):94-99, 1992.

Center for Disease Control: National Immunization Program, *Facts about chickenpox,* Jan 1994.

Chan JC et al: A prospective, double-blind study of growth failure in children with chronic renal insufficiency and the effectiveness of treatment with calcitriol versus dihydrotachysterol. The Growth Failure in Children with Renal Diseases Investigators, *J Pediatr* 124(4):520-528, 1994.

Cherry JD, Flegin RD: Infection in the compromised host. In Stiehm RD (editor): *Immunologic disorders for infants and children,* ed 3, Philadelphia, 1989, WB Saunders.

Chesney RW: Renal osteodystrophy in children: a commentary. In Kher KK, Makker SP (editors): *Clinical pediatric nephrology,* New York, 1992, McGraw Hill, Inc.

Claris-Appiani A et al: Growth in young children with chronic renal failure, *Pediatr Nephrol* 3:301-304, 1989.

Cole JW, Alfrey AC: Aluminum toxicity. In Massey SG and Glassock RJ (editors): *Textbook of Nephrology,* vol 2, ed 3, Baltimore, 1995, Williams & Wilkins.

Committee on Infectious Diseases: *Report of the Committee on Infectious Diseases,* ed 23, Elk Grove Village, IL, 1994, The American Academy of Pediatrics.

Corea AL: Case management of the anemic patient: epoetin alfa focus on cognitive function, *ANNA Jrnl* 20(3):350-353, 1993.

Cunningham C: Tube feeding in the real world: formulas, equipment, finances, and feeding problems, *Advances Peritoneal Dialysis* 6:255-256, 1990.

Currier H: Ethical issues in the neonatal patient with end-stage renal disease, *J Perinatal Neonatal Nurs* 8(1):74-78, 1994.

Daughaday WH, Harvey S: Growth hormone action: clinical significance. In Harvey S, Scanes CG, and Daughaday WH (editors): *Growth hormone,* Boca Raton, FL, 1994, CRC Press.

Drachman R et al: Vaccination against hepatitis B in children and adolescent patients on dialysis, *Nephrol Dial Transplant* 4:372-374, 1987.

Durack DT, Phil D: Prevention of infective endocarditis, *N Engl J Med* 332(1):37-44, 1995.

Elzouki A et al: Improved neurologic outcome in children with chronic renal disease from infancy, *Pediatr Nephrol* 8(2):205-210, 1994.

Eschbach JW, Adamson JW: Anemia of end-stage renal disease, *Kidney Int* 28:1-5, 1985.

Fennell RS et al: Association between renal function and cognition in childhood chronic renal failure, *Pediatr Nephrol* 4:16-20, 1990.

Fine RN: Recent advances in the management of the infant, child, and adolescent with chronic renal failure, *Pediatr Rev* 11:277-283, 1990a.

Fine RN: Recombinant human growth hormone treatment of children with chronic renal failure: update 1990, *Acta Paediatr Scandinavica* 370:S44-S48, 1990b.

Fine RN et al: Growth after recombinant human growth hormone treatment in children with chronic renal failure: report of a multicenter randomized double-blind placebo-controlled study, Genentech Cooperative Study Group, *J Pediatr* 124(3):374-382, 1994.

Fine RN, Salusky IB, and Ettenger RB: The therapeutic approach to the infant, child, and adolescent with end-stage renal disease, *Pediatr Clin North Am* 34:789-801, 1987.

Fine RN, Tejani A: Dialysis in infants and children. In Daugirdas JT, Ing RS (editors): *Handbook of dialysis,* ed 2, Boston, 1988, Little, Brown.

Finney JW, Weist MD: Behavioral assessment of children and adolescents, *Pediatr Cl North Am* 39(3):369-378, 1992.

Fivush BA et al: Defective antibody response to Hemophilus influenzae type b immunization in children receiving peritoneal dialysis, *Pediatr Nephrol* 7(5):548-550, 1993.

Foreman JW, Tsuru N, and Chan JCM: Pathophysiology and management of chronic renal failure. In Chan JCM, Gill JR (editors): *Kidney and electrolyte disorders,* New York, 1990, Churchill Livingstone.

Frauman AC, Gilman CM: Care of the family of the child with end-stage renal disease, *ANNA Jrnl* 17(5):383-386, 401, 1990.

Garvin G: Caring for children with ostomies, *Nurs Clin North Am* 29(4):645-654, 1994.

Grimes DE, Grimes RM, and Hamelink M: *Infectious diseases,* St Louis, 1991, Mosby.

Grupe WE et al: Issues in pediatric dialysis, *Am J Kidney Dis* 7:324-328, 1986.

Haggerty LM, Sigardson-Poor KM: Kidney transplant. In Sigardson-Poor KM, Haggerty LM (editors): *Nursing care of the transplant recipient,* Philadelphia, 1990, WB Saunders.

Hartigan M: Circulatory access for hemodialysis. In Lancaster LE (editor): *Core curriculum for nephrology nursing,* ed 2, Pitman, NJ, 1991, AJ Jannetti, pp 255-275.

Hockenberry B: Multiple drug therapy in the treatment of essential hypertension, *Nurs Clin North Am* 26(2):417-436, 1991.

Josblena M (editor): *Epogen (Epoetin alfa): treatment of the anemic patient with chronic renal failure,* Laurel, MD, 1990, Advenceutics.

Kasiske BL et al: The effect of race on access and outcome of transplantation, *The NEJM* 324(5):302-307, 1991.

Kher KK: Chronic renal failure, conservative management of chronic renal failure, hypertension. In Kher KK, Makker SP (editors): *Clinical pediatric nephrology,* New York, 1992, McGraw-Hill SP.

Khoury S et al: Ambulatory blood pressure monitoring in a nonacademic setting: effects of age and sex, *Am J Hypertension* 5:616-623, 1992.

Kirlin LP: Case management of the anemic patient: epoetin alfa—focus on iron supplementation, *ANNA Jrnl* 20(6):678-681, 1993.

Knight F et al: Hemodialysis of the infant or small child with chronic renal failure, *ANNA Jrnl* 20(3):315-323, 1993.

Koch VH et al: Accelerated growth after recombinant human growth hormone treatment of children with chronic renal failure, *J Pediatr* 115:365-471, 1989.

Korbet SM: Comparison of hemodialysis and peritoneal dialysis in the management of anemia related to chronic renal disease, *Semin Nephrol* 9(suppl 1):9-15, 1989.

Lancaster L: Manifestations of renal failure. In Lancaster LE (editor): *Core curriculum for nephrology nursing,* ed 2, Pitman, NJ, 1991, AJ Jannetti, pp 70-107.

Leichter HE, Kher KK: Management of end-stage renal failure-dialysis therapy. In Kher KK, Makker SP (editors): *Clinical pediatric nephrology,* New York, 1992, McGraw-Hill Inc.

Lindholm B, Bergstrom J: Nutritional management of patients undergoing peritoneal dialysis. In Nolph KD (editor): *Peritoneal dialysis,* ed 3, MA, 1989, Kluwer Academic, pp 230-260.

Locatelli F et al: Prospective, randomized, multicenter trial of effect of protein restriction on progression of chronic renal insufficiency. Northern Italian Cooperative Study Group, *Lancet* 337(8753):1299-1304, 1991.

Lopes AA et al: The excess risk of treated end-stage renal disease in blacks in the United States, *J Am Soc Nephrol* 3(12):1961-1971, 1993.

Lumsden AB et al: Hemodialysis access in the pediatric patient population, *Am J Surgery* 168(2):197-201, 1994.

Lyon RP, Marshall S, and Baskin LS: Normal growth with renal insufficiency owing to posterior urethral valves: value of long-term diversion. A 20-year follow-up, *Urologia Internationalis* 48(2):125-129, 1992.

Mehls O, Ritz E: Renal osteodystrophy. In Holliday MA, Barratt TM, and Paganini EP (editors): Overview of anemia associated with chronic renal disease: primary and secondary mechanisms, *Semin Nephr* 9(suppl 1):3-8, 1989.

Moore LW: Nutrition in end-stage renal disease: a life cycle perspective, *Nephrol Nurs Today* 1(2):1-8, 1991.

Morris KP et al: Cardiovascular abnormalities in end-stage renal failure: the effect of anemia or uremia? *Archiv Dis Child* 71(2):119-122, 1994.

Morris KP et al: Noncardiac benefits of human recombinant erythropoetin in end-stage renal failure and anaemia, *Archiv Dis Child* 69(5):580-586, 1993.

Neff JA: Nursing the child undergoing dialysis, *Issues Compr Pediatr Nurs* 10:173-185, 1987.

Ojo AO et al: Comparative mortality risks of chronic dialysis and cadaveric transplantation in black end-stage renal disease patients, *Am J Kidney Dis* 24(1):59-64, 1994.

O'Regan S, Garel L: Percutaneous gastrojejunostomy for caloric supplementation in children on peritoneal dialysis, *Advances Peritoneal Dialysis* 6:273-275, 1990.

Paganini EP: Overview of anemia associated with chronic renal disease: primary and secondary mechanisms, *Semin Nephrol* 9(1 suppl 1)1-3, 1989.

Painter P, Carlson L: Case study of the anemic patient: epoetin alfa—focus on exercise, *ANNA Jrnl* 23(3):304-307, 1994.

Papadopoulou AL: Chronic renal failure. In Barakat AY (editor): *Renal disease in children,* New York, 1990, Springer-Verlag.

Ponferrada L et al: Home visit effectiveness for peritoneal dialysis patients, *ANNA Jrnl* 20(3):333-336, 1993.

Prowant BF, Gallagher NM: Concepts and principles of peritoneal dialysis. In Lancaster LE (editor): *Core curriculum for nephrology nursing,* ed 2, Pitman, NJ, 1991, AJ Jannetti, pp 277-321.

Raymond NG et al: An approach to protein restriction in children with renal insufficiency, *Pediatr Nephrol* 4(2):125-151, 1990.

Reinberg Y, de Castano I, and Gonzales R: Influence of initial therapy on progression of renal failure and body growth in children with posterior urethral valves, *J Urol* 148(2):532-533, 1992.

Richie MF, Mapes D, and Dailey FD: Psychosocial aspects of renal failure and its treatment. In Lancaster LE (editor): *Core curriculum for nephrology nursing,* ed 2, Pitman, NJ, 1991, AJ Jannetti, pp 109-142.

Ritz EF: Renal insufficiency. In Suki WN, Massry SG (editors): *Therapy of renal diseases and related disorders,* ed 2, Boston, 1991, Kluver Academic Publishers.

Rizzoni G et al: Growth retardation in children with chronic renal disease: scope of the problem, *Am J Kidney Dis* 7:256-261, 1986.

Rodriquez-Soriano J et al: Fluid and electrolyte imbalances in children with chronic renal failure, *Am J Kidney Dis* 7:268-274, 1986.

Rossmann JA, Ingles E, and Brown RS: Multimodal treatment of drug-induced gingival hyperplasia in a kidney transplant patient, *Compendium* 15(10):1266-1274, 1994.

Rotundo A, Nevins TE, and Lipton M: Progressive encephalopathy in children with chronic renal insufficiency in infancy, *Kidney Int* 21:486-491, 1982.

Ruble K, Long C, and Connor K: Pharmacologic treatment of catheter-related thrombus in pediatrics, *Pediatr Nurs* 20(6):553-557, 1994.

Salmon K, Broyan P: Epoetin alfa—issues in self-administration, *Nephrol Nurs Today* 1(5):1-8, 1991.

Salusky IB: The nutritional approach for pediatric patients undergoing CAPD/CCPD, *Advances Peritoneal Dialysis* 6:245-251, 1990.

Salusky IB et al: Aluminum accumulation during treatment with aluminum hydroxide and dialysis in children and young adults with chronic renal disease, *N Engl J Med* 324(8):527-531, 1991.

Salusky IB et al: Prospective evaluation of aluminum loading from formula in infants with uremia, *J Pediatr* 116(5):726-729, 1990.

Scharer K: Growth and development of children with chronic renal failure. Study group on Pubertal Development in Chronic Renal Failure, *Acta Paediatr Scandinavica* 366:S90-S92, 1990.

Scharer K et al: Treatment of renal anemia by subcutaneous erythropoietin in children with preterminal chronic renal failure, *Acta Paediatrica* 82(11):953-958, 1993.

Scharer K, Ulmer H: Cardiovascular complications. In Holliday MA, Barratt TM, and Vernier RL (editors): *Pediatric Nephrology,* ed 2, Baltimore, 1987, Williams & Wilkins, pp 887-896.

Schira MG: The role of cognitive function in education of patients with ESRD, *Nephrol Nurs Today* 4(3):1-8, 1994.

Shusterman N, Singer I: Infectious hepatitis in dialysis patients, *Am J Kidney Dis* 6:447-455, 1987.

Stablein DM: Annual Report 1992: North American Pediatric Renal Transplant Cooperative Study (NAPRTCS), Potomac, MD, 1992.

Summar M, Hakim RNM: The use of computers in clinical nephrology. In Barakat AY (editor): *Renal disease in children—clinical evaluation and diagnosis,* New York, 1990, Springer-Verlag.

Szromba C (editor): *Understanding and managing anemia in the CRF patient,* Pitman, NJ, 1992, ANNA and Ortho Biotech.

Tanner JM: *Growth at adolescence,* ed 2, Oxford, England, 1962, Blackwell.

Taylor JH: A competency-based approach to pediatric hemodialysis. Unpublished lecture presented at ANNA Symposium, Dallas, 1994a.

Taylor JH: Enhancing development in the adolescent with ESRD, Unpublished lecture presented at ANNA Symposium, Dallas, 1994b.

Tonshoff B et al: Growth-stimulating effects of recombinant human growth hormone in children with end-stage renal disease, *J Pediatr* 116(4):561-566, 1990.

Travis G: *Chronic Illness in Children: Its impact on child and family.* Stanford, 1976, Stanford University Press, pp 195-232.

Travis LB, Brouhard BH, and Kalia A: Overview with special emphasis on epidemiologic considerations. In Tune BM, Mendoze SA (editors): *Pediatric nephrology: contemporary issues in nephrology,* New York, 1984, Churchill Livingstone, vol 12, pp 1-19.

Trompeter RS: A review of drug prescribing in children with end-stage renal failure, *Pediatr Nephrol* 1:183-194, 1987.

US Federal Register July 1973, US Health and Human Services, Washington, DC.

US Renal Data System: *USRDS 1994 Annual Data Report,* The National Institutes of Health, National Institute of Diabetes and Digestive and Kidney Diseases, Bethesda, MD, 1994.

Uysal S et al: Neurologic complications in chronic renal failure: a retrospective study, *Clin Pediatr* 29(9):510-514, 1990.

Van EA: Growth hormone treatment in short children with chronic renal failure and after renal transplantation: combined data from European clinical trials. The European Study Group, *Acta Paediatr Scandinavica* 379:S42-S48, 1991.

Weiss R: Management of chronic renal failure, *Pediatr Ann* 17:584-589, 1988.

Wong DL: *Whaley and Wong's nursing care of infants and children,* ed 5, St Louis, 1995, Mosby.

Young EW et al: Socioeconomic status and end-stage renal disease in the United States, *Kidney Int* 45(3):907-911, 1994.

33

Sickle Cell Disease

Barbara A. Carroll*

ETIOLOGY

Sickle cell disease is a term used to describe several inherited sickling hemoglobinopathy syndromes, including sickle-β-thalassemia (HgbS-B° thal or HbgS-B+ thal), sickle-C disease (Hgb SC), and most commonly sickle cell anemia (Hgb SS). Hemoglobin contains two pairs of polypeptide chains, α and β. Each of the hemoglobinopathy syndromes has sickle hemoglobin (Hgb S), which differs from normal hemoglobin (Hgb A) by the substitution of a single amino acid; in Hgb S, valine replaces glutamic acid at the sixth position of the β-chain.

A red blood cell (RBC) containing normal hemoglobin is a very pliable, biconcave disc and has a life span of approximately 120 days. Red blood cells containing predominantly Hgb S will polymerize and form micro tubules (rods) that distort the shape of the cell, characteristically to a crescent or sickle shape. In this form the cell is rigid and friable. Hypoxia and acidosis, which may be caused by fever, infection, dehydration, or other factors, are known to induce this change in shape (see Fig. 33-1). Many times, however, the RBC changes shape without apparent provocation. To a limited degree this change in shape is reversible, though not indefinitely. Eventually the cells become irreversibly sickled cells (ISCs) with a life span of approximately 10 to 20 days. The fragility and shortened life span of these RBCs leads to chronic anemia. This serves as a stimulus to the bone marrow to create new RBCs, resulting in an elevated reticulocyte count.

The sickle "prep" is a solubility test often used to screen infants and children for sickle cell disease. It is inexpensive and rapidly performed but is not very specific. A sickle prep result will be positive for sickle cell trait, sickle cell anemia, and other sickle hemoglobinopathies but will not distinguish between them. The definitive diagnosis of sickle cell disease is made by performing a complete blood count (CBC), peripheral blood smear, and, most importantly, a quantitative hemoglobin electrophoresis. Measurement of hematologic indices are often important in the differential diagnoses of thalassemia syndromes and hemoglobinopathies. Occasionally it is helpful to perform hematologic studies on a child's parents to confirm the diagnosis.

Sickle cell disease has an autosomal recessive inheritance pattern. Both parents must carry some type of abnormal hemoglobin—one or both of them must carry sickle hemoglobin—for the disease to be manifested in their child. Carriers of sickle cell disease are described as having sickle cell trait (Hgb AS). When two individuals, each of whom has sickle cell trait, elect to have a child, there is a 25% chance of having a child with sickle cell anemia (Hgb SS), a 50% chance of having a child with

*The editors and author would like to acknowledge the work done by Maryann E. Lisak on this chapter in the first edition of the book.

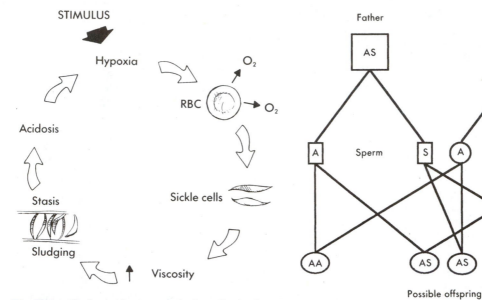

Fig. 33-1.   Cycle causing vasoocclusive episodes in sickle cell anemia. (*From Hockenberry M and Coody D, eds: Pediatric oncology and hematology: perspectives on care, St Louis, 1986, Mosby.*)

Fig. 33-2.   Genetics of sickle cell anemia. Both parents possess one gene for normal hemoglobin *(A)* and one for sickle hemoglobin *(S)*. With each pregnancy, there is a 25% statistical chance that the child will have normal hemoglobin *(AA)* and a 25% chance of sickle cell anemia *(SS);* 50% will have sickle cell trait. (*From Miller D and Baeher R:* Blood diseases of infancy and childhood: in the tradition of CH Smith, *ed 6, St Louis, 1990, Mosby.*)

sickle cell trait (Hgb AS), and a 25% chance of having a child with entirely normal hemoglobin (Hgb AA) with each pregnancy (see Fig. 33-2).

In an effort to decrease morbidity and mortality through early identification and prophylactic treatment, many states are now performing routine newborn screening for hemoglobinopathies. Electrophoresis or high-performance liquid chromatography (HPLC) can be performed on cord blood or heel stick blood, usually at the same time that blood is obtained for other newborn screening tests (phenylketonuria, thyroid function, etc.). Fetal hemoglobin predominates from 10 weeks through the remainder of gestation, beginning to decline at 34 weeks. It comprises 60% to 80% of globin at birth, and reaches low adult levels (<1%) by 2 years of age (Blau and Stamatoyannopoulos, 1994). The remaining globin found on hemoglobin electrophoreses reflects the eventual adult pattern. It is unusual to find clinical manifestations of the disease in the presence of significant amounts of fetal hemoglobin. Therefore, the disease may not be clinically apparent until 4 to 6 months of age or later.

INCIDENCE

Sickle cell disease is one of the most common genetic diseases. It is seen most often in individuals of African descent but is also found in other ethnic groups, including those from the Caribbean, Mediterranean, the Arabian Peninsula, and India. In the United States, 1 in 12 African Americans is a carrier of the sickle cell gene and 1 in 600 actually has the disease (Steinburg and Embury, 1994).

Prenatal diagnosis is available to those couples known to be carriers for a hemoglobinopathy. Diagnosis may be accomplished via chorionic villi sampling during the first trimester or amniocentesis during the second trimester. The choice of method is dependent on the risks and benefits of the techniques involved; both are adequate to determine the diagnosis.

CLINICAL MANIFESTATIONS OF SICKLE CELL ANEMIA

Neonatal:

- Normal birth weight
- No evidence of hemolytic anemia
- Hemoglobin electrophoresis shows no evidence of Hgb A production
- Neonatal jaundice (when present) related to ABO hemolytic disease of the newborn, not to sickle cell disease

Infancy and toddler:

- Development of anemia
- Coliclike symptoms, often associated with feeding difficulties
- Generalized painful episodes of bone or abdomen preceded by acute, febrile infectious disease
- Hand-foot syndrome associated with heat, pain, swelling, erythema
- Splenic hypofunction marked by presence of Howell-Jolly bodies in the blood smear
- Autosplenectomy preceded by splenomegaly in 73% of infants, followed by decrease in size
- Splenomegaly noted frequently during febrile episodes

TREATMENT

- Genetic counseling for individuals with sickle cell trait
- Prenatal diagnosis
- Parental education
- Aggressive treatment of infection
- Maintenance of optimal hydration
- Maintenance of body temperature
- Transfusion with life-threatening events
- Penicillin prophylaxis
- Pneumococcal immunization
- Drug therapy to induce expression of Hgb F
- Bone marrow transplantation in selected subjects

CLINICAL MANIFESTATIONS AT TIME OF DIAGNOSIS

As a result of current newborn screening programs for hemoglobinopathies, infants are now being identified before the onset of acute symptoms. (See Table 33-1.)

Sickle cell anemia in the first two decades of life is marked by periods of clinical quiescence and relative well-being interspersed with intermittent episodes of acute illness. These illnesses are treatable by state-of-the-art medical care and are often preventable. Chronologically, the expression of sickle cell anemia is often characterized by septicemia/meningitis during infancy, followed by cerebral vasculopathy with cerebral infarction during early childhood. Splenic hypofunction is present in nearly 30% of infants with sickle cell anemia by their first birthday and in 90% by age 6, accounting for the high risk of sepsis by polysaccharide encapsulated organisms (Powars, 1994).

TREATMENT

There is no cure for sickle cell disease short of bone marrow transplantation. Despite the thorough understanding that exists among researchers regarding the inheritance, diagnosis, and pathophysiology of sickle cell disease, treatment is essentially supportive and symptomatic. The recent focus of treatment has been on prevention by providing (1) genetic counseling to those individuals with sickle trait, (2) prenatal diagnosis for pregnant women who are at risk for delivering a child with sickle cell disease, and (3) education for parents of children newly diagnosed.

An important consideration in treatment is the prevention of the sickling process whenever possible by preventing hypoxia and acidosis. This includes the aggressive treatment of infection, maintenance of optimal hydration and body temperature, and, when necessary, transfusion.

Table 33-1.   DIFFERENTIAL DIAGNOSIS OF COMMON HEMOGLOBINOPATHIES

Diagnosis	Clinical severity	Hemoglobin (g/dl)	Hematocrit (%)	Mean corpuscular volume (μ^3)	% of reticulocytes	RBC morphology*	Solubility test	Electrophoresis (%)	Distribution of fetal hemoglobin
SS	Moderate-severe	7.5 (6-10)	22 (18-30)	93	11 (4-30)	Many ISCs, target cells, nucleated RBCs	Positive	80-90 S 2-20 F <3.6 A_2	Uneven
SC	Mild-moderate	10 (9-14)	30 (26-40)	80	3 (1.5-6)	Many target cells, rare ISCs	Positive	45-55 S 45-55 C 0.2-8 F	Uneven
S/B° thal	Moderate-severe	8.1 (7-12)	25 (20-36)	69	8 (3-18)	Marked hypochromia, microcytosis and target cells, variable ISCs	Positive	50-85 S 2-30 F >3.6 A_2	Uneven
S/B + thal	Mild-moderate	11 (8-13)	32 (25-40)	76	3 (1.5-6)	Mild microcytosis, hypochromia, rare ISCs	Positive	55-75 S 15-30 A 1-20 F >3.6 A_2	Uneven
S/HPFH†	Asymptomatic	14 (11-15)	40 (32-48)	84	1.5 (.5-3)	No ISCs, occasional target cells, and mild hypochromia	Positive	60-80 S 15-35 F 1-3 A_2	Even
AS	Asymptomatic	Normal	Normal	Normal	Normal	Normal	Positive	38-45 S 60-55 A 1-3 A_2	Uneven

From Vichinsky EP, Lubin BH: *Pediatr Clin North Am* 27:429-447, 1980.
*ICSs, irreversibly sickled cells.
†S/HPFH, sickle hereditary persistence of fetal hemoglobin.

RECENT AND ANTICIPATED ADVANCES IN DIAGNOSIS AND MANAGEMENT

Manipulation of bone marrow through the administration of drugs that induce expression of fetal hemoglobin is now being investigated (Charache, 1994). It is well known that fetal hemoglobin (Hgb F) does not polymerize as does Hgb S. Administration of drugs such as hydroxyurea "turns on" the latent F gene. Expression of Hgb F in combination with the native Hgb S forms a diluted pool of Hgb SF which reduces both the polymerization of the cells and the rate of hemolysis. This in turn reduces the number of sickle cell crises. Hydroxyurea has been approved for adult administration by the FDA and a pilot study is underway for pediatric use (Dover, 1995).

In the future, hydroxyurea may be augmented with butyric acid, granulocyte-macrophage colony-stimulating factor (GM-CSF) and erythropoietin (Rodgers, GP 1993). Further work is needed to establish optimal therapy. Other drugs being studied include Hgb ligands, which work by keeping cells from adhering to one another. Other membrane active drugs work by improving cell structure or by increasing hydration of the sickle erythrocyte. Vasoactive drugs prevent the adherence of sickled cells to the vascular endothelium by blocking cytoadhesion receptors. These agents are currently under study (Orringer, Abraham, and Parker, 1994).

Bone marrow transplantation has effectively cured a small but growing number of individuals with sickle cell anemia. This approach is limited in that only 18% of individuals will have a matched donor (Mentzer et al, 1994). A consideration that limits this approach is the morbidity associated with bone marrow transplantation, including risks of death, organ impairment, curtailed sexual functioning, and impaired motor and psychologic functioning (Secundy, 1994). Other considerations include disturbance of family systems, cost benefit ratios, the rights of siblings, and client compliance (Secundy, 1994). Bone marrow transplantation options must be considered in the arena of shared decision making by the health care workers and the family; differences in cultural background between the two may impede the ability to negotiate informed consent. External factors such as educational level, economic conditions of the family, and quality of life are often more critical in the minority community than they might be in other settings (Secundy, 1994).

The Cooperative Study of Sickle Cell Disease (CSSCD) group has two important studies underway. The Preoperative Transfusion Study group is challenging the aggressive practice of transfusing presurgical clients. It is well known that general anesthesia induction places the client with sickle cell disease at risk for stroke. Standard protocol is to transfuse the client to a hemoglobin of 11 Gm/dl with an Hgb S level of 30%. In the preoperative transfusion study, clients are transfused to a preoperative level of 10 Gm/dl with an Hgb S level of 60%. Early reports indicate no difference in the complication rate (Vichinsky, 1995).

Another study group of the CSSCD, STOP (Stroke Prevention in Sickle Cell Anemia) is looking at genetic markers, laboratory and radiographic indicators, and clinical findings that may prove predictive of stroke in this population. This knowledge would enable those children at increased risk for stroke to be managed more aggressively in hopes of preventing serious complications.

Recent radiographic developments such as transcranial doppler ultrasound (TCD) and magnetic resonance angiography (MRA) have been used in some centers as a predictor of strokes. Both techniques reliably demonstrate flow abnormalities consistent with areas of cerebral infarction (Koqutt et al, 1994). Positive emission tomography (PET) has confirmed areas of irregular brain metabolism in children with sickle cell disease, but this technique is not readily available at most centers.

Genetic engineering is still far off, but must be approached with the same caution exercised in consideration of bone marrow transplantation. Again, cultural considerations must be integral to decision making. In utero hematopoietic stem cell transplants portend to be the next area of investigation for curing sickle cell disease (Cowan and Golbus, 1994).

ASSOCIATED PROBLEMS

Associated problems primarily result from (1) blockage of small blood vessels secondary to the clumping of sickled RBCs that cause tissue is-chemia, and (2) hemolytic anemia and its sequelae (see Fig. 33-3).

Functional Asplenia

Splenic function is normal at birth, but by 6 months of age a state of splenic dysfunction develops, most likely as a result of massive infarction. With the absence of adequate splenic function, children with sickle cell disease are at high risk for infection from polysaccharide encapsulated organisms such as *S. pneumoniae, H. influenzae,* and *Neisseria meningitidis.* Less common causes of bacteremia include other streptocci, *E. coli, S. aureus,* and gram-negative bacilli such as *Klebsiella, Salmonella,* and *Pseudomonas aeruginosa* (American Academy of Pediatrics [AAP] Red Book, 1994).

Intervention should be threefold: (1) aggressive management of infectious episodes; (2) timely immunization including pneumococcal vaccine; and (3) antibiotic prophylaxis.

Because pneumococcal vaccines do not cover all pathogenic strains, antibiotic prophylaxis is the standard of care for all young children with sickle cell disease. It should be started at or before 2 months of age, and it is frequently easiest if started as soon as the diagnosis is made. The usual doses are as follows: penicillin, 125 mg twice daily for children less than age 3 years and 250 mg twice daily for those greater than 3 years of age. For children who are not compliant with oral antibiotic therapy at home, 500,000 to 1.2 million U of a long-acting penicillin may be given intramuscularly each month (Charache, Lubin, and Reid, 1992).

Some experts have recommended amoxicillin (20 mg/kg/day) or trimethoprim-sulfamethoxazole (4 mg/kg/day TMP to 20 mg/kg/day SMX) for children younger than 5 years (AAP Red Book, 1994).

Some experts continue prophylaxis throughout childhood and adulthood in particularly high risk clients. The age at which prophylaxis is discontinued in individuals remains an empirical decision and studies are in progress (AAP Red Book, 1994).

As with other children taking antibiotics, the potential for monilial infections, gastrointestinal (GI) upset, and allergy exists. In the presence of penicillin allergy, other antibiotics may be used. Palpation of a spleen on physical examination is no indication of splenic function. A palpable spleen in

ASSOCIATED PROBLEMS

- Functional asplenia
- Splenic sequestration
- Neurologic problems
- Vasoocclusive crisis
- Pulmonary complications
  - Acute chest syndrome
  - Chronic lung disease
- Hemolysis/anemia
- Priapism
- Aplastic crisis
- Renal problems
- Skeletal changes
- Opthalmologic changes
- Audiologic problems
- Leg ulcers
- Reactions to contrast mediums, anesthesia
- Cardiac problems
- Hepatobiliary problems
- Transfusion complications
  - Iron overload
  - Bloodborne pathogens

the older child is thought to be the result of fibrosis and it is almost exclusively found in individuals with Hgb SC disease. The presence of Howell-Jolley bodies on blood smear confirms the condition of functional asplenia.

Splenic Sequestration

In this condition blood flow into the spleen is adequate, but the vascular outflow system from the spleen to the systemic circulation is occluded. This results in a large collection of blood pooling in the spleen, causing significant enlargement. The systemic circulation may then be deprived of its needed blood volume, causing shock and cardiovascular collapse. The hemoglobin and hematocrit values fall rapidly. Children with Hgb SS are susceptible to this at an early age (<5 years). Those with other variants of the disease may continue to be at risk for this until their teenage years because they maintain splenic circulation longer than children with Hgb SS. Par-

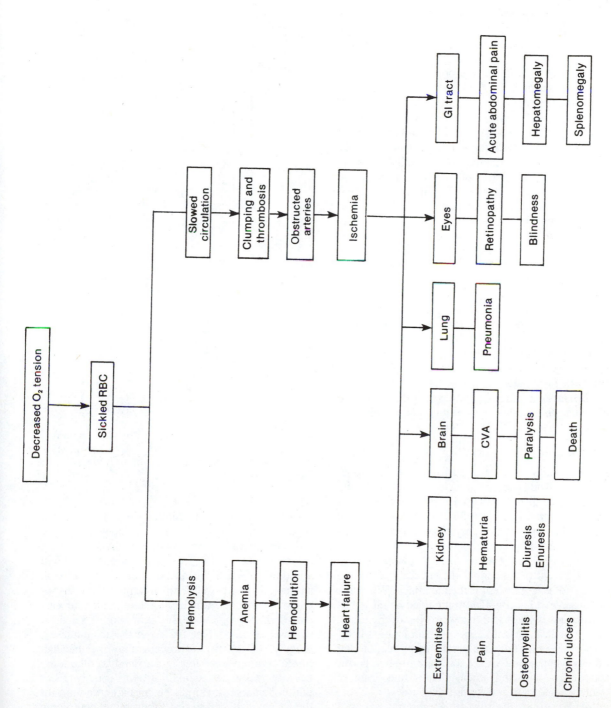

Fig. 33-3. Tissue effects of sickle cell anemia. *(From Wong D: Nursing care of infants and children, ed 5, St Louis, 1995, Mosby.)*

ents can be taught to palpate and measure their child's spleen using a simple measuring device such as a calibrated tongue blade (see Fig. 33-4). Knowledge of the child's steady state spleen size is essential in determining an appropriate diagnosis and treatment during an acute event.

Management of splenic sequestration requires hospitalization with immediate therapy, including transfusion. If shock is present, it will be necessary to support the systemic circulation with fluids. Once adequate circulation is reestablished, however, the volume of fluid previously sequestered in the spleen is returned to the circulation and circulatory overload must be avoided. For children who experience recurrent or severe episodes, splenectomy is indicated and is curative. Splenectomy, however, places the child at an increased risk of infection. It is optimal to splenectomize the child after the age of 2 years and after pneumococcal vaccine has been received. Children younger than 2 years of age who experience recurrent or severe episodes of splenic sequestration may be given regular transfusions in an effort to suppress their body's production of Hgb S and prevent further episodes of sequestration until splenectomy can safely be performed.

Recurrence of sequestration after discontinuing transfusion, however, makes this recommendation controversial (Vichinsky, 1994).

Neurologic Problems

The vasculature of the brain is subject to vasoocclusive episodes in children with sickle cell disease; the frequency varies from 8.5% to 17% of persons attending sickle cell clinics in the United States (Adams, 1994). When a blood vessel is partially occluded by a small embolus or vessel spasm, the manifestations may be focal and last less than 48 hours without residual deficit. This would be classified as a transient ischemic attack. When the affected vessel is completely occluded by thrombus or embolus with or without narrowing of the vessel lining, a CVA, or stroke, occurs. Intracranial hemorrhage is a rare but usually fatal complication that occurs when blood vessel walls are thinned by intravascular sickling then dilate and rupture (Charache, Lubin, and Reid, 1992).

At the time of stroke, most children are at a clinical steady state with no prodrome or symptom

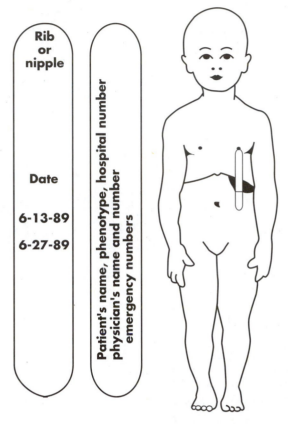

Fig. 33-4. Measurement of spleen size with a spleen stick. *(From Eckman JR and Plott AF: Problem oriented management of sickle syndromes, Atlanta, 1991, Georgia NIH Sickle Cell Center.)*

warning of any impending neurologic event (Ohene-Frempong, 1991). The mean age of the initial cerebral vascular accident is 8 years and is associated with a 4% mortality rate (Smith, 1991). In addition, 10% to 30% will experience seizures with stroke (Adams, 1994). Acute treatment for CVA includes exchange transfusion, stabilization of cardiorespiratory function, and treatment of seizures, if present (see Chapter 19). After the acute phase a lengthy rehabilitation process may be needed. Some children have few or no deficits; others are neurologically devastated. Strokes usually recur within 3 years if there has been no intervention for the sickle cell condition. Progressive neurologic deterioration occurs with each event. The polymerization of Hgb SS is central to development of stroke but is also likely to be a consequence of disruptions of the steady state of flow. Thus stroke is seen as a microcirculatory event in which multiple factors may be involved. These factors include rheologic and microcirculatory behavior of SS erythrocytes, vascular factors, red cell heterogeneity, deoxygenation rates, and red cell-endothelial interactions which all participate in the pathophysiology of sickle cell vasoocclusion (Adams, 1994).

Repeated RBC transfusions of cells containing Hgb A suppress bone marrow production of new RBCs that contain sickle hemoglobin. This is beneficial because it results in a minimal number of circulating RBCs that have the potential to become sickled and create further occlusion in the vascular bed. The necessary duration for transfusion on a regular basis is not known and probably is variable depending on the individual and the vasculature involved. Reports of recurrence of stroke and of silent, undetected central nervous system (CNS) events following cessation of long-term (5 to 12 years) transfusion therapy, suggest indefinite transfusions may be required and that despite compliance with strict criteria, repeated CNS events may occur (Wang et al, 1991).

Vasoocclusive Crisis

Many sources cite painful, vasoocclusive episodes as the most common cause of emergency room visits and hospital admissions for individuals with sickle cell disease. Vasoocclusion is a physiologic process, but the resultant pain is a complex biopsychosocial event. Physiologic factors combined with social considerations such as developmental stage, pain history, and family coping skills contribute to the expression of vasoocclusion. Each client will exhibit his or her own pattern of duration, frequency, severity, and location of vasoocclusive crises. The hallmark of these crises is their unpredictability (Shapiro and Ballas, 1994).

In children who had between 3 and 10 painful episodes per year, 5% of individuals accounted for 30% of crises. Nearly 40% of clients reported no pain in a year (Platt et al, 1991).

The frequency of painful episodes is related indirectly to the Hgb F level and numerous painful crises are a prognostic sign for further complications as a result of sickling (Embury et al, 1994).

The optimal treatment for vasoocclusive crises is multimodal and includes treating any antecedent causes, improving circulation, and providing analgesia. The treatment of antecedent causes includes correcting fever, hypoxia, and acidosis, treating infection, and rehydration. Quite possibly an extraneous illness precipitated a painful episode and the child has two independent problems. The primary care provider must be alert to this when examining the child.

Hydration is an important part of improving circulation to the affected area. The child may be hydrated orally or intravenously with an electrolyte solution. Options for oral hydration include juice, bouillon, water, milk, Gatorade, Pedialyte, or Lytren. Fluids given intravenously may include a normal saline bolus, taking care not to tax the cardiovascular system with too large or rapid a bolus. Maintenance fluids of 5% dextrose with 0.45% normal saline are then given; this solution will replace excess sodium lost in the urine as a result of renal dysfunction in individuals with sickle cell disease. Potassium is added as needed after urinary output is established. The rate of fluids given should be approximately 1.5 times the maintenance dosage, or 2500 ml/m^2 daily. Circulation to infarcted areas may also be improved by the local application of heat (heating pad, warm bath, or whirlpool). Once comfort has been established, passive range of motion and massage may be initiated. The child should be encouraged to be as active as possible.

Analgesia may take several forms, including nonpharmacologic agents, nonnarcotic medicines, oral narcotics, or parenteral narcotics. Multimodel therapy, which includes several of these approaches, proves to be more effective than single agent therapy as each agent targets different pain receptor sites. This combination therapy may also contravene the "ceiling effect" known to opiods such as buprenosphine (Payne, 1989).

There are multiple narcotic agents from which to choose, and each child, health care provider, and institution are likely to have their preferences. At no time are placebos appropriate because they erode the trusting relationship between the health care provider and child. The dose given should begin at a standard therapeutic dose or a dose known to be therapeutic for a given child and then adjusted as needed.

Many narcotics have very brief half-lives, and care must be taken to administer them frequently enough. For example, when a medication with a $1\frac{1}{2}$-hour half-life is used, dosing should be approximately every 2 hours to maintain consistent pain relief. Early in the course of a vasoocclusive episode, the vascular occlusion is constant, not intermittent. Later in the course, collateral circulation may develop or the occlusion may have decreased, improving circulation to the infarcted area. Thus early in the course of a painful episode, pro re nata (prn) dosing is inappropriate. It is preferable to control the child's pain early in the course of the illness and maintain control. Thus scheduled doses of narcotics are given over the first 24 hours after admission.

It is inappropriate to administer intramuscular injections to children for pain relief because an injection alone can be quite painful, unless it is for a single dose and a longer half-life is desired (e.g., for outpatient management) or unless IV access has not been obtained.

The use of intrathecal catheters has been suggested as a route for analgesic administration to the child who is hospitalized with severe, intractable pain (Yaster et al, 1994). This route provides the advantage of pain relief without excessive sedation. Patient-controlled analgesia (PCA) also is recommended if institutions are familiar with its use in children.

For mild pain, nonnarcotic medicines including acetaminophen, aspirin (provided there is no concurrent viral process or other contraindication), ibuprofen, and ketorolac (for adolescents) are appropriate. These may be given at the recommended doses.

Nonpharmacologic forms of pain relief are useful adjuncts to pharmacologic therapy. Self-hypnosis, biofeedback, and distraction are particularly helpful.

If children become significantly uncomfortable they will experience anxiety and subsequently a heightened perception of pain. Ultimately they may develop dysfunctional illness behavior as a result of inadequately treated pain. It is important for the child, family, and health care providers to have realistically attainable goals related to pain control. The goal of pain management should be prompt pain relief. The alleviation of pain provided by narcotics needs to be balanced against known side effects such as pruritus, nausea, constipation, and respiratory depression.

Shapiro (1994) cites several studies that document the low prevalence of drug addiction within this population. Despite these studies, health care providers continue to believe that drug addiction is a major problem among people with sickle cell disease. This is unfortunate because this misperception can interfere with the provision of adequate health care. The causes of this misperception are multiple; they include but are not limited to the rampant illicit drug problems in our society, cultural differences between the health care providers who are often white and clients who are often black, and the desire of most individuals who have chronic conditions to control some aspects of their treatment.

Pulmonary Complications

Acute chest syndrome (ACS) ranks second as a cause for hospitalization and is responsible for 25% of all deaths in sickle cell disease (Vichinsky et al, 1994). The incidence of ACS is seen more commonly in younger children (2 to 4 years old) and is least frequent among adult clients (Castro et al, 1994). ACS is a life-threatening complication that results from occlusions in the pulmonary vasculature, resulting in areas of infarcted lung tissue. The occlusion may be caused by localized sickling, thromboembolism, or embolism with collections of sickled cells, bone marrow, or marrow fat. It can also be induced by respiratory depression caused by narcotics. Special instructions for deep-breathing exercises before surgery can prevent certain episodes (Earles and Dorn, 1994).

ACS is characterized by acute chest pain, a nonproductive cough, leukocytosis, fever, and respiratory distress. It may be difficult to differentiate from, and in fact may be concurrent with, pneumonia. Physical examination usually reveals tachypnea; there may also be evidence of pulmonary consolidation, pleural effusion, a new pulmonary infiltrate, or pleural friction rub. Chest x-ray studies may be normal for the first few days especially if the child is dehydrated. Lung scans may be useful but often are equivocal because a baseline study is rarely available for comparison.

Acute chest syndrome may be a fulminant process; admission to the intensive care unit may be necessary for close monitoring. Arterial blood gas levels should be followed closely; supplemental oxygen and further respiratory support should be provided as needed. Early transfusion may be necessary to prevent progressive problems because hypoxia will induce further sickling; partial or complete exchange transfusion may be needed (Charache, Lubin, and Reid, 1992).

One episode of acute chest syndrome promotes another with progressive lung scarring and pulmonary hypertension (Castro et al, 1994). Because there are no clear clinical or laboratory parameters that differentiate between vasoocclusive disease and pneumonia, the primary care provider should empirically use antibiotics directed against *S. pneumonae* and other pathogens commonly seen in community-acquired pneumonia (Haynes and Kirkpatrick, 1993).

Aplastic Crisis

Periodically the bone marrow does not respond to a fall in hemoglobin and hematocrit values caused by the rapid turnover of RBCs. The hemoglobin and hematocrit values drop, and there is a lack of compensatory rise in the reticulocyte count. This usually happens during or following a viral infection. Human parvovirus B19 has been implicated in most aplastic crises in this population (Sergeant et al, 1993). Children being cared for during a viral illness should be observed for unusual pallor or prolonged lethargy in the face of improvement of other viral symptoms. Therapy includes slow transfusion to a hemoglobin level slightly above the baseline hemoglobin level. Recovery is indicated by a return of reticulocytosis.

Hemolysis

Hemolysis in sickle cell disease is usually of only moderate severity. The symptoms of anemia (pallor, fatigue, dyspnea) are not the hallmark of this disease. Long-term consequences of hemolysis are a high prevalence of gallstones and jaundice (Embury et al, 1994). Increased hemolysis may be triggered by bacterial infections, poisons, or glucose 6-phosphate dehydrogenase (G6PD) deficiency. Hemolysis accompanied by a brisk reticulocytosis requires no treatment.

Renal Problems

The environment within the renal medulla is characterized by low oxygen tension, acidosis, and hypertonicity. As such, intravascular sickling occurs more rapidly in the kidney than in any other organ. This leaves the kidney with a relative inability to concentrate urine (hyposthenuria) or adequately acidify the urine. The relative inability to concentrate urine often leads to enuresis or nocturia. It also results in a relative inability to excrete potassium and uric acid. Gross hematuria may occur in children with sickle cell disease or sickle trait. As with all individuals who have gross hematuria, glomerulonephritis, tumor, renal stones, urinary tract infection, and bleeding disorders need to be excluded. When other diagnoses have been eliminated, hematuria is often attributed to areas of ischemia or necrosis caused by sickled cells (Charache, Lubin, and Reid, 1992).

Priapism

Males with sickle cell anemia are subject to episodes of priapism. Priapism occurs when an accumulation of sickled cells obstructs the venous drainage of the corpora cavernosa of the penis, causing a prolonged and exquisitely painful erection of the penis. Priapism is not associated with sexual desire or excitement. In addition, micturition is often difficult and urinary retention may occur.

One study revealed a history of at least one episode of priapism in 42% of males with sickle cell anemia, with a median onset age of 21 years. Priapism may be seen in boys as young as 7 years. Four general patterns of priapism are described:

1. Recurrent, the "short studdering" attacks lasting <3 hours, several times a week, lasting >4 weeks.
2. Acute "major" attacks lasting >24 hours, followed by partial or complete impotence.
3. Chronic, persistent, usually painless enlargement or induration which persists weeks to years. This pattern develops following a major episode and is associated with partial or complete impotence.
4. Acute-on-chronic priapism is a chronic induration with a superimposed acute attack. This attack may affect only part of the penile shaft (Hakim, Hashmat, and Macchia, 1994).

Treatment of major episodes begins with conservative measures. These include hospitalization, hydration, transfusions, and pain management. Surgical intervention is considered if there is no detumescence after 12 to 24 hours of conservative treatment (Hakim, Hashmat, and Macchia, 1994). Surgical measures aim at the reestablishment of adequate venous outflow and circulation of the corporal body via placement of a shunt. Newer prophylactic regimens include the addition of vasodilatory drugs including hydrolazine and pentoxifylline, calcium channel blockers such as Verapamil, and 6-month transfusion programs. All have been clinically efficacious. (Hakim, Hashmat, and Macchia, 1994).

Skeletal Changes

Skeletal changes as a result of expansion of the bone marrow and recurrent infarction are often seen in children with sickle cell disease. Repeated infarction may lead to avascular necrosis. This most commonly involves the femoral head but may also occur in the head of the humerus or fibula. Treatment initially includes avoidance of weight bearing or bracing of the joint for up to 6 months. Judicious use of local heat and analgesics for pain relief may be employed. If pain persists along with radiographic progression, treatment consists of surgical core decompression of the femoral head. A newer technique, the injection of acrylic cement, has been used to restore the sphericity of the femoral head (Hernigan, Bachir, and Galacteros, 1993). Both of these procedures are seen as temporary measures to forestall an eventual total hip replacement.

Ophthalmologic Changes

Ophthalmologic complications are a direct result of the vasoocclusive process within the eye. These complications include nonproliferative retinopathy, proliferative retinopathy, or elevated intraocular pressure in the presence of hyphema. Nonproliferative retinopathy may not affect visual acuity. Proliferative sickle retinopathy can cause vitreous hemorrhage and subsequent retinal detachment and blindness. The incidence of proliferative sickle retinopathy is dependent on the person's age and type of hemoglobinopathy. It generally begins in the second decade, and increases. It is more common in people with Hgb SC but also occurs in other forms of sickle cell disease. Individuals with sickle hemoglobinopathies who sustain blunt trauma and subsequent hyphema to the eye may quickly develop increased intraocular pressure, which is an ophthalmologic emergency (Charache, Lubin, and Reid, 1992).

Audiologic Problems

Vasoocclusive episodes within the circulation of the inner ear may cause sensorineural hearing loss. This loss may be unilateral or bilateral; it is generally manifested as a high-frequency deficit. Compared to age-matched controls, 22% of children with sickle cell disease as compared to 4% of controls had predominantly high-frequency hearing loss (Adams, 1994).

Leg Ulcers

Leg ulcers are experienced by a significant number of older children and adults with sickle cell disease but have also been reported in children as young as 10 years (Phillips, Eckman, and Hebbel, 1994). The ulcers usually begin as a bite or scratch on the lower portion of the leg or the medial or lateral side of the ankle. The ulcers typically form a shallow depression with a smooth and slightly elevated margin and often have a surrounding area of edema. Bacteria are virtually always recovered from the base of the ulcer. Although this may represent colonization of devitalized tissue, clinical observation suggests that infection contributes to enlargement and maintenance of ulcers (Phillips, Eckman, and Hebbel, 1994). Ulcers can produce significant pain and limitation of movement. The ulcers may take 6 weeks to 6 months to heal. Early, prompt treatment includes bed rest, elevation, and wound care with antibiotics for cellulitic areas; skin grafting and transfusion therapy may be needed. The specific type of wound care is controversial and should be directed by a consultant plastic surgeon. Recurrence is very common and most often results from noncompliance with treatment (Earles and Dorn, 1994).

Preparation for Anesthesia or Contrast Medium

General anesthesia and hyperosmolar contrast medium are both known to induce sickling. If an operative or diagnostic procedure using these agents is anticipated, many primary care providers suggest that the child with sickle cell disease receive repeated transfusions until the percentage of circulating Hgb S is less than 30%. Preliminary reports from the Preoperative Transfusion Safety Study group of the CSSCD suggest a higher level of Hgb S is well tolerated, imposing no excessive risk (Vichinsky, 1995).

Cardiac Problems

Over time the cardiovascular system accommodates to chronic anemia. Cardiac enlargement is often apparent on chest radiograph and a low-grade systolic ejection murmur is often found. Several studies of children and adolescents document a physical work capacity of 60% to 70% of normal. Cardiac output at rest is abnormal. ST depression occurs during exercise in 15% of children with sickle cell disease suggesting endocardial ischemia (Covitz, 1994).

Hepatobiliary Problems

The ongoing elevated rate of RBC hemolysis generates an increase in bilirubin load for metabolism. An elevation of the serum alkaline phosphatase and lactic dehydrogenase levels as a result of bone metabolism and hemolysis is frequently seen. Gallstones made of bile or calcium bilirubinate are a common finding and are easily visualized by ultrasound. They are found in 14% to 30% of children with sickle cell disease and are most common in individuals with Hgb SS (Charache, Lubin, and Reid, 1992).

Surgeons should be aware of the finding that concomitant common bile duct (CBD) stones have been reported in individuals with sickle cell disease and cholethiasis. Both laproscopic and open cholecystectomies are approved for individuals with sickle cell disease.

Transfusion Complications

Individuals with sickle cell disease may need transfusions emergently, episodically, or chronically. The complications of transfusion include possible exposure to bloodborne infectious agents, formation of alloantibodies, and, with chronic or multiple transfusion, iron overload. Individuals with iron overload experience progressive organ dysfunction. Iron chelation with desferoxamine SQ or IV is a difficult process. An efficient, easily administered chelating agent does not currently exist. Oral chelators are currently under investigation (Collins et al, 1994). Several centers have been successful in re-

cruiting minority donors for extended matching for red cell antigens. This practice has markedly decreased the occurrence of alloimmunization and should be the standard for chronically transfused clients (Vichinsky, 1994).

PROGNOSIS

In a classic study done 20 years ago, a group of adults and children was followed longitudinally to determine the natural history of sickle cell disease. It was determined that the disease effects in the adult tended to be chronic and organ related and that the problems during childhood were acute and often infectious. Overall there was a 10% expected death rate during the first decade of life and 5% or less during any subsequent decade (Powars, 1975).

In a large prospective study that followed nearly 3000 children and adolescents for varying periods of time, the following information was obtained:

1. For all hemoglobinopathies the proportion of individuals expected to survive to age 20 years was approximately 89%.
2. Most of the deaths were in children with Hgb SS.
3. Peak incidence of death was between 1 and 3 years of age.
4. The major cause of death in children aged 1 to 3 years was infection.
5. In children greater than 10 years of age, cerebrovascular accident (CVA) and traumatic events were the major causes of death.
6. The survival of children with sickle cell disease is improving (Leikin et al, 1989).

Because of penicillin prophylaxis, mortality for children with sickle cell disease in the first decade of life has decreased from 10% to 1% (Vickinsky, 1991). At least 90% of children with sickle cell anemia are expected to survive into the third decade. As early intervention decreases or eliminates deaths from sepsis, acute sequestration, and acute chest syndrome, the primary issue will be chronic organ damage, notably renal, neurologic, and pulmonary changes.

The decrease in morbidity and mortality has occurred because of the implementation of four principles of comprehensive care:

1. Early diagnosis
2. Preventive health maintenance

3. Early treatment of life-threatening complications

4. Development and implementation of new treatment modalities

Mortality studies further point to increased deaths from infection in children with sickle cell disease in all age groups. Zarkowsky and associates (1986) reporting for the CSSCD confirmed these observations and showed a difference in morbidity between the two most common genotypes, Hgb SS and Hgb SC. Apparently, longer retention of splenic function spared children with SC disease from increased susceptibility to sepsis.

This striking variability between genotypes provides one example of the variable presentation of symptoms and complications which should be considered by the primary care provider. All children with a given genotype (i.e., SS) will present with neither the same symptoms nor the same frequency. Thalassemia is reported to have lower rates of complications and mortality in children who inherit this genetic variant. The β-globin gene cluster haptotype reported by Powers and associates (1994) further modifies the severity of the disorder.

It is now known that 20% of all children with Hgb SS will develop the severe form of the disease characterized by frequent pain crises and ultimate end-organ damage; 40% will display moderate symptomatology. In addition, preliminary data suggest that there may be different prognostic factors for each adverse effect (Piomelli, 1991).

Primary Care Management
HEALTH CARE MAINTENANCE

Growth and Development

Children with sickle cell disease, when matched with controls of similar socioeconomic status, have comparable physical parameters at birth, including weight, length, and head circumference, as well as similar 1-minute and 5-minute Apgar scores. Beginning at approximately 6 months of age, and clearly defined by the preschool years, these children demonstrate a pattern of physical growth that is divergent from that of their nonaffected peers. They are shorter, weigh less, have a smaller percentage of body fat, and have delayed bone age. Muscle mass and head circumference, however, remain comparable with that of their nonaffected peers. Weight is affected more than height, and males are affected more than females. These studies have been repeated with similar findings (Modege and Ifenu, 1993).

These changes are coincident with the usual physiologic waning of fetal hemoglobin levels. It has also been noted that children who, for unknown reasons, persist in producing fetal hemoglobin are usually not as growth retarded as other children with sickle cell disease. Studies finding deficient nutritional intake as a cause of growth delay are sparse. Clients receiving chronic transfusions, however, show significant growth, suggesting a major role of hemolytic anemia in growth retardation in children with sickle cell anemia (Mankad, 1992).

As with standard well-child care, physical growth parameters should be measured and plotted on standardized growth charts at regular intervals. If the pattern of growth begins to plateau or become otherwise abnormal, serial measurements should be obtained more frequently; however, the pattern of growth on their curve is more important than comparison with unaffected children.

Researchers in the psychosocial sciences have long studied the child with sickle cell disease in order to obtain relational information regarding learning abilities, coping skills, anxiety, and self-concept (Hurtig, Koepke, and Park, 1989). Modifying variables such as social supports, socioeconomic status, family structure, education, beliefs, and developmental stage all impact on the child's psychologic adjustment (Midence, Fuggle, and Davies, 1993). Most studies report that children with SCD are well adjusted but vulnerable to experiencing psychosocial difficulties. A benchmark study by Swift and associates (1989) suggested that children with sickle cell anemia had some degree of cognitive impairment but that academic achievement was comparable with intellectual ability. This study examined children aged 7 through 16 years without history of strokes. The data suggest that the onset of impairment occurred before 7 years of age.

Wang and associates (1993) attempted to assess development in children less than 3 years of age as part of the CSSCD. Their data suggest that development is relatively normal before age 3 and that deficits seen in older children may reflect subsequent ischemic events.

Beyond the expected significant psychosocial and intellectual deficits experienced by those children with a history of stroke, researchers are now focusing on the incidence of subclinical deficits resulting from cerebral microvascular occlusion that are not apparent on routine neurologic examinations (Wasserman et al, 1991). Results thus far indicate impairment with fine and visual motor tasks and with short-term memory skills. PET scanners reveal significantly altered frontal lobe metabolism compared with healthy controls (Treadwell and Gil, 1994).

Standardized tools such as the Denver Developmental Screening Test II are helpful when screening for developmental delay. Children found to be at developmental risk should be referred for a more thorough developmental assessment. The involvement of a consistent caregiver and the caregiver's rapport with a consistent health care provider are invaluable tools for monitoring developmental progress in the child with sickle cell disease.

Diet

The child's diet should be well balanced with a generous amount of fluid. Diet during illness or disease exacerbation may include whatever healthy solid foods the child desires with oral fluids at 1½ times his or her usual fluid intake. Maintenance of daily fluid intake is essential in maintaining homeostasis in the child with sickle cell disease. A fluid sheet, outlining times to increase fluids and amounts of oral fluids to be given, provides a handy reference to parents. (See box on fluid requirements.)

Metabolic studies on subjects with sickle cell disease are few but the available ones support the hypothesis that the chronic hemolysis of SCD leads to a state of high protein turnover and increased basal metabolic rate (Gee and Platt, 1994).

Safety

Most children with sickle cell anemia regularly take oral medicines at home, such as folic acid, antibiotics, and narcotics. Ingestion of narcotics could lead to lethargy and respiratory depression or death. All medicines should be safely stored. Adolescents should be cautioned about driving a car or using machinery while taking narcotics and that substances such as alcohol may potentiate the depressant effects of narcotics. Alcohol should also

be avoided because it can cause dehydration and subsequent sickling. Smoking is strongly discouraged as it leads to vasoconstriction and with it concomminant problems.

Recreational activities that involve prolonged exposure to cold, prolonged exertion, or exposure to high altitudes (>10,000 feet) in an unpressurized aircraft should be avoided. Sports injuries should not be treated with ice, because this can cause localized sickling. Adolescents with sickle cell disease often demonstrate the same limit-testing and risk-taking behaviors as other adolescents. Parents must balance their child's need for safety with the child's need to become self-sufficient. An information card or Medic-Alert bracelet is often helpful in emergency situations.

CHILDREN'S CENTER FOR CANCER AND BLOOD DISORDERS SICKLE CELL FLUID REQUIREMENTS

Your child needs more fluids when:
1. He/she has a *fever*
2. He/she has *pain*
3. It's hot *outside*
4. He/she is very *active*
5. He/she is *traveling*

Amount of clear fluids your child needs each day during special times

Child's weight	Number of 8 oz cups per day
10 lb	2 cups
15 lb	3 cups
20 lb	4 cups
25 lb	5 cups
30 lb	5-6 cups
35 lb	6-7 cups
40 lb	7 cups
50 lb	8 cups
60 lb	9 cups
More than 60 lb	10 or more cups

Adapted from "A Parent's Handbook for Sickle Cell Disease (Birth to 6 Years)," National Maternal and Child Health Clearinghouse, 1991.

Immunizations

The conventional schedule may be used for diphtheria-pertussis-tetanus (DPT) vaccine, oral poliomyelitis vaccine (OPV), measles-mumps-rubella (MMR) vaccine, varicella vaccine, and Hib vaccine. The risk of developing invasive *H. influenzae* type b disease is higher for children with sickle cell disease than for unaffected children (American Academy of Pediatrics, 1994). It is important to note that children younger than 6 years of age with sickle cell disease may not develop a reliably immunogenic response to the Hib vaccine (Vichinsky, 1991); therefore, even an immunized child may be vulnerable to infection by this organism.

Protection against hepatitis B is now recommended for all infants born in the United States (American Academy of Pediatrics, 1994). This has not been fully implemented because of lack of resources. Most pediatric hematologists, however, strongly recommend it for children with sickle cell disease because of the empirical risk of infection through blood transfusions (Vichinsky, 1991).

Pneumococcal vaccine (Pneumovax) should be given at age 2 years to all children with sickle cell disease; booster immunization should be given every 3 to 5 years (Wong et al, 1992). It is important to emphasize that even with vigilant immunization and antibiotic prophylaxis, episodes of pneumococcal septicemia have occurred (Vichinsky, 1991). Pneumovax may be given concurrently with the DPT, OPV, and Hib vaccine.

Children with hemoglobinopathies are identified as being at risk for influenza-related complications. Also, children with sickle cell disease are known to be at high risk for bacterial infection, and this risk could be further raised by concurrent viral infection (Vichinsky, 1991). Therefore it is recommended that all children with sickle cell disease receive influenza vaccine on an annual basis. During epidemics of common childhood viral infections, such as respiratory syncytial virus and rotavirus, the child with sickle cell anemia appears to have no increased risk for infection but does appear to have a more severe and protracted course (Powars, 1994).

Opinions regarding the use of meningococcal vaccine are divergent. Some centers suggest administering the vaccine to children more than 2 years of age, but this is not uniform among all comprehensive care centers. The American Academy of Pediatrics (1994) recommends the meningococcal vaccine for all clients with asplenia.

Screening

Vision. During the first decade of life, the child with sickle cell disease requires routine screening. Thereafter the child needs an annual retinal examination by an ophthalmologist to screen for sickle retinopathy.

Hearing. Yearly audiologic evaluations are optimal to screen for hearing loss related to vasoocclusion or hyperviscosity in the inner ear. Sensorineural hearing loss (SNHL) has been well described in this population (Adams, 1994).

Dental. Routine screening is recommended.

Blood pressure. Blood pressure should be measured every year after 2 years of age. Hypertension, although common in African Americans living in the United States, is uncommon in clients with sickle cell disease. The reason for this is unclear. Most clients will have blood pressures lower than unaffected persons in all age groups (Falk and Jennette, 1994).

Hematocrit. Routine hematocrit testing is deferred because a CBC and reticulocyte count is required every 4 to 6 months.

Urinalysis. Routine urinalysis is deferred because of annual renal function testing.

Tuberculosis. Routine screening is recommended.

Condition-specific screening

HEMATOLOGIC SCREENING. A CBC with differential, RBC smear, and reticulocyte count is useful in establishing baseline data and ascertaining bone marrow function. Determining the RBC phenotype and alloantibodies of a well child who has not had a transfusion is very useful to possibly expedite any future transfusions. Repeat quantitative hemoglobin electrophoresis testing at age 5 to 7 years records nadir levels of Hgb F (Rodgers, 1994). Some comprehensive sickle cell centers test at this time in order to correlate Hgb F levels with clinical severity.

RENAL FUNCTION TESTING. A urinalysis should be done and the blood urea nitrogen (BUN) and creatinine levels checked annually after age 3 years to monitor renal function. An inability to concentrate or to acidify urine may be demonstrated in the urinalysis and would be commonly seen in children with sickle cell disease. Urobilinogen, as a by-product of bilirubin metabolism, would also be a frequent finding. Hematuria may be a manifestation of renal dysfunction secondary to sickle cell disease or other, unrelated, pathologic condition. The child should be referred to a nephrologist for further evaluation and treatment if the hematuria is severe or if casts are present in the urine. Proteinuria is the most common clinical manifestation of glomerular injury to the kidney (Falk and Jennette, 1994). Follow-up requires a urine culture and sensitivity, and if negative, a 24-hour collection of urine for protein quantitation. An elevation requires referral to a nephrologist.

LEAD POISONING. Determining erythrocyte protoporphyrin (EP) levels to screen children who may be at high risk for lead intoxication is not valid for children with sickle cell disease. Total EP levels may be elevated with iron deficiency, lead intoxication, or reticulocytosis. In a child with sickle cell disease, an elevated EP level may reflect the process of accelerated reticulocytosis rather than lead intoxication. Rajkumar and associates (1995) concluded that FEP levels are elevated in children with sickle cell disease even in the absence of iron deficiency or lead poisoning. Furthermore, children with Hgb SS have significantly higher FEP as compared with children with Hgb SC, suggesting that higher rates of hemolysis may contribute to higher levels of FEP.

SCOLIOSIS. Scoliosis screening should be done through late adolescence because of the delayed growth spurt of the child with sickle cell disease.

CARDIAC FUNCTION. Electrocardiography (ECG) and echocardiography (ECHO) should be performed every 1 to 2 years to evaluate the impact of chronic anemia on ventricular function. Efforts should be made to establish whether symptoms of chest pain, dyspnea, or decreased exercise tolerance have occurred and significant symptoms should be evaluated with exercise testing (Covitz, 1994).

LIVER FUNCTION. Yearly liver function studies are helpful to evaluate RBC metabolism and liver function. Bilirubin is often elevated as a consequence of hemolysis as well as liver disease. Bilirubin levels rise gradually until the third decade. Alkaline phosphatase levels fall after periods of most rapid growth in adolescence and reach lower levels in females than in males (Steinburg, 1994b).

COMMON ILLNESS MANAGEMENT

Differential Diagnosis

Infections. As a result of functional asplenia, bacterial infection is a significant cause of morbidity and mortality in children with sickle cell disease. The incidence of bacteremia in children with sickle cell disease is highest among those less than 2 years of age, and it declines from age 2 to 6 years. The most common pathogen in children younger than 6 years is *Streptococcus pneumoniae*. Antibiotic resistance to *S. Pneumoniae* has been reported (Pegelow et al, 1991). Some children with sickle cell disease have cultured *S. Pneumoniae* from the tonsilar beds despite appropriate doses of prophylactic penicillin. Therefore, the caregiver must be alert to these exceptions and monitor antibiotic effectiveness closely. The course of *S. pneumoniae* sepsis is often fulminant, with mortality reaching 24% to 50%. *Escherichia coli* bacteremia is often associated with urinary tract infection and *Salmonella* bacteremia with osteomyelitis (Buchanan, 1994).

Fever is a common finding during vasoocclusive episodes, as well as during infectious episodes. There is no test or diagnostic tool to differentiate fever of an infectious origin from fever that results from inflammation secondary to infarction. Again, the primary care provider must be aware of the fact that the child may have two independent problems (e.g., infection and vasoocclusion) and both require aggressive treatment and management.

A child less than 5 years of age who has a low-grade temperature elevation (<38.5° C) may be given appropriate antibiotic coverage and treated as an outpatient, provided a probable cause of temperature elevation can be identified and the child is stable and looks well clinically. There should be a careful follow-up by a clinic visit in 24 and 48 hours.

Current treatment consists of prompt assessment of the child, followed by blood and urine cultures and administration of ceftriaxone. This drug has a half-life of 6 hours and effective bacteriacidal levels persist for 24 hours following a single dose (Buchanan, 1994). Children who appear toxic, who have an extremely high fever, who have an unreliable caretaker, or to whom close outpatient follow-up is not possible should be hospitalized (Wilimas et al, 1993).

Fever is usually high with septicemia, but in 20% of cases studied, the fever was less than 39° C (Buchanan, 1994). All children with sickle cell disease should be considered at risk for fatal sepsis regardless of the fact that they are on penicillin prophylaxis and have received pneumnococcal vaccination.

An aggressive search for the cause should include a CBC count, blood culture, urinalysis, urine culture, chest radiograph, and possibly sinus radiographs. Lumbar puncture should be performed if meningitis is suspected.

In children older than 5 years of age with temperatures more than 38.5° C, an aggressive search for the likely cause should be undertaken and antibiotics administered. The location of treatment, inpatient or outpatient, should depend on the following: the child's clinical condition, anticipated compliance with therapy, and ability to obtain follow-up over the upcoming 24 to 72 hours (Charache, Lubin, and Reid, 1992).

Even common infections such as otitis media or sinusitis may precipitate a vasoocclusive crisis if fluid intake is reduced and dehydration and acidosis result. During periods of illness, the child must be assessed frequently for early signs of crisis. Maintaining fluid intake and controlling fever are critical.

Urinary tract infections. Asymptomatic bacteriuria, symptomatic urinary tract infection, and pyelonephritis occur much more commonly in individuals with sickle cell disease than in the general population. In the presence of urinary tract infection or pyelonephritis, the child should have a blood culture obtained because bacteremia is present in at least 50% of those with urinary tract infection. Appropriate antibiotic therapy should be instituted and adequate follow-up arranged. Follow-up should include a repeat culture. Further diagnostic studies such as renal ultrasound or voiding cystourethrogram should be done to exclude treatable conditions in children with pyelonephritis or recurrent urinary tract infection.

Orthopedic symptoms. Areas of bone infarction may be easily confused with osteomyelitis or rheumatologic disorders. Even after the diagnosis of sickle cell disease is made, it is important to differentiate areas of infarction from areas of infection because children with sickle cell disease have an increased incidence of osteomyelitis. In both pathologic processes the child may have an elevated white blood cell count, fever, and equivocal x-ray findings. Osteomyelitis, however, is more often associated with an increased number of immature granulocytes, bacteremia, and a purulent joint aspirate. Bone scans may be useful in differentiating osteomyelitis from areas of bone infarction. Bone marrow scans have also been used to further discriminate between areas of infection and infarction, especially when the bone scan is equivocal. Opinions regarding the use of the bone marrow scan are somewhat divergent, however, and are largely dependent on the level of expertise available at a given facility.

Lee, Churchill, and Bridges (1995) report confirmation of bone marrow infarction by magnetic resonance imaging (MRI). Normal adult marrow is fatty and has high intensity on T1 images; however, marrow from individuals with sickle cell disease are hematopoetically active and isointense or low intensity on T1 weighted images. MRI scans of extremities with bone marrow infarction show hyperintense signal on T2 weighted images from liquefaction on normally hematopoetic marrow (Lee, Churchill, and Bridges, 1995). MRI now offers a technique to objectively evaluate the extent of bone marrow infarction. Application of this technique to children has not been determined.

Acute gastroenteritis. Vomiting and diarrhea must be carefully evaluated and managed in children with sickle cell disease because these children lack the ability to concentrate urine to compensate for decreased fluid intake or excess losses. Significant dehydration may occur quickly and lead to metabolic acidosis and sickling. If the child's oral fluid intake is less than that needed to maintain hydration, the child must receive IV hydration, often as an inpatient.

Abdominal pain. Episodes of infarction of the abdominal organs such as the liver, spleen, and abdominal lymph nodes occur and may be quite painful. It is important to differentiate these abdominal crises from those problems that would require surgical intervention, such as appendicitis.

Abdominal pain and cramps found commonly in young children are possibly related to mesenteric ischemia (Scott-Conner and Brunson, 1994). Normal bowel sounds and lack of ileus support nonoperative management, with adequate pain control. The duration may last days to weeks, with fluctuations in the severity of the pain.

Achord (1994) states that paralytic ileus is common during acute abdominal pain, making the diagnosis problematic. Right upper quadrant pain creates further complications, because intrahepatic sickling mimics cholecystitis (Scott-Conner and Brunson, 1994). Neither ultrasound nor laboratory values aid in defining the process. Leukocytosis of 30,000 can be seen with both infarction and infection. Most children find that their sickle cell pain has a unique quality or character and they are often able to report whether or not their pain is typical of vasoocclusive pain. Deviation from a characteristic pattern, lower abdominal pain with persistent local tenderness, and symptoms lasting several hours suggest a surgical problem (Scott-Conner, 1994).

Anemia. Virtually all children with sickle cell disease are anemic at baseline. Periodically a child with sickle cell disease may have acute lethargy and pallor. A CBC and reticulocyte count should be obtained. If these reveal a significant drop in the hemoglobin and hematocrit levels, the child is likely experiencing an aplastic crisis or splenic sequestration. Usually a fall in the hemoglobin and hematocrit values serves as a stimulus to the bone marrow, which then produces new RBCs in the form of reticulocytes. If the reticulocyte count is low in the presence of low hemoglobin and hematocrit levels, the child is experiencing an aplastic crisis. If the child has an enlarged spleen, pallor, lethargy and an associated drop in hemoglobin, he or she is likely to be experiencing splenic sequestration. Regardless of exact diagnosis, the child will require immediate hospitalization, with close observation and transfusion.

Respiratory distress. Increased respiratory rate and effort, chest pain, fever, rales, and dullness to percussion may indicate pneumonia or acute chest syndrome. Infiltrates on chest radiograph may reflect either process. With acute chest syndrome the chest radiograph may be clear in the first few days; a pleural effusion is frequently seen. The child should receive antibiotics, hydration, analgesics, and oxygen as needed. Transfusion or partial exchange transfusion may be indicated, de-

pending on the degree of respiratory distress. This is a medical emergency and demands hospitalization.

Neurologic changes. The child who has a seizure, hemiparesis, or changes in speech, gait, level of consciousness, or blurry or double vision should have expedient neurologic and radiologic evaluation for the presence of stroke. This is a medical emergency and requires exchange transfusion as soon as possible.

Drug Interactions

Antihistamines and barbiturates given concurrently with narcotics may cause respiratory depression, hypoxia, and further sickling. Diuretics and some bronchodilators, which have a diuretic effect, may cause dehydration and sickling. They should be used with caution in children with sickle cell disease.

DEVELOPMENTAL ISSUES

Sleep Patterns

Because of chronic anemia, some children with sickle cell disease may fatigue more easily than their nonaffected peers and may desire extra sleep. Parents often report that their child with sickle cell disease naps after coming home from school. This routine can be encouraged.

Toileting

Toilet training should be initiated using the conventional guidelines to assess readiness for training. Bowel training usually progresses without difficulty. Bladder training, however, must take into account the fact that many children with sickle cell disease have difficulty concentrating urine and thus produce a large volume of dilute urine. They may need to be given the opportunity to use the bathroom every 2 to 3 hours during the day. Primary enuresis often occurs in young children and it is not uncommon for it to continue into the teenage years. It is especially troublesome when the child requires extra fluids during a vasoocclusive episode. Some children who previously achieve nighttime continence may develop secondary enuresis as subtle insults to the kidney occur. Typically, a pattern of enuresis emerges as the child begins having more "wet" nights than "dry" nights. This may be reflective of the gradual loss of the kidneys to concentrate urine, although there are no published reports of this phenomenon. Daytime continence is unaffected by these renal changes.

Routine counseling regarding enuresis should be offered. Young children may initially use diapers. By the time the child reaches preschool or school age, however, the use of diapers will often adversely affect the child's self-esteem and sense of mastery. Many families choose to wake the child once or twice during the night to urinate, but severe restriction of fluids is not wise because hydration needs must be met. Careful questioning by the primary care provider may point to a subclinical infectious process that can be treated.

Discipline

The expectations regarding the behavior of children with sickle cell disease should vary little from the expectations held for their siblings or peers. These expectations should be clear and as consistent as possible. Likewise, parents should strive to make discipline fair and consistent. Many parents are fearful of disciplining or setting limits for their children with sickle cell disease, especially because emotional stress is thought to possibly precipitate vasoocclusive crisis. The primary care provider can point out to parents that a lack of or inconsistency in setting limits may, in fact, be more stressful to the child than consistently setting limits. It is also important to encourage parents to note which behaviors the child demonstrates consistently when in pain, such as a certain pitch to his or her cry, a change in activity level, or changes in appetite. This will help parents discriminate episodes of pain from episodes when they are being manipulated.

Child Care

Children with sickle cell disease can participate in normal day care centers, although small group or home-centered day care may be preferable because it provides less exposure to infections. The caregiver will need to be informed of the child's need for extra fluids and need to void frequently. They may also need to administer medications during day care hours and must be instructed in this regard. The caregiver must be able to contact the parent or seek medical care for the child quickly in the event of fever, severely painful vasoocclusive crises, respiratory distress, or stroke, because these events may be life threatening.

Schooling

Parents are encouraged to meet with school officials before the beginning of each school year. This affords an opportunity to communicate about the usual symptoms the child has relative to sickle cell disease. It further allows for a plan to be developed about absences, make-up work, intermittent homebound study (if necessary), and transfer of assignments from school to the home.

Many primary care providers play an active role in educating school officials about the needs of children with sickle cell disease. Some will visit schools and give presentations while others will provide written materials (see resource list at the end of this chapter). The needs for adequate hydration, frequent bathroom breaks, rest, physical education, and appropriate dress are all subject for discussion by the health care team. School officials in turn, can provide information about learning abilities and behavior. This open exchange of information goes a long way in ensuring a successful school year for the student. Knowing whom to call when the parents cannot be reached reduces anxiety on the part of school staff (Earles and Dorn, 1994).

Children with sickle cell disease who have had strokes should be referred for an individualized education plan (IEP). Children with splenomegaly should be cautioned about the risks of injury with contact sports. Modified physical education classes should be offered to keep the child engaged in group activities, which are important in over-all adjustment and well-being. Finally, schools should be counseled about the needs of children affected with chronic orthopedic problems, such as osteomyelitis or avascular necrosis of the femoral head. These children may need additional time to get to classes, or may need to obtain an elevator key during times of bone healing.

Sexuality

Children with sickle cell disease progress through the Tanner stages in an orderly and consistent manner but usually experience puberty several years later than their peers. This can have significant adverse effects on the adolescent's self-concept. Once sexual maturation has occurred, fertility and contraception become important issues that must be addressed by the primary care provider.

For men, impotence is often a problem following a major episode of priapism. For female adolescents, menarche is often delayed by 2 to 2½> years, but fertility is normal. Decisions regarding contraception must take into account the attitudes, lifestyle, and maturity of the adolescent, as well as the hematologic ramifications of the method chosen.

Various contraceptive choices are available to adolescents with sickle cell disease. These include all barrier forms of contraception such as condoms for men and foam, diaphragms, and sponges for women. Women may also use oral contraceptives, preferably those brands containing low levels of estrogen. Progesterone-only pills are useful; it is known that progestins stabilize the red cell membrane. Depo-provera has also been useful in this population (Hatcher, 1994; American College of Obstetricians and Gynecologists, 1995).

Adolescents with sickle cell disease should receive careful, repeated genetic counseling before puberty and during adolescence. They need to understand the pattern of transmission of sickle cell disease and the availability of testing for partners before conceiving a child.

Transition into Adulthood

Early vocational counseling should be offered to the adolescent with sickle cell disease. Consideration should be directed toward the adolescent's interests and intellectual abilities. Work in a climate-controlled environment is preferred over rigorous, outdoor work which might trigger a crisis. Sickle cell disease excludes a person from military service, so technical and academic training is encouraged. Many community-based sickle cell organizations offer scholarships for skilled and academic work. Contacting the Sickle Cell Disease Association of America, Inc can direct families to local resources.

Families should be counseled as to the progressive organ damage that develops as the child ages. Continuity of care by a knowledgeable primary care provider will afford the best quality of life and should be encouraged.

Persons with sickle cell disease may be uninsurable for life insurance and may face waiting periods for insurance. Local sickle cell chapters can counsel such persons regarding options and resources.

SPECIAL FAMILY CONCERNS AND RESOURCES

The families of children with sickle cell disease experience the same psychologic ramifications as do other families of children with chronic conditions. They bear the additional burden of knowing that this disease is genetically transmitted; this knowledge can prompt feelings of overwhelming guilt and responsibility. Exacerbations of the condition often occur without provocation, prompting feelings of helplessness. Many manifestations of the condition are not objectively visible or measurable; therefore, children with sickle cell disease can appear to be well when they are potentially extremely ill. Many parents are fearful that the therapeutic effects of narcotics and blood transfusions will be outweighed by their potentially deleterious effects.

Genetic counseling should be offered to the parents of a child with sickle cell disease at the time of the child's diagnosis and when subsequent pregnancies are contemplated. It is also recommended that the child's siblings be screened to determine their carrier status. The child with sickle cell disease and his or her family incorporates values, attitudes, and beliefs of the "all-American" society while retaining parts of his or her own family's traditional beliefs and practices. Culture cannot be generalized within the entity of sickle cell disease. Beyond the native African-American population, permeations of sickle hemoglobinopathies are found in Hispanics, Central Americans, Greeks, Arabics, Orientals, and Caribbean natives. Each will bring their own view of health, coping, and wellness. The primary care provider must be mindful of these differences within and between cultures. Expections of survival affect both the immediate care the child receives and the amount of effort expended in future care and education (Groce and Zola, 1993). Emphasis should focus on different strengths families bring with them. For example, extended family support is a dominant feature in the African-American community and should be utilized during crisis episodes. Strong church affiliations offer consolation and hope leading to greater acceptance and improved quality of life.

Persons espousing Jehovah's Witness religion will deny blood transfusions to their children, placing stress on the primary care provider. Sensitive, open communication, along with vigilant intensive care management (ICU), may prevent the need for transfusions and thereby support the religious beliefs of the family.

Instructions should be delivered to the head of the household. In contrast to the matriarchal leadership found in many African-American households, Muslin families center their decision making on the father or male head of the household. In all instances, it is best to consult members of a particular ethnic or minority group when actions or choices conflict with those of the medical care team.

Resources

A Brighter Heritage (video, 17 min)
Mississippi State Department of Health
Genetics Division
2423 N State St
PO Box 1700
Jackson, MS 39215 601/960-7619

A Parents' Handbook for Sickle Cell Disease, Part I: Birth to 6 Years, Part II: 6 to 18 years
National Maternal and Child Health Clearinghouse
8201 Greensboro Dr.
McLean, VA 22102

So I have the sickle cell trait (Cat No B050)
National Maternal and Child Health Clearinghouse
2070 Chain Bridge Rd
Suite 450
Vienna, VA 22182/703/821-8955
Help (resource book, listing sources of care for patients with sickle cell disease in the United States, Puerto Rico, and the Virgin Islands)
Sickle Cell Disease—How to help your child to take it in stride
A Parent/Teacher guide
Viewpoints
Also available: Brochures on recent advances, newsletter on chapter activities, fact sheets, and brochures on sickle cell trait, anemia and other topics, home study kit, games, and a video on parenting.
National Association for Sickle Cell Disease, Inc
200 Corporate Pointe, Suite 495
Culver City, CA 90230-7633
800/421-8453

Problem Oriented Management of Sickle Syndromes by James R. Eckman and Allen F. Platt, 1991
PO Box 109 Grady Memorial Hospital
80 Butler St SE
Atlanta, GA 30335 404/616-3572

Sickle Cell Disease Guideline Panel: Sickle cell disease: screening, diagnosis, management, and counseling in newborns and infants. Clinical Practice Guideline No 6 (AHCPR Publication No 93-0562). Rockville, MD, 1993, Agency for Health Care Policy and Research.

Thalassemia Information Sheet
Sickle Cell Anemia Public Health Information Sheet
March of Dimes
Birth Defects Foundation
1275 Mamaroneck Ave
White Plains, NY 10605

The Family Connection—Sickle Cell Trait (English, French, Spanish)
The Family Connection—Hemoglobin C Trait (English, French, Spanish)
Newborn Screening for Your Baby's Health (English, Spanish)
Directory of available sickle cell services in New York State
Sickle Cell Anemia
New York State Department of Health
Newborn Screening Program
Wadsworth Center for Laboratories and Research
PO Box 509
Albany, NY 12201-0509 518/473-7552

The Infant and Young Child with Sickle Cell Anemia, a guide for parents (in English and Spanish)
Pneumococcal Infection and Penicillin
So Your Baby has the Sickle Cell Trait (Spanish and English) Also available: brochures on sickle cell trait, sickle beta-thalassemia, hemoglobin C disease, pain in children, and various complications
Texas Department of Health
Newborn Screening Program
1100 W 49th St
Austin, TX 78756-3199 512/458-7000

Note: The above listings are not all inclusive. Additional material may be available from your own state or local health department, sickle cell agency, or community agency.

SUMMARY OF PRIMARY CARE NEEDS FOR THE CHILD WITH SICKLE CELL DISEASE

Health care maintenance

Growth and development

These children tend to weigh less and be shorter than their peers; weight is affected more than height, and males are affected more than females.

Puberty is delayed for both sexes.

Developmental impairment varies.

Diet

Diet should be well balanced with a generous amount of fluid; fluid intake should be increased during illness.

Safety

Ingestion of narcotics could lead to respiratory depression.

Alcohol may dehydrate and potentiate narcotics.

Narcotics may impair driving or safe use of machinery.

Recreational activities that involve prolonged exposure to cold, prolonged exertion, or exposure to high altitudes should be avoided. Ice should not be used to treat injuries.

A Medic-Alert bracelet may be helpful.

Immunizations

Routine standard immunizations are recommended.

Haemophilus influenzae type b vaccine is given at 2, 4, and 6 months; immunogenic response is not reliable.

Pneumococcal vaccine is given at 24 months, with boosters given every 3 to 5 years thereafter.

Hepatitis B vaccine is routine for infants and recommended for others.

Influenza vaccine given annually is strongly recommended.

Screening

Vision

Routine screening is recommended until 10 years of age, then an annual retinal examination is recommended to rule out sickle retinopathy.

Hearing

Yearly audiologic examination is recommended.

Dental

Routine screening is recommended.

Blood pressure

Blood pressure should be measured yearly after 2 years of age.

Hematocrit

Hematocrit is deferred because of condition-specific screening.

Urinalysis

Urinalysis is deferred because of condition-specific screening.

Tuberculosis

Routine screening is recommended.

Condition-specific screening

HEMATOLOGIC SCREENING

A CBC with differential, platelet count, reticulocyte count, and RBC smear should be checked every 4 to 6 months.

RENAL FUNCTION SCREENING

The BUN and creatinine levels should be checked and a urinalysis done on a yearly basis.

LEAD POISONING

Lead screening using the EP level is unreliable; the serum lead level must be determined.

SCOLIOSIS

Screening should be extended to the late teens because of delayed puberty.

CARDIAC FUNCTION

Both ECG and ECHO should be used every 1 to 2 years after age 5 years.

LIVER FUNCTION

Serum liver function tests should be done yearly. The gallbladder should be assessed using ultrasound every 2 years after age 10 and prn

Common illness management

Differential diagnosis

Infections

AGE 5 YEARS OR LESS

Temperature less than 38.5° C

Outpatient management may be considered if the source of the fever can be identified, appropriate antibiotics are given, and follow-up is ensured.

Temperature more than 38.5° C

Continued.

SUMMARY OF PRIMARY CARE NEEDS FOR THE CHILD WITH SICKLE CELL DISEASE—cont'd

Prompt assessment of the child; cultures taken; administration of Ceftriaxone IM or IV; reassessment in 24 and 48 hours

AGE 5 YEARS OR MORE

The child's condition, compliance with therapy, and ability to obtain follow-up determine whether or not the child should receive inpatient or outpatient care.

Urinary tract infections

Asymptomatic bacteriuria, UTI, and pyelonephritis more common with sickle cell.

Blood cultures should be done if UTI diagnosed to rule out bacteremia.

Treatment must cover cultured organisms and follow-up is essential.

Orthopedic symptoms

Difficult to differentiate bone infarction from osteomyelitis or rheumatologic disorders.

MRI studies used to identify bone marrow infarction in adults.

Acute gastroenteritis

Significant dehydration may occur quickly and lead to acidosis and sickling. If oral intake is inadequate, IV hydration is needed.

Abdominal pain

Abdominal pain crises may be differentiated from surgical problems by evaluating fever, hematologic changes, peristalsis, and response to symptomatic, supportive therapy.

Anemia

Hemoglobin and hematocrit levels significantly lower than baseline levels may reflect aplastic crisis, hyperhemolytic crisis, or splenic sequestration. Splenic sequestration may be life threatening.

Respiratory distress

It is important to evaluate the patient for acute chest syndrome, which may be fulminant and require exchange transfusion.

Neurologic changes

Neurologic changes may indicate stroke. Rapid, thorough evaluation is critical. Exchange transfusion should be performed as quickly as possible if stroke occurs.

Drug interactions

Antihistamines and barbiturates may potentiate narcotics.

Diuretics and bronchodilators, which may have diuretic effects, may cause dehydration and sickling.

Developmental issues

Sleep patterns

Routine care is recommended.

Toileting

Enuresis is frequently a long-term issue because of a large volume of dilute urine.

Nocturia may persist.

Discipline

Expectations should be consistent, fair, and similar to those of peers and siblings.

Child care

The caregiver must be mindful of fluid requirements and the importance of maintaining normal body temperature and must be able to administer medicines.

Schooling

The child may have frequent, unpredictable absences. While at school, the child needs access to fluids and liberal bathroom privileges. He or she may participate in mainstream physical education.

Sexuality

Puberty may be delayed. Women usually have normal fertility but have some special contraceptive concerns.

Transition into adulthood

Early vocational counseling is recommended. Insurance problems may be encountered.

Special family concerns and resources

Because sickle cell disease is genetically transmitted, there is a need for genetic counseling, as well as support for feelings of guilt and responsibility.

REFERENCES

Achord JL: Gastroenterologic and hepatobiliary manifestations. In Embury et al: *Sickle cell disease: basic principles and clinical practice,* 1994, Raven Press, chap 44.

American College of Obstetrics and Gynecology: Report on hormonal contraception. In *American Family Physician,* February 1995.

Adams RJ: Neurologic complications. In Embury et al: *Sickle cell disease: basic principles and clinical practice,* 1994, Raven Press, chap 40.

American Academy of Pediatrics: Red book: Report on the committee on infectious disease, 1994.

Blau CA, Stamatoyannopoulos G: Regulation of fetal hemoglobin. In Embury et al: *Sickle cell disease: basic principles and clinical practice,* 1994, Raven Press, chap 18.

Buchanan GR: Infection. In Embury et al: *Sickle cell disease: basic principles and clinical practice,* 1994, Raven Press, chap 38.

Castro O et al, The Cooperative Study of Sickle Cell Disease: The acute chest syndrome in sickle cell disease: incidence and risk factors, *Blood* 84(2):643-649, 1994.

Charache S: Experimental therapy of sickle cell disease use of hydroxyurea, *Am J Pediatr Hematol Oncol* 16(1):66-66, 1994.

Charache S, Lubin B, and Reid CD: Management and therapy of sickle cell disease, NIH Publication no. 92-2117, Washington, DC, 1992, US Government Printing Office.

Collins AF et al: Iron-balance and dose-response studies of the oral iron chelator 1,2-Dimethyl-3 Hydroxypyrid-4-One (L1) in iron-loaded patients with sickle cell disease, *Blood* 83(8):2329-2333, 1994.

Covitz W: Cardiac disease. In Embury SH et al: *Sickle cell disease: basic principles and clinical practice,* New York, 1994, Raven Press.

Cowan MJ, Golbus M: In utero hematopoietic stem cell transplants for inherited diseases, *Am J Pediatr Hematol Oncol* 16(1):35-42, 1994.

Dover G: Hydroxyurea treatment of sickle cell disease: results of the phase III multicenter trial. Abstract presented at the Annual Meeting of the National Sickle Cell Disease Program, Boston, March 21, 1995.

Earles A, Dorn L: Nursing considerations. In Embury SH et al: *Sickle cell disease: basic principles and clinical practice,* New York, 1994, Raven Press, chap 52.

Eckman JR, Platt AF: Problem oriented management of sickle syndromes, Atlanta, 1991, Georgia NIH Sickle Cell Center.

Embury SH et al, (editors): *Sickle cell disease: basic principles and clinical practice,* New York, 1994, Raven Press.

Falk RJ, Jennette JC: Renal disease. In Embury SH et al: *Sickle cell disease: basic principles and clinical practice,* New York, 1994, Raven Press, chap 45.

Gee B, Platt OS: Growth and development. In Embury SH et al: *Sickle cell disease: basic principles and clinical practice,* New York, 1994, Raven Press, chap 39.

Groce NE, Zola IK: Multiculturalism, chronic illness, and disability, *Pediatrics* 91(5), 1993.

Hakim LS, Hashmat AI, and Macchia RJ: Priapism. In Embury SH et al: *Sickle cell disease: basic principles and clinical practice,* New York, 1994, Raven Press, chap 42.

Hatcher RA: Contraceptive technology, ed 16, 1994, Irvinton Press.

Haynes Jr J, Kirkpatrick MB: The acute chest syndrome of sickle cell disease, *Am J Med Sci* 305(5):326-330, 1993.

Hernigan P, Bachir D, and Galacteros L: Avascular necrosis of the femoral head in sickle cell disease. Treatment of collapse by the injection of acrylic cement, *J Bone Joint Surg* (British vol) 75(6):875-880, 1993.

Hockenberry M, Coody D, (editors): *Pediatric oncology and hematology: perspectives on care,* St Louis, 1986, Mosby.

Hurtig AL, Koepke D, and Park KB: Relation between severity of chronic illness and adjustment in children and adolescents with sickle cell disease, *J Pediatr Psychol* 14(1):117-132, 1989.

Katz JA, Fernback DJ: Guidelines for management of pediatric patients with sickle cell anemia, Houston, 1988, Children's Hospital.

Koqutt MS et al: Correlation of transcranial Doppler ultrasonography with MRI and MRA in the evaluation of sickle cell disease patients with prior stroke, *Pediatr Radiol* 24(3):204-206, 1994.

Lee SJ, Churchill WH, and Bridges KR: Bone marrow infarcts of severe atypical pain in sickle cell crisis: diagnosis by magnetic resonance imaging and treatment with exchange transfusion. Abstract presented at the 20th Annual Meeting of the National Sickle Cell Disease Program, Boston, March 18–21, 1995.

Leikin SL et al: Mortality in children and adolescents with sickle cell disease, *Pediatrics* 84:500-508, 1989.

Mankad VN, (editor): Growth and development in sickle hemoglobinopathies, *Am J Pediatr Hematol Oncol* 14(4):283-284, 1992.

Mentzer WC et al: Availability of related donors for bone marrow transplantation in sickle cell anemia, *Am J Pediatr Hematol Oncol* 16(1):27-29, 1994.

Midence K, Fuggle P, and Davies SC: Psychosocial aspects of sickle cell disease (SCD) in childhood and adolescence: a review, *Brit J Clin Psychol* 32:271-280, 1993.

Miller DR, Baehner RL, (editors): *Blood diseases of infancy and childhood,* St Louis, 1990, Mosby.

Modege O, Ifenu SA: Growth retardation in homozygous sickle cell disease: role of caloric intake and possible gender related differences, *Am J Hematol* 44:149-154, 1993.

Ohene-Frempong K: Stroke in sickle cell disease: demographic, clinical, and therapeutic considerations, *Semin Hematol* 28(3):213-219, 1991.

Orringer EP, Abraham DJ, and Parker JC: Development of drug therapy. In Embury SH et al: *Sickle cell disease: basic principles and clinical practice,* New York, 1994, Raven Press, p 351.

Payne R: Pain management in sickle cell disease: rationale and techniques, *Ann New York Acad Sci* 565, 1989.

Pegelow CH et al: Experience with the use of prophylactic penicillin in children with sickle cell anemia, *J Pediatr* 118(5):736-738, 1991.

Phillips Jr G, Eckman JR, and Hebbel RP: Leg ulcers and myofascial syndromes. In Embury SH et al: *Sickle cell disease: basic principles and clinical practice,* New York, 1994, Raven Press, chap 46.

Piomelli S: Sickle cell diseases in the 1990s: the need for active and preventive intervention, *Semin Hematol* 28(3):227-232, 1991.

Platt OS et al: Pain in sickle cell disease: rates and risk factors, *New Engl J Med* 315:11-16, 1991.

Powars DR: Natural history of disease: the first two decades. In Embury SH et al: *Sickle cell disease: basic principles and clinical practice,* New York, 1994, Raven Press, chap 26.

Powars DR: Natural history of sickle cell disease—the first 10 years, *Semin Hematol* 12:267-281, 1975.

Powars DR et al: Beta-S gene cluster haplotype modulate hematologic and hemorrheologic expression in sickle cell anemia: use in predicting clinical severity, *Am J Pediatr Hematol Oncol* 16(1):55-61, 1994.

Rajkumar K et al: Elevated levels of erythrocyte protoporphyrin (FEP) in children with sickle cell disease in the absence of lead poisoning or iron deficiency. Abstract presented at the 20th Annual Meeting of the National Sickle Cell Disease Program, Boston, March 18–21, 1995.

Rodgers GP: Pharmacologic modulation of fetal hemoglobin. In Embury SH et al: *Sickle cell disease: basic principles and clinical practice,* New York, 1994, Raven Press, chap 56.

Rodgers GP et al: Augmentation by erythropoietin of the fetal hemoglobin response to hydoxyurea in sickle cell disease, *New Engl J Med* 328(2):73-80, 1993.

Scott-Conner CEH, Brunson CD: Surgery and anesthesia. In Embury SH et al: *Sickle cell disease: basic principles and clinical practice,* New York, 1994, Raven Press, chap 55.

Secundy MG: Psychosocial issues: unanswered questions in the use of bone marrow transplantation for treatment of hemoglobinopathies, *Am J Pediatr Hematol Oncol* 16(1):76-79, 1994.

Sergeant GB et al: Human parvo virus infection in homozygous sickle cell disease, *Lancet* 341(8855):1237-1240, 1993.

Shapiro B, Ballas SK: The acute painful episode. In Embury SH et al: *Sickle cell disease: basic principles and clinical practice,* New York, 1994, Raven Press, chap 35.

Smith JA: What do we know about the clinical course of sickle cell disease, *Semin Hematol* 28(3):209-212, 1991.

Steinburg MH, Embury SH: Natural history: overview. In Embury SH et al: *Sickle cell disease: basic principles and clinical practice,* New York, 1994, Raven Press, p 351.

Steinberg MH, Mohandas N: Laboratory values. In Embury SH et al: *Sickle cell disease: basic principles and clinical practice,* New York, 1994, Raven Press, chap 31.

Swift AV et al: Neuropsychologic impairment in children with sickle cell anemia, *Pediatrics* 84:1077-1085, 1989.

Treadwell MJ, Gil KM: Psychosocial aspects. In Embury SH et al: *Sickle cell disease: basic principles and clinical practice,* New York, 1994, Raven Press, chap 34.

Vichinsky EP: Comprehensive care in sickle cell disease: its impact on morbidity and mortality, *Semin Hematol* 28(3):220-226, 1991.

Vichinsky EP: Preoperative transfusion study: results of randomization. Presented at 20th Annual Meeting of the National Sickle Cell Disease Program, Boston, March 18–21, 1995.

Vichinsky EP, Lubin BH: Sickle cell anemia and related hemoglobinopathies, *Pediatr Clin North Am* 27:429-447, 1980.

Vichinsky EP et al: Pulmonary fat embolism: a distinct cause of severe acute chest syndrome in sickle cell anemia, *Blood* 83(11):3107-3112, 1994.

Vichinsky EP: Transfusion therapy. In Embury SH et al: *Sickle cell disease: basic principles and clinical practice,* New York, 1994, Raven Press, chap 53.

Wang WC et al: Developmental screening in young children with sickle cell disease. Results of a cooperative study, *Am J Pediatr Hematol Oncol* (15)1:87-91, 1993.

Wang WC et al: High risk of recurrent stroke after discontinuance of 5 to 12 years of transfusion therapy in patients with sickle cell disease, *J Pediatr* 118:377-382, 1991.

Wasserman AL et al: Subtle neuropsychologic deficits in children with sickle cell disease, *Am J Pediatr Hematol Oncol* 13(1), 1991.

Wilimas JA et al: A randomized study of outpatient treatment with ceftriazone for selected febrile children with sickle cell disease, *New Engl J Med* 329:472-476, 1993.

Wong DL: *Nursing care of infants and children,* ed 5, St Louis, 1995, Mosby.

Wong WY et al: Polysaccharide encapsulated bacterial infection in sickle cell anemia: a 30 year epidemiologic experience, *Am J Hematol* 39:176-182, 1992.

Yaster M et al: Epidural analgesia in the management of severe vasoocclusive sickle cell crisis, *Pediatrics* 93(2), 1994.

Zarkowsky HS et al: Bacteremia in sickle cell hemoglobinopathies, *J Pediatr* 107:579-585, 1986.

Appendix—Additional Resources

AboutFace
99 Crowns Lane, 3rd Floor
Toronto, Ontario
Canada M5R 3P4
(416) 944-3223

The goals of the organization are to link and educate affected individuals, their families, and professionals; educate professionals and the public; and assist in providing advocacy services for those with facial disfigurement.

Allergy Information Center
54 Tromley Drive, Suite 10
Etobicoke, Ontario
Canada M9B 5Y7

This organization is designed to help individuals gain control over their allergy symptoms, thus improving their overall health. A variety of services including periodic reports, a quarterly magazine, and allergy cookbooks (designed for individuals with food allergies) are all published by this organization.

American Brain Tumor Association
2720 River Road
Suite 146
Des Plaines, IL 60018
(708) 827-9910

This organization compiles and distributes relevant information to medical specialists, treatment facilities, and brain tumor support groups. Printed materials including information about diagnosis and treatment options and a triannual newsletter are available. Research support is also provided.

American Juvenile Arthritis Organization
  (AJAO)
Arthritis Foundation
1314 Spring Street, NW
Atlanta, GA 30309
(404) 872-7100

AJAO is a national membership association of the Arthritis Foundation that serves the special needs of young people with arthritis or rheumatic diseases and their families. Videotapes, quarterly newsletters, educational materials for children, parents, and health professionals, as well as information about summer camps, pen pal clubs, and family support groups are available through the national office.

American Trauma Society
8903 Presidential Parkway
Suite 512
Upper Marlboro, MD 20772-2656
(800) 556-7890

This association focuses its activities on public awareness and education. It conducts a yearly symposium and disseminates printed educational materials.

Autism Society of America
7910 Woodmont Avenue
Suite 650
Bethesda, MD 20814
(301) 657-0881
(800) 328-8476

This society has approximately 160 chapters nationwide. Activities include providing information about referral services, publishing selected materials, and lobbying for reform at the local, state, and federal levels.

Beach Center on Families and Disability
University of Kansas
3111 Haworth Hall
Lawrence, KA 66045
(913) 864-7600

This is the only federally funded national research and training center with an exclusive focus on families with members with disabilities. Research findings are disseminated to families and the professionals that serve them through teleworkshops, a newsletter, conferences, training workshops, and publications.

Boy Scouts of America
Scouting for the Handicapped
1325 Walnut Hill Lane
Irving, TX 75062-1296
(214) 580-2000

A program of Boy Scouts of America, it operates in cooperation with numerous national agencies that provide services to youth with chronic conditions. Various services and materials are available to assist in mainstreaming boys into regular scouting events or establishing units for boys who share similar disabilities.

Cancer Information Service
Office of Cancer Communications
National Cancer Institute
Bethesda, MD 20892
(800) 4-CANCER

This service, supported by the National Cancer Institute, provides support and information on cancer prevention, early detection, treatment, and continuing care. Much of this information is available through the cancer hot line, (800) 4-CANCER. Database searches are also available using the PDQ (Physician Data Query). Publications for children and family members may also be obtained.

Candlelighter's Childhood Cancer Foundation
7910 Woodmont Avenue
Suite 460
Bethesda, MD 20814
(301) 657-8401

Candlelighters is a worldwide network of over 400 peer-support groups for parents of children with cancer. Other relatives and professionals working in the field of cancer also belong. Support, information, and socialization opportunities are provided. A newsletter, bibliography, and other print materials are published.

Children in Hospitals, Inc.
31 Wilshire Park
Needham, MA 02192
(617) 482-2915

This organization for parents and professionals seeks to educate concerned individuals about the needs of children and parents when either is hospitalized. It encourages hospitals to adopt family-centered policies whenever possible. Some literature is available.

Children's Defense Fund
25 E St, NW
Washington, DC 20001
(202) 628-8787

This organization serves as a strong voice for children who cannot effectively lobby or speak for themselves. Efforts are made to educate the public about preventive investment in children. Specific attention is paid to children who are poor, of minority descent, or disabled. Technical assistance is provided to other organizations.

Clearinghouse on Disability Information
Office of Special Education and Rehabilitative
  Services
U.S. Department of Education
Room 3132 Switzer Building
Washington, DC 20202-2524
(202) 724-3636
(202) 724-4800

Created by the Rehabilitation Act of 1973, the Clearinghouse responds to inquiries, researches, and documents information in areas of federal program funding, legislation, and programs serving disabled people. Knowledgeable about a variety of information sources, the Clearinghouse refers inquiries as appropriate. A wide variety of publications is also available.

Cleft Palate Foundation
1218 Grandview Avenue
Pittsburgh, PA 15211
(412) 481-1376
(800) 24-CLEFT
(412) 242-5338

The foundation's primary purpose is to educate and assist the public about cleft lip and palate and other craniofacial anomalies and to encourage research in the field. CLEFTLINE, a toll-free service, provides information and referral to parents of newborns with these problems. Parent support groups, client and public educational activities, and research grants are also sponsored.

Coordinating Center for Home and Community
  Care
8258 Veterans Highway
Suite 13
Millersville, MD 21108
(410) 987-1048
(301) 621-7830

The Council for Exceptional Children
1920 Association Drive
Reston, VA 22091-1589
(703) 620-3660

This organization's primary goal is to advance the education of youth who are handicapped and gifted. CEC Information Services is an information broker for educators, students, and parents. In part, this is done through sponsoring the ERIC Clearinghouse on Handicapped and Gifted Children (see ERIC) and the Exceptional Child Education Resources (ECER) data base. Other activities include monitoring and analyzing governmental policies concerning exceptional children, conducting policy research, and disseminating information through conferences, academies, symposia, and other training activities.

Dystonia Medical Research Foundation
8383 Wilshire Boulevard
Suite 800
Beverly Hills, CA 90211
(312) 755-0198

This organization supports research directed toward finding the causes of generalized dystonia, spasmodic torticollis, writer's cramp, blepharospasm, and other focal dystonias. Support for this endeavor is provided through research grants, specialty workshops, and physician-client education.
Free Publication: Dystonia Dialogue

Epilepsy Foundation of America
4351 Garden City Drive
Landover, MD 20785
(301) 459-3700
(800) EFA-1000

This foundation works toward curing epilepsy through a broad range of programs including education, advocacy, research support, and service delivery. An extensive library and resource center with an in-house data base is maintained to answer individualized requests. In addition, the foundation is affiliated with approximately 100 local organizations nationwide.

FACE
The Friends for Aid, Correction, Education of
    Craniofacial Disorders
PO Box 1424
Sarasota, FL 34230
(813) 955-9250

The purpose of FACE is to provide emotional support and referrals for corrective treatment to individuals with craniofacial disorders. Print and audiovisual materials are also available for educational purposes to help dispel prejudice.

FACES
The National Association for the Craniofacially
    Handicapped
Box 11082
Chattanooga, TN 37401
(615) 266-1632

The three purposes are this organization are to (1) provide families with travel money when seeking treatment at comprehensive medical centers, (2) provide information and support to families who have a member with a craniofacial abnormality, and (3) increase public awareness and understanding about facial disfigurement.

Federation for Children with Special Needs
95 Berkeley Street
Suite 104
Boston, MA 02116
(617) 482-2915

A coalition of parent groups, this organization represents children with a variety of disabilities by providing advocacy and information services. Various special projects are sponsored and a wide array of literature is published.

Forward Face
Institute of Reconstructive Surgery, H-148
New York University Medical Center
E 34th Street
Room 901
New York, NY 10016
(212) 263-6656

This organization provides a comprehensive support system for families through referral to self-help groups, networking services, newsletter subscriptions, and other print and audiovisual materials.

Foundation for the Faces of Children
PO Box 1361
Bork, MA 02146
(617) 734-7576

This foundation supports families of children with craniofacial deformities. Support for educational information, clinical work at Boston Children's Hospital, and some financial assistance for families are provided.

Girl Scouts of America
420 5th Avenue
New York, NY 10018
(212) 852-8000

The national organization offers an informal educational program designed to help girls with disabilities develop their own values and sense of individual self-worth. Girls with disabilities participate in the same program as others; mainstreaming is encouraged whenever possible.

Joseph P Kennedy Jr Foundation
1325 G Street, NW
Washington, DC 20005
(202) 393-1250

This foundation funds research, diagnosis, treatment, and education of children and adults with mental retardation. It also meets the physical educational and recreational needs of persons with mental retardation through the Special Olympics program.

Juvenile Diabetes Foundation, International
432 Park Avenue South
New York, NY 10016-8013
(212) 889-7575

The purpose of this organization is to support research into the causes, treatment, prevention, and cure of diabetes and its complications. Support for this mission is provided through research grants, career development awards, fellowships, and new training for established scientists.

Learning Disabilities Association of America
4156 Library Road
Pittsburgh, PA 15234
(412) 341-1515

Dedicated to defining and finding solutions for the broad spectrum of learning problems, this association has more than 775 local chapters throughout the United States. Activities of this association include providing a wide range of materials, serving as a referral center, working with school systems to improve assessment and implementation programs, lobbying for children's rights, and conducting international and state conferences.

The Library of Congress
Division for the Blind and Physically Handicapped
Washington, DC 20542
(202) 707-5100

An extensive program of braille and recorded materials for blind and physically disabled individuals is provided. Books, periodicals, children's publications, music services, and supportive equipment are provided.

Mainstream
3 Bethesda Metro Center
Suite 830
Bethesda, MD 20814
(301) 654-2400

This organization works with employers and service providers to increase employment opportunities for persons with disabilities. Services include print materials, an annual conference, and job placement programs for selected cities.

March of Dimes Birth Defects Foundation
National Headquarters
1275 Mamaroneck Avenue
White Plains, NY 10605
(914) 428-7100

The mission of this organization is to prevent birth defects and related problems of low birth weight and infant death through ongoing programs of research (basic, applied, and clinical), health services, professional and public education, and public affairs.

Muscular Dystrophy Association (MDA)
3300 E Sunrise Drive
Tucson, AZ 85718
(602) 529-2000

This organization provides comprehensive medical services for individuals with a wide range of neuromuscular diseases through a network of nationwide clinics. In addition, research activities, public and professional education, and a wide variety of print and audiovisual materials are supported.

National Association of School Nurses (NASN)
Lamplighter Lane
PO Box 1300
Scarborough, ME 04070
(207) 883-2117

The objectives of this organization are to provide national leadership in the promotion of health services for school children; to promote school health interests to the nursing and health community and the public; and to monitor legislation pertaining to school nursing.

National Adrenal Disease Foundation (NADF)
505 Northern Boulevard
Suite 200
Great Neck, NY 11021
(516) 487-4992

This foundation is dedicated to serving the needs of those with Addison's disease through education, a newsletter, support groups, and, where possible, arranging contact with others with the disease. Formerly (1991) National Addison's Disease Foundation

National Alopecia Areata Foundation (NAAF)
PO Box 150760
San Rafael, CA 94915-0760
(415) 456-4644

This foundation acts as the international center for alopecia areata information. Funding of research, service to individuals with the disease, and ongoing public awareness programs are sponsored. Specific activities include a newsletter, yearly conference, support groups, and print and audiovisual materials.

National Association for the Visually Handicapped (NAVH)
22 West 21st Street
6th Floor
New York, NY 10010
(212) 889-3141

This organization provides public and professional education, client counseling, and a wide array of large print books and visual aids to the partially seeing. It serves as a clearinghouse for related services from public and private sources. Some materials are available in languages other than English.

National Brain Injury Research Foundation (NBIRF)
1612 K Street, NW
Suite 204
Washington, DC 20006
(203) 331-8445

This foundation conducts research on brain injuries; sponsors charitable and educational programs; and publishes the *Journal of Head Injury*, quarterly.

National Brain Tumor Foundation
785 Market Street
Suite 1600
San Francisco, CA 94102
(415) 284-0208

This foundation raises funds for research and provides information and support services to brain tumor survivors and their families. A resource guide, newsletter, and biannual conference are all sponsored.

National Center for Education in Maternal and Child Health (NCEMCH)
2000 15th Street, N
Suite 701
Arlington, VA 22201-2617
(703) 524-7802

This organization serves as a national resource for information, educational services, and technical assistance to organizations, agencies, and individuals with maternal and child health interests.

National Center for Learning Disabilities
99 Park Avenue, 6th Floor
New York, NY 10016
(212) 687-7211

This organization provides legislative advocacy, publications, and training seminars to assist parents, educators, social workers, psychologists, and health care providers in the United States and abroad. Publications and referrals are provided for American families overseas through the Family Liaison Office, US Department of State.

National Coalition for Cancer Survivorship
  (NCCS)
1010 Wayne Avenue
Suite 300
Silver Spring, MD 20910
(301) 585-2616

This organization identifies and addresses issues that affect the quality of living for survivors. Activities include publications, national assemblies and conferences, a speakers' bureau, and advocacy efforts on such issues as insurance coverage and employment rights.

National Down Syndrome Congress (NDSC)
1800 Dempster Street
Park Ridge, IL 60068-1146
(708) 823-7550
(800) 232-6372

This organization for parents and professionals is dedicated to improving education, fostering research, and improving the quality of life for individuals with Down syndrome. It also serves as a clearinghouse for information about Down syndrome.

National Down Syndrome Society (NDSS)
666 Broadway
New York, NY 10012
(212) 460-9330
(800) 221-4602

The major goals of this society are to promote a better understanding of Down syndrome, to support research about this genetic disorder, and to provide services for families and individuals. A variety of print and audiovisual materials is available.

National Easter Seal Society
230 W Monroe Street
Suite 1800
Chicago, IL 60606
(800) 221-6827
(312) 726-6200

Dedicated to increasing the independence of people with disabilities, Easter Seal Society offers a wide range of services, research initiatives, educational programs, and advocacy assistance through a national network of 170 affiliates. Specific services include occupational, physical, and speech therapies; vocational evaluation, training, and placement; camping and recreation; and psychological counseling. Prevention and screening programs are also sponsored.

National Foundation for Facial Reconstruction
317 East 34th Street
New York, NY 10016
(212) 263-6656

The major purposes of this organization are to (1) provide facilities for the treatment and nonsurgical assistance of individuals unable to afford private reconstructive surgical care, (2) assist in training and education of health care personnel involved in reconstructive plastic surgery, and (3) conduct a public education program.

The National Fragile X Foundation (NFXF)
1441 York Street
Suite 215
Denver, CO 80206
(303) 333-6155
(800) 688-8765

The National Fragile X Foundation was established to educate parents, professionals, and the lay public regarding the diagnosis and treatment of fragile X syndrome and other forms of X-linked mental retardation. In addition, the foundation promotes research pertaining to fragile X syndrome in the areas of biochemistry, genetics, and clinical applications.

National Gaucher Foundation (NGF)
19241 Montgomery Village Avenue
Suite E-21
Gaithersburg, MD 20879
(301) 990-3800
(800) 234-6217

This foundation is primarily devoted to funding research for Gaucher disease. A bimonthly newsletter is published and a yearly conference is held for affected individuals and their families.

National Hemophilia Foundation (NHF)
110 Green Street
Suite 303
New York, NY 10012
(212) 219-8180
(800) 42-HANDI

This foundation is dedicated to the treatment and cure of hemophilia, related bleeding disorders, and complications (including HIV infection) and to improving the quality of life for those affected. Services provided include research support, educational programs for professionals and the public, and promotion of beneficial public policies, including the establishment of the comprehensive hemophilia diagnostic and treatment centers. HANDI, the Hemophilia and AIDS/HIV Network for the Dissemination of Information, makes referrals and disseminates resources and materials to those requesting information.

National Hydrocephalus Foundation (NHF)
400 N Michigan Avenue
Suite 1102
Chicago, IL 60611-4102
(800) 431-8093

This organization seeks to educate the lay public and affected individuals about hydrocephalus, lobbies for effective legislation, and has support groups throughout the United States. A wide array of services are provided to its members including numerous publications, videos, and a referral network.

National Information Center for Children and
    Youth with Disabilities
PO Box 1492
Washington, DC 20013
(703) 893-6061
(800) 999-5599

NICHCYD provides free information to assist parents, educators, caregivers, advocates, and others to help children and youth with disabilities become participating members of the community. NICHCYD provides personal responses to specific questions, prepared information packets, publications on current issues, technical assistance to parents and professional groups, and referrals to other organizations/sources of help.

National Neurofibromatosis Foundation, Inc.
95 Pine St, 16th Floor
New York, NY 10005
(212) 344-NNFF
(800) 323-7938

The four purposes of this organization include (1) sponsoring research aimed at finding the cause of and cure for neurofibromatosis, (2) promoting the development of diagnostic protocols, (3) increasing public awareness of the disease through education, and (4) assisting clients and their families by providing information, support, and referrals to specialists.

National Organization for Rare Disorders (NORD)
PO Box 8923
New Fairfield, CT 06812-1783
(203) 746-6518
(800) 999-NORD

This agency is composed of national health organizations, researchers, health care personnel, and interested others dedicated to the identification, control, and cure of rare debilitating disorders. It serves as a clearinghouse for information, encourages research, and accumulates and disseminates information about orphan drugs and devices.

National Rehabilitation Information Center
(NARIC)
8455 Colesville Road
Suite 935
Silver Spring, MD 20910-3319
(301) 588-9284
(800) 346-2742

NARIC is a library and information center on disability and rehabilitation. Funded by the National Institute on Disability and Rehabilitation Research (NIDRR), NARIC collects and disseminates the results of federally funded research projects. The collection also includes commercially available materials.

National Tay-Sachs and Allied Diseases
Association, Inc. (NTSAD)
2001 Beacon Street
Brookline, MA 02146
(617) 277-4463

This association is committed to the elimination of Tay-Sachs and allied diseases, to be accomplished through several avenues: (1) public and professional education, (2) carrier testing, (3) family services, and (4) research support.

ODPHP National Health Information Center
(ONHIC)
PO Box 1133
Washington, DC 20013-1133
(800) 336-4797
(301) 565-4167

This center serves as a clearinghouse for specialty organizations. It maintains an on-line directory of over 1000 health-related organizations that provide health information. Federal and state agencies, private associations, professional societies, and self-help and support groups are all indexed. A special component, the National Information Center for Orphan Drugs and Rare Diseases (NICODARD), responds to inquiries on rare diseases (under 200,000 cases) and little-known drugs.

Osteogenesis Imperfecta Foundation (OIF)
5005 W Laurel Avenue
Suite 210
Tampa, FL 33607-3836
(813) 282-1161

This organization is dedicated to helping people cope with osteogenesis imperfecta. Services offered include literature for lay and professional individuals, a quarterly newsletter, a parent contact network, and a biennial national conference. Some research is also funded.

Phoenix Society for Burn Survivors (PSBS)
11 Rust Hill Road
Levittown, PA 19056
(215) 946-BURN
(800) 888-BURN

Services provided by this society are peer counseling, reentry programs to school, information services, and legislative monitoring. Public education programs, seminars, and conferences for survivors, their families, and professionals are offered. A limited number of scholarships is available to send children who have been burned to specialty camps.

Pike Institute on Law and Disabilities
Boston University School of Law
765 Commonwealth Avenue
Boston, MA 02215
(617) 353-2904

This institute provides services in the areas of individualized and systems advocacy, public policy and legal research, educational seminars about the rights of the disabled, and a variety of publications on these issues.

Prader-Willi Syndrome Association (PWS)
6490 Excelsior Boulevard, E-102
St. Louis Park, MN 55426
(612) 926-1947
(800) 926-4797

This organization promotes communication among parents, professionals, and other interested people through a bimonthly newsletter and a wide variety of publications. Research and selected family services are also supported.

RP Foundation Fighting Blindness (RPFFB)
1401 Mt Royal Avenue, 4th Floor
Baltimore, MD 21217-4245
(401) 225-9400
(800) 638-5555

The RP Foundation supports research into the cause, prevention, and treatment of retinitis pigmentosa and allied inherited retinal degenerative diseases. In addition, related literature is made available to professionals and the public. Services are also provided to affected individuals and their families. A postmortem retina donor program for research is sponsored.

Scleroderma Federation
Peabody Office Building
One Newbury Street
Peabody, MA 01960
(508) 535-6600

The major thrust of this organization is to provide education and support for persons with scleroderma and their families. Activities include providing print information, physician referral, peer counseling, and increasing the public's awareness. In addition, medical information, meetings, and patient education seminars are presented annually. Research into the cause of, and cure for, scleroderma is also supported.

Scoliosis Association (SA)
PO Box 811705
Boca Raton, FL 33481-1705
(407) 994-4435
(800) 800-0669

This association educates the public about scoliosis and other spinal deviations and aids the client in attaining a positive social and emotional adjustment during treatment of scoliosis.

Sibling Information Network
991 Main Street
Suite 3A
East Hartford, CT 06108
(203) 282-7050

This network assists families and professionals, with an emphasis on siblings, interested in the welfare of individuals with disabilities. It serves as a clearinghouse of information, ideas, projects, literature, support groups, and research regarding siblings and other related issues. The network also publishes a quarterly newsletter.

Siblings for Significant Change (SSC)
105 E 22nd Street, 7th Floor
New York, NY 10010
(212) 420-0776

This organization eases the strain of helping individuals with disabilities by providing support and information to their siblings and other caregivers. Conferences, workshops, advocacy training, and counseling services are provided.

Spina Bifida Association of America (SBAA)
4590 MacArthur Blvd, NW
Suite 250
Washington, DC 20007
(800) 621-3141
(202) 944-3285

This association provides information and referral, adult services, advocacy, and public awareness; supports research into the cause of spina bifida; and publishes a quarterly newsletter.

Sturge-Weber Foundation
PO Box 418
Mt Freedom, NJ 07970
(800) 627-5482

This foundation serves as a clearinghouse for information regarding Sturge-Weber syndrome, acts as support group for interested parties, disseminates materials to professionals and the lay public, and facilitates related research.

The Association for Persons with Severe Handicaps (TASH)
11201 Greenwood Avenue, N
Seattle, WA 98133
(206) 361-8870

TASH is concerned with the human dignity, education, and independence for individuals traditionally classified as severely cognitively impaired. Ongoing activities include advocacy services, dissemination of research findings specific to education and rehabilitation, and other educational initiatives.

Tourette Syndrome Association, Inc.
42-40 Bell Boulevard
Bayside, NY 11361-2861
(718) 224-2999
(800) 237-0717

This association develops and disseminates a wide range of print and nonprint educational material to individuals, professionals, and agencies in the fields of health care, education, and the government; operates support groups and other services; and stimulates and funds research toward finding a cure and seeking to improve treatment for Tourette syndrome.

Treacher Collins Foundation (TCF)
PO Box 683
Norwich, VT 05055
(802) 649-3020

The mission of this foundation is to serve affected individuals and their families through providing support, referrals, resources, and networking opportunities.

United Cerebral Palsy Associations, Inc.
1522 K Street
Suite 1112
Washington, DC 20005
(202) 842-1266
(800) USA-5UCP

This organization is a national network of over 170 local affiliates in 45 states. The mission—to improve the quality of life for individuals with cerebral palsy—is operationalized in several ways. A variety of information services about laws and regulations as well as appropriate programs and services are provided. Other services are also offered but may vary among local affiliates.

United Scleroderma Foundation (USF)
PO Box 399
Watsonville, CA 95077-0399
(408) 728-2202

This foundation publishes numerous handbooks, brochures, and newsletters for individuals with scleroderma. A network of local chapters provide workshops and personal contact. Physician referrals are also made from the national office.

Index